THE GREAT
CONTEMPORARY
ISSUES

MEDICINE AND HEALTH CARE

THE GREAT CONTEMPORARY ISSUES

THE GREAT
CONTEMPORARY
ISSUES

MEDICINE AND HEALTH CARE

The New York Times
ARNO PRESS
NEW YORK/1977

SAUL JARCHO, M.D.
Advisory Editor

GENE BROWN
Editor

Library of Congress Cataloging in Publication Data

Main entry under title:

Medicine and health care.

    (The Great contemporary issues)
    Consists of articles which appeared in the New York
times.
    1. Medicine—United States—Addresses, essays,
lectures. 2. Medical care—United States—Addresses, 3. Medicine - U.S. - History
essays, lectures. I. Jarcho, Saul. II. Brown,
Gene. III. New York times. IV. Series. IV. Title.
[DNLM: 1. Medicine—Popular works.
2. Medicine—Collected works. WB130 M4855]
R151.M42   610'.973   76-29724
ISBN 0-405-09850-2

Manufactured in the United States of America

The editors express special thanks to The Associated Press, United Press
International, and Reuters for permission to include in this series of books a
number of dispatches originally distributed by those news services.

Book design by Stuart David

Contents

Publisher's Note About the Series

It would take even an accomplished speed-reader, moving at full throttle, some three and a half solid hours a day to work his way through all the news The New York Times prints. The sad irony, of course, is that even such indefatigable devotion to life's carnival would scarcely assure a decent understanding of what it was really all about. For even the most dutiful reader might easily overlook an occasional long-range trend of importance, or perhaps some of the fragile, elusive relationships between events that sometimes turn out to be more significant than the events themselves.

This is why "The Great Contemporary Issues" was created—to help make sense out of some of the major forces and counterforces at large in today's world. The philosophical conviction behind the series is a simple one: that the past not only can illuminate the present but must. ("Continuity with the past," declared Oliver Wendell Holmes, "is a necessity, not a duty.") Each book in the series, therefore has as its subject some central issue of our time that needs to be viewed in the context of its antecedents if it is to be fully understood. By showing, through a substantial selection of contemporary accounts from The New York Times, the evolution of a subject and its significance, each book in the series offers a perspective that is available in no other way. For while most books on contemporary affairs specialize, for excellent reasons, in predigested facts and neatly drawn conclusions, the books in this series allow the reader to draw his own conclusions on the basis of the facts as they appeared at virtually the moment of their occurrence. This is not to argue that there is no place for events recollected in tranquility; it is simply to say that when fresh, raw truths are allowed to speak for themselves, some quite distinct values often emerge.

For this reason, most of the articles in "The Great Contemporary Issues" are reprinted in their entirety, even in those cases where portions are not central to a given book's theme. Editing has been done only rarely, and in all such cases it is clearly indicated. (Such an excision occasionally occurs, for example, in the case of a Presidential State of the Union Message, where only brief portions are germane to a particular volume, and in the case of some names, where for legal reasons or reasons of taste it is preferable not to republish specific identifications.) Similarly, typographical errors, where they occur, have been allowed to stand as originally printed.

"The Great Contemporary Issues" inevitably encompasses a substantial amount of history. In order to explore their subjects fully, some of the books go back a century or more. Yet their fundamental theme is not the past but the present. In this series the past is of significance insofar as it suggests how we got where we are today. These books, therefore, do not always treat a subject in a purely chronological way. Rather, their material is arranged to point up trends and interrelationships that the editors believe are more illuminating than a chronological listing would be.

"The Great Contemporary Issues" series will ultimately constitute an encyclopedic library of today's major issues. Long before editorial work on the first volume had even begun, some fifty specific titles had already been either scheduled for definite publication or listed as candidates. Since then, events have prompted the inclusion of a number of additional titles, and the editors are, moreover, alert not only for new issues as they emerge but also for issues whose development may call for the publication of sequel volumes. We will, of course, also welcome readers' suggestions for future topics.

Introduction

The text of this volume is composed of articles which appeared in *The New York Times*. In selecting material the compilers have not limited themselves to the news columns but have drawn occasionally on other parts of the newspapers, such as the editorial pages and the book reviews. Necessarily the news columns have made the largest contribution.

Despite the unity imposed by a single theme, such as *Medicine and Health Care,* items gleaned mainly from the news may give a disorderly or bewildering impression, which reproduces the disorderly impression often made by the events as they occur. To offset this it has been thought desirable to supplement the newspaper excerpts by a general exposition, designed to provide at least a modicum of continuity.

For this reason the main text of the volume has been prefaced by the present essay, which undertakes to set before the reader examples of salient tendencies and problems in medicine and health care that appeared in the United States during the present century. The following review is intended to be illustrative and not exhaustive.

Medicine in 1900

Nineteenth-century medicine was rich in technical medical developments, most of which had been initiated beyond the borders of the United States. Most fundamental were the great advances in pathology which are symbolized by the name of Rudolf Virchow (1821-1902) and which were based to a great extent on his recognition of the fact that the unit of life, in health and disease, is the cell. The discoveries of Virchow, his colleagues, and his followers revealed much of the basic mechanism of disease. Late in the nineteenth century an important part of the causal substructure was disclosed by the discovery of bacteria and the revelation of their behavior in infections. Because of these successful researches the late nineteenth century came to be known as the Golden Age of Bacteriology. To these great advances the genius of Konrad Roentgen added the discovery of the ray that bears his name.

At this time the United States was considered to be on the periphery of the medical world, although a few of its contributions and achievements had attracted attention in European centers. These included the discovery of ether anesthesia; the creation of the world's greatest medical library, the Surgeon General's Library (now known as the National Library of Medicine) and of its *Index-Catalogue;* the establishment of the Army Medical Museum (now the Armed Forces Institute of Pathology); and the publication of the *Medical and Surgical History of the War of the Rebellion* in six massive volumes (1870-88), which the Office of the Surgeon General carefully distributed to the principal medical centers and the principal scientists of Europe, thereby building the high reputation of American military medicine.

The Civil War was followed by a great expansion of American commerce and industry. The resultant accumulation of wealth in private hands permitted great development of philanthropy, both nonmedical and medical. In the latter category one of the most important events was the establishment of the Johns Hopkins Hospital (1889) and Medical School (1893), which were responsible for major innovations in medical education and for some important scientific discoveries. Other advances in medical education were Charles Eliot's innovations at the Harvard Medical School in the 1870's, the establishment of a university hospital—the first in the entire country—at the University of Michigan in

1869, the establishment of state boards of medical examination and licensure, and the formation of the Association of American Medical Colleges (1890). These and other events show that the deficiencies of American medical education were widely recognized by responsible citizens. Remedial efforts were predominantly the work of private individuals, freely associated.

By the end of the century many hospitals and outpatient clinics had been established. Physicians were numerous—excessively so, according to some observers. The majority were general practitioners and many of these acted also as part-time specialists. Medical schooling consisted mainly of lectures, supplemented by little or no direct clinical teaching. The best physicians relied on practical experience to compensate for the defects in their training and in this way became highly proficient.

But if industry brought wealth to a few, it meant poverty to many, and poverty was, as always, closely allied to disease. The cities rapidly filled with swarms of poor laborers, most of whom had come from American farms or had immigrated from Europe and Asia. The slums in which they lived could not fail to produce infections and other ills.

At the close of the nineteenth century the war against Spain exacted from the American people a large toll of deaths from dysentery and typhoid fever. Almost at the same moment the microbial causes of these diseases were elucidated. Effective preventive measures were still to come.

As the nineteenth century ended, the main unsolved problems were: the discovery of the causes, mechanisms, treatment, and prevention of many important diseases, i.e. the creation of a technically efficacious body of medical knowledge and skill; the creation of a body of physicians tested and licensed by adequate authority, distributed and equipped with the best available information; and the provision of therapeutic and preventive facilities, adequate in quality and quantity, and situated within easy reach.

It is not intended to imply that the problems of that era were envisioned in these terms at that time. Controversy then existed—and now rages—with respect to almost every item included in the enumeration.

1900-1918

For purposes of description and analysis it is convenient to consider the first eighteen years of the twentieth century as a separate period. At this time the United States, having acquired territories in the Pacific and the Caribbean, began to assume the dimensions of a world power. The new responsibilities involved new obligations in military hygiene and new research in tropical medicine. For these tasks the nation possessed the Army Medical School, established in 1893, a few laboratories

in other government departments, and a very small number in leading universities and hospitals. The successful construction (1904-14) and operation of the Panama Canal evidenced gratifying early success in practical sanitation. Concomitant sanitary achievements in Cuba and Panama were early instances in which public health was used as a weapon of American foreign policy.

The expansion of American political control and influence as yet exerted no great effect on immigration from Latin America. Immigration of Chinese had been suppressed since 1882; that of Japanese was terminated in 1907. Large numbers of immigrants continued to arrive from Europe, especially from the eastern and southeastern parts of that continent. The patterns of health and disease that appeared in the new arrivals tended to represent the conditions of urbanization, poverty, and industrialization that they encountered in the United States rather than diseases imported from the homeland.

Economic and social changes in American life were numerous and varied; many—perhaps the majority—were in some manner connected with the health of the people. A basic change was the steady industrialization of the economy, exemplified by the formation of the Carnegie Steel Corporation (1900), the Ford Motor Company (1903), and the American Tobacco Company (1904). The advance of mechanization and mass production brought the automobile within the reach of almost everyone. It accelerated urbanization, altered the pattern of American daily work and recreation, and fostered the increase of trauma as a cause of disability and death. The automobile also was to extend greatly the accessibility, range, and usefulness of the individual physician.

In 1913 the Sixteenth Amendment to the Constitution legalized the imposition of a federal income tax. The exemptions granted to donations made for charitable and educational purposes were later to act as powerful stimulus to medical schools, laboratories, and hospitals and moreover reinforced the pattern of philanthropy by private individuals unconnected with national or local government. But even before the income-tax laws encouraged the donation of money to charitable causes, many important philanthropic deeds were done. In 1902, for example, Mrs. Collis P. Huntington established the first cancer research fund and in 1913 John D. Rockefeller donated 100 million dollars to the Rockefeller Foundation. Benefactions multiplied, and added to the glory of the nation.

Another important force was the impulse toward reform, which continued the desire for social amelioration that had existed in England and America during the nineteenth century and earlier. The reform movements, highly diverse, were expressions of populism, socialism, egalitarianism, and other trends. Among the more conspicuous, at least temporarily, for its effect on American daily life—and on American health—was prohibitionism; the Eighteenth Amendment to the Constitution was approved in 1917. More fundamental and more durable were social movements which advanced the rights and powers of labor and the rights of women and children. In New York City in 1916 Margaret Sanger and her colleagues opened the first birth control clinic. Other landmarks of reform were the Pure Food and Drugs Act of 1906 and the Meat Inspection Act of the same year.

An outbreak of yellow fever which occurred in 1905 in New Orleans was the last appearance of that scourge in North America; this closed a lurid chapter in American epidemiology. The epidemics of poliomyelitis in 1916 and the pandemic of influenza in 1917 left a long trail of deaths. Both diseases were subsequently to be the subject of notable American researches.

By the beginning of the twentieth century the deficiencies in American medical education were known in influential circles; as has been pointed out in a previous paragraph, several forward steps were taken before 1900. New advances were now launched by the American Medical Association, which established the Council on Medical Education (1904), an agency that in 1907 inspected the medical schools of the country and published educational standards (1906, 1909). Other important events were the establishment of the Rockefeller Institute (1901), of the General Education Board (1902), and of the Carnegie Foundation for the Advancement of Teaching (1905). Laboratory instruction in medical colleges was now observed to be improving, whereas clinical instruction lagged.

During a period of 18 months, beginning late in 1908, Mr. Abraham Flexner, acting under the auspices of the Carnegie Foundation, visited every medical school in the United States and Canada. His frank exposé of educational inadequacies was published in 1910 and caused the immediate collapse of many schools and the modernization and reform of others. In Chicago, designated as a "plague spot", the fifteen schools then extant were reduced to three. The entire country contained 148 medical schools, 116 of which were regular; the remainder were controlled by various cults. The total number of schools declined by about 50% between 1910 and 1940 and began to rise slowly in the early 1950's. All schools now came to have high prerequisites for admission and to exact high scholastic performance.

Many notable physicians and scientists adorned the early decades of the century. Sir William Osler (1849-1919), a Canadian who taught at the University of Pennsylvania and Johns Hopkins, came to be regarded as the physician's ideal of the practitioner and teacher. William Henry Welch (1850-1934) was a leading teacher

and medical statesman. The increasing eminence of the United States in the sciences is shown by three awards of Nobel Prizes: A. A. Michelson (physics, 1907); Alexis Carrel (medicine and physiology, 1912), and Theodore Richards (chemistry, 1914).

1919-1946

This period of less than three decades includes the aftermath of a great war, a period of recovery followed by severe economic depression, and a second world war, unprecedented in its extensiveness.

Many individual events pointed to social change and sociomedical consequences. The Nineteenth Amendment to the Constitution, ratified in 1920, gave nationwide suffrage to women. This act was part of a long campaign toward removal of their social disabilities; its effect on the admission of women to medical schools and to hospital internships was not to reach major proportions for three decades. In 1925 Dr. Florence Sabin became the first woman to be admitted to membership in the National Academy of Sciences. Other landmarks were the establishment of the American Birth Control League in 1921 and the enactment of old-age pensions in Montana and Nevada in 1923.

The year 1929 marked the beginning of a series of catastrophes: the crash of the stock market, the great and protracted economic depression, the agricultural debacle of Dust Bowl, and the resultant impoverishment and migration. Remedial measures were undertaken by the federal government. The resultant increase in the power of central authority was soon to become of major importance in American medicine. Private philanthropy somehow managed to continue and to favor medicine and science with its benefactions.

The American population increased. The birth rate drifted steadily downward until 1933; it rose later, during the years of World War II. The death rate declined slightly. The American people were constantly preoccupied with health, and this tendency was strengthened by the public press and by the radio.

The medical profession received an afflux of refugee practitioners and professors from Europe, including some persons of high distinction. Other arrivals from Europe were American, especially Jews and Catholics, who had been unable to gain entry to American medical schools and had therefore studied medicine overseas. The existence of religious disqualifications and quotas was denied or concealed in American academic circles and almost wholly unreported in American medical books and journals but was clearly established in official investigations undertaken by the State of New York and recognized by several eminent historians.

American medical schools continued to develop affiliation—sometimes nominal rather than genuine—with universities and to elevate their academic effectiveness.

By 1929 they were able to discard the distinction of three grades of quality, which had honored some schools and prodded others; henceforth all schools were in category A. Premedical education continued to be technical rather than humanistic, a fact which left permanent imprint on the attitudes and behavior of the profession.

The development of medical specialists was regularized and greatly improved by the establishment of specialty boards, which imposed the requirement of elaborate training and strict examination. The earliest to be formed were the American Board of Ophthalmology (1916) and the American Board of Otolaryngology (1924). Before many additional years had passed the American public had at its command thoroughly trained and tested specialists in all specialties and in most sub-specialties. As these physicians increased in number, they came to be found even in small and remote cities and towns.

A notable feature of the period was the construction of large medical centers. Several facts were responsible for this development: the invention of increasingly complex and expensive diagnostic and therapeutic equipment; the tendency of medical schools to combine with one or more hospitals; the increase of affiliation between medical schools and universities; the tendency of medical schools to create or acquire affiliates in kindred subjects such as public health, pharmacy, and nursing; and the availability of philanthropic donations. The great size of these institutions brought advantages in efficiency of operation but risked dehumanization. The process was akin to the gigantism that appeared in other aspects of American life.

New technical advances included the "iron lung" or artificial respirator (1927), useful for victims of poliomyelitis, cerebral and spinal injury, and other serious conditions. The cyclotron (1934) opened new possibilities in chemistry, physics, and therapeutics. Both inventions exemplified a growing rapprochement between engineering and biological science; diagnosis and treatment were to be beneficiaries. Other important developments were the introduction of entire classes of new drugs, of which the most notable were the steroids (such as cortisone) and the antibiotics.

An advance of a very different kind was the establishment of Alcoholics Anonymous (1935). While it was not new for laymen to unite their efforts in an attack on a single disease—tuberculosis offered a notable precedent—alcoholism is a disease in which regular medical methods had long scored little success. The new association of laymen soon demonstrated great effectiveness.

World War II. Although actual American participation in the hostilities lasted less than four years, the penumbra which began with the exchange of destroyers for bases and ended with the return of overseas troops extended the temporal dimension of the conflict. Thus the war was notable not only for its duration but also because of the number of military personnel involved, the inclusion of women in armed forces, the number of civilians wounded or killed, the extensiveness of the combat zone (including arctic, desert, tropical, and jungle areas), and the deliberate annihilation of cities. Memorable and infernal was the use of the atomic bomb. Chemical weapons were used also. Bacterial weapons were prepared but not used.

Parallel to the diversity of the military action was the diversity in the training required, and large numbers of civilian physicians and paramedical persons serving temporarily in the armed forces acquired under military auspices a special training in public health, military medicine, tropical medicine, surgery, and surgical specialties. Much of this training was later carried over into civilian medical practice. In addition many medical officers of the regular army and navy were enabled to commence or to complete the training required of specialists in various branches of medicine. The level of practice in the peacetime army and navy was permanently elevated thereby.

As might have been predicted, many technical advances, large and small, resulted from the war. There were great improvements in the promptness and effectiveness of the treatment of wounds, advances in neurological, maxillofacial, and orthopedic surgery, and in anesthesiology, psychiatry, and other specialties. An accidental explosion in Bari, Italy revealed the effectiveness of nitrogen mustard gas in the treatment of lymphoid diseases. The use of antibiotics proved highly effective in the treatment of wounds and in many infections. The use of DDT initiated a revolution in tropical and preventive medicine.

For all these reasons the horrors of the war were, to some extent at least, diluted by such benefits as could be obtained from improved training of civil and military physicians and paramedical personnel and from the technical advance of medicine in all its branches. The medical problems, the medical and medicomilitary efforts, successes, innovations, and failures—are recorded in the multivolume official history, which at this moment is still in process of publication.

1947-1975

In the United States the postwar decades witnessed an increase of population—at a dwindling rate of increase—and a prolongation of longevity. More important, the proportion of aged persons in the nation increased steadily but the old-fashioned extended family, in which three or more generations might live in close proximity, was being replaced by the small nuclear family, which consisted only of parents and their children. To this change was added the factor of geographical dispersal. An important result of these alterations was extrusion of the aged into solitary dwelling-places or nursing homes or hospitals. In the institutions they often were neglected or mistreated. The magnitude and urgency of the problem fostered the development of geriatrics, the creation of special establishments, and the invention of improved systems of domestic care; these innovations were partly subsidized by the government.

The American population, influenced by the press, the radio, and television, continued to be intensely interested in health and aware of disease. More often and more loudly the people claimed that medical care was due them as a matter of right and that the government should intervene at many if not all points in the process of medical care. The citizen was widely but not always correctly informed. The press was flooded with articles on health.

Antibiotics, campaigns of immunization, and improved social conditions robbed the infections and communicable diseases of much of their former importance. Influenza continued to appear in waves, despite the availability of vaccines. Malaria, formerly a great curse of the South, was now limited to cases brought into the United States by travellers and soldiers; autochthonous transmission was at the vanishing point. There was a rise in the incidence of the venereal diseases; this was caused by liberalized social customs. The contraceptive pill was useless in the prevention of venereal infection but engendered a false sense of security.

Characteristic of the era were diseases of the heart and arteries, including arteriosclerosis and hypertension, cancer (including leukemia), disturbances of the psyche, and trauma. During the 1970's the expensiveness of gasoline caused a temporary decline in automotive deaths and injuries. Addiction to narcotics attained terrifying dimensions.

The application of chemistry and physics continued to be fruitful in medicine, as did the application of engineering. Such neologisms as 'biomedical' and 'bioengineering' now joined the older terms 'biochemical' and 'biophysical'. Among the more conspicuous and astounding advances were those in virology, immunology, and genetics. New or virtually new branches of medicine appeared, such as the surgery of transplantation, the surgery of artificial organs, and fetology. The ability to catheterize most parts of the body at will greatly increased the range of roentgen and chemical diagnosis. Another great boon was the mechanization of chemical analysis. The computer contributed its incredible ability to several branches of medicine and created a virtual revolution in some areas of roentgenology.

Requirements for admission to medical schools continued to emphasize technical qualifications rather than humanistic education. A conviction that the country was inadequately supplied with physicians led to increases in the number of medical schools, to enlargement of classes, and abbreviation of curricula. These reforms in part reflected a national addiction to haste and an unwise disregard of thoroughness. Discussants often overlooked the well-known fact that enlargement of classes might involve dilution of desirable personal influences in the classroom. In medical schools and hospitals the relative preponderance of full-time and part-time staff continued to be the subject of vigorous or acrimonious contention.

The internship—especially that in general medicine—dwindled in importance. To an increasing degree it was replaced by the residency in one or other specialty. This meant that more and more physicians were becoming specialists without having learned more than the simplest rudiments of general medicine.

The further spread of specialty boards in all branches of medicine additionally enriched the country with highly qualified specialists, widely if unequally distributed. Medical care of high quality was therefore widely available yet many persons failed to receive it. Further, not all the care that was offered was of high or even passable quality. The need for improved quality control was undeniable.

The question of scarcity and accessibility of physicians continued to be debated. A vexatious complicating factor, the high cost of medical care, had several obvious causes: increasingly costly training, increasingly expensive technology, general inflation of prices, and menacing rises in the costs of insurance against malpractice. The last of these factors was attributable to the litigiousness of the American people, the system of contingency fees, and an alleged deficiency in the ethics of many Americans, both lawyers and clients.

New or revised forms of medical practice became increasingly common: group practice, professional corporations, prepayment insurance plans, hospital-centered ambulatory clinics, and hospital-centered systems of home care. Physicians' aides, nurse-clinicians, midwives, and various other types of partly trained or specially paramedical practitioners had their advocates. The Chinese "barefoot doctors" aroused enthusiasm among some observers who should have known better.

The medical literature grew so rapidly as to embarrass bibliographers and overwhelm the capacities of libraries. The *Index Catalogue of the Library of the Surgeon-General's Office,* an important innovation of the nineteenth century, became inadequate and was abandoned in 1961. It was replaced by the successively more and more powerful computers of the National Library of Medicine, which generate general and special bibliographies at stupendous rates of speed. Concomitantly American medical librarians developed into a body of highly competent professional specialists and exerted worldwide influence.

As was noted in a previous paragraph, the growth and power of American medical philanthropy was favored by the income-tax laws. Some philanthropic organizations were devoted to single diseases. Where these diseases yielded to advances in medicine, such foundations sometimes changed their direction. Thus agencies devoted to tuberculosis became interested in other forms of pulmonary disease and a great agency that had attacked poliomyelitis turned against congenital malformations. Also notable was the establishment of voluntary agencies interested in relatively uncommon ailments such as hemophilia, muscular dystrophy, and cystic fibrosis. Agencies of this kind sometimes originated in the families of the afflicted. Usually they endowed research or established therapeutic institutes.

An important component of the sociomedical panorama was the role of government. In medicine, as in most other spheres of activity, its participation and power were constantly growing. Whether this was a benefit, a menace, or both, was frequently debated.

Military service during World War II had allowed enormous numbers of the military and their dependents to receive efficient medical service from the government and had fostered the easy illusion that such service was free of charge. Moreover, organized associations of veterans had become a powerful, voracious, and apparently permanent part of American life. The vast preoccupation of the American with health and the growth of governmental interest in health were recognized officially by the establishment of a Department of Health, Education, and Welfare in 1953. Even at the federal level this was far from being the only agency concerned with health. Others were the armed forces, the Veterans Administration, and various agencies of the Departments of Labor, Agriculture, Treasury, and Interior. Of agencies concerned with health and with the medical sciences, one of the most famous is the National Institutes of Health (NIH), which administers a large program of intramural, extramural, and international research, the largest that has ever existed. Since 1969 the Chief Executives, it is widely believed, have been less attentive than their predecessors to the advance of science and the NIH has been permitted to decline slightly in eminence. The same has been true of American science in general, according to a reliable survey.

In addition to contributing to the support of medical research, the federal government has contributed large sums to medical education and to medical care. Inevitably it has tended to assume a controlling influence, especially since a general deterioration in economic conditions throughout the country has reduced the flow of contributions from private sources and has increased the need for governmental subvention. There remains great resistance to governmental domination in these areas.

In response to widespread public demand the government, early in the present century, undertook responsibility for the purity and safety of drugs. As the latter increased greatly in number, diversity, and power, the governmental responsibility expanded. This field is now one of great activity.

The drug industry has become large and powerful. Like other business enterprises it has at times attempted to resist reform, while at other times it has fostered medical research, medical education, and medical publication.

The government has been involved also in the sensitive problem of abortion. Recent liberal judicial decisions were followed by a great increase in the number of abortions and a precipitous decline in illegitimacy and in post-abortal infection. The liberalization however encountered organized opposition from some religious sources.

While much has been said in these pages about science and about progress, the existence of anti-scientific and anti-intellectual forces should not be overlooked. In addition to astrology, which has existed since antiquity and which has enormous numbers of devotees, the present decade has shown a marked spread of cults, many of which are of quasi-religious character and some of which involve the use of psychotropic drugs. The young have been preferential but not exclusive victims.

Apart from cults which are involved in eccentricity, mental instability, or even crime, there have been numerous groups which have marshalled effective opposition to valid activities in science, public health, and medicine, such as fluoridation, the use of insecticides, experimental research in genetics, and fetology. Such activities by the ignorant and the fanatical represent Know-Nothingism transferred to science.

Saul Jarcho, M.D.

THE GREAT
CONTEMPORARY
ISSUES

MEDICINE
AND
HEALTH
CARE

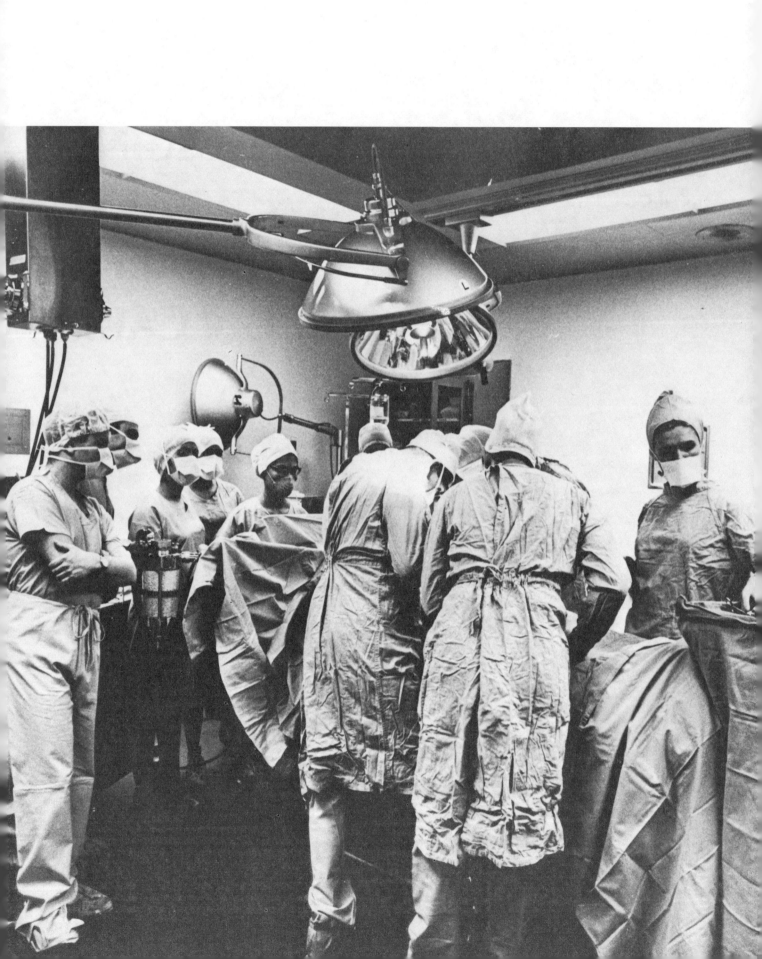

CHAPTER 1

Modern Medicine

An operation at the Albert Einstein College of Medicine Hospital in New York City.

Brower/NYT Pictures

MR. ROCKEFELLER GIVES $200,000 TO SCIENCE

Having conferred with many of the most eminent pathologists in this country as to the best method of setting on foot an original scientific research into the problems of medicine and hygiene, John D. Rockefeller has added to his already long list of benefactions.

Mr. Rockefeller has placed at the disposal of a body of prominent medical men $200,000 to be available for immediate expenditure by an association incorporated under the name of "The Rockefeller Institute for Medical Research." The home of this institute, with such laboratories, staff, and equipment as may be found necessary, will be located in this city.

The officers and Board of Directors have already been chosen. The list of officers is as follows: Dr. William H. Welch, Professor of Pathology at Johns Hopkins University, Baltimore, President; Dr. T. M. Prudden, Professor of Pathology at Columbia University, Vice President; Dr. L. Emmet Holt, Clinical Professor of Children's Diseases at Columbia, Secretary; Dr. C. A. Herter, Professor of Pathological Chemistry at the University of New York and Bellevue Hospital Medical College, Treasurer.

The Directors are Dr. H. M. Biggs, director of laboratories for the Board of Health, New York City; Dr. Theobald Smith of Boston, Professor of Comparative Pathology at Harvard University; Dr. Simon Flexner, Professor of Pathology at the University of Pennsylvania, Philadelphia.

While it is not the purpose of Mr. Rockefeller or the Directors to at once erect buildings, nevertheless it has been decided to begin this Summer the work of scientific research in several places. The present aims of the officers of the institute may be set down as twofold:

First, the endeavor to shape lines of work along which the institute may develop; second, to plan local habitations with an eye to the future needs of the institute. Two kinds of work have been already decided upon. The first will be the study of problems that can be solved by methods such as are now known to medical science; such, for instance, as an investigation, in co-operation with the Board of Health, of the milk supply of New York City. It is intended to thoroughly seek out the sources of danger, and by practical methods safeguard the supply from the danger of infection. It is likely that this field will be at once entered upon.

In the coming Autumn months, according to one of the Directors of the Rockefeller Institute, much more ambitious effort will be entered upon, under the guidance of experienced investigators. It is realized by the men enlisted in the work that the progress along the lines indicated must be slow, carried on with caution, and in a scientific spirit. In this way alone, it is believed, can the results be of undoubted value and of a lasting character.

While in this country medical men have long recognized the necessity for just such an opportunity for research as will now be afforded, no practical steps toward an institute have heretofore been taken. In Europe the achievements of the Koch Institute at Berlin, the Pasteur Institute at Paris, and the Russian Institute, founded by Prince Oldenburg, at St. Petersburg, are possible models for the one just launched.

A well-known physician, when informed last night of the personnel of the Board of Directors of the Rockefeller Institute, said that he regarded it as of the highest order. Of Dr. Welch, the President, he said medical men looked upon him as possessing rare executive ability, and as being one of the most brilliant scientific students of medicine in the United States.

June 2, 1901

ROCKEFELLER INSTITUTE BEGINS ITS GREAT WORK

The Rockefeller Institute for Medical Research, at Sixty-sixth Street and Avenue A, was formally opened yesterday with speeches by President Eliot of Harvard, President Butler of Columbia, Dr. William Henry Welch, President of the Board of Directors of the institute, and Dr. Luther Emmett Holt, Secretary of the board. John D. Rockefeller was not present, but he was represented by his son, John D. Rockefeller, Jr.

The ceremonies were in the presence of a large number of invited guests, many of them physicians and surgeons, with their wives and friends.

The institute as it stands to-day represents $3,000,000 of Rockefeller wealth. Its foundation and endowment were the result of the death of one of the grandchildren of Mr. Rockefeller. The child died as the result of an infant disease beyond the grasp of the medical profession. In founding the institute, Mr. Rockefeller turned over the money to the Directors, writing that it was to be used and administered "in such a way as to accomplish the most for humanity and science."

In the addresses made yesterday little was said of the spirit prompting the establishment of the institute or of the man whose wealth brought it into existence. President Welch referred to Mr. Rockefeller only once, and then only briefly, terming his gift as one of "enlightened munificence."

Looks Like "Business."

The institute building is five stories high. The architecture within and without is severe but dignified, and immediately gives the impression of "business." There is no ornamentation. The building stands on an eminence at the foot of East Sixty-sixth Street, rising boldly against the eastern sky and high above surrounding squares of tenements that skirt the river's edge. It is of buff brick and sandstone.

The land bought by Mr. Rockefeller for the institute covers twenty-six and a half city lots. It was a part of the old Schermerhorn farm. The building overtops everything around. The cost of the building was $350,000.

Dr. William H. Welch, head of the Johns Hopkins Faculty, is the President of the board; Dr. T. Mitchell Prudden of this city is the Vice President, Dr. Holt is the Secretary, and the other Directors are Dr. Christian A. Herter of this city, Dr. Simon Flexner, who is the Director of the laboratories; Dr. Herman M. Biggs of this city, and Dr. Theobald Smith of Boston.

The equipment of the institute is said to be perfect. Every detail for scientific investigation, from a large gathering of live dogs, goats, guinea pigs, rabbits, and monkeys to the most delicate instrument, has been provided. The air used within the building is all filtered and the interior is dust-proof. The laboratories are equipped for experimental pathology, bacteriology, and physiology, and for physiological and pathological chemistry.

The Animal Subjects.

On the roof of the building, in a well-ventilated and well-kept series of inclosures, are cells for many dogs that have been gathered for the first experiments. During the inspection of the building yesterday they leaped eagerly toward the glass upper panels of the doors, giving wild greetings to those who had visited them. One fox terrier bounded up and down like a rubber ball, even neglecting his food, preferring a kindly and friendly glance of a human eye.

In an adjoining building were a lot of monkeys. One of them has already been injected with the virus of so many diseases that he enjoys the term immune. The rest of his life is practically assured for him. He has had in a mild form about everything worth having.

Dr. Holt, who gave a sketch of the preparatory work and the plans for the future in scientific medical study, said that many applications had been made from France, Germany, and England for staff places, but that it had been decided that it would be best to train Americans for the work. Resident scholarships and fellowships will provide the material. The staff will consist of fourteen scientists, and the laboratories will accommodate fifty students. In time, said Dr. Holt, a hospital will be indispensable, and this will be provided, with other buildings. The institute will co-operate with all active agencies for the destruction of disease man, co-operating with Harvard University, to study certain smallpox phases in Manila, and has co-operated with the Health Department of this city. "We hope to have the money and the men of science," he said, "to cope with all emergencies threatening the public health."

Will Be with Europe.

President Welch said that the institute would tend to put America high in rank with Germany, France, and Great Britain for its researches in the interest of man.

President Butler commented on the American happy-go-lucky manner of approaching big problems and the naive egotism and exaltation of the man who does things regardless of how he does them, and said that the American people would soon get down to steadier and soberer methods.

President Eliot discussed the importance of scientific research in medicine, and said that although it might entail pain to the lower order of animals, it was the most humane work that could be done. He referred to the father of Pasteur, who was a private soldier of France and a hard-working tanner, and said that more men like him in America would be good for the Republic. He said that the true democracy was the democracy which permitted the maximum of effort for each individual.

John D. Rockefeller, Jr., made no address. He takes a deep interest in the institute, and, it is said, will continue to aid in its development.

May 12, 1906

EUROPE LOOKS TO AMERICA TO LEAD MEDICAL RESEARCH

War Impoverished Old World Universities and Left Scientists Without Means, Says Dr. Devol, So Their Discoveries Must Be Developed Here

AMERICA is now taking the position that Europe formerly held as the medical centre of the world, according to Dr. Edmund Devol, New York specialist in metabolic diseases. Dr. Devol is just back from a tour of Central Europe, where he made a study of hospitals, laboratories and medical centres generally.

New York, Boston and Baltimore, Dr. Devol says, are now the world's greatest medical centres. The war was the chief cause of the shift. In Europe there are no more great individual gifts to science such as the Rockefeller contributions in America, and one result of this lack of means is that recent scientific discoveries made in Europe are developed here because of the better laboratory facilities.

Dr. Devol visited Berlin, Prague, Vienna and Paris. In Prague he did some work with Professor Biedl, who is looked upon as one of the world's foremost authorities on endocrinology. The researches of Dr. Biedl in the ductless glands are conducted in his own clinic at the German University in Prague.

"Nowadays endocrinology has been popularized by the rejuvenation claims made on its behalf," said Dr. Devol. "Dr. Biedl's clinic is about to publish the latest discoveries through experiments made along this line on men and animals.

Europeans Hampered.

"Medical men there are looking to America for an opportunity to develop their work. Two of Dr. Biedl's ablest assistants, Dr. Robert Weiss and Dr. William Raab, both of whom are doing splendid research work, spoke to me with great earnestness of the advantage of being able to study in America. Dr. Weiss had just finished a year's work at the Rockefeller Institute, where he held a scholarship. He was dazzled by the wealth of material and equipment for scientific research along all lines. He deplored the lack of financial help from individuals in Europe. The universities there must depend on the State for help, and at present this help has been greatly curtailed.

"Europe still has the great medical teachers who appeared in the years when she was supreme; men like Steinach and Biedl. But the withdrawal of needed support from her institutions of learning has dealt European medicine a severe blow. I wish that some of the enthusiastic young doctors I met and some of the splendid professors could be attached to institutions like Johns Hopkins, in Baltimore; the Columbia Medical College and the Rockefeller Institute in New York; and the Harvard Medical School, in Boston. Then truly America would be the greatest centre of medical teaching in the world, with its big endowments, given by American philanthropists, for study in endocrinology, cancer, psychotherapy and other branches."

"What about rejuvenation? Is Europe really going to show us how to postpone old age?"

"I do not believe we can stop old age," replied Dr. Devol. "In theory we ought to be able to keep the secretions of the glands so nicely balanced that old age might be indefinitely deferred. But in practice this is not possible. At the same time valuable results have followed a knowledge of endocrinology. We can make up the deficiencies of certain glands and stimulate others, thereby curing disease and prolonging life."

October 18, 1925

MORE FUNDS FOR RESEARCH.

By charging himself with the cost of establishing and maintaining a great institute for medical research in Cincinnati's Christ Hospital, to which he has already given over half a million dollars, Mr. JAMES N. GAMBLE adds his name to the long list of American philanthropists who have devoted the energies of their declining years and their fortunes to the welfare of humanity. Having witnessed the astounding achievements of research in his own manufacturing enterprise he has every reason to believe that the physical sufferings of mankind can be measurably alleviated if the same organized effort is applied to the study of disease.

Merely to list and state the purposes of the numerous American foundations for social welfare requires forty-eight pages of a phamphlet recently published by the Russell Sage Foundation. Equally impressive is a bulletin which is issued by the National Research Council and which summarizes the funds available in the United States for scientific research alone. Thus in medicine, the subject in which Mr. GAMBLE has displayed so magnificent an interest, we find eighty-eight institutional funds, thirty-one endowed fellowships and scholarships and seven grants. We can only guess at the money that has been given by our men of wealth for social welfare. At the eighth annual dinner of "Better Times" Dr. FREDERICK P. KEPPEL, President of the Carnegie Corporation, estimated that the " total capi- " tal of the American foundations is, " roughly, six hundred millions, and the " income thirty millions, but individuals " each year give away more than a bil- " lion dollars for good works, and give " it voluntarily." Contrast this with the $4,600,000 that the Republic managed to collect as revenue during the first year of its existence.

So huge are the funds now devoted to research and social welfare in its largest sense that giving imposes obligations. Lavishly generous as the donations often are, they are preceded by studies as elaborate as those made by a great manufacturing corporation to determine the selling possibilities of a new product. The impulse to do good is now scientifically directed. Indeed, the entirely new profession of gathering facts for rich men and of managing the institutions established as the result of this fact-gathering has been created.

Thanks to these foundations, we shall hear less of great scientists sacrificing themselves in the cause of humanity. JENNER wrote to his friend Dr. GARDNER: " My experiments move on, but I have " all to do single-handed—not the least " assistance from the quarter where I " had the most right to expect it." In these days of great institutions established by private munificence JENNER would have discovered the benefits of vaccination in some adequately equipped laboratory. We owe to the Rockefeller Foundation the control of the hookworm and a half dozen diseases that held back the onward march of civilization. The spectacle of a LISTER supplementing his private means with fees earned as a medical practitioner in order to pursue his studies in antisepsis or of a ROSS resigning from the Indian Medical Service on a small pension in order to test his anti-malarial measures at his own expense, is not likely to recur when billions are applied in establishing institutions for the protection and the advancement of humanity.

November 27, 1927

3

MEN, ANIMALS AND PLANTS.

Dr. HERTY of the Chemical Foundation in an address in Washington last night called attention to the meager support given by the Federal Government to research studies relating to human health as compared with that voted for studying diseases of plants and animals. More than $13,000,000 was expended last year in fighting plant diseases and pests and more than $8,000,000 in combating diseases of animals. The pitiful sum of $43,000 is asked this year—about the same as last—for the research department of the Public Health Service, which has to do with human beings.

It is estimated by the Public Health authorities that practically 50,000,000 people suffered last year from colds and bronchitis; 17,000,000 from influenza and grippe; 11,000,000 from diseases of the digestive system; 8,000,000 from tonsilitis and sore throat and 5,000,000 from diseases of the nervous system—and so on through a long list of diseases which may be brought under control through intensive study. But the Government, while spending not too much for defense against the enemies of plants and animals, is spending virtually nothing for defense against what brings the greatest economic loss as well as the greatest discomfort to mankind. At present the conservation of the health of the nation is left almost entirely to private interests and to such spasmodic provision as the States or cities may make. It is time that the people as a whole gave attention to conditions with which even the most generous private foundations cannot cope and which in their ravages leap over city limits and State boundaries.

A bill has been introduced in the Senate by Senator RANSDELL of Louisiana providing for the creation of a National Institute of Health within the Public Health Service for the specific purpose of setting a large group of scientists "to work "uninterruptedly upon the funda-"mental causes of sickness, disease "and premature death." It is proposed that $2,000,000 a year be appropriated for a term of five years for the maintenance of a chemo-medical research laboratory. Even so we shall not be giving the health of men, women and children as much governmental attention as we give to that of cattle, hogs, sheep, horses and plants.

April 12, 1928

HOOVER SIGNS HEALTH BILL

Ransdell Measure Provides $750,000 to Establish National Institute.

Special to The New York Times.

WASHINGTON, May 26.—President Hoover today signed a bill providing for the creation of a national health institute here under the auspices of the United States Public Health Service. Present at the signing were Senator Ransdell of Louisiana, author of the measure; Dr. Charles H. Kertz of the Chemical Foundation of New York City, and Dr. J. W. Kerr, assistant surgeon general of the Public Health Service. The measure authorizes an initial appropriation of $750,000 for the construction and equipment of buildings and the Secretary of the Treasury is authorized to accept donations for use in ascertaining the cause, prevention and cure of disease affecting human beings. The establishment of research fellowships within the institute is provided, the scientists to work both in this country and abroad.

"I think the bill is one of the most important ever enacted by Congress in the interest of humanity," Senator Ransdell said.

May 27, 1930

ORGANIZED MEDICAL RESEARCH.

There can be little doubt that the day of the lone inventor, the starving genius of the garret, is over. He gave us great inventions, but he took too long about it. Discoveries and improvements made decades and even generations apart had to be assembled before we had the telegraph, the telephone, the harvester, the flying machine. In the modern industrial laboratory no time is wasted in repeating old experiments. Experimenters are organized into crews. There is team-work, organization, a plan of research, and competent direction.

To Dr. ELLICE MCDONALD of the University of Pennsylvania's Graduate School of Medicine belongs the distinction of first applying in medicine and biology a method which has succeeded brilliantly in industry. He has long been concerned with cancer. It was borne in upon him that the problems presented by that scourge are not likely to be solved by one man. They involve a thorough knowledge of biology, chemistry, physics, cell structure and growth. Yet there is no concerted attack on cancer. Applying the principles that have given us the electric lamp, transatlantic telephoning and synthetic gasoline, he reorganized the Cancer Research Laboratories under his direction so that some twenty-six specialists could work in teams. It was discovered under this system that the nucleus of the cell is the part affected by radiation, that certain ultraviolet rays are deadlier than either X-rays or radiation, that chemicals can be made to fluoresce within the body and give off these very ultraviolet rays, that the spectroscope may yet prove to be an easy means of testing blood for cancer.

The principle of organization and correlation having thus justified itself, the Biochemical Research Foundation of the Franklin Institute has now been established by Dr. MCDONALD to attack what must be regarded as the problem of life itself. Life being a chemical phenomenon, the Foundation will study disease chemically, determine the therapeutic and medical efficacy of new organic compounds, and discover what it can about the chemistry of longevity, with the hope of prolonging the span of life. "Cause and the end result like "the pneumococcus and the resulting "pneumonia would concern us very lit-"tle," Dr. MCDONALD told the Franklin Institute recently. "We are more "interested as to why processes take "place than as to the fact they do take "place." This is precisely the point of view of the industrial laboratory. The prima donna of the microscope, the lone "genius" who depends on trial and error and wastes precious, planless years by following "hunches," gives way to a trained crew concerned with the mechanism of living.

November 17, 1935

ROOSEVELT STARTS DRIVE ON PARALYSIS

From a Staff Correspondent

HYDE PARK, N. Y., Sept. 22.—President Roosevelt announced today the formation of a new national foundation to fight infantile paralysis, in a statement issued before he left on his Western trip.

The function of the new agency would be to coordinate all three phases of the fight against the disease, said Mr. Roosevelt, who is himself a sufferer. These phases are research on the nature and methods of prevention of the disease, such as the new nasal spray recently developed; actual care of those with poliomyelitis, and the care and cure of those suffering from the after effects.

Mr. Roosevelt's statement was written shortly after a conference with Basil J. O'Connor, his former law partner, and Keith Morgan, both of whom are active in the affairs of the Georgia Warm Springs Foundation, of which Mr. Roosevelt is president. The work at Warm Springs, directed toward the after-effects of the disease, will be continued under the new foundation, but will be only one phase of the broad attack on the disease which will include research, an educational campaign and the dissemination of information to the practicing physician, described by the President as "the front-line fighter of this sickness."

Much of the money for the campaign is raised by the annual balls held each year on Mr. Roosevelt's birthday, the proceeds of which go to work in infantile paralysis. The new foundation will continue this work, allocating, as at present, various sums to various hospitals and research organizations.

Mr. Roosevelt said that his official duties would not allow him to head the new foundation, but added that he would remain president of the Warm Springs Foundation.

The personnel of the new foundation is to be announced soon.

THE ROOSEVELT STATEMENT

The text of the President's statement was as follows:

I have been very much concerned over the epidemics of infantile paralysis which have been prevalent in many cities in different parts of the country. I have had reports from many areas in which this disease is again spreading its destruction. And once again there is brought forcibly to my mind the constantly increasing accumulation of ruined lives—which must continue unless this disease can be brought under control and its after effects properly treated.

My own personal experience in the work that we have been doing at the Georgia Warm Springs Foundation for over ten years leads me to the very definite conclusion that the best results in attempting to eradicate this disease cannot be secured by approaching the problem through any single one of its aspects, whether that be preventive studies in the laboratory, emergency work during epidemics, or after treatment.

For over ten years at the foundation at Warm Springs, Ga., we have devoted our effort almost entirely to the study of improved treatment of the after effects of the illness. During these years other agencies, which we have from time to time assisted, have devoted their energies to other phases of the fight.

I firmly believe that the time has now arrived when the whole attack on this plague should be led and directed, though not controlled, by one national body. And it is for this purpose that a new national foundation for infantile paralysis is being created.

Seeks Adequate Financing

As I have said, the general purpose of the new foundation will be to lead, direct and unify the fight on every phase of this sickness. It will make every effort to insure that every responsible research agency in this country is adequately financed to carry on investigations into the cause of infantile paralysis and the methods by which it may be prevented. It will endeavor to eliminate much of the needless after-effects of this disease—wreckage caused by the failure to make early and accurate diagnosis of its presence.

We all know that improper care during the acute stage of the disease, and the use of antiquated treatment, or downright neglect of any treatment, are the cause of thousands of crippled, twisted, powerless bodies now. Much can be done along these lines right now.

The new foundation will carry on a broad-gauged educational campaign, prepared under expert medical supervision, and this will be placed within the reach of the doctors and the hospitals of the country. The practicing physician is in reality the front line fighter of the sickness, and there is much existing valuable knowledge that should be disseminated to him.

And then there is also the tremendous problem as to what is to be done with those hundreds of thousands already ruined by the after-effects of this affliction. To investigate, to study, to develop every medical possibility of enabling those so afflicted to become economically independent in their local communities will be one of the chief aims of the new foundation.

Asks Immediate Action

Those who today are fortunate in being in full possession of their muscular power naturally do not understand what it means to a human being paralyzed by this disease to have that powerlessness lifted even to a small degree. It means the difference between a human being dependent on others and an individual who can be wholly independent.

The public has little conception of the patience and time and expense necessary to accomplish such results. But the results are of the utmost importance to the individual.

The work of the new organization must start immediately. It cannot be delayed. Its activities will include among many others those of the Georgia Warm Springs Foundation, of which I have been president since its inception. I shall continue as president of that foundation. But in fairness to my official responsibilities, I cannot at this time take a very active part in the much broader work that will be carried out by the new foundation, and I therefore do not feel that I should now hold any official position in it.

However, because I am wholeheartedly in this cause, I have enlisted the sincere interest of several representatives and outstanding individuals who are willing to initiate and carry on the work of the new foundation. Its personnel will be announced as soon as it is completed.

New Cases Reach a Peak
By The Associated Press.

WASHINGTON, Sept. 22.—The Public Health Service reported today 879 new cases of infantile paralysis for the week ended Sept. 18, a peak for the year.

Despite the increase in the number of new cases over the total reported for the previous week, officials said that the advent of cooler weather had slowed the rapid gains made by the disease. New cases reported for the week ended Sept. 11 had climbed to 817 in comparison with the 641 new cases reported for the week ended Sept. 4.

Up to Sept. 18 the service had received reports on 6,391 new cases this year, compared with 2,261 for the same period of last year.

September 23, 1937

Curbs on Medical Research In Fund Grants Irk Scientists

By ROBERT K. PLUMB

Some of the nation's most productive medical scientists, and a group of leading medical administrators familiar with research, have said, in reply to questions from THE NEW YORK TIMES, that they are uneasy about the nature of the financial support they now have.

These misgivings are based on a fear that the long-term purposes of medical science—the mastery of human ailments—may be distorted by well-meant but unfortunate plans to stimulate the advance of the science by setting up projects to work toward foreseeable ends.

There is no complaint about the amount of money offered to institutions in the name of research, if research is considered apart from other activities. The amounts actually spent on research in medical schools alone have increased at least 400 per cent since 1941. But this boom has had its drawbacks, it was pointed out to THE TIMES.

Mere Money Not Enough

Many fear the public has been sold the idea that it is necessary merely to spend more money to get more medical "miracles." This is referred to as the "magic-wand theory of medical advance." Most of the new money for research has come from the public through taxes or gifts. The "magic-wand" theory, in the appeal for funds, promises a usable result and in a pretty short time, too. Significant advances are not apt to come that way; the result, many asked by THE TIMES have warned, may be that basic investigations are neglected in the scramble for exploitable scientific "results".

Meanwhile, medical schools and teaching hospitals are, for practical purposes, the only places where clinical material is available for research. And medical schools are in desperate financial condition, being the most expensive functions in the hard-pressed university system. All concerned with medicine and research agree the medical schools need more money. Even the American Medical Association and the Federal Security Agency see eye to eye here, though they disagree as to what should be done. The ten-year boom in research has cost the medical schools more money than was supplied to them by those who wanted their own research projects undertaken, and, paradoxically, the financial plight of medical schools has been aggravated by the gusher of cash earmarked for research.

The first drawback, therefore, is a problem that long has been of concern to scientists. The distinction between "applied" and "basic" research is a subtle one to the layman. Researchers have usually found it easy to interest a wealthy individual in a good-sounding idea, in the past. Now, taxes have changed the situation: the researcher must get his support from the public, through taxes and

5

gifts, or from an endowment, or an industrial concern.

Basic or fundamental research usually is not predicated on an idea that sounds good; it ordinarily cannot be expressed in an "idea" at all. This type of science, those who have experienced it assert, must be something like painting or composing. It must be motivated by a personal desire to extend the area of human knowledge. It cannot be directed or fabricated at will. Basic research may go along for decades without ever "accomplishing" anything. Then, if the findings happen to fit together, a "giant stride" is the result.

The introduction of the germ theory of disease in the last century is one such example in medical science. Another, twenty-two years ago, might be the discovery of penicillin. Two years ago, a demonstration of the role of the adrenal cortical hormones in health and disease was a "giant stride" accomplished by fundamental work.

Studies that can, by chance, lead to such results, cannot be planned in detail in advance, researchers say. Applied work is essential to the success of a striking idea, of course. And everyone cannot be a Nobel Prize winner.

Dangers in Favoritism Seen

The fear expressed by many who replied to THE TIMES inquiry is that medical science may suffer from an excess of planning in which the best-sounding ideas are supported generously and the studies that do not immediately sound so promising are dropped. If the public is to support research, these scientists say, the true significance of "basic" and "applied" studies must be made clear.

That there has been a tendency in the opposite direction is justified, according to some replies, in the effort to raise more money for more research. The emotionalism, and the public response, is increased when the appeal is for cancer, poliomyelitis, heart disease or some other specific goal the public can comprehend. It is impossible to get wide support for basic studies, these men say, if they must appeal to the public.

The second drawback, that the financial situation of the nation's medical schools has been aggravated by the research boom, is based on the observation that research projects cost medical schools more than fund-suppliers usually provide.

That is, it costs just to keep a medical research institution open. Janitors and paper-workers must be paid. Soap and towels, as well as radioactive carbon, must be purchased. And these routine but essential costs, which are not glamorous enough for public attention, are infrequently acknowledged by fund-suppliers, medical school administrators said.

School Financing Important

It was not the intention of THE TIMES inquiry to consider medical school finances, but most respondents stressed the importance of this question in their discussions

of research financing. Research, after all, is a small part of the function of a university medical school. But it is important in engendering an alert and questioning atmosphere favorable to the training of doctors, researchers and instructors.

Financial support for medical research, aside from that which comes through institutionally controlled endowments, is provided principally by private foundations, by public fund-raising organizations and by the Government.

Federal funds, and their effect on medical research, have been reviewed thoroughly in a study recently completed for the Public Health Service by a committee headed by Dr. Lowell J. Reed of the Johns Hopkins University School of Hygiene and Public Health.

A statement on Federal research support was prepared for THE TIMES by Dr. W. H. Sebrell Jr., director of the National Institutes of Health. The Public Health Service, according to Dr. Sebrell, now finances about 25 per cent of all research in medical schools. In 1948, for research, the schools spent $14,000,000 from all sources. In 1941 it was $4,000,000. Other Federal support from research comes from other agencies. Altogether, according to the Reed report, the Government pays for half of all medical school research.

School's Difficulties Recognized

Under Federal law, research grants from the Public Health Service may include an 8 per cent portion allowed for institutional overhead. That this does not actually cover the overhead in a medical school is recognized by the agency. Also, the difficulties in financing basic research through the use of grants designed for a rather specific purpose, as, according to law they must be, are recognized.

The Reed report, which was widely commended by medical school administrators replying to this inquiry, says:

"No matter what problems confront research in medical schools, they fade in the presence of the acute and dangerous general financial stringency faced by the schools."

Dr. Sebrell said, "If the general financial base of the medical schools were more adequate, many of the problems now attributable to the nature of support for research would disappear or decline sharply in significance."

Privately endowed foundations, according to Dr. Alan Gregg, director for the medical sciences of the Rockefeller Foundation, have a special purpose as pathfinders in the finance of research. He commented:

"It is probably sensible for those foundations whose officers and trustees would like to have the financing of some remarkable discovery to their prompt and widely accepted credit, to reflect upon the advantages of not being in too much of a hurry or too avid for justification of their responsibilities. * * * I have personally felt that if the laymen on our funds, foundations and allocations committees could learn more about the

characters of good scientists and the nature of the lives they lead, the terms laid down for various projects would be a great deal more intelligently formulated."

Following are a few excerpts from some of the seventy-three statements received by THE TIMES. No one of these individuals expressed exactly the climate of opinion summarized above, and there were some vigorous denials of specific points that nevertheless seemed to be repeated by many. All were asked the same questions, which were conceived in an effort to lead into a general statement of individual opinion about research financing as it actually works today.

The statements were requested from medical school deans and productive scientists (not mutually exclusive groups) and from a few other individuals, 106 in all. Some asked that their names not be used.

Dr. Vernon W. Lippard, dean of the Department of Medicine, University of Virginia:

"There is an unfortunate tendency on the part of both governmental and private agencies to make funds available for research in restricted areas. As a result, investigators are often required to channel their work into areas where support can be obtained rather than where they have the most fertile ideas * * * the quality of medical research will, in the long run, be dependent upon the quality of medical education."

Dr. Hudson Hoagland, executive director, the Worcester Foundation for Experimental Biology:

"To summarize my own reactions to the situation, we have not found our basic problems to be restricted by the present form of distributing funds. I do believe, however, that there are important aspects of science which are hard to support because they cannot be related to the medical sciences viewed broadly and it is in these fields that very important contributions which should not be overlooked may arise."

Dr. G. H. Whipple, dean, the University of Rochester School of Medicine and Dentistry:

"* * * Funds are frequently designated by an organization or a donor for some particular disease like cancer, infantile paralysis and so on. Medical schools should resist the tendency to take this money unless they have an investigator who is boiling with enthusiasm to work in these fields * * * One fault that is beginning to emerge is the grant without any assignment of funds for overhead to include heat, light, space, technical service and so on. Some schools are actually impoverished because they have a large number of grants * * *"

Dr. Alan M. Chesney, dean, the Johns Hopkins University School of Medicine:

"It is my judgment that in the long run progress in the study of man as a living organism will be most rapidly achieved if we make unrestricted financial support available to the medical schools of the country in fullest measure. Short-term grants for restricted purposes or limited objectives will not achieve the same result."

Dr. James M. Faulkner, dean, Boston University School of Medicine:

"On the whole, the benefit derived from these new sources of income for research has been incalculable, both from the point of view of the results of the research itself and the training and education it has given to many scientific workers. The total benefit derived from these grants has, in my opinion, far outweighed the disadvantages of some of the techniques in their applications."

Dr. Currier McEwen, dean, New York University College of Medicine:

"Much of the research—perhaps two-thirds—in medical schools and research institutes is being supported by short-term grants-in-aid from specifically defined projects. * * * It is doubtful if these agencies can, in the present stage of social thinking, do anything else than operate on a project basis. * * * after all it is the responsibility of institutions not to permit their academic integrity to be diverted by grant bait. * * * by and large institutions match grants more than dollar for dollar in providing facilities, services and the consulting service of senior faculty members to projects. * * * this is another item in the unpaid overhead which agencies owe to the academic world."

Dr. A. C. Furstenberg, dean, University of Michigan Medical School:

"* * * Funds obtained in the name of research by direct appeal to the general public also (should be) consolidated and administered under a nation-wide plan similar to those employed by the National Research Council and the United States Public Health Service."

Dr. Willard C. Rappleye, dean, Columbia University College of Physicians and Surgeons:

"Since we undertake no research activities except those which we do by election, the grants-in-aid have been of enormous value in carrying on our research activities and contributing directly or indirectly to the strengthening of our entire program * * * everyone is in agreement that some device ought to be worked out for permitting forward financing on a more satisfactory basis, especially for key personnel who after all are the nucleus of any research planning."

Dr. H. J. Muller, Department of zoology, Indiana University:

"* * * I am strongly of the opinion that the method at present so prevalent of granting research money for special projects (as for the study of individual diseases) does restrict the range of inquiry unduly and does divert talented workers unduly from basic to popular fields."

Dr. Carl A. Moyer, dean, Southwestern Medical School, University of Texas:

"I think there is little doubt that the practical aspects of research are over-emphasized and that this emphasis will grow as the pressure needs to be increased to obtain funds. * * * It would be distinctly better that all of these fund-raising organizations be joined and that their support go for long-term research projects of basic nature in the fields of biology, chemistry, physics."

May 13, 1951

Increase Is Noted in Funds For Research in Medicine

Public Is Now 'Sold' on Program, Which Has Paid Nation Enormous Dividends

By HOWARD A. RUSK, M.D.

As longevity and good health are among the basic objectives for which each of us strives. it is not surprising that medical research has traditionally attracted financial support from prosperous individuals and groups. Modern medical research had its beginning in the Renaissance, when both the ecclesiastic and merchant princes of the seventeenth century became the patrons of men of science. The cultural stimuli of the times, cumulative technology that made new methods of research possible, and the development of printing, which made the exchange of scientific knowledge possible, were not the only factors that led to this support. The princes saw clearly the utilitarian value of technological advancement, particularly in connection with warfare.

Here in the United States public and private support of medical research to any substantial degree dates back only to the beginning of this century. Previously the American people apparently were much more concerned over their souls than their minds and bodies, for in 1891 American theological schools had endowments of about $18,000,000, while our medical schools had less than $500,000.

This situation, however, began to change at the turn of the century. The discoveries, particularly of Pasteur and Koch, dramatically demonstrated to the public the tremendous possibilities of controlling numerous infectious diseases through medical research.

With the historic report of Flexner in 1910, the standards of medical education rose immeasurably and the public acquired a new and justified confidence in medicine. Under the leadership of Sir William Osler, the Johns Hopkins concept of a great biological-medical center coordinated with clinical departments began to attract national attention. Medical research in the United States was "sold" for the first time on the basis of its financial savings to society rather than simply as a matter of pure humanitarianism.

War Had Pronounced Impact

World War II had a pronounced impact on medical research in the United States, particularly in the scale of expenditures for medical research, and in the relationship between research and educational expenditures of medical schools. In 1941 medical schools spent about $27,000,000 for basic operating costs and $4,000,000 more for research, of which Federal funds for cancer research expended through the Public Health Service amounted to only $83,370. During the war the sum was increased sharply from funds supplied by the Committee on Medical Research of the Office of Scientific Development for projects of direct interest to the success of the war. These reached a peak of $7,000,000 during one year.

There was some apprehension at the war's end that this support might be curtailed at a time when general public policy indicated a marked expansion rather than retrenchment. Fortunately, this did not happen — Federal research grants combined with research support of industry, foundations, voluntary health associations, philanthropic individuals and our medical schools and hospitals reached an unprecedented $181,000,000, or ten times the amount spent in 1941.

Although final tabulations are not yet available, Medical Economics estimates the sources of these funds as follows:

Government, $76,000,000 — Public Health Service, $35,200,000; Atomic Energy Commission, $18,000,000; Army, $6,800,000; Navy, $6,000,000; Air Force, $4,700,000; Veterans Administration, $4,500,000; others, $1,000,000.

Industry, $60,000,000—Drug industry, $52,500,000; industrial foundations, $5,000,000; others, $2,500,000.

Philanthropy. $25,000,000 — Foundations, $10,000,000; voluntary health groups, $10,000,000; personal, $5,000,000.

Professions, $20,000,000 — Hospitals, $15,000,000; medical schools, $5,000,000.

Other Contributions Made

These figures do not, of course, include the millions of man-hours of free-service contributions by physicians and other scientific personnel. Nor do they include indirect expenditures, cash equivalents in service and construction costs for laboratories and other facilities.

As Schifferes points out in that article, although $181,000,000 is a substantial sum of money, it amounts to only 0.3 per cent of the nation's defense budget and only about one-half of the nation's annual expenditure for hair tonics, shampoos and other hair-care items.

Paralleling this increased emphasis of medical research during the past half-century has been the remarkable improvement in the health of the American people. It has been estimated from fossil findings that in prehistoric times the average man lived about 18 years. This had advanced to around 25 during the time of the ancient Romans. By 1900 it had reached 49.2 in the United States, a gain of approximately 100 per cent in 2,000 years. From an average lifetime of 49.2 years in 1900, we have in but a short fifty years increased man's life expectancy in the United States to 67.2 years, a gain of more than eighteen years in less than fifty.

Many of the diseases that claimed their victims with dramatic speed in 1900 -- typhoid fever, scarlet fever, whooping cough, measles, diphtheria, smallpox and malaria—have now been practically eliminated as causes of death. Infant mortality has been reduced to one-quarter of its 1900 rate, and maternal mortality to an even smaller fraction.

Along with medical research, the contributing factors to these advances have included the increase in quantity, quality and availability of medical services; the progress made in public health practices and sanitation, and the rapid rise in our standard of living.

The record speaks for itself. The money the American people have invested in medical research through government, industry, philanthropy and our medical schools and hospitals has paid enormous dividends.

June 29, 1952

Revolutionary Center for Medical Research Dedicated

Special to THE NEW YORK TIMES.

WASHINGTON, July 2—The Federal Government's $64,000,000 Clinical Center, described as a revolutionary stride in medical research, was dedicated today. The fourteen-story building includes a 500-bed hospital section and 1,100 scientific laboratories.

The center, which will be devoted to conquering such killers as cancer and heart disease, is in near-by Bethesda, Md. It will receive on Monday its first patients—eight women who are suffering from cancer. Dr. W. Henry Sebrell Jr., head of the National Institutes of Health, said the women "will be the best studied patients in the world." "This center is not a hospital," he added. "You don't get in by just being sick. You don't get in for medical care. You get in only for research."

"For the first time in history," Dr. Sebrell continued, "we will be able to integrate laboratory and clinical research so that there can be a complete study of the chronic diseases that kill men."

None of the patients will pay for their care.

Mrs. Hobby Leads Dedication

The dedication speech was delivered by Mrs. Oveta Culp Hobby, Secretary of Health, Education and Welfare. The Federal Public Health Service, which will operate the clinic, is a division of her department.

"I proudly dedicate this center to medical research as a symbol of our national concern for the health of our people, for their right to pursue happiness, unhampered by crippling pain and illness," Mrs. Hobby said, adding:

"In freedom, this building and the people who work here are dedicated to the endless struggle against human suffering.

"We are dedicating it today. Dedicating it to the open mind of research. Dedicating it as an example of democracy heeding its obligation to the free men who are together self-governing."

The Secretary said that she felt "tremendous excitement in the face of infinite potentiality," realizing that "each new solution to be found here will mean a new chance at the full and finished life for numberless men, women and children."

"This center," she declared, "will house the widest array of specialists and technicians that has ever, in the history of mankind, been assembled to work in pure and applied science."

The center, for which Congress provided funds for the construction costs and will vote the money required for operation, was five years in building. Its development into full operation will take two to three years as physicians, scientists, laboratory experts and therapists pioneer in new administrative and medical techniques.

Fruition of a Long Dream

The clinic is the fruition of a dream of Public Health Service scientists to bring laboratories and patients together. This dream was expressed in print as long ago as the agency's 1911 annual report. The center will now be the focal point of the seven National Institutes of Health.

These institutes deal with the fields of arthritis and metabolic diseases, cancer, dental research, heart, mental health, microbiological (rheumatic fever) and neu-

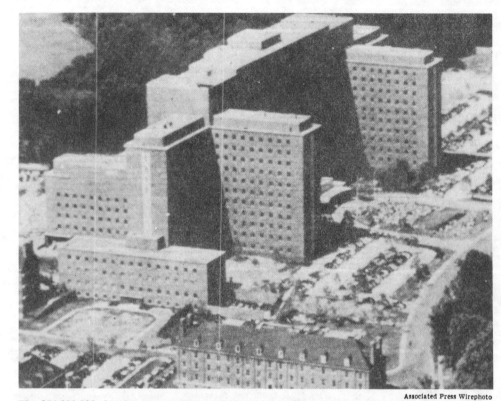

Associated Press Wirephoto

The $64,000,000, fourteen-story Clinical Center Building near Washington. This aerial view was taken yesterday. Other buildings of the National Institutes of Health are in the foreground.

rological diseases and blindness.

Officials recalled that in the past Public Health Service scientists had moved to the scene of the outbreak of diseases as they made progress in conquering cholera, diphtheria, influenza, leprosy, malaria, measles, pellagra, smallpox, tetanus, tuberculosis, typhoid, typhus, venereal disease and yellow fever.

However, today's cripplers and killers—heart diseases, cancers, mental illnesses and chronic diseases—the officials said, are not concentrated in epidemics and must be brought to the scientists for best study.

"This center represents a massive approach to the major killing and crippling diseases," Dr. Sebrell said. "We are not interested in rare, exotic, hard-to-diagnose diseases, but in those that damage and kill the most Americans."

He described how the building had been designed for all the facets of this "massive approach." Ground and top floors of the main building will be used for general services. Included are admission centers, auditoriums and operating rooms.

The in-between floors are divided into three sectors. The southern exposure, overlooking the Maryland countryside, will belong to the patients, with twenty-six to a floor. In the center are the nurses' stations, dietary kitchens and treatment rooms. The northern suites will be used by the scientists for their tests and studies of patients. Each floor has about a hundred laboratories with demountable partitions.

One Wing for Radioactive Study

There also are special purpose wings. One is for animal experimentation. Two are for basic science studies and in another, autopsies will be conducted. In an eight-story wing, three stories of which are underground, will be all radiation facilities.

This wing will not be opened until next January. When finished it will contain all modern atomic energy means of treating patients as well as laboratories to prepare medications containing radioisotopes. An unusual feature of the radiation wing is the provision of rooms for patients, making possible supervised control of radioisotopes for diagnosis and treatment.

Dr. Sebrell emphasized that psychological and spiritual factors in the treatment of patients suffering from often-incurable, long-term diseases had received their place in the Clinical Center. This phase even included the calling in of color experts to supervise the entire decoration.

On the top floor, where the operating rooms are finished in

soft green tile, is a huge gymnasium-like room that will be used for the type of physical rehabilitation pioneered by Dr. Howard A. Rusk, director of the Institute of Physical Medicine and Rehabilitation, New York University-Bellevue Medical Center, and associate editor of THE NEW YORK TIMES.

There also is a dignified chapel, with a revolving stage presenting in turn the altars of the Protestant, Catholic and Jewish faiths. It will be always open for meditation.

More than ninety doctors are now on the staff of the seven research institutes, and there are as many doctors of science.

The first eight patients arriving Monday are cervical cancer cases, which will be treated with large doses of hormones. The second eight, to follow soon, are hypertension heart cases to be treated with new drugs believed to be better for lowering blood pressure than anything now in use. The third eight, sufferers from rheumatoid arthritis, will arrive within a month for further work with ACTH and cortisone.

The patients will continue to arrive at a rate of twenty-five to forty a month until there are about 250 by June, 1954. All will be volunteers.

"Only persons recommended by physicians, hospitals or medical schools will be admitted," Dr. John A. Trautman, director of the Clinical Center, said. "Most of these will come from the Eastern Seaboard [to make follow-up studies easier] and nearly all will come to fullfil a special requirement."

Dr. Sebrell added that "every step of their treatment will be explained to them as we go along," and "they may leave any time they wish."

While the patients will not be charged—their care is regarded as a research cost—they may make voluntary contributions to the Federal Treasury if they desire.

The patients will find dozens of devices and special features in the institution, where some will live for extended periods.

Rooms for the ambulatory are like modern hotel rooms with day beds. Each room, set up for two patients, has its own bathroom. The communications system enables them to talk to the nurse on the floor without her having to walk to the rooms.

July 3, 1953

CHARITY APPEALS RUN INTO REVOLTS

By PHILIP BENJAMIN

The current war over the charity dollar is being fought between the independent fund-raising health agencies on one side and the United Fund on the other. Before examining the major combatants, it might be well to take a look at the "guerrilla fighters" in this war —the housewives.

In the last few years a sporadic, kitchen rebellion has taken hold in some parts of the country.

One of the best known revolts took place in 1956 in Gates Mills, a well-to-do Cleveland suburb. Women there who had formerly served as solicitors for various health agencies practically the year round decided to run a "give-once-for-all" combined drive.

Of the money collected, about $1,300 had been designated by donors for the National Foundation. But the foundation ordered its Cleveland chapter to return the money, in accordance with the national office's policy against federated drives.

Suburbs Join Rebellion

This touched off a series of rebellions in other Cleveland suburbs. At present twenty-three suburbs are linked by a combined health fund, and, according to Mrs. George J. Urban of South Euclid, a leader in the revolt, twenty-one more suburbs want to join.

Mrs. Urban reported recently that the first combined drive had spent only 1.3 per cent of

its income on fund-raising. But this was "to prove a point" about the low cost of combined drives, Mrs. Urban said. The next drive cost somewhat more, but far below that of the independent campaigns.

Last year Mrs. Urban told the National Conference on Solicitations that in most of the suburbs there had been nine independent health campaigns and "rumors of more to come." Things reached the point, she said, "where women found it impossible to recruit workers, and now they are in revolt."

At one point, Mrs. Urban said, the South Euclid chairman

for a national appeal had to make 230 telephone calls before she was able to recruit a captain for house-to-house collections.

Mutterings of discontent have also been heard in New York.

Complaints Voiced Here

"I have reached a point of no return," a woman from Woodmere, L. I., said not long ago, on the matter of the repeated telephone calls asking me, as a public-spirited citizen, to solicit, and the repeated doorbell-ringing asking me, as a community-minded person, to donate."

A Manhattan woman who lives in the Stuyvesant Town housing development said:

"We have been trying to tread water amidst this flood for years. Many of us collect for more than one drive. Many of us have long ceased to collect, because we are given money for our own sake regardless of whose drive we are pushing. Many of us have been forced to bear the abuse from those organizations whom we dare to refuse."

This woman got out her checkbook and ticked off twenty agencies to which she had contributed in a year, not counting a dollar here and there for other little fish."

"Next thing," a woman says, "we'll have an Arthritis of the Big Toe Foundation or a Headache Fund. For a while I was ashamed to say 'no,' but not any more. And the people who do give, generally they're giving 50 cents instead of a dollar."

Combining Prevents Revolt

Last fall civic leaders in northern Westchester formed a United Fund as the answer to signs of a givers' revolt. And in Norwalk, Conn., a citizens' United Fund study group found that residents were in favor of re-establishing a combined fund drive.

Gustave Levy, president of the Federation of Jewish Philanthropies of New York, recently called for a united campaign to "prevent duplication, promote efficiency and economy and actually provide more help for afflicted people."

Four major independent health agencies are in the forefront of the battle over the charity dollar. They are the National Foundation, the American Cancer Society, the American Heart Association and the National Tuberculosis Association.

The New York Times studied reports by and about these agencies, among others, and interviewed officials of these agencies concerning their method, goals and plans.

THE NATIONAL FOUNDATION

Formerly called the National Foundation for Infantile Paralysis, the agency shortened its name and widened its activities last year. Following the decline in polio after the introduction of the Salk vaccine, the foundation's income dropped from a high of nearly $68,000,000 in 1954 to $35,000,000 in 1958.

Last year the foundation announced that henceforth its March of Dimes would march not only against polio but also against rheumatoid arthritis and birth defects. This was an invasion of the field of the Arthritis and Rheumatism Foundation, among others, but Basil O'Connor, president of the National Foundation, remarked that "individual diseases are not the personal property of individual agencies."

The foundation has never been in the United Fund.

Although polio had always had a relatively low incidence —during the worst polio epidemic in 1952 there were 58,000 reported cases compared, for example, with about 10,000,000 cases of heart disease—the National Foundation was the most successful voluntary health agency in the business.

Research Called Neglected

The foundation has been accused of spending too little for research. Of $490,000,000 collected from 1938 to 1958, a total of $34,000,000 went for research, or about 7 cents of every dollar contributed. But 14 cents of every dollar, according to the foundation's figures, went to fund-raising, an activity that produces money but does not go directly to research or medical education or patient care.

There is no arguing with success, however. The foundation did provide the funds that led to the discovery of the Salk vaccine. The question is, Could the vaccine have been discovered earlier had more money gone to research?

The foundation is currently persona non grata at the National Information Bureau. This is a nonprofit organization that issues reports and gives advice on fund-raising organizations to contributors but is in no sense an "official" agency.

The bureau reports that the foundation does not meet its minimum standards because it withholds routine information and has issued "misleading" material.

For example, the foundation's 1957 annual report depicted a dime cut into wedges denoting "How National Headquarters and Chapters Used Funds During the Year." Although all the pieces added up to 100 per cent, there was no wedge denoting an outlay that year of 14.4 per cent for fund-raising, or more than $6,000,000.

Expenses in Footnote

On the following page a "summary of combined funds" of the foundation appeared, listing expenditures. There was no monetary listing of fund-raising expenses. However, at the bottom of the page there appeared a footnote that "fund-raising expenses were approximately 14.4 per cent" of a gross campaign income of $43,987,000.

It should be said, in fairness, that the foundation spent $21,502,000 that year to care for 57,000 polio patients, an average of $377.23 for each patient.

The offices of the foundation are in a new building at 800 Second Avenue. Before reaching the office of Mr. O'Connor, one passes in an outer office an array of fifteen bronze busts of heroes of the fight against polio. The busts are affixed to a wall. In ascending order are the busts of Dr. Jonas E. Salk, Mr. O'Connor and the late President Franklin D. Roosevelt.

Mr. O'Connor, a fresh carnation in his lapel, sits behind a long desk in a quietly elegant office.

In a recent interview he answered many questions. He was asked about the 7 cents of every dollar spent on research as opposed, for example, to the 26 cents for fund-raising, "headquarters expenditures" and "general administrative expenses."

Limit on Research Seen

"What most people don't realize," Mr. O'Connor said, "is that you can't spend an unlimited amount of money on research. There just aren't that many qualified researchers."

He was asked if he thought the multiplicity of fund-raising agencies was not, in the long run, harmful to all because of the public's growing annoyance.

"Not at all," he said. "We know something about the public pulse from the polls we've taken. The real truth is any sound poll would show the public is not annoyed.

"Why, if we went out of business, the other agencies wouldn't benefit a nickel unless they went out for it. You have to go out and sell yourself to the American people.

"Now, you're going to ask, why didn't we go out of business after we licked polio? Well, we had ourselves psychoanalyzed in studies by the American Institute of Public Opinion at Princeton and by the Bureau of Applied Social Research at Columbia.

"We had three choices: to pack up and go home; to confine ourselves to a single disease; or to expand. The foundation had built up experience and an army of volunteers, something belonging to the American people. We decided to go into something where our aptitudes could be used to good effect."

Mr. O'Connor paused.

"As for the United Fund—can't last. They want to take the heart out of giving, combine everything. And it'll lead to a welfare state, Government control.

"Read your de Tocqueville, what he said about the American urge to voluntarily associate for worthy causes."

Count Alexis Charles Henri Maurice Clerel de Tocqueville, a French historian, wrote in "Democracy in America" (1835-1839):

"Americans of all ages, all conditions and all dispositions constantly form associations. Whenever at the head of some new undertaking you see the government of France, or a man of rank in England, in the United States you will be sure to find an association. * * *

"I have often admired the extreme skill with which the inhabitants of the United States succeed in proposing a common object for the exertions of a great many men and in inducing them voluntarily to pursue it."

AMERICAN CANCER SOCIETY

The society was founded in 1913. It has a large but unpretentious office at 521 West Fifty-seventh Street. The society has ordered all its local units to withdraw from United Funds by Jan. 1, 1960, and run separate drives.

The society's "campaign" income for 1958, exclusive of income from investments, legacies and other sources, was $29,796,000. Of each dollar received, 29 cents was spent on research grants, 28 cents on education of the public and of professional men, 25 cents on service to cancer patients, 10 cents on fund-raising and 8 cents on administration.

For this year the society has set no specific goal—its goal is "unlimited."

As at the National Foundation, de Tocqueville was in vogue at the Cancer Society. The other day a public relations man talked about de Tocqueville's rapt description of the American genius for organizing associations.

The executive vice president of the society is Mefford R. Runyon. In a recent interview, he was asked if the society had plans for immortality similar to those of the National Foundation.

Cancer 'the One Problem'

"Definitely not," he said. "The society does not look upon itself as a perpetual organization. We are concerned with one problem: all forms of cancer.

"Now, about fund-raising. We believe in separate campaigns. We believe in the close relationship between the giver handing over a dollar and the solicitor—our 'public health missionary'—handing over educational material on the seven danger signals of cancer.

"That interrelationship is something you can't get when you ask for money for a couple of hundred agencies, all at once."

The multiplicity of health campaigns "has created some resistance in the donors and some fatigue among the volunteers," Mr. Runyon conceded.

He was questioned about the society's policy in Detroit, where its southeastern division had functioned very successfully as a part of Detroit's United Foundation. Ordered by the society to leave the federated drive by Jan. 1, 1960, the southeastern division has refused. The Cancer Society plans to revoke the division's charter and set up a new division.

Mr. Runyon said: "Despite the success of the southeastern division in the Detroit Foundation, we must have a consistent policy. We couldn't be in a federated drive in Detroit and refuse somewhere else. And they were using the success in Detroit as a lever to try to get us in federated drives in other places.

"Our fight is against cancer, not United Fund. There's a place for both of us. We believe the United Fund is geared to local community needs, but cancer is a national disease and must be attacked in a national program like ours."

AMERICAN HEART ASSOCIATION

The association was incorporated in New York State in 1924. In 1955 it voted a ban on the entry of local units into federated drives. Locals already in such drives were advised to withdraw whenever their allocations from the combined drive were not large enough to satisfy them.

In 1958 the association's campaign income was $22,345,-000. Of each dollar received, about 38 cents went to research, 23 cents to education of the public and professionals, 14 cents to community service and 12 cents for fund-raising.

The association's offices are at 44 East Twenty-third Street. The executive director, Rome A. Betts, said recently:

"Our experience with the United Fund dates back to

1948. Until 1955 our policy was to participate, provided chapters felt it was to their best interest.

"By 1954 it was fairly evident that the results in federated drives were not measuring up to our independent campaigns."

On the growing number of independent campaigns, Mr. Betts said:

"We've had to work an awful lot harder this year to maintain our position. One must admit that the growing number of solicitations that employ doorbell techniques are creating a serious problem.

"But one of the reasons for the growing resistance is the United Fund's preaching about the nuisance. 'Aren't you fed up!' Aren't you tired of these campaigns?' They tell the people how they should feel."

NATIONAL TUBERCULOSIS ASSOCIATION

Organized in 1904, the association is the oldest voluntary health agency in the country. It is one of the few that solicits on more or less a "quid pro quo" basis; that is, it mails its familiar Christmas seals to millions of people on its mailing list, hoping to receive a contribution in return.

Of the major agencies, it has

one of the biggest fund-raising costs. The association reports a gross cost of 23½ cents for every dollar in its 1956 campaign.

In fiscal 1958 the association took in $25,959,000 from its seal sales. State and local organizations kept $24,402,000. Of the remainder—the national's income of $1,557,600—about $326,-000 was allocated to medical research. Nevertheless the association's 1958 annual report lists medical research as number one in its field of attack.

Of the major causes of death, tuberculosis ranks twelfth (heart disease is first). The incidence of death from TB is about eight for each 100,000 of population. It used to be 188 for each 100,000. It is estimated that there are about 800,000 active cases in the country.

The drop from 188 in 100,000 to eight in 100,000 is, of course, due in great part to the activities of the National Tuberculosis Association and to new drugs.

Menace Factor Stressed

However, the association's current literature calls TB a "major public health problem" and warns that "millions of Americans have been lulled more and more into a state of

dangerous complacency by the decline in the death rate and by medical advances."

The association's offices are at 1790 Broadway. Dr. James E. Perkins, managing director, said in an interview recently: "Our expenditures for research may be a little low, but we don't need to spend too much."

Dr. Perkins said people were getting too complacent about TB. "We have a long way to go yet," he said. "Two million people have or have had TB, and 40,000,000 people have reacted to the tuberculin test."

He was asked about the association's future.

"We don't plan to go out of business for some time," Dr. Perkins said. "We are interested in all the other respiratory diseases."

Dr. Perkins said that some local chapters of the National Tuberculosis Association were leaving federated drives, having found they could do better alone. No new chapters are now permitted to join the United Fund if they want to continue their contacts with the national association.

"However," Dr. Perkins said, "we are for a live and let live policy as regards the United Fund and the voluntary health agencies."

June 16, 1959

Research and Money

Health Programs Found to Need Continuing Support of Foundations

By HOWARD A. RUSK, M. D.

"Progress of any kind depends first of all on survival and on strength. Because of that, the foundation has had and will continue to have a deep interest in preventing disease, in caring for the sick, in rehabilitating those stricken by illness.

"These are not sentimental considerations. They form the responsibilities and the opportunities of a free society. They cannot be ignored without peril, for it is only the strong who can really be free."

These timely and mature words of wisdom written by Mr. David M. Heyman are from the five-year report of the New York Foundation.

The report was one of three such reports issued last week by major foundations concerned with medical and health-related research. The others were the John A. Hartford Foundation and the Life Insurance

Medical Research Fund.

Continuing, Mr. Heyman pointed out that there has been an "alarming tendency" for individual and institutional philanthropy to reduce its support of medical research on the ground that huge governmental expenditures for such activities have diminished the need for private effort.

Although Mr. Heyman does not name the Rockefeller Foundation, it is obviously one of the organizations to which he refers.

The Rockefeller Foundation, which for 50 years has strongly supported medical research and education, recently announced a change in its policies that will minimize support in this area.

In doing so, it said, "Much of what was once pioneer work by the foundation has now been absorbed, on a vastly increasing scale, into the programs of government and international organizations."

This year, according to a report issued last Thursday by

the National Institutes of Health, non-Federal sources will provide about 40 per cent of the total national expenditure of $1.5 billion for medical and health-related research.

Federal expenditures for such research, which have increased about 25 per cent a year since 1947, will reach about $1.3 billion in 1964. This is about 7 cents out of the total Federal research and development dollar.

Mr. Heyman in his statement admitted that the "vast resources of government dwarf the amount which foundations can appropriate for medicine."

He pointed out, however, that the quantity of money is not the only consideration, for foundations have flexibility and can do many things government is unable to do.

Since the Rockefeller Foundation is reducing its support of medical research, the John A. Hartford Foundation will become the largest foundation in the nation primarily devoted to medical research.

In assets it ranks fourth in size behind the Ford Foundation, Rockefeller Foundation and Duke Endowment.

In 1962 the John A. Hartford Foundation made or paid grants

totaling $17.4 million to institutions and organizations in 28 states. With but few exceptions the grants went to support medical research.

Most research supported by the foundation falls into the category of applied or problem-solving research as opposed to basic research, which is intended purely to add to the sum of man's knowledge.

Although research sponsored by the foundation runs a broad gamut, it has placed particular emphasis on the support of research in open-heart surgery and kidney dialysis, the process by which waste materials are removed through the "artificial kidney."

The Life Insurance Medical Research Fund, which is supported by 113 life insurance companies, made grants of $1.2 million last year to support medical research and fellowships.

The New York Foundation, the John A. Hartford Foundation and the Life Insurance Medical Research Fund are examples of the many voluntary organizations that are concerned with medical research.

As Mr. Heyman has said, "It would be a tragic mistake if foundations now prematurely withdrew from a field to which they have contributed so much and which still needs their special strengths."

October 20, 1963

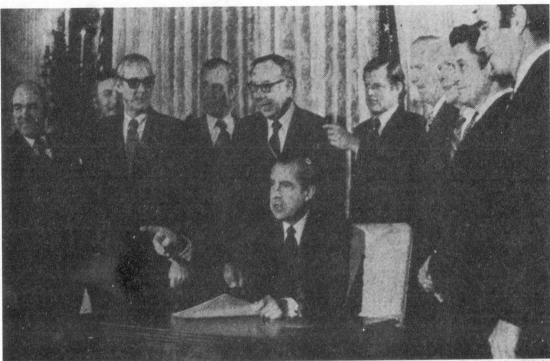

The New York Times/Mike Lien

SPURS CANCER RESEARCH: President Nixon at ceremony at which he signed bill to expand fight on cancer. Behind him, from left: Representative David E. Satterfield, Virginia Democrat; Senator Richard S. Schweiker, Pennsylvania Republican; Representative James F. Hastings, New York Republican; Senator J. Glenn Beall Jr., Maryland Republican; Representative Paul G. Rogers, Florida Democrat; Senator Edward M. Kennedy, Massachusetts Democrat; Representatives William L. Springer, Illinois Republican, Harley O. Staggers, West Virginia Democrat, and William R. Roy, Kansas Democrat, and Senator Harrison A. Williams Jr., New Jersey Democrat.

Nixon Signs Cancer Bill; Cites Commitment to Cure

By HAROLD M. SCHMECK Jr.
Special to The New York Times

WASHINGTON, Dec. 23—President Nixon signed today a bill to implement a much-expanded research attack on cancer, saying it might prove to be the most significant act of his Presidency.

"I hope that in the years ahead that we look back on this as being the most significant action taken during this Administration," Mr. Nixon said at the ceremony in the White House State Dining Room. He said that history might assess it that way because of the importance of the cancer problem.

It was one of the relatively few occasions on which Mr. Nixon has made the signing of a bill a public ceremony.

Some 137 guests were present, including 14 Senators and Representatives, many prominent cancer research scientists and others interested in the bill.

The new law, called the Cancer Act of 1971, authorizes the spending of $1.6-billion over the next three years for research and related activities. The legislation was the fruit of long debate during the last year and a compromise worked out only in the last few weeks.

Schmidt to Head Panel

The President added a final note of compromise today by naming Benno C. Schmidt, of J. H. Whitney & Co. New York, as chairman of a special watchdog committee responsible for keeping him informed on the progress of the cancer effort.

Mr. Schmidt headed a study group, sponsored by the Senate, that made a report about a year ago recommending that a major new independent Federal agency be set up to administer the nation's cancer research program.

The question of whether there should be such an agency was a key issue in the debate over the cancer legislation.

Opponents of the separate agency have argued that the research administration should be kept within the existing Federal framework.

The Senate passed, almost without opposition, a bill that reflected much of the study group's philosophy. The House passed, by an equivalent margin, a bill that took the opposite approach. The final compromise, closer to the House than to the Senate version, centers the responsibility for the expanded cancer program on the National Cancer Institute, a part of the National Institutes of Health. But the cancer institute is given an independent budget and some other attributes of increased stature.

Posing for photographs after he signed the bill, Mr. Nixon was flanked by Representative Paul G. Rogers, Democrat of Florida, chief architect of the House bill, and Senator Edward M. Kennedy, Democrat of Massachusetts, chief sponsor of the Senate bill. They were surrounded by a dozen other members of both houses who had been most active in drafting the legislation.

Mr. Nixon said that the signing of the bill showed that the Administration and Congress were totally committed to a large-scale research effort against cancer and to providing the funds that would make it possible.

The President said that private citizens and voluntary nongovernmental organizations such as the American Cancer Society were also committed to the goal. He said he would not want to raise false hopes simply by the signing of an act.

"But, we can say this," he added, "that for those who have cancer, and who are looking for success in this field, they at least can have the assurance that everything that can be done by Government, everything that can be done by voluntary agencies in this great, powerful, rich country, now will be done and that will give some hope and we hope those hopes will not be disappointed."

Sharp Increases Urged

The bill calls for sharp increases in cancer research funding. For the programs administered and supported by the National Cancer Institute it authorizes $400-million for the current fiscal year, $500-million for the fiscal year 1973 and $600-million for the fiscal year 1974.

The 1972 Health, Education and Welfare appropriation bill contained $337-million for the cancer research programs administered by the institute. Much of the money goes to nongovernmental research programs through grants and contracts.

The new bill also authorizes nonresearch cancer control programs, such as early detection programs, to be supported at the level of $20-million this year; $30-million next year and $40-million in fiscal 1974. Provision for these programs was among the features of the legislation provided in the House bill, but not in the original Senate bill.

December 24, 1971

War on Cancer Stirs A Political Backlash

By HAROLD M. SCHMECK Jr.

Special to The New York Times

WASHINGTON, May 26— Three and half years ago, Congress and President Nixon declared war on cancer. Today some see a backlash emerging, based more on the political than the scientific aspects of the effort.

Critics of the Government's efforts have cited the steady climb of cancer deaths as proof that little if any progress has been made despite the more than $1.7-billion spent on the anti-cancer program since the National Cancer Act of 1971 became law in December of that year.

Prominent scientists have charged that large sums have been spent for the wrong purposes and in the wrong places, and that sometimes too much has been attempted too soon.

Money Called the Key

A few months after his resignation in January as assistant secretary for health in the Department of Health, Education and Welfare, Dr. Charles C. Edwards wrote an article on United States health care for the New England Journal of Medicine.

In it he said that the cancer program had been based on "the politically, attractive, but scientifically dubious premise that a dread and enigmatic disease can, like the surface of the moon, be conquered if we will simply spend enough money to get the job done."

There is no question that political as well as scientific and humanitarian factors played a part in the origin of the program five years ago.

Seeing much of the credit going to Democrats such as Senator Edward M. Kennedy of Massachusetts, Mr. Nixon asserted leadership of the cause himself. When the expanded program got under way, the President promised it unlimited funds, although the promise was never really kept.

Congress Provides Funds

Sponsorship of cancer research has always been good politics. Congress has consistently appropriated more money for it than a succession of administrations really wanted to spend.

Cancer is also a group of dread and deadly diseases whose conquest would, without question, be a milestone in human progress. While the current program was somewhat controversial from its start, neither the original debate over it nor the one causing a flurry of interest now indicates that sides are forming for and against cancer research. On this issue there is virtually no opposition. Everyone favors cancer research.

Furthermore, many agree that the national program, the largest ever undertaken against one category of disease, is generating a great deal of excellent research and is being creditably run.

But critics contend that the effort is getting involved too much in patient care, is gulping money that ought to go to other areas of biomedical research and, through some of its supporters from the outside, is tarred with the image of trying to conquer cancer by feats of research management —such as that of the United States moon program.

The deceptively easy analogy to the moon landing figured in much of the early criticism of the plans for a war on cancer. Some scientists feared the effort would be a rigidly targeted program of research and development that could never unravel one of the most elusive mysteries of biology. Leaders of the effort deny this, pointing to the broad range of basic research being supported. But the stereotype remains to plague them.

Even Benno C. Schmidt, chairman of the President's cancer panel and a stanch advocate of the program, admits that many scientists have been particularly critical of the National Cancer Plan, which is supposed to be the basic strategy document for the "war."

"I suspect that if we took a vote, most scientists would be happier if there were no cancer plan, if there never had been a plan," he said.

Not a Blueprint

Mr. Schmidt insists, however, that the plan is not a blueprint. He says, further, that the cancer program is already proving its worth and that much of the criticism is based on misunderstanding. Even the amount of criticism that exists is far less than some reports in the press suggest, he says.

He and other proponents of the program see the anti-cancer effort as a long fight, and one well worth the effort considering that cancer kills more than 350,000 Americans a year, causing immense suffering at a huge cost.

Most critics concede that the program is supporting a great deal of excellent scientific activity. But they worry that there may be a larger public expectation of quick progress than the facts warrant. They also worry that officials under the pressure of these expectations, may resort to a series of crash programs unlikely to have any significant benefit.

This concern was expressed recently by Dr. James D. Watson, a Nobel Prize winner, who is director of the Cold Spring Harbor Laboratory. In his most recent annual report of that institution on Long Island he said:

"I thus suspect that a major problem now facing cancer research, if not the world of pure biology, is how to be realistic about what we can do for society without seeming to reject the hands that may want to overfeed us."

Early questions concerning the program were partly scientific, partly pragmatic: Was the time really ripe for an all-out research assault on cancer, a scientific problem almost as complex and mysterious as the nature of life? Could large sums be channeled into any such effort abruptly without waste and without damage to the rest of the nation's biomedical research efforts?

The controversy seems more intense now than it was five years ago. The recent complaints are more often linked to the latter question than the former.

Some criticisms are seldom voiced publicly. For example, the charge that large sums were given out early in the program to help finance comprehensive cancer centers at institutions that had received poor ratings by professionals who had evaluated them.

"That's when they really grabbed the money and ran," said one staff member of the National Cancer Institute during a recent conversation.

The institute, the largest and oldest unit of the National Institutes of Health, is the Government agency responsible for the cancer program.

Fruits of Research

The institute has been in existence since the late nineteen-thirties. Until the 1971 act it was devoted almost exclusively to research. The new program also gave it major responsibilities for the task of making the fruits of research available to patients everywhere in the country.

One of the mechanisms designed to do this was the support of comprehensive cancer centers where medical scientists would do clinical research and would, at the same time, bring the latest knowledge to the benefit of local patients and their doctors.

In the 1973 fiscal year—the first after the expanded program came into being—$48-million was awarded in construction grants for comprehensive cancer centers at 10 major institutions. This was a substantial sum for administration by an institute that, just two years previously, had a total budget of little more than $200-million.

This early flowering of the center's program has been criticized on several grounds. One was that in the early days the money had been spent too quickly and, therefore, sometimes accomplished little beyond adding an extra wing or so to an institution.

Ties With Institutions

Another was that the centers were likely to usurp too much highly trained manpower that was already scarce. A third was the risks of conflict of interest when the National Cancer Advisory Board, required to oversee the institutes' spending plans, had members with close ties to many of the institutions receiving the money.

The board members, appointed by the President to oversee the Cancer Institute's programs, include laymen from a wide range of occupations as well as scientists. During the first year of the program, more than half of the institutions' awarded construction grants for comprehensive cancer centers were institutions to which one or another board member had ties.

Some famous institutions, notably Children's Cancer Research Foundation in Boston and Roswell Park Memorial Institute in Buffalo, were awarded major construction grants despite low priority scores given them by scientific review panels.

Spokesmen for the cancer program say stringent precautions are taken to avoid conflict of interest and favoritism in awarding funds. In one area of the program—that having to do with cancer virus research—the board appointed a special committee to investigate reported conflicts of interest. The panel's report last year led to substantial changes.

The committee, headed by Dr. Norton Zinder of Rockefeller University, reported there had been frequent instances of apparent conflict of interest, with officers of the Cancer Institute often awarding contracts to outside laboratories with which the officers were associated.

Environmental Causes

The cancer program in general has also been criticized for not devoting more emphasis to the difficult, but important, problem of environmental causes of cancer and for tending to enter too much into the area of patient care as opposed to research. The latter circumstance, if true, probably reflects the desires of the Congress — which allocates the money.

One major problem worries virtually everyone in the Cancer Institute and many of its well-wishers. This is the institute's shortage of personnel.

In 1971, when the institute was responsible for spending about $233-million for all its programs, the total staff was about 1,600. This year, the staff is only slightly higher—1,836. But this year's expenditures—when the current fiscal year ends next month—will total more than $699-million. In other words, a staff that has grown by less than a third is responsible for administering programs that have more than tripled.

The hold-down on employment is an Administration economy strategy that affects the whole Federal Government. But because Congress and Mr. Nixon vied with each other in espousing an all-out war on cancer, the Cancer Institute has a lot of money and a staff strained to the danger point.

The cancer program is also caught in another bind between politics and science. The promises are made—or implied—by the politicians. The delivery is up to the scientists and physicians.

The politicians—both those of government and of the world of voluntary agency fund raising—want results meaningful to their constituents. Scientists have been reasonably effective in delivering these, but not on anyone's preordained schedule.

Few if any research workers or cancer specialists expected cancer death rates to turn downward within several years of the beginning of the expanded war on cancer. Yet the program is currently under assault because the downturns have not occurred. In fact, most improvements in cancer treatment have origins that go back far before the current program.

At this stage, officers of the Cancer Institute are at a disadvantage in trying to itemize the advances they have made in the past few years because these cannot be translated into lives saved or cancers cured.

Inescapable Lag

Dr. Frank J. Rauscher Jr., director of the Cancer Institute, said that important gains in the ability to treat and cure cancer were made during the past 15 years, but that there was an inescapable lag between improvements and their dissemination.

Dr. Vincent Devita, director of the institute's Cancer Treatment Division, said that some significant improvements in survival in some of the major forms of cancer, including

breast cancer, would probably become apparent soon, based on data being accumulated now.

Dr. Alan S. Rabson, director of the Division of Cancer Biology and Diagnosis, cited a list of scientific advances that have come to fruition during the past few years, some of which could have profound effects not only on cancer but on other diseases.

For example, he cited research with an enzyme called reverse transcriptase, one of the major developments in basic cancer research of the early nineteen-seventies.

Its suspected links to the cancer process might have been discovered without the cancer program, he said, but some of the ways it has been applied already to other research programs would probably have had to wait for years.

It has been used, he said, as a tool for discovering how many copies of a particular piece of genetic information an individual cell makes, a find of great interest to geneticists and one that has already been put to use in studying some hereditary blood diseases.

A scientist at the University of Chicago whose research has been supported by the institute has made a discovery, Dr. Rabson said, that may give doctors an important guide to the post-surgical treatment of breast cancer patients by distinguishing those cancers that are sensitive to hormones from those that are not.

Dr. Thomas Waldmann of the Cancer Institute has found that some patients with immun-

ological deficiencies have hitherto unsuspected suppressor cells in their bodies that may help account for the deficiencies.

None of these advances, nor any of the others Dr. Rabson listed, are likely to have any quick effect on cancer mortality. Indeed it is entirely possible that they may never, themselves, save lives. But they do add pieces to the huge multidimensional jigsaw puzzle of the cancer problem. They are the kinds of advances the nation really "buys" when it supports scientific research. These advances are not readily predictable.

Some make a greater difference to medical practice than others—often in ways that defy advance prediction. And some may even be useless without a long-term, broad-based commitment.

This is essentially what responsible scientists worried about more than five years ago when the groundswell of publicity seemed to suggest an effort to go too big too soon.

Clearly there are many men and women on the nonscientific side of the spectrum who were not misled. But some observers, scientists and laymen alike, fear that escalating budgets may require ever escalating rhetoric and that the whole so-called war against cancer may sink into a Vietnam-like quagmire with inflated promises about "the next few years" and the next few hundred million dollars—all illuminated by the doubtful flickering of "the light at the end of the tunnel."

May 27, 1975

'The Annual Medical Agony'

By Joseph R. Hixson

The Bethesda, Md., campus of the National Institutes of Health lacks only one facility to help mankind cure disease: an official lamentation center to which white-coated researchers and well-tailored lobbyists can return each spring when the President's budget comes out.

Fiscal 1976-77 is proving no exception to the annual medical agony. The Ford Administration is planning a major budget crunch that would severely curtail medical research: Cancer funds would drop from $744-million to $688 million; heart-disease and lung-disease funds from $349-million to $343 million; and maternal and infant-health research would be

Joseph R. Hixson is author of "The Patchwork Mouse: Politics and Intrigue in the Campaign to Conquer Cancer."

cut proportionally from $127 million.

When medical budgets are slashed, anguished cries are heard from various disease parishes: "But not us!"

Benno Schmidt, vice chairman of the Memorial Sloan-Kettering Cancer Center, throws his considerable weight on the side of maintaining or increasing the funding of N.I.H.'s National Cancer Institute. Houston's famed heart surgeon, Michael DeBakey, insists that research on cardiovascular disease at N.I.H.'s Heart and Lung Institute get favored treatment. And Harry E. Green, chairman of the National Foundation March of Dimes, champions the N.I.H. allocation for Child Health and Human Development.

At a recent meeting of anesthesiologists concerned with trauma—the medical term for injury, whether from a gun or an accident—a speaker castigated the Federal Establishment for the scant research attention paid to wounds—the nation's fourth lead-

ing cause of death and the leading cause for citizens under forty. Following a time-worn track, he said the Government spends $122 in research for every cancer patient in the land, $74 for every heart-disease and blood-vessel-disease patient, but only 24 cents for victims of trauma. He meant his field was being shortchanged.

Still others complain that too little money is spent on maternal and child care. Funds for mothers-to-be, appropriated by the Department of Health, Education and Welfare, are scheduled to drop from $322 million to $211-million next year.

It's quite apparent that diseases of the elderly — cancer, and heart and lung disorders—get the bulk of the Federal research dollar. Diseases of the young get one-third of this.

Recently, a professor of law at Brandeis University predicted a backlash as younger citizens came to realize fully how much they were scheduled to contribute to older people via Social Security and other Federal programs for the aged, such as Medicare.

It will be interesting to see whether young parents will mount an attack on Federal health research and health-care delivery systems that favor the diseases of the aged by a two-to-one margin over research on birth defects, mental retardation, and maternal, fetal, and newborn catastrophes that have 30- and 40-year consequences.

Who should decide where the health priorities lie? When Franklin D. Roosevelt was alive, polio had center stage. Mr. Schmidt and Mrs. Mary Lasker have done their best for cancer. The heart people, too, have their heavy artillery.

But the allocation of the nation's health dollars is too important an issue to be left to wealthy influentials, surgeons with vested interests or Presidential intimates.

We have at this moment in Washington an Institute of Medicine, an arm of the National Academy of Sciences. Why shouldn't that distinguished body of medical scientists be asked to counsel us on what part of our health research dollar we should spend on the young, old, crippled, allergic, infected, blind?

I see no reason why the electorate and its politicians shouldn't have a go at the *level* of American health-research expenditures. But once that level has been agreed upon, it does seem odd that lobbyists should have so much influence over what diseases get priority.

The annual and unseemly wrangling over diseased constituencies, or potentially diseased constituencies, ought to yield to some considered judgments.

March 3, 1976

DISEASE: PROBLEMS AND PROGRESS

MOSQUITO CARRIES YELLOW FEVER GERM

Special to The New York Times.

PHILADELPHIA, Oct. 26.—That the mosquito serves as the "intermediate host" for the parasite of yellow fever, and that it is highly probable that the disease is only propagated through the bite of this insect, is the conclusion reached by a board of medical officers who went to Cuba in the Summer of the present year to make a study of the dread disease.

The Philadelphia Medical Journal will to-morrow publish a summary of the results of their investigations. The board was composed of Dr. Walter Reed, surgeon, United States Army, and Dr. James Carroll, Dr. A. Agramonte, and Dr. Jesse W. Lazear, all acting assistant surgeons of the United States Army. A tragic feature of the expedition was that Dr. Lazear himself gave up his life before the work was done, having died of yellow jack on the evening of Sept. 25. Dr. Carroll also contracted the disease, but recovered.

When the board reached Cuba an epidemic of yellow fever was prevailing in the town of Quemados, thus furnishing an opportunity for clinical observations and for bacteriologic and pathologic work. The cases studied during this epidemic had been diagnosed by a board of physicians, selected largely by reason of their familiarity with yellow fever. This board consisted of Drs. Nicolo Silverio, Manuel Herera, Eduardo Angles, Acting Assistant Surgeon Roger P. Ames, and Dr. Lazear.

The board says in the "preliminary note," as the article in The Philadelphia Medical Journal is termed:

" We must call attention to the fact that Dr. Agramonte, whenever he performs an autopsy in this room, [the hospital dead room,] is always attended by a young soldier of the Hospital Corps, United States Army, who is detailed for that purpose, and whose duty it is to assist and afterward to tend to the cleaning of the autopsy table. This soldier, a non-immune American, was present when Dr. Carroll was there, and remained afterward to attend to his duties. He has not contracted yellow fever by his duties in this room from day to day.

" Our own experience would seem to accord with others, viz., that attendance upon autopsies and the handling of portions of organs of yellow fever cases removed to the laboratory is unattended with danger. Certainly the three non-immune members of this board, up to the time of these mosquito inoculations had, during the past three months, come in close contact with the dead bodies and organs of yellow fever cases, freely handling and examining these organs, including the small intestines, even kept at thermostat temperature for twenty-four hours, without contracting the disease."

" Dr. Carroll was bitten at 2 P. M. Aug. 27, 1900, by Culex fasciatus. This particular mosquito had bitten a severe case of yellow fever on the second day of the disease twelve days before; a mild case of yellow fever on the first day of the attack, six days preceding; a severe case of yellow fever on the second day of the attack four days before, and a mild case of yellow fever on the second day of the attack two days before inoculation."

Dr. Carroll remained well until the afternoon of Aug. 29, when he was overcome by lassitude, and developed a very severe case of yellow fever.

An American, twenty-four years old, resident in Cuba, was bitten on the forenoon of Aug. 31 by the same mosquito that had bitten Dr. Carroll four days before. He also contracted a very severe case of the fever.

The story of Dr. Lazear's illness and death is told in the following language:

" Dr. Lozear was bitten on Aug. 16, 1900, by a mosquito, (Culex fasciatus,) which ten days previously had been contaminated by biting a very mild case of yellow fever, (fifth day.) No appreciable disturbance of health followed this inoculation.

" On Sept. 13, 1900, (forenoon,) Dr. Lazear, while on a visit to Las Animas Hospital, and while collecting blood from yellow fever patients for study, was bitten by a Culex mosquito (variety undetermined.) As Dr. Lazear had been previously bitten by a contaminated insect without after-effects, he deliberately allowed this particular mosquito, which had settled on the back of his hand, to remain until it had satisfied its hunger.

" On the evening of Sept. 18, five days after the bite, Dr. Lazear complained of feeling 'out of sorts,' and had a chill at 8 P. M.

" On Sept. 19, 12 o'clock noon, his temperature was 102.4 degrees, pulse 112; his eyes were injected and his face suffused; at 3 P. M. temperature was 103.4 degrees, pulse 104; 6 P. M., temperature 103.8 degrees and pulse 106. Jaundice appeared on the third day. The subsequent history of this case was one of progressive and fatal yellow fever, the death of our much-lamented colleague having occurred on the evening of Sept. 25, 1900.

" As Dr. Lazear was bitten by a mosquito while present in the wards of a yellow fever hospital, one must, at least, admit the possibility of this insect's contamination by a previous bite of a yellow fever patient. This case of accidental infection therefore cannot fail to be of interest."

This is the summing up of the board's preliminary note:

" For ourselves, we have been profoundly impressed with the mode of infection and with the results that followed the bite of the mosquito in these three cases. Our results would appear to throw new light on Carter's (Dr. Henry R. Carter's) observations in Mississippi, as to the period required between the introduction of the first (infecting) case and the occurrence of secondary cases of yellow fever.

" Since we here, for the first time, record a case in which a typical attack of yellow fever has followed the bite of an infected mosquito, within the usual period of incubation of the disease, in which other sources of infection can be excluded, we feel confident that the publication of these observations must excite renewed interest in the mosquito theory of the propagation of yellow fever, as first proposed by Finlay."

October 27, 1900

X RAY CURE FOR CANCER.

Special to The New York Times.

SAN FRANCISCO, Feb. 18.—After suffering from cancer of the face for twenty-five years Dr. J. M. Selfridge, founder of Fabiola Hospital, Oakland, believes he has been almost completely cured by the X-ray. Last October Dr. Selfridge began experimenting with the X-ray in conjunction with his son, Dr. C. M. Selfridge, and Dr. N. H. Chamberlain. So successful have been the trials that numbers of other sufferers have taken the same remedy and have met with astonishing relief. As far as the trial has gone it seems a check has been discovered for the disease.

Dr. Selfridge was led to begin the experiments by noting the powerful irritating effect of the ray on healthy skin. He conceived the idea that the ray might dry up and heal cancerous tissue. He made a face mask of thin sheets of lead, allowing only a small aperture over the cancer. He was placed on the operating table and his face covered with the mask, the cancerous wound only being exposed to the action of the ray.

The beneficial results were noted at once, and since then the cancer began to dry up. Now it is entirely healed, only a scar remaining to show where the sore was.

February 19, 1900

THE TUBERCULOSIS DANGER

The Tenement House Commission of the State of New York, appointed by the Legislature to investigate the tenement-house problem in New York, held its first public hearing yesterday afternoon in the Assembly Hall of the Charities Building, at 105 East Twenty-second Street.

The subject under discussion, "The Relation of Tuberculosis to the Tenement House Problem," was dealt with exhaustively by Dr. John H. Pryor of Buffalo, Dr. Herrman M. Biggs, who has charge of the pathological and bacteriological laboratories of the Board of Health, and is a visiting physician at Bellevue Hospital, as well as several other physicians, who were invited to speak on the subject by the Tenement House Commission. All testified that consumption in this city was almost wholly confined to the tenement-house districts, and that its prevalence was the result of overcrowding and bad sanitary conditions.

Dr. Pryor, when introduced by Chairman Robert W. De Forest, said that he had been a practicing physician in Buffalo for many years, and had been the Chairman of a committee appointed to investigate the tenement houses of that city. In 1893, he said, the conditions of the tenements there were as bad as they are here, but owing to ordinances passed on the recommendation of his committee they have been greatly improved.

"From the facts I have gathered so far," he said, "I should judge that there are always at least 20,000 consumptives among the tenement dwellers of the city. This doesn't show all the cases of tuberculosis, for a great many dying from other diseases have tuberculosis in some form. The two distinctive tenement-house diseases are tuberculosis and rickets. There is at least one case of consumption in almost every tenement house in the city, the reason being that the tenants are so crowded together, without sufficient air or sunlight. They are dirty and careless. The expectorations from consumptive people dry up and are disseminated in the air. While consumption is both preventable and curable in its early stages, the death rate of its victims does not decrease. It remains at 6,000 in the city from year to year. We have no proper accommodations for consumptives. They are the only class of invalids who do not get proper care."

As remedies for the present condition of affairs Dr. Pryor said that at least 500 feet of cubic air should be allowed for each adult in a tenement, and that no rooms without sunlight should be occupied.

"Many houses are infected with the germs," he said, "and every one who lives in them courts death. It would be possible to thoroughly disinfect all these houses, although some of them could not be made sanitary unless they were torn down."

Dr. Herrman M. Biggs produced maps showing the tenement house districts in the city where consumption is most prevalent. According to Dr. Biggs, in one block on Cherry Street 144 out of 1,000 people had died of consumption in the last four years. In the block on Pell Street between the Bowery and Mott Street, and on Mott Street between Pell Street and Chatham Square there have been 318 deaths from consumption out of 2,000 inhabitants in the last four years.

"In regard to remedies," he said, "I think that it is an error to make landlords build very expensive houses for poor people. The cost is ultimately borne by the tenants, and that means overcrowding. The chances of death from fire in a tenement house are infinitely less than the chances of death from consumption. I have no doubt that we can stamp out tuberculosis, for the disease is only transmitted by germs contained in the expectorations of the sufferers. Carpets and wall paper should be prohibited in tenement houses."

Dr. Frankel, manager of the United Hebrew Charities Association, said that in the case of the vast majority of consumptive foreigners who had applied to him for help the disease had been contracted in this country.

"Although these people live an almost unbearable life before they come here," he said, "they very rarely have tuberculosis when they arrive. Out of seventy-two Jews suffering from tuberculosis I found that only one had been in America less than fifteen years."

Dr. Anna Daniel, house physician in the New York Infirmary for Women, said that sweatshop work in the tenement houses was responsible in a great measure for the spread of tuberculosis.

"Frequently a woman is sewing clothes up to the date of her death," she said. "In other places I have seen consumptives manufacturing cigars and expectorating on them. Italian peddlers sort out their fruit every day in their rooms and keep it under their beds. I have known a family living in two rooms to take in as many as nineteen boarders."

"Do you think the present sweatshop law has made any improvement?" asked the Chairman.

"No," said Dr. Daniel, emphatically, "I don't!"

Dr. S. A. Knopf of 11 West Forty-fifth Street next suggested that the roofs of tenement houses should be converted into breathing places, and said that the sills of the windows should be raised to a good distance above the floor, so that the windows could be open without a risk of having children falling out.

November 17, 1900

THE MENACE OF EPIDEMIC.

The annual report of the State Health Commissioner of New York to the Governor makes the startling but not surprising statement that a great many cities and towns are menaced by epidemics of typhoid fever such as have prevailed within the past year or two at Ithaca, West Seneca, Watertown, and other places. Of the economic aspects of this situation the Commissioner says:

If the monetary value of a human life is assumed to be $5,000, the deaths from but five of the preventable diseases during 1903 in this State represent a loss of $94,960,000. These figures seem appalling, and yet millions upon millions can properly be added to this sum, in loss of wages, expense of the care of the sick, and many other expenses incidental to the management of these epidemic and infectious diseases.

The five preventable diseases referred to and the deaths due to each last year are: Pulmonary tuberculosis, 13,173; diphtheria, 3,056; typhoid fever, 1,665; scarlet fever, 1,057; smallpox, 41, a total of 18,992.

It is probably true that the conclusion to be drawn from these gloomy statistics is that the State should make more ample provision for the work of the State Board of Health, but this is not the only one to which they point, nor is it the most important. The State Board cannot safeguard life or health in centres of population where the people are so indifferent to the dangers which menace them that—as at Ithaca, for example—they are content with a weak and inefficient local sanitary administration and deliberately close their eyes to the clearest and most specific warnings of danger to conserve the petty interests of local trade. Whatever is done to protect communities against epidemics must be done where the danger exists. When an epidemic breaks out and reaches proportions which defy concealment, the State Board renders an excellent service in sending an expert to stimulate the local Board of Health to intelligent and efficient activity in dealing with dangerous conditions. To encourage communities to feel that they may safely rely upon the State Board to maintain the vigilance against the consequences of their own negligence which is the price of safety would be to increase the danger which now menaces them. Cities, towns, and villages must be made to appreciate the fact that they must look after their own health, and that unless they do this under good advice and wise guidance and spend the sums needed to clean their neglected places, purify their water supplies, and guard against secondary infection, a calamity may overtake them which will involve the expenditure of thousands to accomplish a small part of what might have been done for as many hundreds if done in time. The inspiration to intelligent activity in such matters must come from public-spirited citizens who are willing to be counted the enemies of local prosperity until such time as their work is appreciated. A revival of the local spirit which found expression in the New England town improvement society movement is much needed, and the missionary who shall preach it effectively will be a public benefactor.

April 18, 1904

INFECTION BY INHALATION.

Special to The New York Times.

WASHINGTON, July 24.—Government pathologists and bacteriologists are following with great interest the general movement under the auspices of the local Boards of Health of the larger cities toward securing better ventilation of street cars, churches, places of public amusement, &c., in connection with sanitation.

Especial interest is felt in the action that the New York Board of Aldermen has taken in making a special appropriation of $10,000 for the New York Board of Health, to be devoted to the study of pneumonia and acute respiratory diseases and the possibility of infection through inhalation.

In this connection Dr. Walter Wyman, Surgeon General of the United States Marine Hospital Service, said:

"We have lately been compelled to modify some of our notions of the causes of contagious and infectious diseases. After the brilliant discoveries by Pasteur and Koch, it was thought that the presence of the pathogenic microbe organism was like the bite of a venomous snake, surely poisonous. But now we know that there are other conditions besides the presence of the microbe necessary to produce disease.

"Many people go about with virulent diplococci of pneumonia in their respiratory tract, but do not have pneumonia. Why? Because their cells are vigorous enough to prevent the diplococci invading the lungs. But put such a person under bad sanitary conditions or depress his vitality, and the microbes are not phagocyted; they invade the lungs and pneumonia and death follow. The same, to a limited degree, occurs with the bacillus diphtheriae.

"In times of cholera epidemics men go about with living, virulent, cholera vibrio in their intestinal canal, yet they are not sick. Why? Because the conditions for the production of the cholera toxins are not favorable. But let such a person eat poor and tainted food or derange his digestion through indiscretion or evil sanitary surroundings, and the disease results.

"Many people live a long and active life with tubercle bacilli encysted in the apex of one lung. As long as they have plenty of fresh air and sunshine and good sanitary surroundings they remain well. But give such a person poor food or bad sanitary surroundings, and see what happens. The battle going on between the bacilli and the cells results in a victory for the bacilli. The cells die and the victorious bacilli spread havoc through the lungs."

July 25, 1904

RATIFIES SANITARY TREATY.

Senate Agrees to Convention Dealing with Plague and Cholera.

WASHINGTON, March 1.—The Senate, in executive session to-day, ratified and made public an international sanitary treaty, adopted by a convention of representatives of practically all nations, held for the purpose of agreeing upon uniform safeguards of the public health against the invasion and propagation of plague and cholera.

The treaty includes the regulations to be observed by the powers signatory to the convention as soon as plague or cholera appear in their territory; the measures of defense by other countries against territories declared infected, and special arrangements for countries outside Europe.

An article in relation to yellow fever is included in the treaty, and is as follows:

"It is recommended to interested countries to modify their sanitary regulations in such a way as to put them in accord with the present position of science, upon the method of transmission of yellow fever, and, above all, upon the rôle of mosquitos as vehicles of the germs of the disease."

March 2, 1905

Flies Are the Great Carriers of Disease Germs

Sickrooms Should Be Made Fly-proof and Foods Kept Under Cover-- But the Microbe Distributer Has His Good Points As a Public Scavenger

ALTHOUGH it is about forty years since it was known that flies were the agents for transmitting disease germs from place to place, it has been but recently that the knowledge has been put to practical uses in the prevention of disease. It is now a matter which should be known by every intelligent man for his own protection. Boards of Health must act in this direction and hospitals must take particular care to prevent flies reaching any infectious material.

Attention has recently been directed to the matter by the success attending a warfare against flies in the Manila prison, to stop an epidemic of cholera which was daily carrying off from two to five of the convicts. The water was free of the infection and so were the foods, yet in spite of all precautions the disease persisted in attacking men who had not been outside the walls for a long time. So it was finally decided that the infection was carried by flies, and the most drastic means were taken to prevent these insects reaching any infectious material in the prison, and especially were they excluded from the foods. Screen doors and windows were placed where necessary, fly paper was used in large amounts to capture occasional intruders—and the epidemic promptly ceased.

+ + +

It has been conclusively proved that flies are responsible for the spread of typhoid fever here and there, where sanitary conditions are not good and it is possible for flies to reach the infectious materials. Of course, in the great majority of cases it is known that the germs are carried from one patient to the next through the drinking water into which they have been introduced in sewage, but there are little local outbreaks in which the water is known to be free of the germs, and in which the foods, particularly the milk, are also pure. In these cases it is found that the local conditions are such as to make it an easy matter for flies to carry the disease germs and deposit them upon foods.

The military camps, both in our recent war and in the Boer war, are examples of this method of the transmission of typhoid fever. To one who has never lived in such conditions it is difficult to appreciate the unsanitary surroundings sure to arise within two or three weeks. Swarms of flies abound, and it is practically impossible to prevent them walking over the foods and spreading infection which they have elsewhere obtained. The commissions of scientists who have investigated this one point have reported that the awful epidemics which disgraced the American and English camps were spread in no other way than by the swarms of flies which pester all military camps in warm weather.

It is generally said that flies do not perform any service which is indispensable, and that the world would move along just as well if they were all exterminated. This mistaken idea would not be mentioned if we would only remember what is called the balance of nature. The world is full of living things, each one serving as a food to some other. It is evident, then, that if any species is killed off there will be a subsequent distress or elimination of others, until a new balance is obtained. So it is quite likely that the elimination of the flies would bring a disaster of some sort.

+ + +

A little investigation of the benefits conferred by flies also shows us that another kind of disaster would result if the world were deprived of their services, and as these services are intimately bound up in the harm incidentally done to a few of us, it is necessary to look into the matter if we are to understand how the flies spread diseases.

In the first place, we must recall the fact that of all the various substances needed by plants and animals in their foods, nitrogen seems to be the central one, without which growth is absolutely impossible. It is the element around which all the others are grouped in that living substance we call protoplasm. The living world is thus composed of complex compounds of nitrogen, together with some carbonaceous materials formed by the living substance.

In a rough sort of way we might divide all living things into two classes—the plants, which require their nitrogen food in solution in water, and the animals, which take theirs in the solid form—grasses, grains, meats, eggs, &c. There are other intermediate forms, such as bacteria and other microscopic beings, some of which require their nitrogen in solution; others require solid forms, and quite a number are able to absorb it in the gaseous form directly from the air.

Now, it has been shown that plants will very quickly absorb, through their tiny rootlets, all the nitrogen compounds in the soil. It is one of the ways land is exhausted, and unless nitrogen is added to the soil all the plants will die. The farmer does this by adding fertilizers containing nitrogen compounds which are soluble, but nature has several ways of accomplishing it. As soon as an animal or plant dies its body is immediately attacked by a host of insects, bacteria and larger animals, and eaten up—which is but one way of saying that the nitrogen compounds in it are burned to a simpler form and made suitable for food for plants.

There are innumerable kinds of bacteria whose only object in life is this destruction of nitrogen compounds and their reduction to a simple, soluble form which is dissolved by the rains and then carried down through the soil, to be taken up by the rootlets of the plants. It is called decay. Thus, if we throw a piece of meat on the ground or bury it in the soil it is soon swarming with bacteria and literally melts away. An atom of nitrogen may thus go on forever, now in a complex substance in a plant, next eaten by an animal, and then, after the animal dies, the bacteria prepare it for some other plant.

Now, we can get back to our flies and understand some of the parts they play in this wonderful endless drama of nature. Most of them—that is, the scavengers among them—require their food in a soluble form, and they are just as much dependent upon the liquifying bacteria as the plants. Only when the meat decays can the fly utilize it, so it seems specially formed for the purpose of distributing bacteria. As it walks over any decaying substance it cannot fail to pick up myriads of bacteria on its feet and the curious bristles on its legs, and when it alights upon another substance it plants the little organisms wherever it goes. This experiment has been made so often in the laboratories by bacteriologists that it is now a very old story.

Of course, the fly does other things besides inoculate everything it touches. It lays its eggs in decaying materials, so that the little larvae or grubs are well provided with food and act as scavengers also. But the rôle of the fly, in transferring bacteria to hasten on the process of decay, seems to have been overlooked. It is thus a part of the great scheme of nature to prepare foods for plants. The importance of flies is so great that they exist in about every part of the world where plants grow, and in such great variety and numbers that we can well assume them to be indispensable. Their elimination would be a disaster whose ultimate consequences we cannot even surmise.

✦ ✦ ✦

Now, a great many of the bacteria which are thus occupied in tearing down decaying substances are capable of producing disease in man, should they be accidentally introduced into his blood or under his skin. Suppose a fly has just been walking over some decaying materials which contain some typhoid germs, and suppose the fly should drop into a pitcher of milk and then crawl out. It has left in the milk some dozens or hundreds or thousands of germs which have an appropriate food and which immediately begin to multiply at an enormous rate. In the course of a few hours, if the milk is at the proper temperature, there are swarms of the germs developed, and the person who drinks them comes down with typhoid fever within the next three weeks.

Suppose the fly merely walks over some fruits or cooked meats exposed for sale, and inoculates them. The germs might develop just the same, and if the food is not cooked to kill them the person who eats it is sure to have typhoid. It is now known that this is the way a great many cases of the disease are contracted, and it is why there is a campaign against the flies in our market places and small stores in the unsanitary parts of cities.

Not all the bacteria of decay can cause diseases in man, indeed only a few of them can; but whenever any of these few species are present the fly transfers them along with the others. It acts as a mere carrier, distributer, and inoculator. Its real business is to do its share in destroying organic matter to keep the living world going. The disease it spreads is a mere incident or side issue.

It can therefore be accepted as proved that the fly can carry every disease whose germ can live outside our bodies—typhoid fever, cholera, dysentery, many of the intestinal diseases of children, perhaps tuberculosis—indeed, we might go through the list of diseases caused by germs, and show that the fly can carry them on its feet and legs. It has also been shown that the bacteria it swallows with the fluids can pass through its digestive apparatus unharmed—but that is another story.

The best way to reduce the fly nuisance is to starve them to death by removing their foods. All such substances must be taken far from our dwellings to places where they can decay harmlessly; in other words, cleanliness of houses and streets is the great modern necessity. It always has been necessary, for that matter, but in the crowding of modern times it is vital.

Above all else, it is necessary to remove infectious material so that flies cannot get at it. Sick rooms must be flyproof, for every fly which touches the sick may carry away with it enough germs to infect another person, either directly or through his food or water—providing, of course, the germs are so situated that the fly can reach them.

✦ ✦ ✦

It is no wonder, then, that sanitarians are beginning a warfare against the fly—not to exterminate it, for that is impossible, but to remove it as far as possible from our foods and keep it from the sick. Wherever there are swarms of flies there we are sure to find unsanitary conditions. The more we learn about these simple truths of prevention of disease the safer will we be.

It must not be supposed that every fly we see has some disease germs concealed about its person. If this were so we would be in a bad way indeed. Only a few of them are thus infected, but if there is any infectious material near by—say, some sputum from a consumptive—we are quite sure to find that a large percentage of the flies have tubercle bacilli on their legs, ready to infect us. It's a suspicious character—that's all. It has a work to do, but it is work which should not be done around our dining rooms or kitchens or sick rooms. It's a good friend to keep at a distance, but if it is too neighborly it is because we are giving it work to do—that is, we are not clean enough in our living arrangements.

CHARLES E. WOODRUFF.

December 24, 1905

X-RAYS BROUGHT DEATH.

Dr. Weigel Caught Cancerous Growth from a Patient.

Special to The New York Times.

ROCHESTER, May 31.—Dr. Louis A. Weigel, the surgeon of this city who became seriously affected by a peculiar disease as the result of continued experiments with X rays, died at his home to-day. He was 52 years of age. His death was due to a recurrence of the disease which first attacked him three years ago, since which time he had undergone half a dozen operations in the hope of stopping the spreading of the disease through his system.

The malady is one that has not been fully diagnosed by physicians. All they know is that it produces a sort of cancerous growth, one which they are powerless to stop. The strange thing about it is that it is while using the X-rays in endeavoring to effect a cure for cancer that the disease itself is produced in the operator.

Dr. Weigel's death is believed to be the fourth that is due to experiments with Roentgen rays. Others were Thomas A. Edison's assistant, a physician of Boston, and Miss Bertha Fleischman of San Francisco.

The disease first manifested itself in Dr. Weigel's hands, and was a puzzle to him for a long time. Early in 1904 he permitted part of the little finger of his right hand to be amputated. It was sent to Dr. Welch of Johns Hopkins University, and he diagnosed it as being affected with cancer.

This convinced Dr. Weigel and his medical friends that the only thing to save his life would be an operation. His right hand was then removed at the wrist and all of the left hand was amputated excepting the thumb and one finger. The operation was attended by many noted physicians from other cities, Dr. Weigel's case having attracted widespread notice.

For a few months he seemed to be improving, and after a tour to the Bermudas he resumed his practice in this city. But soon the disease manifested itself again and more operations became necessary. Part of the right shoulder was removed, and then it was found necessary to cut away a cancerous growth in the chest and part of the muscular covering of the right breast. The last operation was performed in February of this year.

Dr. Weigel realized as well as his medical friends that it was but a question of time when the disease would run throughout the system or attack some vital part, and he calmly and philosophically waited for the end, with the only consolation of knowing that he had done something for the advance of medical science.

None of the doctors who had been in attendance could state to-day what was the exact cause of his death.

June 1, 1906

DIPHTHERIA IN JOHNS HOPKINS

Hospital Quarantined Through Serious Outbreak—Doctors and Nurses Ill.

Special to The New York Times.

BALTIMORE, Md., Feb. 24.—Strange as it may seem, physicians of the famous Johns Hopkins Hospital are fighting an epidemic of diphtheria within its own walls. There are thirty cases of the malady. Those ill include two doctors, six nurses, students of medical school, and patients. The operating rooms have been closed, scores of patients have been removed to other hospitals or to their homes, if residents of Baltimore, and the great hospital with its blocks of buildings, is practically quarantined. All patients excepting those critically ill are being removed. The rapid spread of the contagion has caused great alarm.

One ward has been isolated for the afflicted ones. It is believed that there were several hundred patients in the hospital when the disease broke out. There are from 150 to 200 nurses, including those in the school for nurses. That so malignant a disease should have made such headway in such a perfectly equipped hospital, with its reputed safe sanitary methods, has caused surprise and comment. Whether due to the carelessness, negligence, or incompetency of any of the doctors or nurses has not been determined. Dr. Rupert Norton, acting Superintendent said:

"It is my personal opinion that it was brought in by some one from outside, and I do not believe that it spread through careless handling of the patients in the hospital."

Dr. Henry M. Hurd, who recently resigned as Superintendent, went a few days ago to Palm Beach, Fla., for some weeks rest. The development of the epidemic may bring back both him and Dr. W.H. Smith of the Bellevue Hospital, New York, who is to succeed him.

February 25, 1911

CAUSE OF INFANTILE PARALYSIS A GERM

Animal Experiments Reveal What Even a Microscope Cannot Detect, Says Dr. Flexner.

PREVENTION NOW POSSIBLE

Those Not Suffering from the Disease May Transmit It—Nose Is the Danger Point—Cleanliness the Best Thing.

Dr. Simon Flexner of the Rockefeller Institute declared yesterday that it has now been thoroughly established that infantile paralysis, the disease which has brought so much harm among children in the last few years, is a germ disease. The germ, it is true, is too small to be detected by any microscope, but its presence and nature have been established in other ways through animal experimentation.

Dr. Flexner, who is, as a rule, silent as to the discoveries made at the institute of which he is director, consented to make this statement yesterday to THE NEW YORK TIMES in explanation of one of the arguments he brought forward at a hearing at Albany last week in defense of the use of animals in medical research. He then stated that the means of the prevention of infantile paralysis has already been established, and that it might conservatively be said that the achievement of cure is not far distant.

"Infantile paralysis," said Dr. Flexner, "is a germ disease that attacks the spinal marrow and brain, and by merely injuring or by totally destroying the delicate tissues causes either a temporary or permanent paralysis of the muscles.

"The germ of the disease has been known for a little more than a year. It is so excessively minute that the most powerful microscope fails to reveal it, and yet there are accurate methods through the employment of which the nature and presence of the germ have been determined with certainty.

"The proof that infantile paralysis is a germ disease, and almost all our accurate knowledge concerning the nature of the disease," Dr. Flexner went on, "has

been secured through experiments on animals, and could probably have been obtained in no other way.

Only Human Beings Affected.

"Where does the germ reside?" the doctor was asked. "It is not known to reside anywhere in nature," he replied, "except in connection with human beings, who either have had or have been in contact with some one who has had infantile paralysis, or in relation with some object in close association with patients suffering from the disease."

"How is the disease spread?" was the next question. "By persons sick with the disease or by some one who has been in contact with a patient suffering from the disease. The evidence at present available points to the fact that the germ of the disease can be carried by healthy persons who have come in contact with the sick and themselves will not contract infantile paralysis, but who may transfer the germ to other healthy persons who will develop the disease."

Dr. Flexner went on to explain that the germ of infantile paralysis enters the brain and spinal cord chiefly, if not exclusively, by way of the nasal passages. In the course of the disease, he said, the germ is also thrown off from the brain through the nose and mouth.

Hence, protection can be best secured by disinfecting or destroying the secretions of the nose and mouth of those ill of the disease, and by preventing the contamination of persons or objects with these secretions. Especial pains should be taken to maintain in a state of cleanliness the hands, nose, and mouth of all children exposed to the disease, either directly or indirectly.

Isolation of Patients Essential.

"For how long a time is a patient in danger of spreading the infection?" Dr. Flexner was asked.

"This question cannot be answered with absolute precision at present," he replied, "but it is believed that during the first three or four weeks of the disease the danger of transfer is greatest, and hence patients should be carefully isolated during this period and the discharges from the nose and mouth carefully disinfected or destroyed for the period, and, if possible, for many weeks afterward.

"There is reason for believing that even after the acute symptoms of the disease have passed, the infection may in some instances be still transmitted by the patient by means of the nasal secretions. It is for this reason that the secretions should be cared for over a longer period than is embraced in the acute stages of the malady."

"What are the main sources of infection?"

"Infantile paralysis is chiefly a disease of children, but it sometimes attacks adults," Dr. Flexner said. "Since the germ causing it is carried by those who have been ill, as well as by persons who have been in immediate contact with the patients, it is not surprising to find that the beginnings of many epidemics have been traced to schools where many children are assembled; but any considerable gathering of persons, which includes

many children who are brought together during the prevalence of the disease, may be the means of spreading it widely.

"Thus, it has been observed that country fairs, Fourth of July celebrations, and like events have all proved to be such centres of distribution of the infection.

The period of greatest prevalence of the disease, Dr. Flexner explained, is in the Summer. As an epidemic it is a Summer disease; that is, almost all cases arise in the Summer months, and by far the greatest number in July, August, and September. However, the disease does not wholly disappear at other seasons, but a small number of cases arise in the Spring and Fall months, and even in the Winter months. Whenever a case arises, whether in Summer or in Winter, it should be isolated and treated with great care and promptitude to avoid the infection of others.

Disease Has Spread Insidiously.

"Is infantile paralysis a new disease?"

"It is not a new disease," Dr. Flexner said, "but the epidemics of it are new to this country. The disease has arisen in this country from time to time for almost half a century, but in very rare instances have any considerable number of cases been grouped together until within the last three or four years.

"The present epidemic first appeared around Boston and New York about three years ago, and has gradually, continuously, and insidiously extended over North America from ocean to ocean and from Canada to Cuba. Prior to this period the epidemics were limited to Norway and Sweden, where they have been prevailing regularly for more than a quarter of a century. The present epidemic in America is part of the general epidemic, or pandemic so-called, of the disease affecting a large part of the civilized world. The disease is prevailing in many European countries at the present time, as in the United States and Canada."

Then Dr. Flexner went on to describe the available means of combating the disease: "At the present time," he said, "there is no specific remedy or cure for infantile paralysis. The disease once established cannot, therefore, be controlled by the application of any remedy known to medical science. Luckily, the disease is not a highly fatal one, although it is one of the saddest of diseases because of the large amount of crippling it causes. On the other hand, the outlook has been greatly brightened by reason of the recent knowledge which has been acquired concerning the nature of the cause of the disease and the mode of its transmission.

"This knowledge permits the application of intelligent preventive measures, which, if effectively employed, will serve to diminish the number of persons affected with it. The most scientific, as well as the most humane method of dealing with any disease, is to prevent rather than to attempt to cure it. Hence, the effort to control this terrible disease should be in the direction of prevention. The various States are making a determined effort to deal with the malady through prevention, since they have required notification and quarantining of the disease."

March 12, 1911

PREVENTION OF HOOKWORM.

Physicians Urge That It Be Taken Up by Sanitary Conferences.

Physicians are of the opinion that the international importance of hookworm disease has become so great that its prevention should be taken up by sanitary conference. The editor of American Medicine says:

"It seems that the parasite is an endemic scourge in the whole tropical and sub-tropical belt, and is seriously interfering with industrial efficiency and international trade. Poverty is now recognized as the result of inefficiency, either inherited or acquired, and those who are chronically ill are the feeblest and therefore the poorest of the poor the world over. Social workers have long recog-

nized that the first step in reforming the submerged paupers is to cure them.

"The medical profession, therefore, forms the basis of all modern schemes to lessen poverty and it is justifying the system by the magnificent results in Porto Rico and our South—and even in our slums. The new point now being forced on our traders and manufacturers is the fact that it is not possible to get as much raw materials from the tropics as civilization demands, and that the deficiency is due to the inefficiency of the native workmen, and largely a matter of hookworm.

"Northern races are thus reflexly injured by the filthy habits which make the transfer of the infection so easy in the tropics. It is merely one more illustration of the necessity of controlling the tropics from the north, to force sanitation upon them as we did in Panama.

"The mutual benefit of both controllers and controlled demands the elimination of hookworm."

April 30, 1911

FINDS NEW DISEASE AND THEN ITS CURE

Dr. Simon Flexner, Director of the Rockefeller Institute for Medical Research, announces in the current issue of The Journal of the American Medical Association that it has been discovered that cerebro-spinal meningitis, secondary to influenza or the grip, is far from uncommon and very fatal. At the same time, he announces the outcome of experiments carried on in the institution resulting in the discovery of a cure for the malady.

"That influenzal cerebro-spinal meningitis is by no means a rare affection is being shown by the increasing number of reports of its occurrence," says Dr. Flexner. "Within a few months, in the United States alone, reports dealing with the subject have been published by Wollstein, Dunn, and Davis. Moreover, the disease is highly fatal. All but six of the fifty-eight cases thus far reported in which the influenza bacillus has been detected in the cerebro-spinal membranes have terminated fatally.

"Influenzal meningitis is more frequent among infants and children than among adults. It sometimes follows on undoubted influenza bacillus infections of the respiratory tract, and sometimes develops independently of obvious disease of that tract. Since the influenza bacillus is often present in the secretions of the respiratory mucous membrane in children, suffering from a variety of diseases, during the wide prevalence of influenza, it is probable that the infection of the meninges is always second-

ary to the respiratory infection. Moreover, all or nearly all cases of influenzal meningitis are examples of bacteriemia, since the bacilli have frequently been cultivated in large numbers from the blood during life or at autopsy.

"The fact of the frequency and severity of influenzal meningitis was impressed on us at the Rockefeller Institute, where for a period of several years large numbers of specimens of cerebrospinal fluid have been examined bacteriologically in connection with the studies being conducted there on the serum therapy of epidemic meningitis. All the cases diagnosed by us as influenzal meningitis terminated fatally.

"We undertook therefore, the experimental investigation of this highly fatal disease. Dr. Wollstein was able to show, first, that the injection of virulent cultures of bacillus influenza into the subdural space of several species of monkeys by lumbar puncture would set up a severe and usually fatal form of acute cerebro-spinal meningitis that reproduced the clinical and pathologic effects observed in the spontaneous disease occurring in human beings.

"The effects of the inoculations begin to be apparent about five hours after the injection, and death may result as early as thirty-six hours after the inoculation, or it may be delayed for three or four days. The micro-organisms multiply actively and pus cells are quickly poured into the membranes, but few or none of the bacilli are taken up by the cells. In human cases some of the bacilli are found inside cells, but the greater part also remain free in the fluid. From the subdural space the bacilli pass freely into the blood-stream and sometimes secondary localizations take place in the lungs and pleurae, where inflammations are produced.

"The experimental production of an influenzal meningitis was regarded merely as preliminary to the attempt to influence the course of the infection by means of the local application of a

therapeutic agent. An efficient one for the experimental infection has been found in an immune serum prepared in the goat by the long continued, repeated injection of virulent cultures of bacillus influenzoe.

"It has been found possible to rescue monkeys regularly from the fatal effects of the subdural inoculation of cultures of the influenza bacillus through daily injection, by means of lumbar puncture, of the immune serum for three or four days. Serum injections produce an arrest of the multiplication of the bacilli and bring about a free phagocytosis, with which is connected the cessation of the emigration of leukocytes and a consequent clearing of the cerebro-spinal fluid. The fluid, at first turbid or purulent, tends to return to clear in three or four days, while cultures which are at first abundant become negative in that period or a little later. The bacteriemia is also brought under control and the secondary localization of the bacilli in the organs prevented. Recovery is, therefore, complete.

"In view of the severe conditions surrounding influenzal meningitis in human beings, it would seem desirable to apply the serum to the treatment of the spontaneous disease. If this should be done, then every effort should be directed to the making of the bacteriologic diagnosis at the earliest possible moment, and the employment of a serum that has been prepared with virulent influenza bacilli and that shows a high degree of opsonic value. The manner in which the serum should be employed in human beings is indicated by the manner in which the serum for epidemic meningitis has come to be applied successfully.

"The testing of the anti-influenzal serum will be confined, for the present, to a few places in which its effects can be carefully observed and controlled before it is offered for more general use."

July 3, 1911

'TYPHOID MARY' ASKS $50,000 FROM CITY

"Typhoid Mary," the cook who came by that nickname because of the cases of typhoid fever that seemed to follow her around from family to family, is about to sue the City and its Health Department for $50,000 damages for keeping her in confinement on North Brother Island for three years.

Papers will be served within the next few days on Dr. Lederle, head of the Health Department, and four physicians, Dr. Darlington, Dr. Soper, Dr. Park, and Dr. Westmoreland. Mary Mallon is the name on the complaint. She is forty years old, and says she has never had typhoid fever or any other dangerous disease. She was released from the hospital last February, and since that time she has been unable to follow her trade of cooking, and her chances of making a living have been greatly reduced, she asserts. She will attempt to show that she was not the typhoid germ carrier the city authorities have made her out.

The lawyer who will prosecute Mary's

case against the city is the same one who appeared for her before the Supreme Court in 1909, when her freedom was denied. He is George Francis O'Neil of 5 Beekman Street, and he is a specialist in medico-legal questions.

"If the Board of Health," he said yesterday, "is going to send every cook to jail who happens to come under their designation of 'germ carrier,' it won't be long before we have no cooks left, and the domestic problem will be further complicated. What would the poor jokesmith do then for his stories about the cook who rules the house?"

The story of "Typhoid Mary" has been made the subject of a pamphlet by Dr. George A. Soper, who is mentioned in the complaint. The case goes back to 1906, when an alarming spread of typhoid fever was experienced at Oyster Bay. Six out of a family of eleven had been stricken with typhoid. The water of the well was naturally first suspected, and it was made the subject of a careful analysis. Nothing was wrong with the water. Dr. Soper examined the food supply of the family, but here again he found nothing out of the way. He began to look for some peculiar situation, and focussed his suspicions on the fact that the family had changed cooks about three weeks before the fever began.

Dr. Soper then began to investigate the record of Mary Mallon. He found that in 1904 she had been employed at the home of Henry Gilsey at Sands Point, L. I. The family had eleven persons in it, of whom seven were servants. Within

a month four of the servants were taken with typhoid.

In 1902 Mary was the cook for J. Coleman Drayton at Dark Harbor, Me. Seven persons out of nine were taken ill within a short time. Three other instances are set forth where the fever followed within a short period after the employment of the cook. In all, he laid at her door twenty-six cases of typhoid. And he added that he had traced but fragments of her history during ten years.

The physicians of the Health Department have never been able to discover that Mary herself ever had typhoid. She is described as a robust woman, and weighing about 190 pounds. The Doctor suggested that she undergo an operation. To this she would not submit. In fact, she always insisted that she never gave typhoid to anybody, but that the water was at fault. The case was adjudged one for confinement in March, 1907, and Mary, after a contest of physical strength with five policemen, was taken to North Brother Island. In 1909 she was before the Supreme Court on a writ of habeas corpus. Judge Giegerich sent her back to the hospital, expressing sympathy for the woman, but insisting that she was a menace to the community.

At the time of her release Dr. Lederle made a statement to the effect that Mary had been shut up long enough to learn precautions. She promised the department that she would not again take a place as cook.

December 3, 1911

THE NEW SCHOOL OF MEDICINE.

The celebrated Dr. OSLER has said that he believed in using few, and still fewer, drugs for the treatment of disease. Although there are many medicaments that have been used to alleviate bodily ills and control their symptoms, it is better, Dr. OSLER thought, to treat the sick man by the methods that would keep a well man strong and vigorous, with a regulated diet, fresh air, pure water, light and exercise, and comfortable surroundings. In addition, he and like-minded physicians make a specialty of diagnosing organic diseases which, they say, cannot be cured. Why dose them for a cure? It is more scientific to tell the patient accurately what the autopsy in his case will show.

Those who believe with Dr. OSLER are many, some of them are eminent. Their contempt for drugs is at least excusable, and their despair of finding the cure of ills that have wrought structural changes in the bodily organs is understandable. The drugs they get are often impure, of uncertain quality and strength, and at best they control the symptoms of diseases, they do not heal them. Since the world began, only one chemical compound has been made by man that is an exact specific for a human disease. That is the new drug salvarsan, and it alone serves to confute the nihilists in medicine. It cures an entire class of diseases.

A new school has produced this remedy, and it promises more of them, made to control and destroy, not the symptoms, but the causes of organic disease. Its members discovered, first, that the vital fluids of infected animals might acquire immunity by slight changes of their chemical composition, so that the new principle destroyed the cells of invading parasites. Then it was conceived that chemicals might be found in complexes that would destroy the essentially different cells of the parasites, without harming the normal cell structure of the body. Salvarsan is such a chemical complex. It destroys the pathogenic spirilla of an important group of blood diseases in animals and men, and removes, also, such of the diseased tissue of the body as has undergone a change of structure from the normal tissue.

The next step was clearly indicated. To the extent that the structure of the bodily tissues changes from the normal, it may be successfully attacked by artificially evolved drugs, so that only the tissues that have an original integrity remain. THE TIMES printed on Monday the report of the German chemists working under the leadership of EHRLICH and VON WASSERMANN, which records a second triumph over the nature and causes of the disease of cancer, in one species of animals. They will now proceed upon a solidly based scientific principle, to evolve a remedy to destroy the seat of cancer in man. But their work will continue beyond this. They have set about to combine synthetic drugs, specific remedies for all other organic diseases. This school of medicine flouts the nihilists, it declares boldly that there is no ill that flesh is heir to which may not be cured. The distinction between the new school and the old has been drawn by Dr. S. J. MELTZER, head of the Pharmacological Department of the Rockefeller Institute, in his paper on " The Present Status of Therapeutics and the Significance of Salvarsan," which appeared in the Journal of the American Medical Association of June 10 last. Dr. MELTZER says:

In the past the gifted among clinicians were attracted by pathology and diagnosis. The pharmacologists studied the action of drugs on the organs of healthy animals. Neither of them studied the problem of how to cure diseases. Therapeutics did not attain the dignity of a science. * * * Now this leader of leaders [EHRLICH] for a number of years bent all his energies to do for medicine that which medicine needs mostly, and that is to find remedies which could destroy the cause of diseases. * * * By the scientific position of the master and by his brilliant deed, therapeutics will rise now to a higher level in the estimation of discriminating men.

The young men studying medicine in this country are turning their attention to the brilliant achievements of the masters of this new school of therapeutics. They have leaders here. The biological laboratories are graduating and sending into the larger cities of the country disciples who maintain unflinchingly that what medicine needs most to-day is not simply diagnosis, later confirmed by autopsy, but careful clinical observation of the progress of disease with a view to checking it before organic changes are wrought, and of curing it by the action of drugs precisely formed to stop these harmful changes.

January 10, 1912

OBVIATE '606' DISADVANTAGES

Dr. Ehrlich, Discoverer, Finds Out How to Dissolve It in Water.

By Marconi Transatlantic Wireless Telegraph to The New York Times.

BERLIN, March 18.—THE NEW YORK TIMES correspondent is enabled to make the authoritative announcement that Dr. Ehrlich has succeeded in effecting a remarkable improvement in his famous " 606 " specific, which improvement is regarded as only second in importance to the discovery of the drug itself.

The improvement consists in a method of making the drug completely soluble in plain water without the aid of any other solvent. What is still more vital is that the resulting solution is entirely neutral—that is to say, it is neither acid nor alkali.

The great majority of failures and bad effects which have taken place in connection with the administering of " 606 " were due directly to the difficulty of dissolving the drug and to the fact that the solution derived by the old method was alkaline, causing great pain when injected, and sometimes the destruction of surrounding tissues.

These disadvantages are obviated by the new drug, which will be known as " Neo-salvarsan." It can be given in larger doses than the old " 606 " without fear of producing any discomfort or ill-effects.

Many of the reported failures with " 606 " have been due to the difficulty of mastering the technique of preparing and administering the solution. This difficulty, Prof. Ehrlich asserts, is now completely removed.

Dr. Schreiber, a well-known Magdeburg specialist, has been experimenting exhaustively with Dr. Ehrlich's newest discovery, which has not yet been made public in Europe.

Dr. Ehrlich, in a telegram to THE NEW YORK TIMES correspondent from Frankfort, confirms the statement that he has devised an " easily soluble salvarsan," and adds that Dr. Schreiber will shortly make public details of the new discovery.

March 19, 1912

LEARN MORE ABOUT INFANTILE PARALYSIS

Investigations at the Rockefeller Institute into the nature and treatment of poliomyelitis, or infantile paralysis, have been in progress, but a specific form of treatment for it has not been found. In a bulky monograph Drs. Francis W. Peabody, George Draper, and A. R. Dochez have summed up all that has yet been ascertained as to the causes and treatment of the complaint, and though they cannot announce its conquest, they do make many important suggestions as to the means of infection, the necessity of isolation of the patients, and the best methods of caring for them.

The disease, the report points out, has been identified and studied regularly only in the last seventy years, and the attention of medical investigators has been concentrated upon it for little more than twenty years. It was in 1890 that Medin published the first good clinical account of acute poliomyelitis, and after his work appeared no important addition to existing knowledge was made till 1905. Four years later a great advance was made almost simultaneously by the discovery of the method of producing the disease artificially in Vienna, in Paris, and in this city by Drs. Simon Flexner, and Lewis, and since then the Rockefeller Institute has been studying it steadily and systematically.

It has been established that it is not caused by bacteria, but by a virus, which evinces great tenacity of life. Experiments on monkeys have shown that once an animal has recovered from the disease it is able to resist further inoculations, and fairly satisfactory results have been obtained in the production of active immunity by repeated injections of small amounts of attenuated virus. The authors of the monograph, however, express the opinion that these are not sufficient to warrant the application of this procedure in human beings.

In spite of the terrible nature of many cases of the disease, it has been established that there are many cases of what is known as "abortive" poliomyelitis. The patient is infected with the disease and contains in his body the virus, but he is capable of resisting it and recovers without any of the symptoms that permit of diagnosis. Paralysis is entirely absent, and the patient may be supposed to have nothing but a slight complaint of no particular importance, yet a patient is as dangerous to those with whom he comes in contact as if he had suffered from an acute attack.

This makes an epidemic especially difficult to control, as it is not certain that all who can spread the disease are suspected of harboring it. Consequently, it is declared that the most dangerous centre of infection is the public school, and that the disease is likely to spread through ordinary human contact.

It is believed that in humans the virus is generally found in the upper respiratory tract, and that the nasopharynx in particular is a danger spot. The infection, it is declared, may also be spread by the use of bedding and clothing which have been infected and that the virus may be ground into dust and can conceivably be disseminated by wind.

Some interesting experiments were made at the Rockefeller Institute as to the protective power of human serum. They were not conclusive, but it seemed likely that in typical instances the serum of the infected individual probably always contains, after a certain interval, protective bodies, and that these persist for a very long time. In other cases it was found that the injection of serum from a person who, so far as known, had never had the disease protected a monkey from it, but the authors of the report point out that it cannot be proved certainly that the individuals, from whom the serum was taken had never had an unrecognized abortive attack.

In discussing the predisposing causes of the disease, the authors declare that it seems to have its origin in the open country rather than the cities, and that more of the cases treated in the Rockefeller Institute came from the suburbs and surrounding country than from the densely populated tenement districts. Moreover, a considerable proportion are from families in comparatively well-to-do circumstances, in which the children enjoyed every comfort and care. In general the patients had been perfectly healthy before the attack.

Childhood is the period during which the attacks are likely to occur, but it has been established that adults are by no means immune, as more than one-fifth of the cases recorded by Wickman were of persons more than 15 years of age. The latter half of the second year is the most susceptible period, and boys are a little more susceptible to the complaint than girls.

Permanent paralysis, it has now been established, is by no means an inevitable result of the disease. Wickman shows from a study of 530 cases that from a year to eighteen months after an acute attack 44 per cent. were cured, but the Massachusetts State Board of Inquiry gives a considerably lower percentage of complete recoveries, 16.7 per cent. Complete return of power is more likely to occur in children than in adults, and the authors speak of the surprising return of power after a few weeks or even several months in some cases in which limbs seemed hopelessly paralyzed.

Yet after setting forth the results of all these observations and experiments the investigators are forced to write:

"At the present time there is no specific form of therapy, by which the paralysis in acute poliomyelitis may be prevented, or by means of which resolution of the inflammatory process and consequent return of function may be hastened. The problem of treatment, therefore, consists in preventing the spread of disease to other persons, in applying general symptomatic procedures and in attempting the restoration of muscular efficiency and the prevention of deformities."

July 5, 1912

SOUTHERN HOOKWORM SANITATION

The summary of the forthcoming Third Annual Report of the Rockefeller Sanitary Commission presents impressive figures of the 238,755 persons treated for hookworm disease in eleven States during 1912. That was 762 infected persons a day treated on six days of each week, and during the last quarter of 1912 the Rockefeller doctors remedied the cases of 108,892 individuals. During the three years' life of the Commission upward of 400,000 sufferers have been cured.

What this means for the future physical, moral, and economic welfare of the South can hardly be estimated. Every treatment is preceded by a microscopic examination; of these there were 14,789 in 1910, 90,724 in 1911, and in 1912 the enormous total of 326,951. The number of rural children found affected between the ages of 6 and 18 was 78,572, something over one-half of those examined. They belonged to families in hundreds of communities who were on the edge of pauperism and moral degeneration or had slipped over. A father, mother, and seven children living in a filthy, one-roomed cabin, every member infected with the hookworm disease, barely getting a living from a small, wasted, unproductive farm, and all of them illiterate, have undergone a family transformation. Within two years after the simple cure the father and his older sons have built a neat frame dwelling of two stories; the younger children are in school; the farm is productive, and the whole family is happy and well. This is but one of the Commission's repeated experiences.

The Commission has expended during the past year $184,672, or 77 cents for every human being benefited in health and helped to a better living. That is a small price to pay for rejuvenating the plague-stricken poorer population of the South.

March 24, 1913

WHOOPING COUGH A GERM DISEASE

It has just been definitely established that whooping cough is caused by a germ which has been named the bacillus pertussis by Bordet and Gengou, its discoverers. This organism was suspected some time ago and a vaccine treatment undertaken on this basis. Laboratory findings have confirmed the belief of the two physicians named. Whooping cough is known in medical nomenclature as pertussis.

Commenting editorially on the discovery, The Medical Record says:

"It was over a year ago that we had occasion to call attention to the vaccine treatment of pertussis which had apparently exercised a favorable influence over the course of the disease in a number of instances. At that time the Bordet-Gengou bacillus had been found constantly in certain stages of the disease, and complement fixation tests with this organism were fairly constantly positive. Whether this bacillus was the true causative agent or merely a sec-

ondary invader had not been definitely determined.

"Of late, however, evidence to this end has become conclusive. Mallory and Horner at first demonstrated 'that the primary essential lesion of whooping cough consists in the presence of masses of minute bacilli between the cilia of the epithelial cells lining the trachea and bronchi. Their action is chiefly mechanical; they interfere with the normal movements of the cilia by sticking them together; in this way the microorganisms furnish a continual irritation which results in the symptoms peculiar to the disease.' They used this lesion as a criterion in their later animal experimentation, and they report now some very important results (Journal of Medical Research, XXVII., 391, 1913.)

"It had previously been demonstrated that puppies were susceptible to the disease. These animals were inoculated intratracheally with sputum from patients in the active stage of the disease, and when killed six weeks later the characteristic lesion was found in the trachea. This lesion in all the infected animals corresponds in every way with that found in man. Sections show clearly that the cilia are not destroyed and that the cells are not injured in any noticeable way. Pure cultures of the organism were then obtained from the sputum of suitable patients and a culture

of the original Bordet-Gengou strain was used for comparison and control. They corresponded in every way.

"The authors inoculated several puppies and rabbits with these pure cultures by injecting them into either the nares or the trachea. In practically every instance they were able to demonstrate the characteristic lesion in the trachea of the animal and in several instances were able to recover the organism, not only from the trachea, but also from the nares. It is interesting to note that normal puppies were readily infected if kept in more or less intimate contact with inoculated animals.

"By this work all the demands of Koch's laws are satisfied, and the bacillus pertussis of Bordet and Gengou is definitely and conclusively proved to be the etiological factor in whooping cough. These findings should not only stimulate investigation of the vaccine treatment of the disease, a treatment which has already met with a certain measure of success, but should also arouse the attempt to find a specific antibody which might be suitable for therapeutic purposes.

"In animals and man the bacilli diminish and finally disappear in the course of a few weeks, and the complement deviation tests are regularly positive, two observations which would indicate the presence of some antibody. It should be a fruitful field, and it is to be hoped that it will not be neglected."

August 23, 1913

SERUM AVERTS DIPHTHERIA.

Behring Has Now Made Treatment Preventive as Well as Curative.

Special Cable to THE NEW YORK TIMES.

PARIS, Dec. 6.—Prof. Behring, who, in 1892, created anti-diphtheria serum, has just perfected it so that it is a preventive as well as a curative.

Heretofore this serum had, above all, a curative value. Injected into a person already ill, it arrested the progress of disease in proportion to the promptness of use after the outbreak, but the serum was almost useless as a preventive. In epidemics it was only useful for a few days.

The new serum is obtained by mixing the diphtheria toxin with the antitoxin extracted from the serum of immune animals. This is entirely harmless. Injected into school chil-

dren it will cause to appear in their blood for a long period a quantity of the preservative antitoxin. It has also the advantage of sterilizing bacilli in persons who, while their own systems resist disease, may impart it to other.

Profs. Josué and Bellar have finished their experiments of vaccination against typhoid with results which have caused the French press this week to say that: "Typhoid is vanquished."

They make cultures in blood of the bacilli of eberth, which is the known agent of the disease. After two days this culture generally becomes very fertile and is sterilized by extreme heat, used for six hours. Then the number of the bacilli contained in a centimeter cube, is measured and the vaccination is performed by the

injection three times of 200,000,000 bacilli.

If, after five days, the temperature is above the normal, a new injection is made of 200,000,000, which, in the majority of cases, suffices for rapid amelioration.

This method of treatment of diseases by auto-vaccination has given most satisfactory results. Cases that were very grave have become better after vaccination and recovery has followed in three or four weeks. Milder cases after treatment have improved rapidly.

Heart complications, heretofore, so feared in typhoid, are avoided, or, when they have appeared, have improved rapidly after the first injection.

December 7, 1913

RADIUM WON'T CURE CANCER

Its Value Confined to Superficial Growths, American Society Says.

A warning was issued yesterday by the American Society for the Control of Cancer against putting too much hope in the beneficial results of the treatment of cancer by radium. The society expressed the fear that exaggerated ideas of the power of radium in such cases would lead to deeper despair on the failure of the expected cure after the patients had been put to heavy expense. In its warning bulletin, the society says:

"The curative effects of radium are limited to-day to superficial cancers of the skin, to superficial growths of mucous membrane which are not true cancers, and to some deeper lying tumors of bone, which are not very malignant. The problem of the constitutional treatment of advanced, inoperable cancer is still untouched by any method yet devised or likely to be devised for admin-

istering radium. Even among the so-called radium cures, it still remains to be determined in many cases whether the favorable result is permanent or is to be followed sooner or later by the usual recurrence. The most competent surgeons do not dare to pronounce a case cured until five years have elapsed after an apparently successful operation. The same test must be applied before we can finally determine the real value of radium.

"It should be emphasized especially that radium cannot at present exert any permanent benefit on generalized cancer, and since cancer, in a very large proportion of cases, is widely disseminated in the body early in the course of the disease, this entire group of cases can expect no important relief from radium. Another large group of cancers is comparatively inaccessible to the application of radium, so that the ultimate course of the disease is not affected, although certain portions of the tumor may be reduced in size. Again, many forms of cancer, although localized and accessible to radium, grow very rapidly and resist the curative action of this agent, so that no real benefit can be expected from its use.

"The best results of radium therapy can be secured only when comparatively large amounts are available for use, and the present limited world's supply of

this metal places it out of reach of the great majority of patients. It is to be feared that much harm may result from undue reliance upon small quantities of low-grade radium when other methods of treatment would be more effective.

"Evidence of the possible extent of popular misconception on this subject is found in a pathetic letter recently received at the New York Health Department from a sufferer in California who had somehow obtained the impression that the United States Government was about to purchase large quantities of radium from abroad. Assuming that the 'New York City physician' would have a plentiful supply, the writer asked that some be sent to him C. O. D. without delaying to advise him as to the cost.

"Under the term 'cancer' are commonly grouped several diseases which differ widely in nature, causation, and courses, and in their response to radium. It requires both skill and experience to determine just what type of cancer one has to deal with, as well as the advisability of using radium. Hence, it is extremely difficult to formulate an accurate statement of the true position of radium therapy, but it is quite clear that the exploitation of this remedy as a cure for cancer in general is to be deprecated."

December 26, 1913

MACHINE PURIFIES BLOOD AND RESTORES IT TO THE BODY

Wonderful Apparatus Devised by Johns Hopkins Physicians Is Called the "Artificial Kidney," Because It Removes the Undesirable Constituents of the Blood as That Organ Does.

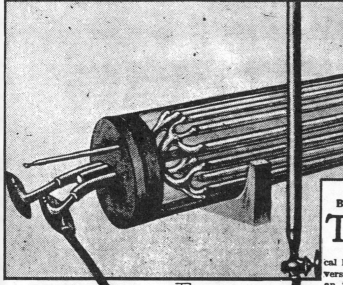

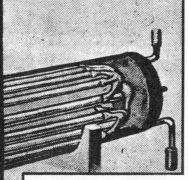

The "Artificial Kidney

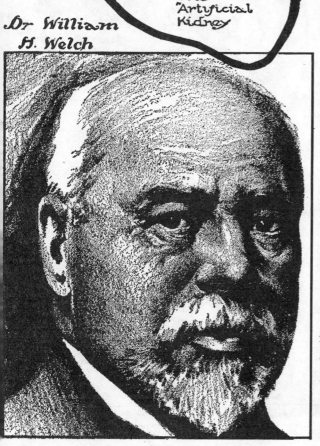

Dr William H. Welch

By Van Buren Thorne, M. D.

THREE physicians, Dr. John J. Abel, Dr. Leonard G. Rowntree, and Dr. B. B. Turner, working in the pharmacological laboratory of Johns Hopkins University, in Baltimore, have elaborated an ingenious theory by which they have succeeded in taking all the blood out of the body of a living animal, "cleansing" it, and restoring it to the body without danger to the animal's life.

The word "cleansing" in this connection means that they are able to remove the diffusible constituents of the blood while it is outside the body. The wonderful apparatus which they have devised is so similar in its action to the kidney that they usually refer to it as the "artificial kidney."

The process of the elimination of undesirable constituents in the blood is called by the investigators "vividiffusion." The first demonstration before a body of physicians was made in Baltimore about fourteen months ago. The method was described in May last, before the Association of American Physicians in Washington, and last Summer demonstrations were given in London and in Groningen. More recently, it was brought to the attention of physicians in Philadelphia, while the current issue of The Journal of Pharmacology and Experimental Therapeutics contains a complete account of the laboratory experiments and a detailed description of the apparatus.

The title of this article, as well as that appearing in The Transactions of the Association of American Physicians, reads: "On the Removal of Diffusible Substances from the Circulating Blood of Living Animals by Dialysis."

Astounding Possibilities.

The physicians so far do not record attempts to apply their principle as a therapeutic measure for the relief of human ailments, but from what they have already made known the possibilities in this direction are astonishing. It is certain that poisons in the blood detrimental to human life, and which are impossible of elimination by inactive or badly diseased kidneys, can be removed from the body by means of this apparatus. Dogs weighing up to forty or fifty pounds have been used in the work, chiefly for the reason that all of the apparatus so far employed was only intended to take care of the quantity of blood contained in a body weighing fifty pounds or less.

The physicians are now constructing a machine capable of doing the work necessitated by a volume of blood circulating in a body weighing up to 200 pounds, and, inasmuch as they have determined to their own satisfaction that the procedure is not inimical to life, there is no reason why it should not be applied to human beings when the occasion arises.

Of course, the impression is not intended to be conveyed that the blood is all out of the body at one time, or that something is not supplied to the body to take the place of that which is temporarily absent. In order to make this point clear it is necessary to give a description of the apparatus and the manner in which it is employed. This will be done in the simplest possible way; and it will be seen that, despite the complicated apparatus used, the theory upon which its employment is based is as plain a physiological proposition as could well be thought of.

Tapping the Arteries.

Although prior to the time of Harvey—not so very long ago, as time is measured—no one was aware that the blood circulated throughout the body, every schoolboy knows nowadays that the heart pumps out blood through the arterial system to the most distant parts of the body; that it next passes through minute vessels called capillaries, and finally returns to the heart again through the venous system. In other words, it leaves the heart through the arteries and returns through the veins. These Johns Hopkins physicians conceived the idea of tapping one of the large arteries, allowing the blood to flow out, and returning it to a large vein when they had finished with it.

There were many difficulties to be overcome, but they finally made a system of tubes of a material porous enough to allow the substances they wished eliminated to escape through the sides as it passed through them. One end of the system of tubes was connected with an artery, which had been opened, by means of a single tube called a cannula. The other end of the system was joined to the receiving vein by another cannula. Now then we have blood coming out of an artery into a cannula, through the cannula into the system of tubes, (whose various branchings and their significance will be explained later,) through the system of tubes to the second cannula, and thence into the vein, and so back to the heart.

So far, we have merely described the method by which blood can be taken out of the body and restored to it without any great difficulty. This in itself is a simple procedure. We have not, however, shown what takes the place in the body of that volume of blood which is temporarily outside of it. The nearest approach to the blood serum of an animal is a mixture of salt and water in certain proportions, referred to in laboratory experimentation as a "normal saline solution." Before circulation in the apparatus is established, the system of tubes is filled with saline solution. When blood flows out of the cannula, through the cannula, and into the tubes, it forces the saline solution in front of it, through the tubes, the second cannula, the vein, and into the circulation in the body.

It will be readily seen, therefore, that as soon as the tubes are filled with blood an equal amount of saline solution is taking the place of the blood absent from the body. For instance, if the system of tubes will hold a volume of liquid equal to one-third of that circulating in an animal body, it will be seen that when circulation in the apparatus is properly established the animal is living minus a third of its blood, which has been replaced by saline solution. This is exactly the proportion of blood that was removed by the investigators in the course of some of their experiments.

It is now in order to explain how the diffusible constituents get out of the tubes while the blood is passing through them. As stated earlier, these tubes are made of a substance which permits certain solids to pass through it. The solids pass into a solution which surrounds the system of tubes, and may be collected therefrom and subjected to analyses which will reveal their nature and quantity. Blood passed through tubes as described, and from which certain constituents have been removed by passage through the walls of these tubes before it again enters the body, has been subjected to dialysis. The walls of the tubes are composed of a "dialyz-

ing membrane," and the substances removed, to use the language of the laboratory, have been "dialyzed out."

Dialysis really means separation. This is a definition of the more formidable word:

The separation of crystalloid from colloid substances in a solution by interposing an animal membrane between the solution and pure water; the crystalloid substances pass through the membrane into the water on the other side, the colloids do not. —(Stedman.)

As the investigators themselves say, the outer fluid may, of course, be water, but this leads very quickly to haemolysis (destruction) of the red corpuscles. If the experimenters desire to prevent any substance in the blood from "dialyzing out" they simply add the same proportion of that substance to the outer fluid as is contained in the blood itself. There is then a complete balance both within and without the system of tubes, so far as that substance is concerned, and, therefore, it will not pass through the walls of the tubes in either direction. The writers say:

Where the object of the experiment is merely to remove from the blood abnormal constituents, as, for example, poisons, or constituents specifically secreted into the blood by a certain organ, normal serum from a similar animal may be used, thus insuring complete balance of all normal constituents, inside and out.

Coagulation Overcome.

One of the problems hitherto arising in connection with the removal of blood with the intention of using it to benefit a second person, as in transfusion, has been overcome by these investigators. It used to be said that blood was never the same once it left its natural environment, the blood vessels, if only for the briefest period. The change most to be feared, especially in blood transfusion, was coagulation. The Johns Hopkins experimenters have effectually overcome any tendency to coagulation by the injection of a substance derived from the medicinal leech and which is called hirulin.

These are some of the remarks of the investigators contained in their summary:

A method has been devised by which diffusible constituents may be removed from the blood of a living animal, which does not involve any procedure prejudicial to life.

Two animals have made rapid and complete recovery after being subjected to the procedure for two or three hours respectively.

The method has been shown to be available for collecting from the blood under the ordinary conditions

Interior View of "Artificial Kidney" Containing 32 Tubes.

of physiological experimentation substances present only in small amount at one time.

As an organ of elimination of abnormal substances (for example, poisons,) quantitative results obtained with salicylic acid show that the apparatus in its present form compares not unfavorably with the kidney. The direction of improvement is indicated and experiments in this direction are in progress.

Material has been collected in large quantity for the study of the nonproteid amino-bodies present in the blood. The chemical separation of these bodies is in progress and only preliminary results are given.

Directions in which the method may be utilized both for the study of problems in physiological chemistry, and as a promising therapeutic agent, have been indicated.

Elsewhere, in indicating the possible use of the apparatus as a thera-

Van Slyke's Amino Apparatus.

peutic agent, the authors say:

Again, there are numerous toxic states in which the eliminating organs, more especially the kidneys, are incapable of removing from the body at an adequate rate, either the autochthonous (aboriginal) or the foreign substances whose presence in excessive amount is detrimental to life processes.

In the hope of providing a substitute in such emergencies, which might tide over a dangerous crisis, as well as for the important information which it might be expected to provide concerning the substances already referred to as normally present in the blood, and also for the light that might thus be thrown on intermediary stages of metabolism, we have devised a method by which the blood of a living animal may be submitted to dialysis outside the body, and again returned to the natural circulation without exposure to air, infection by micro-organisms, or any alteration which would necessarily be prejudicial to life. The process may be appropriately referred to as "vivi-diffusion."

The apparatus constitutes what has been called an artificial kidney in the sense that it allows the escape of the diffusible constituents of the blood, but it differs from the natural organ in that it makes no distinction between these constituents, the rate of their elimination being presumably proportional to the coefficients of diffusion.

It will be shown, however, that any given constituent of the blood, as urea, sugar, or sodium chloride (common salt,) can be retained in the body by a simple expedient when so desired.

The substitution in the animal's body of saline solution for an equal volume of blood leaves the physiological condition as nearly as possible unchanged and chemical results obtained by this method may be expected to represent normal conditions very closely, closer, for example, than when large quantities of blood are drawn off for analysis.

When the circulation in the apparatus is established there is a fall in the blood pressure which is greater or less, according to the size of the apparatus in proportion to that of the animal, but there can be no other immediate symptoms. Rapid and complete recovery after an experiment lasting many hours may be obtained by due regard to asepsis and care in the use of the anaesthetic. Serious loss of blood is avoided by driving the greater part back into the animal's body at the end of the experiment.* * * For purely chemical investigations the experiment is usually performed under complete chloretone anaesthesia.

How Tubes Are Made.

Lack of space does not permit a description of the details of manufacture of the tubes. They are made of a dialyzing substance called celloidin, and are molded inside glass tubes to which they conform. When dry they are pulled out. The dialyzing tubes are attached at the ends to glass tubes of like diameter, and the whole is contained in a glass jacket provided with an inlet and outlet for the outer fluid.

The reason so many tubes are used in the apparatus is to provide the maximum diffusing surface with as small a volume as possible. The apparatus for an animal of moderate size, like a dog, may have from about sixteen tubes up to two or three times that number. Great care is taken in making the apparatus to avoid all sharp angles and sudden bends, and

care must be taken that all branching channels are as nearly as possible of the same width, length and directness. These precautions are necessary in order to maintain a uniformity of flow, which is a very important consideration.

The first apparatus, which consisted of only four tubes, was used on a rabbit, and was connected with the carotid artery (in the neck) and the femoral vein (in the hind leg,) and, consequently, about the length of the animal's body. The experimenters, however, have made a great improvement in practice by causing the blood in the apparatus to turn on itself after the manner of a U-tube, so that inflow and outflow tubes were at the same end and close together. This is the arrangement that is now carried out invariably, the result being that in present experiments the two cannulae are attached to the carotid artery and vein, or femoral artery and vein of the same, or usually of opposite sides.

Chloretone is used as the anaesthetic in these experiments because of its ability to produce prolonged and light anaesthesia with relatively little

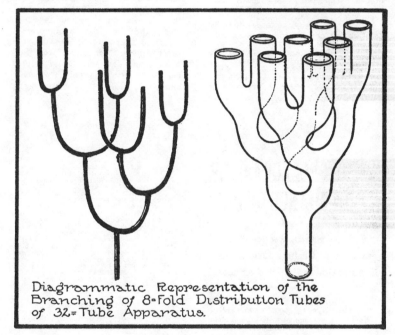

Diagrammatic Representation of the Branching of 8-Fold Distribution Tubes of 32-Tube Apparatus.

depression. The chemical name of this substance is tertiary, trichlorbutyl alcohol. It is administered by stomach tube about two hours before the operation. The powdered crystals are washed down with a little water. This usually produces the desired anaesthesia, but sometimes it is necessary to give a little ether at certain stages.

The investigators found that their experiments were costing a great deal of money on account of the high price of hirudin, the anti-coagulative principle of the medicinal leech. They had to pay $27.50 a gram for it, and sometimes it was necessary to use half a gram in a single experiment. They therefore resolved to extract their own hirudin, after buying leeches by the thousand, and they de-

scribe in detail their method of preparing the agent.

The experimenters declare in the most emphatic manner that the apparatus may be attached to an animal and the blood allowed to course through it for several hours without inducing any untoward effects or injuring the animal in any way. They give the details of two such experiments to prove their contentions. The hirudin is harmless and the substance of which the tubes is composed does not give up to the blood anything that affects the blood pressure.

Quick Recovery.

Both animals in the two experiments mentioned made a quick recovery, and in the weeks following, during which they were kept under observation, nothing abnormal was noted; on the contrary, as is usual in such cases, the animals improved in condition and took on weight because

of the good care they received.

The experimenters selected salicylic acid with which to test the eliminating power of their apparatus, for the reason that quantitative estimations of this drug are easily made; that it is a substance of average diffusibility, and that the time required for its complete elimination by the natural eliminating organ, the kidney, is known. During the first seven hours they recovered by means of the apparatus 19.1 per cent of the total amount given. As the manipulations involved in the separate hourly estimations unavoidably result in some loss, the authors assume that the actual output of salicylates in the apparatus is somewhat higher than that found.

Another interesting fact revealed in the experiments with salicylic acid is that the bladder is entirely free from the drug while the apparatus is dialyzing it out of the blood. A comparison of the rate of elimination of salicylic acid by the authors' apparatus with the rate of elimination by the kidneys of an animal that is not depressed by anaesthetic, or operative, procedures, showed that the animal actually eliminated in the natural way in six hours 1.6 per cent. less than was removed by the dialyzer in seven hours. The writers say:

These data show that the apparatus can already compete with the kidneys on favorable terms, at least, during the early hours of dialysis.

Here are the details of one experiment, as recorded by the physicians, indicating the amount of salicylic acid recorded hour by hour:

Experiment B. May 2, 1913. Dog weighing 11.3 kgm. A small apparatus used, (16 tubes) holding 260 cc. of blood. Apparatus attached to left carotid artery and right external jugular vein.

12.45. Apparatus attached and hirudin solution (0.4 per cent.) allowed to flow slowly into the apparatus the clip on the jugular vein being removed. About 40 cc. of hirudin solution used, more being injected later.

1:02. Arterial clip removed.

2:25. Dialysate removed and fresh solution introduced into the apparatus.

2:30. 0.99 gram sodium salicylate in 20 cc. of water injected slowly into left femoral vein.

3:40. Dialysate removed. Salicylic acid recovered (first hour) equals

24.12 mgm.

4:55. Dialysate removed. Salicylic acid recovered (second hour) equals 15.22 mgm.

5:55. Dialysate removed. Salicylic acid recovered (third hour) equals 13.23 mgm.

6:55. Dialysate removed. Salicylic acid recovered (fourth hour) equals 11.40 mgm.

8:20. Dialysate removed. Salicylic acid recovered (fifth hour) equals 10.50 mgm.

9:05. Dialysate removed. Salicylic acid recovered (sixth period forty-five minutes) equals 9.63 mgm.

It will be seen that the total amount of salicylic acid recovered by dialysis in the above experiment in five and three-quarters hours was 84.10 mgm., equaling 97.5 mgm. sodium salicylate. The average hourly output was, therefore, 17 mgm., which again does not compare so very unfavorably with rate of excretion by the kidney for a similar period when the drug is given by the mouth.

Other Substances Eliminated.

In conclusion, the experimenters mention some of the other substances that are known to be eliminated from the blood by the apparatus. Salicyluric acid is one of them. Many of the well-known constituents of the blood and urine also accumulate in the fluid surrounding the dialyzing tubes, among them sugar, urea, phosphates, and diastase. Ethyl sulphide is also freely eliminated. The writers add:

Of more interest is the fact that we now have at our disposal a method for accumulating the non-proteid nitrogenous constituents of the blood other than urea in any desired amount, the quantity possible to be obtained depending on the size of the animal used, the dialyzing surface of the apparatus and the number of experiments performed.

A wide field of investigation is opened up by the use of this apparatus in a comparative study of the blood flowing to and from various organs with reference both to the substances which they extract from, or add to, the general circulation and to the special active principles (hormones, &c.) which may be present in their internal secretions.

A beginning in this direction has been made by attaching the apparatus to the portal vein (four experiments,) the blood of which gave by diffusion considerably more amino-acids (determined by Van Slyke's method) than that of the carotid.

Work in this direction, as well as in the improvement of the apparatus for the various purposes above outlined and accumulation of the experience necessary along these lines, is being pushed actively forward.

The statement of the investigators to the effect that the apparatus is still in a very imperfect state and is susceptible of great improvement, warrants the belief that ultimately it will aid in solving some of the most vexing problems of medical science.

January 18, 1914

FIND PELLAGRA CURE IN CHANGE OF DIET

Federal Health Service Experiments in Orphan Asylums Remove Odium from Some Foods.

Special to The New York Times.

WASHINGTON, Sept. 7.—An experiment just concluded by the Public Health Service at two orphan asylums at Jackson, Miss., has demonstrated that the disease known as pellagra, the appearance of which in this country caused some alarm and considerable discussion, can be cured by proper dietary measures and has shown apparently that it is not due to any one article of food, but to an " unbalanced " diet. The Public Health Service released the subjects at the two asylums from Governmental observation on Sept. 1, approximately two years after the beginning of the experiment.

The outcome of the experiment is important in view of a statement by the publishers of The American Miller that, as a result of an official publication on the subject of pellagra, last April, the production of highly milled flours had fallen off nearly 25 per cent., and the flour industry had been hit hard in a financial way. At the Public Health Service headquarters the explanation is made that an article in one of the reports of the service was misinterpreted to mean that the use of highly milled flour had been discovered as the cause of pellagra. An entirely erroneous construction was placed on this article, it was said, and in order to correct the misconception the Public Health Service has made a statement reading as follows:

" In the Public Health reports for April 14, 1916, there appeared an article under the following heading: Bread

as 'a Food,' with a sub-heading: 'Changes in Its Vitamine Content and Nutritive Value with Reference to the Occurrence of Pellagra.'

" The facts set forth as regards pellagra have not been challenged, but as some erroneous inferences concerning the value of white flour and of bread made from it have been drawn from the paper, it appears desirable to submit the following statement:

" The paper referred to presented the results of certain of the studies which are being made on pellagra and was designed to demonstrate primarily that when a diet poor in essential food elements, aside from cereals, was constantly used it appeared likely that if the carbohydrate element contained a liberal amount of the accessory food substance known to be contained in whole grains the probability of pellagra developing was less than when the starchy element of food was deficient in these substances.

A Mixed Diet Necessary.

" From the broad view of nutrition, it is very probably immaterial what kind of flour is used in making bread provided that an adequate mixed diet is consumed which will supply sufficient of the essential dietary components outside of the cereals contained in the diet. It may be added that the great majority of people in this country live on a well-balanced, sufficient, mixed diet."

In the early stages of the investigation of pellagra in this country the theory was advanced that the disease was due to the use of corn meal. In the recent experiments of the Public Health Service corn meal has been employed in the curative diet prescribed, and cures have been effected, thus bearing out the conclusion that pellagra is not due to any one article of diet, but to the failure to use a well-balanced diet— that is, a diversified diet.

Perhaps a better illustration of what this means can be obtained from a statement in the article, " Bread as a Food," that pellagra made its appearance in southwestern France in 1850, a period followed by extreme poverty, when the people lived on cereals, fat pork, and a few fresh vegetables, but began to disappear with improved economic conditions in 1860, simultaneously with an improvement in the diet of the people, which now includes more meat, milk, and eggs. At the present time pellagra is practically unknown in France.

In a bulletin on the subject of its observation of the inmates of the two orphan asylums in Jackson, Miss., Surgeon Joseph Goldberger and Assistant Surgeon C. H. Waring of the Public Health Service say:

" The conclusion is drawn that pellagra may be prevented by an appropriate diet without any alteration in the environment, hygienic or sanitary."

The impression, which the Public Health Service says is erroneous, that it made the statement that pellagra was caused by the use of highly milled flour is supposed to have been drawn from an explanation of experiments on fowls made by officers of the service. Fowls, it was said, would live for many months in perfect health on an exclusive diet of wheat, corn, whole-wheat flour, or so-called water-ground corn meal, but if they were fed on highly milled products they would die within a month or two of polyneuritis, a disease very similar to beri beri.

The experiments have shown, however, that chickens can be cured of this disease by giving them a better-balanced diet.

The experiments conducted on the inmates of the two asylums at Jackson were begun two years ago, and the Public Health Service investigators were satisfied after a year of observation that they had demonstrated that the disease, which had existed in the institutions for some time, could be cured by employing a well-balanced diet. But, to make assurance doubly sure, the investigators continued their observation for another year, and have now released their patients from observation with the knowledge that cures are readily effected by proper diet.

Disease Long a Puzzle.

Pellagra has been one of the most puzzling diseases ever studied by medical investigators. For 200 years it has ravaged southern Europe, particularly Italy, where it has been so prevalent that it has often been called " Italian leprosy." The disease in this country has been known for about sixty years; but only in the last decade, when it has attacked thousands of people in the South, has it become a serious problem.

First manifesting itself in lassitude and intestinal disorders, pellagra affects the skin so that it finally becomes thickened and pigmented. Emaciation then sets in. The tongue and mouth later are attacked, swallowing is difficult and painful, and as a result the patient is usually delirious. Likewise the mentality is affected. Melancholia comes with a general retardation of ideas, often accompanied by suicidal tendencies.

Roughly, there have been two different theories as to the cause of pellagra. One group of investigators believed that it was communicated by an insect, while others were convinced that it was of a dietary origin. Italian scientists under Professor Lombroso of Turin asserted that pellagra was due to the consumption of moldy corn. In this country with the alarming increase of pellagra in the South, the Public Health Service established a laboratory for observation of the disease at Columbia, S. C. In 1912, the Thompson-MacFadden Pellagra Commission, organized through the donation of $15,000 by Colonel Robert M. Thompson of New York, and John H. MacFadden of Philadelphia, set up a field headquarters in Spartensburg County, S. C. Some of the members of this commission, particularly Dr. Louis Sambon, lecturer to the London School of Tropical Medicine, arrived at the conclusion that pellagra was due, not to inferior grades of corn, but to some insect carrier.

After careful study of flies and mosquitos Dr. Sambon was led to believe that the buffalo gnat was this carrier. Dr. Sambon's theory receives some support in the September issue of The American Journal of Clinical Medicine in a letter written by Dr. W. J. W. Kerr, who was surgeon in charge of the Andersonville prison hospital, Andersonville, Ga., during the civil war. Dr. Kerr says there were more than 10,000 deaths from pellagra at the prison.

"We examined everything we could conceive as being the possible cause," he writes, "and finally came to the conclusion that the whole thing was produced through the insanitary and crowded condition of the prison. Three regiments of Confederates were guarding the prison, and not one of them ever had pellagra.

"I had from 300 to 500 prisoners out on parole, and not a single case ever occurred outside of the prison after the men had been out a week or ten days. No surgeon or any one on the outside ever took the disease—yet we all had exactly the same diet. We could

not get anything else, so you see that if it had been cornmeal and bad provisions the men on the outside would have had the disease precisely as those on the inside of the prison."

Dr. Edward Jenner Wood of Wilmington, N. C., who has investigated several hundred pellagra cases, came to the conclusion in the May 6 (1916) issue of The Journal of the American Medical Association that pellagra was due to the improper milling of cornmeal, but Dr. George L. Servoss, editor of The Western Medical Times, who was formerly in the milling business, pointed out that the milling process mentioned by Dr. Wood was not the one used in the corn-milling industry, but in the manufacture of brewers' grits.

The new theory is that pellagra should be placed in the same category as beriberi, scurvy, and rickets, which are believed to be caused by a lack of vitamines or the essential constituents necessary for a well-balanced diet.

September 8, 1916

TUBERCULOSIS WAR MAKES BIG STRIDES

Among the various phases of the public health movement in this country of the last decade or two, the effort toward the gradual eradication of tuberculosis stands out prominently in its comprehensive planning and organization. The field that, ten years ago, was almost barren of any organized machinery for the control of the disease, includes at present 1,200 local anti-tuberculosis organizations, 575 hospitals and sanatoriums, 450 special dispensaries, 1,000 dispensary physicians, 4,000 nurses, and 400 open-air schools. The total cost of creating and operating this machinery represents an outlay of over $100,000,000 of public and private funds, according to The Journal of the American Medical Association.

"The results so far achieved," says the writer, "are shown in (1) the steadily growing enlightenment of the people on the subject of tuberculosis, its cause, methods of prevention and treatment; (2) the gradually falling mortality from the disease, (in the registration area in 1902 the rate was 16.3 per 10,000; in 1911, 13.2;) and (3) the impetus given to the entire public health movement through concentration of public attention on a disease, the gradual eradication of which is dependent on the realization of higher general health standards.

"The present lower mortality marks the effect of the intensive educational campaign, of the steadily expanding system of institutional and home control of the disease, and of the general improvement in the sanitary and economic

conditions of the people. Tuberculosis, however, is still with us, with its appalling though reduced mortality, and with some of its fundamental problems still awaiting solution.

"Surgeon F. C. Smith of the United States Public Health Service emphasizes chiefly the following important aspects of a campaign against tuberculosis: (1) Control of sources of 'gross' infection by hospitalization of advanced cases, particularly of those in contact with children; removal from tuberculous surroundings of children under 2 years, preferably under 4, and as much later as possible, and creation of special institutional provision for such children; (2) earlier diagnosis of the disease, rendered possible by the universal application of the principle of periodic physical examinations of children and adults, and a system of industrial insurance permitting the worker to take cognizance of incipient symptoms of disease; (3) reduction in the prevalence of all those diseases which create a predisposition to tuberculosis, and (4) further improvement of industrial sanitation, with removal from industries of conditions causing undue 'stress and depletion.'

"Because of its great prevalence and its baneful effects on the general health standards of this country, tuberculosis must be combated with the active participation of every available agency. The services of the Federal Government should be utilized particularly to establish a national effort against this disease. While the outline of Smith in its entirety is perhaps difficult of attainment, especially with relation to its immediate utilization as a plan of campaign, certainly if put into effect it would tend to decrease greatly the number of new infections through the propagation from old cases."

August 6, 1916

TUBERCULOSIS IN ARMY.

This Disease the Greatest Single Cause of Disability.

A recent report of the Bureau of War Risk Insurance shows that of 27,314 claim cases filed with the bureau, tuberculosis is the greatest single cause of disability. This disease in all its forms is reported as 22 per cent. of the whole. Wounds necessitating amputation of the limbs total only 5 per cent., while wounds not necessitating amputation and miscellaneous wounds all total 51 per cent. Nervous diseases and disorders are 8.3 per cent.

The figures for these diseases on the preceding report show tuberculosis 30.8 per cent.; wounds requiring amputation, 3.0 per cent.; wounds not requiring amputation, 7.9 per cent.; nervous diseases, 9.6 per cent. The changes in these ratios are coincident in time and place in which the disability was incurred, and according to the records 57.7 occurred in camps, 29.7 in battle, 5.7 other sources. The place and source of 6.9 are not stated.

October 5, 1919

SPANISH INFLUENZA MUCH LIKE GRIPPE

EARLY last May dispatches from Madrid told of a mysterious malady which was raging through Spain in the form and of the character of the grippe. Not long after, a similar epidemic took hold in Switzerland and penetrated simultaneously in mild and isolated forms into France, England, and Norway. Early in August this disease, carried from Europe in ocean liners and transports, began to make its appearances in this country, and within the past two weeks the occurrences of the malady in the civilian population and among the soldiers in the cantonments have increased so greatly in number that Government, State, and municipal health bureaus are now mobilizing all their

forces to combat what they recognize to be an approaching epidemic of a so-called "Spanish influenza."

What is Spanish influenza, and what are its symptoms? Although clinical and bacteriological investigations of the disease are still in their early stages, the medical profession believes it has already arrived at certain unshakable conclusions in the matter. In the first place Spanish influenza, if not the grippe itself, is accompanied by all the symptoms of the grippe, and differs from this disease only in that it is more severe and is more likely to lead to pneumonia, if not checked in time, than the less virulent form of influenza which goes by the name of the grippe. As with the grippe, the disease is char-

acterized by excessive sneezing, reddening and running of the eyes, running of the nose, chills followed by fever of from 101 to 103 degrees, aching back and joints, loss of appetite, and a general feeling of debility.

If properly treated, the malady can be overcome without much difficulty. Surgeon General Blue of the Public Health Service, in a report issued several days ago, advises that persons so attacked should go to their homes at once, get to bed without delay, and place themselves under the immediate care of a physician. Treatment under the direction of a physician is simple, but important, consisting principally of rest in bed, fresh air, abundant food, with Dovers powder for the relief of pain. Every case with fever should be regarded as serious, and such a patient should not leave the bed until a normal temperature is restored. Convalescence requires careful treatment to avoid serious complications, such as bronchial pneumonia. During the present outbreak, in foreign countries, quinine and aspirin

Disease: Problems and Progress

have been most generally used during the acute attack.

The history and bacteriological character of Spanish influenza are still uncertain. Few of the cases under observation have revealed the presence of the influenza bacillus which would be required to bear out the contention that Spanish influenza is nothing more than the classified influenza, or grippe, which had its origin in Russia in 1889. The designation of the new malady as "Spanish influenza" is purely arbitrary. The malady has not been definitely tracked to Spain, further than that it was in Spain, early this year, that this particular form first obtained a hold.

Spain disclaimed the unwelcome guest. The people leaped at the conclusion that this new evil, like other evils of the war, must be traced to German origins. Hence two theories presented themselves. One was that a new trench bacteria must have been born in the German lines, where the troops, poorly fed and clothed, were living in a reduced state of vitality, and that this bacteria must have been carried from Flanders into Spain by the strong winds to the Spanish coast last Winter. While this theory would explain the subsequent appearance of the new influenza among the allied troops, it would hardly be as applicable to Spain, because Madrid, a city of the interior, was in the grip of the disease long before any of the coast towns were even touched.

The other theory was that the disease was carried into Spain by the crews of German submarine boats, just as the bacteria of yellow fever were believed to have been created out of the filthy and crowded conditions of the old slave ships.

This theory, in the opinion of medical scientists, must be accepted as ingenious rather than as probable. It has not been definitely concluded that Spanish influenza is anything more than the familiar grippe.

It is fairly certain that the Spanish influenza, if different from the familiar grippe, originated in the German camps. In this connection it may be noted that through all the wars of history diseases generated by unsanitary herding of men in the camps of belligerents have always produced epidemics which before that time had been little or not at all known to many of the populations affected. Going far back, we find that Athens was visited during the Peloponnesian war, 430-425 B. C., by a severe disease known as the Attic sickness, which cost many valuable lives, including that of Pericles. Some historians even ascribe to this epidemic the fall of the Athenian hegemony.

During the Punic wars, the Carthaginian Army was said to have been reduced by smallpox, and Hamilcar was forced thereby to raise the siege of Syracuse. In the year 165, the Roman legions before Seleucia were thinned by a similar scourge, the disease following the banners of the conqueror and conquered and spreading to Rome itself, where it worked havoc under the name of "Antonin's Plague." The Black Death which swept over Europe in the fourteenth century attacked the army of the Black Prince and forced him to abandon the siege of Calais. Syphilis at the end of the fifteenth century spread through the army of Charles VIII., invader of Naples, decimating it after the battle of Fornuovo.

Since the seventeenth century the typhus scourge attached itself to the wake of armies, working its most notable piece of destruction with the Napoleonic hosts. In more recent times typhus has appeared in terrible guise in the Crimean war. According to reliable information typhus cost England 16,000 men, France 80,000, and Russia 200,000. Typhoid fever has repeatedly become a pandemic of wartime, particularly in America during the civil

war and in Europe during the Franco-Prussian war.

In modern times dysentery has been a common affliction of warring armies and still remains a source of serious concern for medical staffs.

Far less dangerous than any of the scourges enumerated above, Spanish influenza has its serious aspect in its possible impairment of an army's offensive efficiency. For this reason the medical staffs of all the allied armies are exerting every precaution to protect the allied front from infection. The disease reduces a soldier's vitality, so that he cannot fight, and makes him a ready carrier of the disease to others, unless he is instantly removed from the ranks.

America was practically exempt from direct contact with the new disease, if it was new, until the arrival in this port on Aug. 12 of the Norwegian liner Bergensfjord, which had during the voyage more than 200 cases of sickness resembling influenza.

Prior to the arrival of this vessel, however, and even prior to the epidemic in Spain, it is worth noting that on April 2, the officials of the Ford plants at Detroit reported that more than 2,000 employes had been suffering from a malady which was very much like the grippe and yet somewhat different from the grippe. At that time "Spanish influenza" was unknown. No observations were made of the Ford cases, and it is only possible to guess at their connection, if any, with what is now known as Spanish influenza.

As to the liner Bergensfjord, however, there was definite investigation. Eleven passengers were transferred immediately to the Norwegian Hospital in Brooklyn.

On Aug. 16, eleven more cases of Spanish influenza were reported at Quarantine from a ship arriving from one of the Scandinavian countries. All of the patients were in a convalescent stage and none of them had developed pneumonia. The ship was passed, but the question was then raised for the first time as to whether the Health Officer of the Port should not be required to quarantine against the disease. At that time Dr. Leland E. Cofer, Health Officer of the Port, and Health Commissioner Copeland, were inclined to take the matter lightly and advanced the opinion that "Spanish influenza" was a misnomer and that the epidemic was not as new to this country as was generally supposed. They regarded it as nothing more than the grippe or at the best a sort of "cousin" to the grippe. At that time also they were firmly convinced that New York was not in danger of an epidemic, a conclusion which fails of justification in light of later developments.

On Aug. 18 a big passenger liner at this port reported that on her voyage twenty-one cases of Spanish influenza developed among the passengers and crews.

The theory that the strange epidemic of influenza attacked only those who were run down because of lack of proper food was exploded in late August when a dispatch from an Irish port told of the occurrence of symptoms of this disease among officers and men stationed at an American destroyer base. Aside from American soldiers, the American sailors are probably the best fed persons in Europe, but the disease attacked several score of them there, and for a week or so disrupted crew assignments completely. All of the cases recovered. It was found in that instance that the disease was not dangerous if taken in hand quickly enough.

Within the last week the so-called Spanish influenza has reaped a harvest in the army cantonments of this country. More than 6,000 cases were reported from Camp Devens alone. Of this number only one case passed from influenza into pneumonia and proved fatal. The cantonment was not placed under quarantine because it had been

decided at Washington that such a step would not check the spread of influenza.

Outbreaks of Spanish influenza at five additional training camps were reported on Friday by Surgeon General Gorgas, making a total number of cases up to noon on Friday 9,313, with 11 deaths. Of these Camp Devens had the greatest number, 6,583; Camp Lee, 1,211, and Camp Upton, 602. Other camps reporting the presence of the epidemic were Camp Gordon, Ga., 138; Camp Syracuse, N. Y., 64; Camp Humphreys, Va., 56; Camp Merritt, N. J., 182, and Camp Lewis, Wash., 11.

Reports received at Washington from European countries indicate that 20 per cent. of the population has been affected this Summer by Spanish influenza, for which reason General Rupert Blue warned the public on Friday against an apparent tendency to underrate the disease. While the epidemic in some places has been mild, he stated that mortality becomes quite common when the Spanish influenza is neglected and allowed to pass into pneumonia.

In view of the fact that the disease is easily communicable from person to person as well as through carriers, precautions are urgent against carelessness in the matter of personal cleanliness. Sneezing, spitting, and coughing should be done always into a handkerchief, as secretions thus released act as carriers. The Health Department has issued a notice suggesting that persons coming in contact with those who sneeze or cough violently in public places should be careful to wash their hands and faces thoroughly with soap and water as soon as possible. Smokers who experience the first symptom of influenza are advised to give up tobacco for a few days until the symptoms disappear, as smoking irritates the mucous membrane.

Inasmuch as the last pandemic of influenza occurred more than twenty-five years ago, physicians who began to practise medicine since 1892 have not had personal experience in handling such a disease as now seems to be spreading through the country. For their benefit Surgeon General Blue has issued a special bulletin setting forth the facts concerning influenza, which physicians must keep in mind in connection with Spanish influenza. The bulletin contains the following points:

Infectious Agent—The bacillus influenza of Pfeiffer.

Sources of Infection—The secretions from the nose, throat, and respiratory passages of cases or of carriers.

Incubation Period—One to four days, generally two.

Mode of Transmission—By direct contact or indirect contact through the use of handkerchiefs, common towels, cups, mess gear, or other objects contaminated with fresh secretions. Droplet infection plays an important part.

Period of Communicability—As long as the person harbors the causative organism in the respiratory tract.

Methods of Control—(a) The infected individual and the environment

Recognition of the Disease—By clinical manifestations and bacteriological findings.

Isolation—Bed isolation of infected individuals during the course of the disease. Screens between beds are to be recommended.

Immunization—Vaccines are used with only partial success.

Quarantine—None; impracticable.

Concurrent Disinfection—The discharger of the mouth, throat, nose, and other respiratory passages.

Terminal Disinfection—Through cleanings, airing, and sunning. The causative is shortlived outside of the host.

(b) General Measures—The attendant of the case should wear a gauze mask. During epidemics persons should avoid crowded assemblages, street cars, and the like. Education as regards the danger of promiscuous coughing and spitting. Patients, because of the tendency to development of broncho-pneumonia, should be treated in well-ventilated, warm rooms.

The local authorities in the last week have taken further steps toward bringing the epidemic under control by placing pneumonia and influenza upon the list of diseases which must be reported as soon as they occur.

September 22, 1918

DRASTIC RULE IN CHICAGO.

Will Arrest Persons Not Using Handkerchiefs in Sneezing.

Special to The New York Times.

CHICAGO, Oct. 3.—In an effort to eradicate influenza in this city, the Health Commissioner and the Chief of Police today issued orders to every member of the Police Department directing him to arrest not only violators of the spitting ordinance, but every person found coughing or sneezing without using a handkerchief. All offenders caught will be taken directly into court.

Theatres, moving-picture shows, courtrooms, and all places where crowds gather are to be invaded by the police in the campaign, which is to be citywide. Dr. Robertson, the Health Commissioner, announced that up to noon 397 new cases of influenza had been reported, as compared with 438 yesterday. There were 297 cases of pneumonia, as compared to 316 yesterday.

October 4, 1918

FEDERAL FORCE READY FOR FIGHT ON EPIDEMIC

WASHINGTON, Oct. 14.—The Public Health Service announced tonight that it now is mobilized for a national campaign against the Spanish influenza epidemic. Additional headquarters for State-wide efforts to control the disease will be established in co-operation with State and local health authorities at Baltimore, Md.; Columbus, Ohio; Richmond, Va., and Columbia, S. C.

Solon Menos, Minister from Haiti, died here of influenza today. Miss Sadie Gompers, daughter of Samuel Gompers, President of the American Federation of Labor, who is now on a mission abroad, also died here. Other victims of the epidemic reported were as follows:

Miss Bessie Porter Edwards of this city, daughter of Major Gen. Clarence Edwards, who died at Camp Meade, Md., Sunday night. She had been a pupil nurse at the cantonment about two weeks, having entered training after her father went to France. General Edwards is in command of the 26th (New England) Division abroad, which recently saw some hard fighting on the western front. His daughter attended boarding school in Dobbs Ferry, N. Y., and completed her education in Paris.

Captain D. F. Shieville of Cincinnati, Ohio, chief of the explosive branch of the Ordnance Department, died in Philadelphia today of pneumonia.

Dr. Admont Halsey Clark, Associate Professor of Pathology of Johns Hopkins University, who died of pneumonia developed from influenza today in Johns Hopkins Hospital, Baltimore, where he was resident pathologist. He was stricken while engaged in experimental work on a cure for the disease, which had been suggested by the officers of the Federal Public Health Service. His friend and associate, Dr. Ernest George Gray of the Johns Hopkins Hospital surgical staff, died of pneumonia on Sunday.

October 15, 1918

TOPICS OF THE TIMES.

Science Has Failed to Guard Us.

When the history of this influenza epidemic comes to be written, it will not reflect much glory on medical science, or, to be more explicit and to recognize the great truth that responsibility is always personal, on the doctors in whom medical science is embodied. It will have to be admitted that though the members of the profession in the United States had long and full warning that the infection would come to this country, though they had read all about its ravages in Europe, and though it is a disease of few or no mysteries either as to its nature or method of distribution, when it arrived they did little more than tell us that among a well-fed people there would be no widespread infection and the cases that did appear would be far milder than under the much different and far worse conditions existing in the war-worn foreign nations.

That makes strange reading, now, with deaths more numerous in our training camps than anywhere else. One recalls, too, that to early suggestions of strict quarantine the reply was made that such measures could not be taken because they would interfere with the movements of our troops and the general conduct of our war business. Would they have done so more than does an epidemic that now covers practically every State in the Union and practically every town in every State?

That the doctors have been either idle or helpless nobody imagines. Widespread as the malady is, and serious as are its effects, it can be claimed without the possibility of contradiction that it would have been worse, the fatalities more numerous, except for the wisdom of our physicians and the labors of the nurses trained by them. That, however, is poor consolation, as the same method of reasoning always is, for what troubles us are the ills we have, not those we might have had, but didn't.

There has been what seems like a lamentable delay everywhere in the adoption of such precautions as the closing of schools, theatres, and churches, and it is only now, when the epidemic is at its height, that we hear, and hear from Washington alone, as yet, of people who go about the streets and in public conveyances, wearing the gauze masks to which resort was long since made by the members of the attendant staff in all well-regulated hospitals. That device certainly has some merit. If it has much, the experts ought to say so and then we would all follow it.

October 17, 1918

PLAGUE CLOSES UP ST. LOUIS

Non-Essential Business to Suspend a Week Because of Influenza.

ST. LOUIS, Nov. 8.—Mayor Kiel today issued a general order closing all business establishments in St. Louis not essential to the prosecution of the war for a period of five to seven days on account of influenza.

November 9, 1918

TEN MILLION DEATHS IN "FLU" PLAGUE A YEAR AGO
Half a Million of Them in This Country

THE accompanying figures on the last previous influenza epidemic were obtained from the Bureau of Vital Statistics of the Department of Commerce in Washington. They have never before been published. In connection with statistics collected from other countries by the bureau, the figures for this country emphasize the supreme importance of discovering, first, the cause of the influenza; second, a means of prevention or control of its spread; third, a means of cure.

Provisional totals of the United States, including the deaths of soldiers, sailors, and marines, indicate that about 500,000 deaths were due to the epidemic at the end of 1918, extending into the early part of 1919. The loss of life in 1919 is estimated at about 45,000. The figures are based on returns covering approximately 80 per cent of the country. The epidemic death rate per thousand was 4.2.

The population of the world during the epidemic was about 1,700,000,000. It was a world epidemic. Applying the death rate in the United States to the world, the grand total would figure 7,000,000. But the number of deaths reported to the bureau from India is 5,000,000; from the British native States, 1,000,000. In India the death rate per thousand reported was 19.8, by far the highest for so large a group. Applying the death rate of the United States to

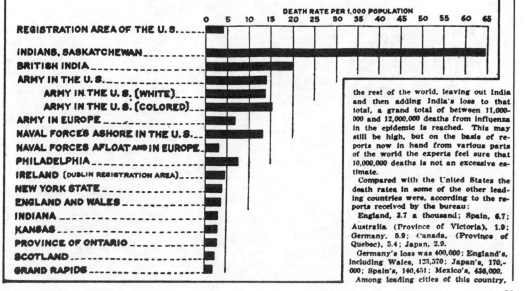

NUMBER OF DEATHS DUE TO INFLUENZA EPIDEMIC PER 1,000 POPULATION, AUTUMN OF 1918

DEATH RATE PER 1,000 POPULATION
0 5 10 15 20 25 30 35 40 45 50 55 60 65

REGISTRATION AREA OF THE U. S.
INDIANS, SASKATCHEWAN
BRITISH INDIA
ARMY IN THE U. S.
ARMY IN THE U. S. (WHITE)
ARMY IN THE U. S. (COLORED)
ARMY IN EUROPE
NAVAL FORCES ASHORE IN THE U. S.
NAVAL FORCES AFLOAT AND IN EUROPE
PHILADELPHIA
IRELAND (DUBLIN REGISTRATION AREA)
NEW YORK STATE
ENGLAND AND WALES
INDIANA
KANSAS
PROVINCE OF ONTARIO
SCOTLAND
GRAND RAPIDS

the rest of the world, leaving out India and then adding India's loss to that total, a grand total of between 11,000,000 and 12,000,000 deaths from influenza in the epidemic is reached. This may still be high, but on the basis of reports now in hand from various parts of the world the experts feel sure that 10,000,000 deaths is not an excessive estimate.

Compared with the United States the death rates in some of the other leading countries were, according to the reports received by the bureau:

England, 3.7 a thousand; Spain, 6.7; Australia (Province of Victoria), 1.9; Germany, 5.9; Canada (Province of Quebec), 5.4; Japan, 2.9.

Germany's loss was 400,000; England's, including Wales, 123,570; Japan's, 170,000; Spain's, 140,451; Mexico's, 436,000. Among leading cities of this country,

Estimated Number of Deaths and Provisional Death Rates from the Epidemic. Cities in the United States, Sept. 8, 1918, to June 1, 1919.

City.	Number of Deaths.	Number of Deaths from the Epidemic per 1000 Persons.	City.	Number of Deaths.	Number of Deaths from the Epidemic per 1000 Persons.
Albany	534	4.7	Milwaukee	1,333	2.9
Atlanta	538	2.7	Minneapolis	1,065	2.8
Baltimore	4,118	6.1	Nashville	1,035	8.7
Birmingham	1,180	6.0	Newark	2,172	5.1
Boston	5,107	6.5	New Haven	860	5.6
Buffalo	2,766	5.8	New Orleans	2,767	7.2
Cambridge	661	5.9	New York	24,329	4.7
Chicago	9,956	3.8	Oakland	1,329	6.2
Cincinnati	1,721	4.1	Omaha	1,133	6.3
Cleveland	3,254	4.0	Philadelphia	12,760	7.3
Columbus	769	3.5	Pittsburgh	4,743	8.0
Dayton	460	2.5	Providence	1,380	5.2
Fall River	749	5.8	Richmond	995	6.2
Grand Rapids	206	1.5	Rochester	703	2.7
Indianapolis	718	2.5	St. Louis	2,323	3.0
Jersey City	974	3.1	St. Paul	907	3.5
Kansas City, Mo.	2,227	7.1	San Francisco	3,621	7.6
Los Angeles	2,968	5.2	Syracuse	1,027	6.4
Louisville	1,133	4.7	Toledo	561	2.1
Lowell	554	5.1	Washington, D. C.	2,637	6.6
Memphis	963	5.8	Worcester	1,287	7.1

Death Rates Per 1,000 of Population According to Ages, Autumn of 1918.

	Indiana.		Kansas.		Philadelphia.	
	Male.	Female.	Male.	Female.	Male.	Female.
All ages	3.0	2.9	3.0	2.8	7.7	7.0
Under 1 year	10.4	7.7	6.3	5.2	19.0	16.6
1 to 4 years	4.4	4.4	2.7	2.6	10.1	10.3
5 to 9 years	1.3	1.4	0.8	1.0	3.3	•3.4
10 to 14 years	1.2	1.3	1.0	1.1	2.1	2.5
15 to 19 years	2.6	2.2	3.0	2.2	4.9	4.7
20 to 24 years	2.8	3.9	3.4	3.6	6.9	9.7
25 to 29 years	4.9	5.3	5.4	5.8	14.0	14.3
30 to 34 years	5.8	5.4	7.1	5.2	16.3	11.3
35 to 39 years	4.4	3.0	4.7	3.5	11.0	6.2
40 to 44 years	2.4	1.9	2.9	2.2	6.1	4.5
45 to 49 years	1.5	1.4	1.5	1.6	5.8	3.7
50 to 54 years	1.2	1.5	1.2	1.4	3.9	4.1
55 to 59 years	1.1	0.9	1.1	1.3	4.3	3.4
60 to 64 years	1.4	1.4	1.2	1.5	3.4	3.2
65 years and over	2.5	3.2	2.2	3.2	5.6	4.8

Nashville, Tenn., showed the highest rate, 8.7 a thousand. Others toward the top of the list were Kansas City, Mo., 7.1; Philadelphia, Pa., 7.3; New Orleans, La., 7.2; San Francisco, Cal., 7.6; Pittsburgh, Pa., 8; and Worcester, Mass., 7.1. New York City was 4.7. Chicago was 3.8. The lowest city in the list was Grand Rapids, Mich., 1.5.

These varying rates are puzzling to students of the disease. Especially puzzling is the varying of the death rates for ages. In this respect the epidemic differed from previous ones of this disease, of which there had been many in the last century. So marked is the contrast that some medical authorities have raised the question whether the cause itself may be different. This dissimilarity stands out not only in previous attacks of influenza, but in comparison with the epidemics of all other diseases. Without exception, so far as medical records show, in all other plagues the death curve had been highest among the young age periods and the old; that is, among the weaker. In the influenza epidemic of 1918-19, the order was reversed in probably the most startling paradox that ever faced the medical profession. In those ages that represent the youthful vigor and prime of life the death curve runs highest; in effect, where resistance would be expected to be the strongest it proved to be the weakest.

Like war, influenza apparently selects the best; on account of this peculiarity, the cost to the world of the epidemic in 1918-19 has not been appreciated in anything like its full meaning. Equally on account of this, the importance of discovering a solution of the problem rises higher and higher.

During the epidemic as above indicated it was noted by physicians that the disease was more virulent in the ages that would be expected to withstand its ravages with less difficulty. Now for the first time comparative figures are published and they bring out the contrast more sharply. They represent complete returns from three different sections of the country, the only ones the Bureau of Vital Statistics has been able to compile, on account of lack of funds. The places represented are Philadelphia, Indiana, and Kansas. A heavy excess of deaths is shown between the ages of 20 and 40. According to the table, the most dangerous age for an attack of influenza is around 30 years; under 20 the least dangerous is from 10 to 14. Above 40 there is not much difference in the low death rate between the ages 55 and 59 and 60 and 64. The high death rate of under one year, as shown in the chart, is accounted for by the large increase in the number of still births caused by the epidemic.

An answer to the two questions—why there was a death rate in inverse ratio to physical vigor and stamina and why it varied so much in different localities—would probably go far toward the solution of the great problem. To illustrate, the difference of death rates in different localities has turned up a clue in England. Returns there show that at places near poison gas plants there was a much lower death rate, and that workers in the gas plants, with the exception of those working where phosgene gas was being manufactured, were practically immune from influenza. This has at least raised the question whether a gas may not be found that destroys the germ.

In this country, owing to the lack of funds by the Bureau of Vital Statistics, it has not yet been possible to discover whether the analogy would hold good. A great mass of statistics is on hand, but because of inadequate clerical help to compile the figures the lessons they hold in throwing light on an immense economic loss to the country have not been read.

Where two towns, close together, have one a high death rate from influenza, and the other a low death rate, some of the questions scientists would like to have answered are: What was the difference in the surroundings? Were the occupations along the same line? Was one better fed than the other? The Joint Influenza Committee representing the Public Health Service, the U. S. Navy, the U. S. Army and the Department of Commerce, has recommended to Congress that an appropriation of $100,000 be made for compiling the statistics. In a report, not yet published, made by the sub-committee on influenza of the American Public Health Association, of which Dr. William H. Davis, head of the Bureau of Vital Statistics, is Chairman, appears the following:

"Much has been learned in the past year about the pandemic. Much more remains to be learned. No easy task lies ahead. The battle for knowledge is on in earnest. More funds and more energy are needed to find the cause of this epidemic, to find out why it affected places, races and ages so differently, and to find effective remedies."

February 1, 1920

MALARIA CONTROL FOUND TO BE EASY

Results in controlling malaria in rural districts of the Southern States are recorded in the fourth chapter of the annual report of the Rockefeller Foundation, made public yesterday.

After telling of destroying the breeding places of mosquitoes and screening houses, immunizing the individual with quinine and destroying the parasites in the blood of human carriers the report reviews its initial experiment at Crossett, a lumber town of 2,129 in Ashley County, Arkansas. Climatic conditions and abundant breeding places favored the offending type of mosquitoes, malaria was widely endemic and physicians of the regions estimated that it was the cause of 60 per cent. of all illness.

The program of eradicating breeding places was restricted to such measures as the community itself well might carry out, and was aimed at a reasonably high high degree of control at minimum cost. The first conspicuous result apparent was the practical elimination of the mosquitos as a pest, the report says. The reduction in malaria as shown by a parasite index taken in May and again in December, 1916, was 72.33 per cent. Physicians calls for the year were reduced 70.36 per cent., compared with the previous year. At the end of the year the community took over the work and carried it on for two years. This table shows the results:

PHYSICIANS' CALLS FOR MALARIA.

Population	2,129
1915 calls (company's records)	2,500
1916 calls (company's records)	741
1917 calls (company's records)	200
1918 calls (company's records)	73
Reduction for the three years	97.1%

PER CAPITA COST.

1916 (omitting overhead)	$1.24
1917 (total cost)	.63
1918 (total cost)	.53

Operations then were transferred to the neighboring town of Hamburg, with these results:

PHYSICIANS' CALLS FOR MALARIA.

Population	1,285
1916 calls	2,312
1917 calls	250
1918 calls	59
Reduction 1916-1918	97.4%

PER CAPITA COST.

1917 (omitting overhead)	$1.45
1918 (total upkeep)	.44

There followed experimental control in four Mississippi towns, the achievements being thus summarized:

	Lake Village	Dermott	Monticello	Bauxits
Population	975	2,760	3,023	2,500
Physicians' call for malaria:				
1916	1,817	1,300	1,413	862
1917	1,388	1,248	1,274	720
1918	83	162	137	172
Per cent. reduction, 1917-1917	94.8	87.8	80.8	78.4
Per capita cost, 1918	$1.25	$0.54	$0.46	$1.11

"Comparison of cost of operations with results accomplished in these six towns tends to show that malaria control in such communities, considered merely as a business proposition, pays," the report continues. "At two dollars per physicians' call. Crossett has been paying annually more than four and one-half times as much in doctors' bills alone for the privilege of having malaria, as it expended in 1918 for the upkeep of the work which kept it practically from malaria and from the mosquito as a pest. Hamburg's annual doctors' bill for malaria had been eight times the cost of protection in 1918. In the four new communities the annual payment for physicians' calls would cover even the relatively heavy cost of first year operations almost one-and-a-half times over. And the doctors' bill is but an insignificant fraction of malaria's total cost to the community."

Turning to a discussion of the work in rural districts where mosquito elimination is not practicable the foundation reports on the first screening experiment on a group of cotton plantations near Lake Village, Ark. The people were taught the importance of maintaining the screens by house to house visits. Most of the population were negroes of average plantation intelligence, yet from the apparent average infection of 11.97 per cent. at the beginning of the work, a parasite index at the end of the year showed a reduction of 70.6 per cent. The average annual per capita cost of screening was found to be $1.75. Similar results were attained on another plantation at a per capita cost of 57 cents.

Setting forth that since all infected mosquitoes have derived their infection from the blood of infected persons, it is possible theoretically to prevent the spread of the infection in a community by destroying the parasites in the blood of the human carrier, the report tells of a two-year field experiment along this line in Bolivar County, Miss. A large number of blood examinations showed that persons who have had clinical attacks may carry the parasites in their blood for months, and demonstrated that the usual physician's treatment does not sterilize the blood.

These tests established the fact that ten grains of quinine a day for eight weeks sterilized the blood of about 90 per cent. of the carriers to whom it was administered.

December 1, 1919

PLAGUE THREATENS 100,000 VICTIMS IN THE COTTON BELT

Special to The New York Times.

WASHINGTON, July 24.—Pellagra, one of the worst scourges known to man, is making alarming headway in parts of the cotton belt States, according to the Public Health Service, which estimates that this year the disease, which is due to semi-starvation, will claim about 100,000 victims, and of these 10 per cent. will, in the opinion of the Government experts, die. This alarming situation, which today presents one of the most grave problems facing the Public Health Service, is due principally to economic conditions in the cotton-growing and cotton-milling sections of the South.

A statement issued from the office of Surgeon General Hugh S. Cumming calls the attention of the country to the pellagra menace, and warns that unless prompt and energetic measures are taken to check the spread of the disease, which is due to lack of proper foods, " it will take a still heavier toll from the already enfeebled population in 1922."

The statement of the Public Health Service follows:

" While the American people have been spending money lavishly to save the Chinese and the Europeans from starvation a veritable famine has been developing in the rural districts of the South, and particularly in those of the cotton belt, which stretches from Eastern Texas to the Carolinas. The tenant farmers, most of whom devote all their land to cotton and allot not even a foot to kitchen gardening or for the use of a cow or even of some hens, have been forced by the failure of the cotton market to adopt a starvation diet that is rapidly decimating them.

Says Thousands Will Die.

" The latest reports to the United States Public Health Service show that pellagra, which results the world around from famine conditions, will this year claim about 100,000 victims, of whom at least 10 per cent. will die; and that, unless radical relief measures are taken, it will take a still heavier toll from the already enfeebled population in 1922.

" That pellagra would show a heavy increase this year was foreseen last Fall, when the cotton market failed. Most American cotton is raised on shares by tenant farmers, who are " carried " by the land-owning planters for about six months each year, during which they are provided with food and clothes for themselves and their families, to be paid for when the crop is sold in the Fall.

" Last year's crop, however, is still unsold, and neither tenant nor planter has received the money on which they had depended. The planters are almost moneyless and are unable to obtain further credit from the banks, which are also hard pressed. Nevertheless, the tenants must be carried till next Fall, with no assurance that the cotton market will come back even then.

" Inevitably there is pressure all down the line, and the tenants, whose credit has been reduced to the disappearing point, are abliged to live on the cheapest foods obtainable.

" These foods, salt pork, cornmeal and molasses, valuable as they are when balanced by other foods, such as lean meat, eggs, and milk and vegetables, lack certain elements that are absolutely essential to the maintenance of health. And the ' other foods ' are away beyond the purses of the tenants.

" Conditions have been getting steadily worse for months, and the cumulative effect is becoming serious. It takes about five months of this particular kind of semi-starvation before pellagra begins to manifest itself, but after that it does so with appalling rapidity. This second stage is now well under way.

" Two remedies are suggested by the Public Health Service—to help the victims directly and to help them to help themselves. Only the first method is immediately applicable. Proper food and medical care are urgently necessary to save the lives of those already ill and to preserve the health of those who will become ill unless they receive aid until the cotton market revives. If it does not revive this Fall aid will probably be necessary for a year or more.

" The second remedy is to induce the farmers to diversify their crops, or at any rate to plant kitchen gardens and to keep pigs, hens and possibly a milch cow. The planters might insist on their tenants doing this. It is, of course, too late to plant this year, and the returns from next year's planting will not be available till next Summer, so this is not a measure of immediate relief.

" However, once established, these things would offer an important protection against the recurrence of outbreaks of pellagra, which ravage the country at every recurrence of hard times.

" The Public Health Service has begun work on both these lines. It is bespeaking the aid of the Red Cross and of other relief agencies in providing immediate local relief; and it will immediately call on the health officers of the Southern States and on other agencies interested to meet for a conference in some central Southern city to consider ways and means for rescue work."

Dr. Joseph Goldberger of the Public Health Service, who is one of the best known pellegra specialists, informs THE NEW YORK TIMES that pellegra appears to have made the greatest headway in the State of Mississippi, where in May last more than 1,700 cases were reported, the victims being chiefly small farmers and tenant planters. Dr. Goldberger added that the May total has undoubtedly been greatly increased, as pellagra is a disease that shows its greatest increases in May, June and July. In one little cotton mill town in the Carolinas thirty-one cases have been reported since May 1.

The sections where the disease made greatest progress are those parts of Mississippi, Arkansas and Tennessee of which the City of Memphis is the centre, parts of Eastern Texas and the Carolinas. It is also in Alabama and Georgia, but the situation in these States is not so serious. A splendid fruit crop in Georgia, in the opinion of the experts of the Public Health Service, is probably the " blessing " that has saved thousands of little farmers and tenant planters in Georgia, the fruit providing the additional element of diet necessary to preserve health.

Southern newspapers have been for some weeks calling the attention of their readers to the spread of the disease, and through these newspapers the Public Health Service has been carrying on educational propaganda in an effort to arouse the people to the menace that faces them.

Senator Dial Asks for Action.

Senator Nathaniel B. Dial in a letter to Surgeon General Cumming calls attention to the situation in that part of South Carolina of which the textile manufacturing city of Spartanburg is the centre. The little cotton mill village previously referred to in this article, where the disease has made alarming progress, is in Spartanburg County. Senator Dial's letter to the Surgeon General read:

Washington, D. C., July 18, 1921.
Surgeon General Hugh S. Cumming, Washington.

My Dear General Cumming—It has just come to my attention that because of the cotton situation in the South, due to the low price of the staple, with the consequent underfeeding of many of the smaller farm tenants, there is likely to be much suffering and disease caused by pellegra in that section in the near future. This information reached me in newspaper accounts which quote your department. If these statements are correct, may I not call your immediate attention to the great necessity that exists for not only informing the people of what may happen, but also for taking such steps as may be necessary to prevent and combat such a situation as would arise should this disease again take hold in the South.

I was under the impression that with the stamping out of pellegra a few years ago the hospital at Spartanburg, S. C., had been discontinued, or was only performing part of its former work. However, this may be, I desire to call your attention to the great necessity of taking such steps now by continuing to work at Spartanburg as may appear proper to prevent a repetition of this disease in that locality.

Yours very truly, N. B. DIAL.

The greatest handicap facing the Public Health Service in its fight against the pellagra scourge is lack of funds. This phase of the situation is expected to be brought to the attention of the President and Congress within the next few days, and it is believed that whatever sum may be necessary to combat the spread of the disease and properly to care for those already afflicted will be promptly voted.

July 25, 1921

ORDERS RELIEF FOR PELLAGRA VICTIMS

President Pledges Every Aid in His Power in Fighting Plague and Famine.

Special to The New York Times.

WASHINGTON, July 25.—President Harding this afternoon directed the Public Health Service to make an immediate and complete report to him of the pellagra situation in the cotton belt States. In a letter to Surgeon General Hugh S. Cumming the President said it was " unthinkable " that any measures necessary to relieve the sufferers on the cotton plantations and in the textile villages should be delayed " for a single day."

The President also wrote to Dr. Livingston Farrand, Chairman of the Central Committee of the American Red Cross, suggesting the complete co-operation of that organization with the Public Health Service in putting into immediate effect any and all relief measures that may be necessary.

In both letters the President stated that Congress will be asked to appropriate promptly any amount of money that may be necessary.

The President gained his first information, as to the gravity of the situation in the cotton belt when he read the Public Health Service statement printed in THE NEW YORK TIMES this morning, in which it was estimated that there are now 100,000 cases of pellagra among the little farmers, cotton tenants and cotton mill workers in the Southern States, and in which the Public Health Service gave warning that unless prompt and energetic measures to control the scourge were taken the indications were that a still more serious situation would exist next year.

Asks for Prompt Report.

President Harding's letter to Surgeon General Cumming read:

The White House,
Washington,
July 25, 1921.

Surgeon General Hugh S. Cumming, the Public Health Service, Washington, D. C.:

Dear General Cumming—I have been greatly concerned to note the public statement from the Public Health Service as to the menace of pellagra and condition of at least semi-famine in a large section of the cotton belt. That such a condition is obviously a temporary incident to the economic dislocation following the war cannot lessen our concern. Famine and plague are words almost foreign to our American vocabulary, save as we have learned their meaning in connection with the afflictions of lands less favored and toward which our people have so many times displayed large and generous charity.

Immediate and effective measures of amelioration are manifestly demanded if conditions even approximate the gravity suggested by the Public Health report. It is unthinkable that we should delay for a single day the institution of such measures. Therefore I am writing to ask you for the most complete possible report that can be made at once—provided there is anything to add to what you have already made public—and especially for suggestion of proper measures to deal with the situation.

I am also writing to Dr. Livingston Farrand, head of the American Red Cross, in the same tenor, and suggesting that co-operation between his organization and your own might be helpful, having in mind the need for haste in making a full survey, and in planning relief measures. I wish you both to be assured of my co-operation and of all aid that can appropriately be given through the Executive departments, and to know that if full information about the situation shall make it apparent that legislative action is necessary, I will, on a proper showing, be prepared to ask the requisite authorization from the Congress.

Most sincerely yours,
WARREN G. HARDING.

Urges Red Cross Co-operation.

The letter of the President to Dr Farrand was as follows:

The White House, Washington.
July 25, 1921.

Dr. Livingston Farrand, Chairman Central Committee American Red Cross, Washington, D. C.:

Dear Dr. Farrand—Recent reports of a distressing condition among the rural population in a large section of the cotton belt are confirmed by a public statement from the Public Health Service. They indicate that, due to the depressed cotton market, many thousands of people are unable to sell their one product for money wherewith to obtain a necessary variety of wholesome food, and that there is grave threat of an epidemic of pellagra.

It must bring a shock to the American people to realize that a great section of their own country, which they are wont to think of as immune from such experiences, is actually menaced with famine and plague. For this is what it would be called if it should befall in any other country, and we may as well give it its right name. It is, of course, a consequence of the economic disorganization following the war, and it demands instant and vigorous attention. Our people, so long and so often moved by splendid charitableness toward the unfortunates of other lands, will never permit such an affliction here at home.

Moved by a realization that there must be no delay in coping with such a condition, I am writing to ask you, if the Red Cross can make an immediate investigation and report the present situation, the outlook for the future and the measures necessary for prompt and effective relief. I am inclosing a copy of report which Surgeon General Cumming has made and am asking to be advised whether the Red Cross possesses the organization and means to make, perhaps in co-operation with the Public Health Service, a survey and outline of necessary measures. Inasmuch as promptness and accuracy are vitally important in such a matter, I will be glad to enlist any public instrumentalities that may properly be employed to assist in the task.

Concurrently with this letter, I am also addressing one of like tenor to General Cumming, suggesting, as I am also taking the liberty to do with you, that you and he confer about the matter. You may be assured of my full co-operation. It is proper for me to add that if your survey shall develop the need of legislative provision for special relief, I will be glad, when the evidence is at hand, to lay it before the Congress and ask the authority that I have no doubt it would promptly grant, once the need be shown.

Please consider me ready and anxious to help in any proper way, by conference or otherwise.

Very sincerely yours,
WARREN G. HARDING.

Immediately upon receipt of the President's letter Surgeon General Cumming called into conference Dr. Joseph Goldberger, who is in charge of the pellagra section of the Public Health Service. At present the scope of the work directed by Dr. Goldberger is very limited, owing to the fact that the total amount of money the Public Health Service has available to fight the pellagra menace is just $18,000. During the last Congress the Public Health Service asked for $30,000 for investigation of the pellagra menace, which then had not assumed the alarming proportions indicated in the report published in today's New York Times.

The Sixty-sixth Congress was in an economical mood, however, when this item was reached in the Sundry Civil bill, and reduced it to $20,000. A short time ago the new budget organization ordered this amount still further reduced by 10 per cent., leaving $18,000 in hand to combat one of the most serious situations that has developed in this country in years. Owing to this lack of funds the Public Health Service is able to maintain only two pellagra experts in the Southern States—Dr. George A. Wheeler, with headquarters in Spartanburg, S. C., and Dr. W. F. Tanner at Milledgeville, Ga. In addition to maintaining Drs. Tanner and Wheeler in the South the pellagra section also has to meet its Washington office expenses out of the $18,000.

Dr. Goldberger said today that the "irreducible minimum" of money immediately needed is about $140,000, which does not include hospitalization or relief supplies for the victims of the disease, their families or other persons who are existing on a semistarvation diet and are therefore in danger of contracting pellagra.

There is immediately needed in every cotton State, according to Dr. Goldberger, at least one pellagra expert operating under the direction of the Public Health Service and in co-operation with the State authorities. There should be also in each State one dietitian acting under directions of the Public Health Service.

It is urgent, Dr. Goldberger holds, that in each of these States a clinic should be established where at least 100 pellagrans who have not reached the serious stages of the disease can be instructed in dietary matters and sent back to their homes to impart the knowledge to their neighbors. It will require about four months to impart the instruction, and on the "irreducible minimum" basis Dr. Goldberger estimated that these pellagrans would be supplied with one wholesome meal a day, to consist of one pint of milk, a portion of lean meat, the best of bread and butter, and vegetables. The cost of such a meal, he said, might possibly be held down to 25 cents per patient.

For One Good Meal a Day.

"We are giving foreigners three meals a day; why not also give our people three meals?" Dr. Goldberger was asked.

"That would take a lot more money," he replied, "and I will say that if we can supply them one good meal it will go a long way in the direction of ameliorating the situation."

The increase of the disease is indicated in a report for the month of June just received from the health authorities of Mississippi. In May, 1,700 new cases were reported in the State. In June the number reported was about 2,400, and it is estimated that the July total will show a still further increase over the June figures. The Health Department of Mississippi is considered the best in the Southern States, and that is why the reports from that State are more complete than those received from other cotton belt States.

Owing to the completeness of the reports from Mississippi an impression has been created that the pellagra situation in that State is more serious than in any other section of the South. As a matter of fact, it is not worse, and State control there is probably the most efficient in the cotton belt.

The States where the disease has made its greatest progress as a result of semifamine conditions among the little farmers and textile workers are the two Carolinas, Georgia, Alabama, Mississippi, Louisiana, Tennessee, Arkansas and Texas. The disease also exists in parts of Virginia, Oklahoma and Kentucky, and it is reported that there are some cases in Southern Missouri.

The great majority of those who have fallen victims of the disease this year have been women and little children. The Public Health Service has made a special study of about 1,100 cases selected at random, and of these only sixty-four were men and boys of more than 14 years of age. Every 100 cases of the disease represent about sixty families in which the disease has found a lodgment, according to the Public Health Service records.

"The real problem that now faces us," said Dr. Goldberger, "is 1922. If economic conditions do not improve I would be loath to prophesy what the 1922 story will be. The disease increases greatest in May, June and July, and from now on we may look for a gradual reduction each month in the number of new cases. Prompt, efficient and energetic precautionary and relief measures if taken now will, without question, simplify the 1922 problem and save thousands of valuable lives."

Dr. Goldberger said he was "in correspondence with the health authorities in all parts of the South, and he hoped that at an early date a conference could be arranged with these officials, to be held in some central Southern city."

July 26, 1921

DENIES PLAGUE IN SOUTH.

But Conference of Health Authorities Admits Pellagra Is Spreading.

WASHINGTON, Aug. 5.—Denial that there is a "condition approaching a famine or plague in the South" was made today in a report unanimously adopted by health officials from a dozen Southern States in conference here with Surgeon General Cumming of the Public Health Service to discuss the pellagra situation. It held that "erroneous and misleading" statement had been made to the public, but the sentence "we do not regard the situation in any sense as more serious at the present time than during the past several years," in the committee draft was eliminated.

The report said the Southern health officials in conference at the request of the Surgeon General "deplore the fact that an impression has been created that famine conditions exist in the South and as a result that pellagra has increased to an alarming extent."

After making an investigation, using all information available, it said, "we do not believe the situation warrants or should occasion any undue alarm. The indications are that there will be an increase in pellagra this year in localities in certain States where the disease has been epidemic, but data in hand shows in an unmistakable way that the number of cases and deaths from pellagra during 1921 will still be less than the annual average during the period of 1914 to 1921."

A resolution pledging "the support of the health authorities and the people they represent in the South" to a constructive program for co-ordination of all Federal Public Health and Welfare activities in one department was adopted today by the conference.

August 6, 1921

F. D. ROOSEVELT ILL OF POLIOMYELITIS

Franklin D. Roosevelt, former Assistant Secretary of the Navy and Democratic candidate for Vice-President in the last election, was brought to this city from Campobello Island, Bay of Fundy, yesterday, suffering from poliomyelitis, or infantile paralysis, which for more than a week has caused the loss of the use of both legs below the knees. Mr. Roosevelt was taken to Presbyterian Hospital, Seventieth Street and Madison Avenue, where it was said that the attack was very mild and that Mr. Roosevelt would not be permanently crippled.

Mr. Roosevelt was brought here on a special car, attached to a train which arrived at the Grand Central at 2:20 P. M. He was carried from the car to an ambulance and was hurried to the hospital.

Dr. George Draper of 116 East Sixty-third Street, Mr. Roosevelt's family physician, said that Mr. Roosevelt's condition was much improved, and that he was regaining control of his legs. He is still unable to walk, however. "I cannot say how long Mr. Roosevelt will be kept in the hospital," said Dr. Draper, "but you can say definitely that he will not be crippled. No one need have any fear of permanent injury from this attack."

Through Dr. Charles H. Young, Superintendent of Presbyterian Hospital, Mr. Roosevelt sent word to reporters that he had had a "comfortable trip" and was "feeling very well."

Mr. Roosevelt's removal to Presbyterian Hospital, it was said at his home at 47 East Sixty-fifth Street, was to enable him to have special treatment which would hasten the return of the control of his legs. His general condition, it was said, was better than at any time in years.

For several weeks Mr. and Mrs. Roosevelt and their children have been at their camp at Campobello. It was there that Mr. Roosevelt was stricken, about Aug. 10. Press reports from St. Stephen, N. B., were to the effect that he had caught cold and was threatened with pneumonia. Dr. R. W. Lovett of Boston, an authority on poliomyelitis, was called into consultation. At that time Mr. Roosevelt's legs and feet were affected. For more than a week he has been recovering control of the affected members and his condition, it is said, was so improved that his removal to this city was planned. A special car brought him from Eastport, Me., to the Grand Central Terminal.

Mr. Roosevelt and their five children accompanied him to this city. The children have gone to Hyde Park, the Roosevelt country home in Dutchess County.

Mr. Roosevelt is 39 years old. He is a lawyer and is a member of the firm of Marvin, Hooker & Roosevelt of this city. He was State Senator from the Dutchess-Putnam-Columbia district, and immediately came into prominence through his fight against the nomination of the late William F. Sheehan, Tammany choice for the United States Senate. He resigned from the Senate to become Assistant Secretary of the Navy under President Wilson and continued in that office through the two Wilson Administrations. Following his defeat for Vice President he became Vice President of the Fidelity and Deposit Company, at the head of the New York office.

September 16, 1921

Canadian Doctors Report Discovery That Checks Diabetes

TORONTO, March 22.—Discovery of an active pancreatic extract, which it is hoped will prolong the lives of persons suffering from diabetes, was announced to the medical profession today from the medical research laboratories of the University of Toronto.

Two young doctors, F. G. Branting and C. H. Best, directing the experiments, first prolonged the life of a diabetic dog fifty-six days beyond previous records. Then, by injecting under the skin of seven human being suffering from the disease a highly potent extract discovered through animal experimentation, a distinct improvement was brought about in the patients, the scientists report.

The experimenters do not claim that the new discovery will effect a cure, but they believe that it will prolong life considerably.

March 23, 1922

FIND SUN PRODUCES THE 4TH VITAMINE

While the study of rickets at Johns Hopkins University has resulted in the discovery reported yesterday of a fourth type of vitamin (Vitamin D), the study of rickets at the College of Physicians and Surgeons of Columbia University has indicated that sunlight may produce vitamins directly in the human blood.

The experiments at the College of Physicians and Surgeons indicated that the frequent exposure of the skin of a child to the direct rays of the sun cured rickets without any change of diet. Copious use of cod liver oil also cured rickets.

Cod liver oil is the richest of substances in the mysterious unidentified objects called vitamins, and its vitamins have commonly been supposed to be the agent which cures the rickets. Sunlight, however, according to the New York experiments, does exactly what cod liver oil does. No definite claim has been made as to the manner in which the sunlight acts, whether it produces new vitamins or increases the activity of those already in existence in the patient or operates in some other way, but X-ray photographs and blood analyses are said to corroborate fully the assertion that the sunlight produces direct chemical changes in the blood, restoring the impaired bones steadily until a complete cure is effected.

The effects of sunlight in the cure of rickety children has been confirmed, according to medical reports by Dr. Alfred F. Hess of the College of Physicians and Surgeons, by experiments on animals. Numbers of rats have been fed on diets which produce rickets. The disease has inevitably appeared in those kept in darkness. It has been invariably prevented in those regularly kept in the sun.

The blood analysis of patients has again confirmed the mysterious effect of sunlight on the blood. Rickets results when something goes wrong with the bone-building process in children. The amount of phosphorus in the blood is always found to be below normal in those afflicted by the rickets. Without any change of diet, the sunlight produces from day to day a steady increase in the amount of inorganic phosphorus in the blood. This effect is believed to be due to the penetration of the ultra-violet rays of the sun through the skin and by its production of some kind of chemical reaction in the blood-stream.

Deficiency of fresh vegetables is one of the chief faults in diet which cause rickets, but the disease may appear in children regardless of diet.

Two further reasons for considering lack of sunlight as a cause are the greater prevalence of the disease in large cities where smoke or the heights of buildings cut off sunlight and the fact that the disease occurs chiefly in Winter, when there is less sunlight.

The treatment of rickety infants involves exposure of their arms and legs and body to the sunlight for regular periods each day. The exposure is direct, because if the light passes through glass a large part of the ultra-violet rays may be absorbed. Cod liver oil or sunlight in sufficient quantities are a perfect cure for rickets, according to Dr. Hess. According to his estimate, $50,000 worth of cod liver oil would be sufficient to cure all of the cases of the disease in the City of New York.

The discovery that sunlight has a very active chemical effect on the blood has caused further interest, because of the possibility that the absence of that effect may produce other diseases than rickets and may be a contributing factor to various complaints.

The discovery of a vitamin in meats by the Department of Agriculture reported yesterday is also paralleled, it was learned, by work done at Columbia University. In investigating the statements of Vilhjalmur Stefansson, the explorer, who reported that his experiences in the Arctic proved that fresh meat of any kind whatsoever would prevent or cure scurvy. That fresh vegetables would cure scurvy was well known, but that fresh meat would have any such effect was disputed.

June 20, 1922

Exploiting Vitamins as Medicines. Something of responsibility rests on the medical profession for allowing, or at any rate for not preventing, the spread among the public of many false notions as to the potency of "vitamins," their nature and their sources. According to two Baltimore physicians, E. V. McCollum and Nina Simmonds, who contribute to The Journal of the American Medical Association the results of elaborate tests made by them, this ignorance is being ruthlessly exploited by certain manufacturers of proprietary drugs.

These have seen, it is said, a chance to revive the moribund patent medicine business by meeting an eager and ignorant demand for isolated and concentrated vitamins as a cure for various maladies. Their nostrums are declared by the writers of the article to have been proved quite incapable of realizing the wild claims set up in their behalf, and there is no reason for believing that anybody, sick or well, needs any more of any vitamin than can be obtained from a well-balanced diet of common foods.

That the usual diet of white flour bread, muscle meat, potatoes and sugar is not well balanced—that it accounts for much malnutrition, especially among children—is declared to be true, but the remedy is the drinking of milk, the eating of salads composed of raw vegetables, including the leafy kinds, and the use of flour more wisely milled, not the swallowing of tablets.

So at least say these Baltimore research workers, and they are in for some fine quarrels, for they do not hesitate to mention the names of manufacturers who are making a lot of money by selling the condemned tablets to a credulous public.

June 30, 1922

EXPECTS DIPHTHERIA SOON TO DISAPPEAR

Dr. Bela Schick Says Results of His Test Here Convince Him of Its Success.

165,000 PUPILS IMMUNIZED

Viennese Expert on Children's Diseases Ranks New York City First in Campaign.

New York City leads the world in the campaign which will eventually stamp out diphtheria, said Dr. Bela Schick, originator of the Schick test which is being used extensively in the public schools, after spending yesterday afternoon at Public School No. 4, Rivington and Pitt Streets, watching the administering of his test to the public under the direction of Dr. Abraham Zingher, Assistant Director of the Research Laboratories of the Department of Health. In Manhattan and the Bronx more than 165,000 pupils have been given the test, which determines a child's susceptibility to diphtheria. Those who have been immunised, even as far back as ten years, are still immune, according to Dr. Zingher. Dr. Schick said that the results obtained here, where his test was first given a fair trial, have convinced him that the disease must soon disappear entirely, when the public fully understands the facts and offers its co-operation.

The noted Viennese physician, an authority on pediatrics, has come to this country to deliver the Harvey Lecture before the New York Academy of Medicine on Jan. 27 and to study the work of the Rockefeller Institute and other institutions in the field of children's diseases. He is especially interested in the work of the Department of Health toward the prevention of diphtheria. This work has been advanced far beyond the point which he has been able to reach in Vienna, due to the unsettled conditions there.

The Schick test is used to determine where it is necessary to immunize by the injection toxin-antitoxin. Experiments have proved that the greatest susceptibility is among the children of the higher classes, while in the congested districts of the city the percentage of children already immune has been found as high as 87, due to the fact that their constant exposure to disease has resulted in an automatic manufacture in their systems of the antitoxin. In the public schools of the better districts it has been found that 80 per cent. of the pupils were susceptible.

The injection is painless and is given only with the parents' consent, but the great ignorance prevailing among the foreigners sometimes makes it difficult to obtain their permission. It is doubly difficult to reach children of pre-school age and it is these who are highly susceptible to the disease. Dr. Schick supported Dr. Zingher's statement that 85 per cent. of all cases, and of deaths were among such children.

January 20, 1923

PROGRESS OF MEDICINE IN A QUARTER CENTURY

Achievements of the Last Twenty-five Years Give Promise of Marvelous Advances in the Science of Healing in the Future Some Recent Gains Against Disease

THE benefits and wonders that the science of medicine will confer upon the world in the near future can be foretold only by the research students working quietly in clinics and laboratories—and they are not the sort of men and women who rush into print with prophesies. But the lay world, by reviewing the important discoveries and developments since 1900, may judge the directions that medicine is taking and the scope of its progress in the years just ahead.

Fatherless frogs, moving pictures of the heart beat, determination of the why and the wherefore of sex, the cultivation of human tissues outside of the body—these are a few of the achievements that mark the first quarter of the twentieth century as one of the most momentous periods the science has ever known.

Of all the experiments conducted in an effort to understand the origin of life the production of fatherless frogs may be called the most interesting, if not the most important. In 1916 Jacques Loeb produced frogs by the Basillon method. He took a glass rod thinner than a human hair. With the point of this rod he nicked the unfertilized eggs of a frog. The result was the hatching of nine tadpoles from eggs that had not been fertilized by the male.

The string galvanometer, invented by W. Einthoven in 1903, is an invention of particular merit and of high importance to the medical profession. A wire only one-third the thickness of a red corpuscle is arranged so that it will be affected by the slight electric current generated by the heart beat. This wire is strung between two magnetic poles, and the current from the heart causes it to execute a series of short jerks. These variations are photographed with a special type of moving picture camera.

The finished film has the appearance of a single jagged line. By measuring the distance between the peaks in this line and the deviations from the centre, physicians are able to tell accurately whether the heart is affected, and frequently what the affection is. This invention has led James McKenzie, Thomas Lewis, Aschoff, Lawrence, Keith and Flack to an entirely new understanding of the irregularities of the heart and the mechanism of the heart beat.

How Sex is Determined

Many pet theories received a death blow when C.E. McClung announced, in 1902, that the X-chromosome is the determinant of sex. This discovery proved conclusively that the mate is solely responsible for the sex of offspring, and that the female has no control over the sex of her child. The X-chromosome is a microscopic formation found only in the male. The female possesses chromosomes which determine the color of the hair of her child, the color of its eyes and other natural characteristics, but the X-chromosome is found only in the male.

Along the same line were the discoveries by T.H. Morgan, in the same year, of sex-limited and sex-linked inheritance. These discoveries showed how characteristics were handed down from one generation to another through the chromosomes, and explained how the offspring of black-haired and black-eyed people might have red hair and blue eyes, inherited from grandparents or great-grandparents. These natural characteristics are transmuted from generation to generation by what are known as accessory chromosomes, found both in the male and the female.

In 1912 and 1913 attention was given to the cultivation of human tissues and organs in glass vessels outside of the body. Ross G. Harrison and Jacques Loeb were exponents of this work and made it possible to study these tissues and organs to much better advantage by cultivating them as one might raise a flower.

How did the "world's tallest man" at the circus ever grow so tall and how did the fat lady manage to accumulate her avoirdupois? W.M. Bayliss and E. H. Starling cleared up these mysteries when, in 1902, they developed the doctrine of the hormones. Hormones are the secretions of the endocrine or ductless glands. Their fluids possess excitatory properties and are responsible for the proper development of different parts of the body, and when they fail to function they cause such things as excessive height or shortness or even bring about abnormal characteristics in the face.

A Life-Saving Drug.

In 1902 Jokichi Takamine succeeded in isolating in crystaline form, adrenalin, the active principle of a small gland situated immediately above the kidney in a calf. When adrenalin is injected into the blood it stimulates heart action; it has been used to such good advantage as almost to be called a life saver. It also checks hemorrhage by its powerful hemostatic action.

The respiration calorimeter, an invention by O.W. Atwater, was introduced in 1904. The calorimeter is a chamber in which a patient may be confined indefinitely. All of the oxygen entering this chamber is carefully measured, as are all the carbon dioxide and other waste materials leaving it. A complete water jacket surrounds the chamber, and the temperature of this water is noted from time to time.

It has been discovered that many diseases literally burn up the tissues of the body. A patient suffering from a disease of this type will give off more body heat than is supplied by the food the patient eats. The use of the respiration calorimeter enables physicians to get accurate information concerning diseases of this kind.

Of a somewhat similar nature is the pneumatic chamber invented by E.F. Bauerbruch in 1904, with negative pressure for use in ultrathoracic surgery. This chamber is simply an operating room where the air pressure may be maintained at such a low point as to keep the lungs of the patient partly collapsed. This invention greatly facilitates thoracic surgery.

New Light on Anti-Toxins.

The complement-fixation test, discovered by Jules Burdet, was an important contribution of 1901. When a disease gains a hold on the body, the system automaically generates an anti-toxin to combat the diseased toxin. This test showed that the complement, a small microscopic formation, brings the disease toxin and the anti-toxin together in such a manner that the anti-toxin, in many cases, destroys the disease toxin and saves the patient serious illness.

The value of sunlight in fighting tuberculosis was demonstrated by Rockeer in 1902. This discovery resulted when physicians noted that raw meat exposed to sunlight in high altitudes showed a strange absence of putrefaction. Different methods of combating the disease with sunlight have since been developed in many countries with good results.

In 1905 Fritz Schaudinn discovered the germ of syphilis. The discovery ranks as one of the most notable in the century, and led to further discoveries in 1907 by August von Wassermann.

An advance in medical knowledge was made in 1905 when A. Binet and T. Simon developed a series of tests to determine mental development and retardation. These tests, which were used extensively during the war and are now employed by Governments as well as by many large business institutions, consist of giving the subject a set of simple sums to do and questions to answer. The time taken to complete the test is considered equally with the accuracy of the results in determining the mental development of the patient.

This period saw the rise of psycho-analysis, fostered by S. Freud and C.G. Jung. Briefly, psycho-analysis is the theory that certain neuroses or psychological ailments are the result of suppressed desires, and that if these desires are dragged out into the light of consciousness and appeased, the condition will automatically correct itself.

Surgical Discoveries.

A technique for joining arteries end to end was evolved in 1902 by Alexis Carrel. Up to this time it had been customary, when a severed artery was to be joined, to lap the two ends over each other, sew them together in this position and than make a hole between them. The new technique made it possible to join the arteries directly and eliminated the bulky result, the irregular blood flow and several other objectional features of the old method.

Dr. Carrel's work also made possible the grafting of glands from animals into the human body. Every one is familiar with the recent experiments with monkey glands.

The stirring days of the World War did not fail to advance medical science, and many discoveries and developments occurred in this period. One of these was the introduction into general use of Dakin's hypochlorite solution in the treatment of burns. This solution was discovered before the war by Barthe de Sandfort while he was in China.

It is a paraffin resin solution which is sprayed on the burn after being heated. When it cools, the solution forms a waxlike covering over the burn. The covering protects the burn and greatly facilitates healing. It also relieves pain to a greater extent than old methods of treatment, and leaves fewer scars when the wound has healed. The practice of cutting away the blackened and diseased flesh in and around a wound was also developed during the war. This operation is known as debridoment.

The allergic skin test for the detection of tuberculosis infection was introduced in 1907 by Clemens von Pirquet. The test is commonly used on children, and consists of injecting under the skin of the patient a quantity of dead tuberculosis germs. If the patient has serious tubercular tendencies, the fact will be indicated at the place of injection.

In 1909 Paul Ehrlich gave to the world his discovery of salvarsan, or 606, as an agent to combat syphilis. Ehrlich made and discarded 605 formulas before he evolved salvarsan, or the 606th formula. It is not a cure, but is the best known method of arresting the progress of the disease.

About Vitamines.

Two important developments came close together in the years 1917 and 1918 when McCollum, Osborne and Mendel conducted experiments to determine the role of vitamines in the diet. These experiments resulted in the realization that a large number of abnormal conditions arise from improper diet, and that corrective dieting may restore health.

The establishment of the National Committee of Mental Hygiene was the other important development of this period. Dr. C.W. Beers and his associates have been responsible for many steps to wipe out unwholesome conditions in institutions for the care of the insane.

Insulin Perfected.

Early last year Dr. E.G. Banting announced his discovery of insulin as a means of fighting diabetes. This announcement was hailed with enthusiasm throughout the world. Treatment of diabetes by insulin is the injection of a fermented secretion of the pancreas in just the right quantities to make up for the deficiency of that secretion in the patient. Insulin is not a cure for diabetes; it is, however, a successful method of fighting the disease, and it has been found that a patient subjecting himself to proper and continued treatment may benefit greatly. The supply of insulin is limited at present, according to C. H. Best, co-worker with Dr. Banting in its discovery. There are already many more patients than can be treated, but rapid progress is being made in increasing the amount of the remedy.

In 1900 an incident occurred which, though sad, was of great importance to the medical profession. Carroll and Lazear, two army officers, died from inoculation with the virus of yellow fever. These two brave men paid with their lives in order that physicians might learn a new method of fighting a disease which once killed thousands of people a year. Their sacrifice proved that a mosquito is the yellow fever carrier and enabled mankind to combat the plague intelligently.

A discovery of 1901 was the germ of African sleeping sickness. The germ is not present in the blood of a man suffering from the new form of "sleeping sickness" which has made its appearance recently, and which is thought to be only a manifestation of influenza. After the discovery of the African germ, Bruce and Nabarro discovered, in the same year, that the tsetse fly is the carrier of the disease. This enabled physicians to carry on a successful campaign against the disease.

A fitting close to the activities of the year 1901 was the opening of the Rockefeller Institute of Medical Research at New York. This institution has since played a great part in medical development.

In 1903 Emil Fischer discovered the synthesis of veronal, a valuable artificial hypnotic. Novacain for use as a local anesthetic was a somewhat similar discovery made by Alfred Einhorn in 1905. The local anesthetic eliminated a number of the bad features of total anesthetics, and has proved of immense benefit in surgery and dentistry.

Studies in vestibular nystagmus by Robert Barany were the outstanding product of the year 1906. It was shown that small glands in the ear govern balance, and without them a patient would be unable to control even the simplest action.

Several developments mark the period between 1910 and 1912 as an important one in medical research. In 1910 Victor Henri, discovered that water can be sterilized by ultra violet rays. The importance of this discovery was seen during the war, when large quantities of water were sterilized by this method for consumption by troops situated where it was difficult to obtain pure water.

In 1910 also Simon Flexner succeeded in producing experimentally the germ of infantile paralysis. The discovery proved that the disease is communicable and greatly aided the fight against it. At the same period Edward B. Veder demonstrated that emetine, a chemical, will kill the amoebae of tropical dysentery.

Many Advances Made.

The year 1910 was marked by a rise in brain surgery, with many important results. A general clean-up also occurred in this year and the following one, and many overnight medical colleges were put out of business.

In 1911 the Nobel prize was awarded to A. Gullstrand for his research work in dioptrics. His work added much to the general knowledge of

the eye and allied subjects. Chemical studies in metabolism in the year 1912 greatly advanced the knowledge of physicians concerning the significance of the waste materials thrown off by the body. The outstanding discovery of 1912 was the cultivation in glass of the malarial parasite, by Charles C. Bass. The parasite had been discovered earlier by Leveran, and the cultivation under glass made a closer study possible.

In 1913 the Phipps Psychiatric Clinic at Johns Hopkins Hospital, Baltimore, was opened, with Dr. Adolph Meyer in charge. The institution has since played a leading role in medical research.

An elaboration of the methods of testing the functional powers of the kidneys was introduced in 1916. This discovery gave rise to the functional diagnosis. Patheline, a chemical is administered to the patient. Under normal conditions, the chemical should act within a few minutes. If it does not act normally, physicians are often able to diagnose the patient's trouble.

In 1917 von Economo reported the new disease known as "sleeping sickness," which has since become prevalent over the world. It is usually followed by a secondary attack within from six months to two years, during which time the patient may lose the use of his limbs and suffer a general disintegration of the nervous system.

A New Anesthetic.

A.B. Luckhart of the University of Chicago introduced ethylene in 1923. The power of ethylene as an anesthetic was discovered some years ago by accident. It was noticed that flowers, when exposed to illuminating gas, "went to sleep." Just what properties in the gas were responsible for this result remained for Dr. Luckhart to find out.

Ethylene, as a new anestetic, has received the endorsement of the leading physicians of the world. Its advantages are many. It has little or no nauseating effect, and the after effects are almost nil. After an operation in which ethylene

was used, patients have been known to eat a substantial meal within two hours. Under ethylene consciousness is regained easily and pleasantly. It is predicted that ethylene will entirely replace nitrous oxide as an anesthetic, and take the place of either in many cases.

Tularemia might be called the "last thing in diseases." It is practically a discovery of 1924. The disease is prevalent in the West, and the microscopic germ is carried by the blood-sucking fly, the stable fly, squirrel fleas and many other insects. It is seldom fatal, but is very contagious and always occasions a long illness. Dr. Edward Francis, who was active in discovering a cure, contracted the disease three times while studying it.

March 2, 1924

NEW X-RAY TUBE SPEEDS TREATMENT OF CANCER

While stressing a warning at the outset that only in certain cases can cancer be cured by X-rays, Dr. Francis C. Wood, director of the Crocker Institute of Cancer Research of Columbia University, announced yesterday an advance in the treatment of this disease. The advance, he said, had been made possible by a new type of X-ray tube.

The improved tube, Dr. Wood said, had no greater curative powers than the old one, its chief importance lying in its radiation of five or six times as many curative rays as the former type, thus lessening the necessary exposure of a patient to the rays from hours to minutes. As a result, Dr. Wood said, physicians will be able to treat a greater number of patients in a day. Thanks to the tube, the cost of treatment is reduced.

The tube is the invention of Dr. C. T. Ulrey, research engineer of the Westinghouse Lamp Company, who has been co-operating with Dr. Wood. They have hopes for an even better tube, now in the experimental stage, which will be able to stand a sufficiently high voltage to give off rays of much shorter wave length, thus approaching the rays of radium. If this tube is perfected, Dr. Wood believes the medical profession will have more success in treating internal cancer.

January 4, 1924

ANNOUNCES PELLAGRA CURE

Health Service Physician Says Scourge Yields to Brewers' Yeast.

WASHINGTON, March 30.—Pellagra, dread disease of rural communities, has been found to yield to dry brewers' yeast. Dr. Joseph Goldberger of the Public Health Service, in announcing the discovery today, said experiments would be conducted this Summer at the Georgia State Sanitarium to determine the element in this yeast which already has brought about cures.

The discovery followed eight years of study, in which Dr. W. F. Tanner, another Health Service physician, was associated with Dr. Goldberger. Dr. Tanner, however, has been assigned to other duties, and Dr. G. A. Wheeler will work with Dr. Goldberger in the continued experiments.

Pellagra, prevalent chiefly in the South, is disclosed in its milder forms by such symptoms as emaciation, lassitude and eruption of the skin, and, in severe cases, by insanity and death.

The brewers' yeast was found to cure black tongue in dogs, Dr. Goldberger said, and further experiments led to the discovery of its effectiveness against pellagra. Dry brewers' yeast, he pointed out, differed somewhat from bakers' yeast, and a much larger quantity of the latter was required to provide the element that cures pellagra.

March 31, 1925

VITAMIN "C."

When JACQUES CARTIER, the French explorer and discoverer, sailed out of St. Malo in 1535 for the northwest passage to Cathay he had three ships. But so many of his men died of scurvy and exposure during their Winter near the present site of Quebec that he had barely crew enough to take one of his ships, the Grande Hermine, back to France. He stated in his account of this adventurous journey that it was probable that not a man would have come back if a specific for scurvy had not been found. This was a decoction, he said, learned of the Indians and made from the bark or leaves of a tree so efficacious that if all the doctors

of Lorraine and Montpelier had been there with all the drugs of Alexandria they could not have done so much in a year as that tree did in six days, for it profited us so much that all those who would use it recovered health and soundness.

What this decoction was CARTIER does not tell us, but it was apparently the chemical forbear of Vitamin " C," which a biochemist in France has obtained in crystalline form from cabbages, as just announced from Washington by Science Service. It is not a startling discovery, for efficacious remedies for scurvy have long been known. It has been both prevented and cured by certain vegetables or fresh fruits, or certain chemicals, or the juice of lime or

lemon, or even vinegar. But the chief value of the isolation and concentration of this new remedy is that it is potent even in minutest amounts. No ship or voyager need be without it. The specific is, moreover, but another illustration of the progress that science is making in fighting disease in every sector of human exposure. Authorities have been at variance as to the cause of scurvy, but it may be due to the absence of what is now known to be its cure—a cure available in great quantities in the very fields around St. Malo, to which JACQUES CARTIER and his men might all have returned had the doctors of France in his day known of Vitamin " C."

June 22, 1925

CANCER TREATMENT BY RADIUM IMPROVES

Memorial Hospital Physicians Announce Gains by Using Gamma Rays.

BETA RAYS FILTERED OUT

More Than 100 Cases Treated With Satisfactory Results in Last Six Months.

PAIN LARGELY ELIMINATED

Heavier Dosage Under New System Will Reduce Recurrences of Disease, It Is Believed.

By The Associated Press.

Physicians of the Memorial Hospital, New York, announce that by filtering out 90 per cent. of the caustic beta rays emanating from radium and the high-voltage X-ray tube, and using principally the healing and stimulating gamma rays, radiation treatment of cancer of the tongue, lips, nose, ears or other part of the head has been improved greatly.

This achievement is regarded by some of the highest cancer authorities in other institutions as one of the most important advances made in the treatment of cancer since radium came into use for that purpose.

In the six months since the new method has been under experimentation more than one hundred cases have been treated with what are considered very satisfactory results. Owing to the elimination of the caustic rays, much stronger applications of the beneficial rays can be used, and painful effects are largely obviated.

Benefits of Heavier Dosage.

How permanent the benefits are cannot be determined without longer observation, but it was said at the hospital that there was reason to believe recurrences would be reduced because of the heavier dosage.

Experiments also are being carried on in the treatment of breast cancer and growths in other parts of the body. Of these, it was asserted, all that could be said was that the filtered gamma rays appeared to have a characteristic effect upon cancerous tissues regardless of their location. The difficulty in treatment in other regions than the head lay in the greater difficulty in reaching the diseased tissues.

The treatment now used at the Memorial Hospital has been developed gradually through the efforts of many physicians. The most important element in this experimentation was worked out fifteen years ago by Dr. Henry H. Janeway, then engaged in research at the Memorial Hospital, who established in a general way a method of implanting in cancerous growths minute glass tubes containing radium. This method was originally employed on skin lesions by Dr. William Duane. It never was entirely satisfactory, because the caustic beta rays penetrated the glass and had a tendency to injure healthy tissue while retarding the cancer.

Gold Tubes Instead of Glass.

The most recent refinement was the employment of gold tubes to replace the glass in which radon, or radium gas, was confined. Although the use of these tubes was reported recently at the London Conference and the Washington Convention of the American Roentgenological Society, the significance of their efficiency was not made clear.

The gold tubes are not inserted into the cancerous tissue until irradiation has been applied externally. The beta rays are electrons or negative charges of electricity traveling away from the radium at approximately 185,000 miles a second—the speed of light waves. The gamma waves are not electrons, but resemble the Hertzian waves of electricity, which carry impulses through the air from one radio station to another, except that the gamma rays have about 10,000 times the frequency of radio waves.

An important part of the external radiation is its application to the lymph nodes of the neck. The lymph system is a circulatory system, in some ways similar to the blood system. In the neck, however, the lymph fluid passes through glandular structures or nodes. These, in a measure, protect the rest of the body, as they check the passage of cancer cells thrown off by cancer in any part of the head. The process by which cancer spreads is called metastasis.

Treatment of Lymph Nodes.

Autopsies have shown that in many cases of cancer occurring in the mouth or other parts of the head the lymph nodes of the neck act as a barrier. In the new treatment these nodes are treated with radium and high voltage X-ray at the same time as the tissue in which the growth first appeared. After several treatments the infected lymph nodes may, if necessary, be removed by surgery. This is the only resort to surgery employed in the present treatment.

At the time of operation the small gold tubes are introduced and allowed to remain permanently in the tissues. The energy of the radon in them gradually diminishes until it ceases to be a factor.

The effect of this treatment upon neoplastic growths is to shrivel them and cause death to their exceedingly active cells. When this happens the tissue surrounding the malignant growth is stimulated to more vigorous activity and replaced with healthy tissue over the area occupied by the cancer.

October 23, 1925

LIVER DIET CALLED A CURE FOR ANEMIA

Doctors Convention Also Hears of Iodine as a Valuable Remedy for Diabetes.

INSULIN HELD TOO COSTLY

Dr. Theobald Smith of Princeton Gets Honor Medal From American Physicians.

Special to The New York Times.

ATLANTIC CITY, N. J., May 5.—Discovery of an effective treatment for pernicious anemia, that iodine is a valuable remedy for diabetes and that dropsical conditions may be entirely relieved by a new injection were announced here today at the closing sessions of the convention of the Association of American Physicians in the Traymore Hotel.

The George M. Kober Medal, awarded annually to the physician judged to have made the most important contribution to medical scientific knowledge during the year, was awarded to Dr. Theobald Smith of Princeton, member of the Rockefeller Institute and discoverers of the fact that diseases of many types are transmitted to human beings by insects.

The new anemia treatment consists of inclusion of liver in large amounts in the diet, according to Drs. George R. Minot, Reginald Fitz, W. P. Murphy and R. D. Monroe of Boston. Thirty-five patients, they said, who were suffering from the disease were put on a diet of liver for from eight months to two years. The red blood-cell count rose rapidly, the physicians said, and the patients recovered.

Would Isolate Tubercular.

Dr. Eugene L. Opie of the Rockefeller Institute, New York, said that the children of tubercular parents could avoid contracting tuberculosis if not exposed to contagion from the parents in the home. As a result, it was advocated that tubercular parents be separated from their children and maintained, if necessary, by the community.

That the human body, like a plant, can obtain and store up energy from the ultra-violet rays of the sun was asserted by Drs. Edward H. Mason and Howard H. Mason of Montreal. They described experiments performed with ten persons whose bodies were shown to have used the sun-ray heat instead of burning up bodily tissue.

Use of iodine permanently cures goitre, according to experiments described by Dr. Charles A. Elliott of Chicago, and Dr. Russell M. Wilder of the Mayo Institute, Rochester, Minn., reported that iodine also lessens and sometimes cures diabetes.

Dr. Wilder described cases in which goitre and a diabetic condition existed simultaneously in the same person. Use of iodine in most of these cases, he said, disposed of both ailments.

"It is highly significant," declared Dr. Wilder, "that treatment with iodine counteracts a diabetic condition."

It was said during the discussion that while insulin was the only positive agency for the cure of diabetes, it was too expensive for general use and became inefficient a short time after preparation.

Pancreas Produces Insulin.

The pancreas is the only organ in the human body which produces insulin, Dr. J. J. R. MacLeod of Toronto declared. It was in Dr. MacLeod's laboratory that Dr. J. Banting discovered insulin as a cure for diabetes. Experiments performed on dogs from which the pancreas glands were removed resulted in the animals developing diabetes. On an insulin diet, however, they thrived, but when this was stopped the animals died.

That an injection of a combination of three drugs—calcium chloride, ammonium chloride and novosaral—dispells all symptoms of dropsy, although not always effecting a permanent cure, was announced by Dr. Norman M. Keith of the Mayor Institute, Rochester, Minn. This discovery was regarded as important toward discovery of a possible cure for dropsy. The injection, Dr. Keith declared, caused all the dropsical evidence, such as pains and swelling, to disappear, but there was no certainty that the ailment would not recur.

That alcoholic cirrhosis of the liver is on the wane in this country was asserted by Dr. Jonathan Meakins of Montreal. The statement caused laughter among the physicians.

"The announcement is apparently a humorous one," said Dr. Meakins, "but it is based on fact. Alcoholic cirrhosis of the liver is becoming more rare in this country today."

Dr. C. F. Hoover of Cleveland was elected President of the association. Other officers chosen were Drs. A. S. Warthin and Arthur Mich, Vice Presidents; Dr. F. W. Peabody, Boston, Secretary; Dr. T. R. Boggs, Baltimore, Recorder; Dr. J. A. Capps, Chicago, Treasurer, and Drs. T. B. Futcher, Baltimore, and G. C. Robinson, Nashville, Councilors.

May 6, 1926

BACTERIA CHANGES AMAZE SCIENTISTS

Congress of Plant Experts in Ithaca Learns One Type Can Be Turned Into Another.

MAY BE CLUE TO EPIDEMICS

Special to The New York Times.

ITHACA, N. Y., Aug. 19.—Intricate and prolonged experiments, which it was believed had demonstrated that the same bacterium may undergo changes during its lifetime so great that the organism seems to be a different species, were described today before the bacteriology section of the International Congress of Plant Sciences now meeting at Cornell University.

Bacteria under miscroscopic observation, it was declared, had been seen to change from the coccus or round form to the radically different filament form characterizing another genus of the general family of bacteria.

Scientists who discussed this subject today threw out the suggestion that medical science might find a profitable field for investigation in the possibility that there were fewer specific germs than was generally believed and that part of the variety in the forms observed was due to variations in the individual germs. It was suggested also that in bacterial variation might be found a clue to some of the mysteries of epidemics. The same bacterium might be harmless in one phase of its development and virulent in another.

May Explain Influenza Epidemics.

The theory of variability in bacteria was developed in detail by Dr. Hilding Bergstrand of Stockholm and Dr. Ralph Mellon, medical bacteriologist of Highland Hospital, Rochester. Dr. Bergstrand applied it specifically to diseases and found in it a possible explanation of certain phenomena of the recent influenza epidemics. He made elaborate studies of the epidemics of 1920 and 1922 in Sweden. The latter epidemic, he said, had spread much more rapidly than the earlier one, but had caused far fewer deaths.

"Evidently we are here dealing with two variants of the virus," he said, "one very infectious but rather mild, and another less infectious but with greater capacity to produce severe forms of the disease."

"It may be mentioned that the study of bacterial variations certainly will change our conception of what are called species and types of bacteria," Dr. Bergstrand continued. "One single example will suffice to show this. For long the bacterium causing lobar pneumonia has been called pneumococcus, or streptococcus lanceolatus and regarded as a fixed species which could even be divided into equally fixed subspecies or varieties. The same has been the case with streptococcus viridans, causing a well-defined heart disease called endocarditis lenta."

Differences Are Not Reliable.

Investigators have found, however, that the differences between the two bacteria are not reliable, he said, and workers in his own laboratory had succeeded in forcing the pneumococcus to take on the characteristics of the typical viridans.

"This investigation seems to me to indicate that pneumococcus, lanceolatus and streptococcus viridans are only different manifestations of the same thing," said the Swedish scientist in conclusion.

Dr. Mellon went into even more detail on the variations and connected it with evidences of sexuality in bacteria. This provoked spirited discussion among other bacteriologists at the meeting today, for it has been almost universally supposed that bacteria propagate by simple cell division.

Dr. Bergstrand said that he had never been able to observe evidences of sexuality in bacteria, but said it was his personal belief that it existed and was similar to the sexuality of yeast plants.

Transformed From Bacilli Types.

"The bacilli or rod forms and the cocci or circular forms, when they have been bred true to type, have been traditionally regarded as distinct genera," said Dr. Mellon. "We seriously question whether they are the equivalent of the genera of the higher forms of plant or animal life. There is no longer any question that they can be under special conditions transformed one to the other and that the hereditary differences in the resulting forms may be relatively slight or quite divergent.

"It is a very well established principle that infectious diseases like tuberculosis, typhoid fever and diphtheria are caused by a single morphological type of micro-organism. Closely allied with this fact is Koch's principal of morphological specificity which states that these types invariably breed true, but as it relates to bacteria the principle is only relatively true. In this event, will it have any modifying influence on the fundamental proposition that an infectious disease is caused by a single type of micro-organism?

"It has been possible to develope ultramicroscopic phases in the life history of some common micro-organisms such as the typhoid bacillus, so that here again the life cycle relations of these organism introduce a situation of great importance from a standpoint of infection and perhaps immunity and ultimate control of the diseases as well.

"Recent observers of the French school indicate that the tubercle bacillus has a filterable phase in its life history which is capable of germinating in forms which make the organism quite unrecognizable at times."

Trees Are Moisture Reservoirs.

In the forestry section today the rôle of trees as reservoirs of moisture was described by Raphael Zon of the United States Forest Service. The old theory that rain was caused by the precipitation of vapor from the ocean carried over the land by air currents has now given way to the knowledge that the forests are the "oceans of the continent." Seven-ninths of the rainfall over the earth is derived from evaporation from land itself, said Mr. Zon.

The time of flowering and fruiting of many plants can be controlled by regulating the number of hours of light received daily, it was asserted by W. W. Garner of the Department of Agriculture.

H. K. Hayes of the University of Minnesota said that the cheapest way of combating the various diseases that afflict crop plants was the development of plant varieties capable of resisting specific diseases. He told of the progress made by Stakman and others in developing types of wheat resistant to rust.

August 20, 1926

100 EXPERTS OUTLINE KNOWN CANCER DATA

Conferees at Lake Mohonk Tell the World How to Combat the Malady.

EARLY TREATMENT URGED

Special to The New York Times.

LAKE MOHONK, N. Y., Sept. 24.—For the first time in the history of medicine, experts from Europe, Canada and the United States agreed here today on an authoritative statement of the present state of scientific knowledge concerning cancer.

The statement, which is designed to aid the medical profession and public generally, was made public by Dr. George A. Soper, managing director of the American Society for the Control of Cancer, at the close of a five-day international cancer symposium held here under the society's auspices.

More than one hundred specialists, leaders in their respective countries, joined in issuing the statement.

It was agreed that cancer is not contagious or infectious, that it is not hereditary and that its cure depends largely upon its early discovery. The only effective treatment known at present, it was declared, is by surgery, radium and X-ray.

The statement follows:

"Although the present state of knowledge of cancer is not sufficient to permit of the formulation of such procedures for the suppression of this malady as have been successfully employed for the control of infectious diseases, there is enough well-established fact and sound working opinion concerning the prevention, diagnosis and treatment of cancer to save many lives, if this information is carried properly into effect.

"Although the causation of cancer is not completely understood, it may be accepted that for all practical purposes cancer is not to be looked upon as contagious or infectious.

"Cancer itself is not hereditary, although a certain predisposition or susceptibility to cancer is apparently transmissible through inheritance. This does not signify that because one's parent or parents or other members of the family have suffered from cancer, cancer will necessarily appear in other persons of the same or succeeding generation.

Prompt Treatment Is Advised.

"The control of cancer, so far as this subject can be understood at the present time, depends upon the employment of measures of personal hygiene and certain preventive and curative measures, the success of which depends upon the intelligent cooperation of patient and physician.

"Persons who have cancer must apply to competent physicians at a sufficiently early stage in the disease in order to have a fair chance of cure. This applies to all forms of cancer. In some forms early treatment affords the only possibility of cure.

"Cancer in some parts of the body can be discovered in a very early stage, and if these cases are treated properly the prospect for a permanent cure is good.

"The cure of cancer depends upon discovering the growth before it has done irreparable injury to a vital part of the body and before it has spread to other parts. Therefore, efforts should be made to improve the methods of diagnosis in these various locations and the treatment of the cancers so discovered.

"The public must be taught the earliest danger signals of cancer which can be recognized by persons without a special knowledge of the subject and induced to seek competent medical attention when any of these indications are believed to be present.

"Practitioners of medicine must keep abreast of the latest advances in the knowledge of cancer and learn signs of cancer in order to diagnose as many as possible of the cases of cancer which come to them.

"Surgeons and radiologists must make constant progress in the refined methods of technic which are necessary for the diagnosis and proper treatment not only of ordinary cases but of the more obscure difficult ones.

"There is much that medical men can do in the prevention of cancer, in the detection of early cases, in the referring of patients to institutions and physicians who can make the proper diagnosis and apply proper treatment, when the physicians themselves are unable to accomplish these results. The more efficient the family doctor is the more ready he is to share responsibility with a specialist.

Dentists Can Aid in Control.

"Dentists can help in the control of cancer by informing themselves about advance in the known cases of cancer of the buccal cavity, especially with relation to the irritations produced by teeth but the condition of the bone dental plates. They can also help by referring cases of cancer which they discover to physicians skilled in the treatment of cancer in this location. It may be doubted whether some dentists fully realize the help which can be obtained from X-ray photographs which reveal not only the state of the teeth but the conditions of the bone surrounding them.

"Medical students should be taught about cancer by the aid of actual demonstration of cancer patients, and this to a sufficient extent to give them a good working knowledge of the subject.

"The most reliable forms of treatment and, in fact, the only ones thus far justified by experience and observation depend upon surgery, radium and X-rays.

"Emphasis should be placed upon the value of the dissemination of the definite, useful and practical knowledge about cancer, and this knowledge should not be confused nor hidden by what is merely theoretical and experimental.

"Efforts toward the control of cancer should be made in two principal directions, the promotion of research in order to increase the existing knowledge of the subject and the practical employment of the information which is at hand.

September 25, 1926

CANCER HELD A GROUP OF SEVERAL DISEASES

Wireless to THE NEW YORK TIMES.

LONDON, Nov. 19.—The official report of the International Conference on Cancer held in London in July was published today. It is the last word on cancer spoken by those who are foremost in the world in combating it and it contains a number of interesting facts about the scourge that now ranks third in the list of fatal diseases.

The chief developments in knowledge of cancer were summed up at the conference by Professor James Ewing, who insisted that cancer was to be regarded more as a group of diseases than as a single disease.

His address was followed by communications from leading authorities on cancer in Europe and America, all of whom appear to agree that cancer is not caused by some single invariable causal agent, but that different causes operate in different cases.

Attempts are being made with some success to ascertain precisely what principal factors are implicated in the "growth substance" which is presumed to exist in cancerous cells and so far to have escaped analysis. Two investigators, by means of experiments with cancerous tumors in fowls, succeeded in disproving the notion that this is a virus or living agent and in showing that it is something like a ferment. Further research will decide whether this discovery will lead to the solution of the nature of the "growth substance" of cancer cells in man and other mammals.

The discussion of the relative values of surgery and radium treatment indicated that surgical operations will not be superseded and that radium has come to stay. Certain cancers, such as those of the tongue and mouth, are being treated for preference by radium, while others are treated by radium and surgery combined. An increased supply of radium to the cancer workers would be a welcome boon to humanity, the report says.

The conference gave little support to the lead treatment of cancer for which a number of Liverpool research workers had claimed considerable success. Several blood tests for cancer were set forth, but of these the most reliable was accurate only in 75 per cent. of the cases.

November 20, 1928

SPEED DETECTION OF TUBERCULOSIS

Special to The New York Times.

ATLANTIC CITY, N. J., May 28.—Two new advances in the war against tuberculosis were marked here today at the twenty-fifth annual meeting of the National Tuberculosis Association at the Chelsea. Both were hailed as of great scientific and social consequence.

Dr. Esmond R. Long and Dr. Florence B. Seibert of the University of Chicago announced the results of research in the last year by which they have been able to produce tuberculin, a substance used in detecting the presence of the disease, in an absolutely pure state.

The second disclosure, in reports submitted by Drs. Florence R. Sabin, C. A. Doan and C. E. Forkner of the Rockefeller Institute, is termed a new mechanism for testing the presence of tuberculosis which reveals the disease within three or four days of infection instead of after two months, as has been formerly the case.

Make Tests More Certain.

Hitherto the presence of impurities in tuberculin rendered the test by it uncertain. In the examination of children, particularly, it was pointed out various impurities might cause a positive reaction, not the tuberculosis germ itself. The new tuberculin will have a good effect on the testing of cattle for the disease, it was said, as many cases had been found in which the animals reacted positively to the test and yet showed no sign of tuberculosis after being slaughtered.

Drs. Long and Seibert declared they planned to continue their research to learn to what extent chicken and cattle tuberculosis might be the cause of the disease in humans.

An application of the method by which tuberculin is freed from any impurities will be of great benefit in the diagnosis of other bacterial diseases, it was declared, the same methods being available to render other testing substances more accurate and dependable. Dr. Kendall Emerson, managing director of the National Tuberculosis Association, praised the work of both groups of scientists, styling the results of the two researches "definite and significant."

Warns of Disease.

Dr. Eugene Opie, president of the association, opened the meeting today with the warning that tuberculosis may still be regarded as the greatest scourge of the human race. He added that control of the disease is in no way assured despite the declining death rate from that source.

"The fact is," he said, "that 100,-000 persons die from tuberculosis in this country every year, and approximately a million suffer from the disease." He termed it one of the greatest dangers of early adult life.

"The mortality from tuberculosis increases rapidly during adolescence," he said, "and in each decade during the last fifty years has been much greater in young girls than in boys. We must have accurate information concerning this problem and the conditions that influence susceptibility at different ages."

Dr. Opie urged an "intelligent program" on behalf of the negro race, to learn whether the negro is particularly susceptible or suffers from the disease as a result of economic conditions.

After his opening speech, the Trudeau Award Board presented its medal to him. The Trudeau medal is given each year for the most outstanding work to combat tuberculosis. The board surveys the work of physicians throughout the world in making its choice. Last year the medal went to Sir Robert Phillips of Edinburgh University.

Dr. Opie's selection was attributed to his "outstanding work during the past twenty-five years, while serving in George Washington University, the Rockefeller Institute, the United States Army and the Henry Phipps Institute, Philadelphia, where he now is. The citation made special mention of his study of tuberculosis as it affects children.

May 29, 1929

NATION'S DEATH RATE HALVED SINCE 1900; DIPHTHERIA CUT 95%

The death rate of the nation has been cut in half since 1900 and in the case of some diseases, notably diphtheria, it has been reduced 95 per cent, it was announced yesterday in the revised report of the joint committee on health problems of the American Medical Association and the National Educational Association.

The report is the first revision of the joint committee's statistics since 1924 and is a summing up of the winning battle which medical science and education are waging against disease. The committee completed its task only last month, after more than a year's extended effort by the eighty authorities in health and education who compose it.

The report will form a new basis for health education in the United States, according to the committee's chairman, Dr. Thomas D. Wood of Teachers College, Columbia.

Fight on Diphtheria Hailed.

The reduction in the death rate of diphtheria is hailed as one of the most striking victories recorded in the report of medical progress in the past fifty years. The factors chiefly responsible for the reduction of 95 per cent in the mortality rate from this disease, according to the report, are the discovery of diphtheria antitoxin and of toxin-antitoxin, used to immunize children.

The decrease in the death rate for diphtheria is matched by that for typhoid and paratyphoid fever, the report reveals.

Despite the tremendous reduction in many diseases, however, the report reveals that the country still pays an appalling toll to sickness in money.

American taxpayers, the report estimates, pay more than $927,000,-000 a year to care for sufferers from tuberculosis and heart disease and to assist those who are physically handicapped. Of this amount $800,000,000 goes to the tubercular, $90,000,000 to cardiac victims and $37,000,000 to the physically handicapped. Deaths from tuberculosis, it is estimated, cost the people of the United States more than $1,500,000,-000 a year.

Since 1900, the report declares, the filtration and chemical treatment of water, the pasteurization of milk, and the control of carriers have cut the death rate for typhoid and paratyphoid from 34 persons per 100,000 to 4.9 per 100,000 in 1928.

The reduction was even more striking in military life, where formerly typhoid took a heavy toll. This the report illustrates by United States Army statistics. During the first two years of the Civil War typhoid caused 1,961 deaths among every 100,000 soldiers, whereas during the first two years of the World War only five soldiers in every 100,000 died of this type of disease.

The committee's report indicates that more than 31,000 soldiers' lives were saved because medical men were more successful in applying their knowledge for the prevention of typhoid during the first two years of our entry in the World War than in the same period of the Civil War.

The almost complete elimination of cholera, typhus and yellow fever, all of which took thousands of lives throughout this country during the last century, is also reported. This success is attributed to the careful studies of the causes and the application of proper preventive measures.

General Death Rate Cut.

A great reduction in the general death rate of the nation is one of the outstanding features of the report. Prior to 1900 the general death rate of the nation ranged between 20 and 30 per 1,000 of population. In 1928 the rate was 12 per thousand. As a result of these and other factors, the report indicates that twenty years have been added to the average expectancy of life in this country in the last seventy-five years. Thus, it declares, a child born in Massachusetts in 1925 was expected to live until it reached the age of 50, whereas such a child born in 1850 was expected to die at 30.

A great reduction in infant mortality was also effected in the last thirty years, the report shows. In 1900 more than sixteen babies of every 100 born died before reaching their first birthday. At present seven of each 100 born die during the first year. A better understanding of baby care has contributed to this, it is asserted.

The fight waged against tuberculosis has similarly been successful, according to the figures in the report. The death rate from consumption has decreased from 194 per 100,-000 in 1900 to 79 per 100,000 in 1928. The causes of the decrease, the report says, include improved economic conditions, particularly among the industrial population, educational campaigns by tuberculosis associations and health departments, and the increased facilities for early diagnosis and hospitalization and care of the sick.

The decrease in tuberculosis mortality has been more pronounced among certain ages than others. Thus the least improvement has occurred among young people, chiefly girls and women between the ages of 15 and 24, according to the report. No explanation is offered for this.

Child's Life Has Greater Value.

Owing to the increased expectancy of life in this country and the decrease in the prevalence of these diseases, the monetary value of newly born children's lives have greatly increased, so that a boy born in 1924 was potentially worth $1,780 more than such a child born in 1901, the report estimates. At that time he would have been worth $7,553, using his life expectancy and earning capacity as a basis for consideration. Thus the report estimates that the results of health education have saved this country more than $3,500,000,000 during the last quarter of a century.

Exclusive of ordinary illness in this country, it is estimated that there are 75,000 blind, 45,000 deaf and dumb, and well over 300,000 mental defectives in the United States at present. More than 700,000 persons in the United States are also crippled to an extent that interferes with their earning a living.

The expense of maintaining these individuals amounts to more than $100,000,000, the report says.

Dr. Wood declared that the 1924 report of the joint committee's work had been entirely revised. A number of new chapters have been added. The chapter on "The Trend of Health," prepared by the subcommittee of biological and public health experts, of which Dr. George T. Palmer, director of research of the American Child Health Association and a member of Hoover's child health committee, is one of the most important additions to the new report, Dr. Wood said.

Other revisions include a more detailed discussion of the immunization against preventable diseases, an elaboration of mouth hygiene, accident prevention, mental hygiene and the applications of psychology to health education.

Another new chapter is the one on "Measurements in Health Education."

Authorities Who Aided.

Among the authorities who aided in the preparation of the work are the following:

Committee of the National Educational Association:

Dr. A. K. ALDINGER, director of health education for the New York City Board of Education.
Dr. EDNA W. BAILEY, University of California.
Dr. WILLIAM BURDICK, Maryland state supervisor of physical education.
Dr. FRANK R. ROGERS, director of health and physical education, New York State Department of Education.

Dr. JOHN M. DODSON, Chicago, chairman committee of the American Medical Association.
Dr. ISAAC ABT, Chicago.
Dr. A. J. CHESLEY, St. Paul.
Dr. R. W. CORWIN, Pueblo, Col.
Dr. EDWARD JACKSON, Denver.

The technical advisory committee which was appointed to aid in the revision was composed of seven subcommittees. The chairmen of these subcommittees were:

Dr. FREDERICK G. BONSER, Columbia, subcommittee of educators.
Dr. L. W. CHILDS, Cleveland, subcommittee of physicians.
Dr. PERCIVAL M. SYMMONDS, subcommittee of educational psychologists.
Dr. PERCY R. HOWE, Boston, subcommittee of dentists.
Dr. MARY S ROSE, Columbia University, subcommittee of nutrition experts.
Miss ETHEL PERRIN, New York, subcommittee of physical educators.
Dr. GEORGE T. PALMER, subcommittee of biological and public health experts.

In addition there was a technical committee of twenty-seven appointed to aid the others in their tasks.

July 6, 1930

Nurse Lives On as Respirator Supplies Air; Chicago Doctors Encouraged by Her Appetite

CHICAGO, Sept. 20 (AP).—Life hovers on tonight within the walls of an aluminum box, and more than hovers, for the doctors say energy is ebbing back into the veins of Frances McCann, the student-nurse whose chest is paralyzed so she cannot breathe alone.

A motor hums regularly. Air swishes in, swishes out. Mrs. Henry L. McGann of Altona, Ill., her mother, sits in a corner of the dimly-lit room.

This is the scene at St. Luke's Hospital. For eight days and eight nights Miss McGann, Knox College graduate, has been encased in the respirator and her body muscles do not function.

Air forced into the case presses gently on her chest. She exhales. The air is withdrawn, a vacuum is created, and she inhales. Last night they turned the machine off for ten minutes. She breathed that long by herself. She moved her hands just a little bit and her feet just a little bit.

"It is not only the machine," said Dr. John Fabill, attending physician. "It's Frances—she wants to live." Her neck is surrounded by an airtight rubber band.

Dr. Fabill thinks she may need the respirator for weeks more. Meanwhile, hope is pinned upon a serum. She had toast, orange juice and coffee for breakfast this morning. That she had the appetite for it is considered a sign for the better.

A little over a week ago Miss McGann was herself attending the ill at St. Luke's Hospital. She suddenly collapsed, the victim of a rare form of infantile paralysis.

The machine, known as the Drinker respirator, is the first of its kind in Chicago. It was donated to the hospital by Samuel Insull Jr. Similar machines have been used recently in Philadelphia and San Francisco.

September 21, 1930

Dying Man Reported Cured in 48 Hours At Mayo Clinic by a New Gland Treatment

COLD SPRING HARBOR, N. Y., Dec. 5 (AP).—Restoration of a man from death's door to apparently perfect health in forty-eight hours was revealed today at the biological laboratory.

The man saved, a patient at the Mayo Clinic at Rochester, Minn., had Addison's disease. At the clinic a purified hormone was injected directly into the veins of the man, who is 39 years old, by Dr. Leonard G. Rowntree and Dr. Carl H. Greene.

"Before its use," they reported, "the patient was excessively weak, bedridden, depressed, nauseated, losing weight and showed evidence of failing circulation. Within forty-eight hours he had taken a new lease of life, his appetite was excellent, his strength was greatly improved and he appeared to be in perfect health."

Addison's disease, due to failure of man's adrenal glands, has been recorded in the past in medical literature as invariably fatal.

The hormone used was an extract of the cortex of the adrenal glands of cattle, obtained in the past few weeks in unusually pure form by Dr. W. W. Swingle and Dr. J. J. Pfiffner of the biological laboratory and of Princeton University.

These scientists first announced the extract in March this year, but it was not then entirely pure, containing some epinephrine, a powerful heart stimulant which is secreted by the same glands.

Presence of this stimulant made it dangerous to inject the new remedy directly into the veins of human beings. It had to be administered by a slower method, subcutaneous injection, which caused considerable irritation.

Drs. Swingle and Pfiffner announced that recently they had found a method of getting the extract so pure that it contains only one part in one or two million of epinephrine.

December 6, 1930

THE ANTIBIOTIC ERA

NEW DRUG SAID TO AID IN PUERPERAL FEVER

Special Cable to THE NEW YORK TIMES.

LONDON, June 5.—Experiments here with the new drug commonly called prontosil, a German aniline compound, in cases of childbed fever have given exceptional results.

Papers by Dr. Leonard Colebrook of the Medical Research Council and by Dr. Meave Kenny of Queen Charlotte's (lying-in) Hospital show that thirty-eight puerperal fever cases infected by haemolytic streptococci have been treated by oral plus intravenous or intramuscular doses of prontosil.

Subject to confirmation by further experience, the impression has been gained that in many of the more severe cases the drug exerted a definitely beneficial effect, manifested by an unexpectedly prompt fall in temperature and remission of symptoms. This impression is supported by a substantial reduction in the case mortality of the whole series.

The medical journal, The Lancet, says:

"It is the first time any drug has been shown to have a specific and regular effect on acute bacterial infection when administered by mouth. All observers are agreed that the effect is limited to infections due to streptococcus pyogenes, although there are slight indications that meningococcus may also prove susceptible.

"The conclusions drawn by Drs. Colebrook and Kenny on the basis of their clinical experience are commendably cautious. It is very much to be hoped that the therapeutic trial they have initiated here will be extended and made to embrace other types of acute streptococcal infection other than puerperal fever."

June 6, 1936

THREE NEW DRUGS COMBAT INFECTION

Sulphur Compounds Found 5 to 30 Times as Effective as Sulfanilamide

TESTED ONLY WITH MICE

U. S. Public Health Service Warns They Are Not Ready Yet for Human Use

The preparation of three new sulphur compounds, which tests on mice have shown to be from five to thirty times as good as sufanilamide for combating bacterial infection, is announced in the current issue of Public Health Reports, published weekly by the United States Public Health Service. The compounds are known to chemists as "sulfones."

The three new chemical weapons against bacteria are described by Dr. Hugo Bauer, research associate, and Dr. Sanford M. Rosenthal, senior pharmacologist of the division of pharmacology, National Institute of Health, Washington.

One of these new chemicals, prepared by Drs. Bauer and Rosenthal, is described technically as a formaldehyde sulfoxylate derivative of the chemical known as di-amino diphenyl-sulfone. On subcutaneous injection, the report states, this new sulphur compound "has a therapeutic index approximately five times as good as sulfanilamide given orally."

"This compound is of interest," the report adds, "in that it is the first water-soluble preparation that we have obtained with high therapeutic activity."

High Therapeutic Index

An acetyl derivative of di-amino diphenyl-sulfone, the report states, "possesses a therapeutic index more than six times as high as sulfanilamide against streptococcal infections in mice." This drug was first introduced by Drs. E. Fourneau, J. Trefouel, F. Nitti and D. Bovet, of France.

The therapeutic action of di-amino diphenyl-sulfone was first studied by Drs. G. A. Buttle, W. H. Gray and D. Stephenson of England in 1937. This drug, the Public Health workers say, "was found [by them] to be approximately thirty times as active against streptococci as sulfanilamide, but its high toxicity makes its therapeutic index only two times as favorable."

Drs. Bauer and Rosenthal also reported having prepared and tested several other new derivatives of sulfanilamide, and of its more recently developed relative known as di-sulfanilamide, as to their action against streptococci and pneumococci.

"Only one compound in this group," the report states, "proved to be slightly superior to sulfanilamide, the sulfanil p-amino anilide.

"It has been confirmed that much more favorable results are obtained with di-sulfanilamide when it is injected in oil than when given orally. By mouth di-sulfanilamide has a therapeutic index only twice as good as sulfanilamide.

"Against pneumococcal infections in mice these three sulfones are all superior to sulfanilamide. However, in mice the action is still considerably less marked than against streptococci; and, while marked prolongation of life can be achieved, few animals permanently survive pneumococcal infections as a result of therapy."

"At their present degree of effectiveness it would seem preferable to consider the use of these sulfones chiefly in conjunction with serum therapy, where a synergism [one drug bolstering up the other] has been shown to exist."

Not Ready for Human Use

The paper cautions that many more comparative studies on other animals must be made before the new drugs could be used on human beings.

"Effects on human beings," the report emphasizes, "are not always predictable from animal experiments and the clinical use of a new drug should be preceded not only by a thorough pharmacological and toxicological study of the drug upon several species of animals, but also by a careful study of its effects on human beings under conditions where they can be closely observed for a considerable period of time.

"It must also be pointed out that the animal toxicity of sulfanilamide and related compounds has not revealed certain manifestations, such as fever, dermatitis, cyanosis and hematological changes, which have been encountered in human beings."

The sulfones were originally described by Drs. E. Fromm and J. Wittmann, German chemists, in 1908, but their therapeutic action had not been previously explored.

January 22, 1938

PNEUMONIA YIELDS TO NEW CHEMICAL

Rockefeller Scientist Tells of Discovery of Powerful Germ Destroyer

TESTS ON ANIMALS ONLY

Drug Extracted From a Soil Bacillus Opens a New Field of Research

A new chemical extracted from an unidentified soil bacillus has proved itself in animal experiments to be the most powerful destroyer yet discovered of all types of pneumonia germs and blood poisoning streptococci, much more potent than sulfanilamide and sulfapyridine, it was reported yesterday before the closing sessions of the third International Congress for Microbiology, at the Waldorf-Astoria, by Dr. René J. Dubos of the Rockefeller Institute for Medical Research.

The new chemical, now in the process of being analyzed as a step toward preparing it synthetically, also has proved itself equally destructive in the test tube against a host of other deadly germs of the group known as Gram-positive bacteria because of their ability to retain a certain blue dye. So far the chemical has been found effective against every Gram-positive bacteria it has been tried on, though it has not yet been tried on all.

Among the Gram-positive bacteria, against which the chemical has proved itself highly potent, is the important staphylococci group. Others belonging to the Gram-positive group, on which the chemical will be loosed, are the bacilli of tetanus (lockjaw), anthrax, and, most important of all, tuberculosis.

Not Yet Tried on Man

So far, it was emphasized, the chemical has been tried only on animals and on germs in the test tube. It has not yet been tried on man.

The discovery that a specific bacillus of the soil, so new that it is still nameless, can manufacture the most powerful chemical germ-destroyer so far to be discovered by man (that is, a destroyer that protects an animal against deadly doses of bacteria without any pronounced toxic effects on the animal), opens up a vast new field in the search for chemical agents for fighting bacterial enemies, it was pointed out. Since there are thousands of types of soil bacteria, it is confidently expected that other types of bacteria manufacture powerful germ-destroying chemicals.

The Rockefeller scientists, it was learned, are busy on two lines of research in this new field of chemotherapy. First, they are seeking to analyze the chemical's composition and structure, in the hope of its synthesis. Secondly, they are in search of a soil bacillus that would provide a similar chemical of use in fighting the important group of microbes known as Gram-negative bacteria, which are unable to retain a blue staining dye, developed by Professor Christian Gram.

Among the Gram-negative bacteria causing serious human diseases are those of typhoid, dysentery, gonorrhea, influenza bacillus and the bacillus of whooping cough.

Another line of research is to determine whether the new soil-bacillus chemical is toxic to other animals, the necessary step-by-step procedure in determining whether the substance is safe for human use. However, it was pointed out, even should this particular chemical prove unsuitable for human application, its chemical structure will furnish a highly important clue to a new vastly important group of chemotherapeutic agents, different from sulfanilamide and sulfapyridine, and promising to be even more powerful than these two miracle drugs of modern medicine.

Tiny Dose Effective

So powerful is the new chemical that one-millionth of a gram protected mice against 10,000 fatal doses of pneumonia bacteria, including the virulent types of I, II, III, V and VIII. Similarly, the mice were protected against fatal doses of hemolytic streptococci.

Dr. Dubos, a young scientist born in a Paris suburb and naturalized here last year, showed members of the congress visiting the institute yesterday a bottle containing 500 grams (about seven-tenths of a pound) of the new chemical, enough to protect five trillion mice against pneumonia and blood-poisoning streptococci. The substance, a whitish gray powder, is separated from the soil bacillus by whirling it in a centrifuge.

Dr. Dubos has grown the specific soil bacillus in pure culture and he now has 5,000 quarts of the culture medium producing the new chemical. This assures an unlimited supply of the new chemical should its use prove as effective in man as it did in animals and in the test tube.

Prairie dogs, chipmunks and thirty-seven other species of rodents scattered over ten Western States have been discovered to harbor the germ of sylvatic plague, another name for bubonic plague, the grim "black death" that decimated half of the world's population in the Middle Ages.

This discovery and the measures being taken to prevent the spread of this plague among humans were reported before the congress by Professor Karl F. Meyer, director of the Hooper Foundation of the University of California, one of the world's leading bacteriologists. A new "flea laboratory" has just been built at the Hooper Foundation, Professor Meyer reported, to study the disease and to prepare a serum against it. The disease is spread by fleas that bite the rodent and then bite man. Recently nine cases were reported in the United States among hunters and trappers.

Foreign members of the congress discussed with their American colleagues yesterday the adoption of measures that would prevent the outbreak of an influenza epidemic during the present European war.

September 9, 1939

'GIANT' GERMICIDE YIELDED BY MOLD

New Non-Toxic Drug Said to Be the Most Powerful Germ Killer Ever Discovered

TRIED ON HUMAN BEINGS

By WILLIAM L. LAURENCE
Special to THE NEW YORK TIMES.

ATLANTIC CITY, N. J., May 5— A new chemical substance elaborated by a special strain of mold in bread and Roquefort cheese that has proved itself in tests on animals and in preliminary clinical trials on human beings as the most powerful non-toxic germ-killer so far discovered, thousands of times more potent than any of the drugs of the sulfanilamide family, was described here today.

Hundreds of leading physicians from the United States and Canada, attending the annual meeting of the American Society for Clinical Investigation, heard Dr. Martin H. Dawson, Associate Professor of Medicine at the College of Physicians and Surgeons, Columbia University, New York City, report on the new germ-killer.

Associated with Professor Dawson in this work, which physicians here hailed as opening a new chapter in the fight of medical science against bacterial infections caused by the vast host of deadly microorganisms known as gram-positive bacteria, were Drs. Gladys L. Hobby, Karl Meyer and Eleanor Chaffee.

Not Available in Pure Form

The new substance, not yet available in pure form, is known as penicillin, after the family of molds known as penicillium. Only one specific strain of it can elaborate the new giant among germ-destroyers, and its final isolation, Professor Dawson said, would depend on a larger supply of the starting material than is now available. However, even in its present crude form, Dr. Dawson reported, minute doses have proved remarkably effective in protecting animals against enormous doses of deadly bacteria of various types.

Recent experiments have shown, Professor Dawson reported, that penicillin is "extremely active" in a dilution of one to 500,000. Mice infected intraperitoneally (through injection of bacteria directly into the peritoneum) with a highly virulent strain of hemolytic (blood destroying) streptococci in amounts up to two cubic centimeters of whole culture, containing from 50,000,000 to 100,000,000 organisms, were protected with a dose of about seven milligrams of a "soluble, impure preparation," given subcutaneously. Control animal receiving the same bacteria in dilutions of one part in 10,000,000, Dr. Dawson reported, died within forty-eight hours.

"In further experiments," Dr. Dawson reported, "it has been shown that penicillin is effective intravenously and intraperitoneally as well as subcutaneously. Animals have also been treated successfully as long as eight hours after infection. Experiments on oral administration are as yet incomplete."

Penicillin, Professor Dawson reported, has been administered to four patients suffering from that deadly form of bacterial heart disease known as sub-acute bacterial endocarditis. "Sufficient material was not available for adequate therapy in these cases," he said. "However," he added, "no serious toxic effects were observed."

"It would appear," Professor Dawson concluded, "that penicillin is a chemotherapeutic agent of great potential significance. Penicillin probably represents a new class of chemotherapeutic agents which may prove as useful, or even more useful, than the sulfonamides."

It was originally observed by Fleming in 1929, Dr. Dawson told the physicians, that staphylococci failed to grow on plates in the neighborhood of a colony of penicillium mold.

New Light on Gramicidin

Last year Dr. René J. Dubos startled the scientific world with the announcement that he had extracted from a special strain of soil bacteria a chemical substance he named gramicidin that had proved the most powerful microbe-killer until then known to man. Unfortunately, gramicidin was found to be highly toxic to animals as well as to bacteria.

At the meeting today there were presented two reports, from the Mayo Clinic, Rochester, Minn., and from the Massachusetts Memorial Hospital, Boston, respectively, announcing studies on the gramicidin that have made it possible to apply it successfully in a number of human infections that had not responded to any other treatment.

Dr. Wallace E. Herrell and Dr. Dorothy Heilman of the Mayo Clinic, set out to determine, by methods of tissue culture the manner in which gramicidin produced its toxic effects on animals. They found that along with its powerful bactericidal action it also possessed the power to break down red blood cells by the process called hemolysis. This at once indicated that the chemical might be used safely in local infections where it was not necessary to introduce it into the blood stream.

Tests on animals proved that this was the case, and that the gramicidin could be used safely in local applications, as it did no harm at all to tissues. It has been used effectively, the Mayo and Boston physicians reported, in the treatment of sinus infections, infections of the bladder, infected but not bleeding wounds, ulcers and empyema from pneumonia.

The Boston report was presented by Drs. Charles H. Rammelkamp and Chester S. Keefer.

Sinus infections were cleared up within forty-eight hours, Drs. Herrell and Heilman reported. Severe bladder infections that the sulfa drugs did not affect were cured within one week.

Infected wounds were freed of all bacteria within twenty-four hours after gramicidin treatment, following which the wounds rapidly healed, Drs. Rammelkamp and Keefer reported.

May 6, 1941

Sulfanilamide Is Put In Kits for the Army

By The Associated Press.

SPRINGFIELD, Mass., July 15 —Sulfanilamide, used in combatting infection, is being put in United States Army kits in a package designed for self-administration with one hand, George A. Mohlman, vice president of the Package Machinery Company, announced today.

Mr. Mohlman said the package was intended to provide means of self-medication for a soldier if he was wounded and separated from his unit.

A simple tape opens the dirt-and-weather protected package.

As the box cover is moved back a single tablet drops forward and can be placed in the mouth without spilling the remainder of the contents.

Wide use of sulfanilamide during the war has been reported by British physicians.

July 16, 1941

SYPHILIS TESTS RECORDED

CHICAGO, Oct. 15 (AP)—Blood tests of the first million selectees and volunteers in the Army showed syphilis infection at the rate of 45.2 per thousand, Dr. R. A. Vonderlehr, assistant surgeon general of the United States Public Health Service, and Lida J. Usilton, statistician, stated today in an article published in The Journal of the American Medical Association.

The report said that out of 1,051,985 men tested, 47,552 had the disease.

"The greatest prevalence of syphilis among the selectees and volunteers was reported by Florida and South Carolina, with rates of 170.1 and 156 cases per thousand, respectively. The lowest rate, 5.8 per thousand, was reported by New Hampshire. Seven Southern States and the District of Columbia reported rates in excess of 100 cases per thousand."

October 16, 1941

Chemicals Excelling Sulfa Drugs As Germ Killers Are Disclosed

By WILLIAM L. LAURENCE

Special to The New York Times.

PITTSBURGH, Sept. 9—A new group of anti-bacterial chemicals approaching in potency the germ-killing powers of that new wonder-drug, penicillin, and providing the first clues to penicillin's chemical identity, believed to hold the key to a new promised land in medicine, was described here today at the meeting of the American Chemical Society.

The isolation from the green cheese mold penicillin notatum, from which penicillin is extracted, of a second substance, named penicillin B, which is nearly ten times as potent a germ-killer as penicillin, was also discussed at the meeting. Penicillin B, isolated by a group of workers at St. Louis University, kills bacteria in dilutions as high as 1,000,000,000 to 1 (billion to one). Unfortunately, it is even more rare than the original penicillin, on the extraction of which America's major chemical houses are now concentrating, with the cooperation of Government agencies. The entire output is reserved for the armed forces.

The new germ-killing chemicals belong to a chemical group known as acridines, composed of three benzene rings joined together and containing one atom of nitrogen in each ring. The nitrogen atom at the lower end of the center ring gives this group a characteristic color.

Aiding Wounded in Africa

One member of the acridine group, proflavine powder, has already been used with great effect on wounded soldiers in North Africa by two British physicians, Drs. G. A. G. Mitchell and G. A. H. Buttle, who use it in the healing of battle wounds that did not respond to sulfa drugs, it was reported.

The bacteria-destroying powers of some of the acridines, it was reported, are as much as a hundred times those of the sulfa drugs. New members of the family recently synthesized, it was stated, are active in dilutions of 10,000,000 parts to one. Penicillin A, in some instances, acts in dilutions of 160,-000,000 to one.

Studies revealing for the first time how these new penicillin-like chemicals produce their effects on germs, opening the way to the synthesis of a host of related chemicals even more potent than those now in existence, were described by Dr. Gustav J. Martin of the Warner Institute for Therapeutic Research, New York City.

The great Paul Ehrlich sought for the "magic bullet" which would destroy bacteria directly without harming the patient, but such direct-acting "magic bullets" are almost impossible to find. The discovery of the sulfa drugs provided a new approach the chemotherapy.

Bacteria Are Surrounded

These drugs do not act as "magic bullets" by destroying bacteria directly. Instead, they act indirectly by surrounding the bacteria with a "chemical magic wall," as it were, which makes it impossible for the bacteria to obtain a food substance vital for their growth. Thus weakened through lack of food, the bacteria fail to multiply. The body's infantry, the white blood cells, then steps in and wipes out the isolated remnants.

The acridines, Dr. Martin found, also exert their effect in an indirect way, but instead of building a chemical wall around the bacteria that deprives them of an essential food factor, the acridines, Dr. Martin found, put the germs in a "chemical vacuum" in which they are deprived of oxygen, the staff of life for most bacteria as it is for other living things. Whereas the sulfa drugs produce starvation, the acridines cause asphyxiation.

The human body as well as bacteria utilize oxygen by means of vital enzyme systems, known as respiratory enzymes, which make possible chemical union between cells and the oxygen from air, water and from food substances. An important group of oxygen-carrying enzymes contains the chemical constellations known as adenines. It is these adenine-containing enzyme systems, Dr. Martin found, that are interfered with by the acridines, and without these adenine enzymes the bacteria are literally suffocated.

Just as too little oxygen is bad for bacteria and man, too much oxygen is equally bad, causing the body's energy fuels to burn too fast, hence, an excess of oxygen-carrying enzymes is also harmful to bacteria, Dr. Martin pointed out.

Penicillin B, the chemical constitution of which has been found by the chemists at St. Louis University to contain an important oxygen-carrying group, acts in exactly the opposite manner from that of the acridines. Instead of depriving bacteria of oxygen, it surrounds them with too much oxygen, in the form of hydrogen peroxide. This results in literally "burning" the bacteria alive.

Thus these new studies of the acridines provide two highly important strategic highways for storming the citadel of disease-producing bacteria. One is to synthesize new members of the acridine family, more potent than those now in existence, to deprive the bacteria of vital oxygen. The other would be to create substances that would produce the same effect as pencillin B, namely, super-carriers of oxygen.

The observation on the manner in which pencillin B produces its death-dealing effect on bacteria, Dr. Martin said, may shed light on the nature of the chemical action of the first member of the family, now known as pencillin A.

When the organism produces two different chemicals, it is often the case that the two act as opposites, one counterbalancing the other. Because of this, it may be reasoned that pencillin A and pencillin B are also two parts of what may be called a "gyroscope of life."

The A May Inhibit the B

Since penicillin B acts as super-carrier of oxygen, it was pointed out, it is not unreasonable to assume that penicillin A acts as an inhibitor to penicillin B, preventing it from supplying too much oxygen. If that is the case, Dr. Martin stated, then penicillin A may produce its effect in the same manner as the acridines, and may even turn out to be a member of the acridine group.

There was excitement here today when the rumor spread among the chemists that penicillin A has already been sythesized by a large pharmaceutical house. No confirmation could be obtained of the report, which, if true, would be one of the greatest milestones in man's age-old struggle against disease, of vast importance to our armed forces and civilians alike.

If such a synthesis has actually been achieved, it was pointed out, it may very likely be kept a military secret for the time being, at least, or until means are available for quantity production of this wonder-chemical, to satisfy civilian as well as military needs.

September 10, 1943

PENICILLIN SAVES FATAL HEART CASES

Six men and a 7-year-old boy who had been doomed by a fatal heart disease stood smiling before a hushed audience of 200 specially invited doctors at Brooklyn Jewish Hospital, where they had been literally snatched from death by the last minute intervention of the new super-drug, penicillin, the most effective disease-fighting chemical so far discovered by man.

All the patients had suffered from subacute bacterial endocarditis, an inflammation of the lining of the heart caused by infection with the streptococcus viridans.

One of the seven, the physicians were informed, had been transferred from St. Elizabeth's Hospital, Manhattan, after the last rites of the Catholic Church had been administered to him.

Ten Hopeless Cases Treated

The report was presented by Dr. Leo Loewe on behalf of himself and his associates at the Brooklyn Jewish Hospital. In all, ten cases that had been given up as hopeless have received the penicillin treatment, along with heparin, a clot-dissolving liver substance.

While refraining from using the word "cure," the report described eight of the patients as being free of the disease-causing bacteria and minus all the other symptoms generally associated with the disease. The patients' temperature, Dr. Loewe reported, was again normal and the blood no longer showed any tendency to form the clots that ultimately prove fatal. Two of the patients, he added, have not responded in the same dramatic manner, while the eighth is still undergoing treatment.

The treatment requires relatively large doses of penicillin, and this factor will make it impossible for the present to make the new life-saving treatment available to the many victims of the disease who will undoubtedly appeal for it, it was pointed out. It takes from ten to eighty times as much penicillin to treat a case of subacute bacterial endocarditis as for a case of pneumonia, and twenty to thirty times the amount now required to treat one case of staphylococcus infection, and there simply is not enough penicillin to meet the needs of both the armed services and civilians.

It takes from 1,000,000 to 8,000,000 units of penicillin (about 100 to 800 grains) to treat effectively one case of subacute bacterial endocarditis, it was learned, as against 100,000 units for one case of pneumonia and 30,000-50,000 for staphylococcus infection. In other words, the lives of ten pneumonia victims and twenty to thirty osteomyelitis cases could be saved as against only one life in the heart disease, taking the million unit as the criterion.

A Difficult Decision Made

Hence it was learned that the special committee of the National Research Council in charge of the distribution of penicillin for civilian use has been forced to make the difficult decision not to release penicillin henceforth for use of victims of subacute bacterial endocarditis, as it must husband the very limited supply for the saving of many more lives in other hopeless cases in which much smaller doses of penicillin are required.

However, the Government has given a 1-A priority for penicillin, which is secreted very slowly in very minute amounts by a soil mold, and has allocated some $20,000,000 to speed up its manufacture. This week Surgeon Gen. Norman T. Kirk announced that an adequate supply of penicillin for both civilian and military uses may be expected in six months. An authoritative source yesterday said that this much-sought-for goal may be reached within three months.

There have been earlier attempts to treat subacute bacterial endocarditis with penicillin. These attempts failed, it is now realized, because the doses were not large enough. The results with much larger doses may lead to a re-examination of the possible use of penicillin in a number of other diseases in which it has so far not proved itself effective, among these being malaria. It has already proved itself highly promising in the treatment of syphilis.

ARMY PENICILLIN TESTS

Special to THE NEW YORK TIMES.

WASHINGTON, Dec. 16—Calling penicillin, the new drug, "neither a miracle nor a cure-all," the War Department reported today that "comprehensive tests" had proved that the drug had "high efficiency" against some types of bacteria but was "almost wholly ineffective" against others.

After conducting tests in thirty-two Army general hospitals and in 313 selected cases, Army medical authorities agreed that penicillin was "most effective when used as a supplement to other types of treatment."

"In some cases," the War Department reported, "bacteria was found to develop a 'fastness' or resistance to the drug, which approached immunization."

Maj. Champ Lyons of the Medical Corps stated in a summary that "the most dramatic results in the use of penicillin are relief from pain and quick restoration of a normal appetite, even in seriously wounded men." These factors, combined with administration of whole blood, have expedited the physical rehabilitation of men, making it possible for major operations to be performed within a few days after injuries.

"Prompt surgery to remove dead issues, bone fragments and foreign bodies, such as bits of metal," the summary continued, "is vitally necessary to insure rapid wound healing * * * the dramatic effectiveness of penicillin in rapidly establishing this phase of convalescence is added proof of the unique position of the drug among anti-bacterial agents."

Maj. Gen. Norman T. Kirk, Surgeon General, commented:

"It remains to be tried in many infections which so far remain unexplored. It has been studied to date almost entirely in conditions in which sulfa drugs have failed. We do not know to what extent it may replace rather than merely supplement these drugs. A huge amount of experimental work on penicillin remains to be done."

December 17, 1943

The Mold That Fights For the Life of Man

Just when it is needed most, penicillin comes along to curb many kinds of infections.

By Daniel Schwarz

USUALLY the first thing doctors say when the subject of penicillin is brought up is, "Please don't call it a 'wonder drug.'" But then they proceed to grow enthusiastic in spite of themselves: "A remarkably effective anti-bacterial agent" . . . "better than the sulfa drugs" . . . "a few months ago in a case like this we'd have been helpless."

Penicillin inspires such enthusiasm partly because it has come on the medical scene at exactly the right time. Army doctors have always searched for a drug that would cure infections in open wounds. The sulfa drugs help, but they aren't always completely effective against pus-forming bacteria. Penicillin has cleared infected wounds that had defied all the usual treatments.

In addition, penicillin has proved extremely useful in treating types of pneumonia that have resisted all other treatment; boils and abscesses, infected burns, the bone disease called osteomyelitis and dozens of other less familiar illnesses. Given in large doses it even conquers the dread sub-acute bacterial endocarditis, formerly "100 per cent fatal." Gonorrhea can't stand up against it—all traces of the germ vanish within a few days—and it shows promise of being effective in treating syphilis, too, though experiments in that field haven't gone far enough to justify positive statements. Moreover, unlike the sulfa drugs, which are sometimes hard on the kidneys, penicillin has the great advantage af being practically non-toxic.

WHAT is penicillin? A rare drug secreted by a greenish-blue mold similar to the familiar mold that forms on cheese, oranges that have spoiled, bread, etc. Molds are fungous growths. Fungi are non-flowering plants, of which mushrooms are the most familiar example. The particular kind of mold from which penicillin is secreted is called technically Penicillium Chrysogenum notatum. Its spores (reproductive bodies) are microscopic; they are carried by the wind.

This particular kind of Penicillium differs from other fungi in one important respect, as Dr. Alexander Fleming, an English bacteriologist, discovered by accident in 1928. While busy with research on influenza he left a culture plate full of staphylococcus colonies out in the open. The next time he looked at the plate he noticed a spot of mold on it, not an uncommon experience, but instead of discarding the contaminated specimen, he studied it more closely. All around the mold, like a moat in a field of bacteria, was a clear ring. He looked at the ring under the microscope. It was completely free of bacteria. For some reason the bacteria died when they entered it. Evidently the Penicillium was giving off some substance that was death to bacteria.

What were Dr. Fleming's first thoughts? He himself reported them just the other day. "Nothing is more certain," he said, "than that when I saw the bacteria fading away, I had no suspicion that I had got a clue to the most powerful therapeutic substance yet used to defeat bacterial infections in the human body. But the appearance of that culture plate was such that I thought it should not be neglected."

Nor did Fleming neglect it. He made pure cultures of the mold, and most of the penicillin produced up to now has been obtained from the descendants of his original colony. He made test-tube experiments on many other types of bacteria, using the strongest solutions he could get of the strange factor Penicillium secreted, and got mixed results. But the thing that surprised him most of all was that the secretion did not damage blood corpuscles. He had been testing all kinds of antiseptics in human blood for years and had never before come across one that did not do more damage to blood corpuscles than it did to bacteria. "Here," as he said with great satisfaction, "was something to bite on."

Fleming gave the name penicillin to the mysterious X that Penicillium produced, published his results and hoped that someone would purify the active substance. But his work attracted little attention because it came at the wrong time—just at the period when the potentialities of the sulfa drugs had first begun to be understood and attention had turned back to Ehrlich's enthralling idea of fighting bacteria with man-made chemicals.

IT was not until 1939, eleven years after Fleming's original discovery, that a group of British scientists at Oxford, led by Dr. H. W. Florey, Professor of Pathology, began work on penicillin in earnest. They knew that if they grew Penicillium in a liquid under favorable conditions something that killed bacteria was somehow added. So they grew Penicillium by the square yard and after a week or two poured off the liquid in which it grew and tried to extract from it the essential compound.

Extraction of one compound from a mixture of several can be very simple: For example, to extract the salt from salt and water all that has to be done is to boil off the water. Or to extract the fat from a piece of meat (a silly idea in times like these) you simply pour ether over the meat, let the ether dissolve the fat and then evaporate the ether from the fat-and-ether mixture. The problem of extracting penicillin was, and is, far more complex. Its properties were unknown, it proved to be exceedingly unstable and it was mixed with a number of other organic materials any of which might have been a part of it or a necessary ally in its work.

So the job was difficult—probably it seemed hopeless at times—but, with the aid of a grant from the Rockefeller Foundation, the Oxford group of bacteriologists pushed it along and began to get results. In time they were able to make a concentrate over 1,000 times the strength of the original fluid. They tried it on mice and it had no poisonous effects. They shot deadly doses of bacteria into other mice, produced infections that were "incurable" —and then cured those infections with their concentrated penicillin. By 1941 they had a pure enough form of penicillin and enough evidence that it was non-toxic to justify experiments with it on human cases, people desperately, hopelessly ill, and it produced amazing results. They came to America and demonstrated their technique here.

FROM all this work some of the advantages of penicillin became clear. Other drugs that killed bacteria worked much faster than penicillin, but they had some nasty toxic effects. Even the sulfa drugs, despite their amazing results, had the disadvantage that a number of people were apparently allergic to the forms of sulfonamides known at the time and some persons even suffered permanent harm. But penicillin singled out the bacteria and left the patient alone. Furthermore, penicillin worked against some bacteria that the sulfa drugs could not cope with, in particular the pus-forming bacteria that gather in open cuts and wounds.

Then came Pearl Harbor. Medicine, like everything else, was mobilized and penicillin research

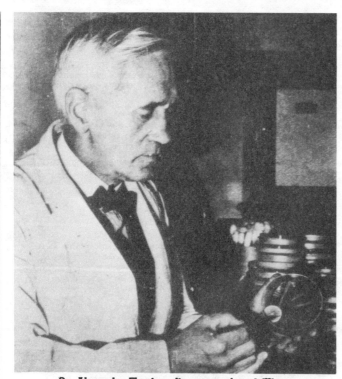

Dr. Alexander Fleming, discoverer of penicillin.

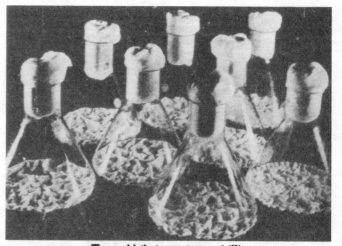

The mold that secretes penicillin.

and production, up to that time conducted only on a laboratory scale, was given an A-1 priority. Manufacture was strictly controlled; a number of chemical houses were encouraged to set up plants for the mass production of penicillin (there are now about twenty such plants in operation); twenty-two groups of investigators were promised supplies of penicillin to carry out experiments in hospitals; and the Army and Navy created penicillin units to do similar work in the armed forces.

COMPLETE authority over every drop of penicillin produced for civilian use was given to a sort of penicillin director, Dr. Chester S. Keefer of Boston. Now requests come to him from doctors all over the country and he doles out the precious stuff on the basis of a set of principles set up by a group of doctors. If previous experience has shown that penicillin won't fight a particular kind of sickness, he is in duty bound to refuse a request for the slightest bit of it. But if penicillin seems likely to help, he rushes the necessary supply and keeps a check on the result.

While penicillin has probably been the most carefully rationed war essential of all, the output is being stepped up so rapidly that a surplus for civilian doctors may be available by next spring or summer. Details of how penicillin is being mass-produced are a military secret, but it isn't revealing anything to Hitler's technicians to say that three methods of growing the temperamental mold are in use: surface culture, bran culture (in which the mold is grown on bran moistened by a liquid nutrient) and submerged culture.

IN submerged culture the mold is grown in huge, covered vats holding hundreds and perhaps thousands of gallons of nutrient fluid (the preferred culture medium is corn steep liquor). The necessary air is pumped through the fluid. After several days, when the mold has produced a sufficient supply of penicillin, the fluid is led through pipes to other containers, where it is concentrated at low temperatures and under high vacuums by a technique somewhat similar to that of drying blood plasma. It has been estimated that the cost of producing penicillin is $18,000 a pound, but the doses needed are so small that each costs only $2.

Penicillin must be concentrated some 20,000 times, or until it is completely dry, before it can be stored without deteriorating. It arrives at the hospital as a yellow or yellow-brown powder and is stored in refrigerators until it is needed. Then it is diluted and jabbed with a hypodermic needle into the muscles (not necessarily near the point of infection) or allowed to drip into a vein in a glucose mixture.

According to an estimate made early this year five gallons of culture fluid were needed to yield a single gram of penicillin. Current production is a secret, but it probably is still a relatively low percentage of the fluid treated. Fortunately the potency of penicillin is extremely high: it requires only one part in 25,000,000 to stop the growth of the pus-forming germ, staphylococcus aureus, which causes boils.

Since penicillin is so powerful, why not simply lay some of the mold on a wound and let it secrete its healing drug? For several reasons. One is that the mold is dirty and would carry more infection than the penicillin could destroy. Another is that

the mold is temperamental; it will grow almost anywhere, but it will not secrete penicillin unless conditions are exactly right. Even under what scientists consider perfect conditions, it sometimes balks. It grows, but it refuses to produce the drug.

ONE object of current penicillin research, and a most important one, is to synthesize the drug with known chemicals, as some of the vitamins have been synthesized. The first step, obviously, is to decide what penicillin is made of, itself an exceedingly difficult thing, and progress has been made on that line. Then, since many houses can be made with the same set of bricks, the particular molecular structure of penicillin will have to be worked out. Biological chemists are convinced that both these things will be done before very long.

Another thing that nobody knows yet is how penicillin does its job. In the case of the sulfa drugs one theory is that the drug is absorbed by the bacteria and that it then (somehow) prevents them from digesting an essential element in their diet (para-amino-benzoic acid). So they starve to death. Other anti-bacterial agents seem to work by upsetting the osmotic balance of the bacteria with this dire result: they absorb so much liquid that they get too big for their skins, like the bullfrog that tried to blow himself up to the size of a bull, and explode.

As for penicillin, it is known to work relatively slowly—in a matter of hours rather than minutes, as some other bactericides do. Therefore one hypothesis is that it doesn't kill the bacteria but simply upsets their process of reproduction. That is enough to do the job. If the total number of bacteria can be kept constant, the white blood cells can be relied on to clean them out. The trouble is that bacteria multiply exceedingly fast (it has been estimated that under proper conditions a single bacterium produces 1,000,000,000 descendants in fifteen hours) and if they aren't stopped they soon become so numerous that the body cannot cope with them.

THE potentialities of penicillin seem even greater than its achievements. It hasn't yet been possible to explore all of penicillin's possibilities because the supply has been so limited and the need so great that even qualified researchers have had difficulty in getting it. Moreover, after penicillin is synthesized, it seems likely that variations of it will be worked out, just as they were in the case of the sulfa drugs, and these derivatives may do miracles as yet unthought of. Finally, the success of penicillin seems certain to lead to extensive research on similar properties of other fungi, a field whose possibilities have hardly been scratched.

But the doctors' warning— "Please don't call it a 'wonder drug' "—is worth remembering. The reason for the warning was explained the other day by a doctor in the "penicillin ward" at Halloran Hospital, the Army's impressive base hospital on Staten Island. "Penicillin is an amazing drug," he said, "but the danger is that people may think of it as a panacea. It isn't. It's only another medical tool.

"LOOK at the boys in this ward," he went on. "They've all had gunshot or shrapnel wounds of one sort or another. They were all brought here because their wounds became infected and the usual treatments, including the sulfa drugs, didn't work. As soon as they were given penicillin their wounds cleared up, their temperatures went down to normal and they began to eat again. Remarkable? Certainly. But that was only the beginning of the job. A four-inch piece of bone in this fellow's right tibia was shot away; we had to graft a new piece of bone there. Penicillin alone couldn't have made it possible for that boy to walk again.

"Don't misunderstand me. Without penicillin we might have had to wait six months before that wound cleared up. Meanwhile that boy's leg would have got weaker and weaker from disuse. With penicillin we could operate quickly so the results were far better. But you see now what I mean when I say it's no panacea." January 2, 1944

Preventing Measles

A new method for treating measles is revealed by Dr. Francis G. Blake, president of the Board for the Investigation and Control of Influenza and Other Epidemic Diseases in the Army. The material, which comes from blood plasma, is the protein known as gamma globulin. It contains antibodies that destroy the germs of measles, for which reason it acts as a prophylactic.

This new weapon against measles is the result of more than a year's work by the Commission on Measles and Mumps, one of ten commissions into which the board is divided. The work on measles grew out of the fundamental studies on blood plasma carried on by Dr. Edwin J. Cohn (Harvard), whose success in separating blood plasma by chemical means into its various fractions or components has been commented upon in this department. Gamma globulin is now being separated from a portion of the blood collected by the Red Cross.

Most of the work was done in Army camps, but one significant study was carried on during an outbreak of measles at a girls' college in the East. Gamma globulin was given to sixty-seven exposed students who had no previous record of measles and who therefore were susceptible to it, but not to thirty-eight other susceptible students. Only one case of average measles developed in the group of the treated sixty-seven students. There were three cases of modified measles and eight cases of mild measles. Among the thirty-eight students who received the gamma globulin there were eighteen cases of average measles and five of mild measles.

May 14, 1944

DOUBLE VACCINE—

A double vaccine against diphtheria and whooping cough has been found to protect children against both these diseases, eliminating the need for separate inoculations, it is reported in the Aug. 5 issue of the Journal of the American Medical Association by Drs. Louis W. Sauer and Winston H. Tucker and Eve Markley, R. N., of Evanston, Ill. In view of the increasing number of immunization procedures required in early life to protect children against various disease hazards this finding is regarded as important. No infant injected with the double vaccine during the last five years is known to have contracted either disease, the report states.

August 6, 1944

ANOTHER GERM-KILLER—

Still another germ-killer extracted from a soil bacterium (Actinomyces), named streptomycin, is announced in Science (Aug. 4) by Dr. Selman A. Waksman, Doris Jones, H. J. Metzger and Albert Schatz of the New Jersey Agricultural Experiment Station. In experiments on embryo chicks streptomycin prevented the growth of several bacterial species, of the gram-positive as well as the gram-negative types, that have been found to be resistant to other antibiotic substances extracted from molds and soil bacteria. Among these were the germs of fowl typhoid and those that cause spontaneous abortion. W. L. L.

August 13, 1944

DISEASE DEATH RATE AT ARMY RECORD LOW

WASHINGTON, Aug. 13 (U.P.)— New techniques developed to safeguard the health of soldiers have cut the Army's death rate from disease to 20 per cent of total deaths, the lowest in history, the War Department said tonight.

In contrast to World War I, when more soldiers were killed by disease than by enemy bullets, only 10,000 of the 49,720 Army dead in the two and one-half years since Pearl Harbor were victims of disease, the department said.

The present health record results from work by the Army board for the investigation and control of influenza and other epidemic diseases, first suggested by Brig. Gen. James S. Simmons of the Surgeon General's office in 1940.

This board has developed procedures ranging from spraying of barracks with an invisible, odorless, non-sticky film of oil that traps germs to injections of a protein substance separated from blood plasma to check measles epidemics. A more recent achievement is perfection of a way to use sulfadiazine in checking the spread of meningococcal meningitis.

"The magnitude of (the board's) accomplishment can be realized when it is remembered that in the Spanish-American War disease killed seven times as many American soldiers as did Spanish bullets," the department declared.

August 14, 1944

ARMY DROPS ISSUE OF SULFA TO MEN

By HOWARD W. BLAKESLEE
Associated Press Science Editor

One of this war's reputed life-saving marvels, the sulfanilamide that men put into their own wounds, has been abandoned for use by the men. Ended by the Army also is issuance of the eight sulfa tablets that wounded men were instructed to swallow immediately.

No more of either the powdered sulfas for wounds or the tablets to swallow are being issued, although the men retain supplies they had on hand.

The change marks the end of a great experiment, good to a certain extent, but which developed disadvantages and which finally was outweighed by the many other life-saving treatments of wounded perfected during the war.

The disadvantages of powdered sulfas in wounds were known at the start of the war, but were outweighed then by the urgent needs of setting up a huge medical organization. The sulfa powders, while they killed some of the infectious germs, failed to stop the decomposition that furnished the material in which blood poisoning ultimately might develop. The powders were a foreign body in wounds and sometimes slowed the natural healing processes.

After three years of study in the combat zones and in hospitals in the United States it was decided that no known drug could sterilize an infected war wound. This decision included penicillin.

The reason for abandoning the eight sulfa tablets was mainly that too many men saved up the issues to use the tablets for gonorrhea. There is one serious risk in self-cures of this venereal disease: If a man does not take enough he not only fails to cure the disease but afterward his germs are likely to have an immunity from the sulfas which makes it difficult to cure him at all.

Another risk is that the sulfas that fail to cure may drive the disease under cover, so that the man shows no symptoms until the trouble comes back in a more serious form.

The sulfas which the soldier took by mouth are effective against some infections of wounds but not against others. In the present care of wounded the surgeons get the men early enough to give them either sulfas or penicillin in time.

August 9, 1945

Cure for Malaria Is Revealed After 4-Year, $7,000,000 Research

By WILLIAM L. LAURENCE
Special to THE NEW YORK TIMES.

ATLANTIC CITY, April 11—A new drug that cures relapsing malaria, the most serious form of the disease that afflicts 800,000,000 of the earth's inhabitants, as well as powerful new drugs that prevent and completely suppress the non-relapsing type, thus promising the eventual eradication of the plague that incapacitates nearly half of the world's population, were described here today at the annual spring meeting of the American Chemical Society.

The curtain of secrecy behind which the multi-million dollar Government anti-malaria program had been operating, in the most concentrated attack in history against this scourge, was completely lifted today for the first time with the revelation of the most potent chemicals so far found out of a total of nearly 15,000 new compounds developed and tested in scores of laboratories, at a cost of about $7,000,000.

The work was carried on during the last four years under contract with the committee on medical research of the Office of Scientific Research and Development. The reports were presented at a symposium on anti-malarial agents that began Tuesday morning, in which a number of leading investigators in the field summarized their findings.

The participants included Dr. Robert C. Elderfield of Columbia University, Dr. Arthur P. Richardson of the Squibb Institute for Medical Research, New Brunswick, N. J.; Dr. L. H. Schmidt, Institute of Medical Research, the Christ Hospital, Cincinnati, and Dr. James A. Shannon of the Department of Medicine, New York University.

There are two principal types of malarial parasites—falciparum and vivax. Falciparum malaria does not systematically relapse, hence a patient once freed of the parasites generally remains free of the disease. Vivax malaria, on the other hand, makes the victim subject to relapses, so that he must continue taking drugs to suppress the parasite when it emerges from its secret hiding places in the tissues.

Until now quinine and atabrine were the two principal drugs available for fighting both types of the disease. While these chemicals effectively suppressed the falciparum type in the great majority of cases and thus rid the patient of the disease, they could only serve as temporary suppressants in vivax malaria.

In the last five years, Dr. Shannon reported, a number of highly effective suppressive drugs have been uncovered considerably more effective than either quinine or atabrine. Because of their greater effectiveness as suppressants against both vivax and falciparum, he pointed out, they can be administered at less frequent intervals. This lessening of the administrative burden, he said, "will place effective suppression within the easy reach of any individual or any organized group of individuals."

In addition to these more effective suppressive drugs, Dr. Shannon reported, "relatively non-toxic curative agents for vivax malaria are now or shortly will be available."

These new curative drugs for relapsing malaria are chemically related to the synthetic anti-malaria known as plasmochin, or pamaquin, originally synthesized in Germany. They are derivatives of a group of compounds known as 8-amino-quinolines.

"The results of study with compounds related to pamaquin, which have been accumulated to date," Dr. Shannon reported, "make it seem quite certain that from this general class of compounds there will be available curative agents for vivax malaria which will be generally tolerated.

"Already it is known that at least one compound of this general series (at present known as SN 13, 27) will cure the virulent forms of vivax malaria at a well tolerated dosage.

"It remains to be demonstrated, however, that this and other promising compounds of this series do not cause the hemolytic anemias which are characteristic of pamaquin administration. These anemias occur more or less exclusively in colored and mixed races, the bulk of the inhabitants of the most hyperendemic areas.

"If it turns out that this is true, then we will have available truly curative agents of a relatively low order of toxicity."

Three of the newly developed suppressant drugs, Dr. Shannon said, "are of sizable importance." They are known as clorquin, oxy-cloroquin and palucrine. The first two were developed in the American program and the third in the British program.

"These drugs," he said, "are important for both practical and theoretical reasons. Each would appear to be sufficiently active and sufficiently nontoxic to ease the administrative burden of suppressive therapy by accomplishing complete suppression of malaria with single, well-tolerated doses of the drug.

"Generally speaking, with active drugs suppressive therapy requires regular administration of the drug throughout the entire period of exposure, which may be for months. The extent to which success is achieved depends largely upon the extent to which a dosage schedule is adhered to. This makes for a serious administrative problem when daily doses of drugs are required, but not when suppression can be effected with doses at weekly, or perhaps longer, intervals."

Among the more promising compounds, Dr. Shannon said, "are some which may be expected to effect complete suppression when administered once weekly in a well-tolerated dose. They will also cause an abrupt termination of a clinical attack of vivax and a cure of falciparum malaria when administration is limited to one or, at most, two days."

"No one of these highly effective agents has, as yet, been fully exploited," he continued. "However, information is at hand which permits the prediction that they will constitute a relatively simple means for the complete control of malaria in many areas due to the lessening of the administrative problem of suppressive therapy."

They may also, in specific areas, contribute to the eradication of the malarias through their ability to curtail transmission of the disease, Dr. Shannon added.

April 12, 1946

DRUG IS EFFECTIVE FOR TUBERCULOSIS

2-Year Test of Streptomycin on 100 Patients Said to Show 'Encouraging Results'

CHICAGO, Nov. 30 (Science Service)—"Definitely and consistently encouraging results" have been obtained with streptomycin treatment of tuberculosis in 100 patients during the past two years.

This is reported by a group of scientists who pioneered in the treatment of tuberculosis with the chemical from bacilli found in soil. They are Drs. H. Corwin Hinshaw and William H. Feldman of the Mayo Clinic and Foundation and Dr. Karl H. Pfuetze of Cannon Falls, Minn.

Streptomycin should have more extensive trials in treatment of many forms of tuberculosis, they recommend in the forthcoming issue of The Journal of the American Medical Association.

Large doses must be given for prolonged periods; they caution against starting streptomycin treatment unless enough of the antibiotic drug is likely to be available for two to four months. This would be close to one pound of the drug.

Most of the patients who get this prolonged treatment will develop toxic symptoms. Their sense of equilibrium is likely to be disturbed, and this will continue for several weeks after the drug has been stopped.

Streptomycin is not a substitute for other and proved effective forms of treatment of tuberculosis, the scientists state. It should not be given to patients who are getting better with other treatment or who are likely to recover under usual treatment.

Actual healing in tuberculosis, they point out, must be accompanied by the slow processes of resorption, fibrosis and calcification, during which the germs are walled off in a calcified area of tissue. The role of streptomycin is to block paths for extension of the disease while the healing forces are operating.

December 1, 1946

RADIOACTIVE IODINE—

Radioactive iodine was effective in the treatment of a patient with a malignant tumor of the thyroid gland, it is reported in the Journal of the American Medical Association by Drs. S. M. Seidlin, L. D. Marinelli and Eleanor Oshry of the Montefiore Hospital and the Memorial Hospital, New York. The patient had his thyroid removed in 1923. In 1939, despite the fact that he had no thyroid gland, he showed all the symptoms of an overactive thyroid. Examination revealed a malignant tumor which had spread from remaining thyroid tissue. Subsequently, other cancerous tumors, of thyroid tissue origin, were found in the lungs, thigh bone, small intestine, skull and second rib on the left side. After X-rays and drugs proved ineffective he was given radioactive iodine, administered by mouth in the form of sodium iodide in water. The iodine has an affinity for thyroid tissue and is drawn to it no matter in what part of the body it is located. By means of periodic treatments with the radioactive iodine any recurrence of the cancer has been quickly detected and kept in check.

December 15, 1946

If a Flu Pandemic Strikes Again—

By FRANCIS RAWDON SMITH

ANOTHER influenza epidemic is expected, possibly this winter, but it will not be like earlier ones. For the first time medical science has weapons with which to fight one of mankind's worst and most widespread scourges. Most authorities believe that flu killed more people immediately after the first World War than were killed by weapons during the war. In three successive waves flu engulfed the entire civilized world, and there was nothing to be done which offered any hope of stopping it. This time there is something to do. Though we have still more to learn, we know a lot more about flu than we did in 1918-19.

Flu is known as a pandemic disease. An epidemic is confined to a relatively small area; flu, when it hits, covers nations, continents, almost the whole world. The word pandemic is an attempt to describe this characteristic; it implies something worse than epidemic, an epidemic on an altogether larger scale.

FLU pandemics occur in cycles—roughly every twenty to thirty years. The regularity of the cycle, however, is not precise, and for this reason the exact time of an outbreak cannot be predicted with certainty. What can be said is that, since the last pandemic was in 1918-19, medical men have been on the alert since 1938—twenty years after 1918. So far, the expected has not happened, this despite the recent war when people moved rapidly from place to place and the nutrition and living conditions of many were such as to reduce resistance materially. This is why an outbreak is feared momentarily; we are very near the "outside edge" of the cycle and have had another war to add to the probabilities.

Influenza is only one of many diseases of the respiratory system, which range from the common cold to pneumonia. With the milder of such diseases, colds and grippes, flu has one characteristic in common — it is caused, primarily, by a virus. The viruses are the lowest form of life, and many of their characteristics are more those of inanimate, physical matter than of biological, living things; but they do resemble all other living things in one fundamental respect—they can reproduce themselves; their colonies grow and expand when their "living conditions" are favorable.

The most important difference between viruses and bacteria, which also reproduce and grow under favorable conditions, is size. Viruses are very much smaller than bacteria, a majority of which can be removed from a solution by a very fine filter. No ordinary filter is fine enough to stop the viruses; for this reason they were first known as filter-passing viruses.

THEIR small size, together with the fact that they cannot be easily grown in the laboratory, has meant that science knows very little about them. Until the development of the electron microscope, no one had ever seen a virus; they are invisi-

FRANCIS RAWDON SMITH, a science writer specializing in physiology and allied medical subjects, was educated at England's Cambridge University and at Harvard. His work has taken him to practically every country in Europe and North and South America.

ble under an optical microscope. Viruses have to live in the cells of living plants or animals; they cannot be grown in dishes like bacteria. Their chemical complexity, too, varies enormously. They are by no means composed of the same things. At one end of the scale they are the simplest of all living things; at the opposite they have all the constituents of protoplasm, of complex biological matter. Along with these differences go immense differences of size; all are minute by man's standards, but by their own they vary from enormous to tiny. All in all, their variations mean that the viruses set medical research a very great problem.

Most people are familiar with the symptoms of flu aches and pains, severe headaches, high temperature, all of sudden onset. One minute a person feels fine, ten minutes later he knows he has influenza. Very often, following the attack (which in duration is usually as short as a week), comes the part which many people dread most—the depression, prolonged debility. After the two big-scale attacks of recent years, that in France in 1891 and the worldwide one from May, 1918, to April, 1919, the suicide rate went up sharply. At least in part this was a result of the depression and melancholia among the convalescent.

IN everyday language the term influenza has come to mean any one of a variety of diseases of widely different degrees of severity, including some which are not influenza at all. Even flu itself varies greatly in its severity and in the number of people it attacks. For this, medical men now believe there are at least two reasons:

First, successive generations of viruses vary in their potency, in their virulence (note the resemblance between the two words, which are of common Latin origin). Because viruses are continually developing, sometimes toward milder, sometimes toward more "severe" characteristics, the character of the diseases they produce also varies from mild to severe.

Secondly, and this is somewhat nearer the realm of conjecture, the potency of the so-called "secondary invaders" which followed the virus also varies from year to year. These secondary invaders are bacteria, and they enter the human body when its resistance is reduced by the initial virus invasion.

A GREAT number of the 1918-19 cases showed, in addition to the viruses themselves, a huge bacteria "count" — streptococci, pneumococci, staphylococci, etc. There is some reason to think that these bacteria were as much respon-

sible for the severity of the last post-war epidemic as the viruses themselves. It just happened that both virus and bacteria had reached a high point in their change of potency at about the same time, so that a body whose resistance had been reduced by the virus attack was then invaded by the potent bacteria. Right here lies the first reason for hoping that no future pandemic need be as bad as those of the past. We can now do something about the secondary invaders.

Against many bacterial types medical men now have a powerful armory. These are the sulfa drugs and the familiar antibiotics, penicillin, streptomycin and others. When given to an influenza sufferer who has been attacked by secondary invaders they can, by helping to take care of the latter, offer the patient a better chance to deal with the virus invasion.

IT often happens that, when faced by many foes, the "antibodies" — the disease-fighting constituents of blood — are temporarily or permanently overwhelmed, in the latter case with fatal results. After the invasion starts, the body calls up all its antibody reserves, sets its antibody-manufacturing plants to work. Like preparation for war, this takes time; if the invasion is too large and too sudden, and the existing antibodies too few, there is no time for additional antibodies to be manufactured and the result may be death.

Obviously, if some of the invaders—in this case the bacterial ones can be taken out of the battle by external means, by administered drugs or antibiotics, the chances of victory over the remainder are vastly improved. But it must be remembered that the drugs and the antibiotics themselves will not kill the primary invaders — the viruses which started the whole thing. These still have to be dealt with by the body's own combat troops.

ALL this means that, if one gets a severe attack of influenza, the chances of survival are far better than they were in 1918-19, when the sulfa drugs and the antibiotics were unknown. An even more promising possibility lies in the fact that there now exists a preventive—something which reduces the chances of contracting flu—which artificially increases the body's resistance to the viruses themselves. This is the anti-influenza vaccine developed during the last war and used on a large scale by the Army. Unlike the familiar smallpox vaccine, which is usually given by scratching

the skin, this is a "shot," administered by hypodermic into a muscle. Seven to fourteen days after the shot, the body's anti-virus resources, stimulated by the vaccination, are so vastly increased that the chances of being infected are greatly reduced.

Neither the Army nor anyone else can yet say just how effective the vaccine is—the carrying out of the necessary controlled experiments and the study of the resulting statistics are a long and difficult job. But it is established that the vaccine does work; people who have been vaccinated are much less likely to contract flu than those who have not. In fact, the Army is sure enough of this to have stored away in St. Louis enough influenza vaccine to give every man and woman in the Army a shot, if a flu wave strikes this winter. The fact that such immunization is now possible is the second reason why, at least if enough people take the shots, there may never be another terrible pandemic like those of recorded history.

RIGHT up to the early Nineteen Thirties it was assumed that influenza was caused by some one specific virus, though it had never been isolated. It is now known that there are, at very least, two types of virus which are responsible, and each exists in many different "strains" having slightly different characteristics.

The two known types are Influenza A and Influenza B. Two strains of A—PR8 (discovered in Puerto Rico, hence the PR) and the Weiss strain—

and one of B—the Lee strain —are included in the vaccine now used, since more than one virus may be present in any one epidemic, and it is desirable to immunize people against as many as possible.

THE way the fluid for these shots is prepared and they are now available to any civilian who wishes to take them makes use of the fact that viruses will grow and multiply in a chick embryo. Ordinary fertile hens' eggs are incubated for around ten days to give the chick time to grow a little. The eggs are then inoculated by means of a hypodermic needle with a little of one of the three virus strains. After a period in which the viruses multiply, the eggs are broken open and the virus-infected fluid is "harvested." The virus is then purified, as far as possible, by separating it from the parent chick-tissue on which it grew. Lastly, it is killed, and the three types from different eggs are mixed together to form the vaccine.

The processes used to remove the chick protein are highly successful. Naturally, however, none removes all of it—a minute fraction always remains. For this reason a very small percentage of human beings with pronounced allergic reactions to eggs or chicken should not, it is held, take these shots without a previous test. Few people are so sensitive, however the Army estimates that less than four persons in a million would encounter a severe result—and anyone who frequently eats and enjoys eggs or chicken need have little fear. Those who do not, for any reason, ever eat these things are cautioned to so advise the doctor before he administers the vaccine.

NO immunization process is 100 per cent successful, and against a complicated disease like flu, caused by so many types of virus and secondary invader, even the remarkable vaccine now available will not certainly prevent one's getting flu. But medical men say it will greatly reduce one's chances of doing so—and if an attack comes, the vaccine will greatly reduce its severity. It will not immunize a person against the common cold, nor yet against the host of grippes, "feverish colds" and the like from which civilized people suffer in a crowded society. Even here, however, it may help indirectly. During a flu wave colds and other minor diseases become far more prevalent—because the general resistance is reduced. By preventing flu, it helps prevent the lesser afflictions.

WE know a lot more about flu than we did, but we need to know more still. Medical research is directed toward isolating more viruses from which vaccines may be prepared. Some day, too, we may hope for a drug or an antibiotic which will effectively kill flu viruses. Preliminary experiments suggest that a substance of this kind is already on the way—Nitroakinidin 3582, still in the laboratory stage. All over the world medical men are seeking to improve and to supplement the weapons now available; a very great deal has been accomplished recently.

Much of civilization's so-called progress has resulted in people moving about more than they did before, moving quickly over great distances. It places them, too, in "congested areas"—offices, restaurants and bars. All these factors have made the diseases of the respiratory system a far worse hazard than they were for our ancestors. The antibiotics and the anti-influenza vaccine are medicine's answer to the fact that here, as always, human "progress" has been backward as well as forward.

January 12, 1947

Artificial Kidney in Use in New York for Treatment of Uremic Poisoning

By WALDEMAR KAEMPFFERT

Dr. W. K. Kolff of Kampen, Holland, turned up by invitation at Mount Sinai Hospital in New York recently and there demonstrated an "artificial kidney" that he invented for the treatment of uremic poisoning. This form of poisoning follows damage to the kidney. Death need not ensue if, during the period required for repair, the kidney can be by-passed to a temporary substitute which will perform the function of excretion. With the artificial kidney as much as 260 grams of urea, which causes the uremic poisoning and death, has been success-fully removed in one treatment of fourteen hours' duration. With improved methods of technique the usual treatment now lasts about six hours.

Kolff's artificial kidney consists of a drum on which are wound fifty yards of cellophane tube. The whole is immersed in a salt solution. The radial artery in the forearm of the patient is connected with the tube and the blood flows through it and diffuses into the salt solution. After the poisonous substances from the kidney are removed the blood is returned from the cellophane tube into a vein in the patient's body.

The Kolff apparatus is useful only when there is hope that a damaged kidney may recover its ability to function if death can be staved off for a few days. Cases of poisoning with bichloride of mercury, toxic reactions to sulfa drugs, reactions after blood transfusions and occasional kidney poisoning after operations are the type in which the artificial kidney would be used. So far, the lives of eight persons have been saved by Kolff's method. His artificial kidney apparatus has been donated to Mount Sinai.

March 30, 1947

LIFE-SAVING FACTOR OF LIVER ISOLATED

By WILLIAM L. LAURENCE

Isolation at last of the mysterious factor in liver that has saved the lives of more than a million victims of pernicious anemia in the United States alone, and millions more in other parts of the world, was announced yesterday by a team of scientists of the research laboratories of Merck & Co., Rahway, N. J.

The announcement, one of the most important of its kind in recent years, marking a new milestone in the fight against disease, is presented in three scientific papers in the current issue of Science, the official organ of the American Association for the Advancement of Science, published today.

Ever since the discovery in 1926 by Dr. G. P. Minot and Dr. W. P. Murphy of Boston that liver con-tained a factor that counteracted pernicious anemia, until then a fatal disease that claimed more than 50,000 each year in this country, usually striking in the victim's most productive years of life, scientists the world over have tried in vain to isolate the life-giving factor. The task seemed so difficult that many had come to the conclusion that the solution was beyond the reach of man's present knowledge.

Team Work Wins

As is usual in such cases, the problem was finally solved by the cooperation of a team of scientists in several fields, including chemistry, microbiology and medicine. The chemical investigations were carried out by Edward L. Rickes, Dr. Norman G. Brink, Frank R. Koniuszy, Dr. Thomas R. Wood and Dr. Karl Folkers of the Merck research laboratories.

The microbiological work was done by Dr. Mary S. Shorb of the University of Maryland and the Maryland Agricultural Experiment Station, whose study was supported by a Merck grant. The medical tests were carried out by Dr. Randolph West, of the Columbia University College of Physicians and Surgeons and the Presbyterian Hospital, New York City.

The compound was isolated in small amounts from enormous quantities of liver in crystalline form, a form that the chemist requires as a sign of a high degree of purity and homogeneity. The crystals are red in color and consist of long, needle-like entities. The matter has been identified as a member of the royal vitamin family of the B complex and, pending further chemical identification of its molecular architecture, has been named vitamin B12.

Vitamin B-12 has been found to be one of the most powerful vitamins in nature. A single administration of as little as three micrograms (about 1/150,000,000th of a pound, or the equivalent of the approximate weight of 1/200th of an inch of human hair of average diameter) has been found by Dr. West to give a positive response in a patient.

Several commercial liver extracts were studied for comparison purposes, and it was found that only 0.001 to 0.014 per cent of the dry weight of such materials consisted of vitamin B-12. Since ten to fifteen grams of liver are required to produce the amount of extract suitable for a single day's dose, it may be calculated that the anti-pernicious-anemia activity in this amount of liver is concentrated at least a million times in the new crystalline vitamin.

Blow at Nerve System

Pernicious anemia is characterized by a decrease in the number of red blood cells, a lack which seriously impairs the functional efficiency of the blood and results in symptoms of weakness and fatigue. It is also characterized by degeneration of the spinal-cord nerve and the nervous system in general. These nerve changes, which may at times precede the anemia, result in loss of sensation and may even extend to partial paralysis.

"Although it is too early to predict the full usefulness of vitamin B-12, a few of its possibilities are already apparent," the Merck announcement states.

"By its use the physician may administer known doses of a pure vitamin so that the exact and reproducible therapy will be insured.

If indicated, potent doses of the new vitamin may be given without physical discomfort to the patient, since it is active in such infinitesimal amounts.

"There is, in fact, preliminary evidence to suggest that by the use of a sufficiently large dose it may be possible to produce a prolonged remission in pernicious anemia and avoid, thereby, the annoyance and expense of the more frequent injections now required."

It appears possible, the announcement adds, that the new vitamin may control, in addition to the blood condition, the other manifestation of the disease, namely, the nerve degeneration. It also may prove to be useful in the treatment of other diseases involving degeneration of nerves, though the latter possibility is at present pure speculation.

Still Difficult to Supply

The announcement also warned that the supplies of the new vitamin are still too small to "replace liver extract at the present time in the routine treatment of pernicious anemia."

The clue to the discovery was provided through studies by Dr. Shorb, which revealed that a milk organism, named lactobacillus lac-tis Dorner, required a factor in liver extracts for its growth and that the activity of this factor paralleled the potency of the extract for the pernicious-anemia patient. This provided at last the long-sought test organism for trying out the various liver fractions for anti-pernicious-anemia activity. Until then no test animal was available.

April 16, 1948

Atom Bomb By-Product Promises To Replace Radium as Cancer Aid

By ANTHONY LEVIERO
Special to THE NEW YORK TIMES.

WASHINGTON, April 21 — The Atomic Energy Commission reported today that irradiated cobalt, a "virtually costless metal," promised in every way to be as effective as radium in the treatment of cancer, and far easier to use.

President Truman, who made the decision to use the atomic bomb for the first time in warfare, was said to be highly gratified at the progress made with one of the many beneficial by-products of atomic energy. It was to Mr. Truman that David E. Lilienthal, chairman of the Atomic Energy Commission, made today's report.

Mr. Lilienthal, while announcing a promised landmark which would have "a profound effect in the treatment of this scourge," warned that the new material was no cure-all.

He emphasized that at best it could not be better than radium and that the cheapness and ease with which cobalt could be used were the only advantages. He stressed that it would be "cruel" to draw any greater promise from what he said.

Nevertheless the new material was regarded as a great advance, as it promised to make treatment and the task of the radiologist easier and to reduce the doctors' bills of cancer victims. Mr. Lilienthal said the new material, known in science as cobalt 60, had not yet been used clinically, although its production was "in the offing."

Mr. Lilienthal went to the White House to report on apparently extremely significant progress on what he himself described as the paradoxical atomic project.

On the one hand, he told of the stride in cancer treatment. On the other, he gave a preliminary report on the highly guarded test of a new atomic weapon at Eniewetok, American atomic laboratory in the Pacific.

The commission chairman visited the President a day after Mr. Truman sent to the Senate the nominations of Mr. Lilienthal and his four fellow commissioners for reappointment. The request for their confirmation threatened to precipitate another long battle along political party lines, as the Republican leadership has proposed that Mr. Lilienthal be renominated for only one year. Mr. Truman has insisted on a five-year term.

Mr. Lilienthal was accompanied by Carroll Wilson, general manager of the commission.

Asked if he would serve out the full five ears if he were confirmed by the Senate, Mr. Lilienthal replied he hoped it would not be necessary. He explained that it was no secret that he desired to return to private life when the atomic project was on a firm footing and he foresaw that this would take place before the term ended.

Mr. Lilienthal told reporters that because Cobalt 60 was "virtually costless," the commission was considering whether it should not be issued free to medical institutions. He explained that cobalt was a metal commonly used in industry and that it could be easily fashioned into a needle or a surgical probe.

The cobalt instrument is then inserted into an atomic furnace at the Oak Ridge, Tenn., atomic laboratory and becomes cobalt 60. In this state it is radioactive and fully as effective as radium itself in the treatment of cancer

By way of contrast, Mr. Lilienthal pointed out that there are only about twenty-six ounces of radium, which is most of the world's supply, in this country. And whereas radium itself is now used, usually in a hollow needle or tube, the new process made the cobalt itself the bearer of the healing rays.

Mr. Lilienthal explained that a great advantage lay in the fact that cobalt, thus irradiated, could be in any shape and more easily applied to disease tissue, with less risk of dangerous burns than from radium.

Cobalt 60 lasts five years while radium has a life of many years, but Mr. Lilienthal emphasized that cobalt instruments could be irradiated in any quantity.

He said that because Mr. Truman felt his responsibility with respect to the atomic bomb he also wished to be kept fully informed of atomic progress of benefit to mankind. Thus Mr. Lilienthal said he also reported that irradi-ated zinc was now being used effectively in studying what happens in the cells in the dread blood disease, leukemia. He stressed that the by-product here was not curative but by showing what went on in the cells might lead to cures.

Additional details on cobalt sixty in relation to cancer were obtained later through the commission, and it was learned that four institutions were using it in research: Memorial Hospital in New York; Ohio State University in Columbus; Washington University Hospital in St. Louis, and the University of California Hospital at Berkeley.

Dr. Shields Warren, director of the division of biology and medicine in the commission, when reached by telephone in Chicago, gave this opinion: "Radioactive cobalt will undoubtedly prove to be as effective as radium but no more so and it will be far more abundant."

General use of irradiated cobalt might be two or three years off, Dr. Warren said, as it would be necessary to establish standardized doses. This period of test was contrasted, however, with the twenty-five or thirty years it took to standardize radium dosage.

Illustrative of the facility of using the new material, was the report that the University of California had fashioned it into tiny beads which were implanted in patterns around a cancer tumor so that the whole tumor was uniformly irradiated. It was not clear here, however, whether the cobalt was being used on humans or experimentally on animals by any of the institutions.

April 22, 1948

4 New Wonder Drugs Are Called Foes of Previously Defiant Diseases

Special to THE NEW YORK TIMES.

LOS ANGELES, Jan. 21—Four new "wonder" drugs that are effective against some diseases that medicine has not been able to overcome in the past were described today by Dr. Perrin H. Long, Professor of Preventive Medicine at Johns Hopkins University Medical School, Baltimore.

Speaking at the midwinter postgraduate clinical convention in ophthalmology and otolaryngology here, Dr. Long, who introduced sulfa drugs in this country in 1936, said that the new curative agents, which might be taken orally, were named aureomycin, chloromycetin, polymyxin and circulis. They are anti-biotics, derived from molds.

Aureomycin was made available on Dec. 11, and chloromycetin is expected to be available next month.

Aureomycin and chloromycetin have been tested with startling results. They are too scarce to be in general use. Increased production with consequent lower prices may put them within reach of all physicians next December, Dr. Long asserted.

"Aureomycin is effective against all typhus-like diseases," Dr. Long said. "It is also effective against Q-fever, staphylococcus, streptococcus, penumococcus, urinary tract infections, certain types of peritonitis, parrot fever and primary atypical, or virus pneumonia.

To date there has been little tendency on the part of organisms to become resistant to 'aureo.'

"Chloromycetin is effective against typhus and typhoid fever. The important thing is that it may be given by mouth. It is essentially nontoxic. Polymyxin is effective in certain types of urinary tract infections, certain types of blood poisoning and some types of peritonitis. Circulis is useful in the same range as polymyxin."

He said that chloromycetin was derived from a mold isolated in soil received from Venezuela. He added that soils were being tested from all parts of the world for molds from which curative preparations might be developed.

"'Aureo' has filled in the gaps that penicillin did not hit," Dr. Long said. "If we had never had penicillin, we would say that it is the most wonderful thing in the world."

The age level of the country is rising because of advances in the field of medicine, and Dr. Long said that he looked for the new drugs to thrust the horizon further away by cutting down the death rate of many ailments. He added that increasing the age level would mean that more persons would live to succumb late to heart ailments and cancer, however.

January 22, 1949

MORE RELIEF FOUND IN ARTHRITIS CASES

By WILLIAM L. LAURENCE

New dramatic triumphs for the recently synthesized adrenal hormone that has enabled rheumatoid arthritis cripples to walk again, and even to run and dance jigs, were reported yesterday at the Seventh International Congress on Rheumatic Diseases in the Waldorf-Astoria Hotel.

The hormone, known until now as "Compound E," was named yesterday by its discoverer, Dr. Edward C. Kendall, world renowned chemist of the Mayo Clinic, as "cortisone," an abbreviation of its long chemical name, 17-hydroxy-11-dehydro-cortico-sterone. Dr. Kendall isolated the hormone from the cortex (bark) of the adrenal glands of cattle in 1935 and played a major role in its partial synthesis, the final stages of which were accomplished after years of effort by Dr. Lewis H. Sarett of the laboratories of Merck & Co., Rahway, N.J.

In addition to its spectacular effect on crippled victims of rheumatoid arthritis, it was announced yesterday for the first time, cortisone also produced similar dramatic effects on the disabling type of arthritis that makes the back as stiff as a board, known as Strumpell Marie spondylitis. "Very significant benefits" were achieved with the hormone after nine days of treatment, it was reported by Prof. Richard H. Freyberg of the Cornell University Medical College and the New York Hospital.

Dr. Philip S. Hench of the Mayo Clinic, Rochester, Minn., who originated the treatment, in association with Dr. Kendall and Dr. Charles H. Slocumb and Dr. Howard F. Polley, reported that the same encouraging results, observed first with the new experimental approach to rheumatoid arthritis, had been observed also on three rheumatic fever victims, a disease of the young responsible for more than a third of all the deaths from heart disease, thus killing annually more than are killed by cancer.

In addition, Dr. Hench reported, cortisone had produced also striking results in the form of arthritis that frequently accompanies psoriasis, a painful and generally incurable skin disease; and in another type associated with the serious skin disease known as lupus erythematosus, characterized by eruptions of scaly red patches, frequently on the face and especially in the region of the nose.

Similar results, Dr. Hench reported, have been obtained on a smaller number of patients with a natural hormone from the pituitary gland of hogs, known as ACTH (adreno-cortico-tropic hormone).

Animal experiments have shown that cortisone influences carbohydrate metabolism (utilization) and that it increases resistance to stress, cold and to toxic substances. There were rumors during the war that the pilots of the German Luftwaffe received injections of extracts of the adrenal cortex (which contains small amounts of natural cortisone) and that this allowed them to fly at ease at an altitude of 40,000 feet or more. This rumor led the medical departments of the Army and Navy to request a large supply of the hormones of the adrenal cortex and acted as a stimulus to work on methods yielding increased quantities of the adrenal cortical hormones, it was made known yesterday.

Observations of patients who received the hormone, also revealed that it produced a state of euphoria (sense of well-being) and also increased mental capacity and activity. Studies have begun therefore, at the Mayo Clinic on the possibility of its usefulness in the treatment of mental ills.

Dr. Hench and Dr. Kendall, who presented their first detailed report on their revolutionary new approach to arthritis in this city, and illustrated it with the dramatic motion picture showing patients before and after the use of cortisone, received an ovation from the several hundred distinguished rheumatologists from this country and abroad unusual at a sedate gathering of men of medicine.

Dr. Hench and Dr. Kendall emphasized, however, that both the partly synthesized cortisone and the natural pituitary hormone (ACTH) existed at present in such minute amounts that it could be given to only a few patients at the time on an experimental basis, and that there was not enough of either substance to give to any single patient for an indefinite time.

They emphasized further that cortisone did not provide a cure, but like insulin for diabetes, or liver extract (or vitamin B-12) for pernicious anemia, it must be given regularly. Withdrawal of the hormone, they declared, causes a return of the original condition in a few days.

"At this stage," Dr. Hench said, "we are not justified even to refer to our method as a treatment, except in the investigative sense." Much work still remains to be done, he added, including determination of the optimum dose, the proper method of administering and the control of some of the "side reactions" observed in some patients to whom the hormone was given over a prolonged period of time.

From Merck & Co., which spent large sums on the final steps of the synthesis of cortisone and on the development of production methods, it was learned that everything possible was being done to speed up production but that it would not be possible to increase the present small yield until 1950, and that even then it would not be possible to meet the demand.

The difficulty arises, Dr. Kendall explained, from the fact that the starting material for the partial synthesis of cortisone is a fraction from bile known as desoxycholic acid, and that it takes sixty-five pounds of bile to yield one-half pound of the acid. Similarly, he said, it takes 1,200 hogs to produce one pound of pituitary gland, and of this only a small fraction constitutes the ACTH.

Dr. Kendall added that they were getting only one week's supply for the treatment of sixteen patients with cortisone and five with ACTH. The material is delivered weekly by plane by Merck.

While Dr. Hench and Dr. Kendall referred to their work as merely "a study," several of their colleagues, who had examined patients at the Mayo Clinic and then treated a total of nine patients themselves, hailed their work as "the real McCoy" and as a great landmark in medicine.

Those who discussed the results included, in addition to Professor Freyberg; Dr. Edward W. Boland of the University of Southern California School of Medicine, Los Angeles; Dr. Edward F. Rosenberg of the Michael Reese Hospital, Chicago; Dr. W. Paul Holbrook, president of the Arthritis and Rheumatism Foundation of Tucson, Ariz., and Prof. Walter Bauer of the Harvard Medical School, Boston.

"This is very important research," Professor Freyberg said. "Its true limit and value is inestimable, but it is the most important contribution to rheumatology. New portals are now opened and we at last have some targets to shoot at. We can give only thanks and praise to the authors of this monumental work."

Dr. Boland reported on two patients he treated with cortisone with dramatic results. One of these, a woman, was unable to lift herself out of bed, or to feed herself. "Within forty-four hours," he reported, "she walked and fed herself. After nine days of treatment she literally danced a jig."

Dr. Rosenberg reported on one patient who received the cortisone. "Within one hour," he reported, "there was extraordinary improvement. In one day he was able to run. This is one of the most significant discoveries of our generation."

Dr. Holbrook reported on two patients, one of seven and the other of two years' duration. In the latter, he said, the recovery was 100 per cent, and in the former about 85 per cent after a short period of treatment.

"This beautiful work of Dr. Hench and his associates," Dr. Holbrook said, "has opened doors wide for the study of the mechanism of the disease."

Prof. Bauer said he had treated two arthritics with cortisone and "could confirm the reports most enthusiastically." "One cannot begin fully to appreciate what really happens," he added, "until one sees the patients for himself."

"This is the real McCoy," Prof. Bauer said. "It will open up immense avenues for study of disease mechanisms."

The treatment requires an initial dose of 300 milligrams and a daily dosage of 100 milligrams. It was learned unofficially at the congress that the cost for a three-week course of treatment reached $18,000.
                                        June 1, 1949

STEROIDS CALLED BIG MEDICAL HOPE

By GLADWIN HILL

Special to THE NEW YORK TIMES.

LOS ANGELES, Sept. 18—While public attention has been focused on the remarkable effects of the hormones ACTH and cortisone ("Compound E") on arthritis, these are only two members of an extensive chemical category of vast potentialities, Dr. Harvey E. Billig Jr. said last week at a meeting of the Southern California section of the International College of Surgeons.

Presenting an informal resume of nation-wide research in this field, Dr. Billig reported "dramatic" results in arresting and correcting the ravages of such ailments as poliomyelitis, rheumatic fever, gout and even dementia praecox (schizophrenia, or split personality).

Dr. Billig is Assistant Professor of Orthopedics at the College of Medical Evangelists here and a staff member of the Hollywood Presbyterian, White Memorial and Long Beach Community Hospitals. He operates a nonprofit physical rehabilitation clinic here and is consultant to a number of large industrial organizations on employe health. In charge of Navy medical research at the California Institute of Technology during the war, he gained nation-wide note with his method of stimulating new growth on moribund nerves by pounding them with a high-speed pneumatic hammer.

The chemical category involved in the current work is steroids, a broad classification of compounds based on their chemical resemblance to cholesterol, a natural fat-like substance found in many parts of the body.

Steroid hormones, Dr. Billig explained in an interview amplifying his talk, are a natural product of human adrenal glands, ovaries and testicles, and are important in the metabolism of connective tissues like ligaments whose functioning characteristically is impaired in the diseases mentioned. Dementia praecox and some other mental disorders are accompanied by a development of fibrous tissues analogous to impaired ligaments, surrounding blood vessels in the brain, Dr. Billig said.

"Polio, for instance," he said, "does other things besides destroying nerve tissue. It inhibits steroid production by its toxic effect on secreting glands."

The deleterious effects of these diseases can be, and in thousands of cases he has treated have been, "corrected," Dr. Billig said, by artificial supply of steroids, preferably by intramuscular injection.

Such administration, he said, restores the "steroid balance" in the afflicted individual: relaxes connective tissues, reviving normal metabolism and preventing fibrosis; and in many cases leads to revival of normal glandular balance.

Such treatment, Dr. Billig emphasized, involved catching ligament deterioration and contraction before it went too far; properly assessing the steroid unbalance in the individual and administering accordingly; and accompanying the medication with proper muscular manipulation treatments and exercise.

If the re-stretching of ligaments contracted by disease and steroid unbalance is too violent, he said, new fibrous tissue may form and make rehabilitation even more difficult.

Because of these factors, Dr. Billig said he was reluctant to go into detail about the steroids he was using, aside from the fact that testosterone, the male sex hormone, and whole adrenal cortex played important parts.

"I don't have any better steroids than anybody else has," he commented. "Everybody is hunting steroids."

Dr. Billig said he had used steroids derived from both plants and animals, and that the cost was within reach of average-income patients.

A typical case of rehabilitating impaired connective tissue might take several months, with steroid injections being gradually "tapered off." Some patients, he said, reported continued well-being after a period of years, while others would revert to steroid unbalance and require a new series of injections, usually at a reduced rate.

In dementia praecox, Dr. Billig said, improvement usually took at least several days "but sometimes it comes within a few hours." He said he had never treated any severe, commitable cases, but had observed remarkable improvement in many "mild" cases.

In polio, he emphasized, steroids did not promise repair on nerve damage which is an important phase of the disease's effects, but only of the concomitant muscle fibre deterioration.

Dr. Billig emphasized also that he was only one of many individuals working along similar lines, there being centers of study at Stanford University, the Mayo Clinic and Harvard University among other places.

His work, he said, had stemmed initially from the report of Dr. F. L. Hisaw, now of Harvard, in 1926 on experimental relaxation of the ligaments in guinea pigs.

The use of steroids to counteract glandular deficiencies in some ailments was a logical outgrowth, he related, of insulin and electric shock treatments for mental disorders, in which one of the main results was stimulation of the pituitary gland. This in turn activated the adrenal, ovarian and testicular glands, with a resultant marked increase in steroid output.

A prominent researcher in this field has been Dr. C. A. G. Wiersma of the California Institute of Technology, with whom Dr. Billig has collaborated.

Dr. Billig, who is 42 years old, graduated from the Stanford University Medical School in 1932, was resident in orthopedics at the Long Island College Medical School Hospital in 1934, and subsequently had a two-year teaching fellowship at the Harvard Medical School.

September 19, 1949

PENICILLIN'S VALUE IN SYPHILIS PROVED

The first four patients treated with penicillin for syphilis were recently re-examined, after a lapse of six years, and found still to be entirely free of symptoms of the disease.

This was reported yesterday by Dr. John F. Mahoney, a medical director of the United States Public Health Service, who six years ago thought penicillin should be effective against syphilis and promptly put his theory to the test with four patients. He re-examined the patients last October after tracing them around the world.

Dr. Mahoney will retire today, after thirty years in the service, to become director of the city Bureau of Laboratories. He has been director of the venereal disease laboratory at the United States Marine Hospital on Staten Island.

The initial disclosure that penicillin might be the long-sought-after, non-toxic compound for use against syphilis was made Oct. 14, 1943. A cautiously worded report written by Dr. Mahoney and his associates, Dr. R. C. Arnold and Dr. Ad Harris, held promise that the search for an anti-syphilitic drug might be at an end.

But the disease is one that naturally tends to reoccur after periods during which no symptoms are evident, and for this reason it was difficult to prove that penicillin "cures" syphilis.

The original four patients were seamen. They received a total of forty-eight injections at four-hour intervals. The period of treatment used at first was eight days. After this course of medication the investigators were able only to affirm that all the symptoms of the disease had disappeared.

After seventy-two months, Dr. Mahoney reported in the December issue of the Journal of Venereal Disease Information, the symptoms were still missing and this had proved that the antibiotic had been effective for at least six years.

With improvements in the technique for using penicillin, the standard treatment for syphilis has been reduced in many cases to a single injection that does not incapacitate the patient.

Wide-spread use of the injections has caused the rate of new cases of the disease to decrease recently and Dr. Mahoney said "we believe that we are getting the disease well under control."

Dr. Mahoney urged that new drugs that are known to be non-toxic be used to treat human patients before they are completely assayed in tests with laboratory animals.

December 16, 1949

SCIENTISTS REPORT NEW 'WONDER DRUG'

Discovery and development of a powerful new drug, effective in animal tests against a wide variety of infectious diseases, is reported in the current issue of Science, official organ of the American Association for the Advancement of Science, by a team of eleven scientists from the research laboratories of Charles Pfizer & Co., Inc., of Brooklyn.

The new chemical, named terramycin, was isolated from a soil organism related to the mold that produces streptomycin, after testing more than 100,000 soil samples from all over the world. It was derived from a new organism of the large family of actinomycetes (soil molds), to which has been given the name streptomyces rimosus.

The newest member of the "wonder drug" family known as antibiotics (germ fighters produced by living micro-organisms) has been found in laboratory and animal tests to be absorbed readily in the body after administration by mouth or by injection. The animal studies also indicate that terramycin has a very low toxicity, being tolerated in large doses.

Preliminary clinical studies on the new drug, the company announced, have been started at the New York Hospital-Cornell University Medical Center and are now being expanded in many hospitals throughout the nation and abroad.

These studies are designed to evaluate the effectiveness of terramycin in man in the treatment of pneumococcal and virus pneumonia, hemolytic streptococcal infections, staphylococcal infections, undulant fever, whooping cough, enteric and urinary tract infections, and certain rickettsial diseases, such as typhus fever.

In high concentrations, the report says, terramycin "appears to inhibit the infection of the chick embryo with the PRS strain of influenza A virus."

"On the basis of experimental data now available, terramycin offers great promise in the treatment of numerous infections," the Pfizer company announcement says, emphasizing, however, that "until the clinical studies have been completed, the true value of the chemical as a chemotherapeutic agent in man will not be known."

The investigations are reported by Dr. Gladys L. Hobby, Dr. S. Y. P'an, Dr. P. P Regna, Dr J. B. Routien, Dr. D. B. Seeley, Dr. G. M. Shull and Dr. B. A. Sobin and Messrs. A. C. Finlay, I. A. Solomons, J. W. Vinson and J. H. Kane. The scientific team consists of bacteriologists, pharmacologists, organic chemists, microbiologists and a virologist.

Charles Pfizer & Co., which celebrated the 100th anniversary of its founding last year, is the world's largest producer of penicillin and streptomycin. The company's background in fermentation chemistry played a major role in producing penicillin in large quantities during the war to satisfy the needs of our armed forces.

January 27, 1950

X-RAY CHAIR—

An advanced type of rotating chair, to be used in the X-ray treatment of deep-seated tumors, has been devised by Dr. V. V. A. Low-Beer of the University of California School of Medicine, and Max Tobi an industrial engineer. The chair, completed after two years of engineering effort, is already being used in the experimental treatment of cancer in selected cases. The chair should make it possible to aim the X-ray beam more accurately, decrease the radiation dose inevitably received by normal tissue, lessen the untoward side effects of X-radiation, and make possible the delivery of higher doses of destructive X-radiation to a tumor. The tumor forms the central rotational axis on which the chair and body turn. As the chair slowly rotates, the X-ray beam is always trained on the tumor. The tumor therefore receives five to ten times as much radiation as any given section of skin and other intervening tissues. The chair can be turned at any desired speed, rotated in a complete circle, made to oscillate on a given arc or reciprocate. The first chair was a western saddle. In the end a tractor seat was selected. W. K.

January 21, 1951

EARLY CANCER DIAGNOSIS

Way Is Given to Spot Malady in Uterus Prior to Symptoms

Special to The New York Times.

WASHINGTON, Nov. 18—The possibility of discovering cancer of the uterine cervix and starting treatment five to seven years before typical symptoms appear was reported today by the Public Health Service.

This diagnosis may be made through the cytologic test and biopsy, the announcement said. Biopsy consists of a laboratory test of a small specimen of tissue for cancer, and the cytologic test is made by taking a smear from the surface of the cervix for laboratory examination. The latter usually indicates whether a biopsy should be made.

The Public Health Service report was based on examination of a group of more than 3,000 women at a clinic that was operated by the Cancer Control Branch of the National Cancer Clinic at Hot Springs, Ark.

Drs. Rodney B. Nelson and Albert W. Hilberg assembled the data.

November 19, 1951

New TB Drugs Are Revealed As Cheap Coal-Tar Synthetics

By WILLIAM L. LAURENCE

The identity of the "wonder drugs" that have given new life to nearly 200 victims of advanced tuberculosis, as well as other facts hitherto kept secret, were revealed yesterday at a special press interview called by Dr. Marcus D. Kogel, Commissioner of Hospitals, in his offices at 125 Worth Street.

Corroboration of the news about the new anti-TB agents, published in THE NEW YORK TIMES yesterday, came from two other authoritative sources at another interview in the offices of the National Tuberculosis Association, 1790 Broadway.

It was learned that the Federal Food and Drug Administration had been requested to study the new compounds for approval of use by physicians generally. That approval, it was said, is expected by May or June, at which time large-scale production of the compounds will start, provided they live up to their early promise. The drugs are pure synthetics that can be made cheaply from coal tar, and it was estimated they might eventually cost about fifty cents a tablet.

It also was estimated that the cost of treating the disease with the new chemicals, should they confirm expectations, might be reduced to less than $100 for each patient. The average cost for treating a case of tuberculosis now is about $3,500.

It was stressed at both conferences that while the results so far were dramatic, they were still far from conclusive and probably several months would be required for further clinical trials. On the other hand, it was made clear that the results indicated powerful new weapons, the first of possibly scores of their kind, had been added to the medical arsenal for the fight against mankind's greatest infectious scourge.

Dr. Kogel said that while the results to date had been "very encouraging," he wished "to emphasize the fact that the use of the drugs is still in the experimental stage."

The pioneer tests, he said, were carried out in the last eight months at Seaview Hospital on Staten Island, one of the municipal tuberculosis institutions, under the direction of Dr. George G. Ornstein, director of the Department of Medicine at Seaview, in close collaboration with Dr. Edward H. Robitzek, acting director of the Seaview Department of Medicine, and Dr. Irving J. Selikoff, associate visiting physician.

Three new chemicals have been tested. All are relatives of niacin, the anti-pellagra vitamin, a member of the vitamin B complex group originally known as vitamin B-3. They were produced independently by two pharmaceutical firms, Hoffmann-La Roche, Inc., of Nutley, N. J., and E. R. Squibb & Sons, New Brunswick, N. J.

The chemicals are known as isomers of niacin. One is isonicotinic acid hydrazine, with the trade names Rimifon, by Hoffmann-La Roche, and Nydrazid, by Squibb. The second, a derivative of the first, is 1-isonicotiny-2-isopropyl hydrazine, with the trade name Marsilid, by La Roche. A third is a glucosyl derivative of the first. Of the three, the first has proved so far the most effective.

These three, it was pointed out, are the forerunners of possibly several hundred similar derivatives to be developed in the future. In this fact lies great hope that these compounds will prove the long-sought weapons against the tough and resourceful TB bacillus, which always has managed to develop a resistance against any drug devised by science to combat it. As was pointed out at one of the conferences yesterday, should the germ develop a resistance against one, other derivatives could be devised to fight these resistant strains.

190 Patients Treated

In all, 190 patients who had not responded to any of the present methods of treatment, including the antibiotic streptomycin and PAS—para-amino-salicylic acid, an anti-TB drug widely used in conjunction with streptomycin—as well as the surgical approaches, and for whom there was no hope, received the niacin derivatives.

In administering the drugs as a last desperate hope, after they had been found to be highly effective against TB germs in the test tube as well as in a series of animal experiments, the Seaview physicians watched them "stop the disease right in its track," Dr. Kogel said.

So far, Dr. Robitzek and Dr. Selikoff reported, no evidence of the development of germ resistance has been observed. Nor have they detected any effect on hearing, as is the case with streptomycin, or any relapses. The evidence so far indicates the chemicals are bactericidal—that is, germ killers—rather than bacteriostatic, or inhibitors of the germs' growth.

Many of the patients had fevers with temperatures ranging from 100 to 105 degrees. In all of these, the Seaview physicians reported, the temperature returned to normal in two to three weeks. In a number of cases the temperature dropped "precipitously."

Within a week, the physicians added, the patients—all of whom were emaciated and had been refusing food—developed "ravenous appetites." One ate as many as eleven eggs for breakfast. A female patient who had declined from 185 pounds to 97, regained 84

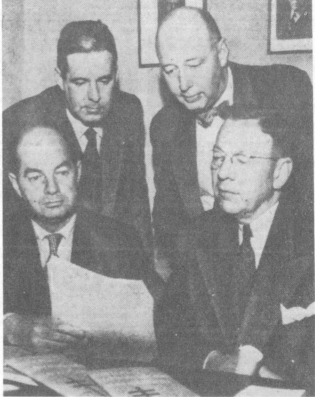

DISCUSSING DISCOVERY OF NEW DRUGS

The New York Times

Research experts conferring on find that raised hopes of eradicating tuberculosis. In the front row are Dr. Geoffrey Rake, left, director of the Squibb Institute for Medical Research, and Dr. Elmer Sevringhaus, director of clinical research of Hoffman-La Roche, Inc. Standing are Dr. Walsh McDermott, left, editor of The American Review of Tuberculosis, and Dr. James E. Perkins, managing director of the National Tuberculosis Association.

pounds in nine weeks. Another gained as much as 95 pounds in a similar period. They then leveled off after reaching normal weight.

The fact that the drugs can be given by mouth, Dr. Kogel pointed out, opens up the possibility of developing a program of home care for the city's tuberculous patients, with a consequent saving of many millions on hospitalized cases. Dr. Kogel said he planned to begin work next month on a home-care program in cooperation with Dr. John F. Mahoney, Commissioner of Health.

There are now more than 5,000 tuberculosis patients in New York City hospitals, each costing the city $8-9 a day, or a total of more than $16,000,000 a year.

The new development, Dr. Kogel said, also may require a revaluation of the city's construction program for additional TB hospitals. Among the projects still in the planning stage are the Seton Hospital, in the Bronx, with 500 beds; a Welfare Island TB unit with 1,500 beds, and a West Side Harlem TB hospital, with 500 beds.

Furthermore, hundreds of beds in existing TB hospitals, it was pointed out, may be made available for victims of other diseases, thus greatly expanding the city's hospital facilities.

The basic niacin derivative, iso-niacin hydrazine, was originally synthesized in Germany in 1912 by two young chemists, H. Meyer and J. Mally, but no one suspected at the time that it was good for anything. It, and the other derivatives, were synthesized again in 1942 in the laboratories of Hoffmann-La Roche by Dr. H. Herbert Fox, J. Lee and Ziering. Even then, however, its value in the treatment of TB was not recognized.

Meantime, a group of chemists working in the Squibb laboratories synthesized the compounds independently.

Experiments Described

Dr. Geoffrey Rake, director of the Squibb Institute for Medical Research, said at the conference in the offices of the National Tuberculosis Association that in the test tube and in mice iso-niacin hydrazine "has demonstrated spectacular activity against tubercle bacilli."

"It appears," he said, "to be many hundreds of times more effective than PAS and, significantly, more effective than streptomycin" (previously the most valuable anti-TB agent). He added that "in extensive animal tests conducted by Squibb Institute workers it was found that the effective dose is reached substantially before a toxic dose."

The compound, Dr. Rake reported, is under clinical investigation by Dr. Walsh McDermott and Dr. Carl Muschenheim at the New York Hospital-Cornell Medical Center. He said that in effective doses "it is well absorbed and well tolerated when given by mouth, according to these investigators."

"The compound is also being investigated for tuberculous meningitis as well as in the more common tuberculosis of the chest," he said.

The studies at the Seaview Hospital have shown, according to Hoffmann-LaRoche, that the chemicals are effective in forms of tuberculosis other than pulmonary or lung infection. Tuberculosis of the throat, the tongue, the intestinal tract and other tissues, it was reported, responds to treatment with these drugs. A beneficial

effect also has been noted in bone tuberculosis, which is the most persistent form of the disease, and in meningitis, the most deadly variety.

Believed to Be Inexpensive

"Up to now," the Hoffmann-LaRoche statement points out, "the compounds have been prepared only in very limited quantities for clinical investigation. If these drugs should prove to be suitable for general use, commercial production will have to be started, and until that time the cost of these compounds will not be definitely known."

However, it is believed that the compounds will be relatively simple and inexpensive and may be expected to become available to physicians within a few months.

Commissioner Mahoney said the new therapy apparently was "a godsend." The Department of Health, he added, "will proceed as rapidly as possible to use this new method of treatment." A precise program for the use of the chemicals, with plans for further study, will be undertaken. "That," he said, "will involve training of the Department of Health tuberculosis clinicians and intensification of Health Department case findings."

Dr. James E. Perkins, man-

aging director of the National Tuberculosis Association, warned that "no drug would solve the TB problem quickly, no matter how good the drug is." Even when drugs work, he emphasized, patients "still must rest and get other treatment, and people with unknown cases of TB still must be discovered to start treatment."

It was pointed out further that while the drugs might destroy TB germs and stop the disease, they could not restore damaged lungs or other tissues ravaged by the disease. Existing lesions would still have to be treated by orthodox medical or surgical methods.

February 22, 1952

CAUTION IS ADVISED IN ANTIBIOTICS' USE

Special to THE NEW YORK TIMES.

CHICAGO, Feb. 26—Serious and sometimes fatal reaction to the use of "miracle drugs" demands that these antibiotics should be used with the utmost caution, Dr. Harold A. Shoemaker, Professor of Pharmacology of the University of Oklahoma School of Medicine, today told a conference of the Academy of Forensic Sciences here.

Dr. Shoemaker warned that "there are no miracle drugs." The true miracle of modern medicine, he added, is in the progress of diagnosis and treatment and in the dissemination of all possible information to the physician who uses this knowledge for the benefit of his patients.

Dr. Shoemaker told the gathering of 100 physicians, toxicologists and teachers in the organic fields of medicine that the antibiotics had saved many lives.

"Many patients are alive today because of their use," he said, "and no physician should hesitate to use the antibiotics when they are indicated."

He said, however, that two recent reports, one of them from the Mayo Clinic in Rochester, Minn., had established that two of the most widely used antibiotics, terramycin and aureomycin, had been responsible for a number of deaths in cases where the drugs themselves encouraged dangerous bacteria to multiply in the intestinal tracts of patients.

In his paper, "Untoward Reactions to Antibiotics," Dr. Shoemaker declared illnesses induced by the antibiotics had resulted from the drug's "superinfections."

This, in turn, he declared, resulted from the fact that a new race of bacteria was able to resist the action of aureomycin and terramycin.

In one group covered by the reports, Dr. Shoemaker said, seven of the ninety-one patients under study had died. In another report, fourteen of 112 cases studied suc-

cumbed to the malady.

Dr. Shoemaker asserted that Dr. P. T. Sloss, Mayo Clinic pathologist, had compared the fatal illness resulting from the use of terramycin and aureomycin to cholera-like symptoms.

When properly used, Dr. Shoemaker declared, the antibiotics were found to be "remarkably safe drugs."

Among other speakers heard at the opening session of the fifth annual meeting of the academy were Dr. R. N. Harger, president of the society, and Dr. Alexander O. Gettler, toxicologist of the office of the Chief Medical Examiner of New York City.

The American Academy membership includes criminologists, pathologists, toxicologists, fingerprints experts, bacteriologists, experts on documents, medical legal authorities and others. It was founded in St. Louis, Mo., in 1948. The conference will continue through Saturday. Dr. Gettler will be cited at a dinner tomorrow night for his accomplishments in the field of toxicology.

Reaction to Penicillin Cited
Special to THE NEW YORK TIMES

BOSTON, Feb. 26—The common use of penicillin contained in ordinary drug store items is creating "explosive reactions" at an accelerated rate, delegates to the annual meeting of the American Academy of Allergy heard today.

Four panelists said that the drug was most popularly found in such items as ointments, nose drops, lozenges and tooth paste. They cautioned against the use of penicillin when its employment was not indicated.

The reactions to excessive use of products containing penicillin were reported as ranging from outbreak of hives to cases of immediate shock. Since 1949, the panelists said, there have been seven fatalities.

The panel participants were Drs. William P. Boger of Philadelphia, Irving W. Schiller of Boston and William B. Sherman and Sheppard Siegal, both of New York. Dr. Bram Rose of Montreal was the moderator.

February 27, 1953

Waging the Hot War on Cancer

A fresh attack on the nation's second greatest killer may be the outgrowth of current research into new chemical agents.

By LEONARD ENGEL

CANCER is now responsible for two of every fifteen deaths in the United States, with a current toll of more than 225,000 victims a year. It far outweighs any other disease as a cause of death, except diseases of the heart and circulatory system.

This is both a mark of progress and a challenge. The success of modern medicine in reducing deaths from many diseases has inevitably made deaths from others go up. When proper allowance is made for the growth of our population and for the increasing proportion of people in older, cancer-susceptible age-groups, there has actually been no change in the rate of deaths from most forms of cancer, and even a slight drop in one form. The single exception to this is cancer of the lung. A real and rapid rise has taken place in recent years in the incidence of lung cancer among men—a rise which is related by one school of cancer specialists to cigarette smoking,

LEONARD ENGEL, a writer who regularly reports on scientific matters, has followed the progress of cancer research for many years.

but which, in the view of others, also involves other and possibly more important factors.

There is indirect, but genuine, evidence of progress on the cancer front. The diagnosis and reporting of deaths due to cancer have greatly improved. Many cases are uncovered now that would have escaped detection two decades ago. Since the reported age- and population-adjusted rates have remained stationary or gone down (except for lung cancer), the real death rates for most forms of cancer must have dropped. So the vast effort against cancer has produced results, even though the cancer problem is essentially unsolved.

AFTER years of disappointment, however, solid hope for a solution is emerging from a somewhat unexpected quarter—the world's chemistry laboratories. In the past, the hopes of cancer researchers have been focused largely on the finding of a simple, universally applicable test for detecting cancer at an early stage, when it might be most amenable to surgery and X-ray. Time has dimmed these particular hopes. A

really simple early detection test seems to many researchers to be as far away as ever. For reasons that will presently become clear, it also seems unlikely that surgery and X-ray can be made much more effective than they now are—which is not effective enough.

But chemists have begun to find chemical agents that cure certain types of cancer in animals and are not too toxic for practical use, and that interfere, or a time at least, with the growth of human cancerous tissue. The Sloan-Kettering Institute recently reported that one anti-cancer chemical cures all cases of a certain type of cancer in rats. Another has cured 83 per cent of a type of bone cancer in mice. Still others cured almost all cases of a mouse leukemia. According to cancer researchers, the chances are good that other and still more effective drugs will be found.

Cancer researchers take this optimistic view because the search for anti-cancer chemicals begins with one of the few things we really know about cancer. By definition, a cancer is a growth. The cells of which it is composed multiply more rapidly than normal cells. Since chemical processes

underlie all events in the living cell, the cancer cell's rapid multiplication bespeaks a chemical difference between cancerous and normal cells.

Modern chemical research has proved itself brilliantly able to exploit just such differences. Examples are the sulfa drugs and antibiotics. These drugs have revolutionized the treatment of infectious disease because they are toxic to germs, but not to the tissues of the patient. (Otherwise, they could not be used.) This "differential toxicity" depends on chemical differences between microbial cells and the cells of man, differences comparable to those that must exist between normal and malignant tissue.

A CONVENIENT starting point for examining the cancer problem is a brief summary of what is known about cancer. Cancerous growths can occur in almost any part of the body, but the most frequent are cancers of the stomach, large intestine and rectum, breast, uterus, prostate gland, lung and skin.

Some cancers grow slowly and kill only when they become large enough to interfere with the functioning of a vital organ; in medical parlance, they are not highly malignant. Highly malignant cancers, on the other hand, grow rapidly and metastasize, or give off daughter cells which are spread widely through the body and give rise to distant growths; such tumors kill by disorganizing wide segments of the body economy.

The intense cancer research effort of recent years has amassed a vast store of information, some of it quite odd, about cancer. For instance, certain animal cancers are caused by viruses, and one cancer-like disease of man, a form of leukemia called Hodgkin's disease, almost surely.

Further, ulcer of the duodenum (the first few inches of small intestine after the stomach) seems to protect against stomach cancer; in any case, individuals who have or who have had a duodenal ulcer seldom develop stomach cancer. And many cancers have the appearance, under the microscope, of embryonic tissue, a fact which has given rise to the theory that some cancers at least stem from unmatured cells or clumps of cells left over, so to speak, from the prenatal life.

BUT what would cause these embryonic tissues to resume growing and turn into cancers after lying dormant for years—or, indeed, what causes any kind of tissue to become cancerous—is another matter. Cancer researchers have bred strains of animals in which hereditary factors precipitate the formation of a particular cancer at a particular time of life in a high proportion of the animals. But heredity has not been found to play any such direct part in human cancer.

Tumors have also been induced in laboratory animals by literally hundreds of other agents, including radioactive materials, X-rays, ultra-violet light, mechanical irritation, certain coal-tar derivatives and the salts of some metals. But only a few of these have been known to induce human cancer, and then in only a relatively small proportion of cases. Thus, carelessness in handling radioactive materials and X-ray equipment is responsible for some cases of

human cancer, and constant exposure to strong sunlight in the wide-open spaces of Texas and the Southwest for a fair number of skin cancers. What is actually responsible for most cancers, though, remains a mystery.

The one thing that is sure is that something present in normal cells is missing or prevented from acting in cancer cells. This is whatever it is that limits the growth of normal cells.

IN one of the most brilliant chapters in the whole history of science, it has been found over the past decade and a half that the body is a simmering cauldron of ceaseless chemical activity. The materials of which the body is made are constantly being torn down and built up, even the material of something as seemingly inert as bone. But all this activity, which goes on to the end of life, stops short of the creation of new cells except when new cells are needed. New cells are formed during growth or to repair wounds and to replace worn tissue, but, under ordinary circumstances, not otherwise.

There are many theories as to what keeps this cell activity within such precisely ordered bounds. Cancer investigators have an obvious interest in the question, and many are studying it. But thus far little has been learned that could lead to a means of re-endowing cancer cells with more normal behavior.

Fortunately, it may not be necessary to find such a means to deal with cancer in a practical way. There is one other point of which researchers may be sure and which provides a lever for attacking the cancer problem.

Every living cell—whether a liver cell or a reproductive germ cell, whether the' cell of

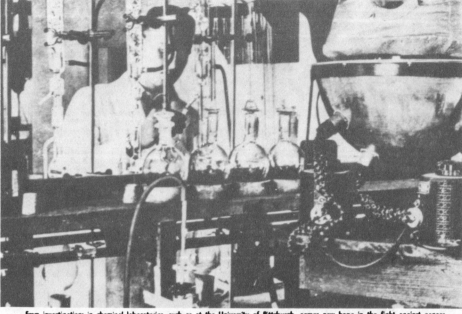

From investigations in chemical laboratories, such as at the University of Pittsburgh, comes new hope in the fight against cancer.

a man or a microbe, and whether normal or malignant - contains a set of genes bearing the hereditary characteristics of the cell and, also, of the organism of which the cell is part. When cells multiply, the genes are reduplicated so that each daughter cell may have a set of genic material. This process proceeds more rapidly in cancerous than in normal cells; in fact, synthesis of genic material does not take place at all in cells that are not multiplying.

A DOZEN or so years ago, it occurred to a young college chemistry instructor named George H. Hitchings that cancer might be fought by blocking the formation of genic material, and thus preventing cancerous cells from multiplying. Dr. Hitchings, who is now at the Wellcome Research Laboratories in Tuckahoe, N. Y., proposed to find agents that would block the formation of a substance named D. N. A. or desoxyribonucleic acid, then thought and now known to be the most important constituent of genes. Since then, the search has been joined by other notable investigators, such as Dr. Howard E. Skipper of the Southern Research Institute in Birmingham, Ala.

Over the years, Dr. Hitchings and his associates alone have fabricated more than 500 compounds resembling one or another of the simpler chemicals out of which D. N. A. (an enormously complex substance) is fashioned in the cell. Many do block the formation of D. N. A. and the multiplication of cancer cells. One, 6-mercaptopurine, has proved one of the most valuable drugs available for treating leukemia. Another, newly discovered thioguanine, promises to be as useful.

The formation of D. N. A. can be blocked not only by supplying false building blocks for D. N. A. itself, but by interfering in the same artful way with the enzymes and other cellular chemical agents that help in forming D. N. A. Indeed, some of the first

chemicals found active against cancer are believed to block D. N. A.-building enzymes rather than D. N. A. itself.

None of the anti-cancer chemicals so far uncovered has cured a case of cancer in man. Dr. Hitchings himself thinks no single one ever will, because of the readiness with which cancer cells become resistant to the present anti-cancer drugs. He and others believe, however, that a highly effective combination of agents can be found, with each blocking D. N. A. formation in a different way and with each contributing its quota of cancer cells destroyed, to the point where the tumor as a whole is eliminated.

One of the attractive features of such a chemical attack on cancer is that it could escape the limitations of both surgery and radiation. The effectiveness of surgery in treating cancer is limited by the difficulty of finding and cutting out the bits and pieces of a tumor that has metastasized. Chemical agents, carried everywhere in the body by the bloodstream, could track them down unerringly, as penicillin tracks invading germs. Radiation's effectiveness is limited by the fact that cancer tissue is not much more sensitive to it than normal tissue; a dose of X-rays strong enough to destroy a cancer will always be dangerous to near-by normal cells.

"Cancer chemotherapy," says Dr. Joseph Burchenall, a Memorial Center physician who has been in the thick of the testing of new anti-cancer agents, "is in its infancy. In certain forms of leukemia among children, in which chemotherapy is most effective, it has lengthened survival from four or five to twelve months or more for only half our cases. In breast and prostate cancer, hormone therapy—which is also a form of chemotherapy — lengthens life by some months. For most forms of cancer, surgery and radiation are still the best method of treatment.

"BUT the chemical attack has provided cancer research

with a powerful and hopeful rationale. Through the work particularly of Dr. Hitchings, we have a definite goal—the exploitation of the great difference between normal and cancer cells in the formation of genic material."

The road to more effective chemotherapy agents for cancer (barring a stroke of luck) seems likely to be long and arduous. In the laboratory of Dr. Chester Stock at Memorial Center, the American Cancer Society is financing a center for the testing of potential anti-cancer drugs prepared by Dr. Hitchings, Dr. Skipper and some of Memorial's own researchers, and in laboratories throughout the U. S.

As of the beginning of April, Dr. Stock's laboratory has had to test more than 12,000 compounds, to find 250 with any sign of anti-cancer activity and a dozen that are good enough and safe enough to be given to patients. The cancer researcher's goal has finally become clearer, but it may still be distant.

IN the meantime, there is much that can be done to reduce the toll of cancer. Cancer specialists like to point, however, to a simple set of figures to show what might be accomplished.

According to a study by Dr. Louis Dublin, recently retired chief statistician of the Metropolitan Life Insurance Company, the death rate from cancer among physicians, who are better able to recognize its early signs than the man in the street, is only 81 per cent of the rate in the general male population. And the rate among surgeons, who are more expert still in recognizing the early signs, is only 81 per cent of the rate among physicians, or 66 per cent of the rate in the general population.

If present efforts for early detection of cancer could be only half as effective among the general public as among surgeons, the number of deaths from cancer in the U. S. would be reduced by no less than 40,000 a year.

Child Polio Immunity Tests Are Assayed as Beneficial

By WILLIAM L. LAURENCE
Special to THE NEW YORK TIMES.

CLEVELAND, Oct. 22 — An army of 55,000 children scored the greatest victory won so far in the relentless war against polio. The story is one of the great epics of modern medicine.

The story was told today at the annual meeting of the American Public Health Association. It was the first report on the results of the far-reaching, large-scale field tests carried out in Utah, Texas and Iowa in 1951 and in this year in the midst of raging polio epidemics with a blood fraction known as gamma globulin, or GG for short. The GG is known to be the blood's precious treasure-house in which the body stores its life-saving immunity factors known as antibodies.

In the history-making tests, one-half of 55,000 children in the three states, in the age group of one to eleven years, received injections of GG by muscle, while to the other half, of the same age group and environment, injections were given of a gelatin solution that contained no protective immunity agents of any kind.

Both solutions looked exactly alike and the doctors administering them did not know which was which. Each vial had a secret code number locked in a safe for purposes of later identification by those in charge of the study.

$1,000,000 Grant for Study

The human field trials, largest ever conducted in medical history, were made possible by a grant of $1,000,000 of the March of Dimes funds by the National Foundation of Infantile Paralysis, for the purpose of determining the value of GG as a preventive of the paralytic form of polio.

Today the report on the results, long awaited, was presented by the scientists who carried out the tests. The invisible antibodies, the tests have revealed, give "marked protection" against all three types of paralytic polio for at least five weeks.

This is the first time, it was asserted, "that any material has been scientifically proved to be effective in preventing human paralytic polio."

The pioneer field study was directed by Dr. William McD. Hammon, Professor of Epidemiology at the University of Pittsburgh's Graduate School of Public Health. He presented the report this morning.

Dr. Lewis L. Coriell, medical director of the Camden (N. J.) Municipal Hospital for Contagious Diseases, was deputy director of the project and Dr. Joseph Stokes Jr., physician-in-chief of the Children's Hospital in Philadelphia, acted as over-all consultant.

Others associated in the tests were Dr. Paul F. Wehrle of the United States Public Health Service, and Dr. Christian R. Klimt, fellow of the Rockefeller Foundation, assisted by physicians and nurses from other institutions and local agencies in the areas involved.

Project Aided by Red Cross

The gamma globulin used in the trials was furnished by the American Red Cross and was prepared from blood collected during World War II from tens of thousands of blood donors in different parts of the country.

Dr. Hammon disclosed that other scientists had determined that one lot of GG contained considerable quantities of antibodies in approximately equal amounts against all three types of polio virus. Whether other stocks of GG, prepared by commercial sources from the plasma of smaller groups of donors contain similar amounts of antibodies is undetermined.

The tests took place during severe polio epidemics in and around Provo, Utah; Houston, Tex., and Sioux City, Iowa. The Provo trials took place in September, 1951. The others were in July of this year.

A total of 5,767 children in the Provo area, aged two to eight years, participated in the tests. The total in the Houston area was 33,137, aged one through six years. In the Sioux City area a total of 15,868 children, aged from one through eleven, were injected.

Thus a grand total of 54,772 children participated in the field tests, 27,386 receiving the gamma globulin and the others, serving as the control group, being injected with the gelatin.

Of the total number injected with the gelatin, sixty-four children, Dr. Hammon reported, came down with paralytic polio, as compared with only twenty-six for those injected with the GG. These figures show that the GG protected thirty-eight children from developing paralytic polio, the only type studied in the tests.

Dr. Hammon reported that in the first week following the GG injection there was little, if any, protection observed. Nearly as many polio cases occurred in the GG group during the first week as in the gelatin control group.

However, the polio cases in the GG group were mild, he added, and within thirty days half of them had recovered completely as compared with no recoveries at all in the control group. While not conclusive, said Dr. Hammon, this indicates that GG may modify the severity of polio during the late stages of the incubation period of the disease, though it may fail to prevent the disease completely if given after the infection had taken hold.

A sharp rise in protection occurred during the second week following injection of GG and was maintained through the fifth week, Dr. Hammon reported.

"During the second week," he said, "there was a marked difference between the number of polio cases in the gamma globulin and the gelatin groups—three and twenty-three cases, respectively. The reduction appears to be great-

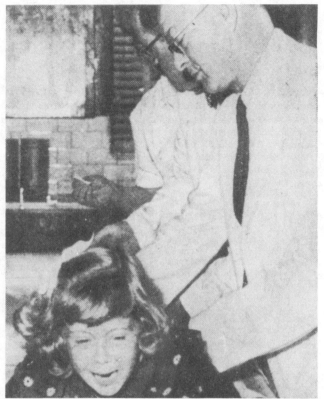

Associated Press

ANTI-POLIO INJECTION: Patricia Ann Burnett, 5 years old, gives some indication of her feelings as she receives first shot in test of gamma globulin for protection against infantile paralysis in Houston last July. Dr. Byron York, president of the Harrison County Medical Association, administers the injection.

est during this week, but protection appears to have continued during the fifth week.

"From the second through the fifth week only six cases occurred among those receiving gamma globulin and thirty-eight among those receiving gelatin. This difference is highly significant."

No one taking part in the local field trials—not even the investigators themselves—knew which child received the blood fraction and which the gelatin until at least thirty days after the onset of polio had occurred through natural exposure. The syringes containing the GG and the gelatin were taken from the carton at random. Both looked exactly alike. The serial number on the syringe was entered on the child's record card for later identification.

The syringes containing the GG and the gelatin were prepared by a pharmaceutical house and packed fifty to the carton—twenty-five of the GG and twenty-five of the placebo. The factory's record of the syringe serial numbers was locked away in a safe and not opened until last Oct. 1, when the analysis was made.

The dosages of the GG and the gelatin varied according to the body weight of the children, averaging 0.14 cubic centimeters a pound of body weight, about one-quarter of an ounce for a fifty-pound child.

Basil O'Connor, president of the National Foundation for Infantile Paralysis, warned that "good as the results are we are still very far from the ultimate goal, an effective and safe vaccine that would provide long term immunity as

compared with the rather brief protection provided by the gamma globulin."

He stressed the fact that there were 46,000,000 children and adolescents in the age group susceptible to polio and that the quantity of gamma globulin available was only a minute fraction of the amount that would be required to give even temporary protection to that number.

The gamma globulin, it was explained, gives only passive immunity, an immunity provided by the introduction into a subject's bloodstream of ready-made immunity bodies produced in an animal, or in another human being who had been exposed to the disease. This type of immunity lasts only a short time.

The most effective form of immunity is that produced by the body either as the result of a natural infection or by the induction of a mild infection by means of a vaccine composed of killed or attenuated germs.

The finding that gamma globulin will afford protection against paralytic polio, Mr. O'Connor asserted, will increase greatly the need for blood donations, with an estimate of at least 2,000,000 additional pints being required for polio alone.

On the other hand, Mr. O'Connor added, the outbreak of polio this year is the worst in history, 60,000 cases, in forty-seven states.

Dr. Hammon cautioned that many further studies must be made to evaluate the role of GG as a protective against paralytic polio.

October 23, 1952

Vaccine for Polio Successful; Use in 1 to 3 Years Is Likely

By WILLIAM L. LAURENCE

A vaccine against polio that has been used safely and successfully in preliminary trials on ninety children and adults, producing protective immunity bodies against all the three viruses causing the disease, was announced last night at a special meeting at the Waldorf-Astoria Hotel under the auspices of the National Foundation for Infantile Paralysis.

The vaccine was described by Dr. Jonas E. Salk, Professor of Research Bacteriology at the University of Pittsburgh, who headed the team of scientists in developing it with the aid of March of Dimes funds. A technical report by Dr. Salk and his associates appears in the issue of The Journal of the American Medical Association out today.

There are three types of polio virus, known as Brunhilde, Lansing and Leon. The vaccine has been found to provide protection against all three. In many cases, Dr. Salk reported, the quantity of antibodies (immunity factors) produced by the vaccine was greater than the number produced naturally in persons who had been exposed to one or more of the viruses.

Dr. Salk warned, however, that further experimentation would be required before the vaccine could be safely given to the general public.

Precise Effectiveness Sought

"Although the results obtained in these studies can be regarded as encouraging," Dr. Salk said, "they should not be interpreted to indicate that a practical vaccine is now at hand.

"However, it does appear that at least one course of further investigation is clear. It will now be necessary to establish precisely the limits within which the effects here described can be reproduced with certainty."

In the medical journal he wrote:

"Because of the great importance of safety factors in studies of this kind, it must be remembered that considerable time is required for the preparation and study of each new batch of experimental vaccine before human inoculations can be considered.

"It is this consideration, above all else, that imposes a limitation on the speed with which this work can be extended. Within these intractable limits every effort is being made to acquire the necessary information that will permit the logical progression of these studies into larger numbers of individuals in specially selected groups."

Discoveries Are Cumulative

These considerations indicate that it may take at least another year, and more likely two to three years, before the vaccine can be made available with safety for general use. There are about 46,000,000 in the United States, 1 to 19 years old, who may require vaccination.

The vaccine is the culmination of one of the greatest concentrated efforts in history. It was made possible by several important discoveries in recent years which, in turn, were made possible by the response of the public to the annual March of Dimes appeal.

One of these discoveries was the recognition that polio could be produced by three species of virus, instead of only one as had been believed, and that protection against one type would not provide protection against the other two.

Another major discovery was that the viruses could be grown on non-nervous tissue, either human or simian.

Another discovery was the fact that the polio viruses might be killed by formaldehyde so that they no longer could produce the disease while they still retained their ability to produce protective antibodies (immunity).

Finally, it was found that emulsification of the killed viruses with mineral oil greatly increased the powers of the vaccine to produce immunity agents.

Process of Preparation

The vaccine is prepared by first growing the viruses of the three types separately in testicular or kidney tissue of the monkey. These are harvested by centrifugation, in which the viruses are separated from the monkey tissues and then killed with formalin.

After tests on animals to make certain that the viruses no longer can produce polio, they are prepared in the form of a mineral oil emulsion for experimental testing on carefully selected human subjects.

The first persons to participate in these studies were patients paralyzed in recent years by a polio infection, who were at D. T. Watson Home for Crippled Children at Leetsdale, Pa. Additional studies were undertaken at the Polk State School, Polk, Pa.

In all, ninety subjects were tested with the multiple emulsified vaccine for all three types while seventy-one others received a single-virus aqueous vaccine.

Success With Emulsion

The tests disclosed that the emulsified vaccine produced antibodies within six weeks and that they were still present after four and a half months, with indications that they would last much longer. The aqueous vaccine was described as spotty, some developing antibodies, while others failed to do so.

Associated with Dr. Salk were Maj. Byron L. Bennett, retired, L. James Lewis, Elsie N. Ward, and J. S. Youngner.

Disease-forming organisms such as bacteria or viruses are known as antigens, that is, they stimulate the body's defensive mechanisms to produce agents to counteract them. These agents are known as antibodies. The immunity agents may last an individual for years, if not a lifetime, depending on the type of organism.

The presence of these immunity bodies in the blood of an individual is determined by taking a sample of the blood and testing it against any organism desired.

For example, a person's serum containing immunity bodies against contracting polio, either by having been exposed to the disease or as the result of vaccination, would inactivate polio viruses in a test tube. Such inactivation could be determined by injecting the virus into a monkey and observing whether or not the animal contracted the disease.

March 27, 1953

SALK POLIO VACCINE PROVES SUCCESS; MILLIONS WILL BE IMMUNIZED SOON; CITY SCHOOLS BEGIN SHOTS APRIL 25

By WILLIAM L. LAURENCE
Special to The New York Times.

ANN ARBOR, Mich., April 12—The world learned today that its hopes for finding an effective weapon against paralytic polio had been realized.

The triple anti-polio vaccine originated by Dr. Jonas E. Salk works. This was revealed in the long-awaited report on the mass field trials of 1954, largest of their kind in medical history.

In these tests the vaccine, designed to protect against the crippling effects of all the three types of virus known to produce paralytic polio, was administered to 440,000 children in forty-four states.

The report, a medical classic, was presented at a special scientific meeting at the University of Michigan by Dr. Thomas Francis Jr. It was he who had directed the evaluation of the vast mass of data provided by the tests, involving the correlation of 144,000,000 separate items of information.

Half Got Dummy Shot

Dr. Francis reported the vaccinations had been 80 to 90 per cent effective on the basis of results in eleven states.

In these states, which included New York, half of the children vaccinated got the Salk vaccine. The other half received a placebo or dummy shot.

These results, Dr. Francis reported, were looked upon with "greater confidence" than the figures in other areas. In these the results indicated an effectiveness of 60 to 80 per cent against paralysis by any polio virus.

Dr. Salk reported at the meeting that new and more potent vaccines and more effective methods of administering them, were ready for the 1955 vaccinations.

Dr. Salk, who is a member of the faculty at the University of Pittsburgh's School of Medicine, said:

"Theoretically, the new 1955

vaccines and vaccination procedures may lead to 100 per cent protection from paralysis of all those vaccinated."

The new procedures he outlined require two inoculations spaced two to four weeks apart, with a third "booster" shot seven months later.

This means that the amount of vaccine immediately available this season is automatically increased by 50 per cent, because in last year's trials the first two inoculations were given a week apart, and the third only one month after the second.

Comparisons Made Possible

There are three distinct types of polio virus, known respectively as Type I, II and III, or Brunhilde, Lansing and Leon. Each is able to produce paralytic polio.

The Salk vaccine is made of the three types of virus, killed by formaldehyde, so that they no longer can produce the disease, but retain their ability to stimulate the production of antibodies (immunity factors) in the recipient's blood stream.

In thirty-three states the vaccine was administered only to children in the second grade. Children in the first and third grades received no injections. The latter served as controls. That is, they were watched for the incidence of paralytic polio among them as compared with the vaccinated second graders.

The areas in these thirty-three states were known as the observed areas, as contrasted with the areas in the eleven states, in which all children in the first three grades were vaccinated. In these latter areas half of those injected were given the placebo. Hence they were known as the placebo areas.

The placebos and the real vaccines looked exactly alike. No one knew which was which until they were decoded by Dr. Francis. The placebos were used to eliminate any possible subjective influence, to make sure of 100 per cent objectivity in the tests.

Results Found to Differ

Dr. Francis' report states, however, that the data show that the vaccine was not equally effective against all the three types of the polio virus, either in the observed or in the placebo areas.

The report adds, "from these data it is not possible to select a single value giving numerical expression in a complete sense to the effectiveness of the vaccine as a total experience."

The results from the observed areas in the thirty-three states, the report states, suggest a lower effectiveness than those in the placebo areas.

"If the results from the observed study are employed," the Francis report declares, "the vaccine could be considered to have been 60 to 80 per cent effective against paralytic poliomye-

litis, 60 per cent against Type I poliomyelitis, and 70 to 80 per cent effective against disease caused by Types II and III.

"There is, however, greater confidence in the results obtained from the strictly controlled and almost identical test populations in the placebo study area.

Effectiveness Calculated

"On this basis it may be suggested that vaccination was 80 to 90 per cent effective against paralytic poliomyelitis; that it was 60 to 70 per cent effective against disease caused by Type I virus and 90 per cent or more effective against that of Type II and Type III virus.

"The estimate would be more secure had a larger number of cases been available."

Type I polio is the most prevalent type of the disease. It accounts for about 65 per cent of all cases of clinical polio. Type II accounts for about 5 per cent of the clinical cases. Type III causes about 30 per cent.

Dr. Salk, talking further about the prospects for the current 1955 tests, said it had been found that a certain chemical that had been used as a preservative for the vaccine had destroyed a great deal of the vaccine potency. This may account for the lack of consistency in the results, the lower figures possibly being due to batches of vaccine that had lost their potency because of the preservative.

The field trials were made possible by $7,500,000 in March of Dimes funds provided by the National Foundation for Infantile Paralysis. The evaluation was carried out at a special center at the University of Michigan by a large staff directed by Dr. Francis, one of the world's outstanding epidemiologists.

Comparable Efficacies Cited

While no official figures are available, authorities here said that the effectiveness of most vaccines was in the neighborhood of 90 to 95 per cent. However, it was pointed out, none of them was 90 per cent efficient the first year it was given.

The two most effective vaccines now known are those against smallpox and yellow fever. Both are made of live attenuated virus. Their effectiveness is in the range of 95 per cent. This means that ninety-five out of every 100 vaccinated are protected against the disease if exposed to it. Effective vaccines, in the form known as toxoids, also exist against diphtheria, about 90 per cent effective, and tetanus, about 95 per cent effective.

Potent vaccines also exist against whooping cough, typhoid fever, typhus fever, Rocky Mountain spotted fever, rabies and influenza. The vaccine against typhus reduces mortality from the disease to zero, but that does not mean it also completely eliminates the sickness. The vaccine against influenza is effective against only the same strain of virus.

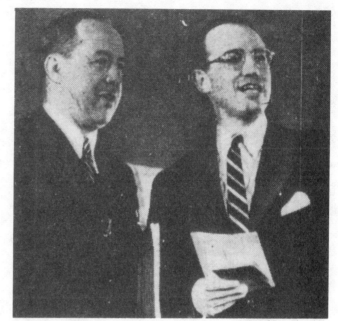

Associated Press Wirephoto

Dr. Thomas Francis Jr., left, and Dr. Jonas E. Salk

The vaccine last year was given in three separate inoculations, of one cubic centimeter each. The first two were given one week apart, while the third, known as the "booster" shot was given one month after the second.

The first two inoculations are the conditioning shots, creating in the blood stream a "memory" that mobilizes the body's defensive forces quickly as it is invaded by the specific microbe against which the vaccine has been designed.

The third "booster" shot is thus the one, aided by the "memory," that produces in the bloodstream the largest amount of anti-bodies.

The effectiveness of the "booster" shot depends on the time interval between it and the conditioning shots, as it takes a definite amount of time for the "memory" to be fully developed.

Dr. Salk's latest studies have revealed, he reported today, that the "booster" shot should properly be given some seven months after the first conditioning shots, as it takes that long for the antipolio "memory" to be fully developed.

These findings, therefore, indicate that the percentage of effectiveness on the mass trials last year would have been considerably greater had the "booster" shot been given seven months after the first two, instead of only one month later.

Would Cut Inoculations

Only two inoculations, spaced two to four weeks apart, should be given in 1955, instead of three over a five-week period, Dr. Salk reported today.

The third shot, should not be given before at least seven months have elapsed, but certainly before the onset of the 1956 polio season, he said.

At present it is known that the National Foundation for Infantile Paralysis has ordered a total of 27,000,000 cubic centimers of the vaccine on the

basis of three shots of one cubic centimer each. This quantity is enough for the immunization of 9,000,000 children.

However, if only two shots of one cubic centimer each are to be given this year, with the third shot to be postponed for seven months, the 27,000,000 cubic centimers would be enough to provide immunization for 13,500,000 individuals.

Basil O'Connor, president of the National Foundation, said no decision had as yet been made as to what course of distribution to follow in the light of Dr. Salk's latest findings.

Reactions to the vaccine were nearly negligible, the Francis report showed. Only 0.4 per cent of the vaccinated children suffered minor reactions. An even smaller percentage suffered more severe reactions.

The persistence of protection appears reasonably good. When good anti-body responses were obtained from vaccination, the report said, "the effect was maintained with but moderate decline after five months."

Distribution of anti-body levels among vaccinated persons was much higher than that in the control population from the same areas.

Out of a total population of 1,829,916 children a total of 1,013 cases of polio developed during the study period and were reported to the center.

In places of control areas, where vaccine was interchanged with an inert substance, 428 out of 749,236 children contracted the disease.

In the observed control areas where only second graders were inoculated, 585 cases developed among 1,080,680 children.

Only One Death Reported

Specifically, thirty-three inoculated children in the placebo areas receiving the complete vaccination series became paralyzed.

This is opposed to 115 uninoculated children who contracted the disease.

Similarly, in the observed areas there were thirty-eight such children who became paralyzed, as opposed to 330 uninoculated children.

There were four deaths among children who received placebo; none among the vaccinated. In observed areas there were eleven fatalities; none among children receiving the vaccine.

Only one child who had been inoculated with the vaccine died of polio, and this death followed a tonsillectomy two days after the second injection of the vaccine in an area where polio was already prevalent.

Other findings were:

¶The vaccine's effectiveness was more clearly seen when measured against the more severe cases of the disease.

¶Although data were limited, findings in Canada and Finland support the report in showing a significant effect of the vaccine among cases from whom virus was isolated.

¶Vaccination protected against family exposure. One out of 233 inoculated children developed the disease, while eight out of 244 children receiving placebo contracted the disease from family contact.

Dr. Salk further urged that all children who had received polio inoculations during the 1954 field trials should be given an additional dose in 1955. This is necessary, he said, because the three doses given in 1954 could not have been expected to produce more than a primary effect.

Dr. Salk explained that the first two inoculations in the three-inoculation series were sufficient to induce a primary stimulation of disease fighters in the blood. Over a period of months, a hyper-reactive state develops. This is simply a state of readiness, somewhat like a revolver that is cocked and ready to fire at a slight pressure on the trigger.

While the amount of measureable anti-body in the blood serum may not be large during this state of readiness, a "booster" shot administered after the required seven months serves as a trigger to explode the anti-body formation to remarkably high levels.

He added that exposure to a natural polio infection also served to induce the rapid production of anti-body once the hyper-reactive state has been developed in the anti-body cells.

In other words, even though anti-body may not be demonstrable in the blood serum at the time of invasion by polio virus, previous vaccination will have so primed the immunologic mechanism that anti-body in good concentration would appear in the serum shortly after the initiation of virus multiplication at the portal of entry.

If such anti-body development occurs prior to invasion of the blood stream and is present in sufficient concentration, access of virus to the central nervous system would be intercepted.

Dr. Salk said that use of vaccine for the first time during the polio season, or even in epidemic areas, might be expected to have a beneficial effect so long as certain time limitations are kept in mind.

He said that measurable anti-body was almost always induced by the fourteenth day after first vaccination. It is conceivable, then, that the probability of contracting paralytic polio would be less if exposure occurred after anti-body was present in the serum in concentration.

April 13, 1955

Safe Polio Vaccine Resulted From '49 Harvard Research in Growth of Disease Virus

The first major scientific breakthrough on the poliomyelitis front came in 1949.

That was the discovery by Dr. John F. Enders and his associates at the Harvard Medical School that polio virus could be grown in test tube culture on monkey tissues of nonnervous origin.

Until Dr. Enders' major discovery it had been universally believed that the polio virus would grow only in the nerve tissues of humans and a few species of monkeys.

On the other hand, it was known that vaccines prepared from virus grown on nerve tissue carried the risk of causing severe damage to the recipient's brain, thus producing a disease worse than polio.

The discovery by Dr. Enders and his associates made possible the unlimited growth in test tubes of polio virus that does not carry the risk of any brain damage. This opened the way at last to a safe polio vaccine.

Invisible Virus Seen

In the course of their studies, Dr. Enders and his Harvard colleagues came upon the highly important observation that the polio virus, as it grows on the monkey tissue in the test tube, caused degenerative changes in the cells upon which it grew.

This made it possible actually to "see" the invisible virus, and thus to tell, by the amount of the degeneration produced, the actual rate of the growth of the virus. Absence of cell degeneration meant absence of growth.

Furthermore, the observation provided a quick and easy test to determine whether or not the serum of an exposed or a vaccinated individual contained antibodies against the virus.

Since polio antibodies (immunity factors) check the growth of the polio virus, the addition of the individual's serum to the test tube virus culture would stop the virus growth and hence the degeneration of the cells on which it grows, the serum contained the specific anti-polio antibodies.

On the contrary, if the serum did not contain the specific antibodies, the growth of the virus, accompanied by the degeneration of the cells, would continue unabated.

The polio virus is about one-millionth of an inch in diameter and cannot be seen even with the most powerful optical microscope. Though it has been photographed recently with the electron microscope, which can magnify objects up to 100,000 times, the viruses thus shown are no longer alive.

Hence, until Dr. Enders and his team made their dramatic observation the only way to determine whether a polio virus was growing was to inject the culture into a living monkey and then wait to see whether the animal became paralyzed. To test for the presence of antibodies also required tedious and costly animal experiments.

Bottlenecks Eliminated

All these bottlenecks, which would have made the production of an anti-polio vaccine on a large scale a practical impossibility, were completely eliminated by the development of the method for growing the virus in test tubes together with the observation that the growth or nongrowth of the virus could be determined by the rate of degeneration of the tissue cells in the test tube.

The progressive destruction of the cells can be observed with the ordinary microscope and serves as a definite visual index of the rate of virus growth: the

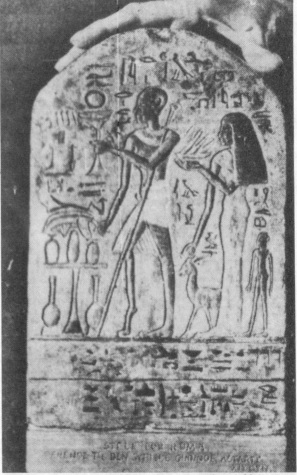

POLIO'S LONG HISTORY: This Egyptian tablet, more than 3,000 years old, is perhaps the earliest pictorial record of the disease. The man's leg was once thought to be badly drawn. Today it is considered representative of polio.

Among the Leaders in the Struggle Against Polio

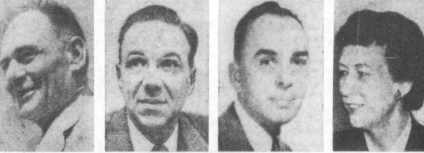

From left: Drs. John F. Enders, William McD. Hammon, David Bodian and Dorothy M. Horstmann. Dr. Enders developed method of growing polio virus in test tube tissue culture. Dr. Hammon demonstrated that small amounts of antibodies were effective in providing protection against paralytic polio. Drs. Bodian and Horstmann, working independently, proved polio virus circulates in blood only briefly before symptoms of disease appear.

greater the destruction the more abundant the growth.

Dr. Harry M. Weaver, former director of research for the National Foundation for Infantile Paralysis, commented that because of the work of Dr. Enders and his Harvard colleagues:

"Today there is no practical limit to the amount of virus that can be produced."

For their epoch-making achievements, which also promises to open the way for vaccines against other virus diseases, Dr. Enders and his colleagues—Drs. Thomas H. Weller and Frederick C. Robbins—received the Nobel Prize in Medicine and Physiology for 1954.

There were two other major discoveries in the field of polio, in the period between 1948 and 1952, of great importance to the development of an effective vac-cine against the crippling effects of the disease.

Three Types Identified

One of these was the isolation and identification of three distinct types of polio virus. This mammoth project was carried out in four major universities from 1948 to 1951, under grants of $1,370,000 by the National Foundation for Infantile Paralysis.

"The solution of this problem," Dr. Weaver said, "necessitated the monotonous repetition of exactly the same technical procedures on virus after virus, seven days a week, fifty-two weeks a year, for three solid years. The number of monkeys utilized in this effort was legion. The physical effort expended by the investigators to cope with the struggles, the lodges and the antics of this horde of primates is almost beyond comprehension."

After three years it was learned that there were three different types of polio virus circulating throughout all parts of the world, each capable of causing paralytic polio in the human being.

It was also found that development of immunity against one of the three virus types—named Brunhilde, Lansing and Leon—does not confer immunity against the other two types. This meant that an individual might contract polio more than once.

These findings also meant, of course, that any polio vaccine, to be fully protective, must produce immunity against all three types of the virus.

The Salk anti-polio vaccine is therefore a triple vaccine, consisting of a mixture of killed viruses of types I, II and III. While they no longer can produce the disease, they are still capable of stimulating the blood serum to produce antibodies against them.

The third major discovery—which came in 1952—was that the virus circulates in the blood for brief periods before the onset of the disease. This removed the earlier misconception that the polio virus attacks the nerve cells without previously passing through the blood stream.

Since antibodies are formed in the blood stream as a defense against germs that circulate in the blood, it seemed unlikely that a vaccine would produce antibodies against a virus that by-passed the blood stream altogether.

All previous efforts to find polio virus in the blood stream of animals infected with it had failed. The 1952 discovery of its presence for a brief period in the blood before it passed into the central nervous system, together with the discovery that small amounts of antibodies introduced in the blood prevent the virus from circulating in the system and from paralyzing the animal, provided strong support to the belief that a triple vaccine would neutralize the virus and prevent paralysis.

All these scientific discoveries formed the basis of the vaccine developed by Dr. Jonas E. Salk, of the University of Pittsburgh Medical School, with the March of Dimes funds.

April 13, 1955

Live-Virus Polio Vaccine Approved for Use in U.S.

By BESS FURMAN
Special to The New York Times.

WASHINGTON, Aug. 24— Live-virus poliomyelitis vaccine was approved today as suitable for use in the United States.

The announcement, ending a long controversy, was made by Dr. Leroy E. Burney, Surgeon General of the Public Health Service.

Simultaneously, he laid down exacting rules under which the live-virus vaccine would be licensed for commercial use in this country. His timetable calls for this to take place next spring. He predicted large supplies by the fall of 1961. He said the winter months were best for live polio vaccinations.

The live-virus vaccine, given by mouth, has already been used to immunize millions of persons in the Soviet Union, South America and other parts of the world. It is a virus so weak-ened as not to cause the disease, but still alive enough to produce antibodies.

In manufacture of the Salk vaccine, used in this country since 1955, the virus is heat-killed to a point where it will not cause disease, but still will produce antibodies. It is given by injection.

Dr. Burney predicted today that the live vaccine would not replace the Salk variety, but that each would complement the other. For instance, live-virus vaccine might be used as "booster" shot for the Salk vaccine.

The rules laid down today permit initial commercial production of only the Sabin types of vaccine—Types I, II and III, developed by Dr. Albert B. Sabin of Cincinnati to protect against the three polio strains.

Ruled out were two other types of live-virus polio vaccines—that developed by Dr. H. R. Cox at the Lederle Labo-ratories in Pearl River, N. Y., and that developed by Dr. Hilary Koprowski, at the Wistar Institute in Philadelphia.

Dr. Burney praised both these scientists for their "great contributions." He said that large-scale field trials of both the Cox and Koprowski vaccines had shown "the hazards to man to be very, very slight."

But he concluded that the Public Health Service had to apply a monkey test for safety in licensing a vaccine—and that the Sabin strains showed least virulence when injected into the brains, spinal cords and muscles of monkeys. Sabin Strain No. 1, the least virulent, was made the laboratory measuring stick for all other strains.

Strains Available to All

Since the Sabin strains were developed with funds furnished by the National Foundation, Dr. Burney added, they will be available to all the drug manufacturers that wish to produce live polio vaccine.

Dr. Burney said he did not know what the cost of the live-virus vaccine would be as com-posed with that of the Salk vaccine. The Salk vaccine now costs about 45 cents a dose, plus the doctor's charge for its injection.

Dr. Burney also said he thought that three or four doses of live virus would be required. This is similar to the Salk vaccine, which ideally is given in three injections with a later booster shot.

There is still some difference of opinion whether the live-virus vaccine confers greater immunity. However, some believe it does because with its passage through the intestine it stimulates formation of more antibodies. Another advantage is that through contact between persons the live virus is spread and immunity may be developed in persons who have not taken the vaccine themselves.

Drug companies already in experimental production of the Sabin vaccine include Wyeth Laboratories of Philadelphia; Pitman-Moore of Indianapolis, and Chas. Pfizer & Co. of Brooklyn.

The American Cyanamid Company, under which the Lederle Laboratories operate, immediately issued a statement that Lederle would start manufacture of the approved strains as soon as all the Public Health Service requirements were met. The company said it had already invested fourteen years and $13,000,000 in its faith in the superiority of live polio vaccine. Other drug companies sending experts to the live virus conference held here last week were the Eli Lilly Company of Indianapolis; Parke, Davis of Detroit, and Merck Sharp & Dohme of Rahway, N. J. Attending as observers were scientists from Connaught Laboratories at the University of Toronto in Canada, where live vaccine is now being produced, and from Chas. Pfizer Laboratories of Kent, England.

The Surgeon General defended his long delay in endorsing the live vaccine by saying:

"It has been stated that we have been ultraconservative. I have no apologies to make for conservatism, which is justified in an issue as important as this."

Dr. Burney said that today's endorsement of the live vaccine resulted from scientific evidence presented at a meeting on polio in Moscow in May; The Pan-American Health Organization-World Health Organization meeting in Washington in June; and the International Congress on Poliomyelitis last month. The final evaluation was made last Saturday by the six-member Public Health Service Committee on live polio virus vaccine.

Dr. Roderick Murray, chairman of that committee and head of the Division of Biologics Standards that will license the vaccine, stressed these points today:

To minimize the possible danger from a wild virus that might develop after repeated trips through the human intestinal tract, use of live virus vaccine should be on a community-wide rather than individual basis.

The claim for immunization through a single dose of live virus has not been borne out by recent experience. Repeated doses must be given at intervals, whether single strain or polyvalent vaccine is used.

Laboratories must be isolated and other special precautions instituted, including tests of both the persons who make the vaccine and the monkeys used in testing it.

The product must be kept under 30 degree centigrade in manufacture, and under refrigeration pending use.

The production regulations will be published in The Federal Register about Nov. 1 and again in late November.

The National Foundation hailed Dr. Burney's announcement as another milestone in the organization's fight against polio.

Basil O'Connor, the foundation president, said here that it had awarded $1,198,000 to Dr. Sabin since 1940 for research that led to his development of the live polio virus vaccine.

Effective in Cincinnati

CINCINNATI, Aug. 24 (UPI) —Dr. Sabin announced tonight that his oral polio vaccine given to 189,000 Cincinnati children in the first widespread test of the vaccine "has proved almost 100 per cent effective."

The first tests of the effectiveness of the vaccine were completed today.

"Of ninety-two children tested—children who had had no immunity to polio before getting the vaccine—all but one showed immunity afterwards," he announced.

August 25, 1960

New Anti-Coagulant Has Great Potential In Dissolving Clots in the Blood

By WILLIAM L. LAURENCE

A new substance, recently made available for clinical use to dissolve dangerous blood clots, is described in a special issue of Angiology as a milestone "opening new vistas of therapeutic potential." The publication is the official journal of the American College of Angiology, the specialty dealing with diseases of the blood vessels.

The new substance, prepared from a fraction of human blood, is known as fibrinolysin or plasmin. Unlike the older anti-coagulant drugs, which merely serve as preventives against the formation of new clots, the fibrinolysin actually dissolves existing clots. It was made available for use in hospitals last June by the Ortho Pharmaceutical Corporation, of Raritan, N. J., under the trade name Actase Fibrinolysin (Human).

Fibrinolysin acts by dissolving the clot-forming blood component named fibrin, acting specifically against that particular protein substance in the blood without affecting other proteins in the blood plasma. In this it differs in a highly important respect from another protein-dissolving substance—trypsin—which dissolves not only fibrin but also other plasma proteins, including important components of the coagulation system, the reduction of which may lead to hemorrhage.

Normal Dissolver

Fibrinolysin is an enzyme (organic catalyst) normally present in the blood. It is the agent by which the body normally dissolves and removes the small deposits of fibrin constantly accumulating as a result of minor injuries. However, the body's normal amount is not sufficient to dissolve blood clots formed as the result of major disorders of the blood vessels. This requires an agent that will enhance the body's normal fibrin-dissolving activity.

The enhancing agent—Actase— is an artificial form of human fibrinolysin. It is prepared from a precursor substance called profibrinolysin or plasminogen derived from human blood. This is converted into active fibrinolysin by combination with streptokinase, extracted from a species of blood-dissolving streptococcus.

So far the biochemically constituted fibrinolysin has been used, with highly effective results, as a specific agent in the treatment of thrombophlebitis (the clotting of veins in the extremities) and pulmonary embolism (the blocking of arteries in the lungs by clots), according to several reports in the special issue of Angiology.

Clinical trials are also being carried out in the treatment of coronary thrombosis, in which a clot cuts off the blood supply to the heart, and in strokes resulting from a clot in one of the arteries in the brain. However, the clinical trials in these conditions are still in the early preliminary stages and no conclusions can as yet be drawn.

400 Patients

In more than 400 patients suffering from a variety of thromboembolic (clot-caused) disorders, a summary of the reports states, "Results significantly superior to standard management were demonstrated in a vast majority of cases. In 367 cases of thrombophlebitis, 330 patients showed excellent response to the material—rapid loss of pain and swelling, and quick return of the affected area to normal size, leading to an average reduction of 50 per cent in length of hospitalization. Excellent response was also reported in fifty-three of sixty-six cases of pulmonary embolism."

In all thromboembolic disorders the reports state, results were significantly better when the material was used within five days of onset of symptoms, because, as clots become organized, their fibrin structure becomes more resistant to dissolution.

Extensive studies have demonstrated, the reports state, that the only significant reaction to Actase therapy is a rise in temperature, which occurs in about half the patients and usually subsides within twenty-four hours. The tests have also shown that Actase does not significantly impair the coagulation system, does not produce hemorrhage, does not interfere with wound healing, and does not lead to any other unacceptable consequences.

Health statisticians estimate that more than a million persons suffer from thromboembolism annually. A number of conditions predispose one toward thrombophlebitis: heart muscle failure, malignancy, obesity, debility, senility, varicosities, injury and surgery. A factor common to all is the tendency to slow circulation, particularly in the veins of the limbs.

Surgery Danger

An above-average incidence is observed among elderly patients, after surgery, and as a complication following childbirth. Patients who have successfully undergone surgery and then died without warning have been found to have died as the result of blood clots that blocked circulation at a vital point. Postoperative thrombosis has been estimated as high as 10.5 per cent by some authorities. It is most common after operations on female pelvic organs for cancer and infection and other long and major operations. Women appear to be more susceptible to it than men.

Pulmonary embolism is the most dreaded complication of thrombophlebitis and the most common serious pulmonary disease in hospital practice, despite widespread use of anti-coagulants. More than 34,000 persons die from it each year—a toll

greater than that from tuberculosis, according to a report by Dr. Harold Israel of the University of Pennsylvania Graduate School of Medicine.

The development of artificially activated fibrinolysin has a history dating back more than a century. Its modern phase began in 1933 with research on streptococcal infections by Dr. William S. Tillett and Dr. Raymond L. Garner at Johns Hopkins University. They were culturing streptococci on blood-covered plates when they noticed the development of certain clear, fluid areas. Either the bacteria themselves or something derived from them was apparently dissolving the clotted blood.

Yale Research

This line of research was carried forward in 1941 by Jacob H. Milstone, a biochemist at Yale, who was then working on blood coagulation at the Rockefeller Institute. He observed that the dissolution of blood clots by the bacteria occurred only in the presence of small amounts of the globulin fraction of human blood protein.

Meantime, in the early Nineteen Forties, spurred by the needs of the armed forces, the late Edwin J. Cohn and his associates at Harvard University were developing their revolutionary method for the fractionation of blood plasma into its different protein components. One of the major blood components that the Harvard group succeeded in separating on a mass-production basis became known as "Cohn Fraction III."

That fraction contains the precursor of fibrinolysin, but Prof. Cohn did not attempt to extract it in concentrated form. This was accomplished by Dr. Daniel Kline in 1952 at the Yale Department of Physiology, and the way was opened for the creation of an artificially activated fibrinolysin by combining the precursor substance from human blood with the "SK" activator from the bacteria.

October 11, 1959

DEFORMED BABIES TRACED TO A DRUG

'Harmless' Tablet Given to Mothers Abroad Is Cited as Infants' Crippler

U. S. GETS PLEA TO ACT

Physician Calls for Stricter Curbs on Introduction of New Pills in Country

By ROBERT K. PLUMB
Special to The New York Times.

PHILADELPHIA, April 11 — The birth of thousands of deformed babies in Europe has led an American physician to appeal for stricter Federal regulations on the introduction of new drugs in this country.

The appeal was made to the American College of Physicians at its annual meeting here. It is based on a new study of several thousand deformed babies born to European mothers who took a common prescription sleeping pill that had long been considered harmless.

The babies are born with useless short stub-like arms and legs to mothers who took, often before they knew they were pregnant, a sleeping compound with the chemical name thalidomide. The drug has been widely sold in West Germany and in Britain since 1958. It was taken off the market last

November. It has not been sold in the United States.

Appeal is Made

The appeal was made last night at a special session of the College of Physicians here by Dr. Helen B. Taussig, Professor of Pediatrics at the Johns Hopkins Hospital, who has just returned from a six-week inspection tour of German and British medical centers. She also held a news conference today.

"This compound [thalidomide] could have passed our present drug laws," Dr. Taussig reported. "There is no question but what we must strengthen our food and drug regulations to include routine testing of new compounds on pregnant animals."

Dr. Taussig said that German estimates were that between 3,500 and 5,000 babies with deformed arms or legs would be born by next August when the last of the mothers who had taken the drug would be delivered. About two-thirds of the babies will live, she said. It is estimated in Britain that there will be 200 to 500 cases there in all by August. A few cases have been reported from other countries, most of them instances in which travelers bought sleeping pills in Europe.

Left no Hangover

Thalidomide, Dr. Taussig said, appeared to be the greatest sleeping pill ever devised. It worked quickly and left no hangover. It was sold by prescription. The trade name in Germany was Contergan. In Britain it was Distaval. The compound was trade-named Kevadon by the American drug company that planned to introduce it here.

However, the American concern, the William S. Merrill Company of Cincinnati, did not

obtain Federal approval to sell the drug here because officials were suspicious of it. Nonetheless, it could have been passed, Dr. Taussig emphasized in demanding stiffer United States drug regulations. American food and drug regulations are stricter than those of either Germany or Britain, Dr. Taussig said.

She pointed out that the drug-caused deformation of the babies, known medically as phocomelia, "is the most ghastly thing you have ever seen." In the malformation, usually both arms fail to grow. Sometimes the affliction causes both legs to fail. Sometimes both arms and legs are afflicted. The babies do not have the normal rate of survival because they often have other malformations as well as the afflictions of the limbs.

Mode of Action Unknown

The precise mechanism by which thalidomide might produce birth abnormalities is not known. In an article appearing in the British medical periodical, The Lancet, for Feb. 10, Dr. A. L. Speirs, consultant pediatrician at the Stirling Royal Infirmary and the Falkirk and District Royal Infirmary, had this to say about it:

"It has been known for some time that certain drugs either used therapeutically in human beings or experimentally in animals can cause malformations. Such agents are insulin, cortisone, progestogens and folic-acid antagonists, and in these instances it is understandable that malformations should result. It is disturbing that such an apparently innocuous drug as thalidomide with no known toxic dose may disturb the growth of limb buds and other tissues at a certain phase of development.

"Further investigation with

the drug and related chemical compounds may demonstrate that they interfere with organizer, or enzyme, function."

Drug Legislation Pressed

WASHINGTON, April 11 (AP)—President Kennedy recommended legislation today for control and inspection of medicines sold over the counter as well as prescription drugs.

He also proposed giving the Department of Health, Education and Welfare power to withdraw approval of a new drug on the basis of "a substantial doubt" of its effectiveness or safety.

The proposals were among a half-dozen that Mr. Kennedy made in a letter to Senator James O. Eastland, Democrat of Mississippi, chairman of the Senate Judiciary Committee. The Administration's bill for consumer protection is awaiting action in that committee.

Mr. Kennedy had discussed the new ideas on drugstore items in his consumer message to Congress and told Mr. Eastland they might be included in the bill.

The President urged Mr. Eastland's committee to work on the measure without delay.

He noted that members of a subcommittee on patents had decided that more study was required on proposed compulsory licensing of other manufacturers to produce new drugs developed by a competitor.

Among the principal additions to the bill proposed by Mr. Kennedy, one would require drug manufacturers to keep records and report to the Department of Welfare any sign of adverse effects from the use of a new drug or antibiotic. Another would create a system that could be enforced to prevent illicit distribution of habit-forming barbiturates and amphetamines.

April 12, 1962

Drug Reform Bill Is Signed at White House, With Dr. Kelsey Present

WASHINGTON, Oct. 10 (AP) — President Kennedy signed a new drug bill today that he said would help to provide safe and more effective drugs to the American people.

Standing by in his White House office were legislators who had helped to pass the bill. With them was Dr. Frances Oldham Kelsey, the Food and Drug Administration medical officer whose vigorous stand prevented the introduction of the sleep-inducing drug thalidomide on the American market.

These are the measure's basic provisions:

¶The Food and Drug Administration will receive new powers for factory inspection and quality control. All drug manufacturers will have to register with the Government.

¶A new drug will have to be proved effective as well as safe and it cannot be marketed without specific approval of the Secretary of Health, Education and Welfare.

¶The Secretary can order a drug

off the market instantly if there is evidence it is unsafe.

¶All antibiotics for human consumption will have to be tested on a batch-by-batch basis for strength and purity.

¶Drug manufacturers will have to list "in brief summary" in their advertising any bad side effects of any prescription drug.

¶The manufacturers will have to print a common, or generic, name for a drug on the label in type at least half as large as its trade name.

Physicians will also be required to obtain the consent of patients before giving them experimental drugs, unless the physician determines that this would not be feasible or not in the patient's interest.

The provision that gives the Secretary authority to halt sale of drugs believed to be dangerous became effective immediately.

Most other sections of the measure become effective in six months.

October 11, 1962

2 Measles Vaccines Licensed; U.S. Sees End of Disease in 1965

Special to The New York Times.

WASHINGTON, March 21— The Government licensed today two vaccines against measles in the hope of eradicating this No. 1 childhood disease.

One variety, a "killed vaccine," will be available immediately in limited amounts. The other, a "live vaccine," is to be on the market within a few weeks. Both were expected to be generally available from the two licensed drug manufacturers within several months.

Surgeon General Luther L. Terry, chief of the Public Health Service, said the first drop in the rate of measles could be expected next year. More than 4,000,000 cases occur annually in the United States, he estimated. There are relatively few deaths—about 400 a year—but sometimes crippling complications of deafness and mental defects occur.

The disease might be eliminated from the nation in two years under ideal conditions, Dr. Terry said. This was an "attainable goal," rather than an expectation, he emphasized.

Measles kill about 50 per cent of the children in other nations who catch it, Dr. Terry said. The disease probably accounts for 25 to 50 per cent of all deaths among children in underdeveloped countries.

The vaccines represent "the most significant advance in recent years toward eliminating this infectious disease from our population," Dr. Terry told a news conference.

The licensed manufacturer for live vaccine, in which the modified measles virus is inactivated to stimulate body defenses without causing the disease, is Merck Sharp, and Dohme. Pfizer & Co. was licensed for the killed vaccine, in which the virus is completely inactivated.

These products have met Federal standards of safety, purity and potency, the Public Health Service said. The vaccines now licensed were manufactured in anticipation of the Federal regulations, which were published last week. The companies knew the regulations in advance.

Both vaccines were outgrowths of pioneering studies by Dr. John Enders, a Nobel prize winner at Harvard University, and an associate, Dr. Thomas Peebles. They isolated the measles virus for the first time in 1954.

Vaccine Actions Differ

The rational reason for licensing both types of vaccines was that they have different characteristics. In general, the live vaccine produces greater and faster protection, but it also has more side effects than the killed type, according to tests on about 50,000 persons.

Live vaccine provided immunity after one injection in more than 95 per cent of the susceptible children tested. This immunity remains for a least four years. However, 30 to 40 per cent of the inoculated children experienced fevers as high as 103 degrees, and 30 to 60 per cent had a modified measles rash.

When the live vaccine is given with a simultaneous injection of gamma globulin, as will probably be the practice, this blood derivative puts down the cases of fever to 15 per cent and reduces the duration of the fever and the rash.

In contrast, injections of the prescribed pre-shot program of killed vaccine over a period of at least two months cause the development of antibodies in 90 per cent of the children. This declines to undetectable levels within a year, and a booster shot may later be required. However, there are no adverse reactions to this vaccine.

It appears that one shot of live vacine and one shot of killed vacine may work best, acording to a report by the Surgeon General's Advisory Committee on Measels. These results must be confirmed with further tests.

Since over 90 per cent of all children get measles, Dr. Terry would like to see infants vaccinated between the age of 9 months and one year. Children usually come down with the disease betwen the age of 2 and 6. Most active cases ocur before the individiual is 15, although some adults also get the disease.

The advisory committe also named groups of people who should not get the vaccine. It said the live-virus type should not be administered to pregnant women; persons with leukemia or other generalized cancers; patients undergoing therapy such as radiation, which reduces their resistance; persons having high fever at the time; persons who have recently received gamma globulin; and persons allergic to eggs. The advice against vaccinating persons who had recent gamma globulin injections was given because presence of this serum might prevent the vaccine from "taking." Persons allergic to eggs were warned against the vaccine because it is grown on chick embryo tissues.

However, some killed virus vaccines are being grown on monkey tissue and could be used in the cases of patients who are sensitive to eggs.

Several other pharmaceutical companies have expresed interest in making measles vaccines, Government officials said, but their licensing is at least several months off.

March 22, 1963

Artificial Kidney Now Being Utilized in the Home

By HAROLD M. SCHMECK Jr.

Patients who would otherwise die of chronic kidney disease are being kept alive and in outward good health by periodic use of artificial kidney machines in their own homes.

In some cases the treatments are being done on a do-it-yourself basis by the patients and their families.

The primary advances that are making this possible are a simplification of the treatment procedure and development of machines with built-in safeguards against any mishaps.

The development promises to reduce the high financial burden of these life-saving treatments and to help overcome a severe shortage of hospital facilities.

One such successful project is reported in the current issue of The Journal of the American Medical Association by specialists in Boston.

Earlier, a specially designed and highly automated artificial kidney for home use was shown by a research team in Seattle.

In Spokane a third group is training patients in the do-it-yourself-at-home techniques used in Seattle.

Removal of Waste

The primary function of the natural kidneys is to remove from the bloodstream the accumulation of waste products and poisons resulting from the multitude of chemical reactions that go on continually in the body.

In a sense these wastes are the ashes of the fires of life. If they are not removed the fire will die. Kidney failure therefore is a grave crisis.

Artificial kidney machines are simply devices to cleanse the blood when the natural kidneys fail to do the job.

Basically all the machines work this way: The patient's blood flows on one side of a sheet of ordinary cellophane, a special chemical bath flows on the other side. Impurities in the blood pass through the tiny pores in the cellophane and are carried away in the bath. The blood cells are too large to pass through. By varying the chemical concentration of the bath, however, virtually any substance with molecules small enough to pass through the pores can be either added to or removed from the blood.

Done 20 Years Ago

The first such device was developed more than 20 years ago to save the lives of patients whose kidney functions had stopped temporarily.

During the last few years, technical developments, principally in Seattle, have made it possible to adapt the treatment for use with patients whose kidney function is permanently lost.

In any artificial kidney apparatus, blood is taken from an artery, usually in the patient's arm, and returned to a nearby vein after passing through the machine.

A key development in Seattle was an attachment worn by the patient through which his artery-to-machine-to-vein linkage can be done simply and without repeated surgery. It is an artery-to-vein shunt that is simply uncoupled when the patient is linked to the machine.

Some patients have now been living for more than four years by the grace of once-or-twice-weekly treatments with an artificial kidney machine.

Many Hold Jobs

Though many of these patients hold full-time jobs and have most of the outward attributes of good health, they would be dead within a matter of weeks if the treatments were stopped.

The very success of this type of treatment has presented the medical profession with a terrible predicament, however, because facilities and trained personnel are extremely scarce and the cost of maintaining a patient for only one year is seldom less than $10,000. Much of the unavoidable cost is in salaries of technical personnel and in the hospital facilities themselves.

It has been estimated that 2,000 patients who would be ideal candidates for this type of treatment die yearly in the United States solely because of the lack of money and facilities for the treatments.

Boston Research

The new report in The Journal of the American Medical Association is by Dr. John P. Merrill and colleagues of Peter Bent Brigham Hospital, one of Harvard University's teaching hospitals and a center for artificial kidney and transplantation research.

Three patients are being treated at home, a physicist, a lawyer and an accountant.

In one case the patient's wife

is supervising the treatment. In another this is being done by a nurse. In the third the patient's wife is being trained for the task.

In all cases the patients received their first treatments in the hospital, where they and their families were trained in the techniques.

In Seattle a team of physicians and engineers of the University of Washington has developed new artificial kidney apparatus which operates through the full treatment cycle on a largely automatic basis.

It was developed through a special grant from the John A. Hartford Foundation.

The device, known to its inventors as "Minnie," is being used by a 17-year-old high-school girl whose parents manage the regular treatments.

Another patient, an insurance underwriter, is using somewhat different equipment at his home with the aid of his wife. Yearly cost is estimated at $5,000 or less. "Minnie" costs about $3,500 to build.

In Spokane, one patient is being trained for home use of artificial kidney apparatus by the Spokane and Inland Empire Artificial Kidney Center, operated as a privately and community supported center by three physicians.

One of the three said yesterday that other patients with the necessary degree of intelligence and responsibility would be trained in home use.

November 2, 1964

Malaria Wins Round 2

By C. P. GILMORE

"WE thought we had malaria under control in World War II," says Col. William D. Tigertt, director of the Walter Reed Army Institute of Research. "But now, 20 years later, we still face the same problems."

The problems Colonel Tigertt refers to exploded violently in Vietnam last fall. United States troops by the hundreds suddenly began coming down with a virulent strain of malaria against which even the most potent wonder drugs were strangely powerless. In October, some 400 men were stricken; in November, more than 700. By the end of the year, 1,801 U.S. servicemen had caught malaria and 12 had died of it. More hospital beds were filled with malaria patients than with those wounded by enemy action. "Next to girls," said Col. Spurgeon Neel Jr., chief medical officer of the U.S. Military Assistance Command in Vietnam, "the thing that American troops talk about most in Vietnam is malaria."

Malaria was eradicated in the United States more than a decade ago. Most Americans, consequently, tend to think of it as one of the world's solved problems. They couldn't be more wrong. Malaria, historically the "king of tropical diseases," is still the world's No. 1 health problem. The World Health Organization, which has waged the most successful campaign in history against this scourge, estimates that it even now strikes 150 million persons a year, killing at least a million of its victims and disabling the rest for long periods. Epidemics still sweep across the world's malarial regions, with effects as deadly as the dreaded plagues of the Middle Ages. As recently as 1958, malaria struck a swath through Ethiopia, infecting three million and killing 150,000. The yearly economic toll and the human misery brought on by the disease are incalculable.

MALARIA is an ancient disease, almost certainly predating man himself. The disease-causing parasite that affects man is almost identical to the one that causes malaria in anthropoid apes. The two parasites appear to be descendants from an earlier strain that affected the common ancestor of man and ape. The earliest written records from Assyria, Egypt and China abound with references to what was clearly malaria.

The disease is transmitted from one individual to another through a complex insect-man cycle, with certain stages of the parasite's life cycle taking place in each. An infected Anopheles mosquito lands on her victim, lifts her tail, shoves her needle-like proboscis through the skin and, to avoid blood clotting, injects a small dose of anticoagulant. Then she begins her meal of warm blood.

Along with the anticoagulant, she injects a parasite called Plasmodium —the one-celled organism that causes malaria. The Plasmodia, at this stage in their life cycle called sporozoites, enter the blood stream and head for the liver, there to develop and grow. Six to 12 days later, in a form called merozoites, they re-enter the blood stream in large numbers, and begin invading red blood cells. In a few days the cells rupture, releasing more merozoites to attack yet more red cells.

Some of the parasites in the blood develop into a sexual form—male and female gametocytes. If a mosquito bites the malaria victim now, while the gametocytes are in the blood, she takes some of them up with her blood meal. In the mosquito's stomach—and only there—the male gametocytes fertilize the female. After a complex series of events, the fertilized gametocytes produce sporozoites which migrate to the salivary glands of the mosquito, there to be ready to be injected into the next victim to start the entire cycle again.

Researchers hypothesize that malaria was once a disease of mosquitoes, since the sexual cycle takes place in the insect. Presumably, at some remote date in prehistory, as mosquitoes fed on warm-blooded animals, certain strains of the parasite injected during feeding began to grow in animal blood, and the complex chain as it now exists was begun. This theory is further supported by the fact that malaria does not seem to make mosquitoes sick; over the millions of years, the insect and the parasite have apparently accommodated to each other.

Man is not so fortunate. As the merozoites in his blood stream mature and burst out of their red cells

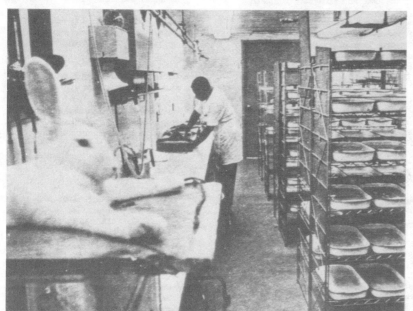

BREEDING GROUND—The trays in this Public Health Service hatchery in Georgia are filled with larvae of malaria-transmitting Anopheles mosquitoes. Rabbits and monkeys, as well as human volunteers, are used in the search for drugs to combat the disease, which remains the world's No. 1 health problem.

C. P. GILMORE specializes in articles on medical and scientific subjects.

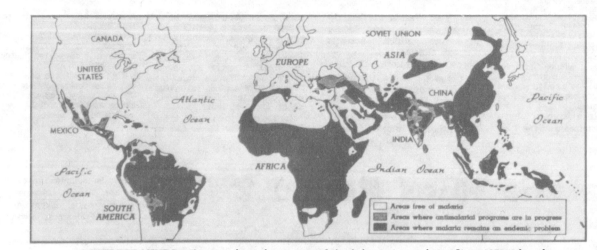

BATTLEGROUNDS—This map shows the progress of the fight against malaria. Since 1955, when the World Health Organization launched a campaign to eradicate the disease, some 250 million cases a year have dropped to 150 million, and deaths, once two million annually, have been cut in half.

in great waves every 48 to 72 hours (depending on which of the four known varieties of malaria he has), he suffers the debilitating effects of the disease. The bursting out destroys the red cells, sometimes faster than the body can replace them. The victim suffers from anemia, high fevers —frequently 104 or 105 degrees—shaking chills, general aches and pains, nausea, convulsions, delirium and, sometimes, death.

The reason for the anemia—the physical bursting of red cells by the emerging merozoites—is well understood. The basic mechanisms by which other symptoms are produced, as is the case with symptoms of most diseases, are not. But the effects are real enough. The attack can go on for weeks; some patients do not regain their strength for months. And the organism may remain in the liver for years after apparent recovery, leading to later relapses.

AS is true of many diseases, man devised an effective treatment for malaria before he had any idea what causes it. In 1632, after the conquest of Peru, explorers took back to Europe the bark of the cinchona tree, the first effective remedy. Some 200 years later, the white, bitter crystals known as quinine were identified as the active substance in the bark.

But quinine, while highly effective, has its drawbacks. It can cause dizziness, ringing of the ears, partial deafness. And it comes from a tropical tree which, in time of need, may not be available. In World War II, in fact, the supply was cut off when the Japanese captured Indonesia, the source of most of the world's supply.

By the beginning of World War II, fortunately, several synthetic antimalarials had been discovered. Atabrine, the most effective, is still remembered by thousands of ex-G.I.'s as the pill that turned their skins a sickly yellow. Men who took it regularly could be bitten by infected mosquitoes, yet not suffer the debilitating symptoms of the disease. Circulating in the blood stream, the Atabrine killed spo-

rozoites as soon as they were injected by the bite of a mosquito, stopping the development of the disease. (The method by which it kills the parasite without harming the host is still unknown. The same is true of most drugs, including quinine and others used against malaria.)

Yet Atabrine's success was far from complete. Malaria, in fact, remained the chief problem of military medicine throughout World War II. Half a million U.S. servicemen fell victim to the disease. In the South Pacific, it took five times as many men out of combat as did enemy action. Of the troops who landed on Sicily, more than 21,000 were hospitalized with malaria, 17,000 with battle wounds.

In the attempt to find even more effective drugs to fight the disease, researchers in the U.S. and elsewhere launched a massive search, during which they screened more than 18,000 drugs and found 80 that seemed to show some promise. Then began the tedious, time-consuming and dangerous part: testing the drugs on human volunteers. The Public Health Service's National Institute of Allergy and Infectious Diseases began a malaria test program at the Federal prison in Atlanta, Ga., in March, 1944. Three months later, the Army Surgeon General's Office set up a project at the Illinois State Penitentiary.

IN the more than two decades since, these units have been responsible for much of the progress, both in antimalarial drugs and in fundamental knowledge of the disease itself. To see how the work with prisoners is carried out, I visited the Atlanta penitentiary in company with the man who set up the project there, Dr. G. Robert Coatney, former chief of the National Institute's chemotherapy laboratory.

Dr. Coatney is a small, dapper man of 63, whose wavy hair shows just a trace of its original color. His small, neatly clipped mustache is completely white. He tends to favor suede shoes, hats with colorful feath-

ers in the band, bow ties, sports jackets. His manner is as lively as his dress. Coatney's walk is so brisk he almost bounces. He shakes hands, slaps backs, laughs, and exchanges cheerful greetings with acquaintances everywhere he goes.

As we walked down a prison corridor toward the malaria unit, he began to fill me in on its background. "In the last 22 years, we've had about 3,000 volunteer subjects, normally about 60 at a time," he said. "A man is usually part of the project for six months, and earns five days off his sentence for each 30 days he spends with us. He also gets $50. Without these guys," added Coatney, "we'd be dead. We couldn't do anything."

The malaria project occupies a long, low - ceilinged room on the ground floor of the prison hospital. A dozen beds line either side of the room. Four or five were occupied, some with men reading or sitting up. Several patients, bare from the waist up, lay still, eyes closed. "Those men are pretty sick," said Coatney. "Malaria is no joke." The others, he explained, were either in the early stages or convalescing.

At one end of the ward was a small dispensary—lined with microscopes, a refrigerator, a sterilizer, medical books and instruments. In the center of the room was a small table that would not look out of place in a kitchen. Around it sat three blue-coated prisoner volunteers and a white-coated technician. On the table were a number of cardboard cylinders, each the size of a spool of thread. Over the end of each was mosquito netting; inside buzzed a single female Anopheles which had recently feasted on a patient with malaria. The technician picked up one of the cylinders and put the mesh end on a prisoner's outstretched arm. The mosquito's rear shot up as she jammed her proboscis into the waiting flesh. After a few minutes, the same mosquito was moved on to the second volunteer, then to the third.

The ritual was repeated with 10 mosquitoes, each biting each of the

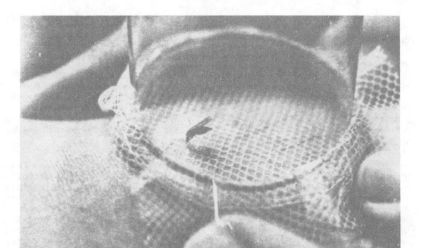

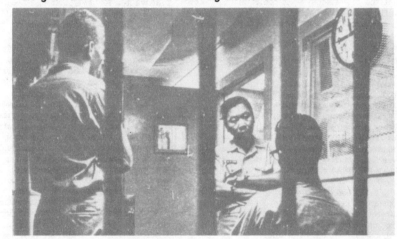

BITER AND BITTEN—An Anopheles mosquito, in a mesh-covered cylinder, above, bites the arm of a malaria-research volunteer. Most U.S. volunteers are convicts. Below, at the Federal penitentiary in Atlanta, Ga., prisoners are given a medical check before allowing themselves to be bitten.

volunteers. Then each mosquito was dissected and examined under a microscope to make sure that her salivary glands showed the characteristic needlelike sporozoites that proved she was infected.

Normally, if a new drug is being tested, two of the prisoners receive it and one—the control—does not. (The prisoners draw lots to see who will be the control.) In testing a single drug, perhaps five such groups—15 men in all—are inoculated. Over the years, hundreds of drugs have been tested. At the same time, various stages of the disease have been studied intensively in volunteers to learn more about malaria and how it may be attacked.

Many valuable discoveries have come from the human volunteer projects, both at Atlanta and elsewhere. Chloroquine, the world's most effective antimalarial for more than 15 years, was tested and found safe and effective at Atlanta in the nineteen-forties. It was given routinely to U.S. troops in Korea. The drug circulates in the blood and kills malaria parasites as soon as they enter the blood stream. Consequently, a man can be bitten by an infected mosquito and not show malaria symptoms at all.

Indeed, so successful was chloroquine in suppressing the symptoms of malaria that it brought on a strange new problem. As soon as men left Korea and returned to the U.S., they started coming down with malaria by the hundreds. While the drug killed the parasites in the blood, researchers found, it did not kill those that lodged in the liver. Thus, as soon as the returnee stopped taking chloroquine, the organism surged into his blood and he became sick.

So investigators came up with a drug called primaquine to kill the parasite in the liver. Military personnel returning from Korea took primaquine for 14 days during the trip home. The sudden rash of malaria in the U.S. stopped as though someone had turned off a faucet.

THE search for new drugs is only one aspect of the continuing battle against malaria. Since the days of Caesar, man has dreamed of eradicating the disease, not merely curing it. The Romans drained swamps to combat it; while they did not know the cause, they knew it was associated with marshy areas. When the mosquito was identified as the carrier late in the 19th century, malaria fighters added insecticides to their weapons.

It was not until shortly before World War II, however, that the discovery of the insecticidal properties of DDT opened the possibility of wide-scale, highly effective antimalarial campaigns. A few years earlier, two workers in Africa had suggested a possible new attack. After a mosquito bites, she usually perches on a wall or ceiling to digest her meal. If a widespread program could be initiated to kill the insects inside homes, the chain of infection might be snapped at that point. DDT was perfect for such use. Sprayed on interior walls, it retains its killing power for months. If every house in an area can be sprayed several times a year, virtually every infected insect will be killed before she can pass on the infection. True eradication of malaria throughout entire regions suddenly became not only theoretically possible, but practical as well.

Large-scale projects got under way shortly after the war. Congress, for example, approved a United States malaria eradication program in 1946, and the Public Health Service set up the National Malaria Eradication Program. By 1950, the disease — which only a few years earlier had been killing between 200,000 and 400,000 Americans annually — was virtually wiped out. Since 1963, not a single indigenous case has been reported in the entire country.

Encouraged by the U.S. success and by similarly effective programs in much of Europe and Russia, the World Health Organization in 1955 set a goal of world eradication of malaria. In the decade since the program started, the W.H.O. and participating countries have thrown almost $1-billion into the fight. As a result, the yearly number of cases in the world has dropped from an estimated 250 million to about 140 million. Deaths, formerly estimated at no fewer than two million a year, have been cut in half. Malaria has been virtually wiped out in the Italian peninsula, Taiwan, Venezuela, Sardinia and Jamaica. Great areas of India, formerly one of the world's worst malarial regions, are now free of this scourge for the first time in history.

The beneficial effects have been spectacular. Rice cultivation was boosted tenfold in Greece, Morocco, Indonesia and Ceylon. (And in Greece, the average height of army recruits has shot up almost 2 inches since the virtual eradication of malaria.) In the Philippines, 20 previously uninhabitable districts have been opened for settlement. In areas of Cambodia, land values have doubled with the suppression of malaria. In French Guiana, infant mortality dropped 50 per cent. Similar stories can be told of Mexico, Thailand, Bolivia, Nigeria and many other countries.

THE program, of course, has not been a string of unbroken successes. In fact, serious — some think insuperable — problems stand in the way of the eventual goal. One, for example, appeared in 1951 — four years before the W.H.O. program got started. Eradication teams in Greece reported that a species of Anopheles there had become immune to DDT. This report and similar scattered ones from other regions, in fact, were partly responsible for the establishing of the worldwide eradication program. If malaria was not totally or nearly eradicated before widespread DDT resistance showed up, experts feared, the goal of total eradication might move forever beyond reach.

The precise chemical or biological method by which insects (or parasites) become drug-resistant is not known, although the general genetic principles are clear enough. As individual human beings differ in their response to drugs, so individual mosquitoes react differently to insecticides. What may be a lethal dose for one mosquito may not be quite enough to kill another. In widespread anti-insect campaigns, those highly susceptible to the chemical being used are quickly killed; those who tend to resist it are not. These surviving resistant individuals produce resistant offspring. Continued application of insecticide kills off susceptible progeny, making the survivors ever more resistant. Quickly, since insect generations come rapidly, almost totally immune strains develop.

With this mechanism in full operation, DDT resistance has been a steadily worsening problem. Today, some 17 of the 60 species of Anopheles that account for most of the world's malaria transmission are resistant not only to DDT but to most other widely used insecticides as well. In addition, the mounting problems of the side effects of DDT on human and animal life have made mosquito eradication teams more cautious about widespread use of the chemical.

The program has run into other snags, too. Political unrest in Laos stopped control programs in 1961, and malaria is now rampant there. Revolts and unsettled governments in certain African countries have made effective programs impossible.

Primitive and illiterate peoples who would benefit tremendously from the programs frequently resist efforts to rid their countries of malaria. In Surinam, for example, there has been widespread objection to the spraying of jungle huts.

Thus, it became clear that anti-mosquito campaigns alone would not achieve the goal of total eradication. Some new approach was needed. "We finally realized that we couldn't kill all the mosquitoes," says Dr. Coatney. "We needed some other weapon."

What was to become one of the most dramatic approaches was first tried a half-dozen years ago by Dr. Mario Pinotti, then Brazil's Minister of Health. Dr. Pinotti's plan was to add chloroquine to the country's supply of table salt. If every Brazilian ate only salt mixed with a small amount of chloroquine—far too little to be noticed—the chloroquine would suppress the parasite in the blood so that mosquitoes biting people would not be infected, and the chain of infection could be broken effectively and rapidly.

It was a good plan, but it bogged down in political and administrative difficulties. Salt supplies were never effectively treated, and the program finally collapsed. But the same plan was yet to prove its worth in a spectacular way.

In the early nineteen-sixties, the Government of British Guiana passed a law making the sale of unmedicated salt illegal. The Government offered to mix wholesalers' supplies with chloroquine free and, as an added inducement, to pack the bulk salt in small bags for resale.

"So they set up the system and began to operate," recalls Dr. Coatney, who, with his prisoner volunteers, had done much of the work in proving that chloroquinated salt would work. "At the end of eight weeks, there was simply no malaria. Not one case.

"Thirty months later, two cases of malaria appeared. Public Health officials got to work and established that the disease had been contracted in Barbados. It's a fantastic story. It works. No mosquito eradication, no nothing. Just the stuff in the salt."

DESPITE the dramatic success of various antimalaria weapons — both drug treatment and mosquito-eradication programs — malaria fighters are still a long way from victory. Either method would be virtually impossible to apply in some areas of the world. "All you have to do is fly over the Amazon basin or go up the rivers of Surinam," says Dr. Coatney. "How are you going to find the people to treat? There are 20,000 aborigines in Malaya. They live in lean-tos. They're here one day; the next day they're gone. Now how in hell are you going to eradicate malaria in people you can't even find?" And such untreated populations continue to be reservoirs of infection that can break out into neighboring regions at any time.

Sometimes it seems to malaria fighters that for every problem they solve, two new ones take its place. One came to light a few years ago in an unlikely setting—a laboratory in Memphis, Tenn.

The late Dr. Donald E. Eyles of the National Institute of Allergy and Infectious Diseases was experimenting with the action of the malaria parasite in the liver by infecting monkeys with a type of simian malaria. The difficulty was that there would frequently be only a few of the parasites in the liver, making them difficult to find. Eyles had an idea as to how to infect the monkeys more heavily.

"Don called to talk about his idea with me," recalled Dr. Coatney. "Now, he was a clever fellow with a dissecting needle and he proposed to get a big bunch of mosquitoes infected with monkey malaria. Then he and Nell Coleman, a technician who had worked for him for years, would sit down for eight hours and dissect mosquitoes as fast as they could, take out the clumps of infectious

sporozoites and inject them into monkeys.

"Don was a heavy cigar smoker," Coatney continued. "And the technique he used was to knock a mosquito down with a puff of cigar smoke, then dissect it before it could recover. But every once in a while, one would get away. And he said, 'Why should we waste time looking for those few, since we can't get infected anyway, because it's simian malaria?'

"Well, bang. Fourteen days later he was sick. He went to the Public Health Service Hospital in Memphis and they decided he had flu and filled him up with penicillin. The next day he was fine. But the third day he was right back sick again with a terrible headache and fever. They gave him another shot of penicillin.

"Suddenly he put it together. An attack every 48 hours. He had a technician make a blood smear, and by that time he was so sick they had to drive him home. But almost before he got in bed the girl called and said, 'Dr. Eyles, you've got malaria.'"

THE next day, feeling better, Eyles went back to the laboratory, had a technician draw blood from him and put it in a clean monkey. Then he took chloroquine.

"Then he called me," said Dr. Coatney. "He said, 'I've got monkey malaria.' I said, 'You're kidding.' He said, 'No, I mean it.'

"I said, 'Pull out some blood and for goodness sake don't take any drugs,'" said Coatney. "He said, 'I knew you'd say that, so I already took some. I'm the one who's sick.'"

Two days later, Miss Coleman, who had done the dissecting with Eyles, came down with the same symptoms. Eyles drew blood from her, but was still too weak to fly to Atlanta with it. When the blood arrived, Coatney's associates injected it into two prison volunteers. By this time, the monkey that had been injected with Eyles's blood had come down with the disease. A couple of days later the prisoners had it. To make sure of what they had, and to prove that it could be transmitted naturally, doctors used mosquitoes to pass the disease back and forth from prisoner to monkey and back to prisoner.

"What we learned," said Coatney, half-jokingly, "is that monkeys and men are more closely related than some of us would like to admit." But there were far more serious implications as well. The discovery was a blow to hopes for total world eradication of malaria. It meant that even if the disease could be totally eradicated in man—by no means a certainty—reservoirs of infection might remain alive in monkey populations in the impenetrable jungles of South America, Africa and Asia.

BUT the crowning blow was yet to fall, and from yet another direction. In 1960, at about the same time malariologists were finding that man was not immune to the monkey version of the disease, two geologists working for an oil company in Colombia showed up with malaria symptoms. The local doctor gave them the usual chloroquine therapy, but, to his surprise, it had no effect. He shipped them off to Dallas for further treatment. There, Drs. Donald Moore and J. E. Lanier tried chloroquine again, with the same lack of results.

"Don Moore called me and asked, 'What do you do when you've got chloroquine-resistant malaria?'" recalled Dr. Coatney. "I said, 'Don, there isn't such a thing.' And he said, 'Well, I've got two cases.'"

Lanier eventually had to resort to the old treatment of quinine to stop the infection. A sample of one patient's blood had meanwhile been sent to Public Health Service investigators who confirmed that it was a strain of falciparum malaria, a virulent type responsible for most malaria deaths. And the strain was able to shrug off chloroquine treatment as easily in prisoners as it had in geologists.

A short time later the Naval Hospital in Bethesda, Md., got a patient who had caught malaria in Bangkok and who failed to respond to chloroquine. His blood went to Atlanta and once again proved to contain a chloroquine-resistant strain of falciparum. A short time later, Don Eyles, then in Malaya, where he had gone to study the monkey malaria in person, reported to headquarters that chloroquine-resistant strains were showing up there and in Cambodia. "I read the note from Don," said Coatney, "and I said, 'Oh, my God, here we go.'" The world's number one antimalaria drug had just been knocked out of the box.

The chloroquine-resistant falciparum strain was the one that hit American servicemen in Vietnam beginning last fall. Supplies of quinine were rushed to Vietnam to control the new menace. In addition, Army doc-

tors decided to try a new drug called diaminodiphenylsufone (DDS) that had been used in the treatment of leprosy since the late nineteen-forties. Tests at the Illinois State Prison had showed it effective against the malaria parasite as well.

Twenty-four hundred troops in Vietnam were put on daily doses of DDS. The drug not only cut the rate of new malaria cases in half but slashed relapses sharply. Given as treatment to those who get malaria, it cuts recovery time. As a result of the tests, officials ordered this July that all troops in Vietnam go on daily doses of the new drug immediately.

DDS will help. So will the continuing antimosquito programs being carried out by the armed forces in Vietnam. But the battle against malaria is far from won. DDS does not stop all cases—only about half. And no one knows how long it will be before malaria strains develop a resistance to it. "This is a sulfa derivative," says one authority, "and malaria has been known to become resistant very rapidly to

this type of drug. So I might stick my neck out and say that if we get six to eight months' good use out of it, we'll be real happy. By that time, we hope we'll have something better."

AND so the fight goes on —in Atlanta, in Army research centers, in drug-company laboratories—screening thousands of new drugs that might be useful in the battle against malaria. But no new drugs of outstanding promise have been identified, and nobody is willing to predict what the outcome may be.

"Every time we think we have this thing pinned to the mat," says Dr. Coatney, "we find that's just the first fall, and it's right back up fighting again. Experience has taught us that we spend more time on our faces than on Cloud 9. We've been up there a few times, and every time we get knocked off. We're not going to do too much talking in the future until we know we can stay up there."

September 25, 1966

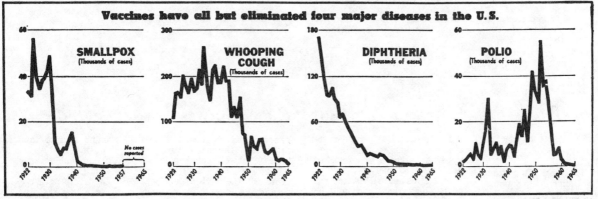

Vaccines have all but eliminated four major diseases in the U.S.

SMALLPOX (Thousands of cases)

WHOOPING COUGH (Thousands of cases)

DIPHTHERIA (Thousands of cases)

POLIO (Thousands of cases)

November 20, 1966

CANCER DETECTION IN BREAST IS SPED

By HAROLD M. SCHMECK Jr.
Special to The New York Times

WASHINGTON, Sept. 26— Radiologists described today a combination method for detecting the early stages of breast cancer, which they say can reduce the death toll from the disease.

Breast cancer is the most common single type of cancer in women in the United States, accounting for almost one-fourth of female cancers. It causes 27,000 deaths a year.

There has been little improvement in the death rate from breast cancer during the last 25 years.

One feature of the new method is to use enlarged veins in

the breast almost as a map to lead the doctors to a cancer that is hidden or too small to be detected by ordinary methods.

This examination of vein size is done by the X-ray procedure called mammography. Veins visible in each breast under X-ray are compared in size.

If veins in one breast are found to be substantially larger in diameter than those in the comparable location in the other, this is considered suggestive of possible cancer.

This detection method is called V.D.R. for Venous Diameter Ratio. In the study reported here today it is coupled with thermography, another relatively new technique, which uses infrared photography.

Cancer generates more heat than normal tissue and often also demands more blood supply from the body.

This produces the two clues —an abnormally warm area and enlarged veins—that are employed in the new screening method.

In the last year, 16 patients have had small tissue specimens—biopsies—taken solely on the basis of these two screening tests. Six were found to have cancers too small to be detected by ordinary examination.

The combination method was described in a report to the American Roentgen Ray Society's 68th annual meeting, now being held in the Washington Hilton Hotel.

The report was given by Dr. Irwin M. Freundlich of Jefferson Medical College in Philadelphia. He said the research had been initiated by his co-authors, John D. Wallace, a physicist and assistant professor of radiology at the school,

and Dr. Gerald D. Dodd, who is now director of the Department of Diagnostic Radiology at M. D. Anderson Hospital and Tumor Clinic in Houston.

The advantage of the combination method is the great rapidity and ease with which screening can be done by thermography, coupled with the precision of tumor location obtained by following up with the vein measurement method, Dr. Freundlich said.

The emphasis is on detecting cancers too small to be felt as lumps or too much obscured by noncancerous material to be found precisely by X-ray or thermography alone.

If more of these extremely small cancers can be detected before they grow, the report said, "it may safely be assumed" that the breast cancer mortality rate will be improved.

September 27, 1967

VACCINE CURBING A BABIES' DISEASE

By JANE E. BRODY

Studies of more than 1,000 women throughout the world have shown that a new, experimental vaccine is both safe and effective in preventing Rh blood disease in infants.

In the studies, described here yesterday at the annual meeting of the American Association of Blood Banks at the Americana Hotel, the vaccine failed in only one case to protect a mother from making antibodies that destroy her baby's blood.

Rh disease, which has the scientific name of erythroblastosis fetalis, occurs in about 10 per cent of the cases when an Rh-negative mother is pregnant with an Rh-positive baby. The Rh factor in the baby's blood is inherited from an Rh-positive father. The baby's Rh factor stimulates the mother, who lacks this factor, to make antibodies to it.

Blamed in Many Deaths

The disease often results in death of the unborn child or serious illness after birth. Rh disease, it is estimated, annually causes the death of 5,000 infants in the United States.

The name Rh is derived from the Rhesus monkey, in which the factor was first discovered.

Once a baby has been seriously affected by Rh disease, it may need exchange transfusions to replace all its blood to save its life. In the last few years, to save a baby that might not survive birth, such transfusions have occasionally been performed while the babies were still in the womb.

The Rh vaccine is designed to prevent onset of the disease by preventing the Rh-negative mother from becoming sensitized by her baby's Rh-positive blood and thus produce antibodies to it.

Doctors have found that the sensitization does not occur until some weeks after an Rh-negative mother has been exposed to Rh-positive blood and may not occur until after several such exposures.

Since exposure to the contrary blood usually occurs during delivery, the first pregnancy is not likely to be affected by Rh-incompatibilities.

The vaccine is given within a few days after the mother has given birth to an Rh-positive baby unaffected by the mother's Rh-negative factor. At that time, the mother has been exposed to the baby's contrary blood but has not become sensitized to it.

Therefore, the vaccine is given within a few days after an Rh-negative mother has given birth to an unaffected Rh-positive baby—before she is sensitized but after she has been exposed to the contrary Rh factor.

The vaccine, a highly concentrated solution of Rh antibodies, is obtained from Rh-negative persons who have been sensitized to the Rh factor. The principle of the vaccine is based on the observation that, when a person with Rh-negative blood is first given Rh antibodies, the person's immune mechanism is blinded and fails to recognize the Rh factor. Without recognition, the immune mechanism does not produce its own Rh antibodies.

In one report yesterday, Dr. William Q. Ascari of the Ortho Research Foundation summarized studies of the vaccine made by 43 researchers throughout the world These researchers used an experimental vaccine called RhoGAM prepared by the Ortho Pharmaceutical Corporation in Raritan, N. J.

Vaccine License Sought

The company has applied to the Division of Biologics Standards of the National Institutes of Health for a license to produce the vaccine commercially. The division said it could not comment about the application until a license had been awarded.

Dr. Ascari said that of 825 Rh-negative women who had been given RhoGAM within three days after the birth of an Rh-positive baby, only one women had become sensitized. But of 578 unvaccinated women, 41 became sensitized. Many of the vaccinated women have since given birth to another Rh-positive baby who was not affected by Rh disease.

Doctors from Liverpool, England, Edinburgh, Scotland, Freiburg, Germany, and New York City also reported at the meeting that hundreds of other women had been adequately protected by vaccine preparations similar to RhoGAM.

In Washington yesterday, Dr. Louis K. Diamond of Harvard Medical School predicted that erythroblastosis fetalis would soon be a "vanishing" disease as a result of the vaccine. Speaking to the 36th annual meeting of the American Academy of Pediatrics, Dr. Diamond estimated that 100,000 American women every year might need this treatment in order to eliminate the disease.

October 25, 1967

Hong Kong Flu: Story of the Close Race Between Man and the Virus

By HAROLD M. SCHMECK Jr.
Special to The New York Times

WASHINGTON, Feb. 8 — It appeared in Hong Kong from Mainland China last summer and washed through the Far East in a silent, invisible wave.

It reached Hawaii at the end of August, the continental United States the next week. Later it produced an epidemic that had hit most states by Christmas. It seems to be fading now, but neither the nation nor the world has seen the last of the Hong Kong flu.

The episode that began in July was a once-in-a-decade phenomenon with elements of a detective story and a race against time. Scientists everywhere are still fighting to catch up with the latest change in the predictably unpredictable flu virus. They have not succeeded, but they have some fresh ideas for the future.

At present the virus type that scientists call A2 Hong Kong 68 still seems to be causing "excess" pneumonia and influenza deaths in major American cities. There is some evidence of a second wave of the infection in Kansas, although no one expects this to spread very far.

In Europe, flu has been inexplicably light so far, although the Hong Kong virus strain has been detected many times.

In the United States, the experts doubt that there will be a widespread second wave this spring even though that was the experience during the big epidemic ten years ago. When the next flu season arrives next winter, it is expected to be light, but mostly of the Hong Kong type.

An estimated total of 15 to 20 per cent of Americans have had the Hong Kong flu since last fall. It is this high attack rate that makes the second wave seem improbable.

So many Americans now have protective antibodies against the virus that only crowded indoor living conditions of midwinter would be likely to permit its rapid spread. When these conditions return next winter, Hong Kong flu will have its second chance. But it will then be the "conventional" strain. Many persons will have acquired natural immunity. Vaccine will be readily available.

The events of the last season reflect the prime advantage the flu virus has always had over human ingenuity. Unlike many viruses that appear to remain the same for centuries, flu is changeable. It probably changes a little every year. By the end of about a decade the cumulative changes are so great that it is a stranger to most of mankind; hardly anyone has natural immunity to it, and the stage is set for another pandemic, an epidemic of worldwide proportions.

Network of 80 Laboratories

A worldwide flu surveillance network of 80 laboratories reporting to the World Health Organization from 55 nations keeps watch for these events. By late June last year none had seen anything unusual. The United States Public Health Service predicted there would be little flu during the coming winter.

But, at just that time, sneezes, coughs, sore throats and fevers were becoming uncommonly common in Hong Kong. By mid-July there was an epidemic, and Dr. W. K. Chang of the flu surveillance laboratory there, captured specimens of the virus from the throats of some of its victims. On July 29, she sent samples to the W.H.O. International Influenza Center in London and to the center for the Americas at the National Communicable Disease Center, Atlanta.

When these were analyzed, it became clear that the virus was substantially different from other current strains. Clinching evidence that another flu pandemic was at hand came from Tokyo where Dr. Hideo Fukumi of Japan's National Institute of Health found that few of his countrymen had antibodies protective against the new strain.

On Aug. 21, the first international alert was sent out by Dr. W. Charles Cockburn of the World Health Organization, but inevitably, the virus had gone out faster.

It had spread to Singapore by the beginning of August and to Malaysia, Vietnam, the Philippines and Taiwan later that month. There also was an outbreak on a ship returning to the American West Coast from Saigon.

Even earlier, on July 31, the 8,783-ton Israeli freighter Teverya entered the port of Nagoya, Japan, from Hong Kong. She was quarantined because 15 members of the crew had influenza. Dr. Fukumi got virus samples from these men and proved that it was the new Hong Kong strain. Some of the samples, adapted for vaccine use by a Japanese pharmaceutical concern, Toshiba Kagaku Koyogo Company, later became a major factor in United States vaccine production.

They were used as seed virus by Merck Sharp & Dohme and helped that company get into early production to make roughly half of the 20 million doses of vaccine available to Americans through the peak of the epidemic this winter.

The rest was produced by five other concerns: Eli Lilly & Co.; Wyeth Laboratories; the Lederle Laboratories Division of the American Cyanamid Company; Parke Davis & Co. and the National Drug Company.

From the start, many American virus experts were doubtful that any substantial amount of vaccine could be produced in time to help counter the epidemic that seemed certain to lie ahead. Only in retrospect could it be seen how close the race between man and virus sometimes was.

Outbreak in Hawaii

On Aug. 27, Dr. Maurice R. Hilleman, internationally known virus expert at Merck, cabled Dr. Fukumi asking for the best of the Japanese virus strains. On the same day, in Hawaii, there was an outbreak of flu at an air force base. Some men stationed there had just returned from a visit to the Philippines, Taiwan and Japan.

The Japanese sent the virus.

The strains also were made available to other manufacturers in this country.

During the second week in September, the United States manufacturers were invited to a meeting on vaccine possibilities by the Division of Biologics Standards of the National Institutes of Health. The division is responsible for judging vaccine safety and effectiveness.

During that same week in Teheran, Iran, medical scientists from all parts of the world were attending a congress on infectious disease. When they left, many of them, including some from the National Institutes of Health in the United States, had Hong Kong flu, presumably brought to the meeting inadvertently by the delegates from the Far East.

Throughout September and October, travelers by ship and airplane brought the infection to the United States and the virus became seeded widely in the country. Outbreaks occurred in several states and, at about the same time, the first batches of vaccine were released.

Work Against Handicaps

The vaccine makers were working against handicaps. Their normal vaccine production season had ended by July and they had shut down. They needed roughly 20 million fertilized eggs on which to grow viruses. These were hard to get. They needed glassware, extra facilities, extra workers. They needed everything in a hurry. Most of all they needed

virus strains that would produce copiously.

The flu won the race against vaccine production, but not as decisively as many had expected. Dr. Roderick Murray, director of the Division of Biologics Standards, noted later that the elapsed time from discovery of the virus to vaccine production was substantially shorter than it had been in 1957 when the most recent of the important new types of flu emerged from the Orient.

But it is also true that man's increasing mobility is making the epidemics more efficient, too. Dr. Bruce Dull, assistant director of the Public Health Service's Communicable Disease Center, Atlanta, said last year the virus seemed to appear almost simultaneously in widely scattered parts of the nation.

Before the day of rapid air travel, the movement was more gradual and in waves.

Scientists at many laboratories are seeking ways to counter-attack the flu virus more effectively. In a recent interview some of these research approaches were listed by Dr. Daniel I. Mullally, chief of the vaccine department branch of the National Institute of Allergy and Infectious Diseases. Included are use of adjuvants — substances that heighten the effectiveness and duration of vaccine effects; antivirus drugs; vaccines that can be sprayed into the nose rather than be given by injection and attempts to capitalize on something virus experts are calling "original antigenic sin."

An antigen is anything that provokes the body to make protective antibodies against it. The theory of original antigenic sin is that the body retains a special memory of the first type of flu virus it encounters. Thereafter, each fresh infection will beget antibodies against the infecting agent—but also some against that original antigenic type of flu.

In theory, if young persons could be vaccinated effectively enough against a broad spectrum of flu viruses, it is possible that in later life they would have some protection against any new strain that would arise.

But today this is theory and no means exists in practice to outwit the changeable flu virus. Some experts think adjuvants offer the best near-future hope, but no flue vaccine that includes one has yet been licensed. There must be abundant proof of safety first.

Meanwhile, the flue experts are haunted by a recollection and a puzzle. The recollection is of the great flu pandemic of 1918-19. For reasons that are still a mystery of it was far more deadly than any flu that has emerged since. During the pandemic, 20 million persons died.

The recollection of that great disaster is a major reason for the worldwide surveillance program that exists today. The thing that puzzles scientists is why it was so deadly then and when—if ever—the same thing will happen again.

February 9, 1969

Venereal Disease Rising; Many U.S. Young Afflicted

By JANE E. BRODY

Gonorrhea, a disease once thought under control, is rampaging through the country, crossing socio-economic lines, making inroads into suburbia and afflicting an overwhelming proportion of youngsters.

The alarm of public health officials over what they regard as a nationwide epidemic of gonorrhea is paralleled somewhat by an increase in the number of reported cases of syphilis in all but one section of the country during the first four months of this year. Syphilis has been on the decline for the last five years and many officials expected this decline to continue.

With more than one and a half million new cases each year, venereal disease is the nation's most common com-

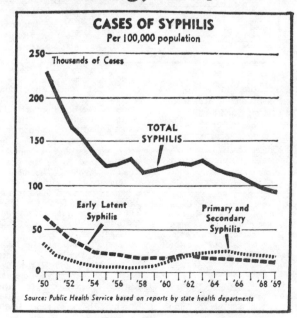

CASES OF SYPHILIS
Per 100,000 population

Thousands of Cases

TOTAL SYPHILIS

Early Latent Syphilis

Primary and Secondary Syphilis

'50 '52 '54 '56 '58 '60 '62 '64 '66 '68 '69

Source: Public Health Service based on reports by state health departments

municable disease, except for the common cold. The reported incidence of gonorrhea is rising at a progressively higher rate, 15 per cent in the last year and more than 200 per cent in some large cities.

In a survey of 30 major American cities conducted by The New York Times, public health officials attributed the rise in gonorrhea to relaxed sexual morality; increased promiscuity, especially among youngsters; abandonment of the condom, which offers some protection against infection, for the birth control pill; greater mobility of the population; general ignorance; lack of cooperation by the medical profession; insufficient funds to trace cases, and ostrich-like behavior on the part of victims who refuse to name their contacts and educational institutions that oppose the teaching of V.D. prevention in the schools.

In some cities, the increase in V.D. has been attributed in part to better reporting of cases to the public health authorities. (Studies have shown that the actual incidence of V.D. is four times the number of cases that are reported.) But most officials interviewed were sure that more and more people are being infected at younger and younger ages.

In Memphis last month, a 5-year-old boy was treated for gonorrhea. Investigation by health officials showed that he had had sexual relations with a 9-year-old girl. The girl refused to name her other sexual partners. End of the investigation.

Although the case is unusual, it illustrates how widely venereal disease is spreading among the young. It occurs most frequently among those between the ages of 20 and 24, followed closely by youngsters 15 to 19 years old. Statistically, a teenager gets V.D. every two minutes somewhere in America.

Last year in Philadelphia, 50 of the city's 13,006 reported cases of gonorrhea occurred among children under 10. And officials in San Francisco estimated that, in some of the city's high schools, a student has a 1-in-5 chance of getting V.D. before graduation.

Dr. Warren Ketterer, head of the venereal disease section of the California Department of Public Health, estimates that one of every 10 persons aged 15 to 24 in San Francisco will have venereal disease this year.

Syphilis Rate Rises

In the United States during the last fiscal year, 18,679 cases of primary and secondary syphilis (representing different stages of disease symptoms), were reported; this was a decline of 7.4 per cent over the total for the previous fiscal year. Thus far this year, however, all regions of the country except the South Central states have reported a higher incidence of syphilis.

Syphilis is caused by a spirochete, a long, tapered, worm-like microscopic organism called Treponema pallidum. The organism, which invades the body through mucous membranes, is spread from one person to another by direct sexual contact. The disease is not transmitted through contact with contaminated articles because the fragile spirochete does not survive outside the human body.

Occasionally, a baby is born with syphilis contracted from its mother during her pregnancy. Nearly 300 cases of congenital syphilis were reported in the country last year. The disease often kills the

CASES OF GONORRHEA AND RATES PER 100,000 POPULATION

Rates/100,000 in Selected Cities

Atlanta, Ga.	2,323.1	Los Angeles, Calif.	473.1
San Francisco, Calif.	1,845.4	New York City	437.9
District of Columbia	1,763.9	Seattle, Wash.	405.3
Norfolk, Va.	1,304.2	Las Vegas, Nev.	358.8
Newark, N. J.	1,259.0	Minneapolis, Minn.	325.6
Chicago, Ill.	1,062.6	Albany, N. Y.	303.9
Houston, Texas	877.4	Miami, Fla.	264.9
Cleveland, Ohio	834.4	Tulsa, Okla.	201.9
New Haven, Conn.	731.5	Pittsburgh, Pa.	114.9
Philadelphia, Pa.	625.4	Atlantic City, N.J.	85.1
St. Louis, Mo.	473.4	Waukesha, Wis.	4.4

Thousands of Cases

'50 '51 '52 '53 '54 '55 '56 '57 '58 '59 '60 '61 '62 '63 '64 '65 '66 '67 '68 '69

RATES → (204.0) (179.5) (161.3) (157.4) (152.0) (149.2) (142.4) (129.8) (129.3) (137.0) (139.6) (147.8) (142.8) (145.7) (154.5) (163.9) (173.6) (192.0) (219.2) (245.9)

Source: Public Health Service based on reports by state health departments

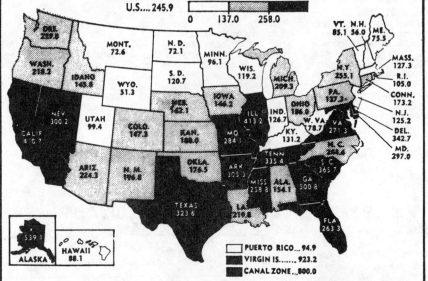

CASES OF GONORRHEA AND RATES PER 100,000 POPULATION
Fiscal year 1969

Median.....187.0
U.S.....245.9

Cases per 100,000 population

0   137.0   258.0

WASH. 218.2
ORE. 259.9
IDAHO 145.8
MONT. 72.6
N. D. 72.1
MINN. 96.1
WIS. 119.2
VT. 85.1 N.H. 56.0
ME. 75.5
WYO. 51.3
S. D. 120.7
MICH. 209.3
N.Y. 255.1
MASS. 127.3
R.I. 105.0
NEV. 300.2
UTAH 99.4
COLO. 147.3
NEB. 142.1
IOWA 146.2
ILL. 413.2
IND. 126.7
OHIO 186.0
PA. 127.3
CONN. 173.2
N.J. 125.2
CALIF. 410.7
KAN. 188.0
MO. 284.1
KY. 131.2
W. VA. 78.7
VA. 271.3
DEL. 342.7
MD. 297.0
ARIZ. 224.3
N. M. 196.8
OKLA. 176.5
ARK. 305.3
TENN. 335.4
N. C. 244.6
S. C. 365.7
MISS. 258.3
ALA. 154.1
GA. 300.8
TEXAS 323.6
LA. 219.8
FLA. 263.3

ALASKA 539.1
HAWAII 88.1

PUERTO RICO... 94.9
VIRGIN IS....... 923.2
CANAL ZONE...800.0

fetus, resulting in a spontaneous abortion, or stillbirth.

The first sign of infection in the adult is a sore, or chancre, on the genital organs. The chancre appears from 10 days to 10 weeks, but most often about three weeks after contact with an infected person. During the next four to six weeks, the chancre may clear up untreated, but a rash and other symptoms of illness may follow. These secondary symptoms may also disappear without treatment, and in about two-thirds of all cases, that is the end of the illness.

Without adequate treatment, however, years later about one-third of the victims develop generalized, debilitating and eventually fatal symptoms, including deterioration of the central nervous system and severe cardiac complications.

The introduction of penicillin after World War II sounded what seemed to be the death knell for syphilis. The number of reported cases dropped from a high of nearly 70,000 cases in 1948 to a low of 6,251 in 1957. Then the Federal Government curtailed funds for the V.D. program.

"That's what usually happens," said Dr. William Holder of the Mississippi Health Department. "When a disease control program reaches the point of near eradication, it's usually the program that's eradicated, not the disease."

The successful eradication of syphilis depends on the complete tracing of all persons who had sexual contact with any potentially infected person.

Last year in San Francisco, where officials interviewed 30,000 V.D. victims and followed up their contacts, an infected woman provided the names of about 300 long-distance truck drivers from all over the country with whom she had had contact.

In St. Louis, a major chain was started by a 20-year-old woman. One of her contacts refused to be treated at first. By the time he was located, he had spread the infection to six other women; eventually, 70 persons were involved.

Gonorrhea Not Traced

Contact tracing is almost solely limited to syphilis. No Federal funds, and in most cases no state funds, are available to do the same for gonorrhea.

Joe Pair of the Texas Health Department's V.D. services division believes that, with 25 more people on the syphilis program, he could eliminate the disease from Texas. He thinks that he would need 150 more people to do the same for gonorrhea.

There were 494,227 cases of gonorrhea reported in the United States during the last fiscal year, an increase of 62,847 over that of the previous year.

Gonorrhea is caused by a bacterium called Neisseria gonorrhoeae, which, like the syphilis spirochete, is transmitted solely by direct sexual contact.

Its short incubation period—three or four days—makes contact tracing far more difficult than with syphilis because by the time a contact is reached the disease is likely to have been spread to many others.

Some Are Resistant

Like syphilis, gonorrhea is readily treated with penicillin, but in recent years forms of the gonorrhea organism that are resistant to penicillin and other antibiotics have appeared in some parts of the country.

But Dr. Frank Gomila, director of the V.D. clinic in New Orleans, said that "the bugs aren't half as resistant to the drugs as patients are to instruction on prevention." Dr. Gomila added that he was plagued by "repeaters" who contract gonorrhea several times a year.

Although gonorrhea is not a fatal disease, it can lead to serious complications, particu-

larly in women. When the infection spreads through the pelvic organs, it can cause sterility.

A man who contracts gonorrhea has a severe burning in the urinary tract and a thick, yellow discharge three to nine days after becoming infected.

Eight out of 10 infected women, however, have no noticeable symptoms and unless they are named as contacts, they may never be treated and may continue to spread the infection for years. Dr. Walter Smartt, head of the V.D. control unit of the Los Angeles County Health Department, estimates that "45,000 women in Los Angeles have gonorrhea and don't know it."

Few Cases Reported

Another problem in bringing gonorrhea under control is the lack of a fairly simple screen-

ing test, such as the Wasserman blood test for syphilis. Gonorrhea can be detected by culturing a specimen from the patient's genital organs, a process that takes a week or more and even then is not 100 per cent accurate.

But by far the greatest deterrent to the eventual eradication of venereal disease is that few cases are reported to public health authorities, precluding the possibility of contact tracing.

A recent national survey found that, although private physicians treat about 80 per cent of the venereal disease cases, they report only one in nine to public health officials.

As one Memphis doctor said, "I'd be crucified by sundown if I reported a case to the health department and a caseworker showed up at the husband's office the next morning."

June 1, 1970

F.D.A. Lists 369 Drugs As Ineffective or Perilous

By HAROLD M. SCHMECK Jr.
Special to The New York Times

WASHINGTON, Nov. 27—The Food and Drug Administration has circulated among Federal agencies a comprehensive list of 369 drug products that it considers either ineffective or unduly hazardous.

The complete list was made available today to newspapers that requested it. A spokesman for the F.D.A.'s Bureau of Drugs said the list would also be sent, on request, to other interested individuals or organizations.

The drug agency has sought to remove each of the products from the market during the last 2½ years and many have been withdrawn, but many others are still in use. Among those on the list are several that have been among the 200 most-prescribed drugs in recent years.

Some of the products on the list have been sold and used for years. They make up somewhat more than 12 per cent of a group of roughly 3,000 products that came on the market between 1938 and 1962.

All these were later evaluated for efficacy by a study group of the National Academy of Sciences National Research Council acting at the request of the drug agency.

All the products on the list

made available today were reviewed and found wanting by the study group and by the F.D.A. In each case the drug agency has taken action to have the product withdrawn from the market.

Some of these actions began as early as mid-1968. In some cases manufacturers had taken the products off the market before-hand or did so after the drug agency acted. In other cases the concerns have contested the F.D.A. decisions. Several of these cases have gone to court, and many are still unresolved.

Because these official actions were taken singly or in small groups no comprehensive list had been available heretofore. It was compiled partly in response to pressure from Congress.

Some Congressmen were concerned over the fact that Government agencies continued to stock and dispense drugs that the drug agency considered useless.

For that reason the list has been sent to the Department of Defense, Veterans Administration, Public Health Service, Agency for International Development and other governmental units that might be concerned.

Because of the large number of products involved and the complicated nature of the legal proceedings, no one knows exactly how many of the drugs are still on the market.

Indeed, a spokesman for the Pharmaceutical Manufacturers Association criticized the list today on the ground that it included some drugs that had been voluntarily removed from the market and others concerning which appeals were still pending or new evidence had been submitted by the drug maker.

Dr. John G. Adams, the association's vice president for scientific and professional relations, said it was unfair to lump all the drugs together with no indication of the present status of any individual product.

He said the association had been trying for almost a month to put all the information on the drugs together in a form that could be used by a computer.

From this the industry group hopes to bring up to date the status of each product.

The drug agency's list includes many prescription drugs as well as products sold "over-the-counter." Among the former are drugs designed to be used against infections, to lower blood pressure, remove excess fluid from the body or to achieve such combination effects as relaxing muscles and relieving inflammation.

Among the over-the-counter drugs listed as ineffective are some mouthwashes, nasal sprays, nose drops, lozenges and several brands of toothpaste.

Inclusion on the list signifies that the drug agency believes the product in question lacks

"substantial evidence of effectiveness" or that its potential hazards outweigh its potential benefits—giving it "an unfavorable benefit-to-risk ratio."

On the list are a large number of fixed-combination drugs designed for use against infections — fixed combinations of penicillin with a sulfa drug, for example.

These have been judged "ineffective as fixed combinations" even though the individual active ingredients are effective. The drug agency's position is that the combination provides no benefits beyond those of the individual ingredients taken separately.

Furthermore, the specialists who reviewed the drugs believe the use of two agents in fixed combination may often either give the patient more of one drug than he needs or else less than is useful for him, thus increasing the risk of the drug treatment without adding any benefit.

The classic case of this sort concerned the widely used antibiotic combination sold under the trade name Panalba. It was finally withdrawn from the market this year after a long court fight. It had been among the 100 most-prescribed drugs in the United States.

In the case of the mouthwashes and toothpaste products on the list, the F.D.A. objected that there was no substantial evidence to support the maker's contention that the products reduced decay or had similar useful therapeutic properties. Presumably the manufacturers could have kept the products on the market without contest if they had withdrawn the advertising claims of effectiveness.

November 28, 1970

Infectious Diseases Rise As Use of Vaccines Lags

By HAROLD M. SCHMECK Jr.

Special to The New York Times

WASHINGTON, Sept. 18—Total victory against some important and all-but-conquered diseases is slipping away in the United States as more and more Americans ignore the vaccines available.

Public health experts consider the trends tragic because the diseases are preventable and, in theory, could be virtually eradicated by vaccines developed at great effort and distributed in major campaigns in communities from coast to coast.

The clearest example is that of measles, which one expert recently called "out of control." Other examples are polio and diphtheria, names that used to evoke terror in American households. They are rarities now, but some children still die because of them and national patterns of immunity are less than rosy.

The communicable disease most seriously out of control in the United States is gonorrhea, but for this disease there is no prospect of eradication by currently available methods. Syphilis is also on the upsurge, but not to the extent of gonorrhea.

The level of immunity to polio has been declining in recent years because of failure to use the vaccine. Public health efforts have been unable to stem the decline, perhaps partly because there have been no large and dramatic outbreaks. Altogether there were only 33 reported cases of polio last year; 20 the year before and this year's toll is about on a comparable plane so far.

But the percentage of American youngsters below the age of four who are adequately immunized against polio has dropped steadily for several years. One report puts the figure at 79 per cent of this age group in 1966 and only 65.9 per cent last year.

"How long this trend can continue before polio will again appear in epidemic form in the United States is impossible to say," one expert said in a report this year. He called poverty areas in some major cities and certain rural areas ripe for a polio outbreak.

Immunity to diphtheria has remained approximately level in recent years, but has been low enough to permit some serious outbreaks. Characteristically these have been in poverty areas.

The bulk of the cases have been concentrated in only a very few communities, but the germ that causes the serious illness is extremely difficult to eliminate from a population. Recent evidence shows that immunization will prevent the disease, but will not prevent a person from carrying and discharging the germ.

Thus it would appear that an extremely high percentage of inoculations in a community would be needed to remove all risk. This has been difficult in those poverty areas of the South where most of the recent local outbreaks have occurred. For reasons that are not clearly known, the South seems to be the major remaining stronghold in the United States of this once common and widespread illness.

The communicable disease situation is incomparably better than it was before vaccines against measles, polio, diphtheria and others were developed. No one foresees a national crisis or a return of the pre-vaccine patterns in any of them, but the end of these serious, and preventable, infections does not seem to be in sight.

"The crisis is in failure when success is totally achievable," said Dr. H. Bruce Dull, assistant director for programs of the Center for Disease Control in Atlanta, during a recent interview there. The center, known universally as the C.D.C., is the Federal Government's main agency for surveillance of communicable diseases.

Dr. Dull's point is well illustrated by the center's figures on measles. Since a vaccine against this virus disease was licensed in 1963 the number of cases and the number of deaths plummeted year by year.

Lines on Graph Up Again

Now the lines on the graph have started back up again. Experts at the C.D.C. think this year's total of measles cases may rise as high as 80,000. That would be almost twice as many as last year and more than any year since 1966.

Many of today's adults, virtually all of whom had measles as children, find it hard to take this erstwhile common childhood infection seriously. But measles can kill.

"This year we will probably be pushing 80 to 100 deaths," said Dr. J. Lyle Conrad of the

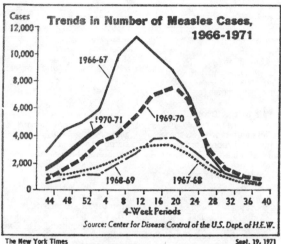

Source: Center for Disease Control of the U.S. Dept. of H.E.W.

The New York Times   Sept. 19, 1971

The measles season occurs between late fall and late spring, which accounts for way weeks are numbered in above chart. The 1970-71 curve has been rising. Its peak is expected to approach or pass that of 1966-67.

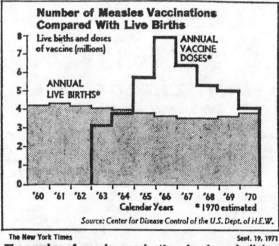

Source: Center for Disease Control of the U.S. Dept. of H.E.W.

The New York Times   Sept. 19, 1971

The number of measles vaccinations has been declining. To eliminate this disease, it would be necessary to vaccinate many more children than are born each year to catch up with the backlog of unvaccinated children.

C.D.C. during an interview earlier this week. The deaths usually result from pneumonia following the original virus infection. Another risk of the disease is encephalitis, inflammation of brain tissue, occurring in about one case in every 1,000. About one-third of the encephalitis victims suffer some permanent brain damage.

As the glamor of the measles vaccine has worn off and as victory over the disease has begun to seem within grasp the number of vaccinations has fallen off too.

Epidemiologists say that, in theory, it would be possible to vaccinate such a high proportion of susceptible people that a point of no return could be reached. Once over that threshold, total eradication might be achieved without a great deal of effort. Indeed, something of that sort may have happened with smallpox. Outbreaks were

once common in this country, but there has not been a documented, nonimported case in the United States in more than 20 years.

"We were heading for the threshhold, or maybe even past it, then we lost ground," Dr. Dull said of the measles situation.

The measles picture illustrates another point: Increasingly, communicable diseases are becoming primarily a problem of unimmunized children living in poverty, particularly nonwhite children. A higher percentage of white children have immunity to measles than do children of other ethnic groups. The central cities tend to lag behind the rest of the country.

"It is apparent that race, resistance and riches are factors affecting immunization status," said Dr. J. D. Millar of the C.D.C. at this year's annual immunization conference. He was speaking not only of measles but also of polio, diphtheria, whooping cough and tetanus. Inoculations against the latter three are given together in a combined vaccine.

He said efforts to maintain high levels of immunization in the population have failed most dramatically among the urban poor, who are predominantly non-white.

"In the United States, our central cities will continue to seethe with immunizable diseases, and thereby create a significant risk to other parts of the society, until these people are regularly included in immunization practice," he said.

Other experts noted that rural poverty areas also had problems with most of these diseases. In both cases the problem is often one of delivery of medical service. For a poor mother with several children a trip to a distant immunization clinic may be a costly all-day episode—unpleasant and seemingly unremunerative unless a disease outbreak is already in progress. But in that latter case the immunization may already be too late.

For some communities the problems have probably been compounded by the fact that funds from a Federal vaccination assistance program ran out in 1969 after being available for most of the decade of the sixties. No substitute program has been enacted to fill its place completely.

Another problem has been that national efforts to vaccinate against one disease seems sometimes to have usurped the impetus needed to complete the work against the previous fashionable illness.

Some experts say, for example, that a major national effort against rubella or German measles has taken attention and effort away from the effort against measles.

This view is not expressed as a criticism of the rubella campaign, which many experts consider highly important in its own right, but a criticism of the American penchant for going continuously from crisis to crisis.

The problem is not so much the crisis campaign, Dr. Dull indicated, but the long-term need for people to persist in getting protection that has become routine even though important.

"The health system doesn't lend itself to the routine in preventive medicine," he said.

September 19, 1971

NERVE TREATMENT CALLED EFFECTIVE

Parkinson's Disease Drug Used in 5-Year Test

By JANE E. BRODY

L-DOPA, a drug first described five years ago as possibly revolutionizing the treatment of Parkinson's disease, has stood the test of time, Dr. Melvin Yahr, medical director of the Parkinson's Disease Foundation, reported yesterday.

Dr. Yahr, a neurologist at Columbia University, said that about 75 per cent of patients who started with the drug were still taking it and getting a "reasonably good response."

He added in an interview that the drug was well tolerated by patients who took it every day for years, and that it had not been found to damage any of the body's main organs.

Dr. Yahr, who spoke in conjunction with the foundation's annual awards dinner, said that a new discovery was making it possible to use much smaller doses of L-DOPA and get faster results. The discovery is a chemical that blocks the use of L-DOPA by all the body's tissues except the brain, where the substance acts to control the symptoms of Parkinson's disease, including muscular rigidity and tremors.

Using this experimental chemical, Dr. Yahr said, 80 per cent less L-DOPA is needed to achieve the same effect and the initial side effects of nausea and vomiting are avoided. Another benefit is a substantial reduction in the usual cost of treatment—about $1 a day.

Available for 2 Years

Five years ago, when Dr. George Cotzias of the Brookhaven National Laboratory first reported his promising results using L-DOPA, his announcement was greeted with disbelief and one medical journal refused to publish the findings.

Today, about half the nation's one and a half million Parkinson's disease patients have been or are being treated with the drug, which was approved for marketing two years ago.

Dr. Yahr emphasized that L-DOPA did not cure the disease. Rather, he likened its action to that of insulin in the treatment of diabetes: it bypasses the function of cells that are "out of order." In Parkinson's disease, the non-functioning cells are believed to be in a region of the brain called the substantia nigra. The cells of this region fail to make dopamine, a crucial transmitter of nerve messages, and the result is uncontrolled tremors.

L-DOPA, which is a precursor of dopamine, serves as a source of supply of this neurotransmitter in the brain.

At the awards dinner last night, Sir John Eccles, a Nobel laureate, was honored for his work in elucidating how the brain controls normal movement. His work is believed to be essential to understanding the cause of abnormal movements in diseases like Parkinson's. Mr. and Mrs. Lawrence A. Harvey received the foundation's award for meritorious service.

May 5, 1972

Cancer Survey Finds Big Gain In Survival Rates Since 1940's

WASHINGTON, Sept. 26 (AP) —The Government reported today that important increases in survival rates from more than a dozen major forms of cancer have been achieved among white American patients since the nineteen-forties.

The National Cancer Institute said results of a new survey show marked improvement in the three-year survival rate for cancers of the bladder, brain, breast, cervix, uterus, larynx, thyroid and prostate gland; chronic leukemia and childhood leukemia; Hodgkin's disease; melanoma cancer of the skin, and multiple myeloma, a cancer that originates in bone marrow.

But the report, summarizing the survival experience of white patients diagnosed with cancer from 1940 through 1969 in more than 100 hospitals throughout the country, said that "there has been little or no improvement in life expectancy for patients with lung cancer and cancer of the pancreas."

Lung Cancer Up

"Lung cancer is the most common male cancer with 62,-000 new cases and 56,000 deaths annually," the report said, "and the incidence is still growing."

The report added that, during the 20 years in which survival rates had shown no improvement, the incidence of pancreas cancer has risen from seven cases for every 100,000 persons to nine for every 100,000.

The report, prepared for presentation today at the seventh National Cancer Conference in Los Angeles, said that similar information on cancer-survival rates among black patients was still being collected and analyzed for future publication.

But an independent study by researchers at Howard University here reported last May an alarming increase in cancer mortality among Negroes in the United States between 1949 and 1967.

The National Cancer Institute report, entitled "End Results in Cancer," said the data for the white patients cover 52 anatomical sites of cancer, treated by surgery, radiation and drugs.

Bladder Malignancies

It said that, while only 48 per cent of patients with cancer of the bladder survived for three years during the 1940-49 period, 62 per cent of patients with the same disease survived for a similar length of time in the 1965-69 period.

Among other findings of the survey are the following:

¶Most cancers are diagnosed after middle age.

¶Women survive longer after cancer diagnosis than men. This is partly because survival is often more favorable for the kinds of cancer found in women.

¶Surgery is the most commonly used form of treatment. Listing similar improvements for other forms of cancer, the report said:

"The one-year survival rate for children under 15 with leukemia indicates continuing progress and provides hope for further improvement.

"The rate has increased from 36 per cent in 1955-64 to 59 per cent in 1965-69. Among children with acute lymphocytic leukemia diagnosed in 1965-69, the one-year survival rate was 67 per cent."

September 27, 1972

L-DOPA Found Not to Slow Parkinson's Disease

By JANE E. BRODY

L-DOPA continues to be highly effective in alleviating the incapacitating symptoms of Parkinson's disease, but pioneers in its use told an international symposium here on Friday that the drug does not seem to slow the underlying progression of the disease.

Parkinson's disease, sometimes called shaking palsy, is an affliction of the nervous system that causes rigidity and muscle tremors, a wide-eyed staring expression and a peculiar shuffling gait. It progressively disables its victims over many years.

Prior to the experimental use of large doses of L-DOPA, which began some seven years ago in studies by Dr. George Cotzias of Brookhaven National Laboratory and others, the only potentially effective therapy was brain surgery.

L-DOPA, an amino acid extracted from velvet beans, was approved for marketing in 1970 and is now being used in the treatment of thousands of Parkinson's disease victims, about 75 per cent of whom benefit from the drug.

The substance acts to increase the brain content of dopamine, a transmitter of nerve messages that has been found to be deficient in a certain area of the brain of Parkinson's disease patients.

However, Dr. Andre Barbeau, a neurologist at the Clinical Research Institute of Montreal, told the symposium at Maimonides Medical Center in Brooklyn that although the drug greatly improved the quality of remaining life, it did not seem to prolong the lives of the patients.

"This shows that the underlying disease is due to something else besides a dopamine deficiency and this something else kills cells," Dr. Barbeau explained.

Throughout L-DOPA treatment, these brain cells continue to die, but those that are still alive are apparently able to function better.

Dr. Martin Mendoza of the Columbia-Presbyterian Medical Center said that a six-year study there of 60 patients treated with L-DOPA supported Dr. Barbeau's view.

"The drug definitely extends the period of independent existence, but makes little difference in life expectancy," Dr. Mendoza reported. The average age of death in the Columbia study has been 63 years.

"L-DOPA is still the best treatment we've got for Parkinson's disease," Dr. Barbeau said.

The research emphasis now is on ways of reducing the drug's unwanted side effects, which include psychiatric symptoms and involuntary movements.

May 21, 1974

A Big Step for Mankind: The End of Smallpox

By LAWRENCE K. ALTMAN

GENEVA — In one of public health's greatest triumphs, the most virulent form of smallpox, a viral killer that also leaves many survivors blinded and scarred for life, has been wiped out of the world.

Statistics from the World Health Organization here show that smallpox now exists in just one country, Ethiopia. In that country the strain of smallpox virus is mild and seldom fatal, according to the W.H.O., the United Nations subagency that over the last decade has brought 180 years of worldwide effort to eradicate smallpox nearly to a conclusion.

Since 1796, when Dr. William Jenner developed the smallpox vaccine, doctors have fought the infection successfully piecemeal. Physicians, by scratching the vaccine into the skin of schoolchildren and travelers, gradually reduced the impact of smallpox. Yet it was only after World War II that the level of health care reached the point at which, through better-organized efforts, the United States and other countries could rid themselves of a disease that has infected populations since ancient times.

Just seven years ago, when smallpox raged in 32 countries, health departments spent millions of dollars mobilizing epidemiologists and vaccination teams on an emergency basis whenever an infected traveler threatened to start an epidemic in a smallpox-free country.

Now, with only Ethiopia infected, chances of spread elsewhere are slim. But the threat remains as long as there is a single case of the disease.

Smallpox spreads primarily by respiratory droplets when a person coughs or sneezes during the initial stages of illness. For a day or two, a victim thinks he or she is coming down with an attack of "the flu." But then, unlike the flu, smallpox proceeds to dot the face and body with hundreds of scabs that often leave deep scars when the rash clears.

Unlike other viral diseases that are transmitted by insects (mosquitos and yellow fever) or animals (dogs and rabies), smallpox spreads through a human chain—each new case is traceable to a previous case. It is a disease only of man.

There are no "healthy" human smallpox carriers as there are of hepatitis, malaria, typhoid and other infections. A vaccinated individual is at no risk of spreading smallpox. Only an unvaccinated person, or one whose vaccination has long expired, can catch smallpox and thereby perpetuate the human-to-human cycle.

Therein rests the theoretical basis for the W.H.O. program to eradicate the disease by 1976, a feat which if achieved will mark the first time that man has made a disease extinct. This program, though laudable for its humanitarian benefits, owes more to the economics of the disease. Once smallpox is eradicated, the world's governments will

Lawrence K. Altman reports on medicine for The New York Times.

The Eradication of Smallpox

Source: World Health Organization

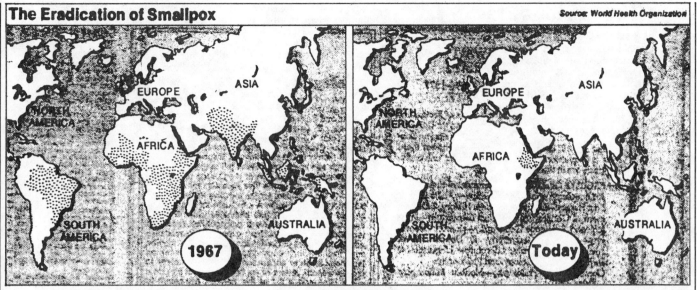

save at least $1 billion they now spend each year to keep themselves smallpox-free.

When the eradication program began in west Africa a decade ago, the strategy was to conquer smallpox primarily by mass vaccination programs that relied on jet immunization guns, with which health workers could squirt measured doses of vaccine into the outstretched arms of hundreds of people an hour.

But the guns often broke down, and spare parts had to be sent wherever the teams vaccinated. W.H.O. simplified the vaccination technique by changing to a needle with two short prongs, adapted from a needle originally used by veterinarians to immunize fowl against viral diseases. The prongs prevented untrained vaccinators from piercing the skin too deeply, minimizing the potential for dangerous secondary infections. And by dipping the needle into a bottle to pick up just a drop of vaccine, workers used less of the drug than the jet gun required.

Dr. Donald A. Henderson, the American epidemiologist who has headed W.H.O.'s smallpox eradication program from the start, said that the original dogma held that smallpox would disappear through the vaccination of about 80 percent of the population in mass campaigns, and the organization of a surveillance system to mop up the last few cases.

The strategy worked to the extent W.H.O. could provide the scores of experts needed to supervise the thousands of non-medically-trained vaccinators.

But a shortage of equipment in eastern Nigeria led, accidentally, to the discovery that by concentrating on the most infected areas, the smallpox cycle could be stopped by vaccinating just half the population.

"It was quite clear," Dr. Henderson recalled, "that we needed to concentrate less on mass vaccination and instead develop a reporting system so we could detect outbreaks, immediately quarantine infected cases and quickly vaccinate susceptible individuals who had been exposed to smallpox."

Where this strategy was applied, epidemiologists turned up record high numbers of cases. In fact, the totals were artificially high, because of the intensive case-finding methods and improved surveillance. But alarmed government officials responded with financial backing that they had previously withheld. In Brazil, for example, officials in 1969 authorized greater expenditures to push a vaccination program that in two years eradicated smallpox from that country, the disease's last focus in South America.

Meanwhile, W.H.O. learned other lessons from earlier mass-vaccination programs in India, where failure had convinced many international health experts that eradication was unattainable.

That failure had been owing largely to use of a technique employing deep circular scratches to administer what often proved to be impotent vaccine. The technique produced scars that were due not to a successful smallpox vaccination, as had been believed, but instead to abscesses and secondary bacterial infections.

And when just a few smallpox cases were being reported in southern India in 1973, Dr. Vladimir Zikmund, a Czechoslovakian epidemiologist who was setting up an active surveillance program there, surprised officials by tracing a case to a raging epidemic that local officials had concealed.

That incident led W.H.O. and higher Indian officials to devise a system whereby 100,000 Indian health workers were mobilized to repeatedly search every house across the country for smallpox cases. In Uttar Pradesh, where about 300 cases were reported weekly, search teams suddenly discovered 7,000 new cases.

"It was a shock when we learned that half the villages that were supposed to have been searched had not been visited," Dr. Henderson said.

News coverage of the newly reported cases made India seem to be suffering one of the world's worst smallpox epidemics. W.H.O. officials, far from being dismayed, pushed on with their effort to eradicate smallpox from India, the last crucial obstacle to the global program.

The key problem was money. The $900,000 that W.H.O. had budgeted for health programs in China, which Chinese officials then said they could finance themselves, were transferred to keep the smallpox program going until the Swedish Government independently donated $6 million in additional funds with which the vaccinators finally stopped smallpox in India and Bangladesh.

Compared to the estimated $85 million that world governments have contributed to W.H.O. over the decade for the smallpox program, the money spent on India and Bangladesh was a small investment that paid huge dividends.

Now that these two countries are smallpox-free, W.H.O. says smallpox apparently has been wiped out of Asia. Now only Ethiopia remains. In that country, health workers armed with two-pronged needles are flying in helicopters to quarantine smallpox cases and vaccinate their contacts to rid the world of what are expected to be the disease's last cases.

February 8, 1976

The Serious Flu

The Federal Government plans to immunize every person in the United States this fall against a flu virus that appeared last month in Fort Dix, N.J., and which seems similar to the virus involved in the 1918-19 world flu epidemic. At that time, an estimated 20 million persons, including 548,-000 Americans, died.

It is the potential for disaster, however remote, that has induced President Ford, with scientists' concurrence and the almost certain approval of Congress, to propose a vaccination program unprecedented in scope and in so brief a time. The vaccine needed will cost $135 million.

The virus, which has been found only in the single outbreak in Fort Dix, appears to be similar to the virus that causes influenza in pigs, the so-called swine flu virus that is blamed for the world epidemic. There is no way of knowing whether the newly found virus is likely to behave like the 1918 virus.

To date only small experimental batches of vaccine against the new virus have been produced. From experience with other flu vaccines, health experts have no doubt that the new vaccine will work. If all goes well, inocculation of high-risk groups, such as persons with heart disease, could begin in late summer.

March 28, 1976

SURGERY

Dissecting Surgery's Past

THE CENTURY OF THE SURGEON. By Jurgen Thorwald. Translated from the German by Richard and Clara Winston. Illustrated. 432 pp. New York: Pantheon Books. $5.95.

By CLAUDE E. FORKNER

USING as a narrative device a fictitious physician who lived through—and witnessed—the various stages of surgical development during the nineteenth century, Jurgen Thorwald takes the reader of his big book straight into the operating room. It is a spellbinding experience.

He shows the early attempts at amputations, plastic surgery and the removal of gallstones; the successful excision of a kidney by Gustav Simon in 1869 is one of the many innovations covered here. Made evident, too, is how swiftly surgery became an art through the tenacious search for advancement over such obstacles as greed, prejudice, sheer ignorance and unsterile methods.

Mr. Thorwald vividly describes the tortures endured by patients prior to the days of anesthesia. Witness the account, for example, of an attempt in 1843 to reset with a pulley-block the dislocated thigh of a fully conscious patient: "When the attendants drew on the rope,

Dr. Forkner is Professor of Clinical Medicine, Cornell University Medical College and attending physician at the New York Hospital.

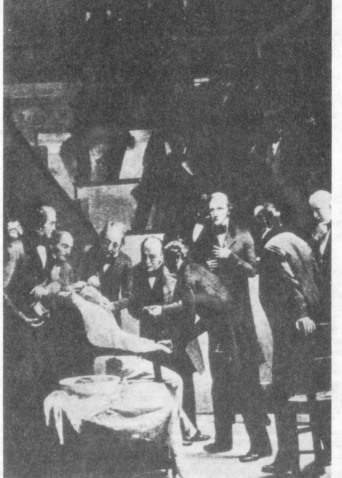

While Dr. William Morton, left, holds the inhaler Dr. J. C. Warren performs the first operation in which ether is used, Boston, Oct. 16, 1846.

Illustrations from "The Century of the Surgeon."

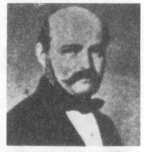

Ignaz Philipp Semmelweis.

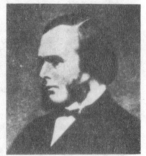

Joseph Lister.

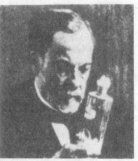

Louis Pasteur.

only the squeaking of the pulley-block was heard at first. But then came the patient's first scream. The attendants continued to pull. The patient tossed his head back and forth. * * * His body seemed to hover above the table as the rope grew tauter. The attendants pulled again. Suddenly the patient swung his arms wildly about, opened his bloodless lips, and bellowed like an animal."

The author, a German journalist with a background of medical study, does leave the impression, perhaps erroneously, that the surgeon of that time was heartless rather than sympathetic and attentive to the pain endured. The narrative soon turns from these early operative scenes, however, to the development of anesthetics. Mr. Thorwald points out that nitrous oxide had been used by Sir Humphrey Davy as early as 1800 for the relief of pain. Later in 1842 Crawford W. Long, a country doctor in Jefferson, Ga., administered ether successfully, but failed to appreciate the importance of his discovery. Other physicians, E. R. Smilie and Horace Wells, anesthetized patients with ether and nitrous oxide, respectively, but it was

William Morton, in 1846, who succeeded in convincing the surgeons at the Massachusetts General Hospital in Boston of the importance of anesthesia with ether. The bitter controversies that arose between Morton, Wells and the chemist Charles Jackson concerning these discoveries are presented in detail.

MR. THORWALD'S descriptions are excellent. There probably is no more dramatic episode in the book than that 1846 operation in Massachusetts General Hospital. After putting the patient, Gilbert Abbott, to sleep, Dr. Morton turned to the surgeon Dr. John Collins Warren of Harvard: "Sir, your patient is ready.' Silently Warren bent over Abbott, his face expressionless as ever. He rolled up his sleeves and took his scalpel in hand. Then, with a lightning motion, he made the first incision * * * the patient did not stir. Warren—astonishment in his face for the first time—stooped closer. He made a second and a third incision, deeper this time, but not a sound emerged from Abbott's slack mouth. Carefully, Warren scraped out the tumor. * * * Still nothing—nothing but si-

lence. Utter silence. Warren straightened up * * * his eyes alight with the glory of an unknown, inconceivable miracle. 'Gentlemen, he exclaimed at last, 'this is no humbug.'"

In spite of the development of anesthesia and the improvement of surgical techniques, the mortality from operations remained extraordinarily high because bacteria, the cause of infections, were not discovered until 1862-63 —and knowledge of their discovery not widely disseminated until much later. For example, until Edoards Porro, of San Matteo, in Pavia, in 1876 developed the method of hysterectomy, the maternal mortality from infection after Caesarian section was near 100 per cent. The perfection of his method reduced the maternal mortality to 56 per cent

There is an excellent description of the birth of the idea that infection was spread by unclean hands and instruments. Here the particular reference is to the studies of Ignaz Philipp Semmelweis at the Vienna General Hospital. Semmelweis, shaken by the epidemic of deaths in his maternity ward, made the discovery that was to drive him mad before it was

generally accepted—a discovery that was translated into a historic notice he posted on the clinic door: "As of today, May 15, 1847, every doctor or student who comes from the dissecting room is required, before entering the maternity wards, to wash his hands thoroughly in a basin of chlorine water which is being placed at the entrance. This order applies to all, without exception."

The subsequent discovery of bacteria by Louis Pasteur and the application of this knowledge by Joseph Lister in 1865-66 to surgical procedures are well presented. The drama inherent in these developments is often quietly evoked. "Suppose," Lister muses after reading Pasteur's paper on microbes, "I covered wounds with dressing soaked in carbolic acid solution—might not this dressing operate * * * as a filter to keep the microbes away from the wound?" Mr. Thorwald graphically sketches in the frustrations, bitterness and prejudice encountered by Pasteur and Lister when their ideas were presented to the scientific societies of their period.

October 20, 1957

REVIVED BY HEART MASSAGE.
Successful Cases Described to Philadelphia Physicians.

From The Philadelphia Public Ledger.

Dr. W. W. Keen declared at a meeting of the Philadelphia County Medical Society last night that a most remarkable field of surgery had been opened in cardiac massage, whereby life apparently extinct had been restored by renewing the heart's pulsation.

"Life apparently extinct has been renewed, or shall we say the dead themselves have been brought back to life," said the doctor, "by continuing the heart's pulsation when it has closed by forcing the physical action through massage."

Dr. Keen made this important assertion when he discussed "a case of abdominal hysterectomy in which massage of the heart for chloroform collapse was employed."

The operation, which the famous surgeons of the world, primarily in Europe, have employed twenty-seven times, has been successful twice. Dr. Keen was himself one of the first to resort to the delicate use of the knife in this country, but was unsuccessful. He reported how, when in operating for "Total Laryngectomy," the heart ceased to beat, respiration was absent, and collapse from chloroform complete, the diaphragm was cut open and the massage method employed. Death in this instance had been apparent for at least five minutes before the operation was undertaken. When at the end of that time the heart had been exposed and massage applied, the heart resumed its pulsation, and the respiration was restored by artificial means, but death occured within thirty minutes.

After the incision in the diaphragm, which should be made within five minutes after life is apparently extinct, Dr. Keen described the

massage method in brief as follows: "Place one hand on the exterior, and with the other apply the massage to the lower lobe of the organ. Within five minutes the pulsation of the heart is restored. While cardiac massage is applied artificial methods of respiration must be applied at the same time."

Dr. Keen mentioned two successful cases, and declared when surgery had perfected the exact method of applying the massage one of the greatest advances of surgery would be achieved.

In explaining the experiment which had given this operation to surgery Dr. Keen related laboratory experiments with dogs' hearts taken from the bodies after death. In these experiments the hearts had been frozen forty hours, and fifty hours after death the pulsation had been restored by massage.

March 25, 1904

HIS HEART SEWN UP, PATIENT STILL LIVING

Physicians in this city are watching with great interest the case of Camillo Detano, a young Italian, who last Sunday night was taken to the Harlem Hospital suffering from a stab wound which had punctured the wall of the heart and penetrated the right auricle. A rare and difficult operation was immediately performed by three of the surgeons attached to the hospital, all of whom are young men, and the wound in the heart was sewn together. At a late hour last night the man was still alive, and there was hope, although a slim one, that he might recover.

That Detano reached the hospital alive was in itself bordering on the miraculous.

He was stabbed in a saloon at One Hundred and Thirteenth Street and First Avenue. He was left for about five minutes sitting in a chair. Then three other Italians walked him up to the Harlem Hospital, about twelve city blocks away. In that walk the man lost so much blood that, according to all preconceived notions of medical science, the loss in itself ought to have been sufficient to kill him.

Finding the man still alive in spite of everything he had undergone, Dr. S. G. Burns and L. A. Parmenter, assisted by Dr. Hazzard, hurried him to the operating room, and began preparations for the operation at once, knowing that every second lost made their task less hopeful. Under the most favorable circumstances the operation they propose to perform does not leave the patient alive after its completion in one case out of a thousand.

While they made their instruments and other paraphernalia ready, a messenger was rushed to the neighboring Church of Our Lady of Mount Carmel, returning with the Rev. Father F. Cardi. The priest administered the last rites to Detano and stayed with him through the operation.

To get at the heart the physicians had to saw off an inch and a half of the third right rib. Their next task was the ligation of two arteries, an operation that in itself involves life and death. Having got that far, and still finding the man breathing, they were able to give their attention to the heart itself.

They found that the right auricle had been seriously punctured, the width of the wound being about one-quarter of an inch. This wound was closed with a single stitch, and the usual dressings applied.

The entire operation consumed thirty-five minutes. Anaesthetics were used. Detano not only survived, but regained partial consciousness during the next night. Last evening he was resting with some ease considering the circumstances, and the physicians were beginning to entertain hopes of his final recovery.

June 20, 1905

MARVELS OF BONE SURGERY.

Surprising Results Obtained in Several Cases of Transplantation.

Dr. John H. Gleason of Manchester, N. H., has summarized, in the International Journal of Surgery, the result of transplanting bones or sections of bone in human beings. He says there is now a general agreement as to the death of the implanted bone. Then it receives a new blood supply and is penetrated by new granular tissue. By this means new canals are formed in the bone and these, the so-called Harversian canals, are lined with new osteoblasts, the "seed" of new bone. The old bone is absorbed and new bone forms in concentric layers around the new vessels. These changes, he declares, depend solely on the regenerative power of the transplanted periosteum and marrow.

Bardenheuer, he says, used half of an ulna, one of the bones of the forearm, to replace a radius, the other bone in the forearm. Kiapp replaced part of the bone of the upper arm with a piece of bone from the leg. H. H. Janeway cut out a piece of an arm bone five and a half inches long, and replaced it with a piece the same length taken from a leg bone, and there was a good functional result and no deformity.

"Of great importance," continues the writer, "is the transplantation of joints by Lexer. In his first publication he reports four functionally successful cases in which portions of bones with adjacent parts of joints have been replaced by bone and cartilage. In a second publication he adds the report of a total transplantation of a knee joint in a girl 18 years of age. In eighteen months' time the patient could walk with only a slight limp and rocking of the knee joint."

January 28, 1911

MIRACLES OF SURGERY SHOWN IN A GREAT CONGRESS

THE efficiency of modern surgery has just been demonstrated in Philadelphia in a striking manner and on a very elaborate scale.

It is certain that no city on this continent has ever before had as its guests at one time such a large and distinguished body of surgeons as that which attended the second annual session of the Clinical Congress of Surgeons of North America from Nov. 7 to and including Nov. 16. More than three thousand of them registered at the headquarters of the congress in the Bellevue-Stratford Hotel.

It is equally certain that a busier lot of surgeons never got together before. The majority of them were busy from 8 o'clock in the morning until nearly midnight. It might be expected that when these men left the fields of private endeavor for a brief period that more or less relaxation could be anticipated. There was no rest for them, however.

Clinics began at a score or more hospitals as early as 8 o'clock, and were continued with brief intermission until 5 o'clock in the afternoon. After dinner papers were read to large gatherings in the auditoriums of the various medical colleges, and were followed by discussions. Nearly all of the surgical ills that human flesh is heir to were dealt with both in the clinics and at the evening meetings.

It may be news to a large number of persons that there are more hospitals and more medical schools in Philadelphia than in any other city of any size in the world. This statement probably will be received with incredulity by some, yet it is boldly stated and apparently without fear of successful contradiction by residents of Philadelphia. Because of the large number of these institutions it was possible to hold fifty or more clinics each day. Half a dozen patients, and in some instances a larger number, were either examined or operated upon at every clinic, and as the work was carried on uninterruptedly for about nine days, it is estimated that between 2,500 and 3,000 persons were attended in one way or another by the most famous surgeons of the United States and Canada.

When Dr. Albert J. Ochsner of Chicago, President of the Congress, called the first meeting to order on Nov. 7 the State of Pennsylvania at large, and Philadelphia in particular, little realized the physical benefit that was about to be derived from the convention. The fact is, the city itself did not have on hand a sufficient clinical material to afford the experts in the various branches of surgery an opportunity to demonstrate their particular methods of procedure for the benefit of their confrères. Hurry calls were sent broadcast, and many a country doctor was enabled to obtain free the services of the best surgeons in the world for needy patients who otherwise would have had to get along without operations necessary to physical rehabilitation.

And, of course, under the critical eyes of his brother craftsmen each surgeon did his best. The results achieved in the rarer and newer operations were notable and called forth the earlier remark that the efficiency of modern surgery was strikingly exemplified. The congress was not distinguished, however, by any startling innovations or radical departures from well-established methods of procedure, if one or two bits of surgery, which were purely experimental and of which the outcome is still in doubt be excepted. One eminent Philadelphia surgeon summed up the work in this laconic fashion:

"We are simply doing an unusually

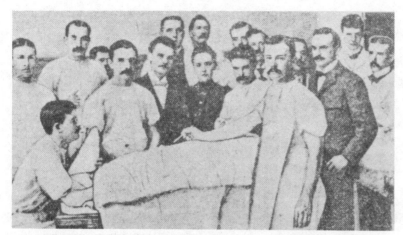

Dr. Howard A. Kelly About to Perform a Serious Operation.

large number of such operations as are being done every day somewhere or other in the world."

It may be mentioned here that every organ and tissue in the human body was subjected to the knife at some time or other during the congress, with the sole exception of the heart.

Before proceeding to a consideration of the details of the work accomplished a brief history of the Clinical Congress of Surgeons is in order. The first annual session was held in Chicago last year. No more than 300 or 400 surgeons attended, but the fame of the body spread, and its popularity was manifested in numbers and enthusiasm at the Philadelphia session. It is planned to hold the third session in this city next year, and the congress can now be regarded as a firmly established institution second to none of its kind.

Dr. J. M. Baldy of Philadelphia, one of the Committee of Arrangements, said that while the attendance had reached the unexpected total of nearly 3,000, probably not more than 1,000 were present at one time.

The clinics most largely attended probably were those of Dr. John B. Deaver, whose fame as an operator is world-wide; Dr. J. M. Baldy, Dr. John H. Gibson, and Dr. W. Wayne Babcock, who has had remarkable success in operating under the influence of spinal anaesthesia and the particular anaesthetic Dr. Babcock employs in stovaine.

The first scientific meeting was held in Egyptian Hall in the Wanamaker Building, on the evening of Wednesday, Nov. 8. Dr. Maurice H. Richardson of Boston, the foremost surgeon of New England, read a paper on "Surgery of the Pancreas," a subject which has not received marked attention except in recent years, although it is now acknowledged to be of prime importance. Dr. J. F. Binnie of Kansas City, read a paper on "Surgical Pathology of the Stomach and Duodenum," and Dr. George E. Brewer of this city, the well-known surgeon of Roosevelt Hospital, read one on "Surgery of the Liver and Bile Ducts."

The assertion is frequently made by the laymen that the surgeon is always ready to use the knife—too ready, the layman often puts it. There is a reason for the surgeon's eagerness, and here it is: When operation is delayed, either through fear of the knife on the part of the patient, his family, or friends, the surgeon often finds, when he is called upon to act, an irremediable condition, due to delay alone, and which would not have confronted him had he been permitted to operate as his judgment dictated.

This point was brought out admirably

by Dr. Deaver when he opened the discussion on Dr. Richardson's paper on "Surgery of the Pancreas."

"I wish to make a plea," he said, "for prompt surgical interference in cases of chronic pancreatitis (inflammation of the pancreas) instead of waiting for the report of the blood diagnosis from the laboratory. I believe in laboratory work, but when it is evident from all the well-recognized symptoms that the trouble lies in the pancreas it is better to operate at once, instead of letting the patient die while the surgeon waits for the blood count from the laboratory to find if the trouble is really what he suspected."

"There is no reason," Dr. Deaver asserted further along in his discussion of the subject, "why any healthy man should have indigestion. In the majority of instances of acute indigestion the trouble arises from enlargement of the pancreas. Chronic pancraeatitis can be averted if the pancreas is treated by the surgeon before it becomes chronic. And cancer can be cured if an operation is performed before it becomes cancer. Too often the trouble develops into cancer while the surgeon is waiting to see if it is really malignant disease he has to deal with. In the same manner diabetes can be averted before it becomes diabetes."

About three years ago the writer described in THE TIMES the astonishing experiments carried on by Dr. Alexis Carrel in the Rockefeller Institute for Medical Research, in the course of which various tissues and organs were transplanted from the bodies of certain animals to those of others, in which they remained and performed their normal functions, as though nature had placed them in their latter environment. Subsequently the transplantation of tissues, such as bone, muscle, and portions of blood vessels, became classic surgical procedures in the human organism. No attempt was made, however, to transplant an entire organ from the body of one human being to another—at least not until the session of the Surgical Congress which has just ended.

The operation referred to was performed last Monday by Dr. L. J. Hammond, chief of staff in the Methodist Episcopal Hospital in Philadelphia. It consisted in the removal of an entire organ, one of the so-called ductless glands, in a male patient, and the substitution of a sound organ taken from another body in its place.

The gland transplanted was taken from the body of a healthy man who had been killed in an automobile accident the previous afternoon, and Dr. Hammond seized upon the opportunity to replace

the pathological gland with a sound one. The patient was anaesthetized and the operation performed in the presence of a considerable number of surgeons who had visited the clinic. In order to prove successful the operation required the exercise of great skill and care, as the most delicate adjustment of blood vessels and tissues was necessary to re-establish an adequate circulation. Dr. Hammond expressed the opinion that this had been accomplished in a satisfactory manner, and sixty hours later informed a reporter for THE TIMES that he had every hope of the ultimate success of the experimental operation.

Dr. Carrel himself attended one of the scientific meetings and told of his latest work in blood-vessel surgery. His talk was illustrated by lantern slides. The details of his experiments in this field have already been presented to the readers of THE TIMES.

One of the many notable features of the congress was the meeting held in the ballroom of the Bellevue-Stratford on the evening of Nov. 9, when Dr. Ochsner delivered his Presidential address. In the course of it he made a strong plea for what might be well termed "free trade" in clinical methods and besought his confrères to free themselves of prejudice, provincialism, and personal conceit.

"The present age has made great strides toward efficiency," he said. "Merchants, manufacturers, and financiers have achieved practical results by the sacrifice of personal conceits and by the use of sound judgment, and practical results in the medical profession have been marvelous.

"Our friends in Philadelphia," he continued, "have furnished for us the most magnificient demonstration that I have ever witnessed in this or any other country. To-day the best thought is for all concerned; prejudice and provincialism are no longer possible as hindrances to progress."

Continuing Dr. Ochsner suggested a system of study for surgeons. He advised them to devote a part of each year to visiting clinics in different sections of the country, and stated that the congress had been organized with a view to carrying out this plan. He also suggested the organization of more surgeons' clubs in the cities, so that the members could meet often and compare notes. The stimulus to good work in the profession, if this plan was followed, would be enormous, he declared. He asserted, moreover, that the working plant for surgeons in this country could be capitalized at half a billion dollars.

Dr. William J. Mayo of Rochester, Minn., one of the two brilliant brothers whose fame as surgeons has spread wherever surgery is known, read a paper at this meeting on cancer of the stomach and its surgical cure. Those who expected to hear determined expressions of opinion from Dr. Mayo were not disappointed, and they were received with warm applause. "Cancer is still a problem," said Dr. Mayo, "and there is no authenticated record of a case of cancer of the stomach being cured by medical means. In spite of this fact, however, this disease continues to be almost entirely treated by physicians, and only rarely gets to the surgeons. This is one form of cancer which should be brought directly to the surgeon. On the other hand, medical men hasten cases of appendicitis to the surgeon, when in the majority of instances the ailment could be cured by means other than surgery.

"Operations on the stomach are no more difficult to perform than on any other organ in the intestinal tract. The mortality resulting from operation for cancer of the stomach has decreased."

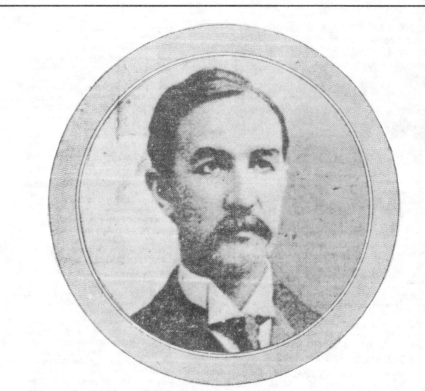

Dr. L. Webster Fox.

Dr. Mayo dwelt at some length on statistics and quoted figures to show that 90 per cent. of patients recover from operations for cancer of the stomach; in more than 36 per cent. of these the patients remain well for three years, while in more than 25 per cent. there is no recurrence in five years.

The speaker also detailed some of the most approved methods of making an early diagnosis, and insisted that when operative interference is resorted to as soon as the diagnosis is established the chances of recovery are quite as good as after operations for cancer in any other part of the body.

At the same meeting addresses were delivered by Dr. John B. Murphy, who is Chicago's foremost surgeon and President of the American Medical Association, and the eminent Dr. Abraham Jacobi of this city, President-elect of the American Medical Association.

Striking improvements in the methods of treating aneurisms have been made in recent years. An aneurism is the dilatation of a blood-vessel at some weak point in the structure. It loses its elasticity and gradually distends until it may become very large. The wall weakens, as in the case of an old, worn out rubber hose. It is a constant menace to life, and interferes with the orderly circulation of the blood to a great extent. In the event of its bursting, death follows with great rapidity.

The most frequent seat of aneurism probably is the aorta, the great parent artery that carries the blood away from the heart. The most helpful method of alleviation in this condition, it naturally follows, is to strengthen the weakened arterial wall. It was discovered a few years ago that a thin wire of silver or gold could be safely introduced into the calibre of the artery and coiled within the cavity of the aneurism. Such a procedure has resulted very frequently in an improvement in the patient's condition. As the heart forces the blood along the artery it must spend some of its force against the new metallic lin-

ing formed by the spiral of wire.

An operation of this sort provided an exhibition of delicate technique on the part of Dr. Charles H. Frazier before several members of the Clinical Congress at the University Hospital last Monday. The patient was a man. After the preliminary incision about six feet of gold wire was introduced into the aneurism of the aorta through a hollow needle. A light current of electricity was passed through the wire to stimulate the arterial wall to contraction and to aid in the coagulation of the blood around the loops of the wire and the wall, thus materially strengthening the aorta at its weakest point.

Another delicate operation performed by Dr. Frazier at the same clinic was the removal of a tumor at the base of the brain and threatening blindness by reason of pressure influence transmitted to the optic nerve.

A hundred or more eye specialists visited the clinic at the Medico-Chirurgical Hospital at different times to watch Dr. L. Webster Fox perform a variety of operations for blindness and other eye defects. The patients operated upon varied in age from six months to eighty-four years.

Some of the women surgeons who attended the congress had an opportunity to show their skill with the knife, and they performed a number of operations at the Woman's Hospital of Philadelphia and the hospital of the Woman's Medical College.

A spectacular operation scheduled as "Resection of the Abdominal Wall for Obesity," an operation, by the way, which was not new to Philadelphia, was performed at Samaritan Hospital on Tuesday by Dr. W. Wayne Babcock, a brilliant young surgeon who has become widely known through his adherence to spinal anaesthesia, a method of procedure which was proved very satisfactory in his hands. The patient was a woman. She wanted to be thin and was willing, as is frequently the case, to submit to the most

heroic treatment to attain that much-desired condition.

Having heard of the wholesale and almost instantaneous reduction of superabundant tissue by the knife, and having the woman's natural curiosity to know what was going on while it was being effected, she selected a painless method, which, at the same time, would not rob her of her senses. So Dr. Babcock employed his favorite anaesthetic—storaine. An injection was made into the spinal canal, and when local anaesthesia had resulted a long incision was made in the median line of the abdominal wall, the skin was carefully dissected back, and several layers of fatty tissue were removed from bewteen the muscles. The external incision was closed with stitches, a dressing applied—and the patient was twelves pounds lighter. While there is no guarantee that the tissue will not accumulate again, this is no indication that the operation will not become popular. At any rate, one who has undergone this operation is furnished with a subject for surgical conversation which ought to last a lifetime.

Only a very few of the hundreds of operations performed during the course of the congress can be mentioned here, but these are sufficient to indicate the latitude of the physical conditions dealt with, as well as to furnish some idea of the degrees of skill which our surgeons of to-day have acquired. The necessity for this skill and the wide application of medical and surgical assistance may be gained from a study of some figures furnished by Dr. Ira S. Wile of this city at the meeting of the American Association of Clinical Research held in Boston a year ago. Here are a few extracts from his report:

"In taking the ordinary history of a patient there are many omissions that are of value when later ascertained. Does the income of a man bear any relation to his illness? Chapin, in his studies, found the following expenditures for health:

"$400 to $500 class spent $14.18, 8.1 per cent.; $500 to $600 class spent $10.30, 1.9 per cent.; $800 to $900 class spent $23.30, 2.6 per cent.; $1,000 to $1,100 class spent $14.80, 1.5 per cent.

"This small expenditure in terms of money indicates a condition of general good health or else the people made good use of gratis service in dispensaries, &c. The percentage of the total income is high enough to receive attention. If one considers the expenditures by nationalities, there is more light shed upon the question:

	$600 to $700 Class	$1,000 to $1,100 Class
United States spent	$11.09, 1.6%	$13.55, 1.3%
Teutonic spent	$15.33, 2.3%	$7.72, 0.7%
Irish spent	$17.05, 2.6%	$21.00, 2.3%
Colored spent	$7.95, 1.2%	$1.00, 0.1%
Russians spent	$14.38, 2.3%	$32.92, 3.1%
Italians spent	$18.75, 2.8%	$11.53, 1.3%

"The Russians, Italians, and the Irish appear to have greater expenditures for health in both groups, but it does not mean that they have more illness than the colored, for example:

"The medical profession is most active in quoting statistics, but the rank and file of its members are extremely passive in the co-operation that is essential for their acquisition. The time must come when every doctor will be engaged in compiling his statistics, so that the problems of health may have a better light shed upon them. Only by this means will morbidity figures be established.

"Ayres investigated the causes of absences of over one week duration among 16,000 children in the New York public schools and found the following cases of illness causing the absences:

Measles	2,108	Accidents	258
Scarlet fever	1,550	Tonsilitis	251
Diphtheria	1,102	Broken bones	221
Pneumonia	621	Typhoid	219
Pertussis	473	Nervousness	217
Varicella	387	Appendicitis	204
Eye troubles	365	Rheumatism	200
Mumps	288	Other diseases	1,562

And here is a paragraph from an article on "Aesthetics of Surgery," by Dr. Antonio M. Crispin of this city, published in the New York Medical Journal:

"We have seen that surgery possesses all the elements which compose the fine arts, besides its highly, altruistic tendencies. It is decidedly utilitarian, increasing the happiness of the individual, relieving him of malformations, repairing and creating new conditions, augmenting their beauty, saving or prolonging life. We also find it to be superior to the other arts in that its aim is not only the weal or woe of the individual but, what is more important still, the betterment and conservation of the race."

An important statement was made by Dr. Deaver in the course of a discussion of a paper read at the meeting of the Pediatric Society last Tuesday evening.

He declared that thousands of infants die because physicians treat them for marasmus and indigestion and other infantile diseases when in reality the trouble is due to tumor at the pylorus, the point of entry from the stomach into the intestine. Dr. Charles L. Scudder of Boston, who had read the paper on "Pyloric Stenosis in Infancy and its Surgical Treatment," quoted statistics to show that since this condition had been recognized, that is, in the last few years, and the proper surgical procedure carried out, the mortality resulting from the operation had been reduced, until now it was about 7 per cent. in the cases which he personally knew.

He declared that the surgeon should take these cases in hand as soon as the diagnosis was made, in order to prevent the starvation of the infants and also in order that the proper procedures could be employed before the patients became too weak to withstand them.

Among the other distinguished surgeons who attended the congress and took part in the proceedings were Dr. Hugh T. Patrick of Chicago, Dr. Harvey Cushing of Baltimore, Dr. Joseph A. Blake of New York, Dr. J. M. T. Finney of Baltimore, Dr. Charles N. Dowd of New York, Dr. R. Tunstall Taylor of Baltimore, Dr. William M. Sweet of Philadelphia, Dr. Edward Reynolds of Boston, Dr. Edward B. Cragin of New York, Dr. John A. Sampson of Albany, Dr. Joseph H. Bryan of Washington, D. C., Dr. Graham Bacon of New York, Dr. John E. Weeks of New York, and Dr. Charles H. Mayo of Rochester, Minn.

Dr. Franklin H. Martin was General Secretary of the congress, and Dr. John G. Clark was Chairman of the Philadelphia Committee on Arrangements.

The following officers were elected for the ensuing year: President, Dr. Edward B. Martin of Philadelphia; Vice President, Dr. George E. Brewer of New York; General Secretary, Dr. Franklin H. Martin of Chicago; Treasurer, Dr. A. D. B. Knabel of Chicago, and General Manager, Dr. A. B. Ballou of Chicago.

November 19, 1911

NEW AID TO SURGERY IN CARREL DISCOVERY

Shows That Almost Any Organ Can Be Patched Up, Says Student of His Work.

STEPS LEADING TO FEAT

Long Experimentation with Keeping Alive Organs After Removal from Living Body.

Physicans and surgeons were of different minds yesterday concerning the practical value of the discovery of Dr. Carrel of the Rockefeller Institute that the viscera can be made to perform their functions after being detached from the living body to which they belonged. Those who discussed the matter at all did so only after stipulating that their names should not be used. Some of these men frankly declared that they did not know what use could be made of the interesting results of Dr. Carrel's experiments. Dr. Freudenthal, of 1,003 Madison Avenue, who was present when Dr. Carrel told something of the story of his most recent achievement, would only say:

"Dr. Carrel's work will add greatly to our knowledge of physiology."

Another physician said:

"Dr. Carrel himself is the only man who can furnish any satisfactory statement of what his discovery will do for, the human race. I know nothing about it, and I will not presume to discuss it."

Other physicians said that there was no doubt but that the knowledge that the organs of the human body could be made to live after the body that held them was dead, or was surviving without them, would be of the greatest possible benefit. One of the surgeons of a big hospital said he had followed the experiments of Dr. Carrel with interest, and had himself studied all that had been written by learned men on the subject. He said he was certain that Dr. Carrel had made it plain that almost any organ in the body or trunk could be patched up and made sound. But he was sure that no organ could be transplanted with any hope that it would do the work that nature demanded of it.

This surgeon was asked to explain what he thought of Dr. Carrel's discovery in words that the lay mind could understand. He replied that he would try to do so.

"Let me say at the beginning," he said, "that no claim is made that this new discovery if it is new, pretends to establish proof that an entire organ can be replaced. That would be manifestly impossible for this reason. Suppose a man had diseased kidneys. One of them could be removed and the man would live until the other petered out, and then he would die. If it was attempted to remove one of them and to put in its place the kidney of a dog or a sheep it would do its work, providing, of course, that the operation was successful, only as long as nature intended a dog or a sheep to live, which is a much shorter period than the life of a man. Therefore, unless nature could absorb the transplanted kidney and finally convert it into a human organ which would be impossible, the man's life would always be hanging by a thread.

"But Dr. Carrel never expected to be able at this time to work such a revolution in the science of surgery as this. That such a big stride as this will be taken is fairly certain, but measured by the pace of other advances in surgery it will take at least thirty years for the accomplishment of such a wonderful result. So the only thing we have gained from this latest discovery is the knowledge that one of the internal organs that is worn around the edges, so to speak, can be patched up."

In order to make his meaning clear, the surgeon told of the work of Dr. Carrel during many years. He said that first Dr. Carrel began working on living tissues, a study that occupied his attention of many years. He would take small bits of the tissue and preserve them in salt solutions of various strengths, in order to observe them under the microscope and see how long they would remain vital. Then he would take a large mass of the tissue and place it in the solution that he had found of the most value, and watch it for a long time in this abnormal condition.

"Dr. Carrel's original idea was," said the surgeon, "to help surgeons in their work, to aid them in getting over obstacles that had always been considered insurmountable. After he had finished with his experiments with the tissues he began experiments with the blood vessels. He found that it was possible to keep the vessels for a number of days in a solution, and that they could then be placed in a dog and be made to work in feeding the surrounding tissues. All of this work was preliminary, for, I believe, Dr. Carrel has always been aiming at some great result, perhaps the prolongation of human life, or perhaps he hopes to make it possible to remove a badly wounded or diseased organ and replace it with a sound one.

"At any rate, after he had completed his experiments with the tissues and blood vessels, he began removing the organs. The first one he removed was from a dog and was a kidney. He found he could remove it with the tube that leads to the bladder. This was done and was placed in a solution where it was kept alive. He was now nearing the master experiment of placing a kidney removed from one animal in another animal.

"Nature has provided all human beings with a certain amount of reserve force. Take the Marathon runners, for instance, and see how the heart responds to the fearful demand made upon it. How it pumps the blood and feeds the body under the terrible strain. This reserve force is always needed in every surgical operation, and if a man has enough of it to stand a big strain he will recover from an operation that would kill a weaker man. This reserve force is always depended upon by surgeons for aid. There are ductless glands in the human body that nobody knows anything about just as nobody really knows much about the chemistry of the body. Some of these ductless glands are so important that if they are injured or prevented in any way from performing the work demanded of them the man will die.

"The thymus gland, the adrenals, and the other ductless glands are of prime importance. Dr. Carrel discovered that by removing the adrenal gland, which lies over the kidneys and in contact with them, he could put another piece of gland in its place to do the work. This operation was a very delicate one. The inserted piece had to be carefully bound around with skin and bits of muscle so that the adhesion with the natural tissues would be as speedy as possible. The operation would have to be made in a very short time or the patient would die. So if it happened that a man's kidneys were diseased because of any fault of this gland or of any other of the attachments or connections of the organ, it could be patched up through this discovery by Dr. Carrel.

"Dr. Carrel's experiments regarding the heart are also of vast importance. He has shown that the heart can be kept pulsating for a long time by placing it in a solution. This solution is made of a mixture of certain salts, such as potassium and sodium. I know what the solution is, but I do not care to describe it, because harm might grow out of making the knowledge public. Dr. Carrel experimented by taking twenty-five hearts and placing them in solutions of varying strengths. The solution in which the heart lived the longest was the one chosen for further experiments.

"Dr. Carrel's latest work has been the removal of several organs such as the stomach, liver, and intestines and connecting them by blood vessels with the heart and in keeping the heart beating. He has also made it possible to cut out pieces of the tendon and replace them by other bits that will serve the same purpose after they have become united. Finally, they will be absorbed and become as human as any other tendon in the body. Dr. Carrel can be described as a man with a transcendant capacity of taking pains."

October 27, 1912

NOTES AND GLEANINGS.

By inserting a tube into the windpipe of a person undergoing a serious operation, Dr. CHARLES H. PECK, M. D., reports in The Journal of the American Medical Association that continuous insufflation of air into the lungs will sustain life for many hours when all respiratory movements have ceased. Dr. PECK presents records of 412 cases treated by this method in the Roosevelt Hospital, following the method invented by Dr. MELTZER and Dr. AUER of the Rockefeller Institute. He finds that the intubation diminishes the surgical shock, and permits more perfect and gentle control of the anaesthesia, so that very old or weak patients are especially benefited by its use.

September 14, 1913

WONDERS IN WAR SURGERY.

Dr. Walton Martin Lectures on Work of Americans Abroad.

Up-to-the-minute war surgery, which finds cloth as dangerous as lead and extracts bullets with the aid of the X-ray and lightning-like calculations of geometry was demonstrated last night before the New York Surgical Society.

The paper of the evening, read in one of the meeting rooms of the Academy of Medicine at 17 West Forty-third Street, was by Dr. Walton Martin of this city. He and his associate, Dr. H. M. Lyle, who also spoke, recently returned from the hospital which Mrs. Harry Payne Whitney maintains as a unit of the American Ambulance in France.

Dr. Martin introduced a chef 55 years old, who keeps busy in his kitchen every day for fourteen hours and yet has had a bullet in his brain these thirty years.

Dr. Martin spoke of bullets which had passed through the limbs of soldiers and disappeared, and yet the surgeon had hard work saving the life of the men on account of tiny threads of infected fibre from the soiled uniforms. These they had laboriously to extract.

Dr. Lyle said that the French surgeons had ingenious ways of finding bullets and pieces of shrapnel with the aid of powerful electro-magnets, but that the palm for ingenuity must be awarded to the Sutton method, which was of American origin.

The wounded man is placed on a bed, beneath which is an X-ray machine, and over him is placed the tube of light used in the photographing process. The bullet is shown on the plate, which is placed beneath the patient. The X-ray has demonstrated that like nearly everything else in France it is "somewhere near a certain locality." But how deep? The tube is placed at another angle. The shadows are made to cross and the bullet is again detected. To find how far to probe the surgeon works out a problem of triangulation.

The surgeon thrusts a hollow, needle-like device into the body, finds the bullet, and puts a piece of slightly barbed piano wire down to hold to the tissue about the bullet. The patient, duly surveyed, is wheeled to the operating room, where the operation of removing the bullet is quickly accomplished. The triangulation is now done within five minutes.

Dr. Lyle said that there were often cases supposed to be tetanus in the base hospitals which were nothing more than small pieces of shell or foreign bodies pressing on the nerves and causing peculiar, convulsive pain.

October 14, 1915

'RAISING THE DEAD' ON THE BATTLE LINE

German military surgeons are now restoring to consciousness soldiers overcome by gas or buried in bombarded trenches by using a device for artificial respiration invented by Dr. Samuel J. Meltzer of the Rockefeller Institute in this city.

A consignment of the mechanisms was sent over last month, and they are coming into use. They are an improvement upon the apparatus which was invented in 1913 by Dr. Meltzer as a result of his investigations for the United States Bureau of Mines. Two dozen of the contrivances were sent several months ago to the Allies, and they have been used on the French side on the western battle front. Germany, however, has received a supply only recently through the Rockefeller Foundation.

The new type is much simpler than any of its predecessors, for it has no delicate valves to get out of order and no glass. The entire apparatus, including the case to carry it in, which is eighteen inches long and twelve high, does not weigh more than fifteen pounds. It can thus readily be used upon the field, and it has advantages over the more elaborate and heavier appliances. The last number of the North German Gazette received in this city has an article describing the demonstration of the device before the Berlin Medical Society, and the Germans are greatly impressed by its practical utility.

Dr. Meltzer is the head of the department of physiology and pharmacology at the Rockefeller Institute for Medical Research. He invented, although he did not patent, several pieces of apparatus for producing artificial respiration and proved their efficacy by experiments on animals and also in the treatment of human beings. His work was popularly spoken of as "raising the dead to life," for he used the apparatus to bring back the breathing function to both men and animals in whom life was practically extinct. The device the Germans are using, which he calls an apparatus restoring respiration through pharyngeal insufflation, consists primarily of a six-foot rubber tube provided with certain contrivances for controlling the flow of air pumped through it into the lungs from a foot bellows. The tube has a nickeled mouthpiece which is inserted deep into the throat.

Each machine is provided with a pair of forceps by which the tongue can be drawn far enough out of the mouth to prevent it interfering with the procedure. The member is tied to the mouthpiece of the machine. A current of air is then forced into the lungs and the functions of taking in breath and exhaling it are imitated by alternately opening and shutting an orifice in the tube by sliding a piece of curved metal back and forth over it. This metal covering is attached to a ring through which the operator can slip a finger and thus easily control the air current.

The abdomen of the unconscious patient is kept flat and rigid by strapping a board upon it, so that all the air goes into the lungs. The pressure of air is also regulated by another tube connected at right angles to the main one the size of the opening of which is varied.

The announcement was made several months ago that a method of treating tetanus with Epson salts injections perfected by Dr. Meltzer had also been employed. Sometimes in this treatment the patient lost consciousness and his breathing was restored by the artificial respiration device. The Germans, according to these last advices, are adopting the method on an extensive scale.

November 25, 1915

WORLD TO BENEFIT BY WAR MEDICINE

New Methods and Discoveries Will Save Lives Henceforth---Some Marvels of Up-to-date Surgery

THE war has taught us how to save more lives than the war has cost."

This is a statement made by Major George A. Stewart of the War Demonstration Hospital of the Rockefeller Institute for Medical Research, who believes that out of the agony and suffering of the recent great struggle will come benefits to humanity that will compensate to a large extent for the lives that were lost and the blood that was shed. Medicine and surgery have taken giant strides during the more than four years of war, and the pressing necessity born through the world's travail has, in the estimation of Major Stewart, developed medical science to such an extent that mankind will be a gainer rather than a loser in the years to come.

"The countless improvements of practice, both in medicine and surgery, made in this war have advanced our science half a century in four years," says Major Stewart. In surgery, the values and technique of 'chlorination'—or the use of some combination of chlorine for the destruction of malignant germs which gave rise to pus—have been learned as never before. There is no longer any good excuse for persistence of pus.

"The development of the 'Carrel-Dakin' method of treating all manner of infected wounds by periodic irrigation with Dakin fluid (a non-caustic hypochlorite) marked an extraordinary advance. And in this the method is as important as the fluid. It is being taught to surgeons the world over.

"Out of forty-five patients in the War Demonstration Hospital suffering from empyema we returned thirty-five to the front. Empyema is pus in the chest cavity. It often follows pneumonia, and hitherto has been highly fatal. There has been an unusual amount of empyema in New York this year of a very serious type. But the death rate has been lessened by the modern treatment.

"Other wonderful advances have been made, for example, in X-ray work, in knowledge of the gas bacillus which causes a form of gangrene, in the serum treatment for prevention or cure of such diseases as typhoid fever, lockjaw, pneumonia, meningitis, &c. These lessons will save far more lives in the long run than the war has cost."

Nor is Major Stewart the only man of repute to hold such views. Josephus Daniels, Secretary of the Navy, also believes that innumerable blessings will arise from the lessons that have been taught by stern necessity in time of storm and stress.

"One of the compensations for the tragedy of the war," he said recently, "is the fact that an enlightened opinion is behind the organized campaign to protect the youth against contagious disease.

"The campaign begun in war to insure the military fitness of men for fighting is quite as necessary to save men for civil efficiency."

Sir Almroth Wright, in The London Lancet, the most famous medical journal in the world, says that "the Carrel-Dakin method (of treating infected wounds) is far the most important contribution to surgical technique since the beginning of the war."

But this is only one of countless other epoch-making methods that have arisen triumphant over the blood and brutality of the boche. There is the famous ambrine treatment for burns that was so successfully administered in the Ambrine Hospital for the French wounded at Compiègne by Miss Elsie de Wolfe and other nurses—a treatment that proved a godsend for agonized poilus suffering from flammenwerfer wounds. Nor should one forget the marvelous anaesthetic discovered by Gordon Edwards, a young American humanitarian, which could be sprayed upon gaping raw wounds and burns, relieving the exquisite agony of the patient and enabling physicians to apply and remove bandages without the wounded man feeling the slightest pain.

Before this war the doctors didn't know much about the habits and habitats of that pest, the louse, which has probably been with us since the first crack of dawn. But the war gave this creature another name, and it wasn't long before all the world was talking of the "cootie," which became the familiar of the soldier in the trench and helped make war even more like Sherman said it was. The "cootie," at first taken somewhat as a joke, became a serious menace, for physicians discovered that he was the greatest little disease carrier on earth, compared with which the New Jersey mosquito was as nothing. It is now generally admitted that the "cootie" transmitted more disease during the war than any other single agency. But now the doctors know all that is to be known about this pest, and have learned to muzzle the "cootie," so to speak.

Disease in time of war has always caused more deaths than shot and shell. This was the case during the brief Spanish-American war, and history has repeated itself during the war that has just ended. In this connection it is interesting to record the established fact that the total death roll of the United States forces in the war was just about one-half of the toll that was exacted of us by the recent epidemic of Spanish influenza. Nor should it be overlooked that, in times of peace, the deaths annually from industrial accidents in this country are estimated to be approximately 30,000. In many accidents where the patient is not killed, he or she emerges from the hospital a hopeless cripple. But the new surgery, the surgery developed during the war, will not only save many of these industrial victims, but will help to restore to usefulness the lame and the halt and the blind.

In a hospital in Milan, Italy, they have been experimenting successfully with a new apparatus which insures immobility of the mouth and jaws, and thus makes it possible for the physician to rebuild, reshape and even to actually restore, lost functions to men who were suffering from mouth wounds. This marvelous jaw-lock consists of two light metal arcs, one of which is placed on the outside of the lower range of teeth and the other on the upper range, the whole being fastened to the teeth by metal ligaments in such fashion that no movement of the mouth can distract the physician at work. And while the work goes on, the patient is fed by means of liquid food inserted between the interstices of the teeth. By means of this contrivance the wonder worker in surgery can practically make over a human face.

Connected with this amazing hospital in Milan, where war remnants are made over into presentable human beings, is a factory where artificial palates, jaw bones and other parts are manufactured. Some of the products that come from this factory are said to be such astounding substitutes for nature's own handiwork that it is often difficult to tell where nature left off and modern science began.

Equally amazing strides have been made in the manufacture of artificial limbs, which are so cunningly substituted by the attending surgeons that the victim of war has all the appearance of being a whole man. In other words, the war has made it necessary for the surgeon to understand the human anatomy as the skilled mechanician understands a machine that he has helped to build from the ground up. And so familiar have the doctors become with every conceivable sort of disfigurement and mutilation, that a gruesome new art has grown up—an art that smacks of miracles and magic but is based on common sense, observation of detail, and a supernormal skill.

The modern hospitals in New York and other cities will bring these benefits to the public. The wizardry of war has made men perform the seemingly unperformable, and wounded doughboys who have fought for world freedom will have every advantage that modern surgery can suggest in the treatment of their wounds by American surgeons, than whom there are no better.

But the war has affected the hospital service in New York very seriously on account of the great need for surgeons on the other side. The recent influenza epidemic proved that. It is a matter of record that only one person in ten who needs hospital care in New York gets it, and the United Hospital Fund is now trying hard to put New York hospitals in a position to do more work for more people. As a matter of fact, the hospitals provided by the city provide only 40 per cent of the total hospital bed capacity of New York.

It has been estimated that under normal conditions about 3 per cent. of the people are sick. Apply these figures to the United States and to New York and the result would show that, out of this country's population of 100,000,000, at least 3,000,000 are sick, and out of New York's population of 6,000,000 approximately 180,000 are sick. Just stop to think what that means in the loss of wages alone, to say nothing of the doctors' bills.

The United Hospital Fund, which is starting a campaign for more money to carry on and amplify the hospital work in New York, collects and publishes full and uniform statistics of the work and finances of the hospitals, and this fund provides a way for every citizen of means to perform a real public service. The strain of war has been keenly felt by the United Hospitals of New York, as large numbers of the profession went to the front. Thirty-six out of the forty-six United Hospitals closed the year with deficits, amounting in the aggregate to $391,341. As a result, some of them have been compelled to reduce their free service.

This United Hospital Fund is the war chest idea in hospital giving, for it collects funds to pay in part for the free work done by the forty-six hospitals that are in the fund, and it is the hope of those interested in this work that at least $1,000,000 will be raised during the coming year for the fund. That hope should be justified when one stops to think that New York is far behind London and the great cities of Europe in its number of hospital beds in proportion to population. For contagious diseases, London, in 1913, had three beds to New York's one. And this shouldn't be so, for, in hospital facilities as well as in other facilities, New York should lead the world.

December 29, 1918

LESSONS LEARNED BY WAR SURGEONS

Dr. Blake Puts Re-establishment of Aseptic Principles Foremost.

DISCOVERIES ABOUT SHOCK

Transfusion of Blood Successful—Nitrous Oxide Likely to Supplant Chloroform.

By WALTER DURANTY.

Copyright, 1919, by The New York Times Company.
Special Cable to THE NEW YORK TIMES

PARIS, April 1.—"There has been little new in the development of surgical knowledge during the war," was the statement of the famous American surgeon, Colonel Joseph A. Blake, to a distinguished medical audience at the Sorbonne today. Colonel Blake has been for several months the chief surgical officer of the American hospitals in Paris.

Previously the French Government had given a striking recognition of his services in putting him in charge of the hospital of the late Dr. Doyen, in the Rue Rossini, in Paris, which is one of the most up-to-date in France. After nearly four years of war work in France, Colonel Blake is about to return to America, where he has been asked to deliver an address before the American Medical Association in New York.

Dr. Blake in his Paris address continued:

"There have been fruitful investigations and observations in regard to the treatment of wound infections and shock. In the first two years of the war a search for novel treatments led surgeons toward a universal panacea for wound infections by antiseptic means. It is only more recently that aseptic principles have become re-established."

Colonel Blake himself was one of the pioneers in wound treatment. At the Doyen Hospital he developed an apparatus of swings and pulleys for fracture cases which has been widely imitated in the allied armies. The point he made in today's speech was that in the early days of the war there was a tendency toward violent antiseptics of the old school, which did kill microbes, but at the same time prevented the surrounding tissue from healing normally.

The latest treatment, which Colonel Blake says began only in the Spring of 1917, is based on the principle that well-nourished tissues cannot only withstand but can eliminate infection. He attributes its success to the methods of the French surgeon Lemaitre, who simply cleansed the wound, removed all devitalized tissues and foreign materials, and then closed it immediately without the use of an antiseptic.

Similarly, in the case of gangrene, whose ravages were very great in the early years of the war, it is now recognized that the ideal treatment consists in removing the conditions favorable to the microbes' growth.

French discoveries have shown that shock is caused by deficient oxidation of red corpuscles, either from loss of blood or body heat. Artificial warmth and transfusion of foreign blood have both been found satisfactory. These remedies enabled the wounded to stand operation for the removal of injured tissue or muscle, which, if allowed to remain, would again bring about weakness through the introduction of acid in the blood. It is in this connection that the use of nitrous oxide, combined with oxygen, has become general as an anaesthetic, because it permits the oxygen contents of the blood to be kept at a high point. Colonel Blake predicts that in future this form of anaesthetic will supplant chloroform.

He concluded his address with the expression of the hope that the interallied surgical work during the war would be continued by a free exchange of ideas, lectures, and visits between the leading allied medical bodies and universities.

April 3, 1919

BROKEN MEN REMADE BY ARMY DOCTORS

American Red Cross Worker Tells of Marvelous Achievements of Reconstructive Surgery.

EASY TO GIVE MAN NEW FACE

Soldiers Brought to Hospital with Countenances Merely Blurs Sent Away with Normal Visages.

Miss Eve Hammond of the American Red Cross, who returned yesterday from Europe after nearly five years' service with the allied armies, and who wears decorations of the British and French Governments, told of the wonderful results achieved in reconstructive surgery by the surgeons of the American and Allied armies. Miss Hammond, whose home is in San Francisco, was attached to the staff of the American Red Cross Hospital in Neuilly, France.

"It is surprising how many things can be done to a man by a shell and leave him still living," Miss Hammond said. "And the things that can be done to make it worth while for him to go on living are even more surprising; they were surprising to us, to whom they were an every day matter and to the uninitiated they were a revelation."

"Dental surgery is one profession that has gone ahead from the impetus of the war in leaps and bounds. The marvels that the doctors of dentistry performed were not entirely unknown before the war, but they were in the theoretical stage. There was no chance to put these theories into practice, except in widely isolated cases. The war proved that those theories were sound and practicable; it afforded them a means of development. There is nothing impossible in dental surgery now."

"I have seen men come into that hospital of ours with bloody blurs where their faces had been. Fed through tubes and kept alive, I have seen their remaining bits of skin stretched over the raw places, which filled with new flesh under careful treatment and finally they have gone out into the world with new faces.

"There was one man, I remember, who came in to us with his entire face gone—nothing left but one eye. We fed him through a tube, built him a metal jaw fitted with teeth, and made him look like a human being again, except that he had no nose—only two nostrils. We found him a false nose with a pair of spectacles attached, hiding the scarred flesh around his missing eye, and making him look so much like other men that one would not have glanced at him a second time to note his deformity.

Another man came to us with the greater part of his face intact, but with no nose. It had been shot off completely, leaving his flesh flat from chin to forehead. We made him a nose to fit him. From the place where his nose had joined to his forehead there hung a little wisp of skin. This was pulled down, stretched every day, and kept dry and healthy by an antiseptic powder. Finally it grew to the correct length for a nose. Then we opened his wrist and grafted a piece of bone to the place where his nose should have been, binding arm and face together until the operation was completed. Then we adjusted the skin, which filled out with healthy flesh, and there was a new nose!"

Easy to Give Man New Face.

A man whose face had been hanging down from below his eyes, Miss Hammond says, was a simple case. His face was sewn back in place.

"I met him on the street in Paris," she says, "just two days before I sailed and his face looked just as usual except for a light scar which ran along under his eyes and across his nose. In time it will almost disappear. A man who had been the victim of a freak shell which had ripped out every one of his teeth, leaving him otherwise unharmed, was supplied with the new gums and complete set of upper and lower false teeth. I have even seen a man with is brain bulging down over his eye from a jagged cut in his skull. The brain has been carefully pressed back in place, and the head fitted with a metal plate. His operation leaves the patient perfectly normal so far as his mental condition is concerned. He is, however, unable to go about much in the hot sun, as strong heat affects him, and he cannot drink because it irritates the brain."

Sometimes, Miss Hammond said a patient would be brought into the hospital with his leg smashed to pieces. Instead of making a hurried amputation, every effort was made to save the injured limb. It was put into a frame, and in a short time the smashed bones would take a position, knit, and begin to grow together, while the splintered bits would gradually work their way out of the leg through the flesh.

Miss Hammond wears three decorations. One is the Star of Mons, the gift of the English Government in recognition of her splendid work among the British wounded; another is the Medaille d'Epidemie, presented to her by the French Government for her efficient care of its wounded, and the other is the Croix de Guerre, with a palm.

July 27, 1919

PIERCED A MAN'S HEART TO BRING HIM TO LIFE

By Wireless to The New York Times.

LONDON, March 25.—How a man was brought back to life by an injection after "the action of the heart had definitely stopped" is told by Dr. Karl Bodon of Budapest. The patient was 70 years old and had heart attacks, for which the doctor first administered morphia, which had no good effect. Reporting the case in The Lancet, he says:

"I resolved to try an intercardiac injection. I hurried to my rooms to provide myself with a long needle and, returning within a few minutes, found that the patient had nearly passed away in the meantime. He lay relaxed and apparently lifeless in a chair, with his head fallen backward. While I was preparing the injection, respiration ceased completely, and the action of the heart definitely stopped.

"I was without medical assistance and considerably agitated," says the doctor, who described his feeling when he plunged the needle containing a solution of adrenalin into the man's heart. "A few seconds later I observed a steady improvement of the heart-beat, which proved regular and effective in less than half a minute."

He reports that the man is now well in every respect.

March 26, 1923

Heart Beats Made Visible by New Device; Promising Great Value in Operations

Special to The New York Times.

CHICAGO, May 30.—Delicate surgical operations on the cardiac valves by which common heart diseases which usually cause death may be cured have been made possible by the use of the cardioscope, an instrument just perfected, which makes heart beats visible. It was announced today at the annual meeting of the American Association of Thoracic Surgeons.

The instrument not only makes possible heretofore impossible operations, it was announced, but it also may be used for observation of the human beating heart and correct diagnosis. It is the invention of Dr. Durff S. Allen, a young surgeon of George Washington University, after two years' research.

So far the cardioscope has been used only on animals, principally dogs, but Dr. Howard Lilienthal of New York, retiring President of the association, declared for Dr. Allen that it was now at the stage of perfection to be used on human beings.

The instrument is about the size of a pocket flash light. A strong lens protrudes from one end and a powerful light is inserted in the other. It is laid against the heart valves through a small incision directly over the heart, and magnifies the valves, acting much like a microscope. It is declared that this may be done while the heart is beating and the valves functioning and without injury to the organs.

"The instrument is particularly valuable in the cases of widening or narrowing of the heart valves, which are so common and have so often ended ultimately in death," Dr. Lilienthal said. "The cardioscope enables us to lay the lens against the valve and observe, and then either cut apart the too narrow valve or tie it with ligatures where it is too wide."

May 31, 1923

NEW ANAESTHETIC TESTED.

Woman Chats With Surgeons as She Has Major Operation.

Anaesthetized locally with a specially prepared novocaine, used for the first time at the United Israel-Zion Hospital, Tenth Avenue and Forty-eighth Street, Brooklyn, a woman patient recently was able to converse with the surgeons and nurses and to feel no pain while undergoing an operation for gallstones and appendicitis, it was announced yesterday.

The operation proved that a surgeon may now operate on almost any part of the body without pain and without using a general anaesthetic. Watching the operation was a gathering of prominent physicians and surgeons, who expressed their satisfaction that serious operations may now be performed without the use of ether or gas.

The patient was perfectly comfortable after the operation and was given liquid nourishment almost immediately.

July 13, 1924

NEW INSTRUMENT IN MEDICINE BUILT LIKE RADIO RECEIVING SET

Electro-Cardiograph Developed by the General Electric Company Renders Heart "Voltage" Visible

A NEW instrument called the electrocardiograph has been developed in the General Electric Laboratory at Schenectady. It offers a new way for electrons, tiny particles of negative electricity, to aid the medical profession.

The cardiograph is, in some respects, much like a radio receiving set. The incoming voltages are considered extremely minute by the medical profession, but radio fans would think them relatively enormous.

The electrical impulse which reaches a receiving antenna is in the neighborhood of microvolt, or one millionth of a volt. One considers that a shock from 110 volts is relatively unimportant, but the antennas of today deal with microvolts and microamperes.

The electro-cardiograph takes the voltage manifestations which come from the heart and makes them visible. Instead of being an audio amplifier, the three amplifying tubes in this set are used to amplify the slight signal current from the heart so that doctors may observe the action of this organ and, by photographing the oscillating light spot, can, at later time, refer to the condition of a patient's heart as indicated on a certain date. In such fashion progress may be noted.

The human body appears to be somewhat similar to a generating station. Every muscular action is accompanied with an electrical manifestation and since the heart is the most active of all muscle groups, the voltage which accompanies its pulsations or beats gives evidence of pathological and physiological conditions.

These voltages are led into the portable cardiograph by means of contacts applied to the forearms and left ankle. They are amplified by using ordinary radio amplifying tubes and the voltage difference is ultimately made visible to the operator and, if desired, recorded on a film.

They are amplified by using ordinary radio amplifying tubes and the voltage difference is ultimately made visible to the operator and, if desired, recorded on a film.

The cardiogram, or trace, which is obtained, is not new. The instrument which has been in use up to this time required an experienced operator and contained a delicate quartz-metal thread in the galvanometer. This thread, many times thinner than a human hair, is eliminated in the electro-cardiograph. Delicate operating parts are replaced by using vacuum tube amplification.

Another improvement in the new instrument is the elimination of what is termed "skin-potential." Inasmuch as an amplifying tube functions only when the voltage charges, the portable cardiograph pays no attention to a constant electric charge. It is ultra-sensitive to a changing voltage. This is important because the old type of apparatus required considerable adjustment to set it correctly for each patient in order to obtain accurate records. The constant potential of the skin, differing in individuals, made necessary a correction each time the apparatus was used.

The power unit in the electro-cardiograph consists of high voltage "B" batteries and a six-volt storage battery.

December 14, 1924

TRANSPLANTS CORNEA TO EYE OF PATIENT

Doctor Performs Operation to Save Life of One Man and Aid Weak Vision of Another.

The Medical Information Bureau of the New York Academy of Medicine and the Medical Society of the County of New York issued yesterday the first authorized statement in connection with an unusual eye operation which took place on Oct. 25 at the New York Eye and Ear Infirmary, accounts of which were published this week in some newspapers. The bureau based its statement on a letter it received yesterday from Dr. Ben Witt Key, who performed the operation.

Dr. Iago Galdston, Executive Secretary of the bureau, of which Dr. Thomas J. Harris is Chairman, explained that the operation had to do with the transplantation of the healthy cornea of an eye, which required enucleation or the operation of extracting a tumor, upon the eye of a patient whose cornea had been rendered entirely opaque by an injury, but which in other respects was apparently normal.

A definite prognosis cannot be given at this time, it was explained, because, in great measure, the procedure was an experiment resorted to only under unusual conditions. It was intimated that a report of the outcome might be expected two weeks from the time of the operation, or about next Thursday. The patient whose sight may be restored as a result of the operation is Bert I Iguson, 32 years old, an inmate of an institution for the blind, who has one glass eye and weak vision in the other due to an opaqueness in its cornea. The cornea in the eye of Charles E. Greenblatt, also 32, of 672 Empire Boulevard, was removed and grafted onto the sclera, or white membrane which, with the cornea in front, forms the outer coating, of Ferguson's eye. Greenblatt had been suffering from a tumor which had to be removed to save his life.

To correct any impression that the eye of one man had been transplanted to another, Dr. Galdston explained that such an operation was impossible. The question to be considered, Dr. Galdston said, is whether this covering tissue, or cornea, will take root and establish nutrition channels. He said the operation had been performed several times before but not quite in the same manner.

November 2, 1928

DOCTOR GETS CATHETER BY A VEIN TO HEART

Special Cable to THE NEW YORK TIMES.

BERLIN, Nov. 3.—Dr. Werner Forssmann, a 25-year-old surgeon, has succeeded in propelling a rubber catheter through a vein in his left arm to the right auricle of his heart.

Applying a local anesthetic only, Dr. Forssmann inserted a highly sterilized and well lubricated rubber catheter, 65 centimeters (about 2 feet 1½ inches) long, into the vein directly above the left elbow. Carefully manipulating it upward and under the collarbone he succeeded in locating the stump artery through which he passed the catheter into his heart.

The course and location of the probe were carefully registered by means of X-ray apparatus which enabled Dr. Forssmann to observe minutely the progress of his experiment. It lasted less than a minute and produced no ill effects on him.

Dr. Forssmann is an assistant surgeon at the Augusta Victoria Hospital, where the experiment was carried out in the presence of his professional colleagues and nurses.

The young surgeon says he now proposes to investigate the practical possibilities of treating heart ailments by injecting drugs through the medium of a catheter propelled through the veins directly into the heart.

November 4, 1929

MEDICAL MEETING CLOSES

Doctors Hear Depression Accidents Developed Traumatic Surgery.

The depression has had a "marked effect" in developing traumatic surgery, that branch of medicine which treats of accidents and injuries, Dr. John J. Moorhead, chairman of the Committee on Graduate Fortnight, declared last night at the close of the ninth graduate fortnight of the Academy of Medicine. About 500 doctors have attended the sessions regularly and several thousand other persons dropped in for occasional lectures, it was announced.

"Traumatic surgery is the oldest form of surgery and yet the newest to be developed," Mr. Moorhead said. "The depression had a marked effect in developing this form of surgery because all other types of surgery were limited to the actual needs of an acute emergency."

October 31, 1936

TELEVISION IS USED TO TEACH SURGERY

Students Watch Operation in an Auditorium in Another Building of Hospital

RESULTS PLEASE DOCTORS

Procedure Followed Even More Closely Than Is Possible in Usual Amphitheatre

A new step in the ancient profession of teaching medicine was taken yesterday when for the first time medical students witnessed an operation by television. Aside from a few experiments within the preceding week with only one or two technicians present, it was the first time that television had carried its visual message of surgical procedure to an unseen audience.

A young man with a hernia was placed on a table in the Izrael Zion Hospital, Brooklyn, and wheeled into an operating room. It was not a room for teaching medical students, for it was small and had no amphitheatre. Instead, a television camera and a microphone were suspended over the operating table amid a cluster of lights.

Some 500 feet away, in the auditorium of another building, a gathering of students, physicians, interns and nurses sat in darkness, which was punctuated by six small panes of light—the screens of the kinets, or television receiving units. A group watched each screen. Suddenly the voice of the operating surgeon was heard and the camera was focused. During the half hour that the operation continued the operator proceeded as if he were demonstrating for students grouped near him.

The pictures of the operation reproduced on the cathode-ray screens were in black and white and the apparatus occasionally got out of focus and made the images hazy. But they were sufficiently clear to follow the course of the operation, with the physician's explanatory comment assisting the audience.

Those in the auditorium followed the operation with interest, physicians among them commenting that it was impossible, when watching an operation from an amphitheatre, to observe the operator's hands so closely.

In one corner of the operating room was the television monitor—the apparatus that changes the picture into electrical impulses for transmission. A robed and masked operator from the American Television Corporation, which manufactured and installed the apparatus, attended it. The surgeon was able to see the picture of his hands and the incision being shown to the audience on a similar screen in the monitor. Occasionally he asked that the camera's focus be sharpened.

The staff surgeon operating, who asked that his name be withheld, declared after the operation that the television transmission of it to students "opens a new leaf in the book of medical science."

March 22, 1939

TREATMENT BALKS SURGICAL SHOCK

Developed by Four Montefiore Hospital Physicians, Who Report 'Striking' Results

The development of a method for the prevention and treatment of what is known as surgical shock, the sometimes fatal condition of prostration and collapse that may occur during or after a major surgical operation, and also in the case of serious accidents, is announced today in the Proceedings of the Society of Experimental Biology and Medicine.

The new method, which promises to eliminate one of the great bugbears of the operating room and the emergency accident ward, and to be of particular importance in the field hospitals on the European battlefields, was developed at the laboratories of the Montefiore Hospital for Chronic Diseases, Gun Hill Road and Bainbridge Avenue, the Bronx, by Drs. David Perla, David G. Friman, Marta Sandberg and Sidney S. Greenberg.

The anti-shock treatment consists of injections of the vital hormone secreted by the outer layer (cortex) of the adrenal gland, in addition to the administration of solutions of common table salt. The cortical hormone is used in its synthetic form, known as desoxycorticosterone acetate.

Results on Animals "Striking"

First tried on rats and mice, the new treatment, Dr. Perla reports, prevented death of the animals from the usual fatal shock following the administration of lethal doses of histamine, a chemical that lowers blood pressure by dilating the small blood vessels. Recent investigations have provided strong evidence that a sudden increase of histamine in the body is the factor most likely responsible for the various forms of shocks, following either major surgical operations, serious accidents, or even mental shock.

The results with the animals were so "striking," Dr. Perla reports, that the method was tried out clinically on human beings suffering from major chronic diseases, such as tuberculosis and cancer, who were in need of surgical treatment but were very poor surgical risks because of their debilitated condition. "Striking benefits" were observed in the case of thirty such patients, Dr. Perla reports. The treatment, Dr. Perla adds, will shortly be adopted in two other New York City hospitals.

Hormone in Significant Role

Studies conducted at Montefiore, Dr. Perla reports, proved that the cortical hormone plays a significant role in the body's fight against intoxications, poisons, shocks and infections. The hormone influences the transfer of water from tissues to cells and the level of salt in the tissues and cells. Disturbance of this glandular balance, which frequently occurs in an exhausting operation, possibly as a result of a sudden increase of histamine, leads to collapse.

"In all instances," Dr. Perla reports, "the patients were strikingly benefited. There was no objective evidence of shock. The blood pressure was maintained or elevated. The temperature in general returned to normal within twenty-four to forty-eight hours. Postoperative exhaustion and toxemia were definitely lessened. Complications did not occur. And operative recovery appeared to the surgeons concerned to be more rapid than in their preceding surgical experience in our hospital."

In the experiments on the animals, Dr. Perla reports, the method was demonstrated also to be useful if applied therapeutically following the administration of the histamine. However, he points out, the method is not as successful as when used as a prophylactic.

March 12, 1940

WAR SHOCK RELIEVED BY CONDENSED BLOOD

Special to THE NEW YORK TIMES.

CHICAGO, Nov. 26—A wartime development in concentrates, a condensed form of human blood plasma, has been found to be highly effective in relieving the shock of battle wounds, says the Journal of the American Medical Association. The substance is the albumin contained in plasma, the liquid of the blood.

The discovery that this albumin could be injected or transfused in a form much more concentrated than the whole plasma provided a new method of selectively combatting shock from injuries, hemorrhages and burns, the Journal says. The new method is regarded as particularly important because it greatly facilitates transfusions to wounded men on the war fronts and thus helps to reduce deaths from shock.

"One-fifth as much human serum albumin is required for a transfusion as is needed when the entire plasma is used," the Journal says. "This not only facilitates shipping and storage but also administration."

The new method resulted from research sponsored by the Bureau of Medicine and Surgery of the Navy Department.

November 27, 1942

CHILD BIRTH TECHNIC HAILED AS PAINLESS

By The Associated Press.

CHICAGO, Jan. 20—Comfortable and painless childbirth safe for both mother and child, is provided by a new type of spinal anesthesia, the Journal of the American Medical Association said today.

Physicians who have used it described it "as the best method yet devised," "100 per cent effective," "perfect painless childbirth," and apparently "the last word in obstetric analgesia."

Both the physicians who developed it and the A. M. A. journal cautioned, however, that the method should be used only in hospitals and only by doctors specially trained in this particular technique, and that there are certain types of cases in which it should not be used.

The new method, which has been in use less than a year, was developed by Dr. Robert A. Hingson and Dr. Waldo B. Edwards, officers of the United States Public Health Service, stationed at the Marine Hospital at Stapleton on Staten Island, N. Y.

"Caudal Analgesia" Used

The technique is called "continuous caudal analgesia" and involves injection of a solution of metycaine, a cocaine substitute, into the cauda, which is at the lower tip of the spine. A special apparatus devised by the physicians is used and the injections are given every thirty or forty minutes throughout the entire course of labor.

The pain-killing drug bathes the nerves at the end of the spine, but does not enter the membranes covering the spinal canal, with the result that the anesthesia does not cause loss of consciousness or hinder muscular movements which have a part in voluntary delivery of the baby.

Physicians have tried many kinds of general, local and spinal anesthesia for childbirth, but virtually all have either failed to kill pain completely or have altered normal labor and increased the difficulties or dangers of birth for the mother or child.

Many Clinics Try Method

The method was first used at Staten Island on Jan. 6, 1942, and since then has been tried in nineteen clinics associated with medical schools and well-established hospitals.

"Altogether some 589 women have been delivered of babies by this method without maternal mortality and with but three instances in which infants died—these without reference to the method of analgesia that was employed," the A. M. A. journal said.

The journal, commenting that relief of childbirth pain has been one of the medical profession's long-sought goals, termed the method "a real advance" and published comments from other physicians who have tried it.

Dr. Norris W. Vaux of Philadelphia Lying-In Hospital said the method was a "100 per cent effective analgesia. It is not dangerous if properly administered, he added, and labor is definitely shortened."

Dr. Francis R. Irving of Syracuse University College of Medicine said:

"There is no question that it is perfect painless childbirth without deleterious effect on mother or child."

Dr. John S. Lundy of the Mayo Clinic, Rochester, Minn., reported:

"We have used continuous caudal analgesia about fifty times and I think it is fine. It has also been used successfully in Brook General Hospital, Fort Sam Houston, Texas; Walter Reed Hospital, Washington, D. C., and many other places."

Attachés of the Marine Hospital, where Drs. Robert A. Hingson and Waldo B. Edwards developed a new painless childbirth technique, said yesterday the cost of the new method should average about $3 per patient, according to The United Press. The cost of the needle used is $1.50. Metycaine, which is injected in solution, costs 30 cents an ampule, and sometimes four or five ampules are required, it was said.

The doctors applied the treatment to their own wives and to the wives of more than 600 Coast Guardsmen, with results which Dr. Donald W. Patrick, executive officer of at the hospital, termed "extremely safe and most satisfactory."

January 21, 1943

AMERICAN DOCTORS HEROES OF TUNISIA

CENTRAL TUNISIA, March 1 (Delayed) (U.P.)—"Fix me up quick, Doc, I want to get back in there," said the soldier with the raw machine-gun wound in his leg as American Army medical men worked over him in the gleaming white operating room of a hospital truck.

And the "doc" did fix him up, for American physicians are saving scores of soldiers' lives daily and have performed some of the most heroic work of the Tunisian war.

The medical unit closest to the enemy line is a battalion aid station usually found about 1,000 yards behind the front, but it is often closer, tucked away in the most sheltered spot available. And, in a barren land like this part of Tunisia, there are not many sheltered spots.

Captain Joseph Nelson of Cleveland, Ohio, surgeon of an armored infantry battalion, said that the foremost job of the front-line medical outpost was to apply morphine and sulfanilamide to relieve pain and prevent infection.

Armored Half-Track Used

"My aid station is an armored half-track carrying Red Cross markings on the top and sides," he said. "The stretcher bearers bring the injured to me and I give them emergency treatment. If they are so injured that they cannot return to the battle immediately, they are sent back to treatment stations in ambulances."

The speed in treatment is often vital in saving lives, so the more quickly the injured are carried to the aid station the better their chances of survival.

At times enemy fire is too heavy to pick up the injured during daylight, so, after dark, Captain Nelson and his men drive their ambulances across the battlefield in a hazardous search for them. Captain Nelson himself has received two slight wounds, but he was able to carry on through the recent Kasserine battle. He said that the bulk of the casualties in his outfit had been shell-fragment cases.

The treatment station is about five miles behind the front, safe from most field artillery fire, but always in bombing range. I visited one station, concealed in a gulch, that consisted of two cleverly arranged operating-room trucks surrounded by a ward tent and several smaller-equipment tents, all of which could be moved to a new location on twenty minutes' notice.

Converted Army Truck

The operation truck is an ordinary two-and-a-half-ton Army truck in which a small but excellently equipped room is set up. The injured are carried directly from the field to the truck, where the doctor is prepared to do anything from dressing a bullet wound in the leg to performing brain surgery. There are no nurses at these advanced units and assistance to the doctor is supplied from the enlisted ranks.

Captain Armand Devittorio of Ridgway, Pa., a treatment station commander, said that many lives had been saved in the operating rooms near the front.

"Each truck has lights and stretcher racks on either side also, so three operations can be performed from it simultaneously," he said. "Once we worked thirteen hours on end and handled fifty-seven operations on our two trucks."

Injections of blood plasma, ample applications of sulfa drugs and seeing that the patients are well covered in blankets are the usual way of dealing with shock, a common battlefield ailment. After treatment, the patients are put in the ward tent until they can be transported to hospitals. Many cases are flown back to base hospital by transport planes.

Captain Robert Beaudet of Franklin, N. H., an operating-truck surgeon, said that his staff was proud because it had not yet had to perform an amputation.

"Today we had a major brought in with his feet shattered when his jeep hit a mine, but we feel confident he will be able to walk again," Captain Beaudet said. "The courage and cheerfulness of the American wounded is remarkable. They never whimper, and tell us to do anything we want just so they will be able to get well quickly.

"A place like this is where morale really shows up. Believe me, these American kids have got all the guts anybody can ask."

March 3, 1943

HELICOPTERS IN A NEW ROLE

Among the many uses of the helicopter which become apparent as this interesting aircraft develops, another was brought out the other day by its designer, Igor I. Sikorsky, at the meeting of the New York section of the Institute of the Aeronautical Sciences. This is the evacuation of wounded men from difficult terrain. Motion pictures of the new Army-type helicopter, a two-man machine, clearly established its adaptability to such service. Over thick jungle country, for example, it can stand still in the air, lower medical assistance by rope-ladder, and thus render invaluably prompt first aid. It can, of course, land in any tiny clearing or on swampy ground and evacuate a severely wounded man. Its smoothness in even rough air insures a high degree of comfort as an ambulance craft.

Although development work for the armed services naturally is of a confidential character, Mr. Sikorsky was able to indicate that speeds of about 140 to 150 miles an hour might be expected of his unique machine. He again made it clear that the helicopter is not expected to supplant the large airplane, but that its inherent abilities to fly slowly, to stand still in the air, to move in any direction, including straight up and down, offer possibilities not only for such military service as anti-submarine patrol, reconnaissance, the landing of "heli-troopers" rather than paratroopers, but for many types of civilian flying.

July 11, 1943

New Surgery Saves 'Blue Babies'; Chicago Doctors Report Method

Special to The New York Times.

CHICAGO, Nov. 12—Three Chicago physicians disclosed today, in the current issue of the Journal of the American Medical Association, the successful development of what has hitherto been considered an impossible operation for saving the lives of so-called "blue babies," whose malformed hearts are unable to pump sufficient blood to their lungs.

Dr. Willis J. Potts, Dr. Sidney Smith and Dr. Stanley Gibson who described the new surgical technique in the publication are all on the staff of the Children's Memorial Hospital, where the operation is credited with saving the lives of three children since Sept. 27.

They related that the procedure, with less danger, gave the same results as the one perfected in 1944 by Dr. Alfred Blalock and Dr. Helen B. Taussig at Johns Hopkins Hospital.

In the Chicago operation Dr. Potts and Dr. Smith, working as a research team, have found a method for joining the body's main artery, the aorta, and the pulmonary artery, which carries the blood from the heart into the lungs.

To accomplish this, they had first to perfect an ingenious clamp, which permits blood to course through the aorta and at the same time prevent it from escaping through an incision, five-sixteenths of an inch long, cut into the outside of the aorta wall.

A similar incision also was made in the side of the paralleling pulmonary artery, which in "blue babies" has an insufficient opening, or stenosis, that obstructs free passage of the vital fluid to the lungs.

After the two incisions were made they were joined together with silk thread, which remained in place and later was covered by new tissue to become a permanent union.

In the Blalock-Taussig operation, doctors explain, there is some danger of paralysis, and also a higher death rate caused by paralysis, which sometimes follows junction of the pulmonary artery with branches of the aorta leading to the brain and arms.

Not all "blue babies" can be saved through the new operation, Dr. Potts said. But those not submitted to surgery cannot hope to survive an average of more than twelve years.

November 13, 1946

New Uses for a Mechanical Heart

It has been known for years that it is possible to suspend the flow of blood to all organs except the brain for ten minutes to half an hour without causing death. One Swedish surgeon, Crafoord, double-clamped the aorta (the big artery that supplies blood from the heart to the entire arterial system) in thirty-three patients who needed operations, and this without causing any disturbances internally. Death is certain if the brain is deprived of oxygen for only a few minutes, and oxygen is carried to the brain by the blood.

It is plain from this that with the aid of a pump outside the body to serve as a heart, an oxygenator to serve as a lung and a perfusion apparatus—that is, a contrivance to send blood to the brain through an artery in the neck—it should be possible to perform operations on a heart from which all blood has been cut off. Reasoning thus, Crafoord and a colleague, Andersson, invented a cardiopulmonary machine, which, in plain English, is a mechanical heart, lung and perfuser.

Experiments on Animals

This invention has been tested on animals with success by Dr. Viking Olov Björk of the Sabbatsberg Hospital, Stockholm. There is little doubt that it will work with human cases.

In a dog Björk clamped the big veins that run down the legs (vena inferior) and up through the chest, neck, head and arms (vena superior) for thirty-three minutes. No blood could pass through the heart. With the aid of the artificial heart the brain was perfused or supplied with blood. The dog showed no sign of damage and later sired eleven puppies.

In the Crafoord-Andersson machine with which Björk experimented the rapidly moving blood is saturated with oxygen. Physico-chemical changes in the blood as well as damage to red cells are avoided. The blood is exposed to oxygen outside the body in thin films. It flows horizontally from one compartment to another in a cylinder through which runs a horizontal shaft with forty to fifty thin steel disks five and a quarter inches in diameter. The disks dip into the blood and, as they rotate, expose new films to the oxygen in the horizontal cylinder. The upper part of the cylinder has a plexiglas lid, so that everything is enclosed. A pump keeps the blood moving.

How the Pump Functions

This pump or artificial heart is connected with a perfusion apparatus; that is, a system of tubes and vessels which conveys venous blood at the right temperature and pressure to the horizontal cylinder of the oxygenator. Warmed oxygen changes the venous into arterial blood, just as in the lungs. After oxygenation the blood enters the main blood stream through an artery.

There is much more to the artificial heart and lung than this, but without a diagram a verbal description is too complex for easy comprehension. The point is that Crafoord and Andersson have provided for everything—prevention of sedimentation, control of temperature, removal of air bubbles, rate of oxygenation, loss of water, separation of the blood's red coloring matter (hemolysis), destruction of white cells, reduction in blood sugar.

Björk says that the apparatus has made it possible to perform bloodless operations on the hearts of dogs. In three dogs the vertebral arteries and veins on both sides were divided at the first stage of a two-stage operation. Ten days later the brain was supplied with blood through the left common carotid artery in the neck, the right being clamped for 25, 63 and 93 minutes. Seven dogs have survived perfusion of the brain with the machine.   W. K.

January 9, 1949

CHILDBIRTH PAINS ARE LAID TO FEARS

Yale Physician Describes New Project to Test 'Natural' Conditions for Mothers

The first comprehensive program in this country for testing "natural" childbirth is proving highly successful, it was reported yesterday. Dr. Frederick W. Goodrich Jr. of the Yale University School of Medicine disclosed details on which no previous announcement had been made.

The project is based, he said, on the concept that virtually all the pain in a normal childbirth is caused by fear.

This concept, advanced in recent years by Dr. Grantly Dick Read, prominent British obstetrician, runs counter to medical teaching and tradition, Dr. Goodrich noted. Consequently, he said, when Yale, with the cooperation of the Maternity Center Association, started its experiment a year ago there was much skepticism on the part of doctors, nurses and mothers.

"Our success has abolished that natural skepticism," Dr. Goodrich asserted.

In his discussion at the thirty-first annual luncheon of the Maternity Center Association in the Cosmopolitan Club, 122 East Sixty-sixth Street, he countered further critical questions with favorable comments quoted from mothers' reports.

Prospective Mothers Schooled

Dr. Goodrich said that the method, as adapted at Yale, involved a course of six sessions for women expecting babies—one lecture and two exercise classes in the early months of pregnancy and three similar meetings in the last month. Women of all degrees of intelligence and education can be taught in this simple manner to face the approaching birth of their child with confidence, the physician asserted.

Further reassurance, provided by specially trained nurses, is the most important factor, however, in teaching each woman as she is brought to the delivery room "what to expect physically and emotionally," Dr. Goodrich said.

He warned against two "misconceptions:" that "natural" childbirth was painless and that no drugs whatever were used.

Only 2 per cent of the 400 women who have had babies in Yale's hospital since the program started have reported absolutely no pain, Dr. Goodrich said.

"The majority say there is some pain," he noted, "but that they are quite willing to tolerate it during the exaltation accompanying childbirth."

50% Use Sedative

Regarding the use of drugs, he said that in slightly more than half the cases a "very mild sedative" helped the mother relax. Stronger drugs are available at all times, he added, if the mother should request them or if abnormal complications should make their administration advisable.

However, in 87 per cent of the cases the mothers were fully conscious at the moment the child was born, Dr. Goodrich reported.

This factor is of extreme importance psychologically, he declared. The other principal reason why the project is considered to have far-reaching implications, he said, is the fact that no absolutely safe drug for "painless" deliveries has yet been found.

As proof of the new program's value, he cited statements from 90 per cent of the 400 mothers. In these the women agreed that "they definitely want" the same method used when they have their next child.

Dr. George W. Kosmak, editor of the American Journal of Obstetrics and Gynecology urged adoption of the method at other teaching centers. He called the Yale project a sign of a "general awakening to the fact that the less artificiality in the childbirth process the better the result."

January 21, 1949

ARTIFICIAL KIDNEY SAVES MANY LIVES

Special to THE NEW YORK TIMES.

WASHINGTON, Jan. 12—A surgical research symposium at the National Institute of Health was told today that patients suffering from extreme post-operative shock had been saved from death by use of the artificial kidney, a comparatively new prosthetic device.

Dr. John P. Merrill, of Peter Bent Brigham Hospital, Boston, said use of the "kidney" in 150 cases in that hospital had given excellent results. A major advancement in surgery was indicated.

He explained that kidney function after surgery is frequently impaired, resulting in urine retention which may be prolonged enough to endanger life. The artificial kidney does not change this anuria, he said, but "can make dramatic improvement of those chemical abnormalities of the body fluids which occur in this condition."

The device was described as a tubing of plastic or cellophane through which blood passes from the arteries into an exterior tank where its chemical contents are changed or "purified."

A case was described in which a 73-year-old woman suffered anuria for eight days after a gallbladder operation. She was in a complete coma. After treatment by the "kidney," she regained consciousness, sat up, and ate and retained 1,300 calories daily in spite of the fact that the anuria continued for four days more.

Another advance described at the symposium was a new spectrometer, capable of analyzing as many as five different gases entering or leaving the lungs during anesthesia. It would take the place of three different instruments now being used.

This mass spectrometer collects and records at twenty-second intervals such data as the concentrations of oxygen, nitrogen, carbon dioxide, and anesthesia being breathed.

Dr. Fletcher Miller of the University of Minnesota, who described it, said that its success during surgery had been amply demonstrated through fifty-five operations.

January 13, 1951

Advances in Lung Surgery Favor Success in Removal

By HOWARD A. RUSK, M. D.

London took on the aura of a hospital waiting room last week, but instead of merely an anxious family waiting the news from the surgery, it was a grieved and anxious population that waited for news from the bedside of George VI. Thousands stood silently about Buckingham Palace quietly hoping for a glimpse of the royal family or medical consultants coming in and out of the palace. As this writer stood among them he could sense the deep grief, devotion and admiration the English people feel for their King. Election talk, which had made the headlines and a good subject for "taxicab conversation," was temporarily forgotten.

The first medical bulletin, signed by all of the King's consultants, announcing "structural changes in the lung" and then the necessity for immediate surgery was the only news that counted. This terse summary, obviously worded with the greatest caution, to the initiated meant serious trouble, most probably a tumor of the lung.

Had the same news been broadcast two decades ago the situation would have been considered hopeless. Today the picture is quite different, for tremendous advances have been made in surgery of the lung. At the turn of the century a French physician reported 400 pneumotomies (simple incision of the lung, primarily for the draining of abscess). This procedure was continued until 1920, often with the actual hot iron cautery method to prevent bleeding.

In the Twenties removal of one or even two lobes of the lung for infection and tumors was accomplished by a number of skillful surgeons. However, it was not until 1933 that the first successful removal of an entire lung for cancer was accomplished in St. Louis by Dr. Evarts Graham, internationally famous surgeon.

This first patient was a physician, 48 years old, who had had a history of repeated attacks of cough, fever and progressive loss of weight. He was thought to have pneumonia, but after the fever was down the X-ray shadow persisted and the diagnosis of a malignant tumor was made. He said to Dr. Graham before the operation, "I hope you will be as radical as you need to be to remove this tumor. I want to be well or I'd rather not get off the table." At surgery it was found the growth had extended to both lobes of the left lung and to hope for a cure the entire lung had to be removed. This was done and after a stormy postoperative course the doctor survived. Today, eighteen years later, he is still practicing medicine in a large Eastern city and has been well ever since.

One interesting anecdote that illustrates the great faith of human beings is worth reporting in this case. When the decision was made to operate, the patient asked to go home for a few days before the operation. This he did and reported on the appointed day for surgery, which was completed. After his recovery he said to Dr. Graham, "I guess you wonder why I wanted to go home before you operated on me. I'll tell you the reason: it wasn't to make my will: I had several fillings in my teeth that needed replacing and I wanted to have this done before the surgery."

Today resection of a portion or a whole lung is common practice. A patient with a lung cancer operated early has twice the chance of complete recovery as those operated for stomach cancer. He has a good chance for complete cure and the operative mortality has been reduced to 5 per cent. In Washington last week a case was reported that involved complete removal of a lung in a 78-year-old woman, the wife of a minister, who recovered entirely and is now at home assisting her husband in his parish duties.

The operation for removal of all or a part of the lung is a delicate one, often requiring several hours. Early ambulation is practiced after the surgery and patients are usually gotten out of bed in a chair within forty-eight hours after the operation. Diagnosis can be accurately made by injection of iodized oil into the windpipe and then followed by X-ray pictures, which will show "filling defects" where the tumor mass may be constricting a branch of the bronchial tree. Diagnosis may also be confirmed by bronchoscopy, in which a tube is passed through the windpipe down to the bronchus where, with small, long-handled forceps, sections of the tumor may be obtained for microscopic examination, a technique developed in the United States by Dr. Chevalier Jackson in Philadelphia.

With mass X-ray examination of the chest these days for the detection of tuberculosis and other pulmonary diseases, the outlook for patients with lung tumors is brighter than ever before, for early diagnosis is necessary for effective therapy. The fact that the King has been under such close medical observation is greatly in his favor, because whatever process was developing, the diagnosis was made extremely early. This is the key to treatment: early diagnosis plus an aggressive, hopeful attitude toward surgery.

The final diagnosis has not been announced in the case of King George, but if the final diagnosis is the most serious, cancer, with the great courage the King has exhibited in the past in overcoming physical handicaps and with every benefit of modern science, it is to be hoped that he will be not only one of the nineteen out of twenty who survived the surgery but one of those who can look for complete recovery.

September 30, 1951

Physiological Monitor

Last week the National Bureau of Standards demonstrated in Washington, D. C., what is calls a "physiological monitor." This is an electronic instrument that measures changes in the blood pressure, heart beat and respiration as they occur on the operating table, and indicates the changes on a panel for interpretation by the surgeon or anesthesiologist.

In the course of the demonstration Dr. George M. Lyon, assistant chief medical director of Veterans Administration research and education, and Admiral Joel T. Boone, chief medical director of the Veterans Administration, expressed the opinion that the "physiological monitor" should prove of great value in the prevention and control of unforeseen surgical emergencies. These opinions were based on preliminary trials in medical wards at Mount Alto V. A. Hospital in Washington, and in an operating room of George Washington University Hospital, also in Washington.

The physiological monitor was developed by Saul R. Gilford and Herbert P. Broida of the Bureau of Standards. Dr. Charles Coakley will carry out more tests in the operating room of George Washington University Hospital and also in the V. A. hospital in Richmond, Va.

During a surgical operation the condition of the patient must be known at all times. Hence the anesthetist measures blood pressure and pulse rate frequently and regularly. If necessary, drugs and additional anesthetics are given or blood plasma is transfused. When the anesthetist is occupied with his other duties the periods between measurements may be longer. The delay is not serious in most cases, but it can have unfortunate consequences. For example, in severe blood loss or heart failure some time may elapse before there is an outward sign of a complete circulatory collapse. It is just in such an emergency that the physiological monitor comes to the surgeon's aid, and this because it records critical changes as they occur in blood pressure, pulse, breathing and the amount of air exhaled in the course of a minute.

June 6, 1954

MAN'S LIFE SAVED BY TWIN'S KIDNEY

Identical Brother Furnishes Organ in First Successful Transplanting Surgery

By ROBERT K. PLUMB
Special to The New York Times.

CHICAGO, Nov. 2—The first known case in medical history in which a man's life was saved because he happened to be one of a set of identical twins was reported here today.

At the annual meeting of the American College of Surgeons it was disclosed that a human kidney transplanted into a young man in Massachusetts last Christmas is still alive and appears to be functioning normally. The donor of the kidney was the victim's identical twin brother.

Never before has such a feat of organ transplanting in man been accomplished. In no other known case in the history of medicine has a human kidney transplant "taken" and lasted so long. Attempts at transplanting other organs have not succeeded, either.

The report was made by Dr. Joseph E. Murray, Dr. John P. Merrill and Dr. J. Hartwell Harrison, all of the department of medicine and surgery, Peter Bent Brigham Hospital, Harvard Medical School.

Former Attempts Failed

In the past failure of kidney transplantings has been attributed to an "antigen-antibodylike" reaction. That is, the tissues of the host pour out disease-fighting antibodies. The antibodies attack the transplanted kidney just as they would any other germ material or "antigen." Dr. Murray reported that recent microscopic studies of kidneys suggest that the kidneys themselves react strongly against the host.

Last December, Dr. Murray reported, one of the twins entered the hospital in a desperately sick condition. A kidney inflamation called glomerulonephritis had severely damaged both kidneys. He suffered high blood pressure convulsions and other symptoms of profound kidney infection.

The patient, a 24-year-old single male, had an identical twin brother. Identical twins grow from one fertilized ovum, in distinction to ordinary twins who, in most cases, are different individuals from different eggs, merely born at the same time.

3 Operations Performed

The evidence suggested that a kidney transplanting between identical twins might "take," Dr. Murray said. Skin grafts between identical twins are successful whereas skin grafts between other individuals are not successful.

The ailing twin's brother had two healthy normal kidneys. Many individuals who have lost one kidney lead normal lives because the other organ takes over the entire kidney burden.

The twins were placed in adjoining operating rooms last Dec. 23. The first operation took five and one-half hours. The left kidney was removed from one twin. It was sutured into the lower right side of the other. The kidney graft was without blood during the operation for an hour and twenty-two minutes. Arteries were sewn in place and the tube leading into the bladder was put in position.

After it seemed that the kidney was going to do well, two other operations were performed to remove the damaged kidneys. The patient is reported now to be without symptoms, carrying on unlimited activity with no apparent disability.

November 3, 1955

New Heart Operations Utilize Intermissions

UNIONDALE, L. I., Oct. 12—(AP)—Intermission heart surgery is making some heart repairs thoroughly safe.

This new technique was described today at the close of the American College of Surgeons' annual congress.

The patient first is chilled to slow body processes and blood flow. The heart then can be opened to direct view.

Under chilling, the blood flow to the heart can be stopped completely for six to eight minutes.

If the surgery takes longer than six minutes, some of the work is done, then clamped arteries are released and the heart is allowed to work again for ten to fifteen minutes. After this intermission, blood flow is halted again and the second part of the operation is carried out.

For the operation the patient is kept at the lowered temperature of about 86 degrees.

Normal oral body temperature is 98.6 degrees.

October 13, 1956

SHOCK TREATMENT FOR HEART URGED

Electric shocks that destroy normal heartbeat need not always be fatal if the victim can be treated in about a minute or less with another shock, an electrical engineer from Johns Hopkins University suggested yesterday.

The speaker was Dr. William B. Kouwenhoven, Professor Emeritus of Engineering and former Dean of Engineering at Johns Hopkins. He spoke at a technical session on safety of the American Institute of Electrical Engineers. The institute is holding its annual winter meeting here this week.

For the last five years, Dr. Kouwenhoven and scientists at the Johns Hopkins School of Medicine have been doing research on the use of electric shock applied to the outside of the chest to stop ventricular fibrillation of the heart.

In ventricular fibrillation, the heart twitches irregularly. Blood circulation stops and there is usually no pulse. It takes only a few minutes of this to produce death. Only in about one case in 100 does the human heart spontaneously stop ventricular fibrillation and resume normal beating, Dr. Kouwenhoven said.

Ventricular fibrillation sometimes develops during surgery. It is also a major cause of unconsciousness in cases of accidental electric shock, according to the paper written by Dr. Kouwenhoven and Dr. W. R. Milnor of the Johns Hopkins School of Medicine.

Equipment for defibrillation in the operating room has been developed and is now employed at Johns Hopkins and several other hospitals, according to Dr. Kouwenhoven, who said that experimental evidence indicated the method was safe, quick and practical. He said he knew of twelve cases in which electric shock applied to the unopened chest had been used successfully to stop ventricular fibrillation. Because of other factors, however, not all of the patients lived.

An alternative to shocking the chest from the outside is the method of opening the chest and applying the electrodes directly to the heart itself. Massage of the heart by the surgeon keeps the blood circulating, but is only occasionally effective in stopping ventricular fibrillation, according to Dr. R. W. Chestnut Jr., a Johns Hopkins medical research fellow who took part with Dr. Kouwenhoven in the presentation yesterday.

The Johns Hopkins research group, with the cooperation of Dr. Paul L. Betz of the Baltimore Gas and Electric Company, is working on the development of defibrillating equipment that might be used in the field to save victims of electric shock.

Shocks ranging in severity between one-tenth of an ampere and three or four amperes will usually cause fibrillation of the human heart, the Johns Hopkins scientists said. Large currents of six or more amperes will hold the heart contracted so long as the current is flowing. However, when the circuit is broken, the heart usually resumes normal beating and re-establishes the body's life-giving circulation, Dr. Kouwenhoven and his colleagues reported.

This ability of a powerful electric shock to stop the heart and hold it contracted is the factor that makes possible the shock defibrillation technique.

Currents of six amperes or larger may temporarily paralyze the respiratory centers and cause breathing to stop, according to the paper, but ventricular fibrillation is not reported likely to occur. The heart will stop, but will usually resume normal beating when the current is broken, the scientists said.

Dr. Kouwenhoven and his colleagues emphasized the importance of quick action in artificial respiration and defibrillating the heart. Experiments have shown that a shock delivered within a minute after the twitching starts is successful in 90 per cent of the case, they said.

The engineers' meeting, with headquarters at the Statler Hotel, will continue through Friday. Registration by yesterday afternoon had totaled more than 3,000.

January 23, 1957

The Healing Knife: A Revolution in Surgery

New operating techniques, along with the great medical advances of the past quarter century, have made possible such dramatic developments as heart surgery.

By LEONARD ENGEL

NOT long ago a 96-year-old woman was brought into a New York hospital with a broken hip. Fifteen years ago she would immediately have been put in a cast and immobilized in bed. And—since old people tolerate immobility poorly—the odds were that she would have been dead in two weeks.

Instead, she was taken to the operating room. There the hip was pinned together with a long nail driven down through the center of the bone. She was out of bed the next day and out of the hospital twelve days later, her hip usable and well on the mend.

This saving of a life was surely wonderful. But it is not unusual. During the past twenty-five years revolutionary advances have taken place in surgery. Surgeons can now even perform the spectacular feat of opening the heart at will—and even stopping it if necessary in order to make repairs deep inside.

Today, literally no part of the human body is beyond the reach of the healing knife. Segments of major arteries, blocked or weakened by disease, can be replaced nearly at will. Removing diseased sections of lung to prevent recurrence of tuberculosis and for other purposes is commonplace. Surgery has developed high skill in treating multiple injuries of appalling severity, as well as the major burns from gasoline that the automobile age has so sharply increased. Even the liver and pancreas, two organs that have been particularly resistant to surgery, can now be operated on successfully.

Surgeons have not only mastered new operative procedures. The benefits of life-saving surgery have also been extended to three great categories of patients largely excluded from this treatment a generation ago—the very old, the very young and the very sick.

CURRENTLY the United States is served by about 30,000 surgeons, of whom over 20,000 have met the stringent requirements for admission to the American College of Surgeons. (Of the others, several thousand are young men who have completed their training as specialists but who have not practiced surgery long enough to be admitted to the college.) They work in some 17,000 operating rooms in more than 6,500 hospitals. They perform well over 10,000,000 operations a year (not counting minor surgery on ambulatory clinic patients).

A far larger proportion of patients than ever before come safely through their operations. An example is the operation for closing a *patent ductus*, a serious and fairly frequent inborn defect of the great blood vessels from the heart. When this operation—one of the first successful heart operations—was first done, as many as one

LEONARD ENGEL is a freelance writer who specializes in medical and scientific subjects.

patient in ten failed to make it; now, 199 of 200 come through. In more routine surgery, such as removal of the appendix, deaths are almost wholly confined to patients with severe complications.

But operative mortality rates do not accurately measure progress in surgery. For, when operations—such as those on the heart—are first performed, they are often accompanied by deaths, both because there are some things that surgeons cannot learn in the animal laboratory and because the first candidates for a hazardous new operation are generally individuals already at death's door.

A truer reflection of surgical progress is given by patients like the 96-year-old lady with the broken hip, or those of Dr. Robert E. Gross of Children's Hospital in Boston. Dr. Gross, although he is even better known for his work in heart surgery, has been a pioneer in surgery upon the newborn. He has even performed major operations upon hundreds of premature infants (usually to correct birth defects incompatible with life). One of Dr. Gross' diminutive patients was a baby girl who weighed but 2 lbs. 6 ozs. at the time he saved her life with a major abdominal operation.

Such patients are, in the language of the operating room, poor risks. They have little or no reserve strength. More deaths are to be expected among them than among older children or adults in good general health except for the illness or injury that brings them to the surgeon. It is a great achievement that the overwhelming majority of even very poor risk patients nowadays recover.

WHAT has made possible the dramatic extension of surgery to new parts of the body and new classes of patients? It isn't greater manual dexterity. For the surgeons of today do not have more dexterous hands than the Theodor Billroths or other great surgeons of the past, any more than modern painters have better

hands than Rembrandt.

The striking advances are primarily the result of a tremendously intensified application of the simple principle underlying all modern surgery. This is to design the operation and conduct both it and associated treatment so as to hold disturbance of the patient and his internal machinery to an absolute minimum.

Surgeons call this the "conservative" approach to surgery. Paradoxically, it is astonishing what radical operations are possible if the operation is designed and executed conservatively.

Rudiments of this concept of surgery are to be found in individual surgeons of many eras. But the real architect of the conservative approach as a systematic method of surgery was William Stewart Halsted, the fastidious genius who came to Johns Hopkins Medical School as teacher of surgery in 1889. Dr. Halsted drank only coffee brewed from beans he himself had selected, one by one; for years he sent his shirts to Paris to be laundered because he could find in Baltimore no laundry that did them to his taste. He exhibited the same fussiness in his surgery.

IN a day when surgeons still worked fast (a hangover from the pre-anesthetic era, when slashing speed was essential), Halsted operated with exasperating deliberation and care. In making an incision, he spent hours tying off blood vessels, one at a time, in order to keep blood loss as low as possible; in closing the wound, he matched layer on layer of muscle, connective tissue and skin with painstaking precision. Where others took an hour for an operation, Halsted took four or six. To the astonishment of his contemporaries, his patients not only survived, they did much better than the patients of other surgeons.

Since Halsted, meticulous care to minimize injury to the patient has been the watchword in the operating room. Thanks to modern research, however, the

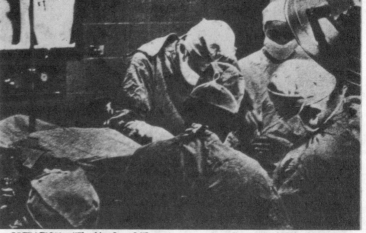

OPERATION—"The benefits of life-saving surgery have been extended to three great categories once largely excluded—the very old, the very young and the very sick."

surgeon today has far greater knowledge than Halsted and his colleagues—or the surgeons of 1930—of what must be done to protect the patient. So the present-day surgeon can do more kinds of surgery on more patients.

THE new ways in which the patient is safeguarded may be summarized under seven main headings. They are:

Advances in diagnosis.

Attention to nutrition.

Safer anesthetics and methods of administering them.

Use of antibiotics and other new antibacterial drugs.

Making up losses of blood and other body fluids and preventing changes in the chemical composition of the blood.

Application of sound physiological principles to the surgery itself, that is, to what the surgeon is trying to do as well as the procedure for carrying it out.

Better post-operative care, especially the development of the recovery room.

When the patient arrives in a hospital for surgery, the surgeon knows, or quickly learns, a good deal more about his illness than the surgeon of a generation ago. Most of the basic tools of diagnosis, such as X-ray, were in existence by 1930. But there has since been a remarkable multiplication of techniques for using them. Almost any region of the body, from the chambers of the heart and the lobes of the brain to blood vessels in the toes, can be studied and troubles diagnosed with precision in advance of surgery. So the surgeon knows far better what he will find when the patient is on the operating table.

MANY patients, especially those needing abdominal sur-

gery, are likely to be extremely undernourished as a result of their illness. Experience has shown that patients weakened by malnutrition are poor surgical risks. So every artifice of nutritional science, from special diets to intravenous feeding, is employed nowadays to build them up before operation. The practice has saved the lives of thousands who at one time could scarcely be considered for surgery.

When the patient entered the operating room twenty-five years ago, he was apt to be deeply anesthetized. Deep anesthesia was the only means by which the muscular relaxation necessary in many operations could be achieved. Today, anesthesia is held to the bare minimum necessary to avoid pain; and such drugs as curare provide muscular relaxation.

The muscle-relaxants are but one of numerous innovations that have strikingly altered anesthesia. In the first place, it's recognized now that all anesthetics are more or less noxious and potentially dangerous to anyone sick or injured enough to need surgery. So anesthetics are used sparingly, and their use is hedged about by special precautions, special instruments and supplementary drugs to offset any possible adverse effects of the anesthetics and to make sure the patient is getting enough oxygen. In the second place, with its ever-widening armory of agents and methods, anesthesia can now be shaped to the requirements of almost any patient or any operation whatever. Thus, there are special procedures for diabetics (who tolerate ether poorly), for such new operative departures as surgery within the chest, and so on.

IN operating rooms today, as in Dr. Halsted's operating

room, blood vessels are painstakingly shut off to minimize blood loss. But the present-day surgeon and his aides also keep track of all blood lost (by drawing it into a measuring glass with a suction machine) and replace it by transfusion, literally as it is lost. Fluid lost by perspiration and evaporation from the wound is carefully replaced, too. Even the chemical composition of the blood is checked—illness, surgery, anesthesia, all may make it more acid than normal or bring about other chemical changes—and immediate steps are taken to correct any alterations detected. As a consequence, surgical shock—once a terror of the operating room—is now uncommon, though desperately sick patients prone to shock are operated on every day.

IN well-run operating rooms, the first line of defense against infection remains the traditional aseptic procedure—rigorous sterilization of everything that may come into contact with the patient's wound.

Antibiotics and other antibacterial drugs are, of course, a powerful modern defense. Curiously, one of their effects has been to do away with much surgery. Operations like mastoidectomy (which once filled children's surgical wards every winter) are now uncommon; penicillin and its partners halt the ear infections that give rise to mastoiditis.

The antibiotics have also greatly simplified some operations (for bone infections, for instance) and made possible others that could not have been done before at all. An example is the removal of tuberculous tissue from the lung—a procedure that has dramatically speeded the restoration of thousands of TB patients to health. Such operations would be too hazardous to be widely attempted without streptomycin and isoniazid to prevent the spread of TB germs to other parts of the body. In addition, antibiotics have proved an invaluable backstop against infection in general surgery; for some wound infections do occur despite the most scrupulous sterile precautions.

The numerous advances we have been discussing have all, of course, had a part in the most spectacular recent development in surgery—open-heart surgery, an achievement all the world has marveled at in the last few years. As with other important new operations, though, success has come because the operations are based on an ever-growing understanding of the workings of the human machine.

TO make repairs inside the heart, Drs. C. Walton Lillehei and Richard L. Varco of the University of Minnesota and

Dr. John W. Kirklin of the Mayo Clinic lay the heart open for periods of from ten or fifteen minutes to an hour or more. This can be done because a heart-lung machine oxygenates and pumps blood for the patient meanwhile. The Minnesota surgeons have a heart-lung machine devised at Minnesota; Dr. Kirklin uses a machine developed by Dr. J. H. Gibbon of Jefferson Medical College in Philadelphia.

The heart-lung machines are a product of the physiology laboratory. They are an example—one of the great ones in medical history—of the basic interrelationship of physiology, medicine and surgery. They were developed successfully because Dr. Lillehei and his colleagues and Dr. Gibbon had a thorough understanding of the heart and circulatory system, and saw clearly what a heart-lung machine must do.

Last but not least, surgery has been significantly advanced by improvements in post-operative care. There have been many of these, but the single most important has been the introduction of the recovery room, a small ward near the operating rooms under the direction of an anesthesiologist or surgeon equipped to deal in seconds with every conceivable emergency that might arise during the first critical hours after an operation.

In nearly all large U. S. hospitals and in many small ones, it is now routine for patients who have undergone general anesthesia (except for those it would be hazardous to move) to spend twenty-four hours or even longer in the recovery room. At first—back in the early Nineteen Forties—hospitals grumbled at the necessity for finding space for such rooms and funds to equip them. They have paid such handsome dividends in lives saved, however, that medical reports glow with satisfaction on the subject.

Conspicuously, surgery in recent years has been steadily transformed into a group undertaking. As many as a dozen-and-a-half people may take part in a long, complex operation. A score of others will be involved in the care of the patient before or after the operation.

THE great increase in operating room and surgical-care personnel is chiefly a reflection of the growth of conservative practices in surgery; there are simply too many ways in which the patient must be safeguarded for the surgeon and a nurse or two to do the job. Burdensome as in some ways they are, the new means of protecting the patient have brought surgery to new heights of daring in saving life and health.

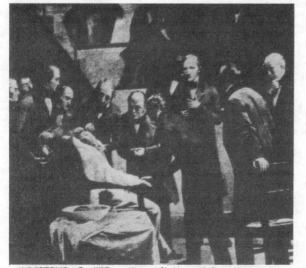

MILESTONE—Dr. William Morton (holding inhaler) demonstrates the use of ether as an anesthetic at an operation in Boston in 1846.

MAN IN BRONX LIVES BY DEVICE IN HEART

A 67-year-old Bronx man will leave Montefiore Hospital today with an electric device implanted in his heart to maintain its rhythm and keep him alive.

He is Herman Nisonoff, a jeweler, of 186 East 164th Street. Mr. Nisonoff entered the hospital last March suffering from an intermittent heart blockage, according to Dr. Seymour Furman, resident surgeon at the hospital.

The heart-rhythm device is portable, weighs two pounds and has a cable with a battery-powered electric shocking tip at its end. The cable enters Mr. Nisonoff's body at his neck, then runs inside a vein into the right side of his heart.

Whenever Mr. Nisonoff's heart falters, the device gives the heart muscle enough of a shock to restore its beat.

Dr. Furman said that seven patients had already benefited from the devices but that previous machines had been the size of a console. He said Mr. Nisonoff could live a "fairly normal life."

June 22, 1959

PROGRESS SLOW ON TISSUE GRAFTS

Body Chemistry Still Defies Most Transplants—New Methods Promising

By JOHN A. OSMUNDSEN

The successful replacement of lost or damaged body parts may depend as much on preventing the graft from destroying the host as on preventing the host from sloughing off the graft.

A report on this field in the Oct. 16 issue of Science did not, however, rule out solutions to these problems.

It suggested that some progress in this direction might have been made already, although what "promise" existed was highly speculative.

Tissue 'Banks' Sought

The prospect of maintaining "banks" for human tissues and organs has already been achieved to a limited extent.

Blood and spermatazoa, for example, are maintained under refrigeration for later use. To some extent, also, some other tissues—skin and bone—can be successfully transplanted.

And cases are on record where whole organs, such as kidneys, have been taken from one person and grafted into another with succes. This has, however, been done only between identical twins.

Tissues and organs cannot be successfully transplanted from one person to another who is not an identical twin because the cells comprising the grafts are incompatible with those of the recipient.

Chemical Differences

More specifically, tissues from individuals of different genetic or hereditary constitution are different chemically. They possess different types of proteins, called antigens.

The appearance of a foreign antigen in an organism stimulates the production of chemicals, called antibodies, that attack and for all purposes destroy the invader.

For this reason, grafts of tissue from one person to another do not "take" except between genetically identical twins.

Only recently, according to the Science report by Dr. R. E. Billingham of the Wistar Institute of Anatomy and Biology in Philadelphia, has it been shown that the graft, too, is capable of developing antibodies for attacking and destroying host tissue.

This means that even if an individual can be prevented from sloughing off a grafted spare part, it will be necessary to treat the transplanted tissue so that it will not attack the substance of its host.

Dr. Billingham indicated that tentative progress had been made.

"It's something we discuss over drinks," he said in a telephone interview.

For example, it has been shown that a potential host to tissue from another, genetically different individual can take a graft if the host is inoculated during the embryonic or fetal stage of development with cells from the potential donor.

Embryo Inoculated

Because the immunological apparatus is not well developed until after the fetal stage, the individual would not reject the injected cells but would then possess their antigens so that the later graft would not be repelled by his tissues.

Another step that may have more practical meaning is the recent discovery that heavy doses of irradiation appear to knock out an individual's resistance to receiving a foreign graft, at least until the transplanted tissue can take hold and establish itself.

Cancer Link Studied

Earlier this year, another scientist suggested that immunological competition between tissues might explain why Hodgkins Disease, lymphatic leukemia and other lymphomas, or cancers of the lymph tissue, are fatal.

Dr. Henry S. Kaplan of Stanford University states in the British Journal, The Lancet, that lymphatic tissue that becomes malignant may have been so changed in its antigens that normal tissue appear foreign to it.

Under those circumstances, the faster-growing lymph cancer tissue would impose an increasing attack on the substance of the normal tissue, eventually destroying it as though it were a transplant from a genetically different individual.

The results of such an interaction, Dr. Kaplan said in a recent interview, would be consistent with what is known to happen in cases of those cancers and is identical with the immunogical effects of incompatible tissue transplants.

October 18, 1959

Doctors Transplant Human Heart Valve

By The Canadian Press.

TORONTO, May 12 — Two medical journals say Toronto surgeons have successfully transplanted parts of dead men's hearts in critically ill heart-disease victims.

The New England Journal of Medicine, one of the oldest of North America's medical publications, says in its latest edition that six persons are alive and well as a result of replacement of aortic valves at Toronto Western Hospital. This valve controls blood flow from the heart to the body.

The Journal of the Canadian Medical Association reports that one man has had his mitral heart valve replaced by the cardiac team at Toronto General Hospital. The mitral valve controls the flow between the blood chambers in the heart.

The operations, reported within a week of each other, are believed to be the first of their kind.

A month after the operation at Toronto General, the Canadian journal reports, the patient died of respiratory complications. A post-mortem examination showed that the replacement heart valve had been working successfully.

A veteran Canadian surgeon, Gordon Murray of Toronto, is credited by both journals with having laid the foundation for the work done by both groups.

Dr. Murray performed the first of the aortic valve transplants nearly seven years ago. The patient, now 29 years old, has married and become the father of four children. He works as a mechanic.

Dr. Murray's work at the time was overshadowed by experiments in the United States with artificial valves. Doubts have since arisen about the durability of the plastic substitutes.

Dr. Murray's work was taken up again two years ago by A. J. Kerwin, a cardiologist; Don R. Wilson, a surgeon, and Susan C. Leinski, a clinical consultant. They comprise the Toronto Western Hospital team.

The three found Dr. Murray's first transplant patient, Norman Perron, who is now living near Victoria, British Columbia, and examined him.

The man, who once could not walk fast without panting, romped through a rigorous test. He was above average in strength and vigor, and every cardiac response was normal.

The Toronto Western team began collecting aortic valves from traffic victims and stored them for as long as two months. The New England Journal says the team then offered the operation to persons with deficient valves. At first only patients with little hope of survival accepted.

Now, less than two years later, nine valve transplants have been performed. Three of the patients died, the journal says, but as a result of complications from pre-operative weaknesses. The six others are healthy.

Dr. Ray O. Heimbecker headed the work with mitral valves at Toronto General Hospital. His team experimented on dogs, the Canadian Journal says. At first it had only limited success.

Then the team performed a transplant on a human who had undergone every accepted treatment without success.

The Canadian journal says Dr. Murray gambled that because heart valves are like the cornea of the eye, which has no internal blood supply, the body will not reject them as it does other transplanted tissue.

May 13, 1962

LASER BEAM USED TO REMOVE TUMOR

By THOMAS O'TOOLE

Laser light has been used to remove bloodlessly a diseased tumor.

Although laser beams had been used previously in operations on the eye, this was not considered bloodless surgery because it did not involve incisions that severed blood vessels.

Surgeons at the Children's Hospital in Cincinnati used a laser beam as a knife to remove a tumor from a man's thigh. Although numerous small blood vessels around the tumor were severed during the 15-minute operation, none of them bled because the intense light of the laser cauterized the blood vessels even as it was cutting through them.

Surgical Ease Hailed

"It's like finding yourself on the threshold of something you've reached for ever since you left medical school," said Dr. Thomas E. Brown, the doctor who devised the operation and one of three who performed it. "I'm absolutely jubilant."

One thing that made Dr. Brown especially jubilant was the relative ease with which he was able to cut out the tumor.

"There's no apparent reason," he said, "why we cannot use the same laser to cut into the liver, the spleen or even the brain without fear of hemorrhage."

Still another possibility envisioned by Dr. Brown is using the laser to cauterize the wounds of hemophiliacs, whose lack of blood-clotting mechanism leads to their losing blood through simple falls that bruise the arteries close to joints and bones.

Laser Devised in 1960

Dr. Brown's work is under the direction of Dr. Leon Goldman, director of the laser laboratory at Children's Hospital, and is being financed by the John A. Hartford Foundation. In his first laser operation, Dr. Brown was assisted by Dr. Goldman and Dr. Bruce Henderson, a fellow in pediatric surgery at the Cincinnati hospital.

If the laser proves to be a significant surgical tool, it will be making something of a medical comeback. Devised in 1960, the light beam of a laser is up to one billion times brighter than ordinary light. This is because ordinary light scatters in all directions. Laser light is so intense that it can be focused through a hole a 50-millionths of an inch in diameter.

This ability to create light or heat in tiny spots led many researchers to forecast a great medical future for the laser. Indeed, it was tried in eye surgery to destroy tumors at the backs of eyeballs and to "spot-weld" detached retinas.

Other techniques, however, proved to be just as effective and less hazardous, so laser surgery drifted into disuse almost from the time it was started.

Before excising a human tumor with the laser, Dr. Brown made countless bloodless incisions on rats, rabbits and dogs. He said he had been so encouraged by the results that he decided to try the technique on a human.

The patient chosen for the operation was a man in his 50s with melanomic skin cancer. Although he had as many as 20 lesions and tumors throughout his body, the tumor in his thigh was selected for surgery because it was the most diseased and one of the easiest to reach.

For the operation, which was performed on Jan. 24, Dr. Brown used a gas laser known as the argon or "green" laser, which was developed at the Bell Telephone Laboratories in Murray Hill, N.J., by Eugene I. Gordon and Edward F. Labuda.

Most lasers emit light in brief, erratic bursts, but the green laser beams out a steady stream of light that can be more easily regulated and controlled by the user. This cuts down the chance that the laser beam will go astray to damage healthy body tissue.

The green laser also has a power output of up to four watts, which is far more than that of other continuous lasers. This enables the user to generate enough heat at the beam's focal point to "cut through" human tissue. Other continuous lasers are not powerful enough to pierce tissue.

The patient's leg was deadened with a local anesthetic, and an incision was made with an ordinary scalpel into the diseased area. Then, the laser beam was directed by a curved mirror onto a portion of tissue adjacent to the tumor, which was about the size of a golf ball and situated about a half inch below the skin.

Slowly, Dr. Brown manipulated the laser beam around the tumor. Each time the beam struck an artery, it coagulated the blood in the vessel on either side of the beam at the same time it sliced through the vessel. An instant later, the heat of the beam cauterized the blood vessel at the very spot where the incision was made, thus preventing bleeding before it could begin.

One reason that the green laser worked so well is that its green light is best absorbed by red objects like blood cells.

'It was like a black box soaking up white light," explained Dr. Brown. "The red blood cells sopped up the green light so well they were able to transfer a maximum amount of the laser's energy to the surrounding body tissue."

February 16, 1966

Booster Pump Used After Heart Surgery

By MARTIN WALDRON
Special to The New York Times

HOUSTON, April 21 — Surgeons successfully implanted what they called an "artificial heart" in a 65-year-old man here today.

The one-pound heart booster was functioning and the patient, Marcel De Rudder of Westville, Ill., was in satisfactory condition tonight.

The team of surgeons and engineers declared that a device of the type attached to Mr. De Rudder could help 75 to 90 per cent of all heart attack victims.

The statement also said "this type of artificial heart could add years of useful life to about half the 900,000 people who succumb to heart disease every year."

Dr. Michael E. DeBakey, the heart surgeon who directed today's operation, said at the conclusion of six hours in the operating room that Mr. De Rudder would surely have died "reasonably soon" without today's operation, and without the heart booster.

If Mr. De Rudder "makes a reasonable recovery, he can look forward to a normal life expectations," Dr. DeBakey said.

He said the device would be left in Mr. De Rudder's body for "a few days, a few weeks at the most," to see how he progresses.

The pump is operated by an outside power supply and for this reason Mr. De Rudder will be confined to bed until the pump is removed.

Mr. De Rudder was suffering from a damaged valve between the upper and lower chambers of the left side of the heart. The lower chamber, the ventricle, pumps blood through the body and is a source of a preponderance of heart trouble.

The machine will do the work of the left ventricle — pumping the blood through the body — giving Mr. DeRudder's heart a chance to heal.

The heart operation was a joint venture of Baylor University College of Medicine and Rice University in a $4.5-million program to develop a complete artificial heart, which could take the place of the human organ entirely.

The device attached to Mr. DeRudder today actually is a pump by-pass. While it will do the bulk of the pumping of blood,

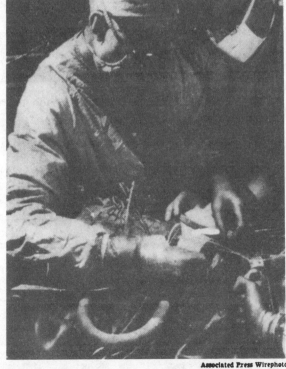

Associated Press Wirephoto

Dr. Michael E. DeBakey, left, implanting heart booster in his patient, Marcel L. DeRudder, at Houston hospital.

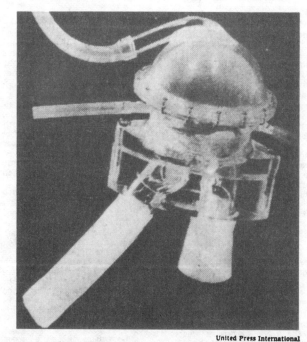

An "artificial heart" or, booster pump, like the one implanted yesterday in a patient by Dr. Michael E. DeBakey.

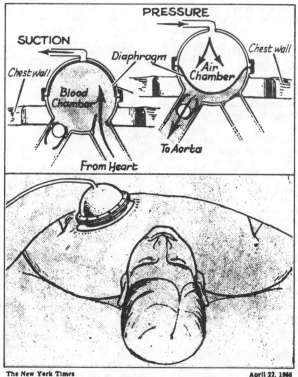

The New York Times   April 22, 1966

Top diagram shows how alternate suction and pressure applied to the pump through a tube leading from a machine outside the body force the blood from the heart and through the aorta to the rest of the body. Pump is placed on patient's chest, as shown in the lower diagram.

Mr. DeRudder's heart will still continue to receive the blood from the lungs, where carbon dioxide is removed and oxygen is added.

The pump will then take over and circulate the blood through the body.

Mr. DeRudder was not considered to be out of danger tonight. "The next 12 to 48 hours will be critical ones," Dr. DeBakey said.

Surgeons Optimistic

The operation itself, however, was adjudged to be a success, and the surgical team was optimistic about Mr. DeRudder's chances of recovery.

In 1963, a Baylor surgical team implanted a rubber pump in the chest of a 43-year-old man who lived for four days thereafter.

The patient's kidneys, brain, liver and lungs were seriously damaged, however, and this damage caused his death, a medical statement said.

The pump still was operating when that patient died.

"This proved its value in a clinical application," said Dr. C. William Hall, coordinator of research on the artifical heart. Dr. Hall, who is Dr. DeBakey's assistant, helped in today's operation.

Today's operation, performed in a 22-by-24-foot operating room, began at 7:45 A.M.

Mr. De Rudder, who had been told last night by Dr. DeBakey what was going to be done, first had to have the damaged heart valve repaired between the upper and lower chambers of the left side of his heart.

This took more than two hours, and it was not until 10:14 A.M. that work was begun on installing the artificial heart.

A planned closed-circuit televising of the operation was canceled because the operating room was too small for the equipment.

However, a physician in the room periodically reported

progress of the operation, and Dr. John Lancaster interpreted reports for a throng of reporters and television and radio technicians who gathered as word of the operation was released.

Mr. DeRudder's wife, Edna, did not know of the operation until newsmen telephoned her. Mrs. DeRudder, who said she was 60 years old and has been married to her husband for 43 years, is a cashier in a supermarket.

"I sure hope he gets along all right," Mrs. DeRudder said. "He's been sick all winter."

Mr. DeRudder, a former coal miner and a former furniture upholsterer, has been unable to work for two and a half years because of his heart condition. He came to the Methodist

Hospital here at Houston last Thursday.

Working with Dr. DeBakey and Dr. Hall today were Dr. Domingo Liotta, 39 years old, a native of Argentina and assistant professor of surgery at Baylor, and Dr. William W. Akers, 43 years old, professor and chairman of the department of chemical engineering at Rice University.

Dr. Akers had directed the bio-engineering aspects of the project to develop an artificial heart.

The $4.5-million grant being used to develop the artificial heart came from the Heart Institute of the National Institutes of Health, United States Public Health Service.

April 22, 1966

Lung Rupture Kills Heart Pump Patient

By MARTIN WALDRON
Special to The New York Times

HOUSTON, April 26—Marcel L. De Rudder, the patient in a heart pump experiment here, died early today of a ruptured lung.

But Dr. Michael E. DeBakey, the surgeon who headed the experiment, said that the heart pump, a device designed to re-

lieve the heart of part of its workload, had proved its worth and that he would not hesitate to use it again.

The heart specialist said, however, that he and his staff of surgeons and engineers would make several modifications in the heart pump before using it again.

Dr. DeBakey, looking worn and tired after almost five days of constant attendance on Mr. De Rudder, said the heart pump had "absolutely no connection" with the patient's death.

Mr. De Rudder died at 4 A.M. Eastern daylight time. An autopsy showed that Mr. De Rudder died from a ruptured lung, Dr. DeBakey said.

He called it a "very unusual occurrence" and said he could not explain what caused the lung to rupture. Methodist Hospital said "an intensive investigation" was under way.

The heart pump, developed after two years of research, is the product of a $4.5-million project to build an artificial heart that could take over the

complete functions of the human heart.

Dr. DeBakey said he was convinced that the pump used on Mr. De Rudder could prove to be of benefit to a majority of heart patients in the future.

"I am deeply grieved at the death of Mr. De Rudder," the surgeon said. "He developed complications over which we had no control. His death had no relation to this particular by-pass pump we have called an artificial heart."

Dr. DeBakey and Methodist Hospital, where the experiment was performed and where Mr.

De Rudder died, said the heart pump — which had been doing up to 80 per cent of the heart's pumping — was working satisfactorily at the time of Mr. De Rudder's death.

The hospital and Dr. DeBakey said the autopsy did not disclose any reason for the lung rupture.

Mr. De Rudder, a 65-year-old former coal miner, had been improving gradually, according to previous hospital bulletins, even though he was in a coma when he died.

Dr. DeBakey said the autopsy showed that the coma had been caused by a blood clot in the middle cerebral artery that probably was a remnant of an old clot surgeons found in Mr. De Rudder's heart last Thursday, when they replaced a valve between the two chambers on the left side.

He said examination showed that the heart pump had not changed Mr. De Rudder's blood in any fashion. There was no evidence of clotting caused by the pump, he said.

The operation of the heart pump was monitored almost constantly for more than 100 hours by Dr. deBakey or a member of the group of surgeons and engineers who developed it. The device, operated by compressed air, times its pulses to coincide with the patient's heartbeat.

He said he would not hesitate to use it on any case in which he felt it could be of some advantage.

Earlier, Dr. DeBakey and other surgeons had said the value of such a pump would be in its giving the heart a chance to rest and heal after surgery.

Dr. DeBakey said the autopsy showed that Mr. De Rudders' heart had been healing as had been expected and had been assuming more of its workload,

an indication that it was getting stronger.

Dr. DeBakey said it would be a matter "of several weeks" before proposed modifications could be made in the heart pump.

The modifications, he said, will be designed to make it easier to attach the one-pound, orange-sized device to a patient's heart.

Dr. DeBakey said the next patient to test a heart pump probably would be one in as critical shape as Mr. De Rudder was.

At the time of the six-hour heart surgery last week, Dr. DeBakey said Mr. De Rudder would die "reasonably soon" without an operation to correct the diseased valve between the chambers of his heart. And, he said, Mr. De Rudder could not survive such an operation without a device to assume part of the workload of his heart.

Respirator Used

In a statement announcing that Mr. De Rudder's death was caused by the lung rupture, Methodist Hospital also revealed that a respirator had been assisting Mr. De Rudder in his breathing since the operation.

The respirator was attached after a tracheostomy was performed on Mr. De Rudder at the same time as his heart was being repaired.

Mr. deBakey said he did not know if the respirator was in any way responsible for the ruptured lung that caused Mr. De Rudder's death.

Mr. De Rudder's body was flown to Westville, Ill., his hometown, tonight for a funeral service and burial.

Mrs. De Rudder, who came to Houston last Friday, was distraught at the news of her husband's death.

April 27, 1966

Heart Transplant Keeps Man Alive in South Africa

By The Associated Press

CAPETOWN, Dec. 3 — The world's first successful human heart transplant was announced today.

In a five-hour operation that began at 1 A.M., surgeons at the Groote Schuur Hospital removed the heart of a young woman who died after an automobile crash and placed it in the chest of a 55-year-old man dying because his own heart was damaged, the announcement said.

When the transplanted heart was in place, it was started beating by an electric shock.

Dr. Jan H. Louw, the hospital's chief surgeon, said:

"It was like turning the ignition switch of a car."

The hospital said that the man was in satisfactory condition but that the next few days would be a critical period.

The heart was removed from the body of Denise Ann Darvall, 24, an accounting machine operator, and transferred to Louis Washkansky, a businessman, the hospital said.

Mr. Washkansky was reported fully conscious, with blood pressure normal.

Doctors around the world hailed the transplant achievement but said the crucial question would be whether the man's body would accept the alien heart.

In the first stage of the operation, Mr. Washkansky and the body of Miss Darvall were put on heart-lung machines, each manned by a team of technicians.

In the second stage, the donor's heart was removed and kept going by a pump.

The third stage was the removal of Mr. Washkansky's heart.

The fourth and most intricate stage was the placing of the donor's heart in Mr. Washkansky's body. When the transplant was completed, electrodes were placed against the heart walls, and a high current was switched on for a fraction of a second.

The heart started beating immediately, Dr. Louw said.

Hospital sources said that the transplant almost took place last Wednesday with another donor but was canceled at the last moment because the donor died too soon.

Miss Darvall's kidneys were also removed and taken to the Karl Bremer Hospital for a successful kidney transplant to Jonathan Van Wyk, 10.

The announcement of the transplant to Mr. Washkansky came from Dr. Jacobus G. Burger, medical supervisor of the Groote Schuur Hospital.

"The operation was his only chance," Dr. Burger said. "Washkansky was dying and wouldn't have lived longer than a few days otherwise."

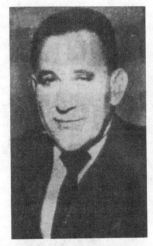

Louis Washkansky, who received transplanted heart.

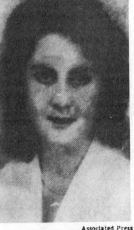

Associated Press

Denise Ann Darval!, whose death made heart available.

Dr. Burger said the next two or three days would be the critical postoperative period.

"The longer Washkansky goes on, the better," he said, "although that does not mean the heart will not be rejected later. The body could decide in five or 10 years' time that it doesn't want this heart."

Mr. Washkansky has a tracheotomy—a tube inserted in his throat through which he is breathing — and is unable to speak, Dr. Burger said. He is being kept absolutely quiet in a special room.

"Even the nurses don't speak to him," Dr. Burger said. "They are doing everything for him and keeping him dead quiet."

Dr. Burger said that apart from the body's natural tendency to reject the heart, the main danger could come from blood clotting and resultant heart failure.

Mr. Washkansky is being fed anticlotting drugs to counter this.

"We are also using steroids to prevent the heart being thrown out rejected," Dr. Burger said.

He said that Mr. Washkansky had been kept alive by using pumps to assist his heart, but this could not have gone on indefinitely.

"The heart muscle was fibrosed, which means that all the muscle was gone and there was only fibrous tissue there," the doctor said. "It wouldn't pump the blood any more, and his condition was deteriorating.

"We thought he was dying a week ago, and he would have died immediately if we had taken the pumps away.

"Washkansky knew what he was going into, but it was his only chance."

Heading the team of five cardiac surgeons was Prof. Chris Barnard.

Dr. Louw assisted with arrangements and advised the surgeons, although he was not operating.

97

Professor Barnard is in Professor Louw's department.

In addition to the cardiac surgeons, there were two neurosurgeons and two anesthetists. Altogether there were about 20 in the theater, including five or six theater nurses, Dr. Burger said. All the surgeons were South Africans.

The woman donor was injured yesterday afternoon. Neurosurgeons, with an electroencephalogram to measure her brain waves, alerted the cardiac surgeons the instant she died, shortly before 1 A.M.

The consent to use her heart was obtained earlier from her father.

"The operation had to begin within half an hour of her death," Dr. Burger said.

The woman's mother was killed instantly in the same auto accident.

Dr. Burger said the heart transplant experiments on cats and dogs had been carried out over the last 10 years at Groote Schuur, which in Afrikaans means big barn.

Mrs. Washkansky said that before the transplant her husband's life was "hanging by a thread." She said he was approached three weeks ago by doctors who told him "in great detail what it would entail."

"I was petrified but my husband had such confidence in medical men he inspired me as well," she said.

She said he had had heart trouble for seven years and in the last two years his condition became progressively worse. She said she and her husband had emigrated from Lithuania as children and married in Capetown in 1946.

The donor's father, Edward George Darvall, said:

"I gave the doctors permission to remove my daughter's heart and kidneys and donate them to other persons if it could have their lives. It was shortly before midnight after I was informed she was dying."

"Professor Barnard has two registrars — young doctors studying for postgraduate degrees—continually experimenting in his animal laboratory," Dr. Burger said. "I know he has successfully transplanted hearts of dogs, but I don't know how long the animal lived afterwards."

United States surgeons at the Stanford Medical Center in California have performed 200 heart transplants in dogs, with a 60-to-70 per cent survival rate.

Surgeons at the center have been reported by The Journal of the American Medical Association to be ready for a heart transplant whenever the ideal donor and ideal recipient appeared at the same time.

Patient's Courage Hailed

CAPETOWN, Dec. 3 (UPI)— Professor Barnard, head of the thoracic surgery department of Capetown University, said today that Mr. Washkansky deserved credit for the operation's apparent success.

"If it had not been for this man's courage and will to live the operation would never have succeeded," he said.

The moment of decision came last night. The doctors told Mr. Washkansky that a heart with blood group and tissue compatible with his own was available. They gave him two days to make up his mind.

"He made up his mind in two minutes," Mrs. Washkansky said.

The surgeons marked one of the high points of their careers when Miss Darvall's heart was set beating anew in Mr. Washkansky's body.

"It's going to work," Professor Barnard was quoted as having said. "I need a cup of tea."

Another doctor said:

"It was the most exciting experience I have ever had. It was like watching a bullfight. Certain classical maneuvers had to be done before the grand finale."

In Chicago, a spokesman for the American Medical Association said that the surgery was "not surprising."

"South African doctors have a fine reputation and there is no reason to suspect they could not be capable of doing such an operation," the spokesman, Frank Chappell, said.

In Houston, Dr. Michael E. De Bakey, a pioneer in surgery implanting artificial heart pumps, called the operation "a great achievement."

Feat Praised in U. S.

STANFORD, Calif., Dec. 3 (AP) — The Stanford Medical Center surgeon who announced plans 13 days ago for transplanting a human heart said today that the world's first heart transplant operation at Capetown was "pretty exciting."

"The thing is it anticipated the artificial heart by possibly three to five years," said the surgeon, Dr. Norman E. Shumway, head of Stanford's division of cardiovascular surgery.

Dr. Shumway said he worked with Prof. Chris Barnard, head of the Capetown surgery team, at the University of Minnesota about 10 years ago.

"We have had numerous reunions since, the most recent in May," Dr. Shumway said. "He is a good man, a well-known, well-respected cardiac surgeon."

He predicted that the heart transplant would become as frequent as the kidney transplant within 10 years.

The surgical team must have the consent of the patient, Dr. Shumway explained.

"It has to be an extreme case, a terminal case, because legally uor are killing the person when you take this heart out and throw it away," he said.

"At the moment he goes into the operating room, he's alive. You have to assume he would be dead without the transplant in a few weeks or a few months."

December 4, 1967

Transplant Patient Dies After 18 Days

By The Associated Press

CAPETOWN, Thursday, Dec. 21—Louis Washkansky, the world's first heart transplant patient, died early today in Groote Schuur Hospital.

He had lived for 18 days with the heart of a 25-year-old woman who was killed in an automobile accident a few hours before the historic operation Dec. 3.

A bulletin issued by Dr. Jacobus Burger, the medical superintendent of the hospital, said the 53-year-old wholesale grocer died about 6:50 A.M. (11:50 P.M. Wednesday, Eastern standard time). No further details were announced immediately.

After almost two weeks of steady progress Mr. Washkansky developed lung complications last weekend and

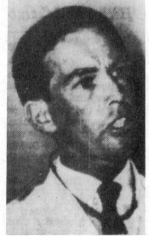

Associated Press
Dr. Christian N. Barnard, who was chief surgeon of the heart transplant team.

his condition slowly deteriorated.

A marked worsening was reported yesterday. During the night the hospital announced there was little hope for him, but doctors continued to administer oxygen in the hope of keeping him alive.

Up to late last night, Mr. Washkansky's doctors were unsure what was causing the deterioration of his condition. His heart was beating comparatively strongly and his pulse rate was good, but the lung complications grew worse.

At first the doctors, led by the chief surgeon, Dr. Christian N. Barnard, had thought this was double pneumonia, then that it was a manifestation of the body's tendency to reject foreign tissue—directed not at the grafted heart but at Mr. Washkansky's own tissues.

A Man Full of Life

CAPETOWN, Thursday, Dec. 21 (Reuters) — Mr. Washkansky was described by friends as a tough, lively and courageous man, full of dry humor.

"Louis is life itself. There's never a dull moment when he is around. If anyone deserves a new lease on life, it is he," a close friend said recently.

Mr. Washkansky's brother-in-law, Solly Sklar, a former South African heavyweight wrestling champion, said they both served in the South African Army Engineers for six years in East and North Africa and in Italy.

Mr. Washkansky came to South Africa from Lithuania when he was a child. He was 5 feet 6 inches tall, but weighed over 170 pounds when he had his first heart attack seven years ago.

Friends say he would not accept his disability until a second and more severe attack occurred two years ago.

He was a keen soccer player, weight-lifter and swimmer in his youth.

'Operation Was Only Chance'

"I'm much better—what kind of operation did I have?"

These were the first words spoken by Mr. Washkansky after the historic operation on Dec. 3 that had attempted to prolong his life substantially by transplanting the heart from a cadaver into his own body.

Mr. Washkansky was unaware at first that the heart that was beating in his chest was not his own, although millions already had heard of the operation that had appeared initially to be successful.

Then the patient, who had been dying because of a progressive cardiac disease, was told that he had become the first man in history to have his life sustained by the heart of another human.

But the revolutionary surgery failed, and Mr. Washkansky did die; sooner than had been hoped, but later than the most pessimistic estimate.

All the hope and effort that was lavished on the South African businessman may not have been completely wasted. The heart transplant may have allowed Mr. Washkansky a few extra days of life.

How much of a new lease on life he gained by virtue of the operation will never be known, although the surgeons who performed the operation had warned him three months before it took place that his heart condition was worsening and that he did not have long to live.

"The operation was his only chance," said Dr. Jacobus G. Burger, medical supervisor of the Groote Schuur Hospital in Capetown where the transplant was performed. "Washkansky was dying and wouldn't have lived longer than a few days otherwise."

Mr. Washkansky's cardiac problems started seven years ago when he suffered a heart attack. Two years ago a second occurred and his condition deteriorated steadily.

Each attack destroyed part of Mr. Washkansky's heart muscle, reducing the effectiveness of the organ's pumping action. Fibrous scar tissue built up near the damaged heart muscle, further complicating his cardiac condition.

Greatly Enlarged Heart

Mr. Washkansky had experienced almost total heart failure three months ago. X-rays disclosed that his heart was more than twice the normal size, and he could hardly breathe.

On Nov. 10 Mr. Washkansky was asked if he would consider undergoing a heart transplant. The surgeon who spoke to him was later to perform the operation. He was Dr. Barnard, a South African who had taken postgraduate medical training in the United States.

Dr. Barnard suggested that Mr. Washkansky take a few days to mull over the hazardous and potential benefits of such an operation. But, according to the patient's wife, Mrs. Anne Washkansky, 53, her husband "made up his mind in two minutes." He remained in the hospital to await the operation.

Twenty-two days later Miss Denise Ann Darvall, a 25-year-old bank clerk was crossing the street near the hospital when she was struck by a car, suffering fatal head injuries.

Miss Darvall was taken to Groote Schuur Hospital, where it became apparent to physicians that she had only a few hours to live.

They asked her father if he would consent to the transplantation of parts of his daughter's body, after her death, to others. He agreed. That night she died.

In a five-hour operation, which started at 1 A.M. the following day, a medical team of 30 surgeons, physicians, nurses and technicians transplanted her heart to Mr. Washkansky. Later one of her kidneys was transplanted to the body of a 10-year-old colored boy, who was in another hospital.

Mr. Washkansky regained consciousness and, less than 24 hours after the operation, started taking liquid nourishment.

"I'm hungry," he said the next day, and he was given breakfast. At first Mr. Washkansky appeared to be regaining his health; he took a few brief steps, chatted with doctors and relatives, including his 15-year-old son, Michael, and sat on the balcony outside his room.

But the drugs and radiation treatments that were being administered to suppress his body's natural immunity to foreign tissue also thwarted Mr. Washkansky's ability to ward off disease.

Almost two weeks after the operation, Mr. Washkansky developed what was at first believed to be pneumonia. But when he failed to respond to antibiotics, his doctors assumed that the condition was not pneumonia but the rejection phenomenon. Although the alien heart appeared to be functioning properly, his condition worsened.

Dr. Barnard, the chief surgeon, and Mr. Washkansky's relatives praised his courage. His brother-in-law, Mr. Sklar, said Mr. Washkansky had shown the same type of courage in battle.

Friends described Mr. Washkansky as a man who had no fear and no enemies; was tough and extroverted, was generous to a fault and lived life to the full.

Mr. Washkansky emigrated from Lithuania with his parents as a child, settling in Capetown, where he went to school.

Although he was Jewish, Mr. Washkansky who was nicknamed "Washy," had told relatives that he hoped to be out of the hospital for Christmas, and that he wanted them to hold a party.

December 21, 1967

5 Get Organs From One Donor In a Series of Transplants Here

By SANDRA BLAKESLEE

One man gave five strangers a chance for longer or better lives yesterday when surgeons transplanted his heart, liver, both kidneys and a cornea in the world's largest multiple transplant operation.

The donor, a 57-year-old man whose identity was not disclosed, died at 3:45 o'clock Wednesday afternoon at Memorial Hospital on York Avenue at 68th Street.

The cause of death was a malignant brain tumor that did not affect other organs in his body, doctors said. The man had been in a coma for over a month.

Two surviving brothers gave permission for the healthy organs in his body to be used, after he had been pronounced dead by a team of doctors, including the man's personal physician, who was not involved in the transplant procedures.

Transplant operations involving three organs from the same person—the heart and both kidneys—have been performed but this was the first to involve more than three internal organs.

Twelve teams of surgeons went into immediate action after the death of the New York donor.

Doctors at Memorial Hospital, who removed the liver for a transplant operation in their own hospital, called colleagues who had done a number of earlier heart and kidney transplants at New York Hospital. The latter institution is on the East River across the street from Memorial and connected to it by tunnel.

Two young surgeons, Drs. Jack Block and Jerry Carlson, from New York Hospital, went to Memorial and removed the donor's heart there at 9:05 P.M. Wednesday in a half hour operation.

They then placed the organ in a large stainless steel bucket, about the size of a flour cannister, which is normally used to stow sterilized scrub brushes. The heart was placed in a saline solution, similar to the liquid part of the blood, and the doctors sprinted with it to their own hospital.

"We had a pre-determined route involving five elevators, a connecting tunnel and guards on relay to help us all along the way," Dr. Carlson said at a news conference yesterday.

The doctors ran and walked through most of the tunnel, described as being "like the sewers of Paris."

"We made it to the operating room in 4.5 minutes flat, by the stop watch," Dr. Carlson said.

At the same news conference, Dr. C. Walton Lillehei, chief of surgery at New York Hospital, hailed this as the first inter-hospital transfer of a heart. Normally, a donor who has died is in a room next to the waiting recipient, and the heart to be transplanted is outside the body for about 20 minutes.

'Time Was of the Essence'

Dog hearts have been "kept outside" for transplantation for up to six to eight hours, Dr. Lillehei said, but this was the longest a human heart has ever been "stored." "Time was of the essence," he said.

The heart transplant operation, which took 53 minutes, ended at 1 A.M. yesterday. The recipient was a 36-year-old man, whose name the hospital has not released.

The heart was kept fresh with the help of a heart-lung machine before and after it was removed and before it was transplanted. It stopped beating for only 20 minutes while it was being transferred from Memorial Hospital to New York Hospital.

The two kidneys were removed after the heart at Memorial Hospital and were also taken to New York Hospital, where they were simultaneously transplanted into a 19-year-old male and a 38-year-old woman. The operations were completed by 1:30 A.M. yesterday.

There was less rush over the kidney operations since the techniques of kidney transplants have become more or less routine, doctors said. According to Dr. Lillihei, a kidney may be kept in storage for 12 to 18 hours.

All three patients at New York Hospital were reported in excellent condition last night.

Meanwhile, Memorial Hospital performed a liver transplant operation on a 27-year-old woman who has been married six months, Mrs. Lynne Varney. Less than 50 such operations have been performed in the world because the liver is such a chemically complex organ, unlike the heart which is a simple pump.

Dr. Edward Beattie, medical director at Memorial, said the names of the surgeons were not available, but that the liver transplant may have been the first on the East Coast. At any rate, it was the first liver transplant performed at Memorial Hospital, which specializes in cancer research and treatment.

A 14-pound cancerous tumor was removed from Mrs. Varney's liver before the new liver was implanted. One problem with liver transplants has been that the special drugs that combat rejection of the new organ also often allow new cancers to grow. Mrs. Varney is taking the drugs despite that.

The cornea was transplanted last night into a male recipient. at New York Hospital. The other cornea is scheduled for transplantation today. Corneas can be frozen and stored for weeks.

Dr. Lillehei said that inter-hospital transfer of an organ was extremely important because it heralded a practice that "inevitably must become" common practice.

"We are in the horse-and-buggy-stage of transplant operations," he said, adding that many organs were often wasted because the right donor and right recipient were not in the same place at the same time.

Donors and recipients must have the same blood type and sympathetic tissue matches for transplant operations to succeed. Many recipients die before the right donor comes to the hospital where the recipient is waiting. Luckily, the recipients at both hospitals yesterday matched the single donor perfectly, doctors said.

Some day soon, Dr. Lillehei said, there may be central clearing houses for donors and recipients, so a recipient from Iowa can be helped by a donor's organ from, say, the West Coast. The center, he went on, would collect and share all vital statistics on potential recipients and donors among hospitals throughout the country.

One donor can give life to as many as 17 people, the surgeon said, "but it is mathematically impossible to have 17 recipients waiting in one hospital who would match one donor."

The 17 vital organs that can be transplanted include the heart, lungs, liver, kidneys, pancreas, adrenal glands, small intestine, and gastrointestinal tract

Yesterday's heart transplant operation was the fourth at New York Hospital and the sixth in New York City.

February 21, 1969

Man Who Got Plastic Heart Dies As Dispute on the Device Looms

By United Press International

HOUSTON, April 8—Haskell Karp, the first person ever to rest his slim chance for life on a manmade heart, died today of complications resulting from that pioneer surgery.

Mr. Karp, 47 years old, of Skokie, Ill., survived three days with a Dacron and plastic heart implanted in his chest, a device that its designer said might have kept the patient alive six months.

But Mr. Karp wanted to "live like a man," with a human heart. He got his chance when Dr. Denton A. Cooley replaced the artificial heart yesterday with that of a Massachusetts woman, who had died of brain damage.

Rejection of the foreign tissues began to set in, however, and early today doctors found a "patch of pneumonia" on Mr. Karp's right lung. He was dead within 18 hours.

The implantation of the artificial heart threatened to stir up a new controversy among the medical profession—particularly in Houston.

Dr. Michael E. DeBakey, president of the Baylor College of Medicine, has drawn up a set of rules that states that none of his staff can use an experimental device in surgery without the approval of a committee of Baylor doctors.

Although he operates at St. Luke's, Dr. Cooley is a member of the Baylor staff. The use of the artificial heart was not brought before the committee.

Dr. Domingo Liotta, the heart's designer, said Dr. DeBakey was not aware that the artificial heart was ready for use until it was placed in Mr. Karp.

Similar guidelines have been established by the National Institutes of Health in Bethesda, Md.

A friend of the family said Mr. Karp's wife, Shirley, had taken the death of her husband "pretty well."

"She was more or less resigned to it," the friend said. "Dr. Cooley told her this morning her husband had developed pneumonia and he broke the news of his death to her this afternoon."

The official cause of death will not be known pending an autopsy, but a spokesman at St. Luke's Hospital said death was apparently caused by rejection complicated by pneumonia and kidney failure.

The artificial heart, which sustained Mr. Karp when his own heart became badly diseased, worked just as it had been intended to.

Dr. Liotta, said the mechanical heart was in good condition even after being removed from Mr. Karp's chest.

"It looked really wonderful," Dr. Liotta said. "It had a real fine lining. I believe he could have lived six months with it. I believe it was possible. For longer periods? For two or three years? I don't know if it was that durable."

Dr. Liotta, who also designed the left ventricle bypass used by Dr. DeBakey almost three years ago in the first major step toward heart transplantation, defended his and Dr. Cooley's use of the mechanical heart.

Dr. Frank Hastings of the National Heart Institute in Bethesda, has criticized use of a mechanical heart, which can be used only as a temporary replacement for a human heart.

"Dr. Hastings is a good friend of mine," said Dr. Liotta, shortly after hearing of Mr. Karp's death. "But for the last five years he has been out of any clinical work and out of contact with the patients."

Dr. Liotta said previously, when Dr. Hastings was still practicing surgery, nothing could be done if a patient's heart failed to begin beating after open heart surgery. Now, Dr. Liotta said, there is the mechanical heart, which can be quickly implanted.

Inquiry About Guidelines

By HAROLD M. SCHMECK Jr.
Special to The New York Times

WASHINGTON, April 8 — Questions have arisen concerning the use of the artificial heart that maintained the life of Mr. Karp for 65 hours.

The main question is whether the Federal guidelines covering human experimentation were followed by the surgical team that installed the artificial heart.

Dr. Theodore Cooper, director of the National Heart Institute, said tonight he had written to Dr. DeBakey for information on the following points:

¶Was research supported by the institute involved in the development of the heart and its use over the weekend?

¶What experimental data provided the basis for the use of the artificial heart?

¶Were the Federal guidelines followed in the decision to use the artificial heart in the attempt to save Mr. Karp?

The Federal guidelines require that the scientific protocol and plans for any experiment involving humans be reviewed and approved by a group of the investigator's peers at the institution where his research is done.

In this case the surgical team that used the artificial heart was led by Dr. Cooley of Baylor. The question that first arose in Houston and elsewhere was whether or not he did obtain approval from a review group before implanting the artificial heart.

But the matter is complicated by further questions.

Dr. Cooper said he wrote the letter today because the ques-

100

tions had been raised. They were not raised initially by the institute.

He noted that the guidelines would apply to the case only if institute funds were involved and if the use of the artificial heart constituted an experiment.

Dr. Cooley is not a principal investigator in any heart institute grant supporting transplantation or development of an artificial heart device.

Dr. Cooper said, however, that he believed Dr. Liotta, who has been credited with designing the heart, had done much of his research under Dr. DeBakey and under the coverage of a grant from the institute.

Therefore the question of whether or not the guidelines apply to this case depends partly on whether the artificial heart was one developed for Dr. DeBakey although first used by Dr. Cooley.

The question of whether the artificial heart was considered an experimental device also has an obvious bearing on the guidelines issue.

If Dr. DeBakey's response indicates that the guidelines do apply and were not followed, Dr. Cooper said he would then have to ask the Baylor College of Medicine what remedial action was being taken.

April 9, 1969

Cooley Ends Tie With DeBakey After Dispute on Artificial Heart

HOUSTON, Sept. 10 (UPI)— Dr. Denton A. Cooley, who has transplanted more human hearts than any other surgeon, cut his ties today with Dr. Michael E. DeBakey and the Baylor College of Medicine, in a professional wrangle over an artificial heart.

Dr. Cooley declined to ask the Baylor research committee for permission whenever he wanted to use the dacron-and-plastic heart in a human being.

Dr. DeBakey, a heart surgeon, who is a pioneer in developing the artificial heart, has complained privately that Dr. Cooley had borrowed the device from him.

Dr. Cooley's new title is physician in chief of the Texas Heart Institute. He retains the title of chief of cardiovascular surgery at St. Luke's and Texas Children's Hospitals.

Dr. Cooley's troubles with Baylor and Dr. DeBakey started last April 4, when he implanted an artificial heart in Haskell Karp, 47 years old, of Skokie, Ill.

Mr. Karp lived for 63 hours with the artificial device. Dr. Cooley replaced the artificial heart with a human heart and Mr. Karp lived an additional 3½ hours. Since then Dr. Cooley has been trying to improve the artificial heart.

Angered over the use of the artificial heart, Dr. DeBakey, then president of Baylor College of Medicine, persuaded the

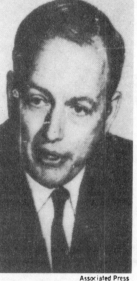

Associated Press

Dr. Denton A. Cooley

trustees to make all members of the faculty sign a pledge that they would seek research committee approval before experimenting on patients with research projects.

A Baylor committee ruled that the heart used in Mr. Karp was basically the one developed by Dr. DeBakey. The committee also said that Dr. Cooley had failed to follow medical protocol.

Dr. DeBakey ousted Dr. Domingo Liotta, an associate, last May for talking to Dr. Cooley. Dr. Liotta was then hired by Dr. Cooley to help him with his artifical heart work. Dr. Liotta did basic research for the artificial heart for both surgeons.

As far as Dr. Cooley is concerned, severing connections with Baylor will mean that he will not be able to draw on the hospital's young physicians for his staff.

September 11, 1969

A World Moratorium On Heart Transplants

Mr. and Mrs. Louis B. Russell Jr. are holding open house in their Indianapolis home today. The occasion: The third anniversary of Mr. Russell's heart transplant. He may also, of course, use the occasion to do some discreet politicking, for he is the Democratic candidate for Councilman-at-Large.

Mr. Russell, a black industrial arts teacher, is the longest-living heart transplant recipient in history. But he is by no means alone in his good fortune. As of late last week, there were 27 survivors of heart transplant operations, a dozen of whom have lived with their new organs for more than two years.

Yet, heart transplants are today among the rarest of surgical procedures, being performed far less frequently now than in the months immediately following Dr. Christiaan N. Barnard's first pioneering effort in late 1967. In the entire world, there were 101 heart transplants in 1968, 47 in 1969, 17 in 1970 and only 10 so far this year.

Three factors have played a role in reducing the frequency of these operations, even for desperately ill patients. The overwhelming majority of heart transplant recipients have died, usually fairly quickly after surgery. The operation and postoperative care have been extremely expensive, mounting quickly to tens of thousands of dollars even for patients who have survived only a few weeks. And a significant percentage of the patients have suffered psychotic episodes after receiving their new hearts.

The result has been what now amounts almost to a complete world moratorium on heart transplants. Only Dr. Norman Shumway's team at the Stanford University Medical School is still doing these operations with any frequency. Last year, Dr. Shumway's group performed eight of the world's 17 heart transplants; so far this year, the Stanford team has accounted for seven of the 10 operations.

Almost all the surgeons who initially flocked into the cardiac transplant field have now abandoned it. They have been frightened off by the high mortality rate caused by the body's rejection of the foreign tissue that the transplanted heart is, and by the infections that result because the patient's defensive immunological system has been weakened by the drugs used to com-

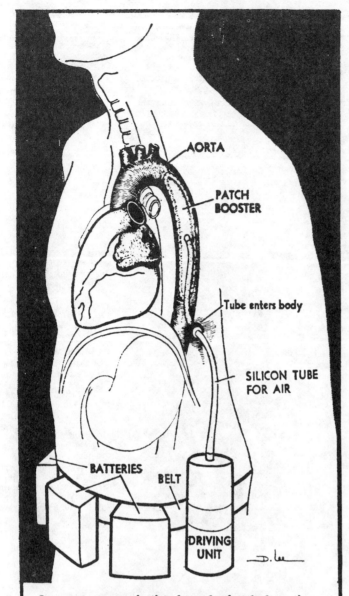

AORTA

PATCH BOOSTER

Tube enters body

SILICON TUBE FOR AIR

BATTERIES

BELT

DRIVING UNIT

D. Lee

In recent years, scientists have developed alternatives to heart transplants for the treatment of some heart ailments. One such (above) was recently installed in a patient by Dr. Adrian Kantrowitz of Detroit, who also devised the pacemaker. A battery-powered unit drives air through a tube to a "booster patch" attached to the aorta; the air pumps the blood along when the heart cannot do the job.

bat rejection. Only a few surgeons—like Dr. Richard R. Lower of the Medical College of Virginia in Richmond, who operated on Mr. Russell—can join Dr. Shumway and Dr. Barnard in claiming to have long-surviving patients.

There is a telling contrast available. Of the 140 or so heart transplants by all surgeons other than Dr. Shumway, only about one patient in 10 is still alive. Of Dr. Shumway's 33 patients, 13 are still living, and one of those who died lived two years with his new heart before he succumbed.

Dr. Shumway himself has often given much of the credit for his superior results to his large and expert team of internists, immunologists and others who help care for his patients post-operatively and who maintain ceaseless guard against rejection, infections and other dangers. Dr. Shumway also attempts meticulous matching of recipient and donor so as to reduce rejection risk. And for many months now, he has done transplants only on patients under 50, thus seeking to avoid deaths caused by the failure of other weakened organs in those receiving new hearts.

Dr. Barnard, the pioneer, is bitter about being shackled by the refusal of South African physicians to send patients to him. "They would rather send [patients] home to die," he complained recently.

Just last week, Dr. Barnard suffered another disappointment when a patient into whom he had transplanted both the heart and lungs of a donor died after a difficult 23 days of post-operative life. But it was only the world's fourth combination heart-lung transplant, and Dr. Barnard's patient lived more than three times as long as the longest-surviving earlier recipient of these organs.

—HARRY SCHWARTZ
August 22, 1971

Bypass Operation for Heart Disease Gains Favor and Stirs a Controversy

By LAWRENCE K. ALTMAN

A coronary bypass operation for arteriosclerotic heart disease that 11 doctors from China saw a Bronx surgeon perform here last week is a promising but controversial recent development that has grown popular and become profitable for surgeons and hospitals.

The controversy involves an operation—if its enthusiastic proponents are proved correct —that millions of men and women now in their twenties and thirties, among others, may need in a decade or later.

Since 1967, surgeons in this country have done about 35,000 such operations—20,000 this

year alone, according to the American Heart Association here. The operation typically costs about $6,000—more when complications develop—for the surgeon's fee and hospital and nursing care.

Experts agree that several more years are needed to analyze the data to evaluate objectively the long-term results

of the open-heart operation. It involves taking one or more veins from a patient's leg and suturing them in the patient's chest to improve blood supply to the heart, which has been damaged by abnormal thickening and hardening caused by fatty deposits in the arterial walls.

The techniques vary among the scores of teams doing the operation at medical centers throughout this country. Few controlled studies are being done in the United States, where no central registry exists despite appeals for its creation.

For these reasons, some experts say that comparable statistics needed to answer questions involved in the controversy will be harder to come by.

Some clues may be given in reports to be presented at the American Heart Association meeting in Dallas next month.

If the long-term results do not support the current wave of enthusiasm, then coronary by-pass surgery may join the fads that have become so familiar to doctors—a burst of publicized, glowing reports followed by a long period of less-publicized disillusionment.

Skepticism on Approach

Medical history is so full of near-misses in the surgical treatment of arteriosclerotic heart disease that doctors have developed skepticism toward this approach, according to Dr. Harvey G. Kemp Jr. of St. Luke's Hospital here, writing in the current issue of the Bulletin of the New York Academy of Medicine.

Also involved in the controversy are major economic, social and ethical questions that cannot be answered until doctors have fully assessed the merits of the coronary by-pass operation.

The key question that doctors are struggling to answer is: Which patients will benefit most from the costly open-heart operation that carries with it perhaps a 10 per cent risk of death?

The mortality statistics vary widely with the severity of the patient's illness and with the skills of the surgical team. Also, a doctor must weigh the risks of surgery to a patient against what is known about the natural course of arteriosclerotic heart disease.

"There are also economic factors at work which make it difficult to be objective," Dr. Richard S. Ross, a Johns Hopkins cardiologist in Baltimore, said.

"There are," he said, "cardiac surgical teams in hospitals in this country which have been doing only an occasional [open heart, non bypass] case —one to two per week—who now, for the first time, see an opportunity to utilize the equipment and personnel and fully to profit economically from them."

As editors of the British Medical Journal emphasized, the excellent results "reported from a few large medical centers cannot quickly be reproduced in units which are just starting up."

Behind the controversy is an "epidemic" of arteriosclerosis that is silently damaging the hearts and arteries of an increasing number of younger people not just in this country but in China and other developed countries of the world.

Crushing Chest Pains

The damage caused by arteriosclerosis is insidious—until the first symptom strikes. This can be the crushing chest pains of angina pectoris, a heart attack—or sudden death.

When the damage appears, the doctor prescribes, for example, nitroglycerine tablets for angina, digitalis pills for congestive heart failure and a coronary care unit for a heart attack.

These and other standard medical therapies are usually sufficient to treat adequately the damage wrought by arteriosclerosis. But sometimes the best of medical therapies do not suffice as the disease progresses daily.

The angina patient, for example, may be forced to slip nitroglycerine tablets under his tongue constantly to control the intractable series of crushing chest pains that evoke a sense of impending doom.

Coronary bypass surgery has dramatically relieved the symptoms of some patients with intractable angina, obviating the need for such pills, allowing the patients to return to work and vastly improving the quality of their lives.

These results, in turn, have led a growing number of cardiac surgeons to perform the operation for a wider variety of problems. It is in this area that most of the controversy is centered.

The Inter-Society Commission for Heart Disease Resources, a federally funded group of experts, said in a report published in the current issue of Circulation, a medical journal published by the American Heart Association here:

"Because there are inadequate data on the course of patients with coronary artery disease with and without operation, it is not yet possible to set down rigid indications for" coronary bypass surgery.

The commission cautioned against needless duplication of expensive facilities that could result as each community hospital, for economic and prestige purposes, bought the X-ray and heart-lung machines needed to start its own program.

The commission also urged that a hospital should begin such programs only if it had an adequately trained team of doctors available on a full-time basis to do the four or more coronary bypass operations each week that it considers necessary to maintain proper minimal skills.

Coronary bypass surgery requires a team of cardiac surgeons, cardiologists, radiologists and other doctors. Each of the specialists must spend years of training after medical school to gain the experience necessary to interpret correctly the data collected in sophisticated tests, called coronary arteriography and heart catheterization, that are needed before the surgeon can perform the surgery.

Each of these procedures carries its own risk of complications, including death. Nationally, the risk involved in coronary arteriography is reported to be lower than 2 per cent, depending on the experience of the team doing the procedure.

Despite the risks, arteriography and catheterization, when done properly, provide the key data that help doctors screen out those patients whose condition cannot be improved by surgery. For those patients who stand to benefit, these tests help determine the precise anatomical location of the blockage and the severity of the physiologic damage caused by arteriosclerosis. Surgeons have pointed out that the grafts of veins achieve little if the heart is already badly damaged.

Because the surgeon knows more precisely where he must suture a vein, he can work more quickly during the few minutes when the patient's heart is purposely stopped.

More Normal Blood Flow

During this period, the surgeon, wearing a pair of magnifying eyeglasses like a watch-maker, sews one end of a vein removed from a leg to a coronary artery at a point beyond the arteriosclerotic obstruction. Then he sews the other end of the vein to the aorta, which is the main artery that carries blood from the heart.

In effect, the surgeon has restored a more normal blood flow to nourish the heart by bypassing the obstruction. Depending on the location and severity of damage, the surgeon may put in more than one such bypass.

Dr. W. Dudley Johnson, a pioneer in bypass surgery at St. Luke's Hospital in Milwaukee, made this appraisal:

"Undoubtedly the major factor contributing to the success of vein graft surgery was the recognition that the heart would tolerate anoxic arrest (total stoppage). By allowing the suturing to be done in a dry, quiet field, vein grafts could be attached to all areas of the coronary system."

Further Complications Seen

Even when surgery goes well in the operating room, complications may develop in the recovery room or in a hospital ward. Doctors have estimated that as many as 25 per cent of patients suffer a heart attack as a consequence of bypass surgery. Hepatitis, a liver infection, can result from blood transfusions.

Good blood flow through the graft occurs in about 90 per cent of the bypass operations. But as time passes, the blood flow can decrease significantly in some cases because fibrosis develops as a natural consequence of subjecting a vein to arterial pressure. Just how long the grafts can be expected to work is a question that doctors say only time can answer.

It is because the risks are so great that Dr. Ross of Johns Hopkins said: "We must expect more of operations than just symptomatic improvement."

To justify the risks, expenses and manpower, Dr. Richard Gorlin of the Peter Bent Brigham Hospital in Boston said, "the only way that we can really assess end results is through long-term follow-up to see whether patients live longer and sustain less angina and less frequent myocardial infarctions [heart attacks] than untreated patients."

October 22, 1972

A Second Opinion Reduces Surgery

By NANCY HICKS

The United Store Workers Union says that it has been able to reduce the amount of surgery performed on its members by having a second doctor review each recommended operation before it is performed.

This "second medical opinion" resulted in the first year of the review in 19 per cent fewer operations than had been recommended, according to Eleanor J. Tilson, the administrator of the health and welfare fund of the union.

Of 289 members who were told by a doctor that their medical conditions required surgery, 51 were later told they need not undergo an operation. The second consultations were held with doctors at a panel at New York Hospital, which provides this service to the union.

Three members sought a third medical opinion, and four elected to have the surgery anyway, with benefits paid in full by the union, Mrs. Tilson said in an interview.

The "second medical opinions" uncovered some diagnoses that were originally incorrect and in some instances the second doctor disagreed with the first on the necessity for an operation.

"We listened to all the discussions about how there is too much surgery performed in this country and how it is pushing up the cost of medical care, and we decided to see if there isn't something to it," Mrs. Tilson said in giving the reason for starting this program 16 months ago.

The cost incentive is great because the union administers its own health and welfare benefits for its 12,000 members and their families. The funds come entirely from contributions from the employers— Gimbels and Bloomingdale's. They reached $2.2-million in 1972.

The medical aspect of the program is the subject of great debate. Many critics of medical services contend that surgeons operate when less radical treatment might suffice.

Whether there is unnecessary surgery has been the subject of numerous articles in professional journals. It is the subject of a book this year written by a surgeon under a pseudonym. It is the subject of a pamphlet released by Herbert S. Denenberg, the insurance commissioner of Pennsylvania.

The American College of Surgeons, the professional accrediting body for the nation's 25,000 qualified surgeons, is studying the issue to see if it really is a problem.

Mrs. Tilson said that the medical profession had been generally cooperative with the union's efffort, although one local medical society denounced the plan before it had even been instituted. Generally, she is pleased with the result.

"All we were trying to do is to give the patient more information on which to make a decision — whether or not he wants to have an operation— and we have provided a means to do that," she said.

June 19, 1973

Breast Cancer Study Finds Radical Surgery Has No Advantage Over Simple Mastectomy

WASHINGTON, Sept. 29 (UPI) —Findings in a nationwide study of breast cancer indicate that the traditional type of radical surgery undergone by Betty Ford offers no advantage over a less-mutilating technique, the director of the National Cancer Institute said today.

Dr. Frank J. Rauscher Jr. said the study also found evidence that chemical therapy could "drastically" reduce the recurrence of breast cancer and that radiation therapy after surgery, with its bad side effects, was unnecessary.

The major "report to the profession," resulting from studies conducted at 37 hospitals around the country since 1971, will be presented tomorrow in a day-long conference of the National Cancer Institute. The conference has been scheduled for many months.

"We consider this to be one of the most important series of findings in the history of cancer research," Dr. Rauscher said in an interview.

Breast cancer is the leading cancer killer of women. But surgical treatment of the disease has changed little in the last 100 years, and scant progress has been made in preventing a recurrence of breast cancer or improving chances of survival.

Officials at the Cancer Institute believe the new discoveries can lead to an important reduction in surgical disfigurement and increase the chances for successful treatment of the 90,000 American women who develop breast cancer every year.

About 95 per cent of the women undergoing surgery for breast cancer receive the kind of radical mastectomy performed on Mrs. Ford—removal of the breast, the underlying chest muscle and the lymph glands extending back under the armpit. This operation, however, often results in lifelong pain, weakness and periodic swelling of the arm.

A less radical form of surgery is the simple mastectomy, in which only the breast is removed.

Dr. Rauscher said that, in a study of almost 1,700 women, it was found that "the more radical procedure in appropriate patients—and that's a key descriptor—is no better than the less radical procedure."

He said surgeons could tell whether to use the more drastic technique by changing present procedures and, with the patient still on the operating table, ordering an immediate laboratory test for cancer cells in the lymph nodes. If the cancer had spread to the lymph tissue, radical surgery would be needed.

"At the present time," Dr. Rauscher said, "I would estimate that well over half of those [undergoing breast cancer surgery] would be candidates for the less radical procedure."

Mrs. Ford's surgeons knew of these findings. But one of her surgeons, Dr. William Fouty, said in a news briefing after the operation that they chose the radical form of the operation as "a solid procedure that we know has worked very well in the past."

"Surgeons don't like to do the radical, Dr. Rauscher said. "But they feel obliged on the part of the patient to do it."

While widespread adoption of the simple mastectomy would reduce the trauma experienced by women who undergo breast surgery, Dr. Rauscher said the other four points to be dealt with in the study could be of greater importance in the fight against cancer.

One of these is the tentative discovery that radiation therapy—which produces such unwanted side effects as loss of appetite, nausea and diarrhea — offers no advantage over surgery alone in preventing the recurrence of cancer.

Another point contributes new strength to the theory that cancer is an "extrinsic" disease, one which arises from a source outside the body rather than from anything a person is born with.

A third indicates that the size of tumors in perhaps 50 per cent of the women who develop cancer can be reduced with a substance that decreases the level of estrogen, the female hormone, in a woman's system.

And the fourth point, to be presented by Dr. Bernard Fisher of the University of Pittsburgh, who directed the study, shows that chemotherapy treatment started two weeks after surgery with either one drug or a combination of three drugs "is drastically reducing the number of women who develop a secondary cancer," Dr. Rauscher said.

September 30, 1974

DISEASE AND MODERN LIFESTYLES

Finds New York Rushing Into Heart Disease; We Hurry Even in Our Sleep, Says Copeland

Everybody being on the run in New York City, deaths from heart diseases are increasing, Dr. Royal S. Copeland, Health Commissioner, said yesterday in comparing deaths from this source last year with those of 1920.

"There can be no doubt that conditions under which people live in this city are conducive to heart disease," said the Commissioner. "They run up the subway stairs two steps at a time; they hurry from their homes and hurry back again; they stand on the transportation lines twice as often as they sit down, and even when in repose they are nervous. Meals are swallowed hastily, and even the evening's entertainment is taken on the rush.

"So far as its increase is concerned heart disease is about the worst disease we have in this city. In 1921 12,006 persons died of diseases of the heart. This was an increase of 664 over the preceding year.

"One factor in connection with heart disease is an increase in the prevalence of dental defects. Adult life begins to show the effects of neglecting the teeth. More and more attention is being paid to children's teeth and tonsils. So I doubt that another generation will show so many cases of heart disease."

January 15, 1922

FINDS CANCER A PERIL TO WOMEN SMOKERS

Dr. Hermann Prinz Tells Dental Session Tobacco Causes Mouth Diseases.

An indirect warning to women smokers was given yesterday by Dr. Hermann Prinz, Professor of Pathology at the University of Pennsylvania, who spoke at the convention of the Dental Society of the State of New York, in session at the Hotel Astor. Dr. Prinz said that with the increase of smoking among women there was grave danger of cancer such as women of the Orient, who are heavy smokers, experienced. He said that in the Orient the deaths from cancer among women were much greater than among men and an overwhelming majority of these deaths were traceable to mouth diseases caused by the use of tobacco.

According to statistics, Dr. Prinz says, 50 per cent. of the cancer cases in this country are due to buccalleucoplakia, which starts on the tongue, and is the most common mouth disease caused by tobacco. He stressed the importance of learning the cancer symptoms so that they might be readily dealt with.

The morning was devoted to clinics and during the afternoon there were lectures in both the north and east ballrooms. Emphasis was placed on the research work done at such places as the Eastman Dental Dispensary at Rochester and the Forsyth Dental Infirmary. An effort will be made to revive the clinics that were conducted in the public schools before the Hylan Administration.

The council appropriated $1,000 to help pay for a motion picture that the New York Tuberculosis and Health Association is preparing to use in propaganda work for clean mouths to prevent tuberculosis. A small amount was also given to the district societies in New York City to aid the work for better teeth among public school pupils.

Dr. Guy M. Fiero of Buffalo was elected President, and the other officers are Vice President, Dr. Gerald C. Burns of Rochester; Secretary, Dr. A. T. Burkhart of Auburn, and Treasurer, Dr. George H. Butler of Syracuse.

The convention ended with a dinner last night at the Astor, attended by 1,000 persons.

May 22, 1926

HOW DUSTY TRADES AFFECT THE HEALTH

Study Indicates That Cement Workers Suffer Abnormally From Respiratory Diseases.

The United States Public Health Service has completed a study of the health of workers in a Portland cement plant, the first of a series covering the dusty trades, according to an announcement recently made by Surgeon General H. S. Cumming. The study was undertaken to ascertain whether persons working in an atmosphere containing numerous minute particles of a calcium dust suffered any harmful effects. The investigation was conducted in one of the older, dustier plants, so that the effect of large quantities of the dust could be observed. Records of all absences from work were kept for three years, and the nature of disabling sickness was ascertained. Physical examinations were made, X-ray films taken, and the character and amounts of dust in the atmosphere of the plant were determined.

"The results of this investigation," says the Public Health Service in a recent bulletin, "indicated that the calcium dusts generated in the process of manufacturing Portland cement do not predispose workers to tuberculosis nor to pneumonia. The workers exposed to dust experienced, however, an abnormal number of attacks of diseases of the upper respiratory tract, especially colds, acute bronchitis, diseases of the pharynx and tonsils, and also influenza, or grippe. Attacks of these diseases serious enough to cause absence for two consecutive working days or longer occurred among the men in the dustier departments at a rate which was about 60 per cent. above that of the men in the comparatively non-dusty departments. Limestone dust appeared to be slightly more deleterious in this respect than cement dust.

"Outdoor work in all kinds of weather, such as was experienced by the quarry workers, appeared to predispose to diseases of the upper respiratory tract even more than did exposure to the calcium dusts. In the outdoor departments of the plant, also, the highest attack rates of rheumatism were found. The study also indicated that work in a cement dusty atmosphere may predispose to certain skin diseases, such as boils, to conjunctivitis, and to deafness when cement dust in combination with ear wax forms plugs in the external ear. When the dust in the atmosphere is less than about 10,000,000 particles per cubic foot of air it is doubtful that the above-mentioned diseases and conditions would be found at greater than average frequency.

"Modernization of plants and installation of ventilating systems are helping to solve the dust problem of the industry."

July 1, 1928

SMOKE REDUCTION URGED IN 2 CITIES

BALTIMORE, Feb. 23 (AP).—New evidence to support the belief that country life is more healthful than city life is offered in results of study of the sunlight cut off by the smoke pall over Baltimore.

The study, made by the United States Public Health Service, shows that smoke from the chimneys of factories, office buildings and homes may at times shut off as much as 50 per cent of the total light from the sun.

A comparison of the amount of sunlight reaching the earth on the roof of Baltimore Police Headquarters with that at a State sanitarium ten miles in the country, where there was little or no smoke, it was found that the city averaged about 14.1 per cent less sunlight than the country.

Moisture in the air helps to cut off sunlight, it was found, the average percentage loss of light increased as the humidity increased. Wind cuts down the loss of sunlight, the study showed, presumably by blowing away the smoke.

Ask Cooperation at Pittsburgh.
Special to The New York Times.

PITTSBURGH, Feb. 23. — The next logical development in the fight on atmospheric pollution must be the creation of air-hygiene districts which will control metropolitan smoke areas, H. B. Meller, head of the air pollution investigation of the Mellon Institute of Industrial Research, declared today in addressing an audience representing boroughs lying outside Pittsburgh.

Restoration of a state of purity the air of the Pittsburgh district, Mr. Meller stated, cannot be accomplished by the enforcement of a city of Pittsburgh ordinance alone. The corporate city is ringed and hemmed in by a score of factory clusters that are beyond its jurisdiction. The big city and the smaller boroughs exchange smoke. Each community pollutes every other community and regulation of any one cannot bring general relief.

February 24, 1933

LUNG CANCER RISE LAID TO CIGARETTES

Increase in Smoking Is Blamed by Ochsner at Session of Surgeons in Chicago

By WILLIAM L. LAURENCE

Special to THE NEW YORK TIMES.

CHICAGO, Oct. 25—An assertion that the increase in the smoking of cigarettes was a cause of the rise in recent years of cancer of the lung, which now ranks with cancer of the stomach as a dominant form of cancer in the United States, was made today at the closing sessions of the Annual Clinical Congress of the American College of Surgeons. The statement was made by Dr. Alton Ochsner, of New Orleans, at one of the group clinical conferences on the diagnosis and treatment of intra-thoracic tumors.

"My contention is that smoking cigarettes is a cause of cancer of the lung because we know that chronic irritation is a factor in the incidence of cancer and we know that smoking causes chronic irritation, as for example, the chronic bronchitis known as 'smokers' cough'," he said.

Since 1920, Dr. Ochsner stated, he had observed a steady progression in cancer of the lung in autopsies at Charity Hospital in New Orleans. In 1931 0.47 of 1 per cent of all the autopsies showed presence of the cancer of the lung. The incidence of cancer of the stomach during that period led all other forms of cancer.

In 1938, Dr. Ochsner declared, the most frequent site of cancer in all autopsies at the hospital was the lung. Lung cancer was found in 2 per cent of all these autopsies, whereas the stomach was found to be the site of cancer in 1.9 per cent of the cases.

Dr. Ochsner said that he and his associates made a study to determine whether a possible increase in the number of automobiles, with the consequent increase of exhaust fumes in the air, might not be a factor in explaining the increase in the incidence of lung cancer.

A check on the sale of automobiles during the period 1920-1936 showed, however, that while there was a rise in such sales up to 1929, the sales showed a distinct drop since the year of the stock market crash, whereas the incidence of lung cancer showed a steady increase since 1929.

The lung cancers, Dr. Ochsner reported, were most prevalent between the ages of 50 and 60, adding further support to the view that chronic irritation over a period of years plays a part in the causation of cancer of the organ irritated by the inhalation of smoke.

Professor Evarts A. Graham of St. Louis, president of the American College of Surgeons, reported at the conference that at his clinic at the Barnes Hospital of the Washington University Medical School the death rate of cancer of the lung cases operated on dropped to 27 per cent from 60 in such operated cases three to four years ago.

October 26, 1940

New Cancer Fight Strategy Stresses Environment Study

By ROBERT PLUMB

A change in strategy for medical scientists in command of the fight against cancer was indicated here yesterday when leading figures in the research field called for new studies on the puzzling relationships between a man's environment and the statistical chance that he will have a cancer.

The National Cancer Institute has begun such a project, it was revealed, and other agencies are cooperating in the work, which will include a study of the cancer hazards encountered by those working in modern industry.

Present indications are that cancer death rates vary from nation to nation, and between areas of a single nation, in a way that cannot be wholly attributed to the local availability of medical facilities to improve diagnosis, treatment of cancer and accuracy in naming the cause of death post-mortem.

Furthermore, the incidence of cancer found in a particular body site, such as cancer of the lung, stomach, skin or mouth, varies in a similarly inexplicable fashion, the authorities reported.

These considerations and the suggestion that medical workers might profitably venture on ecologic studies rather than concentrating entirely on the research for successful cancer therapy were made before scientific sessions of the annual meeting of the American Cancer Society at the Commodore Hotel.

Dr. Charles S. Cameron, medical and scientific director of the society, pointed out that cancer is a "disease of civilization," and where technology is advanced a higher cancer death rate is recorded because of greater organization.

But this factor alone is not enough to account for all observed differences between cancer rates in different areas, and Dr. Cameron said the genesis of a malignant tumor may be identified in habits, social customs, religious practices, occupation, infections, climate and geological influences.

These and a number of other "environmental factors" must be studied more thoroughly throughout the world, he said. In city life it "cannot be categorically denied" that pollution of the air by smoke, chemically treated water supplies and other "artificial" impediments of modern living may increase the incidence of cancer, he declared.

The rate of development of site-specific cancer in varying geological areas is more certainly known, Dr. Cameron said, but it presents an even more fruitful field for exploration.

To initiate comprehensive studies in these fields, Dr. John R. Heller Jr., director of the National Cancer Institute, announced that the institute was establishing an Environmental Cancer Research Laboratory at Georgetown University Medical School in Washington. He termed the new venture "the first of its kind in the world."

The laboratory is one step in a long-range program to study environment and cancer, Dr. Heller said, which began with the authorization of a special section of the institute on the problem and has been extended through the United States Public Health Service by a fund to help study occupational cancer in the field of industrial operations.

Grants have already been made to Ohio, New Jersey and New York, and other states have made requests, he added.

Warns on Industrial Practices

Dr. Heller declared that developments of modern industry have introduced known carcinogenic agents into greater use—though the extent of the danger is not yet known. He listed as examples arsenicals and coal tar products, such metallic compounds as chromates and nickel carbonyl and such chemicals as benzol, soot, tar, paraffin oil, creosote and various dye intermediaries.

"As far as we know, the most dangerous areas are in the field of radioactive substances, the areas of hydrocarbon research and development such as the high-temperature distillation and fractionation of petroleum, and the wide field of organic chemistry which is developing so many new synthetic chemicals," Dr. Heller declared.

Industry is becoming increasingly aware of the danger involved in using agents known to cause predisposition to cancer, Dr. Heller said, and he urged the adoption of the following precautionary measures until more definite facts are accumulated:

The unnecessary use of known carcinogenic agents should be avoided when possible in industrial, civilian or military life and in any case steps should be taken to guard against prolonged exposure.

Safety procedures in all plants should prevent the escape of carcinogenic wastes into the air, water or soil of surrounding communities and workers should be insulated from the manufacturing process.

Periodic and extensive medical supervision of all exposed workers should be provided. The examinations should continue at regular intervals even after the worker is no longer in contact with the carcinogenic agent.

Dr. Heller predicted that the opening of the comparatively new field of environmental cancer "may prove to be the opening of a new era 'in the history of man's efforts to curb one of humanity's worst scourges."

Dr. Daniel A. Blain, medical director of the American Psychiatric Association, urged cancer authorities to shift their emphasis from "scaring" the public to getting an awareness of cancer problems by an approach based on reasonable appeal.

As an undesirable approach, he presented the following:

"Every three minutes someone in the United States dies of cancer. No one is safe. There is one chance in eight that you yourself will be a victim of this deadly killer. Cancer is the greatest and cruelest killer of American women between the ages of 35 and 55. Guard those you love. Give — to conquer cancer."

Instead of this "big club" attitude, public health leaders should concentrate on the advantages of early diagnosis and preventive examinations in the large number of "cured cancer" cases, he said.

Dr. Blain observed that the word "cancer" in the name American Cancer Society conveys unfortunate connotations to the laity and that the emblem of the society, two serpents entwined about a sword, obviously represents a "dangerous weapon" to many minds in spite of the fact that it is derived from the staff of Mercury, the symbol of medicine for many years.

Chairmen for the scientific session were Drs. Frank E. Adair and Cornelius P. Rhoads of Memorial Hospital. Some recent advances in the treatment of cancer were presented in six technical discussions.

November 7, 1948

Tobacco Industry, Upset by Link To Cancer, Starts Own Research

A group of fourteen major tobacco distributors, growers and producers announced yesterday the formation of a Tobacco Industry Research Committee to study all phases of tobacco use.

Assertions have been made in recent months that there is a relation between cigarette smoking and the incidence of lung cancer. The companies took display advertisements today in newspapers over the country to dispute what the advertisements said were recent reports on experiments with mice that linked cigarette smoking with lung cancer in human beings.

The advertisements were headed, "A Frank Statement to Cigarette Smokers."

Of concern also to the industry, but not mentioned in the advertisements, are surveys that show a drop in domestic sales of cigarettes in 1953. The decline is accounted for chiefly by regular-size cigarettes; king-size and filter-tips made large gains.

In charge of the research activities, the announcement said, will be "a scientist of unimpeachable integrity and national repute." In addition, there will be an advisory board of scientists "disinterested in the cigarette industry," made up of "distinguished men from medicine, science and education."

The joint research venture on an industry-wide level was seen as a novel approach to the health problem that has plagued the tobacco industry through the years. It was undertaken, observers felt, in the face of, and perhaps because of, the heavy stress laid recently in radio and television advertising on reducing the supposed deleterious effects of cigarette smoking by the use of king-size and filter-tip brands.

Producers were enjoined from acting in concert by the Federal decree of 1911 that broke up the tobacco trust. However, an industry spokesman said last Thursday that the companies were confident that any action then contemplated "is not in any way in conflict with anti-trust laws or any court decrees now in effect." The contemplated action presumably was the creation of the industry-wide research committee.

In an effort to allay public fears, the committee said that although recent experiments apparently establishing a link with lung cancer had been conducted by doctors of professional standing, "these experiments are not regarded as conclusive in the field of cancer research."

Lack of an Agreement

Authorities have pointed out, the committee said, that there was no agreement concerning the cause of lung cancer, that there was no proof that cigarette smoking was one of the causes, and that the statistics, themselves under question, could apply with equal force to any of many other aspects of modern life.

The industry said its interest in the public health was paramount, and expressed the belief that "the products we make are not injurious to health."

The fact-finding and research committee is supported by the following companies and organizations:

American Tobacco Company, Inc.—Paul M. Hahn, president.
Benson & Hedges—Joseph F. Cullman Jr., president.
Bright Belt Warehouse Association—F. S. Royster, president.
Brown & Williamson Tobacco Corporation—Timothy V. Hartnett, president.
Burley Auction Warehouse Association—Albert Clay, president.
Burley Tobacco Growers Cooperative Association—John W. Jones, president.
Larus & Brother Company—W. T. Reed Jr., president.
P. Lorillard Company—Herbert A. Kent, chairman.
Maryland Tobacco Growers Association—Samuel C. Linton, general manager.
Philip Morris & Co. Ltd., Inc.—O. Parker McComas, president.
R. J. Reynolds Tobacco Company—E. A. Darr, president.
Stephano Brothers, Inc.—C. S. Stephano, Director of Research.
Tobacco Associates, Inc. (an organization of flue-cured tobacco growers)—J. B. Hutson, president.
United States Tobacco Company—J. W. Peterson, president.

January 4, 1954

FAT DIETS LINKED TO HEART DISEASE

Special to The New York Times.

WASHINGTON, Sept. 13 — A world survey of recently discovered facts on coronary thrombosis today showed heart disease to be most common where there was most fat in the diet.

This summary, which included the United States, Italy, Northern Europe, Japan, South Africa and Iraq, was presented here at the Second World Congress on Cardiology.

The heart specialists agreed that a high fat-content diet was more dangerous to men than women. One physician found among 100 unselected cases in a hospital in this country that men predominated in this category in the ratio of 96:4.

In another count, he said, the male preponderance, in 100 cases, was 97:3.

From a world viewpoint, it was brought out, underprivileged countries seem to be the favored ones in the matter of high-fat diets causing heart trouble.

Coronary thrombosis was accorded top importance by Dr. J. N. Morris of London, who called it "the epitome of health problems of this century." The British doctor called it a scourge of Western civilization, linking the condition with arterio-sclerosis, and fatty degeneration of the arteries. The United States has the highest death rate from these causes, he pointed out.

"If high living standards cause this failure of the social system we can expect more in future, and not less," Dr. Morris declared. "We cannot look to society to turn the clock back. A way out of the dilemma of Western civilization must be found."

We may discover a specific agent to treat it with or we can change ways of living. The latter seems more hopeful."

In another presentation, dieting down was decried by Dr. Ancel Keys of Minneapolis. He pointed out that heavyweights were as common in the low fat-diet nations as among the high.

Dr. Paul D. White of Boston declared that the studies, to date, covered only hundreds of cases whereas thousands were needed for study.

A hospital study in Southern Italy, where fat diets are a relative rarity, showed only 2 per cent of coronary cases, against 20 per cent in Massachusetts Hospital, Drs. Keys and White reported.

An analysis of the findings in 10,000 autopsies in Japan showed an incidence of severe coronary disease of only about one-tenth of that in this country, according to Dr. Moboru Kimura of Fukoka, Japan.

Studies also indicated that American service men stationed in Japan had far more heart disease than the native population. Dr. Kimura also said that the incidence of coronary heart disease was 20 to 50 per cent higher among men who used alcohol and tobacco.

Dr. Gunnar Biorck of Malmö, Sweden, said that degenerative heart disease decreased markedly in Scandanavia during the war, rising again when more luxurious living resumed.

Hope for heart patients to be able to hold jobs, except for heavy labor, was advanced at another session. The heart experts were told that almost all physical activities were within the capacity of most people with heart disease.

September 14, 1954

CANCER OF LUNGS CALLED 'EPIDEMIC'

By MURRAY ILLSON
Special to The New York Times.

SAN FRANCISCO, June 2— Lung cancer was declared here today to have become an epidemic disease that still had not reached a peak.

The assertion was by Dr. Lester Breslow, chief of the Bureau of Chronic Diseases, California Department of Public Health. He emphasized that he used the term "epidemic" because of the mounting incidence of lung cancer and not necessarily to imply contagion.

Speaking at the eighty-second annual forum of the National Conference of Social Work, he said that lung cancer was causing more than 22,000 deaths a year in the country and that its frequency had more than quadrupled in twenty-five years.

He added that it was causing more deaths than tuberculosis.

"If this disease had increased in a period of twenty-five weeks instead of twenty-five years," he observed, "consider the excitement that would have occurred. The fact that an epidemic of cancer stretches out over years rather than weeks tends to dull our sensitivity to it."

Increase Declared 'Real'

Dr. Breslow contended that the increase in the disease could not be explained by citing that people were living longer and hence were more likely to develop it or that physicians were better able now to diagnose it, thus increasing its incidence statistically.

The increase is "real and substantial," he asserted.

The available evidence indicates, he said, that lung cancer is "a disease of the environment," that it "must be a reflection of changes" in man's living conditions. Studies in the United States, England and Denmark all indicate, he added, that lung cancer is much more prevalent in urban communities than in rural areas.

He declared that the evidence "incriminates" various occupations. He listed various mining operations, smelting, welding, asbestos work, painting, metal fabrication and restaurant cooking and said that the disease had increased two-and-a-half times more rapidly among men than among women.

As for cigarette smoking as a possible factor in the increase of the disease, he held that it "does not explain all lung cancer."

Dr. Morton L. Levin, assistant commissioner for medical services of the New York State Department of Health, reviewed the evidence on smoking. He said that "some cases of lung cancer occurred in persons who had never smoked."

'Known' Evidence on Smoking

He added that, from what was known, "we can only point to the fact that cigarette smoking is one of the factors which influences the occurrence of lung cancer, that it most probably is not the only factor, and that each person must decide for himself whether the indicated risk is worth taking or not."

Miss Jane Hoey, director of the United States Bureau of Public Assistance in the Administrations of Presidents Franklin D. Roosevelt and Harry S. Truman, was the first recipient tonight of the $1,000 Florina Lasker Social Work Award.

Miss Hoey is now research consultant to the National Tuberculosis Association in New York.

June 3, 1955

BRONCHIAL CHANGES STUDIED IN SMOKERS

Special to The New York Times.

ATLANTIC CITY, June 2—A report by a group of pathologists suggesting the possible discovery of changes in the bronchial tree that might be associated with smoking was presented here tonight.

The report was made at a symposium arranged by the American College of Chest Physicians. It considered recent suggestions that there might be a link between smoking and lung cancer. Medical authorities representing both sides of this question appeared at the meeting.

The pathologists' report was made by Dr. Oscar Auerbach of the Veterans Administration Hospital in East Orange, N. J. Associated with him in the study were five other pathologists.

Dr. Auerbach said they had examined the air tubes leading into the lungs of forty-one patients who died in the veterans' hospital. He said thickening of the basal cell layers was believed to be present in heavy smokers, according to microscopic studies.

He cautioned that forty-one cases were very few, that there was no proper "control" for the study," and that the connection between the thickening observed and the onset of cancer was not established.

Dr. Alton Ochsner, New Orleans surgeon, told the symposium there was a "casual relation" between smoking and lung cancer.

Dr. John J. Phair, Professor of Preventive Medicine in the University of Cincinnati, suggested that air pollution in cities might play a part in the rise of lung cancer.

June 3, 1955

2 New Reports Tie Cancer to Smoking

By ROBERT K. PLUMB

Special to The New York Times.

ATLANTIC CITY, June 6— A majority of cancer researchers, chest surgeons and pathologists believe that heavy cigarette smoking may lead to lung cancer, the American Cancer Society reported here today.

At the opening of the 104th annual meeting of the American Medical Association, the society reported also that its study of 188,000 aging men for thirty-two months suggested that those who stopped smoking cigarettes had a much lower lung-cancer death rate than those who continued to smoke.

Both reports were denounced by Timothy V. Harnett, chairman of the Tobacco Industry Research Committee. He called the poll of doctors "biased, nonscientific and filled with shortcomings." He called the report on the lung cancer study "sweeping generalizations based on a survey that has been criticized by scientists for its limitations and inadequacies."

At the same session Lewis L. Strauss, chairman of the Atomic Energy Commission, said it was "irresponsible" to suggest that our atmosphere was being poisoned by radiation from atomic tests. No one knows the long-range effects by radiation, he emphasized.

Report by Doctors

Dr. E. Cuyler Hammond and Dr. Daniel Horn of the Cancer Society's statistical department reviewed the study of smoking habits and aging men.

To last Nov. 1, they said, 8,105 of the men died. Death certificates were obtained for 7,982 and 285 lung cancers were reported. Of these, 168 were proved by tissue study to have been cancers originating in the breathing tubes of the lungs.

In ninety-three other deaths owing to lung cancer, proof of the cancer depended upon X-ray studies or other less certain diagnostic methods. Twenty-four other cancers were found in the glandular part of the lung.

Men who had a history of cigarette smoking had seven times the reported lung-cancer death rate of men who never smoked. In proved cases of cancer originating in the breathing tubes, the ratio was twenty-nine to one.

The report concerned mainly bronchogenic cancer, which originates in the bronchial "tree," the network of airways that feeds air from the throat into the three lobes of the right lung and the two lobes of the left. This is the most common form of "lung" cancer. Its incidence has been doubling in the United States with each passing decade.

The death rate from lung cancer among two-pack-a-day smokers, Dr. Hammond and Dr. Horn reported, was ninety times as high as it was for nonsmokers. Indeed, they said, only two lung cancers were found among nonsmokers.

The rate for ex-smokers is fourteen times as high as for nonsmokers, the doctors declared. This and other aspects of the report, they said, establishes that those who stop smoking have lower lung cancer rates than those who continue.

Other Observations

Dr. Hammond and Dr. Horn also reported that:

¶So far, after thirty-two months, the study still indicates that there is a connection between cigarette smoking and lung cancer.

¶Those who smoke two or more packs of cigarettes a day have a lung-cancer death rate three times as high as the one-pack-a-day smokers.

¶Cancer of the lung is the second most common cause of death among those who smoke two or more packs a day. Heart disease is the leading cause of death in this group.

¶The lung-cancer death rate increases with the amount of cigarette smoking. The effect is apparent even among those who smoke less than ten cigarettes daily.

¶Lung-cancer death rates are high among cigarette smokers and "very low" among nonsmokers, regardless of whether they live in rural or urban areas.

¶There is no significant association between cigar smoking and lung cancer.

¶Pipe smoking appears to be associated with lung cancer but to a far less degree than cigarette smoking.

Dr. Charles S. Cameron, medical and scientific director of the society, reported that a questionnaire about smoking and cancer had been sent to the members of the American Association for Cancer Research, the American Board of Thoracic Surgery and the American Board of Pathology. About three-fourths responded.

Opinions Registered

In response to the statement, "heavy smoking of cigarettes may lead to lung cancer," 63 per cent of the chest surgeons, 50 per cent of the pathologists and 54 per cent of the cancer researchers answered "yes." Only 7 per cent of the pathologists and researchers answered "no." Thirty per cent of the surgeons, 47 per cent of the pathologists and 43 per cent of the researchers were uncertain.

To the statement that "heavy smoking of cigarettes may have serious effects on body physiology," 89 per cent of the surgeons, 27 per cent of the pathologists and 78 per cent of the cancer researchers agreed. Only 2 per cent disagreed.

Opinion was split as to whether heavy smokers should be advised to reduce smoking or give it up. Few urged the adoption of filter tipped cigarettes. Few advised a switch to pipes or cigars and few recommended that heavy smokers continue smoking as usual.

Dr. Cameron commented that "the present evidence places enormous responsibility on the practicing physician to examine the facts, form an opinion and act in his traditional role as custodian of his patient's health."

Commissioner Strauss emphasized that in the event of war with high-yield nuclear weapons —as opposed to limited controlled testing—the radiation danger to civilian populations would be very great.

June 7, 1955

REPORT IS ATTACKED

Head of Tobacco Industry Unit Holds Study Is Biased

The reports linking cancer to smoking came under heavy fire from the tobacco industry.

Timothy V. Hartnett, chairman of the Tobacco Industry Research Committee, said that "competent opinion-research authorities" considered that the poll of cancer researchers, chest surgeons and pathologists was "biased, nonscientific and filled with shortcomings and defects."

In the poll the doctors were asked whether they agreed with the statement: "There is probably a causal relationship between heavy cigarette smoking and lung cancer."

Commenting on the statement, Mr. Hartnett said:

"The widely known opinion experts, Elmo Roper and Associates, comment that this statement is so phrased that the only way a person could answer 'no' is to be absolutely certain there is no connection between smoking and lung cancer."

In regard to the report on the lung cancer study, he asserted:

"The American public should not be misled by sweeping generalizations based on a survey that has been criticized by scientists for its limitations and inadequacies."

Among the criticisms made by scientists, he said, were these:

"A mere numerical association does not establish any cause-and-effect relationship.

"The survey is limited to smoking habits and therefore does not rule out any number of possible other factors in present-day living that may influence death rates.

"The survey is shown to be non-representative of the national population.

"The small number of deaths from lung cancer—at most, 285 out of 8,105 deaths—makes questionable any conclusions drawn, especially since the sampling methods of the survey are not statistically sound."

Mr. Hartnett also distributed a statement on the study by Dr. Herbert Arkin, head of the business statistics division of City College.

Dr. Arkin said that "from a statistical viewpoint" he considered the study's conclusions "to be of a very dubious character."

June 7, 1955

CANCER IS TRACED TO FOOD ADDITIVES

By ARNALDO CORTESI
Special to The New York Times.

ROME, Aug. 20—A number of food additives used in the United States and Europe as dyes, thickeners, sweeteners preservatives and the like were labeled cancer-producing today by a symposium of the International Union Against Cancer.

Other food additives were put on a suspect list as unsafe until their properties had been more thoroughly tested.

The cancer experts meeting in Rome acknowledged that this created a "serious public health problem." They unanimously recognized the "urgent necessity of international collaboration for the protection of mankind" against such hazards as cancer-producing food additives.

The participants in the symposium also acknowledged that food additives were only one part of the vast problem of environmental cancer, which includes occupational and lung cancers.

The symposium was attended by forty-two cancer experts from twenty-one countries, including seven Americans and four Russians. It was called by the congress of the International Union Against Cancer held in São Paulo, Brazil, in 1954.

Report Subject to Review

The joint report unanimously adopted by the symposium is subject to review by the Executive Committee of the International Union Against Cancer. It is, therefore, possible that some of its conclusions may be modified.

The report laid down the basic principle that no food additives should be used unless specifically permitted by legislation based on lists of substances that have been proved innocuous after stringent laboratory tests.

It went on to give the first lists of food preservatives and dyes that were found either acceptable, dubious or definitely dangerous. Dubious preservatives requiring urgent retesting included ethyl and butyl esters, thiodiprionic acid, sulphureous acid and its derivatives and formic acid.

The dangerous preservatives condemned as "carcinogenous and to be avoided for human use" included thiourea, tioacetamide, 8-hydroxyquinoline and hydroquinone. Most and perhaps all of these are used in the United States and Europe.

The report said certain mineral oils and paraffines used for coating milk containers had produced cancer in man and experimental animals. It issued a warning against foodstuffs sterilized by radiation as potential cancer hazards and against the use of estrogens as fattening agents for poultry and meat animals.

It said that several detergents had "co-carcinogenous and prompting effects" and that their use for cleaning food containers therefore required caution.

Food Dyes Condemned

Food dyes came in for particularly severe condemnation from the symposium. Its report stated that no food dye at present met "agreed criteria of safety." Twenty-nine dyes were listed as "unsuitable" or "potentially dangerous" with the statement that they should on no account "be added to food or drink for men or animals."

Another list contained twenty-three dyes that might prove satisfactory after further tests.

The fundamental paper that formed the basis of the symposium's recommendations was read by Dr. Wilhelm C. Heuper, German-born member of the United States delegation. He is chief of the Environmental Cancer Section of the National Cancer Institute and is co-chairman of the symposium.

Dr. Heuper listed twenty groups of suspect food additives and seventeen groups of suspect food contaminants. Many of these agents, he said, have not been adequately investigated for carcinogenic qualities. The food additives included dyes, thickeners, synthetic sweeteners and flavors, preservatives, shortening, bleaches, oils and fat substitutes. The food contaminants included antibiotics and estrogen for fattening animals, pesticide residues, soot, chemical sterilizers, antisprouting agents, wrapping materials, radiation.

At the end of their labors the symposium and Executive Committee of International Union Against Cancer were received in audience by the Pope at his summer residence of Castel Gandolfo. He delivered a brief address and imparted an apostolic blessing to them and their work.

Ban on Three Dyes Upheld

More than two years ago, in the United States, the Federal Food and Drug Administration prohibited the use of three coal tar dyes on the ground that they were potentially harmful. Ten days ago the United States Court of Appeals upheld the ban on Orange No. 1, Orange No. 2 and Red No. 32.

August 21, 1956

MALE 'RAT RACE' DECRIED

'Suicidal Cult of Manliness' Is Blamed for Early Deaths

CHICAGO, Jan. 17 (UP)—The medical director of a large industrial concern blamed the "suicidal cult of manliness" for the "rat race" in which many American men find themselves today.

Dr. Lemuel C. McGee, Wilmington, Del., of the Hercules Powder Company, writing in the American Medical Association publication, Today's Health, said the average lifetime of men was about four years less than that of women, mainly because of the stress under which men live.

A "little common sense" could eliminate many of the tensions and stresses, providing a healthier and longer life, Dr. McGee said.

"The American male has been indoctrinated, with the philosophy that he must live, work and play at a dizzy pace; that he can and should wade through all emotional and physical situations without flinching and without reflection," he explained.

Dr. McGee said every man and boy must live within his own resources of physical and mental strength, but many fail to do so because of the "cult of manliness."

January 18, 1957

U. S. LINKS CANCER WITH CIGARETTES

By BESS FURMAN
Special to The New York Times.

WASHINGTON, July 12—The Public Health Service took the official position today that there was "increasing and consistent evidence" that "excessive cigarette smoking is one of the causative factors of lung cancer."

This changed an offical pronouncement in 1954 that cited some evidence of statistical association between the two, but left open the question of cause-and-effect relationship.

Leroy E. Burney, the Surgeon General, simultaneously began a nation-wide informational campaign on the subject. He sent to the public health officers of all states and to the American Medical Association copies of his announcement and of two recent scientific reports in the United States that showed "extremely high" association between heavy smoking and lung cancer.

Statement Is Challenged

The Surgeon General's statement was challenged immediately by Dr. Clarence Cook Little, chairman of the Scientific Advisory Board to the Tobacco Industry Research Committee. He said that three years of research by his group "has produced no evidence that cigarette smoking or other tobacco use contributes to the origin of lung cancer."

The action of Surgeon General Burney followed a similar move taken recently by the Ministry of Health in Britain. The British Medical Council reported a high statistical link between smoking and lung cancer on the basis of nineteen studies in seven countries.

The British Government brought these views to the attention of local authorities responsible for health education.

Dr. Burney asked the state health officers and the American Medical Association to consider distributing copies of the United States reports to local health officers, medical societies and other health groups.

Recent Studies Cited

The scientific studies cited in Dr. Burney's statement are:

¶A report of the Study Group on Smoking and Health, made public March 23, which evaluated eighteen independent studies. It found a high degree of statistical association between lung cancer and heavy and prolonged smoking. The Public Health Service was one of the sponsoring agencies of this study.

¶A report by Dr. E. C. Hammond and Dr. Daniel Horn of the American Cancer Society to the American Medical Association, published June 5. This report found "extremely high" associations between smoking and lung-cancer deaths and between smoking and deaths from cancer of the larynx and esophagus and from gastric ulcers. It also raised the question of a link with heart disease.

In his statement today Dr. Burney recommended further research:

¶To identify, isolate, and try to eliminate the factors in excessive cigarette smoking that can cause cancer.

¶To ascertain the role of air pollution and other factors that also may be the cause of lung cancer in man.

¶To determine the meaning and significance of any statistical association between smoking and heart disease.

This research would form a basis for a possible future "cause-and-effect" pronouncement by the Public Health Service.

Dr. Burney stated that while the evidence suggesting cigarette smoking as a cause of cancer was largely epidemiological, some laboratory studies on animals had provided contributory information.

Five Studies Cited

At least five independent studies, he said, have produced malignancies by tobacco-smoke concentrates. It also has been reported that biological changes similar to those that take place in the genesis of cancer had been observed in the lungs of heavy smokers.

Dr. Little said that the Surgeon General's statement had added nothing new to cancer knowledge, and had reflected views of "the relatively few experimental scientists who have actively charged that cigarette smoking is the cause of lung cancer."

"Many experiments on inhalation of cigarette smoke in animals have failed to produce a single cancer similar to the most prevalent type of lung cancer in humans," he declared.

Officials at the National Cancer Institute said that since 1930 the death rate for lung cancer had increased between five and six times for males and between two and three times for females -- a more rapid increase than for deaths for cancer in any other part of the body. These figures were adjusted for increasing population.

Lung-cancer deaths total about 25,000 a year, or about one-tenth of the total cancer death rate. There are about 1,600,000 deaths a year from all causes in this country.

Contradictory Findings Cited

Timothy V. Hartnett, chairman of the Tobacco Industry Research Committee, charged yesterday that the Surgeon General's report "failed to acknowledge" that "many doctors and scientists have publicly expressed their doubts or disbelief in the theory that smoking causes lung cancer."

In a statement issued shortly after the release of the Public Health Service's pronouncement, Dr. Hartnett cited five independent research projects that tended to refute the theory.

He quoted Dr. Joseph Berkson, head of the section of biometry and medical statistics of the Mayo Clinic, as saying:

"It is my personal opinion, and I know as much about it as anyone else, that smoking does not cause cancer of the lung."

Dr. Berkson published a paper on July 27, 1955, questioning the validity of the American Cancer Society's view.

Dr. Hartnett also cited the recently published book, "Science Looks at Smoking," by Dr. Harry S. N. Greene, chairman of the Department of Pathology at the Yale University School of Medicine. Dr. Greene said his experiments with tobacco tar and embryonic human tissue had established no causal relationship between smoking and lung cancer.

Texan's Work Noted

Another work mentioned was an article by Dr. R. H. Rigdon, director of the Laboratory of Experimental Pathology at the University of Texas Medical Branch. Dr. Rigdon wrote:

"A demonstration of carcinogen [a cancer-producing agent] in cigarette tars for the skin of a mouse and a rabbit cannot be accepted scientifically as a carcinogen for the lung of man."

Drs. Milton Rosenblatt and James Lisa, in their book "Cancer of the Lung," published in 1956, were quoted by Dr. Hartnett as saying that the relationship between the increased incidence of lung cancer and the rise in cigarette consumption "is purely speculative." They contended that "the death rate from lung cancer has increased at a far greater pace than has the consumption of tobacco."

Finally, Dr. Hartnett cited a study conducted in 1954 by Edward A. Lew, actuary and statistician for the Metropolitan Life Insurance Company. Mr. Lew wrote that approximately half of the increase in respiratory cancer deaths from 1930 to 1953 "reflects merely the growth and aging of the population, and a considerable part of the remainder represents improved diagnosis and more complete case finding. * * * Data are not available to show how much of it can reasonably be attributed to the effect of specific factors."

July 13, 1957

POULTRY TREATED BY DRUG BARRED

U.S. Says Hormone Induced Cancer in Experiments

By BESS FURMAN
Special to The New York Times.

WASHINGTON, Dec. 10 — The Government announced agreement today with the drug and poultry industries to halt the production and sale of chickens treated with a cancer-inducing hormone.

Arthur S. Flemming, Secretary of Health, Education and Welfare, disclosed that the drug, a synthetic sex hormone called stilbestrol, had been found to induce cancer in test animals when included in their diets over a long period.

Secretary Flemming said recent studies had revealed stilbestrol residues in the skins, livers and kidneys of chickens treated with it. The drug is used on poultry farms to fatten chickens.

Accordingly, he said, voluntary agreements have been reached to stop the use of the drug in chickens.

He said the drug houses making stilbestrol had agreed to quit selling it for use in poultry.

Poultry raisers and retailers have agreed to stop selling the treated birds. The chickens, which have been sold principally in New York and Los Angeles, constitute about 1 per cent of the poultry market.

The Department of Agriculture has agreed to buy all treated birds now ready for market with funds set aside for the purchase of agricultural surpluses.

Stilbestrol, implanted in chickens at the base of the neck and fed to beef cattle or implanted in the ears, has been used for a decade in "finishing" meat. Its effect is to distribute fat evenly and to improve color and texture.

But even with a detection method so sensitive that it reveals traces of the chemical as small as two parts a billion, Secretary Flemming said, no traces of stilbestrol have been found in beef, mutton or lamb. Therefore no action was taken on these meats.

Food and Drug officials said a housewife with several chickens in her refrigerator or freezer could feel safe if she discarded the skin, liver and kidneys.

Last month, Secretary Flemming alerted the country against some cranberries found contaminated with a weed killer suspected of producing cancer. Unlike that situation, he said, no law was violated in the treatment of chickens with the cancer-inducing drug.

After almost two years of study, during which no traces of stilbestrol residue were found in the edible tissue of chickens treated with it, the Food and Drug Administration authorized its use on Jan. 30, 1947. It must now prove its harmfulness before it can take seizure actions.

"We are moving to revoke the licenses," Secretary Flemming said. "Meanwhile we appreciate the willingness of the organizations and firms concerned to take voluntary action."

He listed sixteen organizations and concerns taking part in the recent discussions here, and eight others that consulted by telephone.

The Secretary renewed his vigorous endorsement of the cancer clause in the Food Additives Act. However, he said that the stilbestrol investigation had brought out inequities under it that might cause him to ask some changes in the next Congress.

The additives act now makes mandatory the ruling out of new applications involving any additive "if it is found to induce cancer when ingested by man or animal." But if such a chemical already is in food, the Department of Health, Education and Welfare must prove it unsafe.

Secretary Flemming today protested this clause as "just not good sense" in the health field and said he would ask Congress to change it. He also questioned the mandate that he must rule out new applications for using stilbestrol for cattle when no residue showed up in the meat. He said he might ask Congress to modify this aspect of the cancer clause, which he will also recommend for the pending Color Additives Law. By far the greatest use of stilbestrol is in beef cattles.

Warning on Deadline

In a separate statement the Secretary warned all food manufacturers that March 6 was the deadline on which they must either have cleared their food additives as safe or have secured an extension of time for so doing. He said he would issue no extensions for additives found to have induced cancer when ingested by man or animal.

He also made public a letter written to him by True D. Morse, Acting Secretary of Agriculture, announcing that the department would purchase the treated poultry and would divert it to other uses.

Asked about the uses, the Secretary said he did not know what they were, but he noted that the birds could be made safe by the removal of skins, livers and kidneys.

Jersey Stands By

TRENTON, Dec. 10 (UPI) State officials, recovering from a pre-Thanksgiving cranberry scare, said today that they would operate on a "stand-by basis" on a Federal plan to halt the sale of chickens treated with stilbestrol.

Francis A. Timko, chief sanitarian of the State Health Department, said "these chickens are being sold in New Jersey, but the Federal Government has announced its intent to take care of the sale so we will stand by unless emergency action is necessary.

"I hope this announcement about the chickens doesn't scare people," he said, "because not enough of the chemical is used to harm people."

December 11, 1959

Flemming Scores A.M.A. Article Critical of Crackdown on Drugs

By BESS FURMAN
Special to The New York Times.

WASHINGTON, Jan. 7—The Secretary of Health, Education and Welfare challenged today the truth of an editorial critical of his department in the current issue of The Journal of the American Medical Association.

Secretary Arthur S. Flemming said he hoped The Journal would give the department the opportunity of "presenting the facts as we see them to its readers."

The editorial, written by Dr. John H. Talbott, editor of The Journal, raised questions concerning recent crackdowns by the Food and Drug Administration on the weed killer aminotriazole in cranberries and the drug stilbesterol in chickens. Both drugs were found to have produced cancer in laboratory animals. The editorial also touched on the failure of carbon black used in black jelly beans to make the first "safe" list under the Food Additive Act.

Dr. Talbott ended with the hope that next fall "cranberries will be permitted for festive dinners, that licorice and

jelly beans will be for sale at the candy counter, and that Southern fried chicken will be a permissible menu item."

"On a subject as important as this, feel it is very unfortunate that a reputable professional journal should provide its readers with information that if factually inaccurate," Secretary Flemming said.

He went on:

"Because this is a matter that has a direct bearing on the future health of the American people, I feel it should not be treated lig htly. If a substance induces cancer when included in the diet of test animals, no one knows how much or how little of that substance will induce cancer if included in the human diet.

"Therefore, even though there may be some conflict of opinion on the part of scientists as to a substance causing cancer, the consumer should not be asked to serve as a guinea pig while the conflict is being resolved.."

Secretary Flemming's comment followed an exchange of telegrams.

John L. Harvey, acting commissioner of Food and Drugs, made public today the telegram he had sent to Dr. Talbott and the reply he had received.

Dr. Talbott said in his editorial that "Little stress was placed [by Secretary Flemming and the F. D. A.] on the well-documented evidence that aminotriazole occurs naturally in vegetables, notably cabbage, turnips, broccoli, as well as in mustard, or that anti-thyroid action is described in current text books of therapy."

Mr. Harvey asked Dr. Talbott to wire collect references to substantiate this statement. He told newsmen that his experts had searched in vain for such evidence. He read aloud the telegram ne received from Dr. Talbott in reply:

"Information based upon statements by Dr. Edwin Astwood, Professor of Medicine, Tufts Medical School, Boston, and Dr. H. H. Golz, American Cyanamid Company, and general references in text books to anti-thyroid drugs."

Reached by phone, Dr. Astwood said he had told reporters in Boston that cabbage, turnips, broccoli and mustard contained an anti-thyroid compound that acted like aminotriazole. He said that he had been misquoted in one Boston newspaper as saying that these vegetables contained aminotriazole.

Dr. Astwood reiterated today the testimony he had given at cranberry conferences here—that he did not consider aminotriazole a producer of cancer even in animals.

Mr. Harvey said that since there was no substantiation of aminotriazole in vegetables in the natural state, and no reference to it to be found in medical text books, he would discount the editorial as a whole.

Dr. Talbott conceded yesterday that the information linking aminotriazole to cabbage and other vegetables offered "the opportunity" for a different interpretation. He said, however, that the point "doesn't make a particle of difference" to his editorial argument.

Though the chemical found naturally in vegetables was not aminotriazole, he said, it was a closely related compound with virtually the same biological effects. If the term aminotriazole-like substance had been used, he said, the editorial would have been factually correct.

Dr. Talbott said he would be very happy to give the Department of Health, Education and Welfare a chance to express its views in The Journal of the American Medical Association.

January 8, 1960

Food-Additive Curb Is in Effect; Doubts Over Its Meaning Linger

Industries Back Tighter Law on Use of Chemicals, but Question Its Scope

By JOHN A. OSMUNDSEN

One of the most misunderstood laws on the Federal ledgers goes into full force—or almost—today.

It is the chemical additives amendment to the Federal Food, Drug and Cosmetic Act. Partly in effect for just a year, this law already has thousands of persons throughout the land more than mildly agitated over its consequences, real and imagined.

George P. Larrick, commissioner of the Food and Drug Administration, recently called attention to predictions "that the new law will wreck the food business generally, or the packaging business, or the food equipment business."

"We haven't seen any evidence that this is the case," he said.

But he did say that strong

support by industry, Government and consumers would be required for the new law to get under way smoothly.

The amendment is the first food-law provision specifically to cover such things as flavors, nutrients, preservatives and emulsifiers that are put into foods for various specific purposes. It also covers the traces of container linings, food-processing machinery and inks on food packages that might get into foods unintentionally.

Both the Government and the affected industries have long agreed that such a law was needed. They also concur that the law, as it came to be written over a period of eight years, is basically sound.

Some have even called it one of the most comprehensive insurance policies ever taken out on the nation's health. And yet:

¶Many of the industries affected by the law do not understand it, and some of those that think they do predict it will severely curtail research and development in the field of food technology.

¶The general public, confused by the cranberry, caponette and black jellybean episodes and by misleading information from various sources, is understandably uncertain over just what the so-called "chemicals-in-foods-problem" is all about.

¶The Government agency that is charged with administering and enforcing the new law assumes its enforcement duties at a time when it is almost hopelessly swamped in the early stages of the administrative phase.

Much of the confusion and controversy comes from the uncertainty over which of the more than 1,000 chemicals now used in foods come under the jurisdiction of the new law; who is to assume responsibility for satisfying the Government's demands, and precisely how those demands must be satisfied.

Law Affects 6 Chemicals

As the law goes into force today, only six chemicals have been formally classified by the Food and Drug Administration as food additives. As such, they are subject to control under the additives amendment.

Some 500 other chemicals have been exempted from Federal regulation, being "generally recognized as safe" by qualified experts. Also, 155 have been proposed for this exempt status,

but no decision on them has been made.

This leaves hundreds of other chemicals in foods still unclassified, relegated to a sort of no-man's land of food technology.

Technically, the appearance of any of these unclassified chemicals in food products is illegal as of this morning. The Food and Drug Administration would be within its legal rights to demand the withdrawal from the market of all foods containing such chemicals.

Officials of that agency stated last week, however, that no such action was contemplated except in possibly a few cases where they believed there was sufficient reason to question the safety of the chemicals.

Industry will be given a year's extension in which to satisfy the demands of the new law with regard to the rest of the unclassified chemicals, Food and Drug officials said.

Tests Required

According to the food additives amendment, industry must show through exhaustive laboratory tests that a chemical will be safe to eat in the amounts and under the conditions of its intended use before it may become part of the nation's diet.

Formerly, a food processor could add a certain chemical to a food, and it would be up to the Food and Drug Administration first to find the additive

111

and then to test it on laboratory animals before a harmful one could be pulled off the market.

The large number of additives that have come into use in foods and the thousands of dollars and the years of time usually required for each laboratory test made it extremely difficult for the Food and Drug Administration to carry out its responsibility except in a very limited way.

Food and Drug officials say, however, that even though there was little legal control over the use of chemicals in foods before the new amendment, the public health was probably never seriously threatened. The majority of the food, chemical and related industries ran safety tests of their own on new additives and conferred regularly with Government scientists before using the additives commercially.

Gap Is Closed

Not all members of industry ran such tests, however, and the tests that were run were seldom rigorous enough to show whether a chemical additive might be harmful if eaten over long periods of time. The food additives law has now closed this gap.

The need for more effective controls over the growing use of chemicals in foods to protect the nation's health was only one of the major forces behind the enactment of the new amendment.

Another was aimed at fostering an orderly and safe development of food technology to satisfy the needs of a growing world population.

Food and Drug officials have frequently called attention to the dependency of modern urban society on the chemicals that permit foods to be transported over great distances, stored for long periods, and modified for greater appeal and ease of preparation.

Strange though it may seem, however, some of the very chemicals that have so greatly

improved the quality of the nation's food supply are also capable of damaging animals fed them in large quantities.

For example, sodium nitrate that is used to prevent the color of meat from fading will cause blood damage in animals that eat it in large amounts. And vitamin D, which is used to enrich many foods, damages blood vessels in animals fed much greater than dietary quantities of it.

Those chemicals—and a great many other common ones—were technically outlawed from use in foods before the additives amendment went into effect. The old law held that a chemical must be proved harmless under any conceivable circumstances before it could be used in foods, and sodium nitrite, vitamin D and table salt clearly were not harmless under any conceivable circumstance.

Those substances became legal components of food products only a year ago under the amendment that authorized the Food and Drug Administration to set safe tolerances for food additives according to the amounts and conditions of their intended use. The only exception involved chemicals that were shown to cause cancer in animals or man. No tolerance can be set for those.

At the same time, however, both industry and Food and Drug officials were confronted by the forbidding prospect of having to assess the comparative safety of many hundreds of chemical additives that had never undergone the close laboratory scrutiny now required.

Part of that burden was relieved by two exemptions to the prior-testing requirement of the law. Those exemptions, however, have also been the source of most of the confusion.

The reason for this is that not all chemicals that are added to foods are classified under the new law as food additives.

Some of those "non-additive additives" are chemicals that received sanctions or approvals

for use in foods from Food and Drug before the new amendment became law. These are called "prior sanctions."

Others, comprising a much larger group, include all chemicals that are "generally recognized, among experts qualified * * * to evaluate [their] safety * * * to be safe * * *." These are referred to as "generally recognized as safe," or "GRAS."

Neither the prior sanctions nor the GRAS chemicals are required to undergo further testing. Only those chemicals that fall into neither category are technically food additives and so must be tested for safety.

Industry response to the amendment has been varied.

Some companies began gathering data early on their chemical additives to satisfy Food and Drug requirements. One major producer of food wrapping materials, for example, has started an additives research program involving millions of dollars.

Because the necessary tests are so costly in time and money, competitors in several major food and chemical industries have joined in cooperative research programs. This is an unusual—but legal—activity in a land where anti-trust laws prevail.

Some other members of industry, however, have apparently decided to sit tight. They hope that their chemical additives will either be declared "GRAS" or accepted as additives on the basis of another company's research.

Reading of Law Suggested

And many others are just confused. Einar T. Wulfsberg, who administers the food additives provision for the Food and Drug Administration, said he wants the clause struck from the law.

Industry-wide feeling is that the anti-cancer clause will severely curtail research and development of new products for both agricultural and consumer foods. The argument is,

that the gamble is too great to warrant investing a great deal of time and money in a chemical that is ruled out of use because large quantities of it cause cancer in laboratory rats.

Some Food and Drug officials have privately indicated at least partial agreement with the industry view. Officially, however, their position is that the anti-cancer clause is scientifically expedient and will stay in the additives amendment. If possible, they also say, it will be was still being asked basic questions about the law.

"Also," he said, "we're getting many requests for extensions on chemicals that have already been cleared. Some seem to want us to okay the cream in their coffee. It would help a lot if these people would read the law and keep up with the regulations and orders on it published in the Federal Register."

Above all the confusion, heated controversy rages over one particular clause in the amendment. This clause forbids the use in foods of any amount of a chemical that has been shown to cause cancer in animals or man.

Industry feels this is unreasonable and unscientific and incorporated into legislation pending on the control of ingestible food, drug and cosmetic colors.

That position is supported by the argument that not enough is known about cancer. No data are available to show whether it would be safe for human beings to eat small amounts of a substance that causes cancer in animals when consumed in large quantities.

On this basis, Food and Drug oficials say, if the anti-cancer clause errs, it does so on the side of safety to protect the public health.

The first year of the food additives amendment has been a stormy one, and no break in this climate can be foreseen at this time.

March 6, 1960

U. S. ORDER BANS A FOOD COLORING

Coal Tar Product, Used Also in Drugs and Cosmetics, Is Found Not Safe

Special to The New York Times.

WASHINGTON, Nov. 22—The Food and Drug Administration today ordered an end to the use of F. D. & C. (food-drug-cosmetic) Red No. 1, a water soluble coal tar color that is widely used in food, drugs and cosmetics. It is not used in lipsticks.

In signing the order, John L. Harvey, deputy commissioner of the Food and Drugs Administration, said the action had been taken because preliminary tests showed that the color produced liver damage in experimental animals and because no safe use level had been established.

The test results, he said, do not provide a basis for concluding that the color could cause cancer. The tests will be continued.

Mr. Harvey, however, found that "no action needs to be taken to remove foods, drugs and cosmetics containing this color additive, from the market on the basis of the scientific evidence before him, taking into account that the additive is not an acute toxic substance and that it is only used in small amounts in foods, drugs and cosmetics."

Foods using the color include frankfurter casings, ice cream, and maraschino cherries.

Scope of the Order

The F. D. A. action today included the discontinuance of certification of any further batches of this color and can-

celling of certificates for all previously certified lots.

According to the order, "the Commissioner of Food and Drugs, having concluded that ingestion of this color additive over a long period of time would be unsafe, and in order to protect the public health, hereby terminates the provisional listings of F. D. & C. Red No. 1 for use in foods, drugs and cosmetics."

The F.D.A. said that the lowest amounts of Red No. 1 that have been shown to produce liver damage in test animals were many times greater than the amounts of this color that would be consumed in the human diet.

The F.D.A. action is being taken under the new color additive law, which places on manufacturers the burden of proving that colors are safe before they can be allowed in foods, drugs, and cosmetics. Heretofore there have been no limits on the amount of Red No. 1 that could be used in foods, although in practice the actual amounts have been small.

Results of Tests Given

The experimental results obtained by the F.D.A. from feeding Red No. 1 to rats, dogs, and mice, were as follows:

¶Groups of fifty rats are being fed diets containing F. D. & C. Red No. 1 at levels of 5 per cent, 2 per cent, 1 per cent, 0.5 per cent, and 0 per cent. At this stage of the tests, which have now been in progress for from fifteen months to eighteen months, 116 animals from the 250 being fed F. D. & C. Red No. 1 at various levels and twenty-seven of the 100 controls have died. Of these, eleven being fed at the 5 per cent level, fifteen being fed at the 2 per cent level, eleven being fed at the 1 per cent level, and two being fed at the 0.5 per cent level, have shown liver damage. None of the controls that have died have shown liver damage.

¶Groups of 100 mice are being fed diets containing 2 per cent, 1 per cent, 0.5 per cent, and 0.1 per cent F. D. & C. Red No. 1, with 400 mice as controls. All mice on dosage levels of 2 per cent and 1 per cent died before the seventieth week. Gross liver damage has been observed in all groups fed at the 0.5 per cent diet and above.

¶Groups of four dogs are being fed diets containing 2 per cent, 1 per cent, 0.25 per cent, and 0 per cent F. D. & C. Red No. 1. Three of the dogs on the 2 per cent dosage level died before thirty-two weeks; the other is living. Three of the dogs on the 1 per cent dosage level died or were sacrificed within thirteen months. All autopsies have shown liver damage grossly and/or microscopically. Deceased dogs on the 1 per cent and 2 per cent dosage level showed poor physical condition.

November 23, 1960

A. M. A. SUGGESTS CHOLESTEROL CUT

By DONALD JANSON
Special to The New York Times.

CHICAGO, Aug. 2 — The American Medical Association said today that cholesterol in the blood should be reduced in cases of hardening of the arteries.

It advised doctors to do this by regulating the amount and kind of fat in the diet.

Recommended diets would reduce consumption of saturated fats, contributed principally by dairy products and meat, and substitute unsaturated fats found in such vegetable oils as those made from corn, cottonseed, soybeans and safflower.

The stand was based on a three and a half year study by the association's Council on Foods and Nutrition. It was the medical organization's first official statement on the controversial cholesterol question.

The report will appear in the Aug. 4 issue of The Journal of the association, published here. It is not being made as a recommendation to the general public but as a guide to physicians in treating patients.

The report said there was no clear proof that hardening of the arteries was caused by concentrations of fat in the blood, but continued:

"In the light of present knowledge, it appears logical to attempt to reduce high concentration of cholesterol and other serum lipids [fats in the blood] as an experimental therapeutic procedure."

Studies have established that substitution of unsaturated vegetable oils for animal fats and saturated vegetable fats in the diet has had "marked effects" in reducing blood cholesterol, it said.

Means 'Poorly Understood'

While recommending the diet changes, the report said the ways whereby unsaturated fatty acids lowered blood cholesterol were "poorly understood."

Simply reducing fat intake would lower blood cholesterol concentration, it said, but at the same time would raise blood triglyceride concentration.

Triglyceride is another fat associated with hardening of the arteries. Effective control of both requires not just reduction of saturated fats in the diet, but increasing the ratio of unsaturated fat to saturated fat, the council said.

The report said consumption of the usual fats, an important form of stored energy, was not necessary to replenish fat stores in the body because both carbohydrates and proteins are readily converted to fat.

But it warned that a completely fat-free diet might make the absorption of Vitamins A, D, E and K less effective. And unless skim milk is included, it said, a very low fat diet could be deficient in calcium.

But its recommended diets eliminate whole milk and cream, and limit eggs to four a week.

Only lean meats, fish and poultry are recommended. Commercial bakery goods other than bread are excluded. And so are chocolate and caramel candies made with cocoa butter.

Other fat contributors on the downgraded list are butter, ice cream, some margarines, lard and some other shortenings, cooking oils and salad dressings.

Vegetable oils are favored for use in baking or frying meats, fish and eggs, as well as in salad dressings, on vegetables or in baked products.

August 3, 1962

ANTIFAT DIET FAD ASSAILED BY A.M.A.

By AUSTIN C. WEHRWEIN
Special to The New York Times

CHICAGO, Oct. 11 — The anticholesterol "food fad" is a wasted, dangerous effort, the American Medical Association said today.

The association had in mind widespread fears linking animal fats to heart attacks.

"The antifat, anticholesterol fad is not just foolish and futile; it also carries some risk," the group said.

Its five-page statement was designed as a warning both to what it called "do-it-yourself Americans" and to food processors who have built advertising campaigns on cooking oils, margarine and other foods derived from vegetable oils.

Few medical subjects have aroused more interest among laymen than discussion of the connection between dairy and meat products and heart trouble. Both the meat and the dairy industry have been up in arms about the "antifat" campaign for some time.

Today's statement was a sequel to a report in the Aug. 4 issue of The Journal of the American Medical Association. That report was issued by the 12-member A.M.A. Council on Foods and Nutrition headed by Dr. William J. Darby of the Vanderbilt Medical School.

That report suggested that only physicians ought to consider altering the diets of patients with hardening of the arteries. However, at least one vegetable oil company used portions of the report in a national advertising campaign.

Today's statement, prepared under the supervision of Dr. Phillip L. White, executive secretary of the Council on Foods, said:

"Dieters who believe they can cut down their blood cholesterol without medical supervision are in for a rude awakening. It can't be done. It could even be dangerous to try."

Cholesterol Is Defined

Cholesterol is a white, fatty crystalline alcohol. Produced by the body, it coats the inner surface of arteries somewhat as a pipe would be clogged by minerals in water. This coating tends to restrict blood flow.

The report said that only laboratory tests could show whether an individual had excessive cholesterol in his blood, and whether a change of diet would raise or lower the level.

"Willy-nilly substitution of a few food items without overall control of the diet accomplishes little if anything in reducing cholesterol," the report said, continuing:

"What is more important, the elimination of certain foods of proven nutritional value could be detrimental to health."

Success in reducing blood cholesterol by diet has been achieved only in strictly controlled experimental groups, the report said.

The experiments are not yet of "practical importance to the general public," it said.

"There have been few investi-

113

gations," the report said, "on the effect of different types of fat in the normal diet over a long period of time. It is not known what type of fat, if any, may be beneficial in preventing heart disease, nor is it known that certain fats are harmful."

Generally, it continued, the American diet provides all the nutrients essential to health and a varied diet is the best rule for health.

"Any changes in a diet of such proved worth must await much more study and experience," the report warned.

The statement said that the Council of Foods recommended this diet: milk, cheese, ice cream, beef, veal, lamb, pork, poultry, eggs, fish butter, margarine, fats and oils.

The danger is that when an individual omits certain foods, he runs the risk of depriving his body of essential nutrients, it said. It concluded:

"The current concern about diet reflects a healthy interest on the part of the public. This interest should be directed away from hopeless pursuits to a worthwhile goal that can be attained by most individuals— maintaining normal weight. Overweight plays the villain in many diseases, and overweight can be avoided by not eating more calories than the body needs."

October 12, 1962

THERE'S POISON ALL AROUND US

SILENT SPRING. By Rachel Carson. Drawings by Lois and Louis Darling. 368 pp. Boston: Houghton Mifflin Company. $5.

By LORUS and MARGERY MILNE

POISONING people is wrong. Yet, for the sake of "controlling" all kinds of insects, fungi and weed plants, people today are being poisoned on a scale that the infamous Borgias never dreamed of. Cancer-inducing chemicals remain as residues in virtually everything we eat or drink. A continuation of present programs that use poisonous chemicals will soon exterminate much of our wild life and man as well. So claims Rachel Carson in her provocative new book, "Silent Spring."

"Silent Spring" is similar in only one regard to Miss Carson's earlier books ("Under the Sea Wind," "The Sea Around Us," "The Edge of the Sea"): in it she deals once more, in an accurate, yet popularly written narrative, with the relation of life to environment. Her book is a cry to the reading public to help curb private and public programs which by use of poisons will end by destroying life on earth.

Know the facts and do something about the situation, she urges. To make sure that the facts are known, she recounts them and documents them with 55 pages of references. She intends to shock and hopes for action. She fears the insidious poisons, spread as sprays and dust or put in foods, far more than the radioactive debris from a nuclear war. Miss Carson, with the fervor of an Ezekiel, is trying to save nature and mankind from chemical biocides that John H. Baker (then President of the National Audubon Society) identified in 1958 as "The greatest threat to life on earth."

HER account of the present is dismal. It is not hopeless—at least not yet. But she demands a quick change in "our distorted sense of proportion." How can intelligent beings seek to control a few unwanted species by a method that contaminates the entire environment and brings the threat of disease and death even to our own kind? "For the first time in the history of the world," she writes, "every human being is now subjected to contact with dangerous chemicals from the moment of conception until death. * * * These chemicals are now stored in the bodies of the vast majority of human beings, regardless of age. They occur in the mother's milk, and probably in the tissues of the unborn child."

Albert Schweitzer has said, "Man can hardly even recognize the devils of his own creation." Yet "Silent Spring" will remind some people that a few years ago they went without cranberry sauce at Thanksgiving rather than risk eating berries contaminated with a cancer-inducing chemical used improperly by some growers as a weed-killer in the cranberry bogs. A few others may recall that tax money was paid not only to growers of cranberries, but also (a year or so earlier) to poultry raisers whose chickens retained dangerous amounts of a chemical included in poultry feed upon Government recommendation and had to be condemned.

Miss Carson adds many other instances to the list, and points to programs that cost many millions of tax dollars, yet were doomed at the outset to failure. She gives details about the gypsy-moth campaigns that killed fish, crabs and birds as well as some gypsy moths; about the fire-ant program that killed cows, wiped out pheasants, but not fire ants; and dozens of others that led to *more* of the pest (or of new pests) by destroying the natural means of control.

Miss Carson gives most of her attention to insecticides, herbicides and fungicides, since these are the most dangerous poisons. She shows the futility of relying on them or any new substitutes offered to counteract the swift evolution of immunity to chemical control shown by more and more insects and fungus diseases. She quotes an authority on cancer, Dr. W. C. Hueper of the National Cancer Institute, who has given "DDT the definite rating of a 'chemical carcinogen'"—a cancer inducer. She notes that "storage of DDT [in the body] begins with the smallest conceivable intake of the chemical (which is present as residues on most foodstuffs) and continues until quite high levels are reached. The fatty storage depots act as biological magnifiers, so that an intake of as little as one-tenth of 1 part per million in the diet results in storage of about 10 to 15 parts per million, an increase of one hundredfold or more. * * * In animal experiments, 3 parts per million has been found to inhibit an essential enzyme in heart muscle; only 5 parts per million has brought about necrosis or disintegration of liver cells; only 2.5 parts per million of the closely related chemicals dieldrin and chlordane did the same." Other modern insecticides are still more deadly. Nor did the discovery of their poisonous character "come by chance: insects were widely used [during World War II] to test chemicals as agents of death for man."

IN some of the chapters, Miss Carson does approve of alternatives to the widespread use of poisonous chemicals. She points to the successful controlling of scale insects with ladybird beetles, and Japanese beetles with the "milky disease." So often, harmful species, new to a given area, have ceased to be much of a problem as soon as their natural enemies or their equivalents appear or are introduced. The natural struggle for survival can then keep the numbers of the pests at a fairly low level. This approach, as Miss Carson emphasizes, rarely creates new pests, whereas extermination campaigns often do so.

Those who grow and store food and other products that can be hurt by pests will surely accuse "Silent Spring" of telling only part of the story. They will claim that today efficiency in raising and distributing food and wood depend upon the use of poisons. The traces of chemical compounds left in and on these materials are the price we must pay for such efficiency. If biological control methods were relied upon or hand labor required, the yield would be smaller and the market price higher. They might ask, "Do you want wormy apples and buggy flour, or traces of pesticides that by themselves have not yet been proved harmful?"

Miss Carson can also count on vociferous rebuttal

Mr. and Mrs. Milne, educators and biologists, are authors of "The Senses of Animals and Men," "The Balance of Nature" and other books.

from many pesticide makers and users. Government agencies that have encouraged poisoning campaigns are more likely to remain silent, unwilling to take blame for extensive programs that seem senseless and needless in retrospect. "Silent Spring" is so one-sided that it encourages argument, although little can be done to refute Miss Carson's carefully documented statements. Valiant attempts will certainly be made to defend the motives and methods of biocide users. These arguments will concede that these chemicals *could* be dangerous and that the substances *might* be helpful if used correctly. They are unlikely to cite the calamities that have followed application of the poisons — as "Silent Spring" does.

THE book mentions that in 1960 private citizens of America invested more than $750,-000,000 in poisons to kill insects, rats, unwanted fish, crabgrass and other pests. Federal, state and local governments spent an even larger amount to put poison on public lands (including national forests, parks and roadsides) and on private property (many of whose owners objected vehemently to such treatment). Understandably, the manufacturers, distributors and appliers of all these tons of chemicals hope that the demand for pesticides will increase. To expand their businesses, they are willing to invest a great

---

WHEN The New Yorker published parts of "Silent Spring" during June and July, a gentle author was transformed into a controversial one. The response to Rachel Carson's book shows clearly that one man's pesticide is another man's poison. Hundreds of letters—99 per cent of them favorable—poured into The New Yorker. Newspapers throughout the country published editorial comment. Two Senators and three Representatives read selections into the Congressional Record. Houghton Mifflin ordered 100,000 copies of the book printed.

The reaction of most men in the pesticide industry, according to the trade journal Chemical and Engineering News, was that "Miss Carson presents facts accurately for the most part, but comes to unwarranted conclusions from them and ignores the benefits of pesticides." Parke C. Brinkley, chief executive officer of the National Agricultural Chemicals Association, said: "Any harm that is caused by the use of pesticides is greatly overcompensated by the good they do."

Government agencies criticized by Miss Carson have remained mute, but Chemical and Engineering News found a man in the Food and Drug Administration willing to say anonymously: "The articles are obviously, perhaps also intentionally, one-sided. The cases Miss Carson cites are almost all cases of misuse—but the articles could have a good effect by warning of the dangers of misuse." Another Food-and-Drug source said means were being sought to battle bugs non-chemically. Meanwhile the Federal Council for Science and Technology, composed of representatives of five Federal departments, has begun a study of the problem.

---

many dollars in research and promotion. With so large a financial stake in the continuation of present programs, they can be counted upon to spend even more money to tell the public the other side of the story.

No amendment to the Constitution protects us from this new danger. "If the Bill of Rights contains no guarantee that a citizen shall be secure against lethal poisons distributed either by private individuals or by public officials, it is surely only because our forefathers, despite their considerable wisdom and foresight, could conceive of no such problem," she says.

Nor is Congress likely, unless urged by enough people, to vote appropriations to let the Food and Drug Administration monitor more adequately the poisonous residues in foods. The two criteria that legislators understand are votes and taxes. Few votes and few taxes come from outdoor groups, such as the National Audubon Society. These organizations and their small-circulation magazines have little money to spend on educating and influencing legislators.

About one-third of "Silent Spring" has appeared in The New Yorker; the book itself rounds out and documents the account. In answer to the charge that the balance of nature has been upset, it has been pointed out by some members of the chemical industry that modern medicine is equally upsetting. This sort of defense merely invites a pox on both the biocide and the drug industries. "Silent Spring" offers warnings in this direction too: trivial amounts of one poison often make trivial amounts of another suddenly disastrous; and poisons stored in the body may be tolerated during health, but take effect dramatically as soon as any sickness decreases the body's resistance. It is high time for people to know about these rapid changes in their environment, and to take an effective part in the battle that may shape the future of all life on earth.

September 23, 1962

SCIENTISTS URGE WIDER CONTROLS OVER PESTICIDES

President's Panel Calls for Stiffer Rules to Protect Health of the Nation

KENNEDY BACKS REPORT

A New Drug Agency Study of Chemical Levels in Food Is Already Under Way

By ROBERT C. TOTH
Special to The New York Times

WASHINGTON, May 15—The President's Science Advisory Committee cautioned the nation today on the use of pesticides.

In a critical report that stirred agencies to action even before its official release, the scientists called for changes in laws and regulatory practices to guard against the hazards involved in widespread use of the chemicals.

The committee said that the use of pesticides must be continued if the quality of the nation's food and health is to be maintained.

But it called for more research into potential health hazards and, in the interim, for more judicious use of the substances in homes and the field.

43-Page Document

The 43-page document said application of certain "specially hazardous and persistent materials now registered" by the Government should be modified and new compounds "rigorously evaluated" before being approved.

It urged that the Food and Drug Administration review "as rapidly as possible" the current residue tolerances in foods, particularly those based on "inadequate" evidence.

The scientists all but told the Department of Agriculture to stop its controversial mass sprayings to eradicate gypsy moths, fire ants and two types of beetles. The aim should be control, not eradication, the report suggested.

President Kennedy said without qualification that he had "already requested the responsible agencies to implement the recommendations in the report, including the preparation of legislative and technical proposals which I shall submit to Congress."

The Food and Drug Administration has already begun a reassessment of the tolerance limits of pesticides in foods. The study is largely the result of facts turned up by a special panel of the Science Advisory Committee. The chairman of that committee, which took up the pesticide problem, was Dr. Colin M. MacLeod, professor of medicine at New York University Medical School.

Among its recommendations, the report released today called for Government programs of public education on the poisonous nature of 500 pesticides now registered. These include chemicals to kill insects, weeds, fungi, herbs, and rodents. More than 700,000,000 pounds of the chemicals were produced in the United States in 1961.

Found in Food and Clothes

The substances are detectable in many food items, in some clothing, in man and animals and in natural surroundings, the report said. They travel great distances and persist for long periods of time. One of every 12 acres of land in the 48 contiguous states has been sprayed with pesticides in the last year.

The report said that about 45,000,000 pounds of the pesticides are used annually in urban areas, much of it by home owners. On the average, one "bug bomb" per household is sold each year.

Dishes, utensils and food may inadvertently be contaminated. Citizens come into contact with the chemicals, which can be absorbed through the skin, in their mothproof clothing and blankets as well.

In a tribute to a popular author, the report said that "until publication of 'Silent Spring' by Rachel Carson, people were generally unaware of the toxicity of pesticides."

The book, a study of the dangers inherent in the unchecked use of pesticides, was published last fall by the Houghton Mifflin Company.

The report was critical of both Government agencies with the principal responsibility for pesticides—the Food and Drug Administration and the Depart-

ment of Agriculture. He said the effectiveness of the chemicals was better proved than their safety.

The scientists said that the Department of Health, Education and Welfare should develop a comprehensive system for gathering data on pesticide residues, as well as a national network to monitor residues in air, water, soil, wildlife and fish.

Members of the special committee on pesticides, in addition to Dr. MacLeod, are:

H. Stanley Bennett, Dean of the Division of Biological Sciences, University of Chicago.
Kenneth Clark, Dean of the College of Arts and Sciences, University of Colorado.

Paul M. Doty, professor of chemistry, Harvard University.
William H. Drury Jr., director of the Hatheway School of Conservation Education, Massachusetts Audubon Society.
David R. Goddard, Provost, University of Pennsylvania.
James G. Horsfall, director of the Connecticut Agricultural Experiment Station.
William D. McElroy, chairman of the Department of Biology, The Johns Hopkins University.
James D. Watson, professor of biology, Harvard University.

The chairman of the full advisory committee is Jerome B. Wiesner, special assistant to the President for science and technology.

May 16, 1963

Senate Study Links Fatal Ills to Air Pollution

Respiratory Afflictions Are Traced in Staff Research

Urban Areas Spur Lung Cancer and Empsysema

By PETER KIHSS

A half-dozen types of illnesses have been linked to air pollution in a United States Senate staff study, including one that appears to kill eight times as many men as women.

The 62-page survey was ordered by Senator Edmund S. Muskie, chairman of a special Public Works subcommittee. The Maine Democrat's office in Washington expressed optimism yesterday that the Senate would act this session on legislation to expand Federal air-pollution control efforts, following House passage last July.

The study cited pulmonary emphysema—an increasingly recognized disease that stretches air sacs and interferes with breathing—as causing eight deaths of men as against only one among women for every 100,000 inhabitants in 1959.

Emphysema, the study said, "seems to be increasing especially in urban areas," and "air pollution is suspected of being responsible for much of this." It was the primary medical diagnosis in 6.9 per cent of disability cases receiving Social Security benefits in 1960, exceeded only by the 19.9 per cent for arterio-sclerotic heart disease and costing $60,000,000 in payments a year

Incidence of Diseases

There is "strong evidence that air pollution is associated," the study said, also with the common cold and other upper respiratory tract infections; chronic bronchitis, found in one investigation to affect 21 per

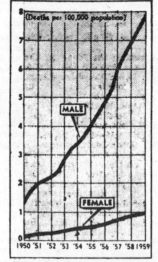

The New York Times   Oct. 25, 1963
Death rates from pulmonary emphysema, by year and sex, in period 1950-59.

cent of men 40 to 59 years old; chronic constrictive ventilatory disease, which causes extra breathing effort; bronchial asthma and lung cancer.

Lung cancer, increasingly frequent, has a higher rate in cities, the study said, and this "cannot be fully explained by other recognizable factors, such as cigarette smoking or nature of occupation."

The study showed how airborne concentration of an important group of cancer-producing agents—benzene-soluble organics—increased with the size of communities. It added that "death rates from respiratory system cancers have a similar relationship."

"A change in air environment," the Senate report went on, "apparently can affect one's chances of getting lung cancer.

"Persons emigrating to New

Zealand or South Africa, after long residence in heavily polluted Great Britain, have greater rates of lung cancer than those of persons of similar ethnic backgrounds and smoking habits who are native to those countries, but lower rates than those who remain in Great Britain.

"Conversely, persons coming to the United States from Norway have lower cancer rates than native Americans of similar backgrounds, but higher rates than among those who remained in the cleaner air of their own country."

Atmospheric Compounds

The study, led by Ron M. Linton, staff director of the Senate Public Works Committee, warned that atmospheric reactions could form secondary chemical compounds "more dangerous or otherwise more objectionable than those originally discharged into the air."

One compound "thought to be responsible for eye irritation in the type of smog first noted in Los Angeles," it said, is peroxyacetyl nitrate, produced in the air by the action of sunlight on automotive exhaust gases.

Thermal inversions—a weather condition in which a layer of warm air acts as a lid over cooler air—occur 10 to 35 per cent of the time along the Atlantic Coast, the study said. The range elsewhere is 10 to 50 per cent, and fall months generally have the most hours of inversions.

Inversions developing over a city during the night, the study went on, frequently persist until three or four hours after sunrise, and then develop again in the evening. This, it said, means that the two daily rush hours with maximum automobile traffic "frequently coincide with the two daily periods least satisfactory for the escape of pollution."

October 25, 1963

CIGARETTES PERIL HEALTH, U.S. REPORT CONCLUDES; 'REMEDIAL ACTION' URGED

CANCER LINK CITED

Smoking Is Also Found 'Important' Cause of Chronic Bronchitis

By WALTER SULLIVAN
Special to The New York Times

WASHINGTON, Jan. 11—The long-awaited Federal report on the effects of smoking found today that the use of cigarettes contributed so substantially to the American death rate that "appropriate remedial action" was called for.

The committee that made the report gave no specific recommendations for action. But health officials said that possible steps might include educational campaigns, the requirement that cigarette packages carry warnings and control of advertising.

The report dealt a severe blow to the rear-guard action fought in recent years by the tobacco industry. It dismissed, one by one, the arguments raised to question the validity of earlier studies.

Role of Smoking in Cancer

Combining the results of many surveys, the study panel found no doubt about the role of cigarette smoking in causing cancer of the lungs.

In men who smoke cigarettes, the death rate from that disease is almost 1,000 per cent higher than in nonsmokers, it said. Lung cancer has become the most frequent form of cancer in men.

Such smoking was also found to be "the most important" cause of chronic bronchitis, increasing the risk of death from that disease and from emphysema, a swelling of the lungs due to the presence of air in the connective tissues. Emphysema is a disease of increasing incidence.

As to coronary artery disease, a frequent cause of heart failure and the leading cause of death in this country, mortality is 70 per cent higher for cigarette smokers than for nonsmokers, the report said.

Relationship Assumed

The role of smoking as a cause of the disease, it said, "is not proved." However, it said, the study committee considers it "prudent" from the public health viewpoint to assume such a cause-and-effect relationship rather than wait until such a relationship has been established beyond doubt.

[The Tobacco Institute rejected the report, saying it was not the last word on smoking and health. The three major broadcasting networks said they would review their policies on tobacco advertising in the light of the report.]

The report was prepared on the initiative of President Kennedy to help the Government decide what to do about the smoking question. The committee was formed by Dr. Luther L. Terry, Surgeon General of the Public Health Service. Its work began in the summer of 1962 and consisted of evaluating and reprocessing earlier studies. No original research was done.

At a press conference in the State Department Auditorium, where the report was released,

Dr. Terry said he did not anticipate any "foot dragging" by the Government in taking the "remedial action" called for in the report. He said the problem was one of "national concern."

Dr. Terry told the committee that the Public Health Service would move "promptly" to determine what steps should be taken. He said that his recommendations would be made to Anthony J. Celebrezze, Secretary of Health, Education and Welfare, after consultation with the Public Health Service staff.

F.T.C. Studies Report

"I am sure that other departments and agencies of the Federal Government, along with non-Federal agencies, will also take the report under consideration promptly," he said. Shortly after the meeting, the Federal Trade Commission said it was studying the report to see what action was necessary.

The committee could find no evidence that nicotine played an important role in causing dis-

ease. Rather, it pointed an accusing finger at the components of tobacco smoke that had been found to produce cancer in animals. These are a series of compounds known as polycyclic aromatic hydrocarbons.

These compounds are complex molecules composed of hydrogen and carbon atoms, the latter arranged in a series of rings.

A spokesman for the committee told the press conference there was no valid evidence that filters helped reduce the harmful effects. The report also said that nicotine substitutes, such as lobeline, used in so-called "withdrawal pills," seemed ineffective in breaking the smoking habit.

The committee said that smoking was a "psychological crutch" for a large part of the 70 million Americans who were smokers in 1963. This posed the question: What would happen if this prop were suddenly pulled out from under them?

'Intangible' Factors

The report said that such factors were "so intangible and elusive, so intricately woven into the whole fabric of human behavior, so subject to moral interpretation and censure, so difficult of medical evaluation and so controversial" that they could not be assessed.

It said that, from time immemorial, men have leaned on props, some harmless, such as the ginseng root of China, some lethal, like opium. So powerful is this human drive, it said, "that man has always been willing to risk and accept the most unpleasant symptoms and signs."

Among these it cited hallucinations, paralysis, convulsions, poverty, malnutrition and even death. If, then, man is bound to continue his dependence on such substances, in the interests of public health this should be done "with substances which carry minimal hazard," it said.

Smoking, the report said, is a habit, rather than a form of addiction. Withdrawal does not produce a characteristic illness, as it does with addicts, and is best accomplished by psychologically replacing the prop, the committee said. However, it added, this invokes "the difficulties attendant upon extinction of any conditioned reflex" — that is, in breaking any habit.

Those who questioned the validity of earlier studies argued that no one had shown how smoking could, for example, cause lung cancer or heart disease. It was said that the statistics were confused by other factors, such as air pollution in large cities, stress and heredity.

Not a Simple Question

The report released today said that no simple cause-and-effect relationship probably existed between a complex product like tobacco smoke and any single disease in so variable an organism as the human body. It also acknowledged that it often seemed to be a combination of factors, rather than any one, that precipitated an illness.

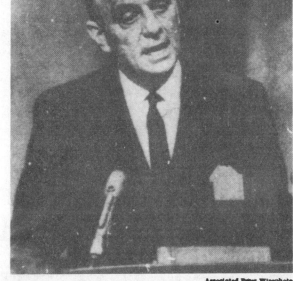

Associated Press Wirephoto
DISCUSSES SMOKING REPORT: Dr. Luther Terry, the Surgeon General, at news conference held in Washington.

Nevertheless, it said, cigarette smokers said they inhaled. A survey of cigar smokers has shown an inhalation rate of 19 per cent. An American study of pipe smokers has indicated 28 per cent inhalation and the figure in a Canadian study was 18 per cent.

The report said that, in men, cigarette smoking "far outweighs all other factors" as a cause of lung cancer. The incidence of this disease has risen dramatically during the years that cigarettes have replaced other forms of smoking.

While the data for women are less extensive, the report said, they "point in the same direction."

Those who questioned such conclusions in the past argued, for example, that in earlier times deaths from lung cancer were incorrectly diagnosed. They said the increase in recorded cases was in part a reflection of better diagnostic procedures. The committee agreed but said that this effect was minor alongside that of smoking.

In the combined results from seven surveys, 1,833 of the deaths among smokers were diagnosed as resulting from lung cancer. Using the rate among nonsmokers as a guide, only 170.3 of those men would have died had they not smoked, the report said.

Thus the rate among smokers was almost 10 times as high.

In coronary artery disease, the deaths among smokers were 11,177, compared with an expected figure of about 6,430, based on the rate among nonsmokers. For smokers, therefore, the rate was less than double that in nonsmokers, but the total number of deaths was far larger.

A "puzzling" discovery in animal studies, the report said, is that all the tarry substances from cigarette smoke, when used together, are far more potent in producing cancer than one would expect from tests with the various constituents. The latter include the seven polycyclic hydrocarbons that have shown varying degrees of potency as causers of cancer.

It seems, therefore, the report said, that "the whole is greater than the sum of the known parts."

Nevertheless, it said, cigarette smoking was clearly the most important factor in some diseases to which it was linked. For example, in chronic diseases of the lungs and bronchial tubes, it was found that the relative importance of cigarette smoking as a causative factor was "much greater" than air pollution or occupational exposure.

"Cigarette smoking is a health hazard of sufficient importance in the United States to warrant appropriate remedial action," said the report, entitled "Smoking and Health."

The conclusions of the committee rested heavily on seven "prospective" studies carried out since 1951, involving 1,123,-000 men. A prospective study is one in which individuals are picked at random and observed, usually until death. In these studies, the deaths of 37,391 participants had been recorded and analyzed.

Number and Age Factors

The committee combined the results of these seven studies and found that for cigarette smokers the death rate per thousand, from all causes, was 68 per cent higher than for nonsmokers.

As in earlier studies, the death rates were strongly affected by such factors as the number of cigarettes smoked daily and the age at which smoking began. Likewise, as others have found, the use of cigars and pipes was far less a factor than cigarette smoking.

The death rates for those who smoke fewer than five cigars a day were found to be almost the same as for nonsmokers. For those smoking five or more cigars, the rate was only "slightly" higher. Even those pipe smokers who smoke 10 or more pipefuls a day and have been smoking more than 30 years did not show a substantially higher death rate.

Inhalation Rates Lower

The reason for lower rates among cigar and pipe smokers is not clear, although some attribute it to less inhalation. The report cited surveys in which 94 per cent of the ciga-

It has been found in various areas of cancer research that the disease may be caused by a combination of "insults" to the body cells, none of which is harmful by itself.

Another factor, as noted in the report, is that smoking seems to impair the function of the cilia, or tiny hairs, whose constant motion cleanses the lungs by sweeping mucous upward into the throat.

The committee found that, as long suspected, pipe smoking is a cause of lip cancer. Cigarette smoking was called a "significant factor" in cancer of the larynx. There was some evidence of a link between smoking and cancer of the food pipe (esophagus) and bladder, the report said, but this has not been proved.

It said that no relationship had been shown between tobacco use and stomach cancer. The same is true, it said, with a dimness of vision commonly attributed to cigar and pipe smoking and known as tobacco amblyopia.

It said smoking during pregnancy seemed to produce smaller babies, but asserted that it was not known whether real damage was done to the child.

Studies have not substantiated the common notion that children take up smoking as a gesture of defiance to authority, the report said.

The change in smoking habits since the turn of the century was charted as follows: In 1900 the average consumption of chewing tobacco, per person each year, was about 4 pounds, and in 1962 it was half a pound. The use of pipe tobacco, 2½ pounds per person in 1910, likewise had dropped to half a pound by 1962. In 1920 the average number of cigars smoked, for every man, woman and child, was 117, but this fell to 55 in 1962.

Rise in Cigarette Smoking

By contrast, the figure for cigarettes at the start of the century was fewer than 50. In

1961 it hit its peak of 3,986 per person per year.

The sequence of events that led to establishing the committee began with a letter sent to President Kennedy on June 1, 1961, by the heads of the American Cancer Society, the American Public Health Association, the American Heart Association and the National Tuberculosis Association.

They urged the formation of Presidential commission to study the "widespread implications of the tobacco problem." The next January they met with Dr. Terry, who proposed to the Secretary of Health, Education and Welfare the formation of a committee of outstanding experts to assess the available knowledge and make recommendations.

Further discussions included representatives of the Tobacco Institute, maintained by the industry, and of various Government agencies. It was agreed that the job should be done in two phases. The first was to be "an objective assessment of the nature and magnitude of the health hazard." This was the report submitted to Dr. Terry today.

The second phase is to include recommendations for action. It was agreed that such proposals should not be a part of the first phase and that they should not be considered until the first report was in.

As stated in today's document, "It was recognized that different competencies would be needed in the second phase and that many possible recommendations for action would extend beyond the health field and into the purview and competence of other Federal agencies."

It was stated at the press conference that the views of the committee were unanimous.

Dr. Terry was listed as chairman of the committee and Dr. James M. Hundley, Assistant Surgeon General, as vice chairman, in addition to the 10 appointed members. The director of the committee's staff was Dr. Eugene H. Guthrie, chief of the Division of Chronic Diseases in the Public Health Service.

January 12, 1964

Tobacco Institute Says Report 'Is Not Final Chapter' in Debate Over Health Issue

By JOHN H. ALLAN

The Tobacco Institute rejected yesterday's Government report on smoking and health as the final word in the 10-year debate over the use of cigarettes.

George V. Allen, president of the institute, which represents most of the industry, declared in Washington: "This report is not the final chapter."

Mr. Allen said he "wholeheartedly" endorsed Surgeon General Luther L. Terry's call at his news conference yesterday "not for less but for more research."

The tobacco industry, Mr. Allen said, is ready to increase its support of health research. Through 1963, the institute invested $6.25 million in scientific research. It has allocated $1 million for research grants in 1964.

Cigarette manufacturers themselves were cautious or noncommittal in their reactions to the tobacco-health report.

'Forward Step'

Zach Toms, president of the Liggett & Myers Tobacco Company, called the report "a forward step toward resolving the honest difference of opinion among scientists."

He said that his company was carefully studying the report and that the findings would be "carefully considered" in planning the company's research and marketing programs.

A spokesman for the R. J. Reynolds Tobacco Company, the largest cigarette manufacturer, said in Winston-Salem, N. C., that "our people will want to digest the report before making any comment." Bowman Gray, chairman of Reynolds, was unavailable for comment.

Reynolds, however, was making considerable effort to get the report. It flew copies from Washington to its headquarters in Winston-Salem in the company's private plane. It said its "top people" were on hand to examine the report when it arrived.

Comment Withheld

A spokesman for Philip Morris, Inc., said his company was studying the report "with our scientific advisers" and had no comment. Officials of the P. Lorillard Company could not be reached.

Robert K. Heimann, assistant to the president of the American Tobacco Company, said his company had no statement to make.

Spokesmen for individual tobacco companies and for the Tobacco Institute did not comment on two key parts of the report. These were the call for "remedial action" and the assertion that there was a lack of evidence that cigarette filters reduce the health hazard.

The president of the Consolidated Cigar Corporation, the nation's largest cigar manufacturer, predicted that the report would cause millions of smokers to switch from cigarettes to cigars.

Stanley S. Keyser, president of Consolidated, made the statement after seeing the Surgeon General's news conference over closed-circuit television.

In his statement on the report, Mr. Allen of the Tobacco Institute said:

"While it is obviously not possible for me to comment in detail on this 387-page report so soon after receiving it, a few observations seem immediately pertinent.

"First, I am sure the report will receive the careful study it so clearly deserves.

"Second, further research is needed. As Surgeon General Terry pointed out, 'There is a great deal yet to be known on the subject.' He specifically rejected a suggestion that there was no longer need for additional research. In short, this report is not the final chapter.

"I endorse wholeheartedly and without any reservation Surgeon General Terry's call at his press conference today, not for less, but for more research—by the Public Health Service, the American Medical Association, and other public and private groups of scientists who are seeking the scientific facts we so urgently need.

"Finally, the tobacco industry, which is already supporting a considerable body of health research, stands ready to increase that support and also to cooperate with the Government and with other groups on any projects which offer possibilities for filling the gaps in knowledge which still exist in this broad field of scientific concern."

Past scientific reports that tobacco is harmful to health have affected only briefly the amount of cigarettes smoked in the United States.

Since December, 1953, when a meeting of New York dentists was told that smoking was a cause of lung cancer, cigarette smoking has risen in all years but 1953 itself and 1954.

Last year Americans smoked 523 billion cigarettes, according to figures published by the Department of Agriculture. That is an increase of more than 25 per cent in 10 years.

Per capita smoking of cigarettes increased in seven of the 10 years. It dropped in 1953 and 1954, then rose each year until 1962, the year the Royal College of Physicians in Britain declared that "cigarette smoking is a cause of lung cancer."

Last year this figure, for Americans over 15 years of age, was 4,005 cigarettes. This amounts to 200 packs, or more than a half a pack a day. Ten years earlier the annual figure per capita was 3,559 cigarettes.

The important years in the decade of debate on tobacco and health are 1953, when the issue was first raised; 1959, when the then Surgeon General, LeRoy E. Burney, warned that risk of lung cancer could best be eliminated by the elimination of smoking; and 1962, when the British report was published.

January 12, 1964

U.S. TO REQUIRE HEALTH WARNING FOR CIGARETTES

Trade Commission Orders That Package Labels Tell of Danger of Cancer

RULE EFFECTIVE JAN. 1

Advertising Curb May Also Be Included in Regulation —Tobacco Stocks Drop

By EILEEN SHANAHAN
Special to The New York Times

WASHINGTON, June 24— The Federal Trade Commission announced today that it would require cigarette packages to carry a warning that cigarette smoking is dangerous to health.

The statement will be required on all packs, boxes and cartons of cigarettes sold, beginning next Jan. 1.

The exact language of the cautionary statement will be left up to cigarette manufacturers. They will be required to state "clearly and prominently" that cigarette smoking "may cause death from cancer and other diseases."

A similar warning will be required in all cigarette advertising beginning July 1, 1965, under the terms of a regulation issued today by the commission. The requirement involving cigarette advertising could be abandoned or postponed, however, the commission said, if the tobacco industry can convince it before the middle of next year that such a warning has become unnecessary.

House Panel Hears Dixon

The circumstances under which the commission would abandon its requirement that cigarette advertisements contain the health warning were not made entirely clear in the announcement. It was indicated, however, that one prerequisite might be that the industry itself participate in campaigns to educate the public concerning the dangers of cigarette smoking.

Changes in the content of cigarette advertisements would clearly be required.

[Prices of tobacco issues took moderate to sharp losses Wednesday on the New York Stock Exchange. Liggett & Myers and Philip Morris were hardest hit, both off 1½. Details on Page 45.]

The commission's decision that the absence of a health warning on cigarette labels was unfair and misleading was based on the findings of a special committee formed by the Surgeon General of the Public Health Service, Dr. Luther L. Terry.

That committee, after reviewing many studies of smoking and health made in recent years, concluded that "smoking is a health hazard of sufficient importance in the United States to warrant appropriate remedial action." The report also found that lung cancer and some respiratory ailments were caused by cigarette smoking.

Paul Rand Dixon, the commission chairman, announced in testimony before the House Interstate Commerce Committee today that the commission had decided to go ahead with its plans to require the health warnings. The text of the commission's proposed rule and a 153-page report, supporting its conclusion that the new rule was necessary, were made public later.

Mr. Dixon told the committee he had no doubt that the commission had the authority to impose the cigarette regulations. Tobacco industry spokesmen indicated, however, that they would immediately challenge this point in the courts.

The commission's rules were first proposed in somewhat different form in January. Its decision to go ahead with the rule caught the industry by surprise, however, and no formal announcements concerning plans for a legal challenge were made immediately.

Gov. Terry Sanford of North Carolina announced that his state would participate in any court action that was taken in the case.

North Carolina's two Senators, Sam J. Ervin Jr. and B.

119

Everett Jordan, both Democrats, said that tobacco growers and cigarette manufacturers had informed them they planned an immediate court test of the commission's regulations.

The Senators said that they would themselves sponsor Congressional action to prohibit the commission from putting its rules into effect should the court test fail and should they be unsuccessful in an attempt to get the Administration to withdraw the regulation.

The Federal Trade Commission, as an independent agency, is not directly subject to the policies of any Administration. However, White House pressure has successfully been exerted on many of these agencies in the past.

The commission's rules, in contrast to the proposal it originally made, do not attempt to limit in any way the affirmative claims that are made in cigarette advertisements.

The commission said that it had dropped this part of its proposed regulation, temporarily at least, because of the industry's plans to act voluntarily to end appeals to young people and other "undesirable practices."

The industry recently named Robert B. Meyner, former Governor of New Jersey, as administrator of its voluntary advertising code. It has received Justice Department assurances that cigarette companies would not be subject to criminal antitrust prosecution for adhering to this code.

The commission's report warned cigarette manufacturers, however, that the commission would "maintain a close surveillance" of the industry's behavior under the voluntary advertising code.

The commission noted that it was not prescribing the precise language of the warning it will require on cigarette packs and cartons. It said it would hold itself available for consultation with the industry and would give advance approval to warning phrases if found acceptable.

While the words "death" and "cancer" do not have to be used, under the commission's rule, Mr. Dixon conceded that he knew of no adequate substitutes.

If the industry, as expected, goes into court to ask that the rule be prohibited from going into effect while the legal power of the commission is tested, the litigation might take up to four years, Mr. Dixon said.

The commission's decision to go ahead with the rule now was made by a 3-to-1 vote. Commissioner A. Everette MacIntyre said that he would have postponed the effective date of the labeling order, as well as other portions of the rule, until July 1, 1965, and would have acted only after giving the industry opportunity to undertake a labeling program voluntarily.

Members of the commission who voted to adopt the rule, in addition to Mr. Dixon, were Philip Elman and John R. Reilly.

June 25, 1964

Obesity Called a Rising Health Hazard

By JANE E. BRODY

Obesity among Americans is a major public health problem that is bound to get worse as the nation eats more and exercises less, a panel of experts concludes. They reach this conclusion in a report soon to be published by the United States Public Health Service.

Although all the statistics are not in, those available indicate that "a high proportion of our population weighs more than is considered desirable for optimum health," the report states.

It points out that obesity is associated with a number of chronic disorders, including diabetes, heart disease and respiratory disorders, and that fat people who are otherwise healthy are more likely to develop major illnesses and die at an early age.

"Regardless of health implications, obesity is an esthetic problem—and thus often a psychological problem —for patients who live in societies where fat people are regarded as unattractive," the report further notes.

The report emphasizes that prevention is the best means of coping with obesity, but it also outlines methods of treating the problem once it exists. It finds most diets and drugs of limited value in weight re-

duction, and instead suggests for long-term success the age-old method of exercising more and eating less.

Exercise and diet have been a perennial concern of the medical profession. Earlier this week, the National Academy of Sciences, in a report on dietary fats and heart disease, noted that many Americans would benefit by exercising more and by eating less food and less fat.

The Public Health Service report, described in the current issue of Medical World News, a magazine for doctors, is scheduled for publication in late August or early September. It will be available free to members of the health professions and may be purchased by other interested persons from the Superintendent of Documents.

The experts note that there is much confusion in deciding who is and who is not obese. They recommend tossing out the old height-weight and age-weight charts and relying instead on better measurements of excess fat. They explain that a person who is "overweight" when compared with some arbitrary standard is not necessarily "obese"—that is, he may not have excess fat tissue in relation to muscle, bone and the like.

"From a practical point of

view, a determination of whether or not any one individual is too fat is rather simple and does not require scientific acumen," the report notes.

"An easy answer without weighing oneself on a scale is to look in the mirror. A realistic appraisal of the nude body is often a more reliable guide for estimating obesity than body weight.

"If sheer appearance fails to give a clear answer, there is the 'pinch test' — particularly helpful for adults under 50," the report continues.

Fat Under the Skin

At least half the body fat of young persons is found directly under the skin. At many parts on the body — the back of the upper arm, the side of the lower chest, the back below the shoulder blade, and others — a fold of skin and underlying fat can be lifted between the thumb and forefinger.

A pinch that is thicker than one inch is an indication of excess body fat, the report explains.

Once the fat determination is made, the next difficulty is how best to get rid of it. The panel does not place much faith in appetite-controlling drugs.

For one thing, "they cannot supplant the need to learn and follow a new pattern of restricted food intake."

For another, in most cases they lose their appetite-reducing effect after about six weeks, the experts note.

As for fad diets, they say, high-fat or carbohydrate diets are potentially hazardous and

"favorable results are usually based on short trials." "A follow-up over a longer period of time would find considerable less enthusiasm," they say.

"Prolonged consumption of formula diets is impractical. Many people find the liquid diet monotonous and unpalatable, and ultimately they must

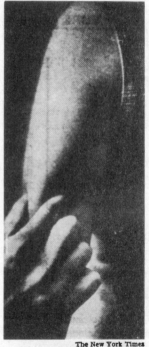

The New York Times

'PINCH TEST': If the fold of skin is thicker than one inch, a person has excess body fat. Here the skin is shown being pinched at the back of the upper arm.

change to conventional sources of food," the study continues.

The experts are cautious, too, about fasting and surgical removal of part of the intestine, since both these "drastic" methods have not been studied long enough.

The best way to lose weight and keep it off, the experts maintain, is to step up physical activity and to make a permanent change in eating habits, preferably under medical supervision.

"The diet should be nutritionally sound and the dieter should not feel too hungry," the report states.

A weight loss of more than two pounds a week is considered "excessive" for persons not under a doctor's care.

Considering the difficulties of taking weight off, the experts say that preventing obesity is the most sensible approach.

They single out four groups of potential "fatties" who should be watched closely: children in families that tend to be obese; persons with heavy builds and a tendency toward corpulence; persons with medical conditions that might be complicated by obesity, and persons who are settling into a more sedentary way of life.

The experts are most concerned about obese children: "They are more likely to remain obese as adults and to have more difficulty in losing fat than people who become obese as adults."

The report was prepared by Dr. Jean Mayer, Harvard nutritionist; Dr. John H. Browe, nutrition director of the New York State Health Depart-

ment; Dr. George J. Christakis, trition director of the New York City Health Department; Dr. Alvan R. Feinstein, associate professor of medicine at Yale; Dr. Charlotte M. Young, Cornell nutritionist; Dr. Robert E. Olson, biochemist and nutritionist at the University of Pittsburgh; Dr. Marvin Plesset, University of Pittsburgh psychiatrist, and Dr. Reuel A. Stallones, public health professor at the University of California, Berkeley.

July 16, 1966

Study Urges Caution in Antibiotic Use

Serious Hazard to Man Seen by an F.D.A. Panel in the Doses Given Animals

By JANE E. BRODY

The Government has been advised in a report being released today to tighten its requirements on the use of antibiotics in food-producing animals and as food preservatives.

Unless it does, an advisory committee formed by the Food and Drug Administration warned, serious hazards to man may arise. It said, for instance, that the presence of residues of penicillin in edible flesh was a "serious public health hazard."

Doctors have noted that persons can develop serious allergies to penicillin. In rare cases the allergies can lead to death. In addition, various researchers have noted that antibiotics in livestock feed can induce a strain of bacteria that is resistant to the antibiotic. This resistance, in turn, can be passed on to man.

Penicillin is one of at least 16 drugs that are routinely added to livestock feed to promote rapid growth or to treat disease or injury. In addition, two antibiotics are now used to prevent spoilage in poultry and fish.

Dr. James L. Goddard, commissioner of the Food and Drug Administration, said that antibiotics have been used for many years, but some questions about their hazards to man have been receiving our renewed attention."

He said that the F.D.A. would "take a closer look" at antibiotics.

"We accept the recommendation to study this problem and will work with other agencies in the Government to investigate the effects," he said.

An antibiotic is a chemical substance that can inhibit or destroy microorganisms. Drug manufacturers who have sought certification for the use of their antibiotics have had to offer information about their persistence in the food in which they are used.

More Data Sought

But in the future, Dr. Goddard said, "we are going to ask the manufacturers for additional data on the drugs we are in doubt about before they are approved for continuing veterinary use."

The committee said that "unauthorized and undesirable" residues of antibiotics had been found in edible parts of animals.

Doctors note that, besides the danger to the growing number of persons with allergies to antibiotics, there is a danger that an antibiotic taken in food may counteract the effectiveness of another antibiotic that is being used to treat an ailment.

The committee said that there was a "paucity of data" on antibiotics in animals. It suggested an inquiry into how antibiotics may change chemically, how much and how quickly they are excreted, and how much may persist in the tissues of animals.

The information gained from these studies, it said, "should be adapted to monitoring procedures for the control of antibiotic residues in edible animal tissues."

No Residue In Food

The committee, which was also charged with examining agricultural pesticides, said they "do not result in antibiotic residues in food."

"Nevertheless," it said, "exposure to antibiotic sprays or dusts may cause sensitization in certain individuals, or may cause the appearance of antibiotic-resistant organisms."

"While no major public health problems resulting from such uses of antibiotics have been reported," it said, "the committee feels that the possibility should not be excluded."

Although the committee said it was "particularly concerned" about the use of antibiotics in animal feeds, it also noted some possible dangers in the use of antibiotics as food preservatives.

"To date, the only registered uses of antibiotics for direct application on food are chlortetracycline on poultry and fish and for oxytetracycline on poultry," the committee said.

But it said that the Food and Drug Administration had received a number of requests for new regulations on food additives to increase the use of antibiotics in food.

"To date," the committee said, "none of the petitions have been granted, but it is expected that there will be additional proposals for the use of antibiotics in various classes of food products."

A Number Reviewed

The committee reviewed a number of proposed food-preserving antibiotics. Among them were nisin, which would inhibit bacteria in certain heat-processed canned foods; pimaricin, to reduce spoilage by fungi in canned and concentrated orange juice, and tylosin, to control various problems in canned mushrooms, dog food and smoked fish.

"Ideally," the committee said, "antibiotics used in food preservation should not be used in human or veterinary medicine."

Furthermore, it said, the antibiotics "should not give rise to the selection of naturally resistant microorganisms, or induce the emergence of resistant strains or cross-resistance to antibiotics approved for treatment of human diseases or antagonize—the activity of such antibiotics."

The committee also urged that antibiotics should not be used as a "substitute for good manufacturing practices with consequent poor sanitation."

Dosage Test Recommended

It suggested that the antibiotic should be studied to determine if it adversely changed the helpful bacterial population in persons eating the food, and it recommended that the antibiotic dosage be tested on a trial commercial basis before it is used widely.

The committee suggested that the Food and Drug Administration examine the way the use of chlortetracycline and oxytetracycline meets these requirements.

A crucial factor in avoiding unwanted residues of antibiotics in foods, the report states, is the "withdrawal period"—the time between the last administration of antibiotics to the animal and its slaughter.

"Since some antibiotics are retained in the body for varying times and in some instances for very long periods, practical withholding times should be established for drugs freely available to farmers, and if a longer than practical period is required for a particular drug it should be available only on the prescription of a veterinarian, with adequate warnings on the label, the committee recommended.

The committee pointed out that some of its recommendations, if adopted, would require the F.D.A. to revise existing regulations, set up new methods of obtaining data, and create "new organizational units and personnel within the F.D.A., and other agencies of the Federal Government."

August 22, 1966

British Publish a U.S. Study of Birth Pills and Cancer After A.M.A. Journal Rejected It

By SANDRA BLAKESLEE

A controversial study, which has found a higher prevalence of early cervical cancers among women who used birth control pills than among women who used diaphragms, has been published in a British medical journal after this country's leading medical journal refused to publish it.

The study concerned itself only with the prevalence of early cervical cancers among women using the two contraceptive methods and did not attempt to incriminate the pill as a possible cause of such cancers. Nor did the report attempt to explain medically the differences observed.

The study, sponsored by Planned Parenthood of New York and Sloan-Kettering Institute-Memorial Hospital, was headed by Dr. Myron R. Melamed, a pathologist at Memorial Hospital.

It was submitted to the Journal of the American Medical Association for publication last February.

After three or four months of deliberation and negotiation, the decision was made not to publish the study.

Author Is Silent

Dr. Melamed and his associates at Memorial Hospital said they were not now at liberty to discuss the study. The public relations department at the hospital, which is handling all queries, said many details were not known to it.

Dr. Melamed was quoted last month in The Medical Tribune, a publication not associated with the A.M.A., as having said that the report had been rejected "because we could not agree on the revisions — if that is what they want to call them."

He was reported to have said that some changes had been made as requested but that "they couldn't seem to decide what they wanted to do with it."

Dr. John H. Talbott, editor of The Journal, was reported to have been unsatisfied with the revisions made by the authors. A spokesman for the magazine said the study would have been published if the authors had been willing to allow criticisms of the report to be printed at the same time.

As a result, Dr. Melamed and his associates sent the study to The British Medical Journal, which published it in its July 26 issue.

The editor of the British journal, reached by telephone last night, said that the time between submission of an article and its appearance in print varied and that he could not recall when the magazine had received Dr. Melamed's article.

The study has been the subject of rumor and speculation for well over a year. References to its contents have cropped up repeatedly in medical journals, newspaper articles and in medical circles, although few people, before its recent publication, were known to have seen a completed draft of the study.

The study was initiated in late 1965 when the Public Health Service gave a five-year grant to Dr. Melamed and Dr. Hilliard Dubrow, an obstetrician-gynecologist at Lenox Hill Hospital. The doctors were to "evaluate the effect of contraceptive devices on cervix cancer incidence."

With the cooperation of Memorial Hospital and Planned Parenthood of New York, the investigators screened about 40,000 patients at 11 Planned Parenthood clinics. Ultimately the subjects included 27,508 women taking the pill and 6,809 women using the diaphragm.

Remarks at Closed Meeting

As the study progressed, the doctors were reported to have alluded to it at various closed medical meetings, although they said the report was not ready for publication.

At a meeting of a New Jersey chapter of the American Cancer Society last September, Dr. Melamed spoke about the study.

Although the meeting had been closed, reports of his remarks were printed in some newspapers.

Following this, little news of the study was given out by officials at Memorial Hospital and Planned Parenthood of New York. They said they had not seen the final draft of the report but added that, on the basis of the preliminary data, there was no reason to stop recommending the pill as a safe contraceptive device.

The national office of Planned Parenthood-World Population sent out telegrams to its affiliates to this effect.

At the same time, the medical committee of Planned Parenthood of New York called in three independent pathologists to review the study.

The pathologists found many things to criticize in the report, including its design, the population segments it studied and the questions it was said to pose.

Questions were raised over the criteria for defining early cancer of the cervix. Pathologists often disagree about what constitutes early cancer and what is merely harmless, although abnormal, cell growth. The pathologists examining the Melamed group slides found many of the smears to be inconclusive as evidence pointing to early cancer.

In essence, they said the report could not confirm or deny a causal relationship between cancer of the cervix and oral contraceptives.

No Causation Hinted

But Dr. Melamed's study, as it appeared in the British Medical Journal, made no hint that a causal relationship between the pill and cervical cancer had ever been suggested.

The study said simply that there was a "small but significant difference" in early evidence of cervical cancers between women who used the pill and women who used the diaphragm.

"The reason for the differences," the report concluded, "is not apparent from these data."

The study said the higher prevalence of early cervical cancer observed among women who used the pill could be attributed to any number of things—perhaps the diaphragm protects against cancer, perhaps the hormonal changes induced by the pill enhance the climate for cancer, perhaps some sociological factors such as frequency of the sex act or the number of partners involved determine the difference in prevalence.

The report concludes that "so long as regular visits to a physician are mandatory for women who are using the steroid contraceptives in order to obtain a prescription, there is a possibility for them to have better medical care, with less danger from cancer of the cervix, than any other group of women."

The types of cancer detected in the women studied were nearly all curable as they were caught at an early stage.

The investigating group is now, according to its report, carrying out a new study that will add two new elements:

First, women who use intrauterine devices will be included in the study. Such women could not be included in the last study, the doctors said, because of early procedural problems.

Second, the new report will attempt to determine the incidence of cervical cancer among women who use the pill as opposed to women who use other contraceptive methods. That is, the doctors will attempt to find out if a woman who starts with one method is more prone to cervical cancer than a woman starting out with another method.

The present report limited its attention to women who had been using one means or another of contraception for some time and who already showed evidence of early cancer of the cervix when first examined at the Planned Parenthood clinics.

July 30, 1969

Federal Heart Panel Asks Public to Eat Fewer Fats

By JANE E. BRODY

A national commission of medical experts recommended in a report released yesterday that Americans make "safe and reasonable" changes in their diets to lower blood cholesterol levels in the hope of stemming the current "epidemic" of heart disease.

At the same time, the commission urged the immediate adoption of a national policy committed to the primary prevention of premature atherosclerosis and its attendant cardiovascular diseases.

Of the 600,000 American deaths attributed to heart disease each year, 165,000 are "premature" deaths occurring in persons under the age of 65. Men are three times more likely than women to be the victims of premature coronary death.

The dietary changes recommended yesterday included a halving of the current average daily consumption of cholesterol and saturated fats and a substantial reduction in total fat intake.

To achieve this, the commission advised Americans to cut down on egg yolks, butter fat, fatty meats, organ meats, shellfish and fat-rich baked goods and candies and to substitute wherever possible products prepared with unsaturated fats. Most vegetable oils are unsaturated.

The commission's recommendation was based on a large body of data gathered from both animals and man that suggest that changes in the typical fat-rich American diet can help prevent or at least delay cardiovascular diseases.

Noting that definitive evidence linking dietary fats and cholesterol to human heart disease is not available, the commission called for large-scale, long-term, Government sponsored studies to determine once and for all the effect that changes in diet and other factors may have on the nation's slowly rising coronary mortality rate.

Such a study would involve perhaps 100,000 persons followed for five to 10 years at an estimated cost of $50-million to $100-million.

The commission said that it was recommending a change in diet despite the lack of definitive evidence because "the American public would probably have to wait at least 10 years for the results of these studies [and] at times urgent public health decisions must be made on the basis of incomplete evidence."

Other 'Risk Factors'

In addition to diet and its effect on blood fat levels, the commission singled out high blood pressure and cigarette smoking as the major "risk factors" leading to premature heart disease and coronary deaths. Accordingly, the report recommended an "orderly phasing out" of the cigarette industry with strict restraints on the sale and advertising of cigarettes and a major national effort to detect and treat victims of high blood pressure.

The commission, called the Intersociety Commission for Heart Disease Resources, consists of 115 leading American medical and nursing personnel. It was set up under the Regional Medical Programs, sponsored by the Federal Government, to formulate policy guidelines to prevent premature heart disease and improve care of coronary patients.

Under the chairmanship of Dr. Irving Wright, professor emeritus at Cornell University, and the direction of Dr. Donald T. Fredrickson, the commission will produce a series of reports in the coming months on other aspects of coronary care.

The current report, considered the commission's major effort, was discussed at a news conference at the Biltmore Hotel here yesterday. The full report will be published in this month's issue of the journal, Circulation.

Dr. Fredrickson summarized the commission's dietary recommendations as follows:

The current American diet, which draws about 40 per cent of its calories from fat, should be cut down to include no more than 35 per cent fats; the saturated fat level, currently at 16 to 20 per cent, should be cut in half, and the cholesterol level, currently at 600 to 750 milligrams a day, should be no more than 300 milligrams daily.

Foods high in cholesterol include egg yolks and dairy and animal fats.

At the same time, Dr. Fredrickson said, intake of polyunsaturated fats (the oils of corn, peanuts, soybeans and the like), which currently averages 7 per cent of calories, should not exceed 10 per cent. The remaining dietary fats should come from monounsaturated fats like olive oil.

Change in Standards

According to Dr. Frederick H. Epstein, epidemiologist at the University of Michigan, such a dietary change "can lower serum cholesterol by 10 to 15 per cent."

"At a conservative estimate," he said, "such an effect on serum cholesterol might lower the incidence of coronary heart disease by as much as 30 per cent."

To help Americans achieve this dietary change, the commission urged that Federal food standards be changed to permit the sale of processed meats and dairy products in which unsaturated fats substitute for saturated fats. Under current standards, for example, milk that has part or all of its butter fat replaced by vegetable oil must be called "imitation milk."

The commission also called upon the Food and Drug Administration to change its labeling laws to permit manufacturers to list the exact fat contents of their products so that Americans would have a better idea of what they were eating in the way of fats and cholesterol.

Other risk factors that the commission linked to premature heart disease were diabetes, obesity, sedentary living, a family history of heart disease and possibly "psychological tensions."

December 16, 1970

DDT Banned in U.S. Almost Totally, Effective Dec. 31

Ruckelshaus Decides After 3-Year Fight That Risk to Environment Is Too High

---

COURT APPEAL IS FILED

Farmers Are Given Time for Instruction in the Use of a Substitute Pesticide

---

By E. W. KENWORTHY
Special to The New York Times

WASHINGTON, June 14 — William D. Ruckelshaus, administrator of the Environmental Protection Agency, banned today almost all uses of DDT, the long-lived toxic pesticide that lodges in the food chain of men, animals, birds and fish.

After almost three years of legal and administrative proceedings, reports by scientific bodies and public hearings, Mr. Ruckelshaus declared in a 40-page decision that the continued use of DDT over the long term, except for limited public health uses, was an unacceptable risk to the environment and, very likely, to the health of man.

"The evidence of record showing storage [of DDT] in man and magnification in the food chain," said Mr. Ruckelshaus, "is a warning to the prudent that man may be exposing himself to a substance that may ultimately have a serious effect on his health."

Three Crops Affected

Mr. Ruckelshaus's order is effective Dec. 31, 1972. In the meantime, he explained, growers of cotton, peanuts and soybeans — the three crops that account for almost the total domestic use of DDT—will get instruction in the handling of a substitute pesticide, methyl parathion. The substitute is toxic, but unlike DDT, it degrades quickly.

Samuel Rotrosen, president of Montrose Chemical Corporation, sole United States manufacturer of DDT, immediately asked the United States Court of Appeals for the Fifth Circuit in New Orleans to set aside the order. Montrose is jointly owned by Chris-Craft Industries, Inc., and the Stauffer Chemical Company.

Formulators Appeal

A parallel appeal in the same court was filed by Robert L. Ackerly, a Washington lawyer who represents a group of formulators of DDT, that is, manufacturers of various commercial pesticides containing DDT.

Mr. Ruckelshaus's order represented a major victory for environmental groups that in October, 1969, petitioned the Secretary of Agriculture to begin the proceedings that would lead to cancellation of DDT for shipment in interstate commerce. At that time the Department of Agriculture had authority to register "economic poisons" for such shipment. The authority was transferred in December, 1970, to the Environmental Protection Agency.

The organizations, which later took their cause to the Federal courts, were the National Audubon Society, the Izaak Walton League, the Sierra Club, the Western Michigan Environmental Council and the Environmental Defense Fund, which also supplied legal counsel for the plaintiffs.

The decision came 10 years after Rachel Carson, the biologist, set off the controversy over DDT with her book "The Silent Spring," in which DDT was called "the elixir of death" for birds, mammals, fish, insects and perhaps for man if it proved to have cancer-causing properties.

The order represented a defeat for the maker and the 31 formulators of DDT; for the Department of Agriculture, which had entered the case on their side, and for Representative Jamie L. Whitten, Democrat of Mississippi, chairman of the House Appropriations subcommittee that handles funds for the environmental agency. Mr. Whitten, a cotton-state Congressman, has maintained that DDT is necessary to combat the boll weevil and boll worm.

Discovered in 1939

The insecticidal properties of DDT were discovered in 1939. During and after World War II it was hailed as a miracle chemical because of its ability to control typhus and malaria in tropical and semitropical countries and the boll weevil and many other agricultural pests in the United States.

In recent years, domestic use of DDT has steadily declined, partly in response to warnings by scientists about its persistence when taken into the food chain, partly as a result of Fed-

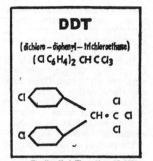

DDT
(dichloro – diphenyl – trichloroethane)
$(Cl\,C_6H_4)_2\,CH\,C\,Cl_3$

The New York Times/June 15, 1972

DDT, as shown in the formula and diagram, is a compound of carbon, hydrogen and chlorine.

eral restrictions and partly because of the discovery of substitutes.

According to the Environmental Protection Agency, domestic use has declined from about 79 million pounds in 1959 to 12 million to 14 million pounds in 1970.

Roughly 86 per cent is used for cotton, 9 per cent on peanuts and 5 per cent on soybeans. Minimal quantities are used on some other vegetable crops.

Exports of DDT, mostly for malaria control by the World Health Organization and under the foreign aid program, total about 26 million pounds a year.

Mr. Ruckelshaus's order will not affect manufacturing for export.

Also, it will permit use for protection of public health — as in outbreak of disease following a flood—and for health quarantine purposes.

The order permits the use of DDT on three minor crops, green peppers, onions and sweet potatoes in storage, for which no effective alternatives are now available. However, certain conditions must be met by applicators.

These three uses now account for less than 1 per cent of domestic sales.

Mr. Ruckelshaus said in his findings that DDT could persist in soils "for years and even decades" and also in aquatic ecosystems, that it could attach to eroding soil particles and so contaminate water supplies and that it could get into the air by vaporizing from soil and crops.

Further, he said, it is toxic to fish and birds and impairs their reproductive processes. The thinning of eggshells through ingestion of DDT, he said, has accelerated the decline of many birds such as eagles and ospreys.

He also said that experiments on laboratory animals had shown that DDT causes tumors and that this raised the possibility that it may cause cancer in human beings.

The chronology of the DDT controversy is as follows:

October, 1969. The environmental groups petitioned the Secretaries of Agriculture to give notice of cancellation of all uses of DDT and to suspend its use as an "imminent hazard" to health pending the cancellation proceedings.

November, 1969. The Secretary, Clifford M. Hardin, issued cancellation notices for use on shade trees, tobacco, around homes and in marshes except to control disease carriers but refused suspension. The environmental groups went to court.

May, 1970. The United States Court of Appeals for the Dis-

trict of Columbia circuit ordered Mr. Hardin to issue cancellation notices on all other uses and suspend all uses pending cancellation proceedings or say why he could not do so.

August, 1970. Mr. Hardin issued cancellation notices on more than 50 uses, but not on cotton spraying, the most important. He still refused to order suspension.

January, 1971. The Court of Appeals ordered Mr. Ruckelshaus to issue cancellation notices on all remaining uses and to consider immediate suspension.

January, 1971. Mr. Ruckelshaus issued the cancellation orders and thus set in motion the long administrative proceedings allowed by law. The companies requested the appointment of a scientific advisory committee to examine the question and also public hearings.

March, 1971. Mr. Ruckelshaus declined to suspend use, finding DDT was not "an imminent hazard."

September, 1971. The scientific advisory board recommended accelerated reduction in use of DDT "with the goal of virtual elimination of any significant additions to the environment."

April, 1972. After seven months of hearings and 8,900 pages of testimony, Edmund S. Sweeney, an Interior Department officer selected by the Civil Service Commission to preside over the hearings, said that benefits of DDT outweighed the risks and recommended reversal of the proposed ban. The Environmental Protection Agency said it would contest the findings.

June 15, 1972

Estrogens:
Disturbing Hints of a Possible Link to Cancer

Thirty-three years ago, a British biochemist, Sir Charles Dodds, accidentally discovered diethylstilbestrol, a manmade chemical that behaved remarkably like the natural female sex hormone, estrogen. This first synthetic estrogenic drug and others that followed paved the way for a whole new range of therapeutics: treatments for menopausal symptoms, estrogen deficiency diseases and certain forms of cancer and, eventually, the development of oral contraceptives. None of them would have been possible on a widespread scale if doctors had had to rely on a limited, costly supply of natural estrogens.

Today, diethylstilbestrol—DES, for short—is mired in a national controversy over its cancer-causing properties, the resolution of which might ultimately spell its demise. Ironically, the controversy is coming to a head at the same time that doctors are proclaiming yet another victory for the drug. Left out of the current oral contraceptives, DES has now shown remarkable effectiveness as an after-the-fact contraceptive, or "morning-after" pill.

Last week, a physician at the University of Michigan Health Service described a study of 1,000 women, most of them university coeds, who had been spared unwanted pregnancies through treatment with DES, starting within three days after sexual intercourse. Under normal circumstances, at least 20 to 40 pregnancies would have occurred, Dr. Lucile Kirkland Kuchera said in her report in the Journal of the American Medical Association. The drug is believed to work by preventing the implantation of the fertilized egg.

According to Dr. Kuchera and Dr. John McLean Morris, Yale University obstetrician who discovered the "morning-after" pill, DES is being used by many physicians as an "emergency" contraceptive for women who are inadvertently or unexpectedly exposed to the risk of pregnancy. These would include rape victims, women who act on impulse and those whose partners' condoms have broken.

A few days after Dr. Kuchera's report, two environmental organizations filed suit in Federal District Court in Washington, D. C., to stop the feeding of DES to beef cattle and sheep. Their charge: Residues of the chemical, which is routinely used to speed the fattening of animals, had been found in meat sold to consumers. And last Friday, the Food and Drug Administration indicated it would order changes in the labeling of DES and related estrogens. Behind both actions was concern over the chemical's carcinogenic potential.

That DES can cause cancer in animals was first demonstrated in the late 1950's. According to Dr. Samuel Epstein, professor of environmental medicine at Case Western Reserve University, the chemical has been shown to produce cancer in a wide range of animals, including rats, hamsters and guinea pigs. According to the two environmental organizations, the Natural Resources Defense Council and the Environmental Defense Fund, mice get cancer when as little as 6.25 parts per billion of DES is included in their diet.

By law, no residues of the chemical are permitted in meat sold to consumers. But the environmental groups say that, among 10 randomly selected animals tested by the Department of Agriculture this month, DES residues up to 15.4 parts per billion were found in cattle and residues as high as 36.9 parts per billion were found in sheep. Routine department tests have indicated that residues above 2 parts per billion

exist in two out of 500 animals slated for the market.

Last February, the Government began criminal prosecutions of farmers who shipped livestock containing DES residues. And this month, the Agriculture Department ordered farmers to stop feeding DES to animals at least seven days before slaughter in an effort to prevent residues in meat. The House Subcommittee on Intergovernmental Relations is scheduled to begin hearings next month on DES residues in food.

DES has been prescribed for the treatment of a variety of human ailments for 30 years with no apparent cancerous effect. It has actually been used to treat prostate cancer and advanced breast cancer in women past menopause. But recently three Boston physicians uncovered an unusual link between DES and cancer in humans.

The doctors reported last April that seven young women, most still in their teens, had developed an extremely rare kind of cancer—adenocarcinoma of the vagina. The physicians traced the apparent cause of the cancer to DES which the mothers of the young women had taken during pregnancy. In the 1940's and early 1950's DES was used frequently in some parts of the country in an effort to prevent threatened miscarriage.

Subsequent to the Boston report, the New York State Health Department found five more such cases. In one, instead of DES, a similar estrogen-like hormone, dienestrol, was used. Nearly 50 additional cases have since come to light.

New York State's health commissioner, Dr. Hollis S. Ingraham, was so alarmed by the findings that last June he issued warnings to doctors throughout New York State and urged the Food and Drug Administration to warn all of the nation's doctors about further use of synthetic estrogens during pregnancy and to tell them to be on

the lookout for cases of vaginal cancer in young women.

The F.D.A. has not taken any action to date, but last Friday a spokesman said the agency was changing the labeling for DES and related estrogens to say that they should not be used during pregnancy.

Although the formulation of DES, produced by Eli Lilly & Co., comes with a warning against its use in pregnant women without the careful weighing of benefits and risks, none of the other synthetic estrogens marketed currently bear such a cautionary statement. And one of the drugs, dienestrol (made by Schering Corporation under the trade name Synestrol), lists as one of its uses the "treatment and prevention of habitual abortion"—i.e. repeated miscarriage.

Dr. Morris explained that he and others use DES mainly because it is commercially available in tablet form at the dosage level required for this purpose. "Other estrogens would probably work just as well, but they would require F.D.A. approval before we could use them clinically," Dr. Morris remarked. He added that even if DES can cause cancer in the fetus, and even if the drug given as a morning-after pill should fail to prevent pregnancy, it would be taken so early in gestation that the chances of affecting the fetus are nil. It is generally believed that to affect the vaginal development in a female fetus, the drug would have to be taken between the eighth and tenth weeks of pregnancy.

The future of DES remains uncertain. But medical authorities are convinced of the need for close surveillance of girls whose mothers received estrogenic drugs during pregnancy. The most common symptom of vaginal cancer—abnormal vaginal bleeding—is easily dismissed as "normal" in adolescent girls, they warn.

—JANE E. BRODY

October 31, 1971

F.D.A. Bans Cattle Feed Drug That Has Been Tied to Cancer

Bar to DES in Cattle Feed Is Likely to Raise Price of Beef 3.5 Cents a Pound

By RICHARD D. LYONS
Special to The New York Times

WASHINGTON, Aug. 2—The Food and Drug Administration halted today the introduction into cattle feed of a growth-stimulating hormone that has been linked to cancer, and banned its use entirely after Jan. 1.

The hormone, diethylstilbestrol, or DES, has been given in small quantities, usually a gram or so over an animal's lifetime, to about three-quarters of the nation's cattle to help fatten them for slaughter.

In the mid-nineteen-sixties, the hormone was suspected of causing vaginal cancer in the daughters of women who had taken a drug containing DES during their pregnancies decades before.

Increase Estimated

Higher beef prices are likely to result from today's action. A spokesman for the Department of Agriculture estimated that when the total ban goes into effect beef will cost 3.5 cents more a pound.

Today's announcement by Dr. Charles C. Edwards, the Commissioner of Food and Drugs, allowed the continued use until the end of the year of those feeds that still contained the hormone.

Three Democratic Senators—William Proxmire of Wisconsin, Edward M. Kennedy of Massachusetts and Abraham A. Ribicoff of Connecticut — complained in statements that the ban should have been total and immediate.

Senator Proxmire noted that 21 nations had completely banned the use of the hormone in animal feeds.

Danger Is Seen

Mr. Proxmire released the text of a letter from Dr. Frank J. Rauscher, head of the National Cancer Institute, that said in part:

"Although a direct connection between the ingestion of

DES in beef and the development of human cancers cannot be documented, the presence of the chemical in food does in my view constitute a danger that should be circumvented."

The Department of Agriculture and the F.D.A. have been criticized for years by consumer groups for what they characterized as foot dragging on the DES issue. However, Dr. Earl L. Butz, Secretary of Agriculture, said he regretted the F.D.A. action although he realized that under the law the agency had had no choice.

The move stemmed from the so-called Delaney amendment to the Food, Drug and Cosmetic Act, which specifically prohibits the use in food products of chemicals that are known to cause cancer in either humans or animals.

DES has been shown to cause cancer in laboratory animals. However, the supporters of the continued use of DES maintained that the residual amount of hormone left in meat sold publicly was either nonexistant or trivial.

Dr. Edwards said that last Friday "new scientific data developed by the United States Department of Agriculture and received by my office casts serious doubt on our ability to set rules for the use of DES in animal feed that will insure against residues remaining in animal livers at the time of slaughter."

The amounts that have been found were in the range of a few parts of DES per billion parts of meat.

Economists at the Agriculture Department have estimated that American consumers would pay $300-million to $460-million additional annually if the use of DES and all other growth stimulators were prohibited.

Food scientists have estimated that an animal given DES will reach a market weight of 1,000 pounds 35 days sooner and will use 500 pounds less feed than a comparable animal without it.

The extra feed required, plus the longer period of feeding the animals, drives up the eventual cost of producing the beef cattle.

Today's ban did not extend to the implanting of DES in cattle, which the F.D.A. and the Department of Agriculture now have under study.

In the implant method, a capsule containing a small amount of DES is inserted in to the animal's ear and it is gradually released into the animal's system. The animal receives a smaller amount of hormone than by the feed method.

In discussing DES in feed and in implantable capsules, Dr. Edwards emphasized that the ban was "not based on any known hazard to human health." However, using more sophisticated sampling techniques, Government scientists have been able to detect four times as much DES residue in animal livers this year as a year ago.

"No human harm has been demonstrated in over 17 years of use," Dr. Edwards said. "Under the law, however, this continued use of the drug may no longer be permitted."

The F.D.A. said it might be possible to fatten cattle almost as well by using implants of DES.

August 3, 1972

ASBESTOS FOUND IN DULUTH WATER

E.P.A. Links Fibers in Lake to Industrial Discharge

By JANE E. BRODY

The Environmental Protection Agency disclosed yesterday that "high concentrations" of potentially dangerous asbestos fibers had been found in the drinking water of Duluth and surrounding Minnesota communities that use Lake Superior for their water supply.

The source of the fibers, the agency said, is believed to be the discharge of waste from the Reserve Mining Company, a taconite processing plant that has been embroiled in an antipollution suit for several years.

The company, whose plant in Silver Bay, Minn., 55 miles northeast of Duluth, has been dumping 67,000 tons of taconite tailings into the lake daily for 16 years, called the charges unfounded and said there was no indication that the tailings presented any hazard to the drinking water.

While there is no health effect known to be associated with the ingestion of asbestos fibers, the Federal agency recommended that communities using Lake Superior water find alternative sources of drinking water for very young children.

In studies over the last two decades, Dr. Irving J. Selikoff, an expert on environmental medicine at Mount Sinai Hospital here, showed that the inhalation of asbestos fibers can cause a chronic lung disease called asbestosis and cancer of the lungs, stomach and colon.

In an interview yesterday, Dr. Selikoff said his laboratory had identified the asbestos fibers in the Duluth water as being the same type (amosite) that has been implicated in half the deaths among workers in a Paterson, N.J., asbestos plant. These workers experienced three times the expected death rate from cancer of the gastrointestinal tract.

"It can be assumed that anyone who inhales asbestos fibers also ingests them, but there have been no pure studies of the effects of ingestion in humans," Dr. Selikoff said.

Dr. Lawrence Plumlee, a physician on the staff of E.P.A., said that limited studies in animals have indicated that when asbestos is placed in the stomach, it rapidly enters the blood stream and is widely distributed to tissues throughout the body.

The agency said it had asked Dr. Selikoff to determined within 60 days the average accumulation of asbestos fibers in the tissues of residents of the Duluth area. Using tissues obtained at an autopsy, Dr. Selikoff and his colleagues from Mount Sinai will compare asbestos accumulation in residents with that of asbestos workers and of persons believed to have minimal exposure to the persistent mineral fibers.

Dr. Selikoff and Dr. E. Cuyler Hammond of the American Cancer Society have already begun outlining studies to determine whether the residents of the Duluth area might have already shown evidence of asbestos-related health effects.

But even if no definite or potential health effect can be readily defined, the finding of asbestos particles in the water supply is expected to strengthen the Government's case against the Reserve Mining Company.

The company is the only major industry dumping anything into Lake Superior, whose waters have long been regarded as the most pristine of the Great Lakes. Besides Duluth, five communities in Minnesota, two in Wisconsin and one in Michigan use the once-thought extremely pure water of the lake for drinking purposes.

The E.P.A. said it was trying to develop treatment methods that would rid the drinking water of asbestos fibers. However, Dr. Flumlee said that with the average concentration of fibers at about 100 billion per liter of water, "we don't know how effective these methods will be."

June 16, 1973

Many Workers Still Face Health Peril Despite Law

The recent discovery of fatal liver cancer among vinyl chloride workers has focused renewed attention of government, labor, industry and medicine on the thousands of known, suspected and as yet unsuspected health hazards that face 60 million working Americans.

Despite the passage three years ago of the Occupational Safety and Health Act, granting every American the right to work without job-induced threats to life and health, the overwhelming majority of workers are not yet protected by the law's provisions. For lack of this protection, hundreds of workers are dying each day from occupational diseases.

The General Accounting Office acknowledges that there has not been nearly enough money and staff allocated to make a dent in the vast problem of occupational health. In addition, fundamental scientific knowledge is lacking upon which to base remedial actions, and without more funds the necessary research is not forthcoming.

Historically, occupational health has been a low-priority item for both government and medicine.

Yet, each year one of every 10 workers suffers a job-related illness or injury. The Public Health Service estimates that prolonged on-the-job exposure to toxic chemicals, dusts, noise, heat, cold, radiation and other industrial conditions each year results in the death of at least 100,000 workers and the development of disabling occupational diseases in 390,000 more.

Researchers in occupational health believe that countless thousands of others succumb to insidious job-related diseases not yet discovered by science.

Industry sources estimate that only between 5 and 15 per cent of workers are covered by comprehensive company medical departments, which have the potential for detecting work-related health threats.

Enforceable Federal standards to protect worker health currently exist for only 450 of the estimated 15,000 chemical and physical agents to which workers are exposed, and experts in occupational health say that most of these standards are inadequate and unenforced.

For vinyl chloride, for example, the existing Federal standard is 10 times higher than what most industrial users themselves adopted years ago, and is infinitely higher than the zero exposure level that labor and university scientists recommend.

New standards developed under the Federal law are being promulgated by the Department of Labor's Occupational Safety and Health Administration (O.S.H.A.) at a rate of only one a year. At the same time, industry is introducing some 400 new chemicals each year, nearly all of which are untested for possible long-term effects on the workers who handle them.

There is virtually no testing of combinations of substances that by themselves may be harmless but become deadly when combined, although a leading occupational hazard—asbestos—is known to greatly increase the risk of lung cancer only in workers who smoke cigarettes.

"The long-term effects of the vast majority of chemical and physical agents used in industry have not been proved, and practically no research is being conducted to find out what these effects are," Dr. Jeanne M. Stillman and Dr. Susan M. Daum state in their new book, "Work Is Dangerous to Your Health."

But Dr. Irving J. Selikoff, director of environmental sciences at Mount Sinai School of Medicine, said, "For scientists to worry about what we don't yet know when nothing is being done about what we already know is a cop-out." He noted that even if there were enough data to develop protective standards for all known and potential dangers, the Labor Department would be hard put to enforce them with only 600 Federal inspectors and hygienists to canvass nearly five million workplaces.

During its first eight months, O.S.H.A. inspectors visited 17,743 workplaces. At this rate, it would take them more than 200 years to visit each one once. If the staff were expanded to the original projection of 2,000 it would still take about 50 years to complete the rounds of workplaces.

In thousands of plants throughout the country, workers do not even know what chemicals they work with since, to protect trade secrets, the substances are given only code numbers. And unless a Federal standard exists, the company is not required to monitor worker exposure to noxious agents or to perform periodic medical examinations of those exposed.

"The act has done a great deal to improve the worker's perceptions about the situation, but it hasn't yet done much to improve the situation," said Anthony Mazzocchi, legislative director of the Oil, Chemical and Atomic Workers International Union.

Franklin Wallick of the United Automobile Workers, who wrote a book called, "The American Worker: An Endangered Species," said that for the most part workers are still "the human guinea pigs for industrial processes."

In interviews last week, labor, industry, government and university sources agreed that although the occupational health law was a giant and essential step in the right direction, the realities of current Administration funding have deprived it of much-needed muscle.

Under the act, the National Institute for Occupational Safety and Health (N.I.O.S.H) was set up to survey industrial health problems, conduct needed research and develop new standards for known and potential occupational hazards.

But in the wide bureaucracy of the Department of Health, Education and Welfare, the institute has thus far been treated like an unwanted stepchild.

According to a recent analysis by the Government Accounting Office, a meager budget of about $24-million and a staff limited in size (600) and professional level have severely hampered the institute's potential accomplishments.

As a result, in its first two and a half years, the institute has been able to develop the criteria for only 16 new standards for hazardous materials, although the institute's list of high priority agents exceeds 400.

To handle "emergencies" like vinyl chloride, the institute has been forced to divert funds and personnel from other essential but less immediate tasks, such as developing standards that might head off other vinyl chlorides before workers succumb to their effects.

Last year, the ordinarily sedate and sober director of the institute, Dr. Marcus Key, exploded with exasperation:

"N.I.O.S.H. is not expanding, it is shrinking. It is getting the proverbial meat ax.... Our present laboratory space isn't even adequate for any kind of research. It is substandard.... We have been frozen on hirings for most of our existence, and we are losing key staff right and left because we don't have the grade points to promote them.... I don't think N.I.O.S.H. is a viable organization at this time."

In an interview last week, Dr. Key said the situation had not yet improved. "If anything, it's worse," he remarked.

The institute's efforts are not aided by the fact that occupational health has been virtually ignored by the medical profession, which regards it as a less-than-glamorous specialty. Only a handful of universities have departments of occupational health and fewer than a dozen physicians enter the field each year, the majority becoming company doctors.

The institute also faces the scientific problem of how to determine when a substance is safe. As Dr. E. Cuyler Hammond of the American Cancer Society said:

"Negative results in testing a substance for cancer-producing properties are meaningless, and a clever-enough researcher can make almost anything induce cancer in animals, but his findings may have no relevance to human exposure."

Rather than recommend "safe" exposure levels, Dr. Hammond and Dr. Key believe that industry should adopt protective work practices that eliminate worker exposure to all agents—whether or not they have been proved harmful.

Such work practices were recommended by the institute for 14 cancer-causing industrial chemicals covered by an emergency standard issued last spring. The institute advocates a similar approach to vinyl chloride, a gaseous chemical in the plastics industry that in the last month has been linked to angiosarcoma of the liver, an extremely rare cancer, in nine workers at four different plants.

A further problem in gaining worker protection under the act has been the slowness of the Labor Department in issuing new exposure standards and its reluctance to assume full enforcement responsibilities. Thus far, the institute has acted on only two of the institute's 16 proposed standards — asbestos and carcinogens — and in both cases the action resulted in a weaker standard than the institute had recommended.

Under Administration pressure — and to the distress of occupational health activists — the Labor Department has been seeking to turn enforcement of the Federal regulations back to state occupational safety and health divisions.

Robert E. Nagle, general counsel for the Senate Labor and Public Welfare Committee who is the main author of the Occupational Safety and Health Act, said that the states traditionally have had little interest or expertise in occupational health (as opposed to safety), and that state officials are likely to be more susceptible to pressure from local industry than Federal enforcement agents would.

March 4, 1974

U.S. Banned 11 Coal-Tar-Derivative Dyes Since 1919

Benzyl Violet of FD&C Violet No. 1, which like Red No. 2 is a coal-tar derivative, was abruptly banned by the Food and Drug Administration in April, 1973, after two Japanese studies showed that it caused cancer in female rats.

The F.D.A., which had confined its testing of the color to male rats, certified 20 times as much Violet No. 1 in 1972 as in 1971 because manufacturers had used it to replace Red No. 2 when it came into question.

Dr. Virgil Wodicka of the F.D.A.'s Bureau of Foods said the Japanese studies were convincing enough to dictate an immediate ban on the color, which was used to stamp meat, and in candy, beverages and cakes. The bureau is now doing its own tests on the dye, Dr. Wodicka said, and "if it comes out clean on our tests, then we'll bring Violet No. 1 back."

Since 1919, 11 coal-tar-derivative dyes have been banned because of possible harmful effects; some scientists say that the 11 still remaining on the F.D.A.'s approved list are also suspect.

Five of those banned were found to cause cancer, two caused organ damage and, at high dosages, two caused intestinal lesions, and two caused heart damage.

Two others are presently severely restricted. Citrus Red No. 2 is used only to color the skins of Florida oranges because there is evidence it is a weak carcinogen. The use of Red No. 4, which caused adrenal damage in dogs, is confined to maraschino cherries.

Most of the artificial colorings on the market are coal-tar derivatives. Originally made from compounds derived from coal tar, they are now made with synthetic chemicals identical to the original coal-tar compounds.

Besides Red No. 2, at least one other widely-used coal-tar dye has become controversial. Tartrazine, or FD&C Yellow No. 5, has been proven to cause allergic reactions in some people, especially those who are sensitive to aspirin. Because Tartrazine, whose production has almost doubled in the past 13 years, is sometimes used to disguise products (egg or butter bread look as if they contain more of those ingredients if the coloring is used), it is a special target of consumer groups.

Richard Ronk, head of the F.D.A.'s Department of Color Additives, said that the agency recognizes the studies that have been done on the allergic responses and the recommendations by some scientist that the dye be eliminated from medications that use it for coloring.

He said the F.D.A. has no forseseable plans to restrict it, although it might consider requiring food and drug manufacturers to disclose the presence of the dye on the label.

Tartrazine is found in pickles, gelatin desserts, powdered drink mixes, breakfast cereals, margarine, salt butter, cakes, cake and pudding mixes, candies, noncola soft drinks, puddings and custards and many other yellow-colored products.

December 19, 1974

2 Heart Experts Dispute Personality-Type of Risk

By JANE E. BRODY
Special to The New York Times

MARCO ISLAND, Fla., Jan. 21 —Two leading experts in heart disease challenged today the widely publicized theory of a fellow cardiologist that an aggressive, competitive, impatient personality pattern is the main cause of heart attacks in this country.

The theory was described and defended here today by Dr. Ray H. Rosenman, a cardiologist at Mount Zion Hospital and Medical Center in San Francisco who is co-author with Dr. Meyer Friedman of the recently published book "Type A Behavior and Your Heart."

Dr. Rosenman described the Type A person as someone who is always racing even when he does not have to—an overly concientious, constantly busy, obsessively punctual and highly competitive person who wages a continual battle against time and other people.

His critics — Dr. Jeremiah Stamler, chief of preventive medicine at Northwestern University, and Dr. Richard S. Ross, immediate past president of the American Heart Association who is chief of cardiology at Johns Hopkins University— agreed that Type A behavior patterns may play some role in coronary heart disease.

But they argued that the case for personality as a risk factor had not yet been proved, maintaining that other well-established coronary risks, such as high blood cholesterol, cigarette smoking, high blood pressure, overweight and lack of exercise, are robably more important.

Dr. Ross and Dr. Stamler said that until more was known about the importance of behavior and until widely applicable methods of changing such behavior were found, controlling the other known risks remained the only rational way of trying to curb the nation's current epidemic of heart disease.

"To the extent that [Doctors Rosenman and Friedman] have distorted the issue, they have done a disservice to the public," Dr. Stamler said. He continued:

"We in science have a major responsibility to bring our data to the public carefully and soberly and not in a way to add grist to the mill of selfish interests that want to obscure, obfuscate and bury knowledge, particularly the food and cigarette industries."

Doctor Stamler was referring to the tendency of commercial interests to support theories that detract from public health recommendations that are potentially damaging to sales.

With regard to heart disease, such recommendations have included stopping smoking and cutting back on consumption of fatty meats, dairy products and eggs.

The debate with Dr. Rosenman was conducted here at the American Heart Association's second science writers' forum.

Dr. Ross said he objected to Dr. Rosenman's attempt to push the personality factor by putting down the importance of blood pressure, diet and smoking, all of which are well-established.

In response to questions, Dr. Rosenman said he was "not down-playing the role of other risk factors" but maintaining that these were only "contributory [to] not the primary cause" of the modern epidemic of heart diseas.

He said that his studies, which have been conducted primarily among 3,500 California men who have been followed since 19617, had shown that Type A persons tended to be heavier smokers and have higher cholesterol levels than Type B persons, whom he described as "more relaxed, unhurried and more easily satisfied."

At the meeting, as in the book, Dr. Rosenman insisted that Type A behavior is the "No. 1 cause" of heart attacks, and that 90 per cent of men who have heart attacks before the age of 60 are Type A personalities.

He said that heart disease rarely occurs at such a young age among persons with a Type B personality, regardless of whether they smoke, eat fatty foods or fail to exercise.

However, Dr. Rosenman said, in treating patients, he recommends control of all the known risk factors as well as modfying Type A behavior traits.

Changing Type A behavior is "very difficult," Dr. Rosenman conceded. In an interview, he suggested starting with a personal inventory—"a self-audit of one's aims in life." He said that Type A persons must realize that there is more to life than constant achievement.

"They have to stop rushing around, stop over-committing themselves and eliminate deadlines that are not important," he said, adding that such persons should also train themselves to "relax and do nothing? without feeling guilty.

In his own life, Dr. Rosenman said, he has cut down on the number of patients he sees each day and he has stopped playing golf because his companions had made the game too competitive by "betting on every hole."

January 22, 1975

Drop Reported in Coronary Death Rate

By JANE E. BRODY

New statistics indicate that the nation has passed the peak of an epidemic of coronary heart disease that for decades has taken the lives of an ever-increasing proportion of middle-aged American men, a leading heart expert said yesterday.

The new data suggest that years of public health efforts to change American lifestyles that increase coronary risk have begun to show results.

The drop in the coronary death rate, first noted last year in data from the nineteen-sixties, has continued through 1972, indicating that "the downtrend is real, not a statistical fluke," Dr. Jeremiah B. Stamler concluded after analyzing the new Government statistics.

In essence, the new data mean that a man in his 40's or 50's is less likely to die of a heart attack than his counterpart of a decade ago.

The decline in coronary deaths since the peak rates of the last decade means that "roughly 10,000 lives are being saved each year among persons under age 65," Dr. Stamler said

Coronary heart disease, which accounts for from 80 to 90 per cent of total heart disease mortality in the United States, refers specifically to heart disease caused by severe hardening, or atherosclerosis, of the arteries feeding the heart, as distinguished from diseases like rheumatic heart disease. It is usually manifested by a heart attack.

From 1968 to 1972, the coronary death rate for white men aged 35 to 64 dropped 8.7 per cent, with similar trends for black men and for white and black women, Dr. Stamler reported.

"We're not exactly home free—coronary death rates are still quite high compared to 1950—but it looks as if we're beginning to control the epidemic of premature heart attacks," he added in an interview. "I'm cautiously optimistic that at long last we are over the hump."

Dr. Stamler, an internationally known cardiologist who is chief of preventive medicine at Northwestern University Medical School in Chicago, presented the as yet unpublished statistics on coronary death rates for men and women of different ages and races to the closing session Wednesday of the American Heart Association's science writers' forum in Marco Island, Fla.

These data emerged recently from the computerized records of the National Center for Health Statistics.

Last year, the center released data for the population as a whole that showed that death rates from all diseases of the heart declined during the nineteen-fifties and nineteen-sixties. The data did not distinguish between different categories of heart disease.

A second hint at a decline in heart disease came from a study, published in 1973, of Metropolitan Life Insurance Company policyholders, whose coronary mortality rate in 1972 was only 93 per cent that of previous years. However, most heart experts remained puzzled by the earlier data and were dubious of a turn-around in the epidemic.

Dr. Stamler attributed the apparent downturn in coronary heart disease to significant changes in the heart-attack-inducing habits of Americans and, to a lesser extent, improved health care during recent decades.

A major factor, he said, has probably been the dramatic decline in the percentage of men who smoke cigarettes—from a high of 60 per cent in 1955 to 40 per cent in 1970. During this period, the percentage of women smokers hovered around 30, declining slightly in recent years.

Numerous studies have shown that stopping smoking can begin to reduce a person's risk of death from heart disease within one year after giving up cigarettes. On the average, after five to 10 years, former smokers have half the coronary heart disease rates as those who continue to smoke.

Another factor Dr. Stamler cited is the change in American eating habits, with a decline in saturated fats from animal sources and an increase in polyunsaturated fats from vegetable sources. Saturated fats tend to increase blood levels of artery-clogging cholesterol. He said that studies indicate that the average level of cholesterol found in middle-aged American men has dropped from about 240 milligrams per 100 milliliters of blood in the nineteen-fifties to about 220 now.

Dr. Stamler added that a third coronary risk factor—high blood pressure—had also changed for the better, with 30 per cent or more of high blood pressure victims currently receiving adequate treatment, as against 10 or 15 per cent in the 1960's.

Other possible contributors to the downturn in deaths include the use of heart pacemakers and the widespread establishment of hospital coronary care units. However, since the overwhelming majority of coronary heart disease deaths occur outside the hospital, such changes are thought to have had a relatively small effect on coronary deaths, Dr. Stamler said.

January 24, 1975

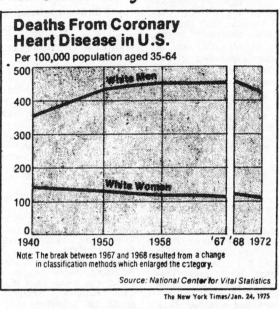

Deaths From Coronary Heart Disease in U.S.

Per 100,000 population aged 35-64

White Men

White Women

1940 — 1950 — 1958 — '67 '68 1972

Note: The break between 1967 and 1968 resulted from a change in classification methods which enlarged the category.

Source: National Center for Vital Statistics

The New York Times/Jan. 24, 1975

Study of Japanese-Americans Indicates Stress Can Be a Major Factor in Heart Disease

By SANDRA BLAKESLEE
Special to The New York Times

BERKELEY, Calif., Aug. 4—A new study indicates that stress, American style, is a major contributing factor in heart disease, a group of epidemiologists announced last week.

In an extensive study of Japanese men living in the San Francisco Bay area, the researchers found that Japanese-Americans who cling to their traditional cultural values have the same low incidence of heart disease as do men in Japan.

But, according to the study, Japanese-Americans who become Westernized in their habits have a heart disease rate two and a half times higher than that of those who live more traditional lives.

Moreover, the study found, those Japanese-Americans who plunge most fully into the American life-style have five times the heart disease rate found in the more traditional group.

Competition and Haste

The stresses of the American way of life, especially competition and haste, seem to account for the differences among groups more than the other major heart disease factors, such as diet, smoking and exercise, the researchers said. While all the factors are important, they added, stress in this study seems to lead the pack.

The study lends some support to the theories espoused by Dr. Meyer Friedman and Dr. Ray Rosenman, both of San Francisco, in their book, "Type A Behavior and Your Heart," published last year. In their book, the doctors said that people with certain personality traits, including "aggressiveness, impatience and a harrying sense of time urgency," are most likely to develop heart disease.

American men have one of the highest heart disease rates in the world. Three hundred fifty of every 100,000 men in the United States die of coronary disease every year, and more than a million have a serious coronary attack every year.

The heart disease rate in Japan is the lowest in the world for an industrialized nation. Only 50 out of every 100,000 Japanese men die each year of coronary diseases.

Why Rates Differ

Dr. Michael G. Marmot, the project director, said the study was undertaken to find out why the rates in coronary disease differed so much between American and Japanese men. Also, the study sought to explain why the rate of heart disease increased so dramatically among Westernized Japanese.

The researchers first looked at several established risk factors in heart disease, including diet, smoking and lack of exercise. According to Dr. Marmot, many researchers had long believed that diet alone would explain the increase in heart disease among Japanese moving to the United States. Stress was considered an unlikely factor, he said, because Japan seemed to be as modernized and hectic as the United States.

In the study, nearly 4,000 Japanese men living in the San Francisco Bay area were given a 24-page questionnaire. They were asked about the number of years spent in Japan, whether they had attended Japanese or American schools, what religion they had practiced while growing up, the ethnic background of their friends, and their wives' cultural background. All were given comprehensive physical examinations.

2 Groups Selected

From their answers, the Japanese men were divided into traditional and nontraditional groups.

The nontraditional group, the researchers observed, seemed to have adopted the characteristic American cultural traits of being competitive, aggressive and impatient.

The traditional group, on the other hand, apparently kept to Japanese cultural norms of staying within a close-knit group, living quiet lives and being noncompetitive.

In Japan, groups may compete but individuals generally do not, Dr. Marmot said. Thus, individuals in the Japanese culture undergo much less stress than Americans.

When the data on Japanese-Americans were finally analyzed, the researchers said, a clear relationship emerged between heart disease and the degree of change from Japanese customs to American lifestyles.

The researchers then set out to discover which factors in life-style played the most important role in heart disease.

Diet Not a Factor

To their surprise, they said, they found that differences in diet did not prove to be the main factor. When comparing Japanese in Japan and Japanese in the United States who had equivalent high-fat diets, the men in Japan still had a lower rate of heart disease than Japanese-Americans.

Dr. Marmot said the research group also studied the usual coronary risk factors of smoking, cholesterol, blood pressure and weight. Again, none of these risks established a pattern that could completely explain the increased rate of heart disease among Japanese-Americans.

Heading the project with Dr. Marmot are S. Leonard Syme, professor of epidemiology, and Warren Winkelstein Jr., dean of the school of public health.

The study is being funded by the National Institutes of Health, the American Heart Association and the Bay Area Heart Association. The current findings are about to be submitted for scientific publication.

August 5, 1975

NEW DATA LINK CANCER AND DIET

By JANE E. BRODY

Cancer specialists are finding increasing evidence that ingredients of the daily diet may be causing, directly or indirectly, half of all cancers among women and 30 percent of those among men.

The evidence, in a 300-page report published this week in the November issue of the journal Cancer Research, suggests that nutritional factors — including a diet high in animal fat, excessive alcohol intake, deficiencies in vitamins A and C, certain food additives and natural as well as man-made contaminants of food—are related to the development of cancer of the colon, stomach, esophagus, breast, liver and uterus.

These hints have sparked a new research program sponsored by the National Cancer Institute, which expects to spend between $4 million and $6 million this year toward further investigation of the links between died and cancer

Although this effort is relatively minor compared with other institute research programs (more than $50 million is spent annually to explore the links between viruses and cancer, for example), it represents an unmistakable revival of interest in a long-neglected aspect of cancer causes. Some research was focused on the relationship between diet and cancer in the 1940's and early 1950's, but it fell by the wayside in recent decades when more specific items such as viruses and cancer-causing chemicals captured research attention.

Recent studies, while emphasizing the complexities of the nutrition and cancer picture, nevertheless suggest that a large portion of the cancer problem around the world—and especially in the United States—may be preventable by making certain modifications in the diet.

These studies were outlined at a closed conference held last May in Key Biscayne, Fla., by the National Cancer Institute and the American Cancer Society. The new report contains the proceedings of that conference.

"Nutritional factors are harder to pinpoint than, say, a chemical like vinyl chloride, but they seem to affect the major types of human cancers," according to Dr. Ernst L. Wynder, epidemiologist at the American Health Foundation here, who was chairman of the May conference.

Thus far it appears that, for the most part, nutritional factors have an indirect cancer-causing effect, setting the stage for the action of other more direct carcinogens. Some nutrients may enhance the activity of carcinogens or act as carriers of carcinogens to their site of action.

Other nutritional factors, such as animal fat, may change the body's hormone pattern, increasing the output of hormones that are cancer-causing. The diet may also work by changing digestive microbes, resulting in the formation of cancer-causing metabolites.

In addition, some foods contain substances that are directly cancer-causing such as pesticide residues, certain food additives, trace elements picked up from the soil, and a poison called aflatoxin produced by a mold.

Overnutrition—the consumption of too much of certain foodstuffs as well as too many calories—and undernutrition—the deficiency of some vitamins and trace elements—have also been found to increase the risk of developing various cancers.

The findings and suggestions presented in the report that have direct implications for the prevention of human cancer include the following:

¶Cancer of the colon, the most common life-threatening cancer among Americans, is related to an "affluent" diet, particularly the excessive consumption of animal fats and the relatively low consumption of fibrous foods. For example, a study of Seventh-day Adventists showed that those who at one time ate meat had two to three times the risk of developing colon cancer as those who were strict vegetarians all their lives.

¶Breast cancer has been linked to a fatty diet in human studies and in animal experiments. Throughout the world there is a five-fold to ten-fold difference in the death rate from breast cancer between countries with low-fat diets and those with high-fat diets, such as the typical American diet. It is thought the rich diet in the United States overstimulates the body's hormonal system "producing the same effect that one would obtain running a diesel engine on high-octane airplane fuel," Dr. John Berg of the University of Iowa told the conference. The hormones, in turn, overstimulate the breast tissue and may set the stage for cancer.

¶Nitrates which are used to preserve certain foods, including some meats and fish, and contaminate food plants grown on heavily fertilized soils, may be an indirect cause of stomach cancer. Stomach cancer is ex-

ceedingly common in Japan, where preserved foods are frequently consumed, and in parts of South America where the soil is rich in nitrate. The disease has become increasingly less common in the United States. Dr. John Weisburger of the American Health Foundation has found that refrigeration inhibits the conversion of

nitrates into potential cancer-causing substances.

¶Certain substances, including vitamin A and vitamin C, the trace element selenium and the artificial preservatives BHA and BHT, inhibit the action of cancer - causing chemicals and thus may help protect against the development of cancer.

The heavy consumption of alcohol is associated with a greatly increased risk of developing cancer of the esophagus. In this case, the alcohol is thought to work indirectly, causing certain nutritional deficiencies that enhance the action of carcinogens like tobacco smoke.

December 3, 1975

Physicians' Views Unchanged On Use of Estrogen Therapy

By JANE E. BRODY

Gynecologists around the country indicated in a spot check yesterday that the new reports linking estrogen therapy during and after menopause to an increased risk of uterine cancer have had little effect on the doctors' attitudes toward the drug or their treatment of patients who take it.

Each of the dozen doctors in private practice questioned pointed out that the reports, published this week in The New England Journal of Medicine, did not prove that the estrogens, which are given to alleviate the symptons and aftereffects of the menopause, directly cause cancer. In the absence of such proof, they said, no drastic change in practice is warranted.

Those doctors who have been liberal in their prescription of estrogens, giving them to virtually all menopausal women for indefinite periods, said that in their views the benefits of the hormones still outweigh the risks.

The doctors who traditionally have been more conservative in prescribing estrogens, restricting them to women with severe menopausal symptoms, for a period of one to four years, said that the drug is clearly useful for such women even

if it may increase their risk of developing cancer of the endometrium, or lining of the uterus.

However, all the doctors interviewed emphasized that every patient treated with estrogens should be thoroughly examined every six months and that if a postmenopausal woman experiences vaginal bleeding while taking the drug, she should receive an endometrial biopsy or a D and C, to check for possible cancer.

The doctors said that semi-annual checkups should include a breast and pelvic exam, Pap smear (which can detect about two-thirds of endometrial cancers) and blood pressure check.

"Everything in life is a tradeoff—there are risks and benefits and you must weigh one against the other," remarked Dr. Frederick H. Berman, a San Francisco gynecologist.

Dr. Malcolm Margolin, a Beverly Hills gynecologist, said, "When we drive the freeways here we take a risk in order to get there faster." But he and most of the other doctors questioned said that the patient should participate in the evaluation of benefit versus risk and that such participation meant that the women must be told of the possible hazards of estrogen

therapy.

Increased Risk

The journal reports said that menopausal and post-menopausal women who take estrogens (the vast majority take a drug called Premarin, produced by Averst Laboratories from the urine of pregnant horses) face a 5 to 14 times increased risk of developing endometrial cancer.

Various cancer registries have reported that this disease has been rising in frequency greatly in recent years. Doctors say that the increase has occurred not in the typical kinds of endometrial cancer patients— women in the 60's or 70's who are obese, diabetic or have high blood pressure— but in younger, slender otherwise healthy women.

Most of the new victims of the disease are women in the upper socio-economic brackets, those most likely to be treated with replacement estrogens.

The sales of estrogens, which are prescribed to replace the hormones that the ovaries stop producing at menopause, have quadrupled since 1972. While some women take estrogens only to relieve such menopausal symptoms as night sweats, hot flashes and insomnia or postmenopausal vaginal dis-

comfort, others take the drug for years in the hopes of delaying the aging process. There is no proof, however, that estrogens can keep women youthful forever.

"I think of the menopause as a deficiency disease, like diabetes," said Dr. Rubin Clay, a San Francisco gynecologist. "Most women develop some symptoms whether they are aware of them or not, so I prescribe estrogens for virtually all menopausal women for an indefinite period."

However, Dr. Clay added, he has lowered the dosage for some women who requested it and before he prescribes the drug for a newly menopausal patient he discusses the new findings with her.

Another physician who prescribes estrogens routinely for menopausal patients, Dr. Brandon C. Chenault of San Antonio, Tex., said he simply reassured his patients who are worried about the cancer report that the findings were "highly preliminary" and that he did not believe "there's much in it."

Dr. John B. Martin of St. Louis said he was already conservative in prescribing estrogens but that in light of the new findings, he would be even more reluctant to place a new patient on replacement estrogens. However, he said, he does not intend to stop using the drug for women who are already taking it.

December 5, 1975

U.S. Finds Nation Is Generally Healthy

By NANCY HICKS

WASHINGTON, Jan. 12 — The Federal Government said today in its first comprehensive report on the state of health of Americans that the population was generally healthy but the American life style continued

to be a major health hazard.

"The data suggest that much improvement in health status could come from individual action," said Dr. Theodore Cooper, Assistant Secretary for Health, whose staff prepared the report.

Excessive use of alcohol and tobacco and the lack of proper exercise and diet contribute heavily to cancer, heart and respiratory ailments, kidney and liver disease and accidents (a major killer among young people), according to the fig-

ures gathered by the Department of Health, Education and Welfare.

The infant mortality rate declined from 29.2 per 1,000 live births in 1950 to an estimated 16.5 in 1974, the report said. Even with the drop in the United States, there still are 14 other countries with lower infant death rates.

Deaths from heart disease are falling, the report said, and life expectancy has risen by almost four years since 1950.

At the same time, cancer deaths and chronic and venereal diseases are on the rise, according to the report.

The three-volume report, entitled "Health, United States, 1975," was required by law. This first annual report to Congress and the President attempted to merge health statistics with figures on population trends and health costs so that planners and policymakers could make decisions with some knowledge of potential impact.

While the trends for particular diseases may not be new—infant mortality rates have been falling for years—their presentation together gave a more complete view of health and how well the health care system functions.

"The report shows considerable achievement as well as need for improvement," Dr. Cooper said.

"Virtually every area touched upon is marked with contrasts. For example, the death rate for heart disease among persons aged 55 to 64 dropped almost 15 percent over the past six years. In the same age group, the death rate from cancer rose almost 4 percent.

"Among younger people, accidents and homicide are major causes of death," he said.

The report said in the nonwhite population the infant death rate was almost twice that of whites.

White women are expected to live to be 75.9 years old and nonwhite women 72 years, according to the report. For men, the gap is greater between races, reflecting socioeconomic factors, the report says.

Nonwhite males have a life expectancy about five years lower than the 67.4 year average of white males.

The increasing life expectancy is producing an increasingly elderly population that suffers from a number of chronic diseases, such as arthritis and diabetes, which should receive better medical management, the report said.

The findings also show that despite the continuing rise in health care costs, the use of health services by poor people has increased. Twenty-eight percent of poor people had not seen a physician within two years in 1964. The number fell to 17 percent in 1974.

"As a people, we are receiving more medical care now than 10 years ago, and we have made considerable progress in lowering the income barrier to care," Dr. Cooper said in a statement.

Yet, the poor pay a disproportionate share of their income for health services, the report said. About 13 percent of the income of families earning less than $2,000 a year goes to health care. For most families, however, insurance companies pay two-thirds of those health costs—a reversal since 1950, when individuals paid that much.

While access to care has improved, and the number of physicians practicing "has been growing far more rapidly than the population," the uneven distributions of those doctors and the clumping of physicians in similar specialties has not meant ready access to everyone, the report said.

The report, which will be published Feb. 1, was prepared by the National Center for Health Statistics and the National Center for Health Services Research, all parts of the Public Health Service, which Dr. Cooper heads.

January 13, 1976

Cancer Death Rate Rose in 1974 and 1975

By HAROLD M. SCHMECK Jr.

WASHINGTON, March 5 — Government experts on health statistics now estimate that the United States death rate from cancer rose more sharply last year than in any previous year since World War II.

The new estimate, based on more complete figures, is for an increase less dramatic than one indicated by early figures available late last year and then somewhat discounted. But the situation is highly unusual and is made even more so by the fact that the 1974 increase in cancer death rate was also abnormally large.

No one knows what these rises mean or how long the trend will continue, if at all. Specialists are intensely interested in such figures, however, because the large majority of human cancers are believed to depend on environmental factors. Changes in the death rate could be viewed as a case in which nature is trying to tell the human race something for its own good.

Complete figures for 1975 are not yet available, but specialists at the National Center for Health Statistics estimate that the rise in the death rate from 1974 to 1975 will be 2 to 3 percent, and perhaps even slightly above 3 percent. The provisional figure for the year through November was 3.2 percent, but this rate of increase is expected to drop somewhat when the full year's figures are analyzed.

The increase from 1973 to 1974 was 1.9 percent. The rate at which people die of cancer has steadily increased for many years. Not since 1950 has the increase in the cancer death rate gone as high as 2 percent, the center's figures show. It has not risen above 2 percent since 1945, when the increase over the previous year was 4 percent.

Specialists believe the World War II figures may be somewhat distorted, however. Millions of young men and women were overseas and were not used in calculating the resident death rate. Since more older people than young ones die of cancer, the wartime situation would favor an apparently high death rate.

The 2 percent figure was exceeded several times in the late 1930's, and in 1948. The latter case, however, results partly from a change in the statisticians' classification of cancer and did not represent a true picture of a changing death rate.

Specialists at the center do not take an alarmist view of the new high rates of increase. Whatever factors influenced the 1975 death rate were likely to be multiple and diverse and were probably exerting their influence 20 years or more ago. Many cancers are believed to take decades to develop.

The cancer death rate represents the number of persons per 100,000 of the population who die of cancer during a given year. For 1974, the latest year for which complete figures are available, the rate was 170.5 per 100,000.

Robert J. Armstrong, chief of the national center's mortality statistics branch, said today that cancer was the only leading cause of death for which the death rate has been steadily increasing in recent decades.

Over the last two decades, the rate of increase has been about 1 percent a year on the average, according to the national center's figures. A substantial part of this is attributed to the increasing average age of the population. The rest of the annual rise is of unknown cause. It is the "unknown" part that is of great public health interest.

In recent years there has been a cyclical pattern, Mr. Armstrong said, in which a relatively sharp rise would be seen one year, followed by a lull involving hardly any rise the next.

The reason for these cycles is unknown, but the center's experts believe the pattern of rise and fall in influenza incidence is probably a contributing factor. Their theory is that flu is likely to weaken persons already near death from a chronic disease such as cancer and thus hasten deaths that might otherwise have occurred weeks or months later.

Provisional monthly figures from the National Center for Health Statistics began to show unusually high rates early in 1975. When figures for the first seven months of the year became available, the rise in rate appeared to be 5.2 percent—a dramatic increase. Earlier figures covering shorter portions of the year had shown even higher apparent rates.

The 52 percent figure was published without comment in November in a routine monthly vital-statistics report of the center. The startling size of the increase immediately brought much publicity to the figure and speculation as to the causes of the rise. In January, a biostatistician of the National Cancer Institute gave a talk to the institute staff on the subject, emphasizing that the seemingly dramatic trend for part of the year was returning toward normal as more and more months were added.

He described the seemingly threatened one-year rise of 5.2 percent as "the increase that wasn't there."

While that great an increase has not occurred over the full year, the final figure is nevertheless expected to be far above the trend experienced during recent decades.

"We will certainly be watching the monthly figures in 1976 with great interest," one expert said.

March 6, 1976

PREVENTIVE MEDICINE AND PUBLIC HEALTH

MICROBES IN THE MILK.

As Many as 516,000,000 Bacteria Per Cubic Centimeter Found in Milk Used In This City.

Members of the Medical Society of the County of New York met last evening in regular session at the New York Academy of Medicine at 17 West Forty-third Street. President George B. Fowler was in the chair.

The chief interest of the meeting was the report of the Milk Commission appointed in January, 1900, consisting of Drs. Henry Dwight Chapin, Abraham Jacobi, W. L. Carr, and Joseph E. Winters.

The report was read by Dr. Chapin, the Chairman of the committee. He first spoke of what the committee had done, having made over 800 bacteriological tests, thirty visits to farms, many of them more than 200 miles from the city, and having had two conferences with milk dealers.

"From a chemical point of view," he said, " we found the milk good. Out of twenty samples which we examined all showed at least 4 per cent., and some 5 per cent., of fat, while the law requires but 3 per cent. So we devoted our attention to the bacteriological conditions of milk and the question as to its proper handling and preservation.

"It has seemed wise to establish a standard of cleanliness for a bacteria standard to which dealers must conform. The standard prescribed by the commission is that the acidity must not be higher than 3 per cent. and that the milk must not contain more than 30,000 germs or bacteria of any kind per cubic centimeter, and that butter fat must reach 3.5 per cent.

"The amount of bacteria in the milk used in the city is something alarming. Out of twenty samples examined on a Winter day, Nov. 19, the lowest was 90,000 germs and the highest 2,280,000, while on June 29, with the thermometer at 90 degrees, out of twenty samples examined the lowest contained 240,000 and the highest 516,000,000 per cubic centimeter. The prevalence of bacteria, to a great extent, arises from the dirt in the milk.

" There are seven conditions on which the amount of bacteria depends—the cleanliness of the barn, condition of the cow, condition of the milker, condition of the utensils, the cooling process, the transportation, and the cleaning of the milk bottles before they are returned."

Aeration, he said, is not a success to-day as used by the ordinary farmer. In good hands it might work all right, but in many cases as at present used it resulted in an increase of germs.

The three things which are absolutely necessary to secure milk comparatively free from germs are strict cleanliness, rapid and sufficient cooling, and thorough icing of milk until it reaches the consumers.

In the transportation of milk, ordinary freight cars should not be used, and the ends of the cars should be kept closed, thus preventing the heated air from passing through the car and breeding the germs.

The railroads could be asked to co-operate and furnish refrigerating cars in which the milk could be kept constantly on ice, and after being unloaded it should be re-iced before reaching the dealers.

The Milk Commissioners, he said, agree to guarantee or certify the milk of all dealers desiring such certificates, a special label having been printed for this purpose.

Officers for the ensuing year were nominated as follows:

President—Dr. Frank Van Fleet.
First Vice President—Dr. Charles N. Dowd.
Second Vice President—Robert Lewis, Jr.
Treasurer—Dr. E. W. Peet.
Secretary—Dr. John Vandoren Young.
Assistant Secretary—Dr. E. P. Fowler.
Censors—Dr. George B. Fowler, Dr. H. S. Sterns, Dr. Wendell C. Phillips, Dr. Robert F. Morris, and Dr. James F. McKernon.

One hundred and seventy-five delegates were elected to the State Medical Society and a committee was appointed to arrange for a reception to the State Society when it meets at the Academy of Medicine here for its semi-annual session, Oct. 15 and 16.

September 24, 1901

CANNED FOODS DENOUNCED.

Members of Medical Association Blame Them for Many Ills.

Foods and nutrition were the subjects of a series of addresses given at a meeting of the Medical Association of New York, held in Hosack Hall, 17 West Forty-third Street, last night, by some widely known physicians and surgeons. The general opinion was that canned meats and vegetables were highly injurious to the human system and should be strictly avoided by those who esteem their health. In his remarks on preserved foods containing chemicals, Dr. Harvey W. Wiley, Chief of the Bureau of Chemistry, United States Department of Agriculture, said: "Some scientists tell us that teeth are now no longer necessary, as the new methods of preparing food have done away with mastication. When some other scientists discover the hunger microbe, we shall reduce the cost of living to a minimum.

" In the last 25 years it has been quite unusual to find any preserved animal or vegetable foods free from chemicals. My investigations into the effect these drugs have upon nutrition is distinctly unfavorable to their use. Chemicals have no taste and do not reveal themselves, and are often eaten without knowledge of the consumer.

"We ought to be able to choose our food," continued Dr. Wiley, " the same as we do our politics and religion. The introduction of chemicals into food without the knowledge of the consumer is a crime. When taken in food for a long time these chemicals are prejudicial to health and digestion. They cause loss of appetite, weight, and malaria, and are unnecessary. Kidney disease is very much on the increase in this country, and all these chemicals act directly upon the kidneys, especially borax, which is one of the drugs most commonly used in canned goods.

" Let us keep the pharmacopoeia out of the family groceries."

Col. Valery Harvard, M. D., Assistant Surgeon General, United States Army, said that on a black bread and meat diet the Russian soldiers had enjoyed excellent health in the Far East, and the percentage of deaths from disease had been less than those from wounds in battle, for the first time in the world's history.

Major Louis L. Seaman, M. D., late First Surgeon First Regiment of Engineers, United States Volunteers, denounced can goods as the cause of dysentery and catarrh among the troops in Cuba in '98. He said that his regiment lost five tons in weight in that Summer in Cuba and Porto Rico.

Prof. La Fayette B. Mendel of Yale University, said that man could exist on a strictly vegetable régime, but in his opinion a mixed diet of meat and vegetables was best for the human system. In regulating diet it was best to regulate quantity rather than kind. The chair was taken by Dr. Thomas Satherwaite and the hall was well filled with members of the medical profession, a number of them women.

Dr. Carl Van Noorden, the eminent German physician, who was present at the meeting, was called upon by the Chairman for a speech. He said that America was ahead of the whole world in the study of nutrition. He said that the work of the Department of Agriculture was without an equal.

October 10, 1905

RESULTS OF THE FIGHT AGAINST FOOD AND DRUG FAKERS

What the Courts Have Done With Adulterators and Misbranders Since Dr. Wiley Began His Crusade---Almost Everything Edible or Drinkable Affected by the Decisions.

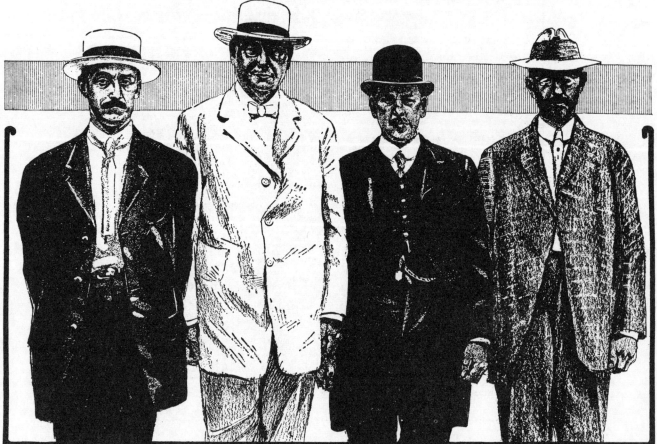

Dr. H. W. Wiley and His Associates. From Left to Right Are L. F. Kebler, Chief of the Bureau of Drugs; Dr. Wiley, Dr. H. H. Rusby, Chief of the Bureau of Chemistry, and W. W. Bigelow, Assistant Chief of the Bureau of Chemistry.

NOW that the searchlights are to be turned on Dr. Harvey W. Wiley, Chief Chemist of the Department of Agriculture, and on those who have been after his scalp for several years and seem now to have some chance to make good, because of what at worst is a technical infraction of a rule that has been broken thousands of times in every other Government Department, a glance at the concrete work that he has accomplished will be of interest.

While a great deal of publicity has been given to the pure food law regulations, and many of the more important cases which have been decided under them have been written up at some length, yet it is doubtful whether the public generally is well informed as to the manner in which the law has worked out and the direct and immediate benefits which have resulted to the consumer from its enforcement.

By direct benefits is meant the effect of the judgments obtained in specific cases of inter-State shipments—the only ones to which the pure food law is applicable—in the Supreme Court of the District of Columbia and the various United States District Courts before which criminal information was laid, with reference merely to the subject matter directly in-

volved and without regard to the future deterrent results of the judgments.

The decisions of the courts in the cases brought before them as a result of the activities of the Board of Food and Drug Inspection are published by the Government in a series of pamphlets, issued by the Department of Agriculture, pursuant to Section 4 of the pure food and drug law, as " Notices of Judgment." The board is composed of Dr. Harvey W. Wiley, Chief Chemist; Frederick E. Dunlap, Associate Chemist, and George P. McCabe, Solicitor—the two latter being now active in their opposition to Dr. Wiley, it is stated.

The first of these pamphlets was issued on May 2, 1908, the judgment, which covered a case of misbranding of apple cider to which sugar had been added to increase the alcoholic content, being rendered on April 22, 1908. No. 894, which ordered the destruction of a tomato paste as putrid, filthy, and decomposed and unfit for human consumption, is dated May 21, 1911, and was issued on June 16, 1911. That is, the Board of Food and Drug Inspection has in the short space of three years and twenty-seven days presented to the courts 894 distinct cases.

As might have been expected, there were more cases of adulteration than of any other offense, 401 matters of this na-

ture having come up. Misbranding by the use of false statements as to the contents or effect of the article, particularly in the case of drug products and preparations, was the cause of complaint in 273 instances; misbranding as to the quality of the goods occupied the attention of the board 130 times; misbranding as to the place of manufacture or origin of the article was the least common, occurring only 56 times in the entire list, and there were 75 cases of shortage in quantity.

Speaking generally, the courts imposed 490 fines, amounting in the aggregate to $21,296.01, and ranging from $500 for a so-called " headache cure," which was both misbranded and adulterated, to a fine of 1 cent as a penalty for a shortage in weight of two dozen cans of peas. In addition to the two fines mentioned, there were three of $400 each, sixteen of $200, one of $185, eight of $150, three of $125, fifty-seven of $100, four of $3, and six of $1 each, the balance ranging from $5 to $75, the greater number being fines of $10 or $25. Costs were assessed in every instance of the 1,206, and the amount ranged apparently from $11 upward, but it is given in so few instances that the total cannot even be estimated.

But it is when one comes to examine the individual cases and groups of cases affecting the same food or drug product that the great value of the work of the board becomes more readily apparent. In 1,000 of these cases there were, of course, many duplications of the same offense, and sometimes by the same offender.

Taking up the food products first, for there is the greatest general interest in them, it appears that all of the shortages, most of the adulteration, and not a little of the misbranding affected articles of daily consumption. For instance, there were 100 separate cases of milk brought, as were all the others, on "criminal information" laid before the courts by or through the board. In most of these the only adulterant used was water, and the abstraction of the butter fats, and a small fine was imposed as a warning. Five of the dealers were twice before the courts, and one of them came up four times. In only two cases, however, did the board discover the use of any chemical preservative, and in these cases, where the presence of formaldehyde was detected, fines of $100 were imposed, as was also done in one instance where it was felt that entirely too much water had been used.

There were two cases of powdered milk, two of milk flour, and two of condensed milk considered, but in these cases only small fines were levied, and the goods released under bond to be properly relabeled before being sold. In twenty-two cases where cream was the subject matter, the general complaint was the absence of butter fats, and the adulteration with water or skim milk. Small fines, the largest being $50, were imposed, and the goods ordered destroyed, no quantity being mentioned in the judgment.

Next to milk the most popular single article for adulteration and misbranding seems to have been vinegar, for there were 78 judgments affecting this article, seven of the manufacturers being before the courts twice each, three of them three times, and two of them no less than four times apiece. Fines of $100 each were assessed against three of the offenders who were guilty of both misbranding and adulteration. Acetic acid and citric acid were the favorite adulterants, and "Pure Cider Vinegar" and "Apple Cider Vinegar" the favorite forms of misbranding. Considerable of this vinegar, 140 barrels in all, was ordered destroyed, the rest being released on bond, to be properly relabeled before sale.

Flavoring extracts, considered as one subject, required 106 judgments to dispose of, and these present some curious features. In 52 instances the adulterated and misbranded article was passing as lemon, in 30 as vanilla, in 8 as strawberry, in 7 as orange, while almond, banana, peach, peppermint, pineapple, raspberry, rose, and wintergreen appeared only once each. One fine of $400 covering several kinds of extract, one of $200, and thirteen fines of $100 each were imposed on manufacturers of these alleged extracts; and in only four instances did the same manufacturer appear a second time. The adulterants were many and various, and most of the alleged extracts were the basest kind of an imitation, being colored artificially as well as having the flavor chemically faked. In one case the "Compound Lemon Flavoring" was made up of an "imitation lemon flavoring, containing no oil of lemon," and "a dye, known as naphthol yellow S." This flavoring, so the label stated, was "a compound prepared from oil of lemon grass, citral and diluted alcohol." The quantity of these imitation extracts destroyed is not given, but was undoubtedly very considerable.

In forty-eight cases eggs were decided to be a fit subject for absolute condemnation. Four fines of $200 each and one of $150 were imposed on the worst offenders, and in every instance the eggs were seized and ordered destroyed as being filthy, putrid, decomposed, and unfit for human consumption. The total of fines for bad eggs was $985, and costs were collected, of course, in each of the forty-eight cases; two of the offenders repeated their offense twice each, one of

them three times, and one of them was hailed up by the board on four separate occasions. The eggs were declared in every instance to be full of bacteria and streptococci and absolutely unfit for food purposes. The following shows the quantity ordered destroyed:

Plain eggs, 4,560 dozen.
Frozen eggs, 319 tubs, 10 cases, 3,700 pounds.
Liquid eggs, 877 cans or 52,260 pounds.
Desiccated eggs, 27 drums, 16 barrels.
Crystal eggs, 2 barrels.
Evaporated eggs, 1 barrel, 10,080 pounds.

A fair estimate of the eggs thus destroyed would be 84,000 dozen, or about 2,800 cases, and the value of these, figured from the consumer's average price at the present time, would be $25,200.

Out of the forty-one cases of syrup of all kinds that demanded and received the attention of the board and the courts, nineteen were so-called maple syrup of various brands and the other twenty-two included ordinary and fruit syrups. Four makers had to face the courts on two occasions each, and one of them three times, the remaining twenty-seven cases involving as many different makers. Fines of $100 each were imposed in five instances, all for adulteration either as to artificial coloring, imitation of chemical fruit flavoring, or the use of glucose. Mere misbranding was common, but was largely confined to the use of the words "Pure Maple" on syrups that were never nearer the real maple sap than perhaps to be packed in a barrel that had a maple stave. No syrups were ordered destroyed, and in most of the cases the goods were released under bond and only a fine of the costs imposed.

Feeds of various kinds, mainly for chickens or horses, were the subject of consideration by the courts on thirty-nine occasions; in three instances the same makers were haled up twice, and one manufacturer tried it a third time. Only one fine of any amount was imposed and that was $150 in a case where some chicken feed was both adulterated and misbranded. A large quantity of horse feed was destroyed as being unfit for food purposes, but in a majority of the thirty-nine cases the feed was released to the maker or owner under a proper bond that it would be correctly labeled as to its compositions and not sold as originally put out.

In thirty-six cases there was trouble over olive oil, it being either adulterated or misbranded, or both. Five of the packers were before the courts twice. Most of the cases were those of adulteration by the use of cottonseed oil, and in at least one instance the cottonseed oil was not only the chief adulterant, but constituted the only substance in the barrels involved, there being no olive oil in the entire shipment complained of. Many of the cases were also misbranded as to place of origin, the idea being conveyed that it was imported olive oil. Two fines of $200 each and seven of $100 were the heaviest penalties imposed, with costs in every case, of course, and in addition the goods involved were only released under heavy bonds; 330 gallons of oil were ordered destroyed as unfit for food purposes, and some of it was ordered reshipped abroad.

There were twenty-eight cases where canned corn was the subject matter before the court, two packers having two complaints each against them and two others three each. These goods were mainly misbranded as to weight, the shortage ranging from five to eleven ounces in a can supposed to contain two pounds. One lot of 850 cases was found to be adulterated by the use of saccharin instead of sugar, but were released under bond, to be properly relabeled before sale. One fine of $200 and one of $100 was imposed, and costs were taxed in every instance. The shortage, as shown by the table printed elsewhere, was exceedingly heavy.

In each of the twenty-three judgments affecting cheese, of which one firm had

two and another three cases, the complaint was misbranding, the great majority of the cases being a question of weight, and the cheese showing a shortage of about 3 per cent. There were also a few cases of misbranding as to place of origin, but none as to quality. But one fine of any amount, $125, was imposed, and but one lot of cheese was ordered destroyed, this being a case where sodium borate was used as a preservative in forty-two cases of a so-called "imperial" cheese.

Coffee was another fruitful subject, there being twenty-five judgments concerning it, and three firms having two cases each. The complaint was almost invariably misbranding, and particularly as to the country of origin. Almost every packer haled up by the board had put the goods on the market as "Mocha and Java," or used these names in some form or other, whereas with but one exception the coffees were Brazilian grown and contained neither Mocha nor Java. In only one instance was there any real adulteration, and only one lot of coffee was ordered destroyed, that being because the beans were found to be coated with lead chromate, a poison.

Apples, canned and evaporated, occupied the attention of the board and the courts in seventeen instances, and forty-two boxes of evaporated apples were ordered destroyed as being filthy and unfit for human consumption. But two of the packers repeated their offense.

Canned vegetables, that is, peas, beans, and tomatoes, were the subject of thirty judgments, eighteen of them being devoted to tomatoes, eight to peas, and four to beans. No other vegetable, except corn, which is referred to above, appears in the list. These were practically all cases of misbranding as to shortage in weight, only one lot, that of a shipment of 2,000 cases of tomatoes, being found to be unfit for consumption as a food product because they were filthy and decomposed, and this lot was ordered destroyed. Only one packer was complained of twice, his cases both being shortages in weight, and there were no large fines levied, the goods, with the exception noted, being released under bond.

Canned fruit, including apricots, blackberries, blueberries, cherries, pears, pineapple, and plums came up for examination in thirty-eight cases, and again the main question involved was one of shortage in weight, save in one instance, where nineteen cases of pineapple from Hawaii were condemned for destruction as being filthy, decomposed, putrid, and unfit for human consumption.

Jams, jellies and preserves, grouped together for the purpose of this article, account for thirty-eight notices of judgment. In this group three manufacturers had two cases each, one had three cases, and another came up even for the fourth time. The offense in every case but one was misbranding so as to represent a perfectly good apple jelly as being made of some other fruit.

Flour came in for some considerable notice on the part of the board, and there were enough instances of adulteration, largely in the case of wheat flour by bleaching processes, and of misbranding, with two small cases of shortage, to bring the total up to thirty-five cases. Of these nineteen were wheat flour, eleven buckwheat, three rye, and two corn flour.

No fines were imposed in these cases, and the flour was ordered destroyed only in two instances of bleaching, the goods in all the other cases being released under bond. But one offender appeared a second time. The question of the bleaching process was fought out at considerable length, and one of the largest of the pamphlets is devoted to a decision and a review of the evidence taken in that matter. The subject has been written up at length several times, and the final decision was against the use of dioxide fumes as a bleaching agent.

In two of the twenty-two cases involving

oats fines of $100 were imposed. These cases were all of adulteration, barley, chaff, weed seeds, &c., being used to fill out the quantity. There was some misbranding. Two of the offenders appeared twice each, and one of them four times.

Black pepper was probably the most completely and variously adulterated article in the entire list of food products. There were thirteen cases before the courts and none of the offenders returned a second time. Only two fines of $100 each were imposed, but quite a lot of so-called pepper was destroyed, though the notices of judgment are silent as to the exact quantity. The list of adulterants is a long one, and includes cracker crumbs, ground nutshells, ground fruit pits, wheat meal, flaxseed meal, wheat flour, as well as cocoatnut shells, leguminous seeds, and coffee.

Because of the presence of worms and other filthy and decomposed matter in the packages 522 boxes of raisins which the board examined, and on which they laid an information with the court, were ordered destroyed as unfit for human consumption in the twelve actions involving that article. These goods were all from the same packer. No large fines were imposed on the raisin men, the general complaint being misbranding as to place of origin, and the goods, except as above stated, were released under bond.

The packers of currants were not so fortunate as the raisin men, because while they only had four cases before the courts 302 packages and 6 barrels were found to be so wormy and generally filthy and decomposed as to render them unfit for food purposes, and as a consequence they were ordered to be destroyed. Here again the fines imposed were small ones, the costs being far the greater portion of the penalty other than the loss of the goods.

Practically the most guilty packers and manufacturers whom the board hauled before the courts were the packers of tomato ketchup or catsup. As will be seen by the table given below, a very large quantity of this article was ordered to be destroyed. It was found to be filthy, putrid, made of decomposed vegetable matter, to contain chemical preservatives, to be filled with bacteria, and to be utterly unfit for food purposes of any kind. Only two of the packers had the temerity to appear a second time, and one fine of $150, which was imposed in a particularly flagrant case, appeared to have a good effect. There were twenty-three judgments on this product.

Fish, including herring, sardines, and "Italian" codfish, formed the subject of eighteen decisions altogether. Much of this was misbranded, as well as adulterated; the bulk of it was destroyed as unfit for food, being filthy and putrid; the sardines were adulterated with tin in one case and rotten in another; and the so-called Italian codfish was misbranded as to quality and place of origin, as well as being adulterated. The great bulk of this latter fish was released under a heavy bond. The fines imposed were nominal.

There were seventeen judgments rendered, affecting macaroni, spaghetti, and noodles, these being mainly cases of misbranding as to place of origin, although two large shipments of macaroni were ordered destroyed as unfit for food. Two of the makers were caught a second time each, but escaped with nominal fines and took their goods back under bond to properly relabel them before selling. Not even water was free from the fine work of the misbranding packer or the adulterating manufacturer. Thirteen times water of some particular description was the subject of judgment, and in four instances it was ordered destroyed; two of the bottlers appeared twice each to answer charges; and two fines of $100 were imposed in the case of a water that contained bacteria and was unfit for human consumption.

Butter was the subject of thirteen judg-

ments, the general complaint being misbranding as to place of origin. In one case a fine of $200 was imposed, in the others the fines were small and the goods released under bond, none of it being found unfit for food. Beer was misbranded three times. Six fines of $100 each were imposed for calling alcoholic liquids "apricot" and "peach" brandy when they were nothing of the sort; and two bottlers misbranded brandy as to the place of origin. There were nine cases of misbranded and adulterated whisky, two of them from the same distillery; and in two cases the alleged whisky was made from molasses and water. One of the seven judgments in the cases of misbranded wine imposed a fine of $100. Of the five cider cases none was of a nature to call for extended comment, the trouble in each instance being misbranding as to the quality of the goods involved.

In the eight cases in which olives were the subject matter a very considerable quantity of the goods was permitted to be reshipped to Italy at the expense of the importer to avoid the payment of heavy duties as well as to prevent the destruction of the olives by order of the court as unfit for food purposes.

The packers of tomato paste and tomato pulp were every whit as careless of the quality of their product as were the makers of tomato catsup. One packer of tomato paste was haled before the courts twice, and four firms who put up tomato pulp got into difficulty. A large quantity was destroyed of each product, the court saying practically in every instance that the material was "in a filthy, decomposed and putrid condition and wholly unfit for human consumption."

Other food products which the board found to be adulterated and misbranded, and whose makers or packers were brought before the courts, were baking powder, of which there were four cases, one of which was a shortage in weight, and the others were adulteration and misstatement as to the composition of the goods; cereals, three judgments; cornmeal, two cases; cottonseed meal, of which there were ten cases, one firm being proceeded against no less than six times, and fined on four occasions for adulteration with hulls, &c. There was one judgment as to the misbranding of curacao; six cases involving honey, of which a large quantity was ordered destroyed, four judgments being against the same packer; and ten cases where the subject matter was molasses, with a fine of $100 on one offender for misbranding as to quantity and having a considerable shortage.

Quite a quantity of oysters was ordered destroyed in the four judgments affecting that article, two of the lots being "shucked" oysters, and all being condemned as filthy, putrid, decomposed, and unfit for human consumption. The fines imposed are all small. One of the two lots of peanuts, both shelled, which received attention and formed the subject of judgments, was ordered destroyed because of the presence of worms and other filthy matter. Eighty-three boxes of figs were destroyed also as unfit for food. There were two cases of sugar, one being maple sugar and the other the straight article; two judgments affecting salt, both simply misbranding as to place of origin. Two judgments against ice dealers for disposing of ice which contained filthy and putrid vegetable and animal matter are to be noted, and in one case a fine of $150 was imposed on the company responsible for the article. The ice in both cases was ordered to be destroyed. There were also two cases involving ice cream and six judgments against makers of ice cream cones. These last were the boric acid cases which were so much commented on in the newspapers last Summer, and three of the complaints were against the same manufacturer. A very large quantity of these goods were ordered destroyed.

There were only two cases which came

under the head of confectionery, and they were both of so-called silver dragees. These goods which were coated with metallic silver were ordered destroyed, and fines of $100 imposed in each instance. The adulteration of bran with rice hulls cost one maker of feeds a fine of $200; and one dealer in spices lost forty-eight bales of cloves and paid costs because the cloves were found to be "colored, coated, and stained" to a degree that unfitted them altogether for use as a food product.

There were three judgments rendered affecting mince meat, two against the same maker. In each instance the goods were destroyed, and were described as filthy, putrid, decomposed, and unfit for human consumption. No fines were imposed, but costs were assessed against the offenders.

The following is a list of the food products which were the subject matter of judgments and which have not been mentioned above in more detail. There was but one judgment in practically every case:

Alfalfa meal,	Linseed meal,
Apple butter,	Mapleine,
Biscuits,	Phosphate,
Butterol,	Rice,
Custard,	Rice meal,
Grape juice,	Rusk, Holland.

Of the food products destroyed there was a very large qauntity, as will be seen by the following table, which includes everything the quantity of which is given in the notices of judgment, with the exception of eggs, a list of which was given above. The value of these goods can hardly be estimated, but it is away up in the thousands of dollars in the aggregate. In every instance the adulteration was such as to render the article unfit for food purposes:

Articles and quantities destroyed:
Apples, evaporated, 42 boxes; beer, 7 cases; cheese, 42 cases; cloves, 48 bales; coffee, 166 sacks; corn, 850 cases; currants, 6 barrels, 302 packages; figs, 83 boxes; 64 barrels codfish, 1,000 pounds codfish, 705 cases sardines, 55 barrels herring; flour, 140 barrels, 420 sacks; honey, 14 barrels, 210 cases; horse feed, 200 sacks; ice cream cones, 285,550; macaroni, 9,110 boxes; maple syrup, 36 gallons; mincemeat, 6,852 pounds; olives, 5 casks, 59 barrels, 290 gallons; oysters, 23 barrels, 45 gallons; peaches, dried, 1,750 pounds; peanuts, 900 pounds; pineapple, 19 cases; prunes, 19 boxes; raisins, 522 boxes; tea, 200 pounds; tomatoes, canned, 2,009 cases; tomato catsup, 3,550 gallons, 2,676 cases, 233 barrels, 15 half barrels; tomato paste, 4,150 boxes, 262 barrels; tomato pulp, 180 barrels, 60 cases; vinegar, 140 barrels; water, 96 bottles, 100 demijohns, 383 cases; whisky, 50 barrels.

Before passing to the consideration of the judgments affecting drugs and drug products, a few words should be devoted to the question of shortages. It is hard to realize to what an extent this system of cheating by means of short weights has grown. The most noticeable shortages were in the canned goods, and they ranged from two ounces per two-pound can to as high as eleven ounces in the same sized can. It may not mean much when you speak of one can, but consider these figures as taken from the notices of judgment and grouped together as to subject matter:

Apples, canned, in 17,040 three-pound cans, as labeled, the total shortage was 7,875 pounds, or the equivalent of a steal from the consumer, since he was paying for what he did not get, of 2,625 cans.

Apples, evaporated, the shortage on 2,736 packages was the equivalent of 342 packages.

Apricots, canned, 11,880 labeled 2½-pound cans were shy just 5,655 pounds, or the equivalent of 1,502 cans, and 1,200 so-called gallon cans were 25 per cent short, or 300 gallons less than they should have been.

Baked beans, 2,116 cans showed a shortage equal to 252 cans.

Beans, string, in 20,010 so-called 2-pound cans, were shy 8,979 pounds, or the equivalent of 4,490 cans.

Baking powder, 45,600 pound packages, as labeled, were lacking to the extent of 4,275 pounds, and 150 so-called 5-ounce packages were short just 20 per cent., or 30 packages.

Blackberries, canned, 19,200 cans, 2 pounds, according to the label, were 9,600 pounds short, or 4,800 cans.

Blueberries, 7,920 "2-pound" cans, lacked 1,548 pounds of being honest weight, or 774 cans were deducted from the consumer; and in 3,000 labeled one-half-gallon tins a shortage of 15 per cent., or 450 half gallons, added to the packer's profit.

In cheese the shortage was not large in any one instance, but in the aggregate it looms up considerably, being, in 535 boxes of cheese, the very respectable amount of 779 pounds.

Cherries showed also a considerable shortage, for in 3,022 cans the quantity less than the labeled figures was 1,408 pounds, or the equivalent of 589 cans.

Corn shows a large shortage, because one of the most common canned goods in table use; 137,368 cans were found lacking over the marked "two-pound" figures 78,371 pounds, or the equivalent of 37,185 cans, or more than 25 per cent.

Fruit, lumped together under one head, 3,600 cans showed a shortage of 1,350 pounds, or the equivalent of 540 cans.

Flour was almost a negligible article in the shortage line, since 100 barrels showed a shortage only of 2 per cent., or two barrels.

Grape juice was also packed in the same dishonest manner, 6,114 points of it lacking 461 pints of the quantity shown on the label.

Milk, condensed, was shy about 20 per cent., and 2,400 cans contained the equivalent of 480 cans less than it should have done.

In molasses the shortage in quantity is given as 21.51 per cent., but the total quantity is not given, so the shortage cannot be accurately estimated.

Peaches were also packed short, 19,408 cans containing 6,914 pounds less than the declared quantity, being 2,765 cans short of what the consumer had to pay for.

Peas betrayed a shortage in 62,948 cans of 13,210 pounds, or 6,605 cans taken out of the consumer without his knowledge or consent.

Pineapple also ran up heavily, 125,424

cans containing 76,695 pounds less than the advertised quantity, being 38,519 cans shy of living up to the label declaration.

Preserves as a class had fallen under the same form of graft, 45,648 cans or packages being shy the equivalent of 5,197 properly labeled packages.

Tomatoes were treated in the same way, the shortage in 77,904 cans being 50,931 pounds, or 17,100 cans; and in 13,800 alleged gallons the amount that was missing was 2,760 gallons.

Syrup, like molasses, one cannot estimate on because no quantities are given, but it is stated that the shortage runs from 3 per cent. to 28 per cent., giving an average that meant much increased profit and dishonest profit to the packer.

Water was even the subject of shortage, 816 quarts of a mineral water being exactly 163 quarts shy of its declared content.

Comment on these shortages would be superfluous; the figures speak for themselves in tones that should reach every housekeeper in the land.

Passing on to the subject of drugs and drug products, there are 222 distinct judgments affecting these. Four thousand one hundred and five dollars was collected as fines from the offenders in this class, and a very considerable quantity of drug preparations was destroyed, though the figures are not given save in two instances. The fines ranged downward from $500, which was chalked up against one of the headache cure firms which misbranded as well as adulterated its product, the misbranding taking both the form of false statements as to the effect on the system of preparation and the form of deception as to the component parts of the preparation. This was the common form of misbranding. The facts speak for themselves.

Of all the drug products affected by the judgments of the courts in cases brought by the board, the group classed as "headache remedies" is by far the most numerous. No less than fifty-one judgments affect some form of cure, tablet or powder, alleged to instantly cure headaches. Fines to the amount of $850 were imposed on the offenders who misbranded their goods and deceived the public thereby, the first fine, $500, being the largest yet imposed in any of these cases. Only one of the offenders

came back a second time. The general concealment as to the composition of the drug was a deception as to the quantity or even the presence of acetanilid.

There were just twenty-one cases involving bitters of various kinds. One fine of $100 was imposed, and 110 cases of bitters in all were ordered destroyed.

Twenty-four judgments, equally divided as to number, deal with hair tonics and hair stain, the same trouble being present in each case—that of false statements on the labels as to the effect of the use of the contents. Most of these goods were released under bond. One of the five concerns putting up an alleged cancer cure which the board had its attention called to, and which the board in turn presented to the courts, was fined $100 for similar false statements; as were also a catarrh cure maker, a soda-water flavor maker, a dealer in camphor, and one in cocaine, a putter up of liquor sulphur, the proprietor of a teething syrup, and a bottler of gin and strychnine.

A concern that puts up a belladonna root preparation was fined $400 because its labels contained untrue statements; and for the same reason the owners of an aniseed syrup and a febrisol preparation were each fined $150, and the same fine was paid by a man who tried to make persons believe by a very high-sounding label that he was disposing of radium-impregnated water, which he declared was possessed of wonderful curative qualities.

Few of the drug product people came back a second time, only two of them being listed twice, and but one had a third offence charged against him. Six different concerns adulterated their spirits of turpentine with too much mineral oil, but they all gave bonds to relabel it properly before sale, and had the goods released to them.

Of the goods stated to be destroyed, in but four instances is the quantity mentioned, as follows:

Cough cure.....................41 boxes
Microbe killer.................37 cases
Make-man tablets.........180 packages
Bitters (various kinds).......110 cases

It would be difficult to give a list of the different drug products for the misbranding or adulteration of which the board brought action in the courts, but they ranged from Aceton and Anadol, all the way through cocaine preparations and plaster pads to saltpetre. None of the remaining cases are especially worthy of note, for the reason that the greatest punishment the offenders received was the publicity they got at the time of the trial, except in the instances noted of fairly heavy fines. By long odds, the food product decisions far outweigh the drug product judgments in every possible way as interesting and as immediately valuable to the American household.

July 23, 1911

MUST PASTEURIZE MILK.

All City Dealers Ordered to Put in Plants—New Grades Fixed.

After the lapse of a short period especially granted to milk dealers so that they may equip their bottling plants with pasteurization appliances, the sale of raw milk in New York except from inspected and certified farms will be prohibited by the Health Department.

The pasteurization proposed, according to Dr. William H. Park, director of the Health Board's research laboratory, who joined Commissioner Lederle in making the department's plans public, is not of an extreme type. Heat will be applied well below the point at which chemical changes begin in the milk, and this, Dr. Park believes, will eliminate any question

as to the effect of the pasteurization on the milk's quality as a food.

To further aid in obtaining the richest and best milk for mothers who are using it as children's food, the present grading of milk will be abolished, and instead will be created three classes—"infants' feeding," "drinking," and "cooking."

Dr. Park said that almost any milk that is not sour is safe to use for cooking, as the heat does all that pasteurization would do to rid it of germs. The grade to be known as "infants' feeding," according to the new plan, will closely approximate in richness, purity, and sanitary handling the milk now sold as "certified" at a material advance over the standard price.

The "drinking milk" will be that of known origin, but not of the highest percentage of fats, while the "cooking milk" will be all that is of questionable pedigree, or from dairies about which the Inspectors have doubts.

January 31, 1911

SOLDIERS PROTECTED BY NEW HEALTH LAW

A health law, described as being the tic ever enacted in any State in this country and which was passed by the Legislature at the request of the Federal Government for the protection of soldiers and sailors, went into effect yesterday. It provides for the arrest and detention during treatment of persons afflicted with blood diseases.

Officials of the Health Department were sent to the Night Court last night for the purpose of enforcing the law, the administration of which is placed by the law mainly in the hands of the Health Department. The law was Bill 1,097, introduced at the last session of the Legislature by Senator Whitney.

Health Commissioner Copeland said yesterday that this was a wonderful law and that the part which the Federal Government had played in its enactment foreshadowed a time when the Federal Health Department would control and direct the work of local health departments in all cities. The law resembles the Page act, which was in effect some years ago until it was declared unconstitutional by the State Court of Appeals. The law was held to be class legislation because it applied to women only, but the Whitney act applies equally to men and women.

The Health Department intimated yesterday that arrests would be made under this act at the beginning at the rate of twelve a night. The prisoners will be held for a diagnosis. After that only those will be held who are suffering from a communicable form of the diseases specified in the act. They will be held in city hospitals, or may be released at the discretion of the health authorities upon guarantees that they will receive treatment. Those who are detained will be kept in hospitals for a period generally of from two to four weeks, at the end of which time they cease to be sources of contagion.

The Federal health authorities have turned over to the Department of Health a list of "suspects," who have been named by soldiers who have been questioned at army hospitals. The complaint may be made by any person, soldier or civilian. It was announced at the Health Department that men were to be arrested as well as women.

May 4, 1918

SAVING MORE BABIES

IT is an accepted fact that maternal instinct is not, and never can be, a substitute for training in the care of babies. Responsibility for the welfare of the child is now, therefore, shared with the mother by the State, the physician, and the sanitary expert.

The development of the child at present constitutes a scientific problem to be solved for the good of the race. The value of infant life has but lately been appreciated, and perhaps the most striking evidence of what has been brought about by modern measures in preventive medicine is shown by the reduced infant mortality statistics. But, although many agencies now co-operate in the care of the child, the latter still spends most of its time with its mother. Therefore, no matter how much knowledge there is which is of benefit to the child, if there were no one to convey this information to the mother she would be none the wiser and the child none the healthier.

The visiting nurse of the Henry Street Settlement forms a connecting link between the tenements of the east side or the flat in Manhattan or the Bronx, on the one hand, and the advanced teachings of the medical schools and the investigations of the laboratories on the other. The instruction given by them has been an important factor in helping to reduce infant mortality. It is the visiting nurse chiefly who has taught the mother the health possibilities of the small apartment or flat, who has initiated the mother into what would otherwise have been mysteries of nutrition and sanitation. It is she who has helped to clear away the rubbish of tradition and superstition.

It is not just a happy coincidence that infant mortality has decreased as the intelligence of the mother has increased.

"It is on the intelligence of the mothers that the conservation of our babies depends," said Dr. L. Emmett Holt recently. Dr. Holt is Professor of the Diseases of Children at Columbia University, and as he sketched the rapid strides made in the rearing of infants he emphasized three things: The general education of the community, the growing intelligence of the mother, and the important part played by the visiting nurse in the home.

"There are two things which every American woman was once supposed to know how to do without previous preparation or instruction. One was to teach school and the other to bring up children. Long ago the error of the first assumption was discovered and more recently we have come to realize that the second was a mistake also and to appreciate its serious consequences.

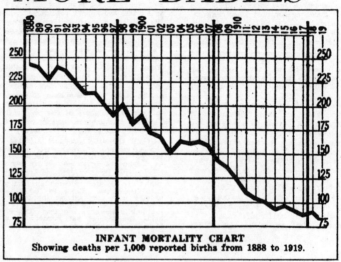

INFANT MORTALITY CHART
Showing deaths per 1,000 reported births from 1888 to 1919.

"A generation ago for every 1,000 infants born there were 280 deaths a year. In 1919 the figures show only 82 deaths per 1,000 births, a reduction of the infant death rate to less than one-third of what it was. This has been brought about largely by a campaign of education. At the present time one of the most important agencies in touch with the mother is the visiting nurse in the home, and it is largely owing to her efforts that so much has been accomplished in the education of the mother. The reduced infant mortality statistics show that educating the mother is the most effective means of saving the babies. The Bureau of Vital Statistics of the City of New York gives the following figures on the infant death rate per 1,000 births:

1890	182 Deaths.
1900	144 "
1913	102 "
1919	82 "

"For July, 1907, the bureau has recorded 2,292 deaths, and in July, 1919, only 873. As recently as 1890 26 per cent. of all deaths were among infants under 1 year. Today the bureau reports that they comprise only 14 per cent.

"The result of a well-organized and well-administered campaign of education in connection with infants is illustrated by the decreasing infant mortality in New York State. When Dr. Biggs became State Health Commissioner he introduced throughout the State the same general plan that had been inaugurated in the city, and the result has been that the mortality in the State has steadily fallen, although it is still a little above that of the city where the educational work has been going on a longer time.

"Those who question the ultimate value of the saving of infant life and look upon these measures as simply a means of saving the unfit are answered by the figures. There has been a greater reduction in the mortality rate of the children under 5 years of age than of infants, as is shown by the following table, based on a child population of 1,000 under 5, prepared by the Bureau of Vital Statistics:

1890	61.1 deaths
1908	50 "
1913	37.6 "
1919	24.7 "

"The same agencies which so materially reduced infant mortality brought about also a corresponding reduction in the mortality of adults as well as of older children. Again quoting the figures of the bureau, 'In 1890, out of a total population of 3,356,722, the death rate was 19.5 per 1,000, while in 1919, with a total population of 6,008,724, the death rate was only 12.4 per thousand.'

The decrease in the infant mortality rate can be traced in a measure to the visiting nurse of the Henry Street Settlement, who in her visits to all parts of New York acts as an individual instructor to the mother, for Dr. Holt believes that one cannot emphasize too strongly the unique place that the visiting nurse as a health teacher occupies.

"It is the individual work that counts," he says. January 25, 1920

THE NEW PARADOX IN MEDICINE.

Without precisely acknowledging the fact, the Rockefeller Foundation subscribes to the Chinese opinion, formerly held a paradox, that the physician earns his fee only when his patient is well, forfeiting it straightway in every case of sickness. "Who knows but the doctor of the future," writes the President of the Foundation in his current report, "will receive an annual retaining fee from his clients and feel no embarrassment in taking the initiative and in keeping a watchful eye on them?" With equal fearlessness, though again not crediting the originator of the thought, Dr. VINCENT echoes the paradox of SAMUEL BUTLER of Erewhon. A "vertical rather than a horizontal position," he says, is not a satisfactory criterion of health. "Being ' up and around ' or ' I can't complain ' represents a far from stimulating conception of bodily prosperity." In the 'philosophy of Erewhon a proclivity toward crime, being hereditary, was a subject of neighborly condolence, whereas seasonal illnesses, being preventable by sound hygiene, were a flagrant offense to the community. Thus a banker discovered in embezzlement received friendly visits of sympathy; but when it was discovered that he had contracted a cold he became socially ostracized.

BUTLER wrote before the need and the possibilities of community sanitation were understood. If his paradox has meaning for us, it is because we are approaching the end of an era of progress. "The presence of smallpox is now a disgrace to any civilized community or country; cholera and plague have disappeared from the leading nations; typhoid fever has been enormously reduced; malaria and hookworm disease are giving ground; yellow fever is being narrowly restricted; typhus is practically unknown among a cleanly people; the fear of diphtheria has been largely allayed." The emphasis of the future must of necessity be laid upon personal hygiene. "It is roughly estimated that 80 per cent. of the maladies which produce the total death rate cannot be directly controlled by the sanitarian." The present need is thus for something beyond community prevention—for "more positive and constructive ideals." The tendency is toward "education in personal hygiene, nutrition for old and young, physical exercise and mass athletics, provision for mental and emotional satisfactions through social and recreational activities."

Here, obviously, is a new field for trained leadership in medicine. The laboratory researcher and the old family doctor who holds aloof from his patients until he is "called in" must give way to the administrator of personal hygiene. As yet, the traditionally minded will see in this at best a wild paradox and at worst an insufferable inquisition. But the Rockefeller Foundation takes the situation very seriously and in its schools of hygiene at Johns Hopkins and Harvard provides instruction of the first order for the intending administrator. Eventually, such work must be well paid. Those who enter the new field now will find an escape from the accustomed walks of the medical profession, which are yearly more crowded.

June 12, 1922

REPORT VITAMINE SYRUP.

Scientists Describe Formula for Use in White Bread.

Discovery of a method of extracting the vitamines and mineral salts from the germ of the wheat berry and wheat bran, in fluid form, so that they may be introduced into foods lacking in those important elements, was announced yesterday.

The process was perfected by scientists of Yale, Harvard, Johns Hopkins, Mellon Institute of Industrial Research, and other American universities working in co-operation with a group of chemists employed by George S. Ward, the baker. The research workers were seeking primarily for a method whereby all the food elements of wheat could be combined in a white loaf of bread, thus eliminating the dark whole wheat loaf to which many persons objected.

The vitamine syrup which resulted, however, can be used for increasing the food value of other articles of diet which lack the important elements, it was asserted.

Tests of the syrup were made on pigeons, rats, mice and guinea pigs. It was found, the investigators reported, that animals fed on a sole diet of water and ordinary white bread died within three weeks. Those fed on water and white bread containing the vitamine syrup thrived and lived to natural ages.

November 6, 1922

ATTACKS MEDICAL SERVICE.

Dr. Biggs Says Only a Few Are Aided by Recent Discoveries.

The majority of the people of New York State and the nation are not enjoying the advantages of the most recent medical discoveries, but are getting the same kind of medical service that prevailed twenty-five years ago, said Dr. Hermann Biggs, State Health Commissioner, yesterday afternoon in an address on "The State and Public Health" in the new Central Administration Building of the Henry Street Settlement, 99 Park Avenue. The new structure, opened for inspection yesterday, is for the use of its Visiting Nurse Service, and is the gift of Mrs. Jacob H. Schiff as a memorial to her husband.

One of the great problems of the medical authorities, Dr. Biggs said, is to bring all the advantages of modern medicine within reach of the whole nation. At present, he said, the newest discoveries are within reach only of those who can afford to consult specialists or live near the great teaching centres. He said he regarded the work for public health of Miss Lillian D. Wald, Chairman of the settlement, as having had "a more far reaching effect than that of any other person in the country."

January 12, 1923

NEW CLINIC TO SORT OUT MISFITS

A MENTAL hygiene clinic which promises in its scope to vie with clinics of psychiatry in Detroit, Boston and St. Louis is to be opened this month in Cincinnati. It is to be financed the first year, at least, by the City Community Chest as an experiment in city betterment.

Other cities already supporting mental hygiene clinics have centred their attacks upon city problems through the Juvenile Courts. Cincinnati plans to reduce criminality and poor dependency and to give its youth a maximum chance for normal development through coordinated work with the Juvenile Courts, the public schools, social agencies, Board of Health and Vocational Bureaus.

Supporters of the Cincinnati clinic are determined to set a world precedent in reaching every type of defective or delinquent man, woman and child. It is said to be an established fact that many defectives are found among the so-called better class of families. The clinic will not be class-bound.

The director of the clinic is to be Dr. Emerson E. North, former head of Longview, an Ohio State institution for the insane. Dr. North is a national authority on mental disorders. In connection with being head of the clinic, he will hold a chair in the Cincinnati Medical College.

Starting with $15,000 from the Cincinnati Community Chest for the first six months, with the understanding that $30,000 will be forthcoming for the year, the Board of Directors and staff of the clinic propose to show a large economic

saving. It is argued that there is a large loss in confining a mental delinquent without having attempted to cure the cause of criminality or delinquency. The clinic promises to see to it that such persons are either cured or helped, or kept apart from society where they may not continuously repeat their acts of delinquency. If hopelessly affected and they must be kept in an institution, it is planned to fit them for what ever work they are able to do.

Dr. V. V. Anderson, Associate Medical Director of the National Committee for Mental Hygiene, is to be the chief adviser of the Cincinnati Psychiatry Clinic. Dr. Anderson has found that three-fourths of the persons dependent upon charity organizations show mental deficieny, feeble mindedness, unstable emotions, and the like. It has been proved that by adjusting such lives, through unraveling their mental differences, many have been made self-supporting members of society.

" There will be first a general examination of the individual, whether he be brought in from the schools, the courts or the social agencies," said Dr. North in describing the procedure which will be undergone in caring for a patient at the psychiatry clinc.

" It will be determined, whether there are any mental deficiencies, then cases will be analyzed, first to ascertain the sociological conditions of the patient; that is, the conditions in his home which might lead to his dependency, his vagrancy or criminality, and, secondly, to ascertain his physical state. Next, the psychology department will determine an individual's intel-

lectual level through tests."

The important point is that the varying casses of social misfits now punished or supported by the people will be divided and treated accordingly. For instance, two boys may be brought into Juvenile Court. At present, unless they happen to come before a Judge who deems it necessary to investigate further than the elementary facts, both are likely to be sent to a school of correction, although one perhaps should go to a school for the feeble-minded.

" In other words," said Dr. North, " both with children and adults we have been guilty of the same mistake sometimes made in the schools of the country, that of depending too much on curriculum and not enough on individuality."

Other cities are watching Cincinnati's clinical program for diminishng criminality and giving its youth a better chance for normal citzenship. At the recent annual congress of the American College of Surgeons in Cincinnati there was much interest in the clinic plans. Dr. William D. Haggard, professor of surgery at Vanderbilt University, said he knew of no mental hygiene program which had approached this one.

" Education being the greatest phase of public health, a clinic organized as I understand this to be planned is bound to have a new road toward general public health," said Dr. Allen Craig of Chicago, former Health Commissioner of Canada. " Children who are laggards in school or inclined toward ordinary criminality will be found out through this clinic at the age when real curative work can be done." He added that he believed no person should let a year pass without consulting his family physician for a general examination any more than a great corporation would let a year pass without having has a council meeting with its attorney.

January 14, 1923

PROTECTING HEALTH OF WORKERS SEEN AS INDUSTRY'S BIG NEED

More Study of How to Keep Fit Expected to Yield Greater Dividends Than Mechanical Efficiency—Executives as Well as Employes Affected

By DONALD B. ARMSTRONG, M. D.
Executive Officer, National Health Council.

THE " Safety First Campaign " has sold itself to industry. The " Health First Campaign " has not yet done so, although " safety first " saves only what industry had to start with. " Health First " creates a new value. It is possible to spend $10,000 in health work and make $50,000—measured in decreased labor unrest, decreased turn-over, increased production, decreased loss of time for illness, and such things. Still, most business men are not yet convinced.

The reason for the feeling that there is a definite return on money spent in safety work and not in health work is because safety bookkeeping keeps itself. If you spend $250 on the installation of

safety devices and save $1200 in compensation costs in a year, you can see that it is a profitable investment. But if you install medical service and keep no records of money made by increased production or decreased absenteeism, you don't know whether it pays or not. Compensation for accidents is required by law, but the law does not require compensation for illnesses that it would be 50 per cent cheaper to prevent.

Why not recognize that the object of industry is profitable production and invest in health only as it increases profits? The owner of Port Sunlight did this. Although he had a model village, mid-morning lunches and all the health work with frills, he insisted that he never spent a cent on his workmen. Well, he was Mr. Lever when he started investing in health work, and he is Lord Leverhulme now, so it must have paid.

Installing medical service will pay if we stop trying to amuse, edify and pacify the worker with the idea of taking his mind off his troubles. Let us keep our minds on our own troubles. Large labor turn-over, absenteeism, discontented workers are factors in the cost of production, and ill-health is an important factor in their cause.

The time is coming when we will select a community for industrial development, not only because of its railroad facilities and labor market and availability of raw materials. We shall also take into consideration health conditions and death rates and illness prevalence. Is it better to pay high wages to a group of workers, two per cent. of whom are ill at any one time, or is it better to take a chance with low wages in a population with a much higher continuous illness rate and the

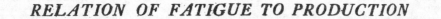

RELATION OF FATIGUE TO PRODUCTION

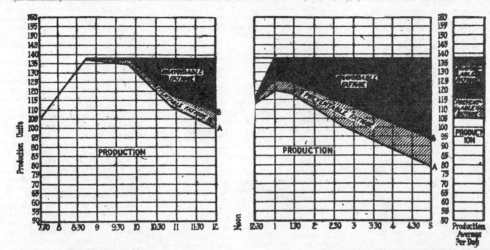

The Two Charts Cover a Day's Work; the First Covering the Period From 7:30 in the Morning to Noon; the Second Covering the Period From 12:30 to 5. They Show That Production Reaches Its Peak at About 8:45 in the Morning and then Declines; and That Fatigue Is Much Greater in the Afternoon. Line A Represents Production in an Old Factory With Poor Seating; Line B Production in a New Plan With Correct Seating. The Heavy Shading Indicates the Drop in Production Due to Fatigue That Cannot Be Avoided; the Area in Lighter Shading Indicates a Gain in Production That Can Be Attained by Proper Seating. Thus the Chart Shows That a Greater Saving Through Preventing Fatigue Can Be Made in the Afternoon Than in the Morning. The Figures in the Vertical Column Represent Units of Production; the Figures Arranged Horizontally at the Bottom of the Chart Show the Hours of the Day.

coincident low production, inefficiency and time loss? If the health index is at all a safe guide, the former represents the better investment. Is the establishment of an automobile plant in a New York city contemplated, or a factory employing hundreds of men and women in the south? Then important questions are: What is the death rate from tuberculosis, or the morbidity rate from typhoid fever? Tuberculosis control in the urban centers, the tremendous strides in southern communities toward the elimination of chronic, partially incapacitating illnesses, such as malaria and hookworm, — these rank high as community assets upon which securely to project industrial expansion.

"Poor old Brown is losing his punch. He worries too much and is taking no care of his health." Thus say Brown's associates among the executives in his industry. What would his fellow-executives have said if he had embezzled the firm's money? Yet his salary is based on his best service. His ill-health may make his services worth only a fraction of what they cost the company. Embezzling would cost the firm less than prolonged ill-health on the part of this key-man. No one speaks of pitying the man who embezzles the firm's money, but if an executive, through ill-health, lets his department go bad, we pity the poor fellow—"He never took any proper care of his health."

He is paid for his best service, and his best service demands that he take care of his health as a matter of common honesty. Very little sympathy would be spent on the production manager who employed no master mechanic to keep his machinery always at maximum production, and to prevent unnecessary deterioration. We would say that he was not onto his job. But executives neglect their own machinery, which costs every year large sums of money, and they are pitied instead of condemned. Usually, business men seem to be no more businesslike about their own health than about that of their employes. Of course there are exceptions.

A Western fuel and iron company insists on the regular medical examination of executives and necessary follow-up work. This medical examination is both free and compulsory. Other employes may obtain it on a voluntary basis by the payment of a monthly fee.

This distinction probably is based on the idea that it is more important to take care of a dynamo than a screw driver. However, in most industries there are a great many more screwdrivers than dynamoes, and it would seem good business to take care of the screwdrivers, too. After all, according to conservative estimates, every man employed represents between $1,000 and $20,000 invested each year.

How It Works Out.

A considerable number of examples could be given of increased production following installation of the simplest measures of industrial hygiene. I have seen an interesting graph showing the curve of production by units for each half hour in morning and afternoon work periods. The peak was reached in the middle of each period and then fell back at the end. In the afternoon the fall was 50 per cent. greater than in the morning owing to accumulated fatigue. By the installation of better seating, by this single change alone, ten production units were gained in the morning and fifteen in the afternoon. There was still the decline from unavoidable fatigue, but the continued rate of production was maintained at a higher speed.

How many employers have installed seats, either to be kind or to obey the law, and have no idea whether the seats paid for themselves? Records are kept of how long it takes to stamp an envelope, but records of whether it pays to do health work are often ignored. There are many conditions hampering health which do not result in a man's stopping work entirely, but which constantly and progressively curtail his production. If to normal fatigue be added the strain of high humidity, high temperature or lack of moving air, less work is done. Would you play your best game of golf in New Orleans in the Summer?

Health is an asset, and the sick worker has to compete with the well worker in job getting and keeping. Incidentally, if he blames the conditions under which he works for his ill health he naturally will feel resentful toward whoever is responsible for those conditions.

You, as an executive, wake up feeling fine. It is a snappy, clear day. You walk into your office ready to "eat your work." You do a tremendous day's work. You go home and tell your wife, "Well, today was a big day!"

And perhaps one of your employes with more natural physical vigor walked to work that day feeling fine too. Then, as he opened the workroom door he was heard to remark, "How this place smells!" Did the smell decrease the output of his first hour? It did.

There is the obvious money loss from sickness, absenteeism and turnover, but there also is the less easily computable loss from the inhibition of production following lowered attention. If your worker is thinking how tired he is, he is not working at his maximum speed. Fatigue, inattention, lack of concentration, cost money. A healthy man likes to work and the man who likes his job does a good job. The healthy worker is the contented worker; the diseased worker is an apostle of unrest.

It would be absurd to point out that the training of a new man is a factor in labor costs. It is said to run from $15 to $300 a job or more. A comfortable man is less likely to change his job than a uncomfortable one. And comfort depends on the care given to physical conditions of work. Where obvious physical hazards exist, of which the worker himself is conscious, he is naturally more inclined to change his job. He has invested his health in industry and he does not care to lose his investment—his chief asset.

The output of one worker supplies the material for another. Any factor that lowers production makes for "unemployment within employment." The overtired, coughing, aching worker is the one who spoils and wastes material and who lowers a firm's reputation for high quality.

The Way to Start.

A man in lowered physical health is more subject to industrial diseases and accident than a well man. This also may result in increased surgical and medical charges, compensation costs, &c., and whatever increases the cost of the product in the plant, increases the cost to the public and decreases the goods absorbed by the public. This, in turn, decreases wages, and with lowered wages goes lowered health and increased doctor's bills for workers, with decreased buying power. That in general is the economic base for improving health in industry.

What, then, can we do by increasing the health of the worker, to lower the cost of production, and how can we do it? Suppose a concern started to assemble automobiles and bought from various manufacturers sample wheels, tires, seats, radiators and engine parts, and hired any available workers to put these together. Probably the car would not run. Health work in which the parts are assembled from samples here and there and are put together by inexperienced or second-rate workers will not run either.

The health service division of any plant should be built according to careful specifications; the individual needs of a given plant run by top-notch experts. Naturally there, should be a physician in charge. But there is not an overabundant supply of trained industrial physicians. The man who wants to turn a factory into a hospital will not do. The finger-wrapper who reads his paper until some one gets hurt will not do either, and the man who thinks his job is curing sick employes will not do. The man who has no knowledge of industrial conditions, and out of several hundred industrial diseases can name five, is not wanted. The man who lacks human appeal also is out of place. Men will not take their problems to a hurried, inaccessible, uninterested physician. The cheap man is equally bad. A doctor who will work for much less than he could make outside ought not to arouse gratitude, but suspicion. The man who expects to be told what his job is never will do. The real industrial physician makes his own job and knows that he must make his job make money for the firm. Among other things, he and his staff should succeed in this way:

Diminish employment of the unfit; assign men to suitable jobs; run a regular clinic service and treat accidents; study and eliminate unhygienic conditions throughout the plant as to ventilation, light, cleanliness and accident

hazards; diagnose chronic affections and refer them to the patient's own physician for treatment; promote health education by posters and talks; provide a special personnel service for the executives, a sort of life extension in industry; examine new employes and old employes periodically.

We must remember that the basis of all future health work is personal hygiene, and the keynote of personal hygiene is the health examination. We overhaul our automobiles periodically—why not the same thing for the most delicate of machines—the human body? We go to the dentist regularly, but we can still buy a set of store teeth. Let us remember that we cannot buy a set of store kidneys. The human machine is the only machine for which there are no extra parts.

In one large plant in Schenectady they have found that compulsory health examinations, coupled with an effort to fit the right man to the right job, resulted in not more than 2 per cent. rejections. Many industrially trained but physically defective men are eligible for continued employment. It certainly pays to keep them on their jobs if they know their jobs, for the cost of correcting health or making special occupational provision is often less than the cost of training new workers.

A human machine should be used with sagacity and not permitted to depreciate through improper use or lack of care. Putting a nervous, tuberculous little man in a boiler factory is improper use of a human machine. The conservation of health has a direct connection with the duration and value of service rendered.

Here is an example of the way men are picked. In two optical goods factories in a single street one employer stated that he always employed Swedes, as they have particularly steady eyes. The other employer stated that he avoided Swedes, as their eyes were no good. There are firms which think it pays to get facts, instead of using old wives' tales and traditions based on generalizations from perhaps a single experience of a single foreman.

It is difficult to specify just how much health service is necessary for any plant. However, if I would generalize at all, I would say that not more than 3,000 workers could be taken care of by a single full-time physician, at least two full-time nurses, one or two medical assistants, one clerical worker, and perhaps some provision for dental service.

After all, to get health we must get facts. To get facts we must study our problems. To study our problems we must keep accurate statistics. To compile our statistics we must have trained health workers. To begin or to continue health work, we must be willing to invest money in health in order to get returns.

The chief point seems to be that health in industry has thus far been largely ignored by those responsible for industry. I find that a widely read periodical dealing with industrial management has begun a functional index to save time for the busy man and to tell him what subjects are covered by what articles. The subject headings include mechanical engineering, office, management, personnel and other subjects. But the subject of health or medical engineering is not included.

It is necessary to develop a respect for health and a will for health among employers and employes. Health is the prevention of sickness. Its theory in industry is based on the economy of prevention. We all more or less believe that "a stitch in time saves nine" and that "an ounce of prevention is worth a pound of cure." How beautifully and how convincingly this same sentiment is expressed by the great playwright:

"A little fire is easily trodden out
Which, being suffered, rivers cannot
    quench."

Health is the creation of physical vigor. It is the basis of economic and social welfare. It is our greatest individual and national asset. It is the foundation of happiness and the keystone of life.

April 8, 1923

DEATH RATE OF INFANTS RESTS ON MOTHERS' HEALTH

RESULTS of an extensive investigation into infant mortality and its causes in Baltimore have just been made public by the Department of Labor, through the Children's Bureau. In many respects the investigation is regarded as the most important of the bureau's infant mortality studies. Previous investigations were made in Johnstown, Pa., Manchester, N. H., Waterbury, Conn., Brockton, Mass., Saginaw, Mich., New Bedford, Mass., Akron, Ohio, Pittsburgh, Pa., and Gary, Ind.

Poverty, employment of mothers outside the home, housing below the proper standard, short intervals between births, and the death of mothers at or soon after childbirth were among the conditions causing high death rates among certain groups of babies under one year of age in Baltimore. Similar conditions were found responsible for high infant mortality rates in other cities. A summary of the Baltimore report contains the following observations:

The mortality in the entire group of 10,797 legitimate births studied was approximately the same as the infant mortality in the cities of the United States birth-registration area for the same year. Mortality rates markedly above the average for the entire Baltimore

group occurred among the colored families, foreign-born Polish families and the very poor native white families.

Low mortality rates, approximating those in New Zealand, which has the lowest in the world, were found among the babies of foreign-born Jewish mothers and in families of the highest earning groups.

Breast-fed babies in every group of the population had lower mortality than artificially-fed babies in the same group. In the poorest families studied, about one baby in six died within the year; in the most prosperous families, about one baby in twenty-six died within the year.

Employment of the mother away from home during the period of approaching motherhood, chiefly in factory work, was accompanied by a high percentage of premature births and high infant mortality. Employment of mothers away from home during the first year of their babies' lives also markedly increased the hazard to the baby. Room congestion and lack of sanitary equipment in the house were accompanied by death rates above the average.

First-born babies had a mortality slightly higher than second or third babies.

September 9, 1923

SCHOOL NURSES.

EMPLOYMENT of a school nurse in a community adds point to health teachings in the schools. The number of cities in the United States employing nurses has more than doubled in ten years, and the proportionate figure for rural schools is even greater.

No uniformity has yet been reached as to terms of contact or duties required of the school nurse, but in 116 out of 179 cities having a population of 30,000 or more, from which information could be obtained, the nurse is employed for the school year, and in fifty-eight for the calendar year.

The average number of children per nurse is about 3,000, varying from 800 to as many as 7,000. In some cities the applicant must stand examination, in others a certificate as registered nurse is required. The salary ranges from $637 to $2,700. In 110 of the cities sick leave with pay is granted, in 102 vacation with pay, and in forty-one benefit of the retirement fund.

March 14, 1926

LIFE LENGTHENED BY HEALTH WORK

Movement to Reduce Disease Has Extended Average Span of Years From 40 to 56— Many Ailments Conquered

THIS survey of the public health movement indicates what diseases have been eradicated, subdued to control or reduced in prevalence. In two generations science has added fifteen years to the average life span.

By MARY ROSS.

HUMAN life is safer and healthier and, on the average, longer, in the United States today than ever before. Not even the most determined pessimist who chatters about the decadence of the race can read the health record and fail to acknowledge that thousands of men and women and children are alive and well today who would have been lost in any previous American generation. The public health movement of the last century, and particularly of the last twenty-five years, has spread lifelines about us on which we rely unthinkingly. The effect of that movement is little short of a revolution in American life.

You can put it in terms of lives saved. In the New York of the '60s one baby in three died before it was a year old; last year one in sixteen. In those good old days a family had to have five or six children to make sure of bringing up two or three. You can put it in terms of lives lengthened. In 1880 the average life span in New York and other large cities was about 40 years; now it is 55 or 56. Or you can put it in terms of diseases. Some of them have been abolished.

Who ever thinks now of danger from yellow fever? Yet there have been epidemics of it in the United States which swept as far north as Philadelphia. The outbreak in New Orleans in 1878 took 8,000 lives. Yellow fever has been suppressed in this country, and, largely through the efforts of the International Health Board, almost abolished in the rest of the Western Hemisphere, till it has only a handful of refuges in the whole world, one of them the African Gold Coast, from which it may have come here originally in the slave ships.

Conquered Diseases.

In this same class are typhus, Asiatic cholera, bubonic plague, and, for most of New York and New England, smallpox. These have killed their thousands of Americans, but now, thanks to an intelligent and alert public health service, they have well-nigh ceased to exist. An exception to this statement must be made regarding smallpox for those parts of the country where popular prejudice still prefers a few thousand deaths and many thousand disfiguring illnesses each year to the tested alternative of universal vaccination.

There are other diseases no one need have if he is willing to take a little trouble to avoid them. Last year 12,000 people, most of them children,

died quite needlessly from diphtheria. Yet there are few city communities, and not so many country ones, where a parent cannot have his children immunized against diphtheria for the asking. New York State has just started on a five-year campaign to banish diphtheria by 1930, and in the opinion of experienced and conservative leaders in public health work that is a perfectly possible ideal.

Then there is typhoid fever. It is not difficult to get typhoid even in these salubrious days, particularly if you go on camping and motor trips. "Vacation typhoid," they sometimes call it in the health reports. Cities have protected themselves from disastrous epidemics. New York, for example, may well take pride in the chart which shows a downward slide from 1870, when typhoid killed forty or so each year in each 10,000 of population, to the present time, when the rate is scarcely one-twentieth of the earlier rate.

The conquest of typhoid fever is one of the great victories of sanitary science, and mass measures protect large aggregations of people. Furthermore, if you travel away from the mass, you can carry that protection with you by taking the precaution of that anti-typhoid vaccination which made the disease almost a curiosity among our soldiers in France. Death still lurks in many an innocent clear spring or quaint roadside well.

Scarlet fever may be added to the list of diseases to which one can be made immune, and possibly measles, though for measles the preventives are still to be proved by experiment.

Wages and Tuberculosis.

One of the first great battles of the public health movement (it is still a major part of any public health campaign) was against tuberculosis. There is no sure preventive of tuberculosis, no certain cure. Yet within fifty years the New York death rate from tuberculosis has been halved, then halved again. It has been pushed from a place at the head of the list down to fifth place, below heart disease, the pneumonias, cancer and violence.

Yet it remains the deadliest of the foes of women and men—especially men—in their most productive years. Probably it is accountable in general for 30 per cent. of all deaths between 15 and 60.

Tuberculosis is not a disease that attacks suddenly. Many persons are infected with it in childhood, without knowing it or suffering appreciably from it. The infection stays there, harmless unless the body is put to some severe overstrain that wears down its resistance. Such a strain seems to come most often in a man's life when the burden of family support is heaviest—that is, in his late twenties, his thirties and his early forties. For women it comes a little earlier.

Improved facilities for the diagnosis

and care of tuberculosis have been an important factor in bringing about the sensational decline in its death rate; when treated early, tuberculosis is one of the curable diseases. Yet possibly more important than the organized movement to fight it have been general improvement in living conditions, better wages, better houses and a shorter working day with more leisure to spend in the open air.

Studies of statistics have proved that the year-old baby may expect fifteen more years of life than his grandfather could reasonably have looked for at the same age. But the gain does not stop there. The expectation of life for the average 5-year-old is materially longer than it was two generations ago, and for the 10-year-old, and the boys and girls in their teens, and young adults, and so on straight through middle age, though in the later decades the gains are less. Out of 100,000 babies born in 1901, Dr. Dublin calculated for the Metropolitan Life Insurance Company, 40,911 might be expected to live to the age of 65. Out of 100,000 born in 1924, 52,466, or nearly a third more, may be expected to live to be old people.

Diabetes a Trouble of the Rich.

Diabetes is one of the ailments in which progress has gone the wrong way. Dr. Haven Emerson, who has made a special study of it, estimates that in the last two generations it has caused fifteen times as many deaths as it did in the times of our grandfathers; that is, the rate rose from 1.4 for each 100,000 of population in 1866 to 22.9 in 1923.

The disease is common among wealthy city merchant groups; rare among the manual workers. It is the disease of the rich, that is, of people who habitually, over long periods of time, have been able to afford to eat, and have eaten more than they needed to keep themselves going. Diabetes assails persons of middle age; it is especially prevalent in women, who sit back after the children are reared and "plan menus for exercise." In all these particulars it is exactly the antithesis of tuberculosis. That disease shows low rates among the well-to-do city folk and high among laborers, developing most easily in the young, where there is under-nutrition. The moral is that which the doctors have repeated again and again—cherish a reasonable plumpness before 30—avoid it afterward. Insulin helps to make the diabetic more comfortable, and in many cases prolongs life; but in our present state of knowledge it cannot be considered a cure.

No Proved Cure for Cancer.

As increasing hundreds of thousands of people are living to be middle-aged or old, there is inevitably an increase in the diseases which are especially associated with those ages. Of these the most important is heart disease.

Some kinds of heart disease are preventable—they result from infections in childhood or later, such as scarlet fever, diphtheria or rheumatism. They can be prevented by avoiding these ailments. Some kinds of heart disease are curable under the care of specialists, though it sometimes requires a long period of time. Many other cases can be so helped by a carefully planned régime of work and play that patients can lead almost normal lives despite their handicap.

More dreaded than heart disease is cancer. Cancer begins to appear in the death records in the twenties, but it becomes important in the forties, and reaches the crest of its destructiveness in the early sixties. Probably nothing has given more ground for the popular delusion about the physical decadence of civilization than the increase in the cases of cancer. Yet there is a question as to whether or not there are more cases among persons of 50, let us say, than in earlier years, or merely a larger proportion of people who have reached the age of 50 and are ripe to have it.

Several promising lines of research have been directed against cancer, but so far no proved cure for cancer has been found, unless early diagnosis and immediate operation for operable cases can be called a cure. That method can save many lives and much suffering.

Can't Produce Methuselahs.

All those unpleasantly named "degenerative diseases" of heart, kidney, arteries and the like, the cause of the majority of deaths in middle and later life, point to a wearing out of the physical machine, inevitable some time, tragic when it comes too soon. The best recipe man has devised for making life safe for middle age and old age is a regular yearly health examination by a qualified physician to check up the weak places and reinforce them when possible, so that no one part may give way and wreck the whole machine.

But eventually that machine will go to pieces. Despite the great gains in the years of life which young people may expect, statistically, to attain, there is no evidence to show that med-

ical science is on the way to produce a race of Methuselahs. In the aged groups the gain in life expectancy is negligible. There is an engaging theory that longevity is an inherited characteristic, like blue eyes.

According to that theory, some newborn babies might be considered clocks, made to go for, say, sixty years, while others are wound up for eighty or so. A clock will stop before it runs down if you knock it off the shelf, or it may refuse to keep time if you treat it roughly. According to this analogy the public health movement can prevent those knocks—infections, illnesses—which will hamper the efficient working of the best human constitutions or stop them altogether.

The Future Contest.

Where lies the fight of the future? All along the line, one must answer, if one looks over the program discussed by that first important American Health Congress which brought together 5,000 nurses, doctors, health officers, public health workers of all kinds at Atlantic City late in May.

In addressing that Congress Dr. Samuel J. Crumbine, Executive Director of the American Child Health Association, asserted that there were more than 60,000 preventable deaths from the so-called preventable diseases in the registration area of the United States in 1923. In that year the fire losses in this country, he reported, reached nearly $160,000,000, and the cities of more than 30,000 population spent $114,000,000, or $2.93 per capita, to prevent fire. Yet the total loss from preventable deaths, figuring the average to be $6,000, was

$384,816,000. And for health protection, the protection of life, those selfsame cities spent 45 cents per capita, as compared to the $2.93 for fire protection, protection of property.

Some sanitarians now consider that the easiest group of lives to save in this country are those of women who die needlessly at childbirth. It is startling to find that the record of the United States in this respect is below most of the European countries and Japan.

The public health movement, too, is making intensive studies of that most prevalent and probably most costly of all illnesses, the common cold; of diseases such as rickets, which makes children liable to many sorts of infection; of the mental and emotional quirks and twists that take the joy out of life and efficiency out of work; of fatigue, food and the effect of sunlight.

Pneumonia runs a deadly course through all the ages of man, especially the youngest and the oldest. A leader in the public health movement said recently that if the influenza epidemic were to come again we should know little better how to treat it than we knew before. Possibly something helpful regarding those deadly weeks in later Winter may be derived from the reading of the riddle of the sun, and from learning more about the ultra-violet rays, essential to life and growth. Careful scientists are working in laboratories all over the world in an endeavor to conquer the group of respiratory diseases as they have conquered others.

August 1, 1926

GROWTH OF RURAL HEALTH MOVEMENT

Country Health Is Beginning to Receive Adequate Protection, Says Rockefeller Foundation.

Concerning the growth of the rural public health movement, the Rockefeller Foundation says:

"The appropriations for the support of county health units by State, county, and town have gradually grown. The standard of the personnel employed has been raised and the number of workers has been increased so that the health of the public in the rural areas is beginning to receive adequate protection.

"As early as 1910 there was a definite trend toward organization for rural sanitation, but up to the close of 1916 only thirteen full-time county health units were functioning in the United States. At the close of 1925, there were 299 full-time county health units in operation in thirty-three States, and 80 per cent. of these had

been established in the preceding six years. The establishment of the work in about eight additional States will be contingent upon the passage of State laws which will permit counties to make appropriations for health purposes. Pennsylvania adopted permissive legislation in 1925.

"There has been a rapid expansion in county health work in 1925 in several States, notably in, Mississippi, Oklahoma and Missouri. In certain States, such as Ohio, North Carolina, and Alabama, the period of rapid expansion has passed, and the State Boards of Health are devoting their energies to strengthening the health units already organized; to the improvement of the service rendered, and to the standardization of procedure. In North Carolina, Alabama, and Ohio over 50 per cent. of the total population is served by full-time county health units.

"The board, since 1916, has contributed to the organization of seventy county health units. In 1925 it aided ninety-two units in twenty-three States. It also gave assistance to central supervision of county health work in 123 counties in fifteen States, and aided in the training of twenty-eight men representing sixteen States.

"The counties that have been selected for county health unit activities as a

rule have been above the average in wealth, population, schools, roads, and in progressive spirit, and have been willing in conjunction with the State to appropriate from 25 to 50 cents per capita, or approximately a half-mill tax on the assessed value of the property of the county, for the support of the work.

"In 1925, the board continued to cooperate in Brazil in the operation of five county health units in the State of Minas Geraes and four units in the State of Sao Paulo. In the latter State four additional posts were installed during the year. In the State of Bahia personnel was lent to help in the establishment of two units.

"A rural health service was started in the district of Hartberg, Austria, on July 1, with assistance from the board.

"The rural hygiene demonstration in the district of Kvasice in Moravia, Czechoslovakia, was continued.

"In Poland two local health services were aided.

"The health service which was initiated in 1924 in the Department of Hérault in France was continued with the board's cooperation. The chief advance during 1925 has been the creation of a central public health office in Montpelier."

August 8, 1926

EMERSON STRESSES DISEASE PREVENTION

Special to The New York Times.

NEW HAVEN, Conn., Sept. 21.—Individual periodical medical examinations are the next indispensable step to be universally taken in the public health program, according to Dr. Haven Emerson, Professor of Health Administration at Columbia University and formerly Health Commissioner of New York City, who gave the chief address tonight at the second annual clinical congress, held at Yale College, which brought nearly 600 physicians from all parts of the country here.

"We have passed through eras of sanitation and of law enforcement and through a period of popular education in the elements of personal hygiene," he said, "and we are now at the point where individual and universal participation in preventive medicine is indispensable for both patients and for physicians.

"The periodic health examination, as proposed by the American Medical Association, when widely employed and used as seriously and effectively as the services of physicians for the care of the disease can be relief upon to have a greater influence in reducing sick and death rates than all the powers and expenditure of public and private health agencies combined.

"A reasonably adequate program of personal protective services for health includes prenatal and infant care, supervision of the pre-school and the school child, of the wage earner and men and women of mature and advanced years, based always upon an exact direction of their manner of life by the family physician, whose diagnostic skill will be matched against incipient rather than against advanced disease or disorder of function and structure of body, and whose treatments will be directed toward the use of physiological measures, rather than upon operative and medicinal procedure."

September 22, 1926

INSURANCE COMPANIES TEACH HEALTH GOSPEL

By ROSE C. FELD.

INSURANCE companies are no longer interested solely in the business of adding policyholders to their lists. Their work has branched out until it includes the greater field of conservation. Through educational matter, welfare bureaus, surveys, experimental stations and in many other ways, a program of conservation is carried on, the purpose of which is to inform, to protect and keep safe the life, limb and property of the public.

It goes further than that. Many of the insurance companies, both life and fire, maintain national clearing houses of information where any one can obtain the information necessary to put himself and his personal property or business in good order. It may be information that will aid him in paying off mortgage on his house, help him install the most modern safety devices in his industry, suggest methods of introducing pension plans. The insurance companies will provide him with such information if they have it; if they have not they will get it for him.

In 1909, the Metropolitan Life Insurance Company, one of the forerunners of the movement for greater health and safety, announced a policy worded as follows: "Insurance not merely as a business proposition but as a social program."

The main purpose of the campaign was to educate policyholders in personal hygiene, proper living conditions, disease prevention, better housing and in the reduction of personal hazards. The campaign started primarily with policyholders. It has grown until it now includes the general public.

Disseminating facts about tuberculosis was the first step undertaken by this company. As time went on other diseases were carefully studied and the material put into form for distribution. In 1916, during the epidemic of infantile paralysis, all forces were directed toward helping the public cope with this disease. In 1918, the influenza epidemic brought out a similar campaign. The health publications of this organization alone are sufficient to fill a library. They include scores of pamphlets for layman and scientist. Their various subjects are classified under headings such as the Health of the Mother and Baby, Child Health, School Health, Family Health, Personal and Community Health, Home Nursing.

Tuberculosis Experiments.

Often the surveys are conducted in cooperation with existing civic health bodies. In 1916, for instance, the Metropolitan Life Insurance Company worked with the National Tuberculosis Association in inaugurating a seven-year experiment in tuberculosis control in the town of Framingham, Mass. For ten years prior to 1916 the death rate from this disease had averaged 121 per 100,000. At the end of seven years' work the death rate had dropped to thirty-eight per 100,0000. So satisfactory was this experiment that other cities throughout the country have taken up the work.

In 1920 the company made a grant to the American Public Health Association to cover the expense of a committee organized to study health department practices in the larger American cities. The chief purpose of the study was to determine the relative effectiveness of various methods employed and to standardize and improve municipal health machinery. As a result of this survey, the American Public Health Survey has established a permanent field service for advising and assisting health officers of cities, counties and States in their problems of administration and of public health procedures.

A study made of the infant death rate in the Province of Quebec showed a high percentage of mortality. A demonstration was undertaken at Thetford Mines, and a maternity centre with a French physician and a nurse who spoke French was opened. Instruction was given to mothers in pre-natal and post-natal care. At the end of three years the infant death rate had dropped from 200 per 1,000 born to 96 per 1,000 As a result of this work the Provincial Government appropriated a large sum to be used in other communities.

Group Insurance.

Figures given out by the Metropolitan Company show that the death rate from tuberculosis in 1926 among their policyholders was 55.8 per cent. lower than in 1911; from typhoid, 81.6 lower; from communicable diseases of children, 56.2 lower. Of course, it is not their work alone that is responsible for this great improvement. The country as a whole has taken a stronger interest in health and in disease prevention. But the fact remains that insurance companies have done and are doing a great deal to stimulate constructive work along these lines. That it is good business for them certainly is not an argument against them. It is also good business for the family to avoid disease and to cut its doctor's bills.

Nor is it in health alone that insurance companies maintain a service that does more than take care of periodic premiums and eventual reimbursement. American insurance companies have in ten years built up a total of about $3,000,000,000 of group insurance. A group insurance policy is one taken out by an employer to cover his employes. Sometimes he pays the entire premium; sometimes it is shared with the workers. The plan is one of many adopted by modern employers in an effort to humanize their working relationship with the people they employ.

Companies that write group insurance policies today act as an advisory body to the industrial organizations they cover. Their educational work in disease prevention is but one of the many services they offer. If John Jones, who is President of a large plant turning out machine parts, wants to know what are the latest safety devices to protect his men at work, he gets in touch with his insurance company and asks that an expert be sent to his shops to make suggestions for changes and repairs. The man who is sent will also prepare accident prevention programs and cooperate with the employer and employes in putting them successfully into effect.

If this same John Jones, after installing all the modern machinery he needs, and after putting in all the safety devices necessary, finds that his shop's production is unsatisfactory, he may again turn to his insurance company and ask for help. An expert on production engineering will discuss with him such questions as plant organization, labor saving devices, scheduling of work, heating, lighting, ventilating, records, layout —everything, in fact, that has a direct bearing on successful labor relations and costs and on the conservation of man and machine power.

Industrial Service.

The same procedure on any one of a hundred questions that an employer has to face is considered part of the service that insurance companies are now prepared to offer.

They are clearing houses of information for industrial relations which include employment management, employe organizations, pensions, plans, profit sharing, stock ownership plans. They are clearing houses for information gained by Federal and State departments, trade associations, statistical companies, conference boards, educational institutions.

There is little, as a matter of fact, that the insurance company will not do in an effort to make the business of the policy holder stronger, more modern, more successful. To the insurance company the health of an industrial organization is just as important as is the health of an individual. Whatever can affect the health of a plant, whether it be the pay envelope or the Summer vacation, is considered a subject worthy of expert attention. Conservation is the keynote of this service.

Strictly speaking, the very word insurance means conservation. It means preparing today for tomorrow; using foresight today so that tomorrow may be protected. Life insurance, health insurance, accident insurance, endowment insurance, all are recognized to be good business methods of conserving one's funds in a manner calculated to avoid future embarrassment. More recent aspects of insurance go even further in the field of individual conservation. The New York Life Insurance Company, for instance, made a survey of the longevity of women and found that those with assured incomes live longer than do those who do not know what the future offers. Pension policies have the same effect; so have unemployment insurance plans.

October 2, 1927

VITAMINS THEORY CHANGES OUR DIET

By EUNICE FULLER BARNARD.

WITHIN a single decade, unhonored, unsung and—still more extraordinary—unadvertised, a revolution has come over the general food habits of America. Into the time-hallowed huddle of meat, potatoes and coffee on the average home dinner table and restaurant menu has crept another year-round staple: salad. The once casual lettuce and tomato and their sisters of the vegetable kingdom have come into a new popularity, which has changed the aspect of our markets, enlarged our docks, perfected refrigerator transportation and planted new gardens throughout the United States and her neighboring islands.

With the overweening growth of the city has come an urge for the products of the soil the city dweller has abandoned. In New York, for instance, for every head of lettuce and every bunch of celery on the grocer's stands in 1919, today there are four. For every tomato and box of strawberries are now three, and for every cabbage, onion and grapefruit, two. New York's shopping thoroughfares, from the pushcarts of Avenue A to the gilded groceries of Madison Avenue, have been transformed since the war into bowers of greenery and glowing fruits. The city, in fact, consumes the enormous total of 500 carloads a day of fresh produce, as against about half that amount ten years ago.

The Pennsylvania Railroad has just tripled the capacity of its produce-receiving piers in downtown Manhattan, and the Erie has similar extensions under construction. In announcing its new plans for electrification recently the Pennsylvania cited the increasing demand for fresh vegetables as a compelling factor in the necessity for higher speed freight service. Meanwhile the City Markets Department has completed a new wholesale terminal market in the Bronx and is to spend millions more for similar ones in the other boroughs.

Democratizing the Vegetable.

Gastronomically, New York already lives the year round in a fruit and vegetable paradise that the South Sea Islands themselves could not equal. Delicacies with which Ward McAllister coaxed the appetites of the Four Hundred in the banqueting '90s are the not uncommon fare of messenger boys today. Twenty, even ten years ago perhaps, the mushroom, the artichoke and the grapefruit had a slight patrician flavor, which is all but forgotten now. And later comers on the vegetable list have been still more rapidly democratized.

Broccoli, for instance, was introduced to America with flourishes a few years ago by a Waldorf-Astoria steward, who remembered it in the Italy of his childhood. As recently as 1926 it was still a vegetable of the few. Not enough was brought into New York to be noted on the market reports of the Agriculture Department. Last year 151 carloads were used here, and this year the department estimates that they will total about five hundred.

More than seventy-five different fruits and vegetables, from anise to watermelon, pour yearly into New York by carload lots, as well as a dozen others that come in smaller quantities. To get them the city ransacks the globe. Cauliflower comes in from Holland; cucumbers, eggplant, grapefruit and okra from Cuba, oranges from Porto Rico. Onions are pouring in from Spain, Holland, Belgium and Italy. By Spring they will be coming also from Egypt, Chile, Bermuda, Cuba, other West Indian islands and a score of our States. All in all, New York eats farm and orchard produce from forty-two States and fifteen foreign countries.

Fed by the World's Gardens.

For almost half of its various fruits and vegetables New York knows no season. They come steadily, month in and month out, the year round. Take the metropolitan urge for fresh tomatoes. To satisfy it come refrigerator cars, successively, from West, South and East—as the seasons change—at the rate of twenty a day. Just now New York's tomatoes come mainly from California. In the next three months they will come, largely, by steamer from Cuba and the Bahamas, which a decade ago sent none at all. Then from March on, Florida will hold an enormous lead until June, when Mississippi ships her crop. With our own Summer comes the turn of Tennessee, then of Maryland and New Jersey and their sister States of the Atlantic seaboard.

Old standbys like potatoes and apples have barely held their own in proportion to the increase in population. Potatoes, to be sure, are still New York's favorite vegetable, being consumed at the rate of sixty-one carloads a day and making up more than one-tenth of all our fresh produce. But they are relatively no more popular than they were a decade ago. Indeed, M. P. Rasmussen, marketing specialist at Cornell University, questions whether potato eating is not on the decline. With the immense new variety of fruits and vegetables now eaten in New York he believes it is only logical to conclude that they "compete with or displace potatoes to some degree."

"The buyer for a large chain of fashionable hotels," he said, "insists that his patrons are not eating half as many potatoes as a decade ago, while the manager of a low-priced chain of restaurants states that he sees no difference. Buyers for more than a dozen chain grocery store systems all over the United States are unanimous in stating that people are eating less starchy foods, particularly potatoes, and eating foods of a lighter type, especially leafy and succulent fruits and vegetables.

"Potato-consuming habits have apparently changed since the World War, due probably to the increased prosperity of wage earners, which has enabled them to afford a more varied diet and to regard potatoes as less of a staple food. Perishable fruits and vegetables have been abundant and relatively cheap since the war. The rapid replacement of man power by machinery and the sedentary habits of many consumers, accompanying the wide use of motor vehicles, are both factors that would seem to decrease the demand for heavy food and increase the desire for a smaller and more varied diet than formerly."

Fruit Distances Potatoes.

Last year for the first time potatoes were outranked in New York's favor by fruit. Grapes, in consequence, it is suggested, of the "noble experiment," were consumed here at the rate of seventy-two carloads a day. Bananas too, as may have been guessed from an erstwhile popular song, are another metropolitan fruit favorite, and apples and oranges are practically tied for third place. Rather surprisingly, the fourth fruit in rank in the city taste is the cantaloupe, which far outclasses the pear and the grapefruit, its nearest competitors. And its use, too, has doubled in the decade.

As for the vegetables, lettuce has all but caught up with onions for second place. Fresh tomatoes are next, having—though probably no child could believe it—about twice the use of spinach, which, as a matter of fact, is far down the list, being outranked by green beans, celery and cabbage.

What has caused this immense new craving? Mr. Rasmussen believes that it is a kind of unconscious economic and physiological reaction to prosperity and the physically easier ways of life. Dr. Arthur E. Albrecht, city director of the State Department of Agriculture and Markets, on the other hand, believes the new food habits are far more deliberate.

Dietetics in the Home.

"The increase in the use of the lighter vegetables and fruits," he said, "is in large part due to the fact that the housewife is more interested in the dietetic principles of feeding the family than she used to be. Newspapers, radio speakers and school and college courses are calling attention to the necessity of vitamins in a balanced diet. Hotels, restaurants and householders alike are becoming more discriminating and scientific in food selection. And the trend is most marked in the salad vegetables, which have been recommended for their vitamin content.

"Again, consumers have enough income today to diversify their purchases, and fruits that were luxuries a few years ago are necessities in most families now. Growers and dealers also have been alert to see that New York City tables show no evidences of the changing of the seasons. At most New York grocers it is Summer the year round, and their shelves are often greenest in midwinter, when vegetables are coming

all the way across the continent.

"Indeed, almost a third of the city's fresh produce comes from California, about a sixth from Florida and only a tenth from our own State, which is the third largest contributor. This means, too, of course, a great development in the building and use of refrigerator cars. There is a far greater attention to service than there was a decade ago, and to such essential details as re-icing en route."

Thus, it is believed that there are five causes, all doubtless working together, which have brought about the recent apotheosis of the green vegetable. These and prosperity, which means more money to buy variety in food; the machine, which in lightening labor has removed much of the necessity for the more substantial foods; improved methods of transportation, and the competition among dealers to increase variety and lengthen the season of fresh produce; and most basic of all, probably, what might be termed America's new philosophy of food, inspired by the discovery of vitamins and the campaign of education based upon it.

The New Family Chemist.

Eating in the last fifteen years, the fact is, has been evolving from the good old Victorian orgy into a kind of chemical game, with doctor, dietitian or mother of the family as hit-or-miss score keeper among the vitamins, calories, proteins and carbohydrates. A well-known chain of restaurants has each item on the menu rated according to vitamin and caloric value. At the recent height of its health fervor this chain went temporarily vegetarian. Many sanatoria of the Middle West are full of health foods and green vegetables, and there is an increasing number of vegetarian restaurants in New York and tourist roadhouses outside it. Many of these, it is said, cater to Jews, who in the absence of kosher meat have learned to substitute vegetables. And the popular restaurant window displays offer succulent mushrooms, strawberries and grapefruit, where once the éclair and the tart reigned in permanent and dusty splendor.

In an age devoted to health and slimness the fresh vegetable has few peers. For it, almost alone in the whole culinary category, has been found to yield the mysterious vitamins without adding superfluous pounds. Its vogue owes its birth to the health cult and the chemical laboratory, having been almost coincident with the popularization of knowledge of the vitamins.

Indeed, it is little more than two decades since the existence of vitamins was first foreshadowed. In 1906 Dr. F. Gowland Hopkins of Cambridge University, England, found that white rats on a diet apparently nutritionally complete would die unless fed small amounts of milk. He therefore suggested that there must be in diet certain factors essential to life and growth which are too small to be classed as foods.

Five years later in the same laboratory Casimir Funk, discovering one such factor in whole cereals and vegetables and fruits which he found was necessary to prevent beri-beri, named it "vitamin." And it was not until 1915 that E. V. McCollum and Miss Davis in Baltimore, distin-

guished several already known vitamins and discovered the growth factor they called vitamin A. They located it in butter and egg yolk and the green leaves of plants. For less than thirteen years, therefore, have the five vitamins now usually referred to as A, B, C, D and E, been known, though almost from the first they have received wide, if somewhat cryptic, publicity.

Three Other Vitamins.

Vitamin C, which is present notably in oranges and tomatoes, prevents scurvy. Vitamin D, contained especially in fish oils, prevents rickets. Vitamin E, the anti-sterility element, is contained in wheat germ and lettuce.

Now, as will be noted, for four out of five of these vitamins green vegetables and fruits are an important source. In a general way for a decade the public has been getting it in mind that a diet properly garnished with vitamins must have fruit and vegetables at practically every meal. Recent discoveries have emphasized rather than weakened the theory. At Michigan State College of Agriculture, this year, it was announced that green color in vegetables is an actual guarantee of the presence of vitamin A. Rats fed on white asparagus tips, cut before reaching the surface of the ground, died in six weeks. Rats fed on green tips were healthy, gaining at the rate of five grams a week.

"In some mysterious way," said the investigators, J. W. Crist and Marie Dye, "chlorophyll [the green coloring matter of the leaves] manages to capture, transform and render available the energy contained in rays of sunlight." Carrots, beets and radishes contain vitamins because they are produced as parts of plants whose tops are green. The vitamins built up in these tops are transported to the roots for storage. Similarly, milk, butter and cheese have this same vitamin A from the herbs the cattle eat. Therefore, they advise, "Eat fresh vegetables, and those decidedly green in color."

Meat Holds Its Own.

Whether in this decade of glorifying the vitamin and more or less shunning the calory, meat as well as potatoes has been neglected in favor of the fruits and green vegetables is an interesting inquiry. Apparently it has not. To be sure, meat-eating shows no such enormous increase as that in the consumption of salad greens, but with the exception of beef, it has about held its own, and in the case of pork shows a substantial gain.

In 1919 the per capita consumption of beef was 61.6 pounds, last year it was only 58 pounds. But the figures for pork-eating are the reverse: 68.5 pounds last year as against 54.8 pounds in 1919. Lamb and veal showed very slight decreases, but the gain in pork more than counterbalanced them, so that taking all meats together, the average American is eating nine pounds more than he did a decade ago. Though we are becoming a salad-eating, nation. And the shades of Plato, Shelley and Bronson Alcott, or the more substantial Bernard Shaw, cannot yet rejoice.

December 16, 1928

ADVANCE IN SOCIAL HYGIENE

Dr. M. J. Exner Reports Grade Schools Are Adopting Courses.

Parents have surprised the principals and teachers of many American schools by requesting a greater measure of instruction for their children in elementary social hygiene than the authorities were willing to give the latter, thinking that the parents might object to it, according to Dr. M. J. Exner, director of the educational work of the American Social Hygiene Association, which opened its two-day annual meeting with a discussion conference yesterday afternoon at the Hotel Pennsylvania.

The effort of the association is to make this instruction an integral part of college and school courses in biology, sociology and natural science, he said. Particular emphasis is now shifting from the colleges and high schools, where this program is being adopted, into the grade schools. The benefit of this,

according to Dr. Exner, is that the child receives a scientific background of knowledge as a part of his regular instruction in general science before the time when the material becomes of pressing importance in his personal problems. The eventual ideal of the workers, he said, is to have this teaching done in the home and merely supplemented by the courses given at school. Teachers, especially in high schools and colleges, it was reported, are showing an ever increasing interest in the subject and are enrolling in large numbers in courses designed to fit them to teach it.

Dr. Charles W. Margold, Professor of Sociology at Michigan State Normal College, told of his experiences during a year spent observing conditions in Russia. The complete freedom of moral practice there for a time went further "than I believe Havelock Ellis or others of the most advanced philosophers would go in actual practice," he said. "But there is evidence of an increasing change of opinion among the lead-

ers and a realization, as expressed in discussions in the press, that the family must and will again be the fundamental institution."

Dr. Walter M. Brunet of the social hygiene committee of the New York Tuberculosis and Health Association told of a survey of social diseases and their spread which his group is conducting throughout Greater New York. Of 6,200 physicians approached only 10 refused to cooperate, he said. Ray H. Everett, editor of The Journal of Social Hygiene, presided at the meeting.

A report read at the dinner last night at the Town Hall Club announced that the association has 10,372 members, drawn from almost every profession and occupation, an increase of more than 3,000 over 1927. The report also says that there were 324,525 cases of social diseases reported by State health departments to the United States Public Health Service during 1928.

January 19, 1929

Yearly Medical Examination Urged by Governor for Safety

Governor Roosevelt urges annual medical examinations in a message published over his signature in Health News, the bulletin published by the Bellevue-Yorkville Health Demonstration, it was announced yesterday. The Governor's message stresses the need of medical attention, begun in time, in the case of many illnesses whose beginnings are imperceptible to the victim.

"Instead of waiting," the Governor writes, "to send for a doctor in great haste when we can no longer avoid the knowledge that we are really ill, how much better it would be to go to our doctor from time to time to be looked over. A general medical examination once a year is the soundest kind of insurance against serious illness and possible death."

June 10, 1929

TRAVELING CLINICS EMPLOYED IN THE FIGHT ON DIPHTHERIA

FOR the use of the already large staff to which has been assigned the task of combating diphtheria in the city, the Health Department is using three "health-mobiles"—large trucks rebuilt and specially equipped. They are to serve in the free-treatment campaign the department is waging with the aid of the toxin-antitoxin that prevents diphtheria. These "health-mobiles," now being used for the first time in a municipal health campaign, are making regular rounds of the parks and playgrounds where doctors immunize children, give advice on diphtheria and advertise their program by means of pamphlets printed in ten different languages.

Traveling clinics are the most recent devices to be used in the intensive campaign which the city, with the aid of private funds, has been waging against diphtheria since the first of the year. In seven months the special Diphtheria Prevention Commission has effected the immunization of 125,000 children and distributed millions of pieces of literature explaining the necessity and value of the treatment.

Death Rate Decreased.

The first semi-annual report of the commission showed that the death rate had decreased 28.5 per cent, or from 560 to 329, for the first six

months of 1929, as compared with the same period in 1928. The case rate also had decreased 19.4 per cent, or from 7,659 cases to 6,171 cases. These decreases are traced directly to the efforts of the commission, and Dr. Shirley W. Wynne, Commissioner of Health, is convinced that the mortality from diphtheria would be cut down to zero if every child between the ages of 9 months and 10 years were treated with the standardized toxin-antitoxin.

The treatment, which is simple and painless, is given by injecting three small doses of the serum, with a period of a week allowed to intervene after each dose in order to make sure that the inoculation "takes" effectively. By this method hundreds of thousands of children have been treated without one fatality or serious illness. The explanation offered for this success is that the mixture of toxin and antitoxin injected is not itself toxic, since the antitoxin neutralizes the toxin; and yet the preparation retains the property of stimulating the cells to produce the natural antitoxin which serves to protect the body from future threats of the disease.

The Diphtheria Prevention Committee recommends that all children between the ages of 9 months and 10 years receive these three treatments. The child inherits from its mother a temporary immunity which sometimes persists for almost a year. From that time until the age of 3,

almost all children are helpless to defend themselves against diphtheria. Half of all the children between the ages of 5 and 10 years and one-quarter of those between 10 and 15 need the treatments. The Schick test for determining whether children are naturally immune is seldom used for those under 10 years, because the immunization treatments are not much more difficult and cannot hurt them.

Educating the Public.

The chief task facing the commission has been that of educating parents as to the necessity of having their children immunized. This is being accomplished by an enormous advertising campaign: 2,000,000 pieces of literature have been distributed, 500,000 pastoral letters have been issued by Cardinal Hayes and 4,000,000 circulars have been sent out with the statements of gas and electric companies.

A diphtheria movietone and placards in subways and street cars have also helped to bring information to the general public. As each child born in the city reaches the age of 9 months its mother receives a letter urging her to have her baby protected against diphtheria. No effort is being spared to drive home the fact that doctors believe every death from diphtheria and a large number of the cases can be prevented by treatment with toxin-antitoxin.

September 8, 1929

HEALTH WORK HALVES INFANT DEATH RATE

Many Mothers Also Saved by Commonwealth Fund in Rural Experiments.

Deaths of infants and mothers due to childbirth were reduced on an average of more than one-half in experimental groups in widely separated rural communities where public health care was given mothers before the births of their children, the Commonwealth Fund, of 578 Madison Avenue, which conducted the tests, announced yesterday.

Of 10,000 children born in these communities, the fund announced, about 2,500 were born under the auspices of public health workers.

"Expressed in terms of deaths per 1,000 births," the report stated, "the maternal death rate among the mothers cared for was 3.2, as compared with 7.6 for those not cared for. The stillborth was 25.8 in the group under care and 48.4 in the group not cared for. The infant death rate under one month of age was 16.3 per 1,000 live births among those cared for and 39.4 among those not reached by this service."

Public health service also reduced materially the death rate among babies between 1 month and 1 year of age, the report added, the death rate in this class being only 18.1 per 1,000 among 6,000 children reached by that service, compared with 47.6 per 1,000 among 3,500 infants who did not have the benefit of that care.

The experiments were conducted in Fargo, N. D.; Athens, Clarke County, Ga.; Rutherford County, Tenn., and Salem, Marion County, Ore. They have been conducted by Courtenay Dinwiddie, and the last demonstration by the fund was announced to end on Dec. 31.

December 16, 1929

COST OF DEPRESSION IN HEALTH REVEALED

Surveys of Public Health Service Disclose Waste of Unemployment In Terms of Human Resources

By JOSEPHINE ROCHE, Assistant Secretary of the Treasury in Charge of Public Health Service.

WASHINGTON, Sept. 13.—There has been in recent months much speculation on the effect of the depression on health. Certain dramatic statements have been made indicating a severe breakdown, but on the whole the assumption has prevailed that the declining general death rate of the past few years has meant a state of physical well-being among our people. In fact, there have been not infrequent comments that "the depression was good for our health." The mortality rate has popularly been taken as the barometer of our people's physical condition. Analysis shows it to be a very poor index.

The death rate does not indicate the extent or nature of the 90 per cent of illnesses that are not fatal, nor the physical impairments such as malnutrition. It is not affected immediately by unfavorable living conditions unless starvation and pestilence are actually present. It does not properly measure decreased resistance to disease.

Figures Not Final.

Furthermore, an actual increase in mortality among the unemployed and their families could have taken place but have been entirely masked by the downward trend among the more prosperous elements of the population.

That such may well be the case is indicated by facts reported in a recent survey by the United States Public Health Service and the Milbank Fund of the wage-earning population in ten industrial localities. It was found that the death rate during the period 1929-1932 declined in families with full-time employed wage earners, but in families with no employed members or only part-time wage earners, it increased 20 per cent.

A death rate that does not increase, or even one that declines, does not tell the health story. For every case of sickness resulting in death there are from 50 to 100 cases which recover.

An assessment of the nation's health requires, therefore, that illnesses rather than deaths should be the basis from which to draw conclusions. The sickness rate, unfortunately, shows that the physical well-being at least of that portion of the nation most affected by the depression has been harmed by the lowering of the standard of living, worry and other by-products of the depression.

Recent Studies Made.

Recent studies indicate a high rate of acute and chronic diseases and serious physical impairments among families on relief rolls. In a number of communities severely affected by unemployment the United States Public Health Service, in a house-to-house canvass made in collaboration with the Milbank Memorial Fund, found distressing conditions.

The surveyed localities included seven large cities—Baltimore, Birmingham, Cleveland, Detroit, New York (the Boroughs of Manhattan and Brooklyn), Pittsburgh and Syracuse—a group of coal-mining communities in the vicinity of Morgantown, W. Va., and a number of cotton-mill villages in the neighborhood of Greenville, S. C. Districts were selected in the poorer sections of the cities, but not in strictly slum areas. A record was obtained of the illnesses of each member of the family for the three months before the visit.

Twelve thousand families were visited during this study. The incomes of these families showed that their standard of living must have been very low. It was found that 66 per cent had incomes of less than $1,200 in 1932 and 32 per cent had less than $600. One-fifth of all the families were depending on public relief. In 1929 three-fourths of these people had been in reasonably comfortable circumstances.

Illness Rate High.

The illness rate was 56 per cent higher in families hardest hit by the depression than it was among their more fortunate neighbors. Sickness among these "new poor" was more prevalent than among the "chronic poor" who had been poverty stricken even in 1929, a fact which suggests that ill health is associated with sudden drop in the standard of living.

The direct effect of unemployment is indicated by the fact that the sickness rate of families having no employed workers was 48 per cent higher than the sickness rate of families with full-time workers and 14 per cent higher than that of families with part-time workers only. These higher illness rates appeared among the children as well as among the adults.

There was proportionately more disabling illness among persons on relief than in any other class. Those who had dropped from reasonable comfort to the relief rolls had the highest illness rate. Among both relief and non-relief families, more illness occurred in the groups that had suffered the severest economic change during the depression.

Further data were collected recently by the Federal Emergency Relief Administration on physical impairments and chronic diseases among the relief and non-relief populations of a large city. This survey indicated that the portion of persons on relief who had serious physical defects or chronic diseases was three times that in the same occupational class not on relief.

Group Is Analyzed.

Analyzing the group of persons reporting no physical impairments or chronic diseases, the survey showed only 12 per cent were on relief, whereas 30 per cent of those who had some impairment or chronic disease were on relief. Also, the survey indicated that within the non-relief population, the proportion of persons with disease or impairment increases definitely from the lowest rate in the professional, proprietary and clerical classes to the highest among unskilled laborers.

In contrast, within the relief population, which had a proportion of handicapped persons far in excess of the non-relief figure, there was little variation of the rate of disease or impairment between occupational groups.

Obviously facts such as these reveal not only conditions of human suffering and wretchedness but economic waste, and challenge us to a swift-moving program of conservation of one of our most valued national resources—the health and vitality of our people.

September 15, 1935

HEALTH SERVICE EXPANDS DUTIES

Special Correspondence, THE NEW YORK TIMES.

WASHINGTON, April 11. — Dr. Thomas Parran Jr., formerly Health Commissioner of New York State, became guardian of the entire nation's health this week, taking up the duties of Surgeon General which Dr. Hugh S. Cumming had laid down after sixteen years of service.

Dr. Parran, nominated by President Roosevelt on March 23, was confirmed by the Senate four days later. His commission, signed by the President during his fishing trip off the Florida coast, was flown back to the capital and presented to him on Monday.

During Dr. Cumming's administration Congress has added to the duties of the Public Health Service, broadened its research program and enlarged its assistance to State and city health authorities. Dr. Parran, in taking over the task, will direct the work of approximately 400 commissioned officers, many of them specialists in the control of particular diseases.

Dr. Parran, a close friend of President Roosevelt, had been an Assistant Surgeon General of the Public Health Service, from which post he had had leave since 1930, when the then Governor Roosevelt asked Dr. Cumming that the officer be lent to New York State.

Strides Forward

Advances made by the service under Dr. Cumming include the completion of the national quarantine system, establishment of a national leprosarium and Federal narcotic farms, health supervision over international air navigation and medical examination at American consulates abroad of aliens seeking admission to the United States.

Previously existing activities have been expanded to keep pace with the health problems of a growing nation. Greater emphasis has been laid on research, both as to specific diseases and community sanitation. Public health officers have been active in giving assistance to local health agencies in the prevention and control of epidemics.

Officers collect data on the outbreak of disease dangerous to public health and assemble statistics on the current prevalence of diseases in all parts of the country. They inspect incoming vessels and airplanes to prevent the introduction of disease from foreign countries. They keep watch, for the same reason, on the Mexican and Canadian borders, and with the cooperation of local organizations examine the sources of water used by interstate transportation lines. They inspect vaccines and serums.

New Work Imposed

The Social Security Law authorized an $8,000,000 appropriation annually to assist State and city governments to maintain public health services. Under the law the Surgeon General determines the conditions under which these payments will be made. These funds will be allocated to the States on the basis of three factors—population, financial need and special health problems.

To carry out its assignments under the Social Security Act the Public Health Service will establish five regional offices, with Federal officers available in each for consultation with State officers.

April 12, 1936

CHOLERA DECLINE LAID TO PASTEURIZED MILK

Acting City Health Chief Tells of 25-Year Results in Guarding Children.

Commenting on the twenty-fifth anniversary this year of the enactment of the Compulsory Milk Pasteurization Law, Dr. William H. Best, Acting Commissioner of Health, declared yesterday that pasteurization virtually had eliminated cholera infantum. He gave figures showing that last Summer only 166 infants had died from this disease while in 1910, the year before the Pasteurization Law was adopted, 3,598 children had died in three months.

"When one considers that upward of 3,000,000 quarts of milk are consumed in New York City daily," Dr. Best said, "he will realize what a vast job the Department of Health has in controlling this important food supply. Many of us still in the department recall the violent opposition which arose at the time Commissioner Ernst J. Lederle began to enforce pasteurization.

"The control of the city's milk supply has been one of the major functions of the Department of Health and, by drawing the strings tighter each year, we have succeeded in giving the City of New York the safest, cleanest and best milk possible."

Dr. Best made public the following table, showing how cholera infantum deaths have decreased over five-year periods:

Summer of 1910 3,598
Summer of 1915 2,287
Summer of 1920 1,280
Summer of 1925 477
Summer of 1930 302
Summer of 1935 166

July 19, 1936

GOOD WATER AIDING HEALTH

Special Correspondence, THE NEW YORK TIMES.

WASHINGTON. — The National Resources Committee in a recent report to the President declares that the improvement in the nation's drinking water has brought not only a decline in water-borne diseases but a general improvement in health and comfort as well. "In less than half a century, typhoid fever, once the leading captain of death," the report says, "has declined to a point where it is not unusual for a medical student to graduate without having seen a typhoid fever germ."

Some 80,000,000 Americans now obtain their drinking water through 10,000 public water supply systems, the National Resources Committee estimates. Of these, about 37,000,000 use filtered and chlorinated water, 26,000,000 partially purified water and 17,000,000 untreated water.

Although public water supply systems serve most of the cities with populations of 5,000 and over, the smaller communities in which millions of Americans live must still depend upon private wells and cisterns.

The report declared that about 72,000,000 Americans today live in communities which have sewerage facilities; five years ago, about 30 per cent of the urban population was provided with sewerage equipment; today, approximately half the urban population has the protection of such facilities; progress has been due to increased public interest and to Federal programs of public works.

March 27, 1938

VAST HEALTH PLAN URGED FOR COUNTRY

By WILLIAM L. LAURENCE

Special to THE NEW YORK TIMES.

WASHINGTON, July 18.—A comprehensive and far-reaching national health program for providing more adequate distribution of medical care to the American people, calling for the expenditure of $850,000,000 a year for a ten-year period, was submitted in outline here today before the National Health Conference.

The conference, called at the suggestion of President Roosevelt by the President's Interdepartmental Committee to Coordinate Health and Welfare Activities, is the first of its kind ever held. It brings together representatives of the various important medical bodies and leaders of organized labor, agriculture and other important lay groups who have a direct interest in bringing the present high cost of medical care within the means of the majority of the population.

The $850,000,000-a-year program was submitted to the Interdepartmental Committee by its technical committee on medical care and was presented to President Roosevelt last February, it was revealed.

The President thereupon, it was stated by Miss Josephine Roche, former assistant secretary of the Treasury and chairman of the conference, suggested calling this conference for the purpose of submitting the various recommendations of the program for discussion by the representatives of the groups most vitally concerned, before taking final action.

Cabot and A. M. A. Heads Clash

The national public health plan brought from Dr. Irvin Abell of Louisville, president of the American Medical Association, the criticism that it was impractical.

Dr. Hugh Cabot of the Mayo Clinic in turn assailed the attitude of organized medicine toward public health services. Dr. Cabot, a member of the Committee of Physicians, who are "rebels" against the policy of the American Medical Association, exchanged caustic words with Dr. Olin West, secretary of the A. M. A.

Dr. Abell told the conference that no practical health administrator could possibly approve a centrally controlled medical service plan which failed to take into account "varying conditions of the States, counties and cities of this country."

"The medical profession and the allied health agencies throughout the country are exerting every effort to determine the needs and the demands for medical care," said Dr. Abell. "Changes to meet health needs must be consistent with local conditions and requirements and must be judged by the effect which such changes will have on the quality of the medical care for the individual sick person."

Dr. Cabot charged that, "as at present organized," medicine was a "competitive business."

"The maintenance of standards of medical practice by the medical profession as at present organized has been grossly unsatisfactory," he said. "There are very large areas in this country where the practice of medicine as at present carried on is medieval."

Thousands of persons in the country wanted doctors and a lot of doctors wanted patients, he added, and were "starving to death."

Dr. Cabot hailed the conference as the first real action on the "mass demand of the consumer of medical aid" for a way out of the economic difficulty.

Dr. West Retorts

In reply to Dr. Cabot Dr. West said that the American Medical Association spent hundreds of thousands of dollars yearly in the interests of the people as a whole.

"I am here," Dr. West added, "in defense of the medical profession of the United States, which one member saw fit to ridicule. I doubt if the medical profession has any more pride in him than he has pride in the profession."

The tenor of the conference and of President Roosevelt's message indicated that, while the Federal Government sought the cooperation of organized medicine, it intended nevertheless to embark on a comprehensive program for the expansion of the public health services.

"Need" Stressed by Roosevelt

The conference was opened in the morning by Miss Roche with the reading of a message from President Roosevelt stating that "there is nothing more important to a nation than the health of its people" and that "there is a need for a coordinated national program of action."

Following the reading of the President's message, dated July 15, the purposes of the Conference were outlined further by Miss Roche, Miss Katharine F. Lenroot, chief of the Children's Bureau of the Department of Labor, and by Dr. Thomas Parran, Surgeon General of the United States Public Health Service.

Other groups were represented by William Green, president of the American Federation of Labor; Dorothy C. Kahn, director Philadelphia County Relief Board; Dorothy J. Bellanca, vice president Amalgamated Clothing Workers of America; Benjamin W. Kilgore, executive secretary Kentucky Farm Bureau Federation; Mrs. H. W. Ahart, president Associated Women, American Farm Bureau Federation.

Outline of National Program

The ten-year national health program, the Technical Committee on Medical Care suggests, should be supported by the Federal, State and local governments, with the Federal Government contributing one-half the cost, or a maximum of $425,000,000 a year over the period. Details of the report will be further revealed during the remaining two days of the conference.

The committee stated that it "is firm in its conviction that, as progress is made toward the control of various diseases and conditions, as facilities and services commensurate with the high standards of American medical practice are made more generally available, the coming decade, under a national health program, will see a major reduction in needless loss of life and suffering—an increasing prospective for longer years of productive, self-supporting life in our population."

The committee's study of health and medical services in the United States, the report states, indicates that deficiencies in the present health services fall into four broad categories, as follows:

1. Preventive health services for the nation as a whole are grossly insufficient.
2. Hospital and other institutional facilities are inadequate in many communities, especially in rural areas, and financial support for hospital care and for professional services in hospitals is both insufficient and precarious, especially for services to people who cannot pay the costs of the care they need.
3. One-third of the population, including persons with or without income, is receiving inadequate or no medical service.
4. An even larger fraction of the population suffers from economic burdens created by illness.

The committee then submits five recommendations for meeting "with reasonable adequacy existing deficiencies in the nation's health service."

It is the first three of these recommendations that, it is estimated by the committee, will require additional expenditures of $850,000,000 a year by the Federal, State and local governments. The remaining two recommendations, the report states, "involve chiefly a revision of present methods of making certain expenditures, rather than increase in these expenditures."

The first recommendation includes two items, expansion of the general public health services for the purpose of eradication of tuberculosis, venereal diseases and malaria; the control of mortality from pneumonia and from cancer, mental hygiene and industrial hygiene. The additional expenditure for this part of the program was estimated at $200,000,000 annually.

The second item of this recommendation calls for the expansion of maternal and child health services, at an added cost of $165,000,000.

"The objective sought in this phase of the committee's proposed program," the report says, "is to make available to mothers and children of all income groups and in all parts of the United States minimum medical services essential for the reduction of our needlessly high maternal mortality rates and death rates among infants, and for the prevention in childhood of diseases and conditions leading to serious disabilities in later years."

The second recommendation calls for an annual added expenditure of $146,050,000, to provide 360,000 new hospital beds in rural and urban areas and 500 health and diagnostic centers in areas inaccessible to hospitals.

Care for the Medically Needy

The third recommendation calls for the "provision of medical care for the medically needy."

This part of the program, the committee states, "might be begun with the expenditure of $50,000,000 the first year and gradually expanded until it reaches the estimated level of $400,000,000, which would be needed to provide minimum care to the medically needy groups."

The fourth recommendation deals with a general program of medical care aimed to lighten the burdens of sickness for the self-supporting groups. To finance this, the report states, two sources of funds could be drawn upon: (a) General taxation or special tax assessments, and, (b) specific insurance contributions from the potential beneficiaries of an insurance system.

"The committee recommends both, recognizing that they may be used separately or in combination," it was stated.

The fifth recommendation deals with insurance against loss of wages during sickness.

President Green of the A. F. of L. suggested amending the present Workmen's Compension Laws "to provide compensation for loss of time and hospital and medical services for workers and families during sickness."

Dr. Parran told the gathering that he believed "this conference marks the ridge of the hill between the old indifference to health as a matter of national concern and a new understanding that health is the first and most appropriate object for national action."

Roosevelt Message to Meeting

President Roosevelt's message to the conference read as follows:

"I am glad that your committee has had such an excellent response to its invitations to representatives of the public and of the medical and other professions to participate in the National Health Conference. I regret that because I shall be on a cruise I shall be unable to speak to the conference.

"I am glad that the conference includes so many representatives of the general public. The professional experts can, and, I feel sure, will do their part. But the problems before you are in a real sense public problems. The ways and means of dealing with them must be determined with a view to the best interests of all our citizens.

"I hope that your technical committee's report on the need for a national health program and its tentative proposals will be read and studied, not only by the participants in the conference but by every citizen.

"Nothing is more important to a nation than the health of its people. Medical science has made remarkable strides, and in cooperation with government and voluntary agencies it has made substantial progress in the control of various diseases.

Cites Gains Being Made

"During the last few years we have taken several additional steps forward through the extension of public health and maternal and child welfare services under the Social Security Act, the launching of a special campaign to control syphilis, the establishment of a national cancer institute, and the use of Federal emergency funds for the expansion of hospital and sanitation facilities, the control of malaria and many related purposes.

"But when we see what we know how to do, yet have not done, it is clear that there is need for a coordinated national program of action. Such a program necessarily must take account of the fact that millions of citizens lack the individual means to pay for adequate medical care. The economic loss due to sickness is a very serious matter, not only for many families with and without incomes, but for the nation as a whole.

"We cannot do all at once everything we should do.

"But we can advance more surely if we have before us a comprehensive, long-range program providing for the most efficient cooperation of Federal, State and local governments, voluntary agencies, professional groups, mediums of public information and individual citizens.

"I hope that at the National Health Conference a chart for continuing concerted action will begin to take form."

July 19, 1938

Social Hygiene Aids Children

Increase in Knowledge and New Laws Have Removed a Menace to Health

By WALTER CLARKE, M. D.,
Executive Director American Social Hygiene Association

Next Wednesday, Feb. 1, is National Social Hygiene Day. Five thousand meetings to be held all over the country under the auspices of the American Social Hygiene Association will help to safeguard the common birthright of all our children—good health.

Parents everywhere know that pure milk, a clean water supply, vaccination and protection against diphtheria are among the common safeguards of childhood, which are demanded in modern communities for the protection of boys and girls.

Public health education in recent years has made it equally plain that syphilis is another threat to the health and lives of children against which we have ample measures of safety. It is the purpose of Social Hygiene Day to direct attention to this fact.

Public Opinion Aroused

In twenty-five years we have come a long way in our thinking on social hygiene. A quarter of a century ago it was known that the use of a few drops of silver nitrate solution in the eyes at birth prevented much of the blindness among babies. But there was a hard fight to get this simple precaution into the statute books. The law is now taken for granted. And infant blindness from infection at birth has been almost entirely wiped out.

Widespread education has made the task of social hygiene legislation easier than it was in the days when drops in a new-born baby's eyes was a new-fangled notion. It is now clear that the public is eager to know of protective measures and ready to endorse laws in their support. A vote overwhelmingly in favor of pre-marital laws—requiring a physical examination and blood test of all applicants for marriage licenses—was recorded two years ago by the American Institute of Public Opinion. A poll on the question, "Would you favor such a law in your State?" indicated that 92 per cent of the people in the country were ready to answer "Yes."

This popular acceptance of a social hygiene program is also shown by enlightened legislation now existing in many States.

Laws requiring examinations for all those about to marry (so-called pre-marital laws) have been passed in ten States—New York, New Jersey, Connecticut, Illinois, Michigan, Kentucky, Wisconsin, New Hampshire, Rhode Island and Oregon. Three States—New York, New Jersey and Rhode Island—have enacted legislation requiring every physician attending an expectant mother to include a blood test in the pre-natal examination.

Important Precaution

This, in many ways, is of greater importance than the pre-marital law, insuring as it does against the appearance of syphilis in the unborn child. With correct treatment, begun not later than the middle of pregnancy, and continued to the day of delivery, we obtain more than 90 per cent of satisfactory results, that is, a child free from syphilis. In other words, nine out of ten of the babies now born suffering from this disease could be healthy if expectant mothers insisted upon blood tests and full treatment, when needed, at least during the last five months of pregnancy.

This I believe to be one of the most brilliant achievements of modern medicine. From the point of view of any parent it may be considered one of the greatest contributions preventive medicine has made to child health.

Protection of childhood is, of course, only a part of the larger problem of protecting the whole population, young and old. As a result of twenty-five years of educational work of the American Social Hygiene Association and its affiliated organizations, the fight on this needless scourge gains in effectiveness every day.

January 29, 1939

SCIENTISTS CHART A DIET 'YARDSTICK' TO GIVE US HEALTH

New Food Guide for the Nation Is 'a Challenge to Us All,' Dr. Parran Says

HAILED AS A DEFENSE AID

Chart, Presented on Eve of Nutrition Parley, Gives Units of 10 Basic Food Needs

By WILLIAM L. LAURENCE
Special to THE NEW YORK TIMES.

WASHINGTON, May 25—A new yardstick for nutrition, to serve from now on as the "nutritional gold standard" for the American people, was announced here tonight on the eve of the opening of the three-day National Nutrition Conference for Defense, called by President Roosevelt.

The new food guide, described by Dr. Thomas Parran, Surgeon General of the United States Public Health Service, as "a yardstick which is a challenge to all of us," was worked out in accordance with the latest discoveries in the science of nutrition by a special committee composed of the country's leading authorities on the subject.

The new standard for adequate human feeding is aimed to bring the physical and mental health of America up to a new "par" never before attained by any nation. It consists of a carefully worked out chart giving the basic amounts of ten essential food requirements for men and women of all ages and types of work, as well as for children and growing boys and girls and for expectant and nursing mothers.

Required Food Intake Charted

The chart gives the total required daily food intake for the various groups in calories, the minimum required daily amount of proteins, the minimum daily needs for Vitamins A, C and D, as well as for three members of the highly important Vitamin B family, and the minimum daily requisite, for good health, of the minerals iron and calcium.

The three B-complex vitamins are thiamin, known as the "morale vitamin"; riboflavin, the vitamin necessary for growth and for maintaining the integrity of the eyes and skin; and nicotinic acid (not to be confused with either nicotine or acid in the ordinary sense), which is necessary for the maintenance of normal mental balance and for the prevention of pellagra, the dread disease afflicting many of the poor of the South and also found to be widespread as a precursor of other diseases among wider segments of the population.

Other minerals and vitamins that the human body needs for the prevention of ill-health and for the maintenance of optimum health as distinguished from merely border line health, are provided for.

These include such minerals as iodine, supplied in iodized table salt; copper, necessary with iron for maintaining the supply of red blood corpuscles; phosphorus, needed for healthy bones and teeth; manganese, the mineral without which the love of mother for offspring has been found to vanish; Vitamin E, the fertility factor; Vitamin K, necessary for blood coagulation; about nine, and possibly more, vitamins of the B group; as well as zinc, cobalt, boron and a number of other minerals.

Typical Daily Diet Is Given

Dr. Lydia J. Roberts, head of the Department of Home Economics of the University of Chicago and chairman of a subcommittee which assembled the data for the food standard from hundreds of nutritional studies and from experts in the field, presented a typical daily diet which would meet the standard.

A good diet of natural foods, such as Dr. Roberts suggests as an illustration, will not only meet the requirements of the ten elements in the chart but will also provide the other minerals, the requirements for which are less well known.

Speaking among a number of leaders on the American Forum of the Air on the Mutual Broadcasting System's coast-to-coast network, over which the new food guide was presented, Dr. Roberts explained that "the recommended allowances for foods which this committee has agreed upon are expressed in laboratory terms." She continued:

"Here is a diet which would measure up to these proposals:

"One pint of milk for an adult and more for a child; a serving of meat, of which the cheaper cuts are just as nutritious; one egg, or some suitable substitute, such as navy beans; two vegetables, one of which should be green or yellow; two fruits, one of which should be rich in Vitamin C, found abundantly in citrus fruits and tomatoes; breads, flour and cereal, most, or preferably all, whole grain or enriched with minerals and vitamins; some butter or oleomargarine with Vitamin A added; other foods to satisfy the appetite.

"There are many combinations of food which meet these new requirements. America is fortunate today that it has a large number of trained nutritionists who can translate these allowances into terms of foods available and practical in many parts of the country."

Goal Set, McNutt Asserts

Paul V. McNutt, Federal Security Administrator, said that the new diet standard would set the goal for which the whole country and its organized groups must work "if America is to realize her full strength for defense."

People were healthy only if they were adequately fed, he said, declaring that America was not fed nearly well enough for our own security.

Dr. Parran commented on the practicability of the new food guide,

New Dietary Yardstick

Special to THE NEW YORK TIMES.

WASHINGTON, May 25—*The new dietary yardstick for America, made public tonight by the food and nutrition committee of the National Research Council, recommends daily allowances of specific nutrients as follows:*

CALORIES

Man weighing 154 pounds:
Moderately active—3,000.
Very active—4,500.
Sedentary—2,500.
Woman weighing 123 pounds:
Moderately active—2,500.
Very active—3,000.
Sedentary—2,100.
Children up to twelve years:
Under one year—100 calories per kilogram.
1-3 years—1,200.
4-6 years—1,600.
7-9 years—2,000.
10-12 years—2,500.
Children over twelve years:
Girls, 13-15 years—2,800.
16-20 years—2,400.
Boys, 13-15 years—3,200.
16-20 years—3,800.
Pregnancy (latter half, for 56 kilogram weight)—2,500.
Lactation period—3,000.

PROTEINS

Man—70 grams.
Woman—60 grams.
Pregnancy—85 grams.
Lactation Period—100 grams.
Children up to 12 years:
Under 1 year—3 to 4 grams per kilogram weight.
1-3 years—40 grams.
4-6 years—50 grams.
7-9 years—60 grams.
10-12 years—70 grams.
Children over 12 years:
Girls, 13-15 years—80 grams.
16-20 years—75 grams.
Boys, 13-15 years—85 grams.
16-20 years—100 grams.

CALCIUM

Man—0.8 gram.
Woman—0.8 gram.
Pregnancy—1.5 grams.
Lactation—2.0 grams.
Children up to 9 years—1.0 gram.
10-12 years—1.2 grams.
Girls, 13-15 years—1.3 grams.
16-20 years—1.0 gram.
Boys, 13-20 years—1.4 grams.

IRON

Man and woman—12 grams.
Pregnant woman—15 grams.
Children under 1 year—6 grams.
1-3 years—7 grams.
4-6 years—8 grams.
7-9 years—10 grams.
10-12 years—12 grams.
Boys and girls, 15-20 years—15 grams.

VITAMIN A
(International Units)

Man or woman—5,000.
Pregnancy—6,000.
Lactation—8,000.
Children under 1 year—1,500.
1-3 years—2,000.
4-6 years—2,500.
7-9 years—3,500.
10-12 years—4,500.
Girls, 13-20 years—5,000.
Boys, 13-15 years—5,000.
16-20 years—6,000.

THIAMIN

Vitamin B-1 for "Morale"
(Milligrams)

Man weighing 154 pounds:
Moderately active—1.8.
Very active—2.3.
Sedentary—1.5.
Woman weighing 123 pounds:
Moderately active—1.5.
Very active—1.8.
Sedentary—1.2.
Pregnancy (later half)—1.8.
Lactation—2.3.
Children under 1 year—0.4.
1-3 years—0.6.
4-6 years—0.8.
7-9 years—1.0.
10-12 years—1.2.
Girls, 13-15 years—1.4.
16-20 years—1.2.

Boys, 13-15 years—1.6.
16-20 years—2.0.

RIBOFLAVIN

Vitamin B-2, for Growth, Healthy Eyes, Normal Skin
(Milligrams)

Man weighing 154 pounds:
Moderately active—2.7.
Very active—3.3.
Sedentary—2.2.
Woman weighing 123 pounds:
Moderately active—2.2.
Very active—2.7.
Sedentary—1.8.
Pregnancy—2.5.
Lactation—3.0.
Children under 1 year—0.6.
1-3 years—0.9.
4-6 years—1.2.
7-9 years—1.5.
10-12 years—1.8.
Girls, 13-15 years—2.0.
16-20 years—1.8.
Boys, 13-15 years—2.4.
16-20 years—3.0.

NICOTINIC ACID

Third member of Vitamin B family, preventive of pellagra and mental symptoms.
(Milligrams)

Man weighing 154 pounds:
Moderately active—18.
Very active—23.
Sedentary—15.
Woman weighing 123 pounds:
Moderately active—15.
Very active—18.
Sedentary—12.
Pregnancy—18.
Lactation—23.
Children under 1 year—4.
1-3 years—6.
4-6 years—8.
7-9 years—10.
10-12 years—12.
Girls, 13-15 years—14.
16-20 years—12.
Boys, 13-15 years—16.
16-20 years—20.

VITAMIN C

For healthy teeth and to prevent scurvy; present in citrus fruits, also in tomatoes and potatoes.
(Milligrams)

Man weighing 154 pounds—75.
Woman weighing 123 pounds—70.
Pregnancy (later half)—100.
Lactation—150.
Children under 1 year—30.
One-three years—35.
Four-six years—50.
Seven-nine years—60.
Ten-twelve years—75.
Girls, 13-20 years—80.
Boys, 13-15 years—90.
Sixteen-twenty years—100.

VITAMIN D

"Sunshine Vitamin"

Pregnancy, lactation and children under 1 year—400-800 international units.

Older children and adults also need it in similar amounts when it is not available from sunshine.

The committee states that the quantities in the above chart "are tentative allowances toward which to aim in planning practical dietaries and which can be met by a good diet of natural foods." Such a diet, it adds, "will also provide other minerals and vitamins, the requirements for which are less well known."

Terms used in the table are explained as follows: A gram in the international metric system of weights and measures is about one-twenty-eighth of an ounce. A kilogram, which is 1,000 grams, is equal to 2.2 pounds avoirdupois. A milligram is one-thousandth of a gram. A calory is a unit of measurement used to express the heat-producing or energy-producing value of food.

which he said could be attained immediately by all except families of the lowest incomes.

"Now, for the first time, the United States has definite nutrition recommendations from an authoritative national committee which has pooled all the available knowledge on foods and drawn a blueprint of the amounts and kinds of dietary essentials for good health," the Surgeon General said.

"This is a yardstick which is a challenge to all of us. With the exception of families of the lowest income groups, this yardstick can be attained now.

"There is no narrow list of foods from which to draw. Ample allowance is made for geographical differences in prices of foods. Many diets today do not reach these standards. This is a dangerous situation. Our work is to bring the story of good nutrition to every American family.

"Those who can afford the foods recommended will want to include all of them. Those whose budgets do not permit them to buy what they need are the responsibility of all of us. I expect the Nutrition Conference for Defense to outline ways in which this new dietary yardstick can become a reality."

League Gave a Guide in 1935

Nutrition standards were set by the League of Nations in 1935 as the result of a study to which scientists in various parts of the world contributed. However, much has been added to knowledge in this field since that time, said Professor Russell M. Wilder of the Mayo Clinic, chairman of the Food and Nutrition Committee of the Division of Medical Sciences of the National Research Council, a committee composed of thirty of the country's leaders in the science of nutrition and which prepared the new food guide.

"The food allowance recommendations we now make are higher in vitamin content, especially in thiamin, riboflavin and nicotinic acid, about which much has been learned in the past four years," Dr. Wilder said. Nicotinic acid was not even known as a vitamin until 1937, while the role of riboflavin was known only vaguely in 1935.

"If America is to have the healthy people we need in this national emergency, we must improve our diets so that they more nearly measure up to this new yardstick for nutrition," Dr. Wilder declared.

Mr. McNutt hailed the significance of the committee's work.

"These standards are the result of far-reaching work by the food and nutrition committee of the National Research Council," he said. "They will set the nutrition goal for which government, industry, labor, science, education and every organized group and every citizen must work if America is to realize her full strength for defense.

Others who participated in the forum included Claude R. Wickard, Secretary of Agriculture; Dr. M. L. Wilson, director of extension work, United States Department of Agriculture, who is chairman of the Interdepartmental Government Planning Committee for the national nutrition program; David Dietz, science editor of the Scripps-Howard newspaper, and this correspondent.

The compilation of the data, the work of Dr. Robert's subcommittee, will serve as the basis of discussion by the 900 delegates from all parts of the United States who are gathered here for the National Nutrition Conference for Defense, the first of its kind ever held on a nation-wide scale.

May 26, 1941

ARMY TO BUILD UP HEALTH OF 200,000 DROPPED IN DRAFT

President Tells Rehabilitation Plan and Says Our Health Conditions Indict America

Special to THE NEW YORK TIMES.

WASHINGTON, Oct. 10—Plans for rehabilitating 200,000 of the 1,000,000 youths who have been rejected for military service because of physical or mental deficiencies were announced by President Roosevelt at his press conference today.

The program will apply immediately to the 200,000 who were certified by local draft boards as susceptible of physical rehabilitation for the Army. Local physicians and dentists will give the treatments, for which the Federal Government will pay as part of the cost of national defense. When in proper condition, the men will be inducted into the service.

While this is the immediate program, Mr. Roosevelt said that it was only the first objective, adding that something should be done along broader lines, and declaring that he considered the existence of the conditions revealed by the selective service examinations as an indictment of America. Nearly 50 per cent of 2,000,000 men examined for selective service were found unfit mentally or physically.

The President said that he would start a long-range program calling for cooperation of States, counties, cities, townships and individuals to remedy the underlying causes of the situation.

The plan for rehabilitating the 200,000 men was adopted on the basis of a report to the President from Brig. Gen. Hershey, director of the selective service system. The President could not estimate how much it would cost but said that it would be much less than if the men had been inducted and rehabilitation had then been attempted.

The plans are already far advanced for helping the 200,000 men. Those suffering from heart diseases, musculo-skeletal defects and mental and nervous disorders will be put in a special category and will be examined by traveling boards or teams of specialists who will recommend curable cases for immediate treatment at government cost.

Of those rejected under the Selective Service Act, 100,000 were found mentally unequipped for service, since they did not have the equivalent of a fourth-grade education. The other 900,000 rejections were due to physical defects or mental and nervous diseases. The largest category of physical defects came under the dental classification, representing nearly 21 per cent of the whole. Defective eyes were another major cause of rejection.

Commenting on this, the President said that we did not want men in the Army with false teeth. This remark prompted an interjection from one of his listeners that General Grant had false teeth.

The report of General Hershey was as follows:

"About 50 per cent of the approximately two million registrants who have been examined for induction into the Army of the United States under the Selective Training and Service Act of 1940 have been disqualified because of physical, mental or education reasons. Of the approximately one million rejected, 900,000, or about 90 per cent, were found to be physically or mentally unfit.

"The physical rejections of registrants were distributed as follows:

Cause.	No. of Cases.	Percentage.
Dental defects	188,000	20.9
Defective eyes	123,000	13.7
Cardiovascular diseases	96,000	10.6
Musculo-skeletal defects	61,000	6.8
Venereal diseases	57,000	6.3
Mental and nervous diseases	57,000	6.3
Hernia	56,000	6.2
Defects of ears	41,000	4.6
Defective lungs, including tuberculosis	26,000	2.9
Miscellaneous	159,000	17.7
Total	900,000	100.0

"Of this number, about 200,000 can be completely rehabilitated and made available for general service in our armed forces. The remainder can be rehabilitated to perform only limited service or because of mental, nervous, cardiovascular and pulmonary diseases, and musculo-skeletal defects are incapable of rehabilitation for even limited service and are, therefore, not being considered under the present rehabilitation program for Selective Service registrants.

"Our initial objective in this rehabilitation program will be the 200,000 registrants who can be completely rehabilitated and made available for general military service in the armed forces at a small cost and in a reasonably short period of time.

"Certain types of venereal diseases, operable hernias, deficiencies in teeth and vision and other minor defects will be corrected in cases where the Army determines that the registrant will then be acceptable for general military service.

"The registrant will have the privilege of having the services performed by his family physician or dentist in his own community.

"The cost of this rehabilitation program will be borne by the Federal Government as a necessary part of our national defense program, and additional funds will be made available to the Selective Service System for this purpose."

Asked whether the men could be compelled to undergo the treatment, President Roosevelt said that when a registrant appeared before an examining board he was under its jurisdiction and could be directed to undergo such treatment. If he should refuse, he could be inducted into the Army and compelled to undergo the treatment there.

Mr. Roosevelt said that he had rejected an alternative plan suggested by the Army for the defectives to be inducted and then rehabilitated as enlisted men in Army medical centers. When housing, food, clothing, Army pay and medical care were considered, this would have cost some $500,000,000, he explained, whereas the salvage program by local physicians and dentists would cost much less than that.

October 11, 1941

SIGNS BROADENING OF HEALTH SERVICE

President Hails Public Gains— Law Provides Research Aid and Tuberculosis Drive

WASHINGTON, July 3 (AP)—President Roosevelt approved today legislation broadening the scope of the United States Public Health Service and in a statement commended the department for "its excellent record in protecting the health of the nation."

The act authorizes Federal grants for research by non-Government institutions, larger appropriations to aid State public health work and establishment of a national tuberculosis program. It provides commissions for public health nurses.

President's Statement

The text of the statement was as follows:

"The Public Health Service Act is an important step toward the goal of better national health. A constituent of the Federal Security Agency since 1939, the United States Public Health Service is one of the oldest Federal agencies— and one in which the people have great confidence because of its excellent record in protecting the health of the nation.

"The act signed today gives authority to make grants-in-aid for research to public or private institutions for investigations in any field related to the public health. It authorizes increased appropriations for grants to the States for general public health work.

Army-Navy Plan Adopted

"It strengthens the commissioned corps of the public health service for the enormous tasks of the war and the peace to come. Authority is granted to commission the nurses of the public health service, just as the nurses of the Army and Navy are commissioned.

"It provides for the establishment of a national tuberculosis program in the public health service. Since adequate public health facilities must be organized on a nation-wide scale, it is proper that the Federal Government should exercise responsibility of leadership and assistance to the States.

"In establishing a national program of war and post-war prevention, we will be making as sound an investment as any government can make; the dividends are payable in human life and health."

July 4, 1944

INFANT DEATH RATE CUT 31% IN DECADE

Maternal Mortality Falls 61% From 1933—Federal Study Also Shows Births Up 30%

Special to THE NEW YORK TIMES.

WASHINGTON, Dec. 6—In issuing findings of a comparative study of the country's birth rate from 1933 to 1943, the Children's Bureau of the Department of Labor said today that babies and their mothers had a better chance of survival now than they did ten years ago.

The birth rate, which was at an all-time low in 1933, rose 30 per cent in the succeeding decade, the survey showed. The infant mortality rate was cut 31 per cent, from 58 to 40 deaths per 1,000 live births. The maternal mortality rate in the same period fell from 62 to 24 deaths per 10,000 live births, a decline of 61 per cent.

In an analysis of statistics by States, the bureau reported that infant mortality rates, for every 1,000 of live births, declined 38.4 per cent in Connecticut, 27.2 per cent in New Jersey and 39 per cent in New York during the 1933-43 decade. The greatest decline, 41.8 per cent, was reported from North Dakota.

On the basis of every 10,000 live births, the maternal mortality rate fell 67.9 per cent in Connecticut; 63.7 per cent in New Jersey and 66.1 per cent in New York. Nevada's 75.6 per cent decline was the greatest in this category.

Major Credit Is Given Doctors

"The major credit for this remarkable record," said Dr. Martha M. Eliot, associate chief of the bureau, "goes to the doctors, those in private practice and in public service, for the work they have done in their care of women during pregnancy and the improved care they are able to give at childbirth and after delivery and in the dangerous early days and months of the baby's life. Improvements in hospital care also come in for a large part of the credit.

"Improvement in the economic status of many families is also an important factor. Many women have been able to have a better diet during pregnancy and the diet of the mother affects her child's well-being as well as her own. More women were able to have their babies in hospitals, and hospitals are the safest place for a baby to be born."

Still another important factor, Dr. Eliot emphasized, has been the extension of maternal and child-health services under the Social Security program.

"Record Still Not Good Enough"

"But, great as the reduction has been," said Dr. Eliot, "the record is still not good enough, for thousands of the 118,000 babies and of the 7,000 mothers whose lives are lost each year die needlessly. If the care we know so well how to give were available to all groups of the population in all parts of the country then we could cut still further the present tragic loss of life."

Among the facts revealed in the survey were these:

Although the actual number of births reached its all-time high for the country in 1943, with 3,000,000 live births—and the number was almost as high in 1944—at no time did the birth rate during 1933 to 1943 reach the high levels of 1915 and 1916, when the rate was twenty-five per 1,000 of population. In 1933 it had reached a low of seventeen live births per 1,000. By 1943 the birth rate was 21.5.

Far more babies are being born in hospitals—72 per cent of today's babies, as compared with as estimate of 35 per cent ten years ago.

Slightly fewer Negro babies, proportionately, are being born. In 1933 the number of live Negro births was about one out of eight of all live births; today it is closer to one out of nine. Their risk of birth, and that of their mothers, is greater than that for the white group.

December 7, 1945

TELL 37-YEAR RISE IN BETTER EATING

U. S. Economists Report Wide Advances in Civilians' Nutrition During War

Special to THE NEW YORK TIMES.

WASHINGTON, July 19 — Important advances in civilian nutrition in this country during the war years were reported today by the Bureau of Human Nutrition and Home Economics on the basis of a thirity-seven-year study of the per capita food supply, 1909 to 1945.

American gains in consuming during the war years more of the vitamins and minerals which scientists have prescribed for protecting health and promoting growth, calcium, iron, B vitamins and vitamins A and C, than in any other equal span in the thirty-seven-year period was ascribed to changing food habits which resulted in increased eating of milk, eggs, meat, poultry, vegetables and fruit.

The enrichment of white bread and flour was also given great credit for general better eating in this country. Said the report:

"Because of the enrichment program, grain products now furnish a much greater share of the total available supply of iron, and B vitamins, thiamine and niacin, than before World War II."

The rise of calicum and riboflavin in the diet was ascribed largely to greater consumption of milk. This rise was from a per capita of 169 quarts in 1909 to 212 quarts in 1939, a 205-quart average for the thirty years; followed by a quick jump from 215 quarts in 1940 to 257 in 1944. The early gradual increase in milk consumption was ascribed to increased use of manufactured dairy products other than butter. During World War II, the report said, fluid milk consumption reached new highs because of substitution for other foods, greater consumer purchasing power, and emphasis on the nutritive value of milk.

The rise in consumption of vitamins A and C was said to be due to increased use of fruits and vegetables. Citrus fruit and tomatoes jumped from a 44-pound per person average annual consumption in 1909 to 119 pounds in 1945; leafy green and yellow vegetables from 77 pounds in 1909 to 134 in 1945. The consumption in citrus fruit alone was a 400 per cent increase in the thirty-seven years.

Changing eating habits were also shown in the fact that there was a 30 per cent decrease in the consumption of potatoes and grain products.

The thirty-five-page report represents the longest-range study of the nutritional value of this country's diet ever made, and is probably the one such study for any nation. All figures given are national averages, and do not give regional variations or diet differences by income levels.

July 20, 1946

60 DELEGATES SIGN HEALTH 'CHARTER'

Constitution for a New World Organization Wins Wide Acclaim at Assembly

"A Magna Carta for health" is provided in the World Health Organization Constitution, signed yesterday here by sixty national delegates, Dr. Thomas Parran, president of the Constitutional Assembly, declared at the ceremony.

The United Kingdom and Chinese delegates affixed the only signatures to the Constitution that were tantamount to ratification, at the last meeting of the United Nations Health Assembly in the Henry Hudson Hotel.

Eighteen other delegates empowered to sign without reservation the new international health charter declined at the last moment to exercise their full powers. As a rule, their reservation was the result of domestic political considerations rather than any sudden loss of faith in the new health organization.

Stress on Psychiatry

Dr. Parran upheld the organization (to be created when twenty-six United Nations States have ratified the Constitution) as "a powerful instrument for peace," in which psychiatry would play its "urgent" part in removing the seeds of war. He said:

"The World Health Organization will * * * help to heal the wounds of war and to eliminate the ancient human plagues, such as malaria and cholera, tuberculosis and syphilis. Prevention of disease is a first objective.

"But this is only a first step. Hunger and malnutrition stunt the bodies and warp the minds of a large part of the world's population. To attain freedom from want of food is another goal which we may hope to reach by pooling our nutritional knowledge with the food and agriculture efforts of the United Nations."

Since the United States and the Soviet Union are expected to follow the United Kingdom in ratifying the World Health Constitution, through their respective legislative procedures, the Health Organization appeared to be the first of the United Nations specialized agencies to which all members of the "Big Three" would belong.

Russian Action Expected

Dr. Lev Medved, Ukrainian delegate to the Assembly, declared that Russia "undoubtedly" would ratify the Constitution "as soon as possible"; taking such action directly after the ending of the peace conference in Paris. Dr. Parran, too, as chief United States delegate, believed the Senate also would ratify the health charter, creating the first fully empowered international public health agency. He observed that the Senate had unanimously endorsed the idea and even had recommend that this nation sponsor the health conference.

However, the United Nations sponsored the international conference, the first it has held. The fact that the conference was served by an international secretariat, and attended by representatives of sixteen non-United Nations States and ten non governmental organizations lent it noteworthy "universality," Arkady M. Sobolev, Acting Secretary General of the United Nations, pointed out.

Ratification Urged

Congratulating the Health Assembly, on behalf of Secretary General Trygve Lie, absent in Europe, Mr. Sobolev urged all member Governments to ratify the Health Constitution speedily. "No time is to be wasted in relieving world suffering," he said.

Excepting the Hungarian, Icelandic, Swedish and Finnish delegates, who were absent from the last meeting of this constitutional session of the Assembly, and excepting delegates of Afghanistan, Rumania and Yemen who did not attend the entire conference, the Health Charter was signed by representatives of all the invited fifty-one United Nations States and sixteen non-United Nations States (excluding Spain).

Italy and Austria were among the signatory States, participating for the first time since the war in such a conference. The only woman delegate to take part in the signing was Dr. Martha. M. Eliot, vice chairman of the United States delegation. She is associate chief of the Children's Bureau of the United States Department of Labor.

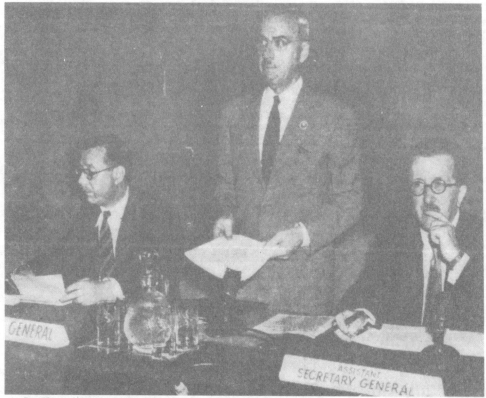

Dr. Thomas Parran of the United States addressing the session at the Henry Hudson Hotel yesterday. Also seen are Arkady M. Sobolev (left), acting Secretary General of the United Nations, and Henri Laugier, Assistant Secretary General for Social Affairs.
The New York Times

July 23, 1946

Survey Shows Vast Health Gains; 1900's Death Rate Cut Nearly 50%

By BESS FURMAN
Special to THE NEW YORK TIMES.

WASHINGTON, Aug. 10—The Brookings Institution reported today that the average death rate in the United States had been cut nearly in half in the past fifty years—from 17.2 per 1,000 persons in 1900 to 9.6 in 1950—and that individuals of all ages in the nation had enjoyed increasingly good health in that period.

"The factors primarily responsible for the over-all improvements in health since 1900," the report said, "are advances in medical science, the increased use of medical facilities, and the control of communicable diseases.

"Health progress is a story of the improved treatment of disease on the one hand and prevention of disease on the other."

The survey is published as a book entitled "Health Resources in the United States."

Where, in 1901, an infant had three chances in four to reach the age of 25, in 1940 he had nine chances out of ten, the report stated. In 1901, 39 per cent of the adults of 50 reached the age of 75, while in 1940 the number had risen to 46 per cent.

The death rate for infants under one year of age dropped from 162.4 per 1,000 live births in 1900 to 31.3 in 1949, it was found. Sharp drops were also noted in the death rates for children between 5 and 19, and for adults from 20 to 25.

Viewing the population as a whole, the book said that 80 per cent of all individuals had, in 1950, an expectancy of attaining the age of 50, compared to only 59 per cent in 1901.

"The tremendous advances in the field of health since the beginning of this century," the report said, "which are reflected by all mortality figures, not only give cause for pride in what has been done but also indications of what can be done in the future.

"Essential to further advances is the belief that the still existing differences in the health of broad social groups, or sections of the country, are not immutable."

The report was the product of three years of study by a staff of a dozen research experts under the direction of Dr. George W. Bachman, a specialist in experimental medicine and public health. More than 700 private and public agencies contributed to the compilation.

Particularly complete is its analysis of health personnel, which shows that both physicians and registered nurses have decreased in the last ten years in proportion to all health personnel and that one physician in three devotes his entire time to a specialty.

The civilian population has least access to physicians, dentists, and nurses in the South Atlantic, West South Central, and East South Central States, the survey finds.

The book reported that "with the exception of a few cities" drug addiction was not increasing among adolescents. Addicts, on a national basis, number about one in every 3,000 persons, or a total of 50,000 to 60,000, but it is as low as one in 25,000 in the West North Central states, the report said.

It noted that draft rejections for drug addiction fell from six in 10,000 in World War I to one in 10,000 in World War II.

A comparison of health personnel in 1940 and 1950 showed that physicians had increased from 175,-163 to 204,400 in the last ten years; dentists from 70,121 to 82,575; nurses from 270,630 to 318,880.

However, these three groups have decreased proportionally to a point where, the study said, "the major professionals make up a smaller proportion of the health labor force than ever before."

The over-all increase in health personnel was 40 per cent. The average increase of 17 per cent for the three major professional groups compared with an average increase of 70 per cent among the other health occupations. Auxiliary nursing personnel increased by 98 per cent, from 196,656 in 1940 to 368,-735 in 1950.

The report found that, exclusive of inactive and Federal physicians, there was a ratio of 121 physicians per 100,000 population. However, this varies from 267 in the District of Columbia and 196 in New York to a low of 64 in Mississippi.

Specialists Increase Sharply

The number of full-time specialists was found to have increased from 36,800 physicians in 1940 to 62,688 in 1950, and to include now about one of three physicians in active practice.

"The effect of specialization within the profession has been to increase the disparities in physician-population ratios between different parts of the country," the report said.

In nursing, called "almost entirely a profession for females" it was found that "a substantial proportion drop out within the first three years after graduation, and do not re-enter the labor force until they are 45 years of age or older, if indeed they do then."

A chapter on medical group practice, which gave the Mayo Clinic at Rochester, Minn., credit

as the trail-blazer, said that Minnesota, Wisconsin, California and Texas had the most groups in the order given.

A survey of more than 4,000 industrial plants shows that accident prevention programs have led to a reduction of accident rates. Reduction in incidence of occupation-

al diseases was found due to health and safety programs.

More than 86 per cent of the companies studied said their health programs had contributed to better employer-employe relationships. Medical costs per employe increased in ten years from $8.81 to $25.90.

Voluntary agencies receive credit

for great advances in treatment of mental cases, which were given as totaling 9,000,000, and cancer and heart diseases. Alcoholics Anonymous was termed as a "most successful attempt" at alcoholic rehabilitation. Alcoholics total 4,000,000.

August 11, 1952

CITY MODERNIZES ITS HEALTH CODE

By MILDRED MURPHY

A modernized health code for this city, the first extensive revision since 1914, was enacted yesterday by the Board of Health.

The document, which covers 500 pages, will be filed this morning with the City Clerk, thus ending three and a half years of work in which the board had the collaboration of representatives of medicine, industry, labor and the public.

Introduced under a new title, the New York City Health Code, it will become effective Oct. 1.

The new name distinguishes

it from the former Sanitary Code. The revision of that code in 1914 was made on the basis of regulations formulated by the Board of Health in 1866. Health Commissioner Dr. Leona Baumgartner said yesterday that the Health Code presented up-to-date concepts of medical science.

A typical example, under the new code, is in the section on communicable diseases. The section deletes the requirement for posting a sign on the door of the ill person's home. It also eliminates the period of quarantine that formerly was required for certain highly contagious diseases that are now readily combated.

Scarlet Fever Rules

Under the old code a person with scarlet fever was required by law to be isolated for a week, even though he might be fully recovered. The new code

enforces isolation only in the case of acute illness accompanied by fever.

Other deletions from the old regulations are many requirements remindful of the customs of generations past.

Midwifery becomes, henceforth, a thing of the past. Although the new regulations will permit the only two remaining midwives in the city to continue their practice until they retire, midwifery permits will be issued only to professional nurses who work under the supervision of an obstetrician.

An entirely new provision covers the use of chemical food additives. It also makes their safety the responsibility of the manufacturer instead of regulatory agencies.

The only section of the code left temporarily open for continued study by the board is

the one concerning milk, milk products and frozen desserts. The board announced last month that it intended to review certain provisions that no longer affected public health, but that related to current economic, trade and labor practices. It said that decisions on new milk legislation would be made by the end of the year.

The code's five main sections cover the Health Department's general regulatory powers, communicable diseases, maternal, infant, child and school health; regulations on the handling, sale and distribution of food and drugs, and rules on birth and death records.

The new code was formulated at a cost of $160,000, provided by the Board of Estimate, the Rockefeller Brothers Fund and the W. K. Kellogg Foundation.

March 24, 1959

HIGH COURT BACKS SEARCH OF HOMES FOR HEALTH CHECK

By ANTHONY LEWIS
Special to The New York Times

WASHINGTON, May 4—The Supreme Court held today, over strong dissent, that health inspectors may enter a private home without a warrant to search for unsanitary conditions.

The vote was 5 to 4. Justice Felix Frankfurter wrote the opinion of the court and was joined by Justices Tom C. Clark, John Marshall Harlan, Charles Evans Whittaker and Potter Stewart.

"Time and experience have forcefully taught," Justice Frankfurter wrote, "that the power to inspect dwelling places, either as a matter of systematic area-by-area search, or, as here, to treat a specific problem, is of indispensable importance to the maintenance of community health; a power that would be greatly hobbled by the blanket requirement of the safeguards necessary for a search of evidence of criminal acts."

Fourth Amendment Is Issue

For the dissenters, Justice William O. Douglas said:

"The decision today greatly dilutes the right of privacy

which every home owner had the right to believe was part of our American heritage."

With him in dissent were Chief Justice Earl Warren and Justices Hugo L. Black and William J. Brennan Jr.

In another case, the court upheld a Quaker who had refused to answer questions by a Virginia legislative committee about race relations, and reversed a contempt conviction.

The central issue in the health inspection case was the Fourth Amendment to the Constitution, which prohibits "unreasonable searches and seizures," by Federal officials. The Fourteenth Amendment has been held to apply similar restrictions to state and local officials.

Baltimore Case

The case arose in Baltimore, when the City Health Department got a complaint about rats in a neighborhood. An inspector looked through a number of houses and eventually reached the home of Aaron D. Frank.

The inspector looked outside and found evidence of infestation by rats. When he asked for permission to inspect the basement, Mr. Frank refused.

A Baltimore ordinance authorizes health inspectors to enter any house during the daytime and makes it an offense to deny an inspector admission. Mr. Frank was found guilty of violating this law and was fined $20.

Justice Frankfurter reviewed the history of the Fourth Amendment and concluded that its primary aim was to protect a man's home against indiscriminate searches "for evidence to be used in criminal prosecutions" or for illegal goods, such as smuggled merchandise.

In this case, he said, there was no search for criminal evidence. The Justice wrote:

"Appellant is simply directed to do what he could have been ordered to do without any inspection, and what he cannot properly resist, namely, act in a manner consistent with minimum community standards of health and well-being, including his own."

The opinion noted that the Baltimore code strictly limited the inspection power. The inspector must come in the daytime and must show valid grounds for believing unsanitary conditions exist. He may not force entry into a house.

That procedure, Justice Frankfurter said, makes "the least possible demand on the individual" and his right of privacy. The opinion then measured that demand against "the needs which have produced it."

"The problems which gave rise to," [city health] ordinances," Justice Frankfurter said, "have multiplied, as have the difficulties of enforcement.

"The need for preventive action is great, and city after city has seen this need and granted the power of inspection to its health officials; and these inspections are apparently welcomed by all but an insignificant few."

Justice Whittaker joined Jus-

tice Frankfurter's opinion. He added a brief concurrence saying that he did so because he was convinced that a daylight inspection for the habitat of disease-carrying rats was not "an unreasonable search."

Justice Douglas, stating his dissent orally in the courtroom, called the decision "a rather sad one" that took "a long backward step in constitutional law."

His opinion differed sharply from the majority view that the Fourth Amendment was aimed primarily at searches for evidence in criminal cases. Justice Douglas said the aim was to protect the privacy of the home against any official intrusion without a warrant.

Now, he said, "if officials come to inspect sanitary conditions they may come without a warrant and demand entry as of right. This is a strange deletion to make from the Fourth Amendment."

Justice Douglas noted, finally, that in England search warrants were required for health inspections. He saw no enforcement problem because, he said, Baltimore has prosecuted only about one person a year for resisting inspections. He went on:

"One rebel a year is not too great a price to pay for maintaining our guarantee of civil rights in full vigor."

The case was argued for Maryland by Attorney General C. Ferdinand Sybert and by a special assistant attorney general, James H. Norris Jr. Benjamin Lipsitz of Baltimore represented Mr. Frank.

May 5, 1959

Food and Drug Businesses Gird For War Over Use of Vitamins

By PETER BART

A curious struggle appears to be developing over the consumption of vitmans in the United States. The question at issue: Do people take too many vitamin pills or too few?

On one side is the powerful drug industry, which is eager to increase its $500,000,000-a-year vitamin sales. On the other is the food industry and allied interests, who prefer that people eat better instead of gulping so many vitamins.

Both sides are getting set to wage campaigns to win the public to their particular views. The resulting tussle may have a significant impact on this country's nutrition habits. It also may affect the profits of the two principal industries involved — the drug and food businesses.

"This is basically not a scientific battle but an economic one," acknowledges Dr. Robert S. Goodhart, a noted nutritionist, who is executive vice president and scientific director of the National Vitamin Foundation. Dr. Goodhart's organization has just hired a prominent public relations concern and allocated $100,000 for the development of an education program aimed at demonstrating the value of supplemental vitamins.

The Vitamin Foundation's member companies include such important producers as Hoffmann-La Roche, Inc., Chas. Pfizer & Co., Inc., Merck & Co., Inc., and E. R. Squibb & Sons.

Meanwhile, the Nutrition Foundation, a group whose members include many of the biggest food companies, also is starting an education program and has hired a director of public information to lead the drive. The group, which was organized in 1941 mainly to sponsor research in the field of nutrition, believes that there is an abundance of food available from which all persons can select a balanced diet.

"Last year, Americans were robbed of $500,000,000 through food fads, extreme diets and cure-alls," said Dr. Charles Glen King, executive director of the nutrition group. "We hope to prevent some of this loss."

In addition to the two foundations, a number of food and drug companies also have been encouraging the publication of articles and pamphlets to publicize their causes. Some magazine articles, for example, have cited the possible dangers of an overdose of vitamins and argued that most people in this country have a balanced diet and do not need supplementary vitamins. Others have contended that our eating habits have deteriorated rather than improved and that people with vitamin deficiencies are vulnerable to all sorts of ailments.

As a result of this crossfire, some nutritionists fear that "the great vitamin war" may have little impact other than to scare the public.

The vitamin industry, however, is in no mood to let things ride. Vitamin producers have been stung not only by anti-vitamin propaganda but also by rising imports of bulk vitamins, higher production costs and the rapid growth of vitamin discount houses.

In the light of these economic headaches, the vitamin producers are particularly sensitive to attack. Perhaps the most nettling was an article in The Journal of the American Medical Association last November, written by the A. M. A.'s president, Dr. E. Vincent Askey, which deplored the emergence of "vitamania."

"Ingenious advertising and misleading claims have helped to cram Americans full of vitamins which they don't need," Dr. Askey stated. The tragedy is that "masked organic disease may be the basic cause of the symptoms that are being treated erroneously with vitamins," he warned.

According to Dr. Goodhart of the National Vitamin Foundation, the A. M. A. editorial mirrors the physician's conventional suspicion of all forms of self-medication. He argues, however, that between 70 and 80 per cent of the 75,600,000 people who occasionally take vitamins take them at the recommendation of a doctor.

April 25, 1961

DUAL DRUG PRICES HELD MISLEADING

By RICHARD D. LYONS

The American consumer often pays too much for the drugs he buys, a Harvard Medical School physician observes in a new book being published today that offers specific advice on methods to reduce pharmaceutical costs.

The author, Dr. Richard Burack, provides in his book, lists of manufacturers' brand names and the official chemical names of about 162 of the pharmaceutical agents most commonly prescribed by American doctors.

Comparisons of prices show, Dr. Burack contends in his book, that in most cases brand names cost more, often many times more, than the same drugs purchased by their chemical names. Pharmacists usually refer to the chemical names as generics.

Titled "The Handbook of Prescription Drugs, Official Names, Prices and Sources for Patient and Doctor," the book is being published by Pantheon Books and sells for $4.95 in hardcover and $1.95 in paperback. The book cites many examples of sharp differences in brand and chemical name drug prices.

"For example, CIBA, the enormous Switzerland-based company, offered to sell to the United States Government for about 60 cents a quantity and quality of reserpine [a drug to lower blood pressure] for which the corner pharmacist must pay $39.50," Dr. Burack writes. "The Government buys it as reserpine; the corner pharmacist buys and dispenses it as Serpasil."

"There are no important differences between the two; only the name and $39," Dr. Burack contends. "Ironically, CIBA did not win the contract, for they were underbid by a company willing to sell the same drug for 51 cents."

Asked for comment on the example, Donald J. Storch, a public relations representative of CIBA, said, "I don't believe it's incorrect."

"But it should be remembered," Mr. Storch said, "that the Government order was for a large quantity and trying to compare it with a small order is like comparing apples and eggs."

He said that CIBA had developed and holds a patent on reserpine, but licenses it for manufacture by other companies.

"We question whether generic manufacturers stand behind their product the way CIBA does," Mr. Storch commented.

In another example, Dr. Burack cites the case of a 10-year-old boy who developed rheumatic fever and had to take two penicillin tablets a day for at least 20 years.

A prescription for a brand product of 250 tablets of Pentids of 200,000 units "will cost about $27.50 at most drugstores," Dr. Burack writes. But a prescription reading merely potassium penicillin G tablets "need cost only about $6.25, sometimes as little as $5," Dr. Burack says. Over 20 years, he adds, the saving would amount to $1,275.

Edward H. Beckwith, president of the Squibb Pharmaceutical Company, which makes Pentids, said in a statement:

"There is no quarreling with the figures that Dr. Burack uses in this rather extreme example of the use of penicillin. One can find cheaper drugs if one looks for them because some companies do not invest as heavily in quality, research and a national distribution system."

Mr. Beckwith noted that the price of Pentids "has been reduced recently and the cost of penicillin from Squibb has gone through many price declines since it was introduced in 1945."

Prices of the commonly prescribed drug digitalis, an old remedy to increase the contraction of the heart muscle, may range from $1.36 to $18.40 for a bottle containing 1,000 tablets, Dr. Burack writes. The only difference, he holds, is that the lower-priced drug is made by a small company and lacks a brand name.

The price of an antihistamine with the generic name of chlorpheniramine maleate may range from $1.95 to $20.59 for a bottle containing 1,000 tablets. The difference again, according to the author, is merely manufacturer and brand name.

"A patient should shop around for drugs because he is a captive consumer and has the right to know what he is buying and how much it costs," Dr. Burack said in a telephone interview from his home in West Newton, Mass.

Dr. Burack urged patients to ask their physician to make prescriptions by generic name so that the patient may be able to pay less for the drugs. He said most pharmacists would fill orders by generic names, at a cheaper price, if specially requested to do so.

"I've found druggists are most cooperative and will order generically from the wholesaler if they are asked," Dr. Burack said, adding that in four years of private practice he had found only one pharmacist who would not fill generic orders.

Spokesmen for the drug industry have repeatedly stated that the buying of brand name products, while they may cost more, insures better quality, which is partly responsible for the price difference. Another factor, they have added, is that the companies marketing drugs under brand names spend more money for research to develop new agents.

Dr. Burack challenged the idea that brand names mean a higher quality product by saying that "there is absolutely no difference between generic and brand names, except price."

He pointed out that most Federal, state and municipal agencies buy drugs through competitive bidding in which generic names, rather than trade, or brand, names, are used.

Senator Gaylord A. Nelson, Democrat of Wisconsin, in a speech on April 27, cited Dr. Burack's book as evidence that the American people are being outrageously overcharged for prescription drugs.

The Senate Monopoly and Antitrust subcommittee is planning another investigation of drug prices. Public hearings are scheduled to start next Monday. The investigation is the latest in an eight-year series of Congressional hearings first started by the late Senator Estes Kefauver.

May 8, 1967

DRUG TESTS FIND 'GENERICS' DIFFER

WASHINGTON, Aug. 20 (AP) — Five university scientists say they have found differences in the way brand-name and generic drugs behave in the body.

"Our findings raise serious doubts about the equality of different products of the same drug in the treatment of disease," said Dr. Christopher M. Martin, head of the five-man research team at Georgetown University.

But Dr. Herbert L. Ley Jr., commissioner of the Food and Drug Administration, which authorized the university to do the research, issued a statement on the findings cautioning that:

"The Food and Drug Administration has in no sense concluded that 'generic' drugs are less effective as a class than 'brand-name' products."

Dr. Ley said: "In my opinion,

there are fewer than two dozen drugs where therapeutic differences among competing products may be a problem."

A brand-name drug generally is defined as one put out by the company that originated it. A generic drug is another company's version of the same chemical compound.

Generics can be made when the originator's 17-year patent runs out or when the originator "licenses out" the drug to other companies.

Generic drugs often sell for less than the brand version— sometimes for a fraction as much. It has been contended in some quarters that there was no significant difference in the performance of generic and brand-name drugs.

Dr. Martin said in a paper that his team found that some generic drugs were absorbed in the blood streams of healthy volunteers more slowly than brand-name versions. And he said at least one generic product was absorbed much faster than the brand-name drug.

He emphasized however that the findings do not answer the final question of how drugs perform when given to sick patients.

The Georgetown tests were conducted with chloramphenicol, a powerful antibiotic used for combating serious infections; with sulfisoxazole, a sulfa drug used for urinary infestions, and with diphenylhydantoin, a drug used for treatment of epilepsy.

Dr. Martin presented the findings in a paper prepared for a meeting in Minneapolis of the American Society for Pharmacology and Experimental Therapeutics The paper also was released here, and Dr. Martin elaborated on the findings in an interview. Dr. Martin is professor of medicine and pharmacology at Georgetown's medical school.

With chloramphenicol, Dr. Martin said, two generic versions were found to enter the bloodstream more slowly and unreliably than an identical amount of a brand drug.

He said it was partly on the basis of the Georgetown studies that the F.D.A. ordered generic versions of chloramphenicol off the market. The F.D.A. took the action in January, saying there was substantial doubt about the safety and efficacy of the generic chloramphenicols.

With sulfisoxazole, the studies found "similar but less striking differences" than with the chloramphenicol tests. Dr. Martin said certain evidence from the tests made it doubtful, however, whether the differences were significant medically.

He said in the interview that the findings indicated further tests with sulfisoxazoles might turn up medically significant differences.

With diphenylhydantoin, the tests indicated that a generic product was absorbed in the blood much more rapidly and completely than the brand name drug.

August 21, 1968

Health of the Nation Lagging Behind Great Advances of Medical Science

By HAROLD M. SCHMECK Jr.

Special to The New York Times

WASHINGTON, July 15 — American medical science has made spectacular advances in the last quarter-century, but improvements in the over-all American death rate and the infant and maternal mortality rates have leveled off and the United States still lags behind many other nations.

This phenomenon, along with rising medical costs and bottlenecks in the delivery of health care, are key factors in a growing national debate that is likely to spill over into the 1972 political campaign and is causing pressure for health care reforms. It is prompting new interest in such questions as: How healthy are Americans? And how good is the care they receive?

This interest was demonstrated today with the issuance of a statistical analysis of health problems by the National Health Education Committee, which brought together many of the findings of the public health authorities in government and private agencies.

Like other analyses, this report showed there were no easy answers to the question of health care.

Despite all the scientific advances, the country is in the grip of at least two vast epi-

Some Statistical Gauges of the Health of Americans

Life Expectancy (in years)

Year	Total	White Male	White Female	Nonwhite Male	Nonwhite Female
1930	59.7	59.7	63.5	47.3	49.2
1932	62.1	62.0	64.5	52.8	54.6
1933	63.3	62.7	66.3	53.5	56.0
1934	61.1	60.5	64.6	50.2	53.7
1935	61.7	61.0	65.0	51.3	55.2
1936	58.5	58.0	61.9	47.0	51.4
1937	60.0	59.3	63.5	48.3	52.5
1938	63.5	63.2	66.8	51.7	54.3
1939	63.7	63.3	66.6	53.2	56.0
1940	62.9	62.1	66.6	51.5	54.9
1941	64.8	64.4	68.5	52.5	55.3
1942	66.2	65.9	69.4	55.4	58.2
1943	63.3	63.2	65.7	55.4	56.1
1944	65.2	64.5	68.4	55.8	57.7
1945	65.9	64.4	69.5	56.1	59.6
1946	66.7	65.1	70.3	57.5	61.0
1947	66.8	65.2	70.5	57.9	61.9
1948	67.2	65.5	71.0	58.1	62.5
1949	68.0	66.2	71.9	58.9	62.7
1950	68.2	66.5	72.2	59.1	62.9
1951	68.4	66.5	72.4	59.1	63.3
1952	68.6	66.6	72.7	59.1	63.7
1953	68.8	66.8	72.9	59.7	64.4
1954	69.6	67.4	73.6	61.0	65.8
1955	69.5	67.3	73.6	61.2	65.9
1956	69.6	67.3	73.7	61.1	65.9
1957	69.3	67.1	73.5	60.3	65.2
1958	69.4	67.2	73.7	60.6	65.5
1959	69.9	67.6	74.2	61.4	66.5
1960	69.7	67.4	74.1	61.1	66.3
1961	70.2	67.8	74.5	61.9	67.0
1962	70.0	67.6	74.4	61.5	66.8
1963	69.9	67.5	74.4	60.9	66.5
1964	70.2	67.7	74.6	61.1	67.2
1965	70.2	67.6	74.7	61.1	67.4
1966	70.1	67.6	74.7	60.7	67.4
1967	70.5	67.8	75.1	61.1	68.2
1968	70.2	—	—	—	—

Infant Mortality (Under 1 year, per 1,000 live births)

Total Deaths (Per 1,000 population)

Maternal Mortality (Per 1,000 live births)

Source: U.S. Public Health Service

The New York Times

July 16, 1971

The health gains achieved in the 1930-1968 period have leveled off in some categories

demics — venereal disease, which in its most widespread form, gonorrhea, has doubled frequency in the last six years, and heart disease, which is the nation's No. 1 cause of death.

However, medical science has made tremendous strides in transplanting hearts, in curing polio and curbing infectious disease with antibiotics.

The truth is, no one really wants health care at all; what everyone wants is health. But in the United States, health is a mosaic of contrasts and contradictions. Obesity rubs elbows with malnutrition. Many old killers have been vanquished, but some remain and others have come forward.

Moreover, in American society a person's state of health and chances of getting good medical care depend a lot on who he is, how much money he has and where he lives. This has always been true, but today the best of care can do so much that it makes the worst seem doubly hard.

The middle-aged man who has his heart attack near a hospital equipped with a special coronary care unit has a much better chance of survival than the man whose hospital lacks one.

The young person with early Hodgkin's disease has a good chance of cure or control of that usually fatal illness—if he goes to one of a handful of major cancer centers that most patients never reach.

The kidney patient whose family—or community—can afford the huge expense of the artificial kidney machine may live. The patient without such resources will probably die.

Several Americans have lived for more than a year with transplanted hearts. Several thousand have had kidney transplants. Yet between 100 and 200 persons each year die of tetanus, an infection that should be totally preventable by inoculations that have been available for decades.

Statistically, American children are among the largest in the world and probably among the healthiest. But a few of them have kwashiorkor, a form of infant malnutrition so severe that it is often fatal. The cause is simple lack of good protein food. The underlying cause is almost always poverty.

Indeed, throughout American life, the problems of poverty and ill health tend to be closely linked. Often, too, they are compounded by geography.

Some of the most acute health problems are in rural areas where isolated communities simply have no care at all.

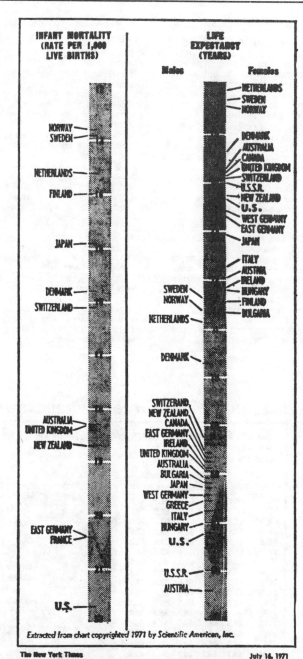

INFANT MORTALITY (RATE PER 1,000 LIVE BIRTHS)

NORWAY
SWEDEN

NETHERLANDS

FINLAND

JAPAN

DENMARK
SWITZERLAND

AUSTRALIA
UNITED KINGDOM
NEW ZEALAND

EAST GERMANY
FRANCE

U.S.

LIFE EXPECTANCY (YEARS)

Males — Females

NETHERLANDS
SWEDEN
NORWAY

DENMARK
AUSTRALIA
CANADA
UNITED KINGDOM
SWITZERLAND
U.S.S.R.
NEW ZEALAND
U.S.
WEST GERMANY
EAST GERMANY
JAPAN

ITALY
AUSTRIA
IRELAND
HUNGARY
FINLAND
BULGARIA

SWEDEN
NORWAY

NETHERLANDS

DENMARK

SWITZERLAND
NEW ZEALAND
CANADA
EAST GERMANY
IRELAND
UNITED KINGDOM
AUSTRALIA
BULGARIA
JAPAN
WEST GERMANY
GREECE
ITALY
HUNGARY
U.S.

U.S.S.R.
AUSTRIA

Extracted from chart copyrighted 1971 by Scientific American, Inc.

The New York Times   July 16, 1971

United States lags behind some industrialized countries in standard health indicators. The figures on infant mortality are for 1968, while the life expectancy statistics are for different years in the nineteen-sixties.

To Government bureaucrats this is a "failure of the delivery of health care." To the sick person far from the nearest doctor or hospital it may mean a minor illness made grave through neglect. It may mean death. Throughout the United States there are 134 counties, with a total population of nearly 500,000, that have no doctors at all in private practice.

In general, Americans are almost certainly healthier and far less prey to disease than they were a few decades ago. The dread infections that used to rage through whole communities are muted. Diphtheria,

typhoid fever, paralytic polio, whooping cough, undulant fever and rheumatic fever are no longer among the common risks of life. Their retreat has been rapid since the advent of antibiotics and new vaccines after World War II. Death and disease rates from tuberculosis have been declining steadily for more than 50 years.

But tuberculosis has not vanished, nor have the others. There are nearly 40,000 cases of tuberculosis a year, most of them among the poor, the down-and-out. Paralytic polio and diphtheria still occur in small outbreaks that seem all the more tragic because they

need not have occurred. The chief cause is lack of immunization; and the chief cause of that, again, is poverty.

The nation's infant mortality rate has dropped from about 65 deaths per 1,000 live births in 1930 to less than a third of that toll today. Maternal death rates and over-all death rates have also declined steadily during most of the last 40 years.

But in those indexes of health the United States is behind many of the other highly developed nations. At least a dozen countries have lower infant mortality rates than this, according to figures from the National Center for Health Statistics. The rate at which American mothers die in childbirth exceeds that of 100 other countries and the women of six other countries live longer than their American sisters.

There has been a lot of debate over the worth of this kind of score keeping. Some critics say true comparisons are impossible because of differences between populations and methods of record keeping. Other public health specialists doubt that these factors account entirely for the poor showing of the United States.

The differences are particularly striking when infant mortality rates are compared. For many decades these rates declined steadily in virtually all of the world's economically advanced countries. Then, about mid-century, the progress slowed and there was a general leveling off. A comparative study done by the National Center for Health Statistics showed that this unfavorable new trend started five years earlier in the United States than in six countries of Northern Europe—England and Wales, the Netherlands, Scotland, Denmark, Norway and Sweden. No one knows why. In general our rates were less favorable than theirs before the leveling off and we still lag behind them.

Some experts think it more useful to consider trends in the United States over time than to compare this country with others. This exercise is not entirely reassuring either.

In 1949 the average 35-year-old American could look forward to 37.3 more years of life. During the two decades of medical miracles that followed, the outlook for the 35-year-old age group improved only little more than a year.

That improvement was less than it was between the years 1900 and 1919—before antibiotics, sulfa drugs, heart surgery and intensive care units in hospitals. There were improvements in health care during those first two decades of the twentieth century, but, from the evidence, there must have been other factors too. Better sanitation of all kinds was probably one such factor.

In fact, the over-all American death rate declined steadily from 1900 to about 1950. About then the improvement slowed to a virtual halt, for reasons that are still obscure.

"This failure to experience a decline in mortality rates in the United States since about 1950 is little known, unexpected and extremely important," according to Dr. William H. Stewart, former Surgeon General of the Public Health Service. He blames two factors for the new trend.

The first of these is the success of the last few decades in treating infectious disease. The degree of success was so marked and so rapid, he believes, that there simply has not been room for enough further improvement to make dramatic changes in mortality.

The second factor, he says, was the emergence of chronic diseases and accidents as "the great undertone of mortality" today. These causes of death are certainly not new, but their impact was less when so many died of acute infections.

Paradoxically, the improvements in medical care and public health are also bringing into sharper focus some of the effects on personal health that are more related to life style and socio-economic status than to medical care itself.

Experts guess that there are probably more than 200,000 narcotics addicts in the United States today, many of whom will die young after years of poverty, degradation and pain. The number of alcoholics and problem drinkers runs into the millions. Their final problems are always medical, but it was not failure of health care that first lured these men and women into the grim quicksand of the drug world.

Even in more fortunate circumstances, life style probably puts a strong imprint on state of health. This is an area of many complexities and contra-

dictions but some salient points emerge.

We kill 50,000 fellow citizens a year with that prime American weapon of violence, the automobile.

Heart specialists say millions of Americans eat too much and exercise too little, and that many die early because of this.

Some cancer specialists say we have virtually created our own epidemic of lung cancer, killing ourselves at the rate of more than 60,000 a year while we debate new gimmicks for breaking the smoking habit.

Americans today are also widely believed to be the most over-medicated society that has ever existed. An official of the Food and Drug Administration estimated recently that about two billion drug prescriptions a year are written in this country.

Recent studies suggest that a significant part of all this drug dosage does the patient little or no good and that many of the prescriptions are for drugs of doubtful value.

Furthermore, it has been estimated that 1.5 million hospital admissions a year are caused by bad reactions to medicinal drugs.

While such things put their stamp on the quality of the nation's health care, the total picture revealed by national statistics is no more than a rough approximation.

Dr. Theodore D. Woolsey, director of the National Center for Health Statistics, said recently his organization was trying to develop better ways of measuring the state of American health. The center has started a continuing nutrition survey, for example, and is looking into ways of gauging an important aspect of health that seldom finds its way into the statistics—the population's unmet needs. It is also looking into a relatively new notion in health statistics, the concept of a person's years of disability-free life.

It is clear, for example, that American life expectancy has

increased markedly since the early years of this century. The child born in 1900 lived, on the average, 49.24 years. The child born in 1970 had an average chance of 70.2 years.

Much of the difference reflects the drop in the nation's infant mortality rate over those years, but the longevity figures do not tell the whole story. How much of the person's later years are impaired by serious chronic illness? That is the important factor the national center is seeking now.

Even with the conventional data available today it is clear that great inequities exist in American health.

"Some care in this country is superb," said Dr. Lester Breslow of the University of California at Los Angeles, during a recent interview. "Other aspects are mediocre, some is very bad—and the poor tend to get the worst."

Indeed, migrant workers, Indians and blacks have more than their share of ill health. Although not all of the reasons are known, evidence points to poverty as a major factor.

Nonwhite American babies die at a rate nearly twice that of white babies. Nonwhite mothers die at a rate four times that for white mothers. On the average, nonwhite Americans can expect to die seven years earlier than whites.

An indication of the poverty factor in this is information showing that infant death rates in urban slums tend to be markedly higher than in prosperous neighborhoods in the same cities.

Yet, in Denver, Dr. Thomas Sbarbaro said his community's neighborhood health centers had been able to reduce the infant mortality rate among the poor to the level of the city's prosperous residential areas. The program appears to have done so simply by providing proper health care for people who never had it before.

On the other hand, a study in another city showed that chronic disease rates among

adults varied with the amount of air pollution in the neighborhood, and that the poor lived in the most polluted areas, another hint that health care is by no means the whole of the health story.

Among the most difficult of the nation's unsolved health problems is heart disease. Few specialists think any changes in the health care system would have profound impact on this huge American health hazard. Recent data from the long-term Framingham heart study, now closed down for lack of Federal funds, shows why.

The study disclosed that half of all persons who died suddenly, presumably from heart disease, had no previous evidence of that disease detectable by doctors. Even among those with known heart disease, almost half of all deaths occurred quickly and outside the hospital.

The authors concluded that the only road to any substantial reduction in premature death from heart attack would be prevention of the underlying disease itself.

Some experts think this goal would require major changes in American life style. Others doubt that anyone knows with certainty what those changes ought to be. Few, if any, think the goal could be achieved without a major commitment to long-term research.

Even in heart disease, poverty emerges as a health factor. Rheumatic heart disease tends to be more common among the poor. Even coronary heart disease, the kind that often culminates in a heart attack, seems to hit hardest in the lower income groups. The statistics show that it is not really a rich man's disease, despite popular opinion to the contrary.

Not only in that health problem, but in most others, poverty and illness are intertwined in the whole fabric of life. Poverty begets disease and illness begets poverty.

July 16, 1971

Facts About Killing and Crippling Diseases

By ROBERT REINHOLD

Despite great advances in medical science, heart attacks, strokes and cancer continue to exact a heavy toll among Americans. Details on these and other major killers and cripplers were listed yesterday in a study released by the National Health Education Committee.

Its chairman, Mrs. Albert D. Lasker, the philanthropist, said that the $1.5-billion-a-year Federal outlay on medical research was insufficient

and urged again that more money be spent for research to solve the remaining health problems.

The study, a compilation of Government and private statistics published under the title "Facts on the Major Killing and Crippling Diseases in the United States," lists four major disorders—heart attack, stroke, cancer and mental illness.

Other once-dreaded diseases, such as tuberculosis, polio, diphtheria and rheumatic heart disease, have been all but eliminated as

causes of death among Americans.

A summary of the facts about some of the major illnesses today follows. In most cases, the study is based on figures for 1968, the latest year for which figures are readily available.

ARTERIOSCLEROSIS

Sometimes called hardening of the arteries, arteriosclerosis is the condition that underlies heart attacks and strokes and is the leading cause of death in the United States. In 1968, 927,660 Americans died of arterio-

sclerosis—more than 48 per cent of all deaths from all causes that year. It is estimated that one-quarter of all American adults have "either definite or suspected" heart disease.

CANCER

The second leading cause of death, cancer, killed 313,910 persons in 1968. This was about one in every six deaths. It is estimated that 625,000 new cancer cases are diagnosed every year, and that one of every four Americans will contract cancer at some time in his life unless preventive measures are devised. Of all cancer deaths in 1967, 44 per cent were among persons under 65 and 56 per cent over 65.

MENTAL ILLNESS

One in every 10 persons, or about 20 million Americans suffers from some form of mental or emotional illness. Some 2,579,600 persons were treated in various psychiatric facilities in 1968. The largest number of first admissions to hospitals was for alcoholism and schizophrenia.

MENTAL RETARDATION

With 126,000 infants born with mental retardation every year, there are about 6 million retardates in the United States. Of these, about 248,000 in 1968 were confined to residential institutions. Experts believe that as many as 75 or 85 per cent of retardates are capable of becoming self-supporting with proper training.

ARTHRITIS

Second only to heart disease as the most widespread chronic disease in the United States, arthritis and rheumatic diseases afflict about 17 million Americans. They cause 12.2 million days of lost work and 205 million

1968 Death Rates, by State, in the U.S.
(Per 1,000 population)
■ 11 to 11.4 ▨ 10 to 10.9 ▧ 9 to 9.8 ▥ 8.3 to 8.9 ☐ 4.9 to 7.9

Source: National Center for Health Statistics

The New York Times   July 16, 1971

For reasons not entirely clear, death rates differ markedly from region to region. In 1968, latest year for which statistics are available, state with highest rate was Maine, with 11.4 deaths per thousand persons. Lowest rate was in Alaska, with 4.9. New York rate was 10.7.

days of restricted activity annually.

BLINDNESS

It is estimated that 5,390,000 Americans have some form of visual impairment; 435,000 of them are legally blind. A condition found largely among the elderly, visual impairment is caused chiefly by such aging-connected diseases as glaucoma and cataracts. More than 10 per cent of all hospital patients are eye patients.

CEREBRAL PALSY

A severe nervous disorder, cerebral palsy afflicts 750,000 Americans and 25,000 palsied infants are born annually. Only one of every five victims of the disease can be trained to be independent enough to hold a competitive job.

EPILEPSY

Experts estimate that from 1 to 2 million Americans suffer from some type of epileptic seizures. Anti-convulsant drugs are effective in arresting many seizures, but large numbers of epileptics do not get treatment.

DEAFNESS

There are 236,000 totally deaf Americans, and one of every 10 has some degree of hearing loss. The incidence is increasing as Americans live longer.

MULTIPLE SCLEROSIS

A debilitating neurological disease of adults, multiple sclerosis afflicts about 250,000 persons. Of all multiple sclerosis patients, 70 per cent are first diagnosed between ages 20 and 40.

MUSCULAR DYSTROPHY

A wasting disease, muscular dystrophy afflicts more than 200,000 persons. Nearly two-thirds of these are children between 3 and 13—and they almost all die before adulthood.

PARKINSONISM

Another neurological condition, Parkinsonism claims about 50,000 new victims every year. Altogether there are 1 million to 1.5 million patients in the United States. A new drug, called L-DOPA, was recently found to help patients in many cases.

July 16, 1971

A Billion in Health Funds Found Unspent by H.E.W.

By HAROLD M. SCHMECK Jr.
Special to The New York Times

WASHINGTON, July 26—During the last year, the Nixon Administration did not spend nearly $1.1-billion in funds Congress had intended for major health programs, according to figures obtained by the House Commerce Committee.

The total withheld was more than one-fifth of the roughly $4.759-billion allotted to the Health Services and Mental Health Administration and the National Institutes of Health, the two largest health-related agencies of the Department of Health, Education and Welfare.

The discrepancies between funds available for spending and funds spent were found in the mass of data sent to Congress by the department.

This led to an exchange of letters between the Commerce Committee chairman, Representative Harley O. Staggers, Democrat of West Virginia, and Caspar W. Weinberger, Secretary of Health, Education and Welfare.

"I am dismayed that you have felt it appropriate to impound the billion dollars your letter describes," Mr. Staggers said in the latest letter, which he made public. "I am not convinced that this is legal, necessary, or in the best interests of the people of our nation."

He asked the Secretary for program-by-program justification for not spending the money that was allocated in the continuing Congressional resolution under which the department's spending was authorized during the 1973 fiscal year.

The funds authorized by the resolution were, in effect, appropriations. They were handled through the resolution mechanism because of the President's veto of the health appropriation bill for 1973.

In a letter to Mr. Staggers, Secretary Weinberger defended the withholding of the funds as legal, but a spokesman for the Commerce Committee said there had not yet been a reply to the request for a program-by program analysis.

A detailed breakdown of the unspent funds showed that even some of the programs given special public emphasis by the President were affected. For example, the National Cancer Institute left 58,859,000 unspent in a total budget authority of $492,205,000.

The National Heart and Lung Institute left unspent $44,217,000 from its permissible spending level of $300-million.

Most severely hit were Federal mental health programs. Of $743,723,000 available, $199,209,000 was unspent.

The Administration's decision not to spend such large sums that had, in effect, been appropriated was criticized sharply today by Representative Paul G. Rogers, chairman of the Commerce Committee's Health and Environment subcommittee.

Mr. Rogers, Democrat of Florida, said the Administration was not carrying out the laws passed by the Congress and was thus distorting the constitutional premise of the separation of powers.

Saying he considered it a "very serious situation," Mr. Rogers suggested it might be necessary to hold hearings on the subject and even to call for the resignations of officials who refuse to carry out the laws involved.

In his letter to Secretary Weinberger, Mr. Staggers said the programs in question had been created to meet specific needs, such as protection from disease, health manpower, biomedical research and improved health services of many kinds.

"Unless these needs in fact do not exist, or have been met, or are being met by alternative superior programs, then these impoundments must be considered a sad failure of our Government's commitment to serve its people," the letter said.

A spokesman for the Department of Health, Education and Welfare said there would be no comment until Mr. Weinberger had replied to Mr. Staggers's latest letter.

July 27, 1973

F.D.A. EASES RULES ON SOME VITAMINS

Agency Changes '73 Decision to Control Them as Drugs —A and D Still Curbed

By DAVID BURNHAM
Special to The New York Times

WASHINGTON, May 27—The Food and Drug Administration backed away today from its decision of 1973 that superpotent vitamins and minerals should be regulated as drugs.

The F.D.A. proposed instead a new regulation that would treat most such products as foods when they are generally recognized as safe and sold as dietary supplements.

The F.D.A. said its latest proposal was developed in response to a Court of Appeals decision on a number of suits challenging the regulation of 1973.

The original plan had proposed classifying as a drug any preparation that contained more than 150 per cent of the recommended daily allowance of the vitamin or mineral included in the preparation. The agency argued that such super vitamins could sometimes be dangerous and were sometimes promoted to treat illnesses in which they should not be used.

The decision today was immediately criticized by Dr. Sidney M. Wolfe and Amita Johnson, both with the Public Citizen Health Research Group.

"Vitamins are the patent medicine—the snake oil—of our age," said Miss Johnson, "and the F.D.A. has backed down under terrific pressure from the health food industry, some segments of phamaceutical industry, and Congress."

According to recent Congressional testimony, there has been a 42.7 per cent increase in vitamin sales in the United States since 1969. Total sales for 1973, according to trade reports, come to $434-million.

Though most vitamin and mineral preparations would be considered as food under the proposal, high potency vitamins A and D would continue to be regulated as drugs because of their demonstrated toxicity, the F.D.A. announcement said.

Alexander M. Schmidt, commissioner of the F.D.A., said in a statement that "we believe the revised regulations are a substantial improvement over the original approach because they will be less subject to misinterpretation and misrepresentation."

He said the proposal would provide the consumers with more and better information about the vitamins and minerals they buy, deter misleading claims and eliminate nutritionally useless ingredients from dietary supplement products."

But Dr. Wolf and Miss Johnson, whose health research group had supported the original plan, said today's proposal would mean that the old and poor people who look to vitamins as essential would never receive complete information about the preparations.

'No Information'

"The point is that people are popping huge numbers of pills with no information about what they will do," said Miss Johnson. "If the vitamins and minerals had been classified as drugs, the manufacturers would have had to submit tests showing their safety and efficacy. As a food, the F.D.A. has authority to make such tests itself but not the necessary staff or money."

The F.D.A.'s 1973 proposal, announced after extensive hearings, met with broad support from a variety of groups such as the American Association of Retired Persons, the National Retired Teachers Association, and the American Institute of Nutrition.

But 15 lawsuits were filed against the agency by vitamin and mineral manufacturers and others who disagreed with the proposal. Thes 15 suits were consolidated and the United States Court of Appeals in New York City issued a decision that generally sustained the regulations, but called for revisions that would have required many months of additional hearings.

The F.D.A. said today's proposals—open to public comment for 45 days—were issued in response to the court decision. Another factor, however, was believed to have been legislation proposed by Senator William Proxmire, Democrat of Wisconsin, that would remove even more of the F.D.A.'s power over vitamins and minerals.

Because of a flood of mail to Congress from passionate users of vitamins and minerals, some observers felt the bill of Senator Proxmire had a chance of becoming law.

May 28, 1975

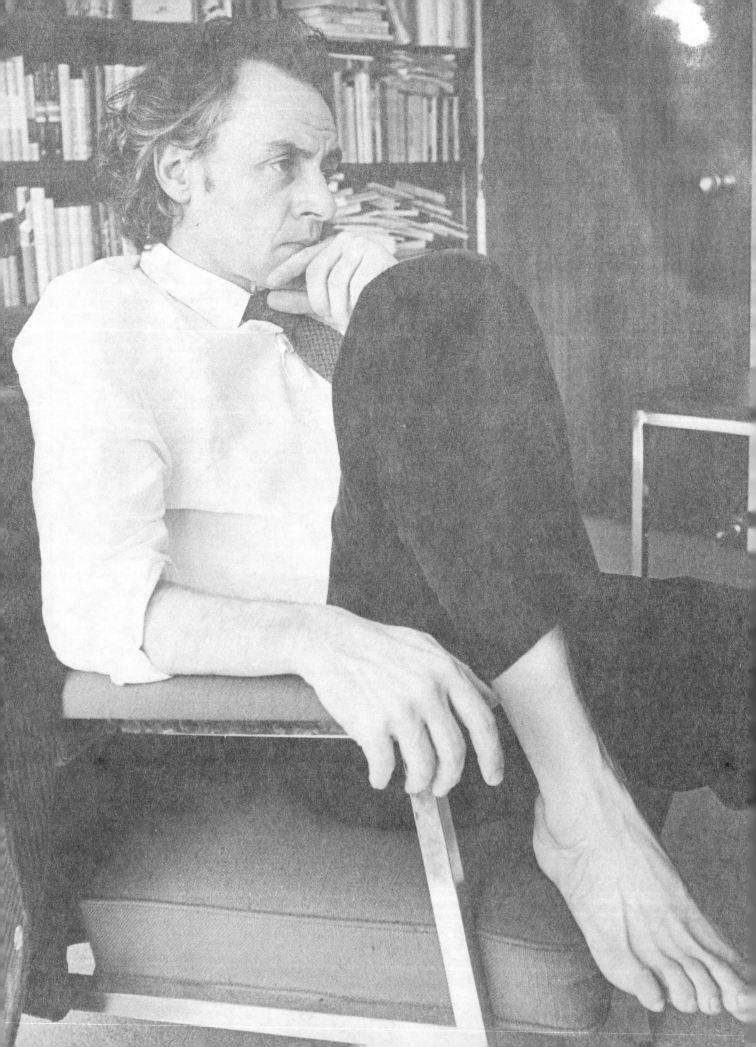

CHAPTER 2

Mental Illness

R.D. Laing, proponent of some controversial ideas
on the treatment of schizophrenia.

Hausner/NYT Pictures

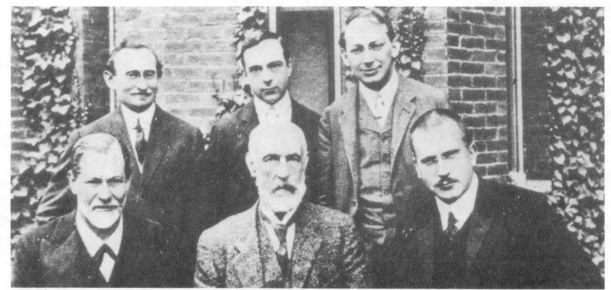

Freud, seated at left, at Clark University in 1909. Standing from left, A. A. Brill, Ernest Jones and Sandor Ferenczi. Right of Freud, Stanley Hall and Dr. Carl G. Jung.

Freud And the Americans

The Beginnings of Psychoanalysis in the United States, 1876-1917. By Nathan G. Hale Jr. 574 pp. New York: Oxford University Press. $15.

By PAUL A. ROBINSON

America has been remarkably generous to Freud. Both as the author of an elaborate intellectual system and as the founder of a lucrative psychiatric business, he has achieved more spectacular success in the United States than anywhere else in the world. Among Europeans perhaps only the English have rivaled the Americans in their enthusiasm for psychoanalysis, while Freud's native Austria, ironically, has turned into a psychoanalytic wasteland.

Clearly the diverse national receptions accorded Freud's thought constitute one of the important unsolved mysteries of 20th-century intellectual and medical history, deserving at least as much attention as has been devoted to the various national fates of Darwinism and Marxism. Nathan Hale's "Freud and the Americans," one hopes, marks the beginnings of just such a scholarly enterprise. While the book makes no attempt at a genuinely comparative examination of national psychoanalytic traditions, it does offer the most detailed and, on balance, persuasive

Paul A. Robinson is author of "The Freudian Left" and teaches history at Stanford.

account of the initial Freudian invasion of America. Moreover, Hale promises to undertake in a second volume an equally exhaustive investigation of the psychoanalytic triumphs of the 1920's.

Like previous historians of Freudianism, Hale traces the origins of the American psychoanalytic movement to the conference Freud attended in 1909 celebrating the 20th anniversary of Clark University in Worcester, Mass. At Clark, Freud delivered five popular lectures on psychoanalysis to an audience that included such luminaries as G. Stanley Hall, James Jackson Putnam, William James and Emma Goldman. However, in contrast to earlier historians, Hale insists that Freud's American reception in the years following the Clark conference can be understood only against the background of indigenous American developments in psychiatry and sexual morality. Accordingly, more than a third of this long volume is devoted to the pre-Freudian American setting.

In the period after 1870, American psychiatry came to be dominated by a set of essentially materialist assumptions. Almost all mental disorders were thought to result from organic causes, usually brain lesions, and it was further believed that these disorders would respond to some form of physical therapy—either electric shock, improved diet or simple rest.

Hale nicely documents the rise and fall of this somatic tradition in psychiatry, which between 1890 and 1910 saw a number of its basic doctrines challenged and was confronted with a distressing increase in therapeutic failures. As the "somatic style" entered its period of crisis, there emerged, well before Freud's arrival, a native American tradition of psychotherapy associated with

such figures as William James, Adolf Meyer and Morton Prince. Against the somaticists, the American psychotherapists argued that mental illness might have psychological causes, and they experimented with a number of psychic therapeutic methods including hypnosis and suggestion. They thereby paved the way for what was in effect the most radically psychological of European therapies, Freud's psychoanalysis.

Paralleling these developments in psychiatry and in some sense complementing them were certain changes in American sexual attitudes. The late 19th century marked the ascendancy of what Hale calls "civilized morality," a phrase he borrows from Freud's great revolutionary essay of 1908, " 'Civilized' Sexual Morality and Modern Nervousness." Civilized morality deemed only one form of sexual expression permissible: adult, genital intercourse, indulged solely for the sake of procreation. In fact, civilized morality sought to outlaw even the mention of sexual topics, demanding an extraordinary degree of reticence on the part of both men and women.

Without being fully explicit, Hale makes the ingenious suggestion that civilized sexual morality represented an appropriate response to the needs of the American middle classes during a period of rapid economic growth. Abstinence meant fewer children. It therefore freed both psychic energies and financial resources for deployment in the economic struggle.

This line of reasoning is in a sense supported by Gordon Rattray Taylor's historical analysis of English sexual mores. In a little-known book, "The Angel-Makers," published over a decade ago, Taylor showed that the high-water mark of civilized morality (or, if you prefer, Victorianism) in England came in the late 18th and early 19th centuries—that is, in precisely those years when England was undergoing the kind of economic revolution that occurred in the United States after the Civil War. Both Hale and Taylor would thus seem to confirm Herbert Marcuse's contention that sexual repression in the West is intimately connected with the development of capitalism.

Like the somatic tradition in psychiatry, American civilized morality came under severe criticism in the two decades preceding Freud's American visit. Its critics were not apologists for sexual release, such as emerged in several European countries during this period, but Progressive moralists who argued that sexual reticence had to be overcome if such problems as venereal disease and prostitution were to be honestly confronted and eliminated. Despite their puritanism, however, the American reformers, by repealing the established tradition of reticence, anticipated the Freudian ethic of complete sexual frankness.

In demonstrating the presence of native American psychiatric styles and sexual attitudes remarkably similar to those supposedly introduced by Freud, Hale, of course, has not solved the riddle of Freud's American success. He has merely given it a new form. Now the question becomes, why

did the Americans need Freud when they had already achieved a quasi-Freudian revolution of their own?

Hale does not answer this question in as definite a fashion as one might wish. In part he attributes the Freudian takeover to the energy, intelligence and collective discipline of Freud's earliest American disciples. He also suggests, correctly I think, that psychoanalysis enjoyed the advantage of being more extreme, more dramatic and thus more marketable than the indigenous American psychotherapies—which is another way of saying that Freud, after all, was a genius. In the end, however, Hale places heaviest emphasis on the therapeutic effectiveness of psychoanalysis. In 1917, for example, the American analyst Isador Coriat published a statistical analysis of 93 psychoanalytic cases. Coriat's criteria of recovery seem to have been very demanding. Yet he reported that 46 of his 93 patients had completely overcome their difficulties, while 38 showed improvement, and only nine failed to respond to treatment.

Hale accounts for these remarkable results by suggesting that of all competing psycho-

therapies, only Freud's systematically sought the origin of mental disorders in repressed sexual traumas and attempted to relieve those disorders by bringing their sexual nature to light. This procedure succeeded, he surmises, because the generation of neurotics treated by the first American analysts were in fact victims of the 19th-century regime of civilized morality. It was as if psychoanalysis had been expressly designed to cope with the psychological problems created by America's peculiarly repressive sexual order—an ironic comment on the frequently aired criticism that Freud's theories represented little more than a grandiose projection of the sexual difficulties experienced by certain Viennese women at the turn of the century.

I fear that this highly schematic summary of Hale's argument will convey a false impression of the book's texture. For all its concern with presenting a thesis, "Freud and the Americans" is essentially a richly detailed history of the American psychoanalytic movement in the decade following Freud's Clark lectures. Hale is particularly successful in describing the manner in which

the American analysts shaped Freud's doctrines to suit the native environment—their muting of Freud's sexual radicalism, their enthusiasm for sublimation, their tendency to ignore the finer points of psychoanalytic technique such as transference. The book also pays considerable attention to the wider impact of Freud's ideas, as reflected in newspaper articles, popular literature and medical textbooks.

"Freud and the Americans" is unquestionably a major achievement. Its scholarship is prodigious, its analytic categories arresting, often brilliant. Regrettably I must also report that it is not a particularly well-made or readable book. In fact, it is exasperatingly repetitious (we need not, for example, be told three times that Boris Sidis was a student of William James) and it is made overlong by an indiscriminate use of quotations. There is also a certain opacity about the book's organization. I hope, therefore, that before the publication of the second volume of this important study, Mr. Hale obtains the services of a genuinely tyrannical editor.

December 26, 1971

ATTACKS DR. FREUD'S THEORY

Clash In Academy of Medicine When Vienna Physician Was Honored.

Dr. M. Allen Starr, specialist in nervous diseases, created a sensation at a crowded meeting of the Neurological Section of the Academy of Medicine last night by denouncing the theories of Sigmund Freud, the Viennese psychologist, whose conclusion that all the psychological life of human beings is based on the sex instinct has gained considerable hold on American physicians, and whom all the doctors in last night's meeting had gathered to praise.

Dr. Starr warned his fellow physicians that the doctors of this country should be careful before accepting wholly and entirely a theory which probably depended for its existence largely on the environment of the man who had originated it.

"I knew Dr. Sigmund Freud well in Vienna some years ago," Dr. Starr said. "Vienna is not a particularly moral city, and working side by side with Freud in the laboratory all through one Winter, I learned that he enjoyed Viennese life thoroughly. Freud was not a man who lived on a particularly high plane. He was not self-repressed. He was not an ascetic. I think his scientific theory is

largely the result of his environment and of the peculiar life he led.

"As a matter of fact I believe that Freud, in the theory which all you gentlemen have praised so highly, has turned into a frivolous vein the really serious new science of psychanalysis, by which we neurologists are enabled to study the mental processes of our patients as exactly and as mathematically, as we have previously been able to study the human body by the use of the microscope and the scalpel. There are many other influences which give rise to complex psychoses in human life, besides the sex instinct. An equally strong instinct, for example, is the self-preservative instinct. In America this self-preservative instinct is represented by the struggle for wealth. It is my opinion that if we American physicians recognize the equal value of the self-preservative instinct in shaping our patients' lives and mental states, we will have much greater success."

Dr. Starr's speech had been preceded by addresses by Dr. William A. White, Superintendent of the Government Hospital of the Insane at Washington. D. C. Prof James I. Putnam of Harvard University, Dr. A. A. Brill, and Dr. C. MacFie Campbell of Bloomingdale Hospital. All these physicians had stated that Freud's theory that the root of all psychological states lay solely in the sex instinct was absolutely correct according to their experience. Prof Putnam had gone so far indeed as to state that he

had always found that persons who denied the accuracy of Freud's theory were generally the best example of its absolute truth. Although these and the other Freudians in the crowded room seemed to be considerably startled by Dr. Starr's remonstrance, other physicians in the room applauded Dr. Starr warmly.

Dr. Starr concluded his speech by asking Drs. Putnam and White to state categorically whether, even if Freud's theory was true, it was going to be of any practical benefit to physicians in diagnosing a case. In the confusion which followed, Drs. White and Putnam did not reply.

Dr. E. W. Scripture described to the big meeting of physicians the practical uses which the new science of psychanalysis is being put.

"Ask a thief, for example, to name the first word which comes into his mind, or is associated with a number of harmless words, and you will always find his mind going instinctively to words representing various forms of dishonesty," said Dr. Scripture. "The word 'find,' for example, will suggest the word 'steal.' After mentioning the dishonest words, too, the thief's mind will become disturbed, and after making the break, so to speak, he will hesitate a long time before finding an association for the succeeding words, and even fail to find them at all."

Dr. August Hoch and Dr. Smith Ely Jelliffe were other speakers in favor of the Freudian theory.

April 5, 1912

Doctors and Dreams.

A significant and important point in the history of science is marked by the formal recognition by the British Medical Association, at its recent annual convention in Newcastle, of psychoanalytic and psychotherapeutic methods as legitimate and effective in the treatment of certain mental and nervous diseases.

This action deserves attention, not because all the doctors of England and other countries, including the United States, hitherto have refused to countenance these methods, and have ignored or condemned Freud and all his works, but because it gives a certain regularity or warrant of high medical authority which psychoanalysis up to this time has lacked.

Here and elsewhere the reputable medical journals long since stopped the constant ridiculing and denouncing of the Viennese psychologist and began to take him and his theories seriously. They are printing innumerable articles on the subject, some by doctors who doubt or deny

his soundness, but of late these journals have contained many more articles whose authors have learned in daily practice the utility of the new device for the exploration of the human mind and that "readjustment to environment" which is its aim. Its antagonists are not yet all dead by any means, but they obviously are carrying on a losing fight—one that in reality was lost some time ago.

As was to be expected from such a body, the British Medical Association, in making the announcement of its ap-

proval, emphasized the fact that psychoanalysis is a worse than worthless, a dangerous, tool in other than skilled hands, and that the only right preparation for its use is a thorough medical education. It is a field into which too many charlatans have entered, some of them vicious, the others merely ignorant, and it is hard to tell which of the two classes is doing the more harm and the more to bring into disrepute discoveries that potentially are of almost incalculable value.

September 12, 1921

FREUD REACHES SEVENTY STILL HARD AT WORK

Father of Psychoanalysis Continues to Expand and Alter The Theories That Have Made Him a Storm Centre

By JOSEPH WOOD KRUTCH.

SIGMUND FREUD, father of the theory of psychoanalysis, who is, with the possible exception of Einstein, perhaps the most talked of scientist alive today, celebrated his seventieth birthday in Vienna on Thursday. Threescore and ten found him still at work. Age has necessitated some curtailment of his physical activities, but his mental processes go on at the old impetuous rate.

He takes few patients now and appears in public, even to lecture, but little, yet he continues to elaborate his theories and to add steadily to his already voluminous works. Additions to and modifications of his theories continue to absorb him, and this year he has already published a small volume dealing particularly with the origin of anxieties which is considered by his disciples to constitute a considerable advance in his work.

The mere outline of Freud's career gives little indication of its stormy character. He was born at Freiburg, in Moravia, and he took his doctor's degree at Vienna in 1881. Having been particularly interested in psychiatry there he proceeded to France to study in the famous school of Charcot and Janet, the virtual founders of modern abnormal psychology. After remaining there for a year he returned to Vienna, where he became a professor extraordinary in 1902.

Broke From French Teachers.

But he was never one to follow the routine course of orderly progress under the patronage of his masters. He left his Paris teachers, plunged into a wholly new investigation of neurotic disorders and emerged with a theory and a method so new that Janet remains his most uncompromising enemy, accusing him of perverting the orthodox doctrine of the schools and of introducing wholly unwarranted assumptions.

Several of his own most famous pupils in their turn, notably C. G. Jung and Alfred Adler, have diverged from him almost as widely as he diverged from the French school. The entire subsequent development of psychoanalysis has proceeded in the midst of controversies often acrimonious in the extreme.

This fact, which has not been without its unfortunate consequences, is in part the inevitable result of the development of any new, far reaching science and in part the result of Freud's own boldly speculative mind. Though a physician and a psychiatrist, it is said that he had little knowledge of academic psychology proper and that he built his system with little reference to it. He is charged with introducing a bewildering number of new terms and conceptions with little regard to their relationship to either the language or ideas of conventional psychology,

thereby angering the academic psychologists, who saw their systems somewhat cavalierly ignored.

Certain of his fundamental conceptions—for example the famous "Censor" supposed to stand before the door leading from unconsciousness to the conscious—were declared to be, at best, mere metaphors. No sanction could be found for them in what was known of the nervous system on the physical side. And so in general he met with the resistance generally accorded to the heretic.

Twofold Criticism of Him.

Freud was not by temperament, however, a man inclined to compromise. He has won his way largely by a stubborn insistence which usually had the tendency either completely to alienate his associates or to transform them almost into disciples.

The history of the criticism of Freud and his theories may be divided into two periods. The first was marked by violent prejudice, due partly to the natural inertia which resists new conceptions and partly to an outraged moral sense. The second stage, which is still in progress, is marked essentially by critical study which has as its aim the perfection rather than the destruction of the method which he initiated.

There are, of course, even today, the behaviorists and other uncompromising anti-Freudians; but it is safe to say that the influence of his chief conceptions is reflected more and more strongly in the writings of most of the important psychologists and psychiatrists. Certain phases of his theory are under constant fire, but the debt owed to him by the majority of the workers in the field of abnormal psychology is readily acknowledged.

Freud Stresses the Will.

The layman, aware of the attacks on Freud, is not likely to realize fully the extent to which a fundamental agreement exists. Just as it was said that "scientists disagree about evolution" so it might be said that scientists disagree about Freudianism," without proper acknowledgment of the fact that in most cases the things accepted are more fundamental than those in dispute.

The central fact of Freud's psychological system is the stress which it lays upon the element of will or desire in determining the processes of the mind. Previous to his entrance into the field, psychology had been overwhelmingly "intellectual." It had regarded images, perceptions and ideas as the fundamental factors in mental life, and it had gathered much information concerning them; but it did not progress. There seemed to be no perceptible link between ideas on one hand and action or conduct on the other. Knowledge of ideas threw little light upon a man's behavior.

But when Freud approached the

study of the mind of an individual from the standpoint of its needs and desires he introduced a dynamic element which set the whole in motion. He conceived of man as a willing rather than a thinking animal. The fruitfulness of his conception was immediately revealed by the ease with which it made possible the formulation of illuminating theories in many other fields of thought.

It made clear the meaning of the delusions and phantasies of the deranged mind by showing how they represented the fulfillment of desires. It gave a key to the significance of dreams, which up to that time had remained as completely a mystery as it had been for thousands of years, and it proved equally useful in understanding the processes of the normal mind.

Combined with the theory of the unconscious it made plain the solution of some of the most baffling problems of personality, and it afforded a new approach to the study of all the products of the human mind, including, especially, mythology and literature.

Rapid Spread of Doctrine.

The almost incredibly rapid spread of the Freudian conceptions, their adoption by workers in fields apparently widely separated from that of psychiatry, in which they were first developed; and even the widespread, if superficial, popular interest in them, is now held up as proof not only of their fundamental importance but of the fact that they fit in with the general drift of thought in many different departments today. Whether or not Freud was directly influenced by them, both Schopenhauer and Von Hartmann perceived the importance of both the will and the unconsciousness. Their philosophic conceptions were to some extent taken up by Nietzsche, and through him they were popularized. So Freud's contributions served to bring many scattered thoughts to a focus and to provide the world with an intellectual tool the need of which it had already perceived.

Time alone can arbitrate between Freud and those who have introduced modifications into his theory; whether or not he has, as many maintain, overstressed the sexual and underestimated other sources of desire. But whether his doctrines are modified much or little, his name must continue to be the one most closely associated with the development of one of the great conceptions of science.

Freud has himself seen with some alarm the too rapid spread and too reckless use of his theory. He has warned the world against the quack analyst by declaring that an analysis is "a major surgical operation performed without an anesthetic," and he has not always viewed with favor attempts to extend the application of his doctrines.

It must be said, however, that the movement with which his name is the one most generally associated is of too far-reaching importance to remain under his exclusive control. He declared upon one occasion that he had never dreamed that he would attract during his own lifetime more than a very modest following; but he has, in a way, paid the penalty of succeeding better than he had hoped. Instead of merely founding another school of psychopathology he planted a seed from which in a marvelously short time has sprung up a whole forest. He is thus in the position of a man who can no longer control what was once him. He has, however, shown some disposition to wish to maintain such control, and it is undoubtedly one of his defects that though he is not averse to modifying his own conceptions from time to time he shows little disposition to accept either criticism or suggestion from others.

Two Other Chief Schools.

Aside from his own there are today two chief schools of psychoanalysis. One is headed by Adler, whose system of "Individual Psychology" is particularly concerned with the study of the effects in the individual of conflict between a sense of inferiority and the egotistic impulses. Another, headed by Jung, has devoted itself to an investigation of the chief psychological types into which humanity may be divided.

To the general public it is probably less the applications of psychoanalysis to the abnormal than to the normal mental phenomena which is of the greatest interest, and one may not read much contemporary history, biography, criticism, sociology or even belles lettres without meeting many examples of its influence. Aside from the studies in all these fields, which are definitely Freudian, influences of his work are strongly present in the most diverse kinds of writing. In criticism, for example, one may mention the studies made by Van Wyck Brooks of Mark Twain and of Henry James; in the broad field of sociology James Harvey Robinson's widely-read book, "The Mind in the Making," in which the stress laid upon the process of rationalization and the difference between our "good reasons" and our "real reasons" is important; and in the field of philosophy John Dewey's "Reconstruction in Philosophy," which, if not directly influenced by Freud, at least follows an analogous line of thought in tracing idealistic philosophies to the rationalizing processes of the unconscious mind.

Goethe on one occasion said that it was in her moments of abnormality that nature revealed the secrets of her laws. The truth of this idea was never more strikingly asserted than it has been in the development of Freudianism. Beginning as the study of the deranged mind, it found a key to the understanding of the normal mind, because it found in insanity normal mental processes exaggerated in such a way as to force themselves upon the attention of the observer. Passing from the clinic into the study and into the market place, it seems destined finally to be absorbed into the general thought of the world and to become one of the tools which the thinker unconsciously uses.

Many implications of the theory of evolution have already been so absorbed. Without being consciously aware of the fact we think of religions, governments and institutions as parts of an evolution, a development. In a similar way we are already making wide use of the Freudian conceptions, and in the course of time they will probably become, like the conception of evolution, a part of the mental equipment which every thinker takes for granted.

May 9, 1926

EX-DISCIPLE ACCUSES FREUD OF INTOLERANCE
Dr. Stekel's Attack Stirs Interest of Vienna in Quarrels of Psycho-Analysts

SCIENTIFIC, literary and intellectual Vienna has been aroused to renewed interest in Freudianism. This has been largely brought about by disclosures of how Freud and some of his disciples dealt with insurgents within the Freudian movement, and purports to explain, furthermore, the cause of many of the leader's broken friendships.

One of the leading spirits in this revolt against Freud is Dr. W. Stekel, who wields a trenchant pen. He has been recounting the story of his relationship to Freud and other lights of the psychoanalytical movement in the days before it became so widespread.

Dr. Stekel writes in an objective and restrained manner, even when there are obvious signs that he is hard put to it to restrain himself. His little book upon sex impulses in children first attracted the attention of Freud. They soon became friends and Stekel was one of his champions and disciples. Stekel is said to have been the only psychoanalyst beside Freud who was engaged in active practice at this time. A number of pupils had gathered about Freud and weekly Wednesday sessions of this small circle often partook of the oracular, every participant feeling the gift of tongues descend on him.

Pupils Broke Away.

In time some of these pupils went their own ways. This gave rise to the first tensions and differences. Stekel describes with dramatic effect how it grew steadily more difficult for him to keep on working with Freud, how Freud sacrificed one friend after another—Adler, Jung, Bleuler, Breuer—his paternal friend, to whom he owed much of his own introduction to psychoanalysis—then Fliess, Kahane and others.

Dr. Adler's withdrawal from the inner circle is discussed. Stekel describes an evening devoted to discussion, during which he had read his latest work, "The Speech of Dreams." He had noticed a marked hostility on the part of Freud and some of the others, though this hostility had expressed itself chiefly in the criticism of details without attack on the scientific value of the work.

"I left the room and pondered upon human pettiness and revengefulness," continues Stekel. "But Dr. Adler saw further than I. He kept on saying: 'This enmity is directed not against you, but against me.'

His Friendship With Adler.

"I thought he was mistaken, for Freud simply overwhelmed Adler with friendly attentions and kindnesses. H. flattered him and sought to win him completely for himself. Adler called him a 'catcher of souls' and remained suspicious. Adler was finally requested to explain his new theories in full. He had just worked out a thesis for the understanding of neuroses.

" 'We are all anxious to learn, said Freud, 'let us have an account of your theory.'

"Adler was incredibly happy and full of self-reliance. He was going to speak for three whole evenings upon his new views and researches. And then they were to be brought up and subjected to open discussion. A whole month devoted to the theories of Adler!—this was something new in the annals of these psychoanalytical sessions—in which hitherto only Freud and things Freudian had been discussed.

"Adler was not at all skeptical on this occasion and believed that Freud had really changed his attitude. Why not? Why should the master not be willing to accept something new—and correct and alter and extend his own theories? Many discussions took place, though none of us had any intimation of the storm that was preparing itself.

"Adler spoke during three evenings and gave a logical exposition of his views—which he afterward embodied in his book 'The Nervous Character.' The fourth evening was devoted to the debate. Reitler fired the opening gun. He had prepared his answer and read it from the manuscript. His conclusion was that all that Adler presented as new was in reality old, and that what was really new was worthless. He was followed by Rosenstein who spoke in the same strain. And so it went on, one condemnation and adverse criticism after another.

Friend Also Against Him.

"Professor Freud also took the floor and refused to extend any recognition to the new ideas which Adler had promulgated. His repudiation was unnecessarily sarcastic and forceful. The master was also very much excited and it was clear that he had prepared himself very thoroughly.

"A small number of Adler's supporters put in a word for him, and as for myself, I distributed praise and blame, as I thought, in a measure that seemed just to me. Then came the surprise.

"Dr. Maximilian Steiner took the

floor. He declared that the theories of Dr. Adler no longer represented any kind of analysis. Adler was an opponent of Freud's and had no right to belong to this society. And it was suddenly clear that this was the gist of the whole matter. Adler was to be expelled from the Verein.

"The final decision was postponed until the next meeting. This took place in a coffee house (Café Arkaden) in rooms belonging to a medical club. Everybody was very much wrought up. I came out strongly in favor of Adler and for the freedom of scientific research, but I was voted down and out—along with the other supporters of Adler. And thereupon Adler and his friends left the room. Most of his friends were Socialists, comrades of his party. Among them were Professor Oppenheim, Furtmüller, the two Grüner brothers and others, some eight or ten in all.

"My first impulse was to join them. But I had just made a move in respect to my profession which made this step particularly difficult for me. I had given up my general practice and taken up a specialized practice for psychoanalysis. Freud had promised to give me his support. I was once more dependent upon him and he knew this quite well.

"It would also have been most difficult for me to give up the official organ for physical research which I had founded. And so I remained and for a time Freud overwhelmed me with kindnesses. During a session which took place after Adler's resignation, Professor Freud told me that he regarded Adler as a paranoiac.

"And now I must touch upon the most important point—and describe what led to my separation from the great Sigmund Freud. Freud, in his history of the psychoanalytical movement, writes as follows concerning this point: 'Herr Stekel is alone responsible for the contents of the official organ from the third number of the second volume on. His conduct, which it would be difficult to describe in public, has forced me to resign from the editorship of the magazine.'

"Freud fights shy of the truth in this matter, and the same charge holds good with regard to what he writes of Adler in the same publication, namely, that 'Dr. Alfred Adler had decided, because of scientific differences with the editor,' to resign voluntarily from the editorial staff.'"

Stekel does not merely attempt to make charges and to establish facts; he seems also striving to understand and to forgive.

May 23, 1926

REVIEWS STUDIES IN HUMAN BEHAVIOR

In the form of a proposed "reconditioning plant" for the cure of psychological maladjustments, Dr. John B. Watson, behaviorist psychologist, who lectured last night at Town Hall at a showing of the Russian film "Mechanics of the Brain," gave a direct, practical application of his theories to the problems of the nervously and emotionally maladjusted adult.

According to Dr. Watson's theories of human behavior, which he links closely with the work of Professor Ivan P. Pavlov, on whose work the film is based, the adult human consists of nothing but a mass of acquired responses to stimuli, built on the comparatively few primary responses found in every new-born infant. Many of these, such as unnecessary fears, are unsatisfactory and can only be removed by a process of "unconditioning."

To try to uncondition yourself," said Dr. Watson, "is as impossible as trying to pull yourself up by your own boot straps. But if we could establish large reconditioning plants where all the stimuli were determined for a person by the psychologists in charge we could start the reconditioning with the simple unconditional reflex. In a place where it would be entirely determined for a person not only how his thoughts and emotions would be stimulated, but whether he was to have food or not to have it, to have sex or not to have it, there might be some hope for rebuilding the adult in the same manner as we have shown we can take the new-born child and practically determine what manner of man he shall be."

He intimated that psychoanalysis loses a great deal of its beneficial value because it ignores the physical basis of the emotions. He said:

"It gives mental release and is of some good, but it does not give complete physical release."

Dr. Watson acknowledged the great debt his work in behaviorism on the study of emotions owes to the researches of Professor Pavlov. It is to him, he said, that he owes the concept of the "conditioned response," which he applies to emotions, which are based, he says, on gland action. An illustration of this is the fear produced in a child by the mere sight of an animal if the animal has been previously present in association with some loud noise. Dr. Watson's use of the principle was illustrated in the showing of a film depicting his observations and experiments on children, made at the Johns Hopkins University.

Arthur Garfield Hays presided at the showing, which was under the auspices of the American Society for Cultural Relations with Russia.

May 24, 1928

REFUSES TO PUT BAN ON PSYCHOANALYSTS

Special Cable to THE NEW YORK TIMES.

LONDON, July 22.—A motion which, in the opinion of some doctors seemed to suggest that psychoanalysts were charlatans, was rejected by the British Medical Association at its annual conference in Manchester today. The representative body of doctors, drawn from all parts of the country, instead accepted the report of its committee which, for two and a half years, has been investigating this form of treatment and which found itself "unable to express any collective opinion either in favor of the practice or in opposition to it."

Its claims, the committee found, must "be tested by time, experience and discussion."

The committee's report presented the following six general conclusions:

Six Conclusions Made.

1. Freud's use and definition of the term, psychoanalysis, is one to be accepted.

2. Psychoanalysis should not be held responsible for the opinions or actions those not, in the proper sense, psychoanalysts.

3. Other misconceptions, in relation to the subject, are to be recognized and removed.

4. There is a disposition, even among those hostile to psychoanalysis, to accept the existence of the unconscious mind as a reasonable hypothesis.

5. The committee cannot pronounce between the psychoanalysts and the most important criticisms of their theory and method.

6. The committees expressed failure to express a collective opinion either for or against it.

Vigorous dissentions marked the debate today.

Dr. C. E. Douglas, a Scottish physician, said that psychoanalysis was really an "old story" and that if Freud had asked any Roman Catholic Priest in the last thousand years he would have been told that in the confessional something like 90 per cent of all confessions made dealt with sex subjects. "The gravity of the whole charge against psychoanalysis is," said Dr. Douglas, "that it is a bad thing, morally, to direct a patient's attention to such things as it deals with. Can we, as doctors, entrust our patients to such a revolting method of treatment?"

Dr. L. A. Parry then offered a motion regretting that the committee had not "laid more emphasis on the very real and serious dangers, especially to children and adolescents," and Dr. Manson, in reply, said that this appealed to prejudice.

"Doubtless," he said, "there are abuses of this process and doubtless there are untrained people practicing it, but that is not the subject of the report. Let us avoid condemning this thing merely because of its repugnance."

Dr. Parry retorted:

"Psychoanalysts are men who are soaked year in and year out in nothing but sex and it must be obvious that there must be great dangers in any system of treatment so based. In my four years of study of this subject and in listening to protagonists of the psychoanalytical school, I have not a single fact before me which convinces me that there is anything whatever in this theory. I say the theory has no basis in fact and I ask you to realize there is a danger of bringing discredit on ourselves, as a profession, if we leave the public unwarned."

Dr. Peter MacDonald said the committee's report showed that psychoanalysts were not charlatans and that many dangers disappeared on investigation.

The association rejected Dr. Parry's motion and adopted the committee's report.

July 23, 1929

DR. SIGMUND FREUD DIES IN EXILE AT 83

Founder of Psychoanalysis Theory Succumbs at His Home Near London

Special Cable to THE NEW YORK TIMES.
LONDON, Sept. 23—Dr. Sigmund Freud, originator of the theory of psychoanalysis, died shortly before midnight tonight at his son's home in Hampstead at the age of 83.

Dr. Freud fled from Austria last year when the country was invaded by Germany and had been living with his son, Dr. Ernst Freud, ever since. He had been in ill health for more than a year and yesterday he passed into a coma from which he never rallied.

His Methods Widely Discussed

One of the most widely discussed scientists of the present day and originator of countless new ideas in the field of psychology, Dr. Sigmund Freud was a man who never compromised but often modified. In his long and stormy career he set the entire world talking about psychoanalysis, the method which he originated and in which he dramatized for mankind the hampering force of inhibitions.

"The mind is an iceberg—it floats with, only one-seventh of its bulk above water," was one of his metaphorical statements on the vast preponderance of the subconscious element in human life. Another was, "The conscious mind may be compared to a fountain playing in the sun and falling back into the great subterranean pool of the subconscious from which it rises."

Probably the most radical departure from the old psychology introduced in Dr. Freud's science of psychoanalysis was that man is a willing rather than a thinking animal. Previous to his time psychology had been overwhelmingly "intellectual," regarding images, perceptions and ideas as the fundamental factors in mental life. But Dr. Freud, not satisfied with this non-progressing view of man's actions, laid the main stress of his system on the element of will or desire, relegating intellect to the background.

Brought New Words to Science

It was under this new system that Dr. Freud was able to explain many of the old "mysteries" of life, particularly regarding the fantasies and delusions of the deranged mind, and to shed a ray of light on the significance of dreams. It was also natural that, with this new basis of desire, sex should occupy the focal point of the system and that a new vocabulary of "Freudian" words should arise, among them "complex, inhibition, neurosis, psychosis, repression, resistance and transference."

The early critics of Freud's theories were filled with violent prejudice and moral indignation and sought to tear to pieces his entire system. The later critics, among whom are many present-day psychologists and scientists, acknowledged many of his theories to be valuable and devoted themselves to critical studies of his plan with a view to perfection rather than destruction. Dr. Freud himself believed that his ideas were harmed by their excessive popularity, which led to a reckless use of his theory and an exaggeration of his doctrines.

Although known as a Viennese, Dr. Freud was a Moravian by birth. He was born in this old Austro-Hungarian province on May 6, 1856, in the town of Freiberg. His parents moved to Vienna while he was still young and he received his education there, taking his degree of Doctor of Medicine at the university there in 1881. His parents had hoped he would follow a literary career, finding ability as a poet in him, but once he chose science he renounced all thought of literary aspirations. After his graduation he served in turn as demonstrator in the physiological institute, Vienna; assistant physician in the general hospital and lecturer on nervous diseases.

Studied in Charcot School.

After becoming intensely interested in psychiatry he went on to Paris in 1885 to study in the famous school of Charcot and Janet, known as the virtual founders of modern abnormal psychology. The influence of his masters, however, was largely one of provoking thought on his own part. He plunged into a wholly new investigation of neurotic disorders and delevoped a method so new that he made Janet one of his bitterest professional enemies, being accused by him of introducing unwarranted assumptions into the orthodox doctrine. Several of Dr. Freud's pupils in turn, among them C. G. Jung and Alfred Adler, diverged from him as widely as he did from his own teachers.

In forming his ideas about psychoanalysis Freud proceeded with an independence and uncompromising attitude which served either to alienate his associates completely or to win them over as virtual disciples.

After remaining in Paris a year he returned to Vienna, where he became a Professor Extraordinary of Neurology in 1902. He also used his apartment in Berggasse as a clinic and received daily many patients who came to him with all types and varieties of mental ailments. Later in life, age and illness forced him to cut down the number of his patients to a minimum and to make but few public appearances, but he continued to develop his theories and to write treatises on his chosen subject.

Deeply Interested in Soviet Russia.

The Communist experiment in Russia was of great interest to the psychoanalyst, but the United States failed to attract him, even though he had visited this country in 1909, when he received an honorary LL. D degree from Clark University. Probably the only American whom he held in high esteem was William James, who he said was "one of the most charming men I have ever met." Professor James, however, was to him the one exception in a country which has produced only "an unthinking optimism and a shallow philosophy of activity."

The United States, on the other hand, was scarcely more tolerant in many ways toward Dr. Freud, and many of Dr. Freud's conceptions of this country were based on exaggerated or burlesqued writings on his principles. "America is vulgarizing too extensively," he once said. "The newspapers seem too prone to popularize the lewd instead of the intellectual fact." Probably the most predominant criticism in America of the Freudian theory is that the element of sex is grossly overplayed in his explanations of human actions and reactions.

Even the defenders of Dr. Freud have from time to time admitted that, like most specialists, he had carried many of his ideas too far and that he saw sex, where its presence was debatable or even completely absent. They have also deplored the development of the original therapeutic system into one of philosophy and almost religion, placing the responsibility for this more on Dr. Freud's followers and rivals than on Dr. Freud himself.

Was a Prolific Writer.

Dr. Freud was a prolific writer. His books have won popularity in many countries and have put before the world his wealth of ideas, startling and even sensational during the pre-war conservatism. His works on hysteria and the interpretation of dreams were probably his most widely known writings. In these he brought out the theory that hysteria is the result of a nervous shock, emotional and usually sexual in nature, and that the ideas involved have been suppressed or inhibited until they can no longer be recalled. By a use of the principle of psychoanalysis and the employment of the patient's free-will associations these ideas can be recalled, he wrote, and the cause of the hysteria removed.

One of his outstanding works was an incidental writing which appeared near the close of the war, entitled "Reflections on War and Death."

"The history of the world is essentially a series of race murders," he wrote. "The individual does not believe in his own death. On the other hand, we recognize the death of strangers and of enemies, and sentence them to it just as willingly and unhesitatingly as primitive man did. In our unconscious mind we daily and hourly do away with all those who stand in our way, all those who have insulted or harmed us."

In August, 1930, Freud received the Goethe prize for the year, awarded by the city of Frankfort, Germany. The prize at that time was the greatest scientific and literary distinction in Germany. Illness prevented his accepting the honor in person.

Despite the ravages of cancer and infirmities of age, Dr. Freud continued active until after his eightieth birthday on May 6, 1936.

At that time, declining a request for an interview, he wrote: "What I had to tell the world I have told. I place the last period after my work."

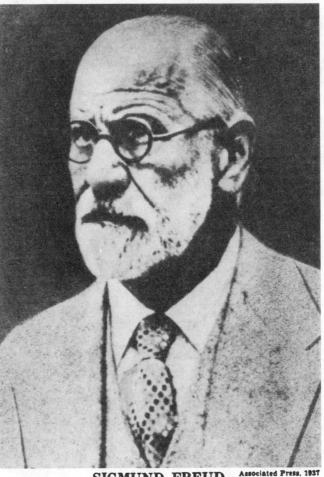

SIGMUND FREUD   Associated Press, 1937

Many who had been the bitterest critics of his psychoanalysis theories gathered in Vienna on his eightieth birthday to do him honor. He himself was not there, but his wife and family were, and they wept as Dr. Julius Wagneur-Jauregg, president of the Viennese Psychiatrists Association, said in opening the meeting:

"Viennese psychiatrists followed the trail blazed by Freud to worldwide fame and greatness. We are proud and happy to congratulate him as one of the great figures of the Viennese school of medicine."

One of Dr. Freud's last writings was a revision in 1936 of an article for the Psychiatric Almanac. A year earlier he had completed and published his "Autobiography," and three years before he had issued a small book, "A New Series of Introductory Lectures on Psychoanalysis."

He still received a few patients after 1930, but most of the questioning was done by his daughter Anna, whom he recognized as his successor, the aged, bearded, stoop-shouldered doctor merely nodding agreement from time to time. He made no public appearances and received only a few old friends, who called on Wednesday nights to talk and on Fridays to play cards.

To the last he remained intolerant of criticism or disagreement with his theories and he could not understand why he should be censured for his bitterness.

"What claims are to be made on us in the name of tolerance?" he wrote in his 1932 lectures. "That when somebody has expressed an opinion that we consider fundamentally false we should say, 'Thanks for the contradiction.'"

His last years also were disturbed by the pogroms against the Jews. When his books were burned by the Nazis in the bonfire which also consumed the works of Heine and other non-Aryan authors he remarked, "Well, at least I have been burned in good company."

Although egotistical in his professional contacts—he told the story himself that a peasant woman had told his mother when he was born that she had given birth to a great man—Freud was described by his family and his friends as gentle and considerate, a delightful companion when not talking "shop."

Soon after his eighty-first birthday, when he was suffering not only from cancer but also from a painful heart malady, he said despairingly, "It is tragic when a man outlives his body."

Dark Days Under the Nazis

During his last years, when he was to taste the bitterness of exile, Dr. Freud had been in retirement, engaged upon writing books to which all his research and study would have been but a preliminary. He had completed his last work in the development of his theory and now only a few patients were admitted to him.

He had retired into his library and was seeking, in the few years left to him, to make a pioneering study of the nature of religion. As the annexation of Austria appeared more and more a menace, he was urged by his friends to seek refuge abroad, but he refused to go. If the Nazis invaded the refuge of his library, he told them, he was prepared to kill himself.

He was ill, a shadow of his former self at 82, when Nazi Germany moved her army into Austria and absorbed his homeland and he was not at once told about it. His family was obliged to burn a whole truckload of his books they had sent to Switzerland. He was virtually penniless and the news came as a great shock to him.

He remained in seclusion in his five-room apartment, "dreading insults if he emerged—because he is a Jew," friends said. A delegation of Netherlands admirers went to Vienna to offer him the hospitality of their country, but the authorities

forbade him to go, refusing him a passport. Soon the reason was disclosed. Not satisfied with having destroyed his income, as well as his family firm's stock of books, the Nazis were demanding that he be ransomed.

Huge Fund Raised for Passport

A fund had been raised quietly by American admirers to pay his and his family's living expenses once they left Vienna, but it was sadly inadequate to meet the demand. Princess George of Greece, who as Princess Marie Bonaparte had studied under Freud, induced the Nazi authorities after lengthy negotiations to accept a quarter million of Austrian schillings she had on deposit in Vienna to restore his passport. The American, British and French Psychoanalytical Associations and scientists all over the world brought pressure to aid her.

In June, 1938, he was able to leave with his family and some personal books and papers. He went to Paris and then to London, the Nazi press sending after him a parting gibe, calling his school a "pornographic Jewish specialty." A condition of his release was that he keep silence, and he was not able to tell how frequently Nazi officials upbraided him in the months before. Settling in London, he finished a book, "Moses and Monotheism" (published here last June), a study of the Moses legend and its relation to the development of Judaism and Christianity.

The book, a first effort to use his psychoanalytic system to explain the origins of the institution of religion, origins shrouded in the obscurity of ages, aroused a storm of controversy. Although he had long wanted to make such an investigation of the Bible, he had delayed its completion while in Vienna, he explained in an accompanying manuscript, because he had not wanted to affront the religious sensibilities of the Catholic authorities, who had treated him well and had protected his fellow-Jews.

Bulwark Against Barbarism

"Catholic Austria seemed the last bulwark against an impending danger," he wrote, "and even those who are opposed to the results of Catholicism have learned to submit to the lesser evil."

The book was bitterly attacked, no less for such beliefs as that Moses was an Egyptian, than for such suggestions as that ethical monotheism was not a cultural achievement evolved in the course of the spiritual development of the Jews but rather an amplification of the idea of one God Moses brought to the Jewish people from the religion of an Egyptian king, Ikhnaton.

But it also found admirers. Thomas Mann hailed it as showing that the Freudian theory had become "a world movement embracing every possible field of learning and science," as, for future generations, one of the most important foundation stones for "the dwelling of a freer and wiser humanity."

In London he spent a contented year in a house a few hundred yards north of Regent's Park. Leaving further development of his psychological theories to his daughter, Anna, and his disciples, he concentrated on his monumental study of the Old Testament, which he estimated would take him five years to complete, a work of which "Moses and Monotheism" was only to have been the first fruit.

He had stated its theme, that all religions only reflect the hopes and fears of man's own deepest nature, in "Totem and Taboo" twenty-five years before, but now he sought to buttress his speculations with supporting evidence. This work, which he believed would have a far-reaching effect on religion, is now left uncompleted, it is believed.

September 24, 1939

CURBING ASSAILED IN PSYCHOTHERAPY

Psychologist Argues Fitness of Non-Medical Group but Doctor Would Restrict It

The medical profession is holding back the development of psychotherapy in this country by insisting that a medical degree is necessary for the practice of "the art of psychotherapy," it was charged last night by Dr. Robert Lindner, a prominent psychologist. Declaring that some of "the most eminent architects" of present-day psychotherapy have been and are holders "of other than the medical degree," he said that the present campaign to exclude the non-medical psychotherapist from practice was, in his opinion, "an ill-advised and foredoomed adventure of those who have little understanding of the nature of psychotherapy, little love for the work and little respect for its future."

He presented the psychologist's point of view in a discussion of

who shall practice psychotherapy held at the New York Academy of Medicine under the sponsorship of the Association for the Advancement of Psychotherapy.

Normal and Abnormal Line

Dr. Iago Galdston, executive secretary of the academy's committee on medical information, upheld the medical point of view, saying that his opinions, however, were solely his own.

Declaring that the issue of "what is and what is not psychotherapy" must first be settled, he offered the definition that "psychotherapy is the treatment of the abnormal" as distinguished from the giving of guidance and counsel to help normal individuals resolve the difficulties that they encounter "in normal living."

"In the treatment of the abnormal there cannot be any such thing as lay psychotherapy," he said. "The layman can perform other functions than psychotherapy, but if he attempts psychotherapy, he must be and must be considered to be—a quack."

He gave the following as example: "An embarrassed, shy, self-deprecating adolescent girl out on her first formal dance may be very unhappy and very gauche. She most certainly needs help, but not necessarily that of a psychiatrist.

On the other hand, should she become so shy that she remains indoors for weeks, doesn't dress, etc., she would very much be in need of psychiatric help."

"The treatment of the sick requires a thorough training in, and the absorption into one's thinking patterns of, biologic realities and dynamics," he contended.

The medical profession is opposed to the practice of lay psychotherapy and "includes the clinical psychologist among the laity," he said. The clinical psychologists are, however, valuable in diagnostic work, he added.

Psychology as Basis

Dr. Lindner, who is also a lay analyst, declared that he regarded as "arrant and unscientific nonsense any claim that a medical education in any way better suits" a person for the practice of psychotherapy, which he described as "less science than art" and as such, "predominantly unteachable."

He called it "a process of education as much, and more, than of healing," and said that psychology was "the scientific well from which psychotherapy takes its beginnings and draws its sustenance."

The community at large is paying the price for the "ill-advised and poorly motivated disregard of the facts," he said.

Among the medical practitioners of psychotherapy, the majority are "but spottily educated and informed," he held, possessing "a handful of clinical facts wrapped about with terminological vagaries and ill-considered generalizations; while the non-medical therapist denied access to the clinic and dieting on the crumbs that fall from the medical table, has little opportunity to round off his own education in the manner required for achieving scientific and professional virtue."

Out of the misguided allegiance of the practitioners who assume the office of psychotherapist on the license of a medical education and "hew strongly and strictly to the alleviative goals of medicine," have come "the twin abortions of the shock therapies and psychosurgery," he said.

Calling them "desperate remedies," he described their objective as "relief for the individual patient and the attending physician," and said that, "in some cases, it is obtained at the expense of the total reduction of the personality to a state of inhuman robotism."

Dr. Clarence P. Oberndorf and Theodor Reik, psychoanalyst, were the discussants.

January 28, 1950

After Fifty Years–An Analysis of Analysis

By LAWRENCE GALTON

ONE February night fifty years ago, sixteen men gathered in the New York City home of Dr. A. A. Brill, translator of the writings of Sigmund Freud and the first psychiatrist in America to treat patients by Freud's psychoanalytic methods. The fifteen other men were psychiatrists who had followed Brill into the practice of psychoanalysis. That night, the New York Psychoanalytic Society was formed. Only a few months later, in May, 1911, a national organization, the American Psychoanalytic Association, was founded. Psychoanalysis had come to America.

It is not too much to say that America has never been the same since.

This year, as it celebrates its anniversary, the New York society, a leader of American and even world-wide psychoanalytic thought, has a membership of 287; the national organization a membership of 923. Even now, by no stretch of the imagination does the total number of people under treatment at any one time by these analysts, and by hundreds of other physicians in training to become analysts, exceed 15,000.

But psychoanalysis has had — and continues to have — an influence totally unlimited by the limited number of its practitioners and patients. It has permeated the rest of psychiatry and, indeed, virtually all of medicine.

Psychotherapeutic techniques based upon analytic principles are now used to treat many scores of thousands of people yearly. A medical specialty, psychosomatic medicine, which takes into account the mind's capability for producing bodily symptoms, has been sparked by psychoanalysis. Analytic ideas and language have been borrowed for novels and poetry and, of course, jokes. To a considerable extent, they guide the upbringing of our children. They are reflected in current views on education and philosophy and on crime and delinquency as well.

And yet, with all this, in the year 1961 psychoanalysis remains, to much of the general public, a matter of mystery and even misunderstanding and, to no small number, a seeming mumbo-jumbo collection of far-fetched and off-color theories and strange, even occult rituals.

Moreover, it remains today a hotly controversial issue — perhaps more controversial than ever before — among scientists, some of whom assert that, whatever analysis may be, it cannot lay claim to being scientific.

JUST what is psychoanalysis? And how effective is it? And what are the major criticisms against it?

A basic theory of mind as well as a method of treatment, analysis began with the studies, mostly made about the turn of the century, of Sigmund Freud, a Viennese physician, showing that the human mind is like an iceberg in the sense that most of it is out of sight, hidden in what Freud called the unconscious.

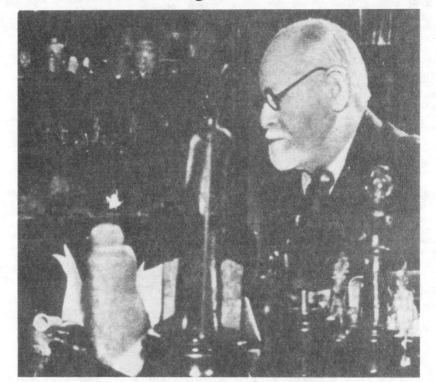

Freud in his consulting room in Vienna—"Since psychoanalysis' advent it is not too much to say that we have never been the same."

Freud mapped out three basic functional areas of the mind. One, the id, in the unconscious, is completely out of touch with the outer world; it is the seat of the instincts, of such powerful, primeval drives as sex, hunger, thirst. A second is the ego in the conscious mind, developed from the outer layer of the id, in contact with the world, sensitive to society's rules, and meant to act as a brake on the id. The third, the super-ego, arises out of rules of behavior imposed early in life.

In a nutshell, the child is born with the id, acquires the ego, and has thrust upon him the super-ego. And it is the gist of analytic theory that the ego all too often is weakened, particularly during childhood, as it tries to deal with the demands of both id and super-ego.

The child has instincts—basically destructive and sexual—demanding to be satisfied. Under the influence of his parents, the instincts are brought under control. If the child is overly intimidated in the process, he may repress his forbidden impulses and ideas to a far greater extent than in normal situations.

BUT repressed impulses don't cease to exist. They are ever present, ever active through life. They appear in disguise in dreams. They are behind slips of the tongue. They influence behavior, produce seemingly irrational fears, are the causes of neurotic symptoms ranging from heart palpitations to procrastination, from work difficulties to sexual impotence, from facial tics to paralysis of limbs.

The aim of psychoanalysis is to bring repressed material into the conscious mind where it can be comprehended and mastered, and, in the process, to strengthen the ego. The repressed material is disclosed to the patient through his dreams and through free association in which he reports all ideas flowing through his mind. To further the process, the patient lies upon a couch and the analyst sits behind him, out of sight.

To Freud, psychoanalysis was not necessarily the final answer—either as therapy or theory. "Psychoanalysis has never," he said, "claimed to give a perfect theory of human psychic life."

And he added: "The future may teach us how to exercise a direct influence, by means of particular chemical substances, upon the * * * apparatus of the mind. It may be that there are other undreamed-of possibilities of therapy. But for the moment we have nothing better at our disposal than the technique of psychoanalysis, and for that reason, in spite of its limitations, it is not to be despised."

AS it has been from the start, analysis today is an extensive and expensive procedure. It involves four to five sessions a week, each running forty-five to fifty minutes. It continues for two to six years—and, not rarely, even longer. The fee ranges from $15 to $35 a session, or more—high, but necessarily so. It is difficult for any analyst to have more than eight or nine patients in analysis at one time, whereas many medical practitioners may see that many patients in one hour.

Not only is the number of patients who can be treated by analysis sharply limited; it is likely to remain so. No great multiplication of analysts is in sight. Analytic training is long and stringent. To be admitted to one of the eighteen training facilities approved by the American Psychoanalytic Association, the potential analyst must have a medical degree, a year of general internship, and two years of full-time psychiatric residence.

His analytic education then requires another four or more years. He must himself undergo analysis, running on the average to 700 hours, in order to be freed of personality factors that might interfere with his ability to treat others. On top of the cost of all his previous education, the cost of his analytic training averages $19,200. Currently, only some 100 new analysts are graduated each year.

Analysis over the years has been credited by its practitioners with helping thousands to overcome unhealthy, neurotic adjustments to life, to rid themselves of inhibiting anxieties and compulsions, to minimize or eliminate many bodily symptoms. But from the very start it has been criticized on some grounds, and it is being sharply criticized today on broader grounds.

When, in 1910, a distinguished German neurologist whipped himself into a frenzy at a psychiatric convention and screamed that psychoanalysis "is not a matter for discussion at a scientific meeting; it is a matter for the police," the reason was the seeming overconcern of analysis with sex.

FREUD had ranked libido, or sexual instinct, as the major force in psychic development. All neuroses, he believed when he started, stemmed from unfilled or unfillable sexual desires. Later, he amplified the term libido to include other forms of pleasure-seeking.

It wasn't long before Adler and Jung, early Freud collaborators, and then others, were stressing that conflicts associated with "drive to power" and with various social and cultural factors in the individual's environment were as important as sex.

Today, criticism is not limited to the libido theory; it is directed against the emphasis, by *all* analytic schools, on conflicts, *whatever* the type, to the neglect of other possible factors. Certainly, critics grant, conflicts may produce neuroses, but constitutional factors also must be considered. It is obvious enough that people have different intellectual endowments. They may, no less, have different emotional endowments which can enter into the development of emotional disorders.

Recent research—notably, investigations showing that some hormones can create psychic disturbances and that normal people, when given injections of certain substances, develop symptoms of mental disease—indicates that mental illness may be associated with specific physical and chemical changes.

Dr. Linus Pauling, Nobel Prize-winning chemist, has suggested that mental disorders may be due to deranged molecules in the genes, the carriers of heredity, and that some day out of the chemist's laboratory may come means to correct the abnormalities.

PRIOR to analysis, organic disorders were overstressed as the causes of mental disease. Analysis performed a great service in showing that people don't live in a vacuum and that environment can affect mental functioning, its critics agree, but there is no basis for going to the extreme of negating organic factors.

Moreover, critics of analysis today question its therapeutic effectiveness. Analytic treatment has been of little value, they charge, for the severely disturbed, the psychotics who fill our mental hospitals.

It has had some success in neuroses, they grant. But how often? Many emotionally ill people recover without any treatment at all. Is analysis a better healer than time?

And when analysis is effective, is it for the reasons analysts think? When changes occur in an individual over the course of years of analysis, is it really because basic conflicts are eliminated? Could it be only a matter of repeated suggestion? Could it sometimes be the result of forces that operate independently of analysis?

At a recent critical symposium on psychoanalysis, one participant remarked: "If, as a priest of some Mithraic cult, I give an ailing penitent moldy bread and say a prayer over him, he may recover. If the recovery takes place several times when penitents are treated in this fashion, I am justified in continuing to use the technique. But the success of the treatment is not decisive with respect to the validity of the theory that prayer is efficacious." (Not, that is, until every other possible explanation has been eliminated.)

Analysts hold that their interpretations—of dreams and material produced by free association—are important in the treatment process. But could it be that some patients, without help from interpretations, benefit simply from insight they gain into some of their own maneuverings simply by talking about them and thus recognizing them?

The fact is, say some critics, interpretations vary considerably between analysts. It would be enlightening, they suggest, to make studies to see how many patients improve after being given false interpretations.

MANY analysts believe that the key to therapeutic success is transference. During the long, intense relationship with the analyst, the patient reproduces earlier disturbing relationships in his life —with mother, father, siblings or others—and transfers his conscious and unconscious emotions and feelings onto the analyst.

Where is the proof, some critics demand, that this is essential? How come, one asks, that some patients, after years

of analysis without benefit, are helped by some short form of psychotherapy which does not provide any such intense relationship with the therapist as does analysis?

A prime reason why so few analysts use tranquilizing drugs in analysis is the belief that the drugs would interfere with transference and would reduce the patient's motivation for continuing. But is there any proof of this?

One well-known psychiatrist says: "I do not believe that the use of a drug necessarily interferes with the transference relationship * * * Many patients are very appreciative of the fact that their considerable suffering is made more bearable. This usually leads to an enhancement of the transference relationship and not the opposite."

Drugs, he goes on to say, introduce what may be a basically important new approach into psychiatry.

THE fact is that psychotherapy by itself often can reduce anxiety and tension. But beyond a certain level of severity, it may not do so, while drugs may. On the other hand, psychotherapy may work in some instances where drugs do not.

Drugs, of course, have their limitations. They do not reveal to the patient why he has conflicts or why he is anxious in some situations and not in others. Psychotherapy does this. But it is possible that proper integration of the two approaches could make for better results. Given the job of reducing the emotional intensity of symptoms, drugs might well permit a less anxiety-ridden psychotherapeutic elucidation of conflicts, making psychotherapy at once more effective and more economical.

"The idea that the patient has to be profoundly uncomfortable for effective psychotherapy," says the doctor quoted above, "is an old shibboleth which-has never been proved and which should be carefully reexamined in the light of newer knowledge. I do not believe that theoretical ballast of this sort should be carried year after year without the re-examination of the correctness of the foundations."

TO a large extent, this last statement epitomizes much of the criticism against analysis. It has tended to stand still.

Analysts have been too busy with endless ruminations and rhapsodizings, with variations on original analytic themes and theories. They have not been busy enough devising adequate scientific tests to see if the theories are really valid. They have failed to experiment

enough with techniques of treatment, seeking ways to shorten it and make it more effective. Analysis, to this day, remains a hit-or-miss affair, with no effective method for clearly forecasting which patients will be helped. And there is not even proof, it is charged, that long-drawn-out analysis is any better than short-term psychotherapy.

There are many forms of psychotherapy. They vary considerably, but have two things in common: the establishment of rapport, or a harmonious relationship, between therapist and patient; and an attempt to influence the patient.

Psychotherapy may make use of dreams and free association, but not with anything like the detail of analysis. And it may forgo dreams and free association entirely.

One form—ventilation psychotherapy—begins with taking the patient's history and continues with unhurried interviews in which the patient is given opportunities "to confess" his problems and discuss his life history.

Another form—supportive psychotherapy—may start with a physical examination and reassurance about physical health and be followed by suggestions and the giving of illuminating information. Treatment may also include the use of drugs where necessary.

A THIRD form—manipulative psychotherapy—may consist of vocational guidance and establishing a daily routine, including diversion and entertainment—all designed to produce a change in the patient's environmental attitudes. Still another form, explanatory psychotherapy, includes efforts to reduce the patient's oversensitivity to difficult situations and to re-educate him by means of suggestion.

There is also group psychotherapy, in which half a dozen or more patients with somewhat similar problems meet one or more times a week under the guidance of a psychiatrist and talk out their problems.

Can analysts prove, critics ask, that their technique is any more effective than any one, or all, of these forms of psychotherapy?

Analysts are hardly without answers to the critical needlings.

To begin with, they don't dispute the fact that many people recover from emotional disturbances without any treatment. Indeed, as one of the most distinguished said:

"Life cures more neuroses than all psychoanalysts combined. For a neurosis is a reaction of a susceptible individual to difficulties and pressures in life. Conditions change

174

and the change may be enough to re-establish the individual's equilibrium. This is no evidence for or against the validity of psychoanalysis."

FREUD himself, analysts point out, remarked that one of the most effective cures for neurosis is to fall in love. Religion, they also say, affords the opportunity to find forgiveness or penance which may help to control anxiety and guilt feelings. And even hobbies may have a therapeutic effect by serving as acceptable substitutes for the expression of impulses that could cause too much guilt if given direct expression.

But they also point out that it is rarely the person who might be cured spontaneously or by other means who seeks analytic treatment or, for that matter, psychotherapy. Hunting up a psychiatrist, they point out, isn't quite like going to a physician for a sore throat. People don't enter into psychiatric treatment lightly. They wait. They often wait for many years and there is no spontaneous improvement.

As to short-term psychotherapy, analysts are quick to respond that it is decidedly valuable. They deplore any tendency of the public to overrate analysis as treatment, to think that it is invariably better because it is longer and more expensive.

Anaylsis cannot now, nor is it ever likely to be able to, meet the huge demand for help for the emotionally troubled. Nor is it necessary for it to do so. Analysis may be required in certain deep-rooted disturbances that short-term therapy might not reach. But, at most, only one of every ten people with mental or emotional problems is suitable for, or needs, deep analysis. The others, say analysts, not only may do just as well with psychotherapy, but sometimes, even better.

Analysts themselves rarely confine their work entirely to deep analysis; most also engage in psychotherapy, as do thousands of nonanalytic psychiatrists and, increasingly now, even family doctors who have been learning the techniques in courses taught by analysts and other psychiatrists.

HAS analysis—and psychotherapy as well — failed psychotics? The techniques depend upon communication and it is difficult to communicate effectively with many severely ill psychotics, some of whom speak only in gibberish or even refuse to speak at all. But these techniques are frequently used to help further the improvement of psychotics who have made some response to electro-shock, insulin shock or drug treatments.

It is no difficult matter today to find analysts willing to concede that analysis has definite limitations as a therapy. Its real strength, some emphasize, lies in its value as an investigative tool. It is, they say, the most effective instrument yet devised to study the total functioning of the human mind, to conduct microscopic psychological investigations.

At least one analyst has recently publicly expressed regret that analysis ever had to become a therapeutic instrument, instead of remaining a tool for basic research. "Freud," he notes, "repeatedly predicted that in the retrospective view of history psychoanalysis would be regarded as more important as a method of psychological investigation and as a theory of human psychology than as a therapy."

NEVERTHELESS, there is increasing concern among analysts now over improving analytic therapy. There is increasing concern among them that some of the basic therapeutic concepts of analysis — such as the importance of interpretation — have not been clearly validated as yet; that precise criteria of change in patients undergoing analysis are lacking.

Some analysts are outspoken about the need for analysis to try to find ways to sharpen its treatment measures; to make thorough tests to find out which are really effective and which are not, and for which patients; to determine more precisely the type and amount of therapy the individual patient needs for recovery. Many efforts to achieve these goals now are being made under the direction of the New York Psychoanalytic Society.

In the past, analysis had to depend for its data on what individual analysts heard and reported. There were no witnesses to analytic sessions. Recently, however, tape recording techniques have been developed.

"Here," one analyst says, "analysis stands on the frontier of new developments, based on a precise study of the raw material of analytic communications * * * Auditory data, particularly susceptible to distortions of memory, no longer must be relied on exclusively. With data recorded. it can be re-examined, reheard and rethought, not by one observer alone but by many."

RECENTLY, some analysts, impressed with cybernetics, "thinking machines" and similar developments and the possible light they may throw on some aspects of mental activity, have begun working in this area. One remarks:

"I venture to say that in the long run the application of principles based on models derived from modern electronic engineering, communications engineering, mathematical machinery, digital and analogic computers, and electronic devices in general, will clarify much that at present is confused and muddy in psychoanalytic theory, concepts and terminology, and eventually will furnish us with further techniques for critical self-examination."

If, on the fiftieth anniversary of organized psychoanalysis in America, analysis remains, as some of its critics aver, more prescientific than scientific, still it might be said that half a century is not very long when it comes to developing a science dealing with the most elusive of problems — the human mind and emotions.

February 12, 1961

NEW UNIT FORMED ON SCHIZOPHRENIA

By JOHN A. OSMUNDSEN

The formation of a foundation to study schizophrenia along biological rather than purely psychological lines was announced here yesterday.

Called the American Schizophrenia Foundation, it will be the first to concentrate all its efforts on schizophrenia. It will focus on mounting evidence that the mental disease is a metabolic disorder—as diabetes and arteriosclerosis are thought to be—and not merely a manifestation of psychological and sociological trauma.

The foundation was formed partly in recognition of this growing trend of thought on the disease, its officials said in a press briefing at the Waldorf Astoria Hotel, and partly because there has been little coordination of effort along biochemical lines on this major public health problem.

It has been estimated that one in every four hospital beds in this country is occupied by a schizophrenic.

"The recovery rate remains low and the rate of re-admission is high," said Dr. Abram Hoffer, a trustee of the new foundation and director of psychiatric research at University Hospital, Saskatoon, Sask.

Brain Poison Suspected

"There is now overwhelming evidence," Dr. Hoffer said, "that schizophrenics are victims of a subtle brain poison that produces the bizarre psychological changes in perception, thought, mood, personality and behavior so common to the disease."

Dr. Humphrey Osmond, another trustee of the foundation and director of the bureau of research in neurology and psychiatry at the New Jersey Neuro-Psychiatric Institute in Princeton, said "the disease has not received the attenton it deserves."

Up to now, he said, there has been no agency solely and totally devoted to schizophrenia.

Some estimates place the number of schizophrenics in the United States and Canada at two million. Victims perceive the world differently from the way normal people do, often experiencing a distorted vision of life and alien tastes, smells and tactile sensations. The experiences often produce what victims describe as "terrifying fears."

Dr. Osmond declared that the belief was not new, that schizophrenia was a metabolic, or biochemical and probably hereditary disorder. That idea was born in the mid-17th century, he said, was resurrected and reached a peak of interest about 1945, declined almost to oblivion in 1951 and then began to rise again a few years later.

In the last few years, Dr. Osmond said, scientists in several laboratories in this country and abroad have reported evidence of a chemical difference in the composition of the blood or urine of schizophrenics and those of normal persons.

Although the professional attitude toward the disease in the United States is predominantly psychiatric in its orientation, he said, it may not remain this way for long, but may swing toward regarding schizophrenia more as the expression of a physical disorder rather than a psychosociological confusion.

It is not a germ that scientists are now looking for in schizophrenia, but a gene, or carrier of heredity. Support for the possibility that there is a genetic basis for this mental disorder was rcently reported by Dr. Osmond, Dr. Hoffer, Dr. Ernst Mayr, who is a Harvard zoologist and member of the foundation's advisory board, and Sir Julian Huxley, the noted British biologist.

Attending the foundation's news briefing were John D.J. Moore, of W.R. Grace & Co., its vice president; Robert B. Ross, an attorney with the law firm of Burke & Burke, secretary; and Kahlil Samra, vice president and executive director of the foundation, which has offices in Ann Arbor, Mich. The foundation's president is Bernard P. McDonough of the McDonough Company, in Parkersburg, W.Va.

November 27, 1965

A Quiet Revolution In Mental Care

BOSTON—For most of this century, "talk" therapy has dominated the psychotherapeutic scene.

A patient visits the psychiatrist's office one or more times a week, often for several years, to explore the depths of his problem from birth onward. Hopefully, through this exploration the patient gains insight into his problem, and through the insight resolves it. He is then considered "cured."

But it was readily apparent at the annual meeting of the American Psychiatric Association here last week that many psychiatrists, who are disenchanted with the slow, plodding, often ineffective results of traditional psychotherapy, are looking for a new thing.

Attendance surpassed all expectations at sessions on drug treatment of mental disorders, on biochemical theories of mental illness and on behavior therapy —a conditioning technique that is designed to eliminate the symptoms of mental illness rather than its supposed cause.

The growing forum for these approaches may quietly revolutionize the management of mental illness in this country. For it may result in more direct, effective, faster-acting and farther-reaching care for more people.

Not New

Drug and behavior therapies and biochemical theories of mental illness have been around for 15 years or more, but until now they have generally been regarded with suspicion, defensiveness and denial by the psychiatric community at large.

But if, as someone once said, "Maturity is the ability to tolerate conflict," then it seems as if psychiatry has come of age.

It is no longer hard to find people like Dr. R. Bruce Sloane, chairman of psychiatry at Temple University, who said in an interview:

"It's very nice to have insight psychotherapy—if you can afford the time and money and are appropriately introspective. Some patients eventually say 'Eureka' and they're cured. But when you analyze the results of treatment, you find that this doesn't happen too often."

Dr. Sloane, who said he himself is not a behavior therapist, predicted that "some of the techniques of behavior therapy may ultimately be found more effective than those of orthodox psychotherapy.

Indeed, Dr. Joseph Wolpe, speaking to a capacity audience of more than 1,000 psychiatrists, reported that among 618 neurotic patients "about 87 per cent were either apparently recovered or much improved" through this method.

Dr. Wolpe is a professor of psychiatry at Temple University and the father of behavior therapy in this country. Dr. Wolpe said he was trained in the analytic technique, but that he soon became disillusioned with how long it took to achieve good results and sought a more direct route to the same end.

Behavior therapists direct their attention to such psychiatric problems as phobias, obsessions and compulsions, impotence and frigidity, psychosomatic ailments and homosexuality.

They view these problems as growing from a learned set of inappropriate responses to particular situations—responses which can readily be unlearned.

The unlearning is achieved through a variety of techniques that have their roots in Pavlovian conditioning.

According to Dr. Wolpe, a neurotic person becomes anxious under circumstances that for most people would not be associated with anxiety. Thus, a person with acrophobia becomes anxious when he is in a high place even though there is no danger of falling, and a homosexual becomes anxious when faced by the possibility of intimate contact with a member of the opposite sex.

Almost Hypnotic

Behavior therapy, then, is aimed at desensitizing a person to the circumstances which make him anxious. This is often done while the patient is in a state of deep relaxation—almost a mild hypnotic state.

During relaxation he is exposed to a graduated series of anxiety - arousing circumstances —the least arousing first and the most arousing last—until none of the circumstances produces anxiety.

According to Dr. Wolpe, the patient usually is then able to face the same circumstances in the real world without suffering from anxiety. He reported that relapses and substitutions of other neurosis are rare.

Other techniques of desensitizing a neurotic patient include rewarding him for the right behavior or punishing him for the wrong.

A hospitalized woman who always wore 25 pounds of clothing was weighed before every meal and told she couldn't enter the dining room unless she weighed three pounds less than she did at the particular weigh-in. She soon discovered that the fastest way to lose weight was to take off some of her clothing.

It was not long before she was wearing the normal three pounds of clothing.

Some male homosexuals have been successfully treated by subjecting them to electric shocks while they viewed a picture of an attractive man. When the shocks were stopped a picture of a female was flashed.

The homosexuals gradually learned to associate the male figure with punishment and the female figure with reward.

Fast Treatment

The major advantage of behavior therapy is that it is fast— requiring an average of 30 sessions with a therapist instead of 200 as in traditional psychotherapy and 700 as in psychoanalysis.

The treatment method therefore costs less and is potentially available to more people.

The use of tranquilizing, stimulating or otherwise mind-affecting drugs to treat mental illness has risen tremendously in the last few years as psychiatrists have found that through drugs they are often able to keep patients on their feet, at home and sometimes working, whereas formerly they might have been hospitalized for life.

Drug therapy has stimulated a fast-growing interest in the biochemistry of mental illness, a notion long discussed by analytically trained psychiatrists. At last week's meeting, psychiatrists stood and sat on the floor for three hours to hear discussions of research on body chemicals associated with such disorders as depression and schizophrenia.

Although the chemical approach to mental illness may one day explain its causes and provide a cure, the immediate goal is rehabilitating the patient.

As Dr. Nathan S. Kline, research director at Rockland State Hospital, said in an interview: "Eighty per cent of general medical patients are treated and rehabilitated, not cured. If psychiatrists could adopt that approach, many patients could spend their lives at home instead of in state mental hospitals."

JANE BRODY

May 19, 1968

Psychoanalysis Reaches a Crossroad

By JOHN LEO

"Psychoanalysis is vanishing," says Dr. Thomas Szasz, a psychoanalyst and professor of psychiatry at the Upstate Medical Center in Syracuse. "It's as moribund and irrelevant as the Liberal party in England."

The psychoanalytic movement, says Dr. Judd Marmor, former president of the American Academy of Psychoanalysis, is in danger of 'receding into an unimportant sidestream" of psychiatry.

These are two responses to what many in the field call "the crisis of psychoanalysis," a growing feeling that the most glamorous form of psychical treatment reached a peak of influence and prestige in the early nineteen-fifties and may now be in serious decline.

After 50 years of profound impact on art, medicine, literature, child-rearing and the social sciences, psychoanalysis is beset by internal dissension, rising criticism and evidence that talent and money are flowing toward newer therapies.

But if some see the future of psychoanalysis in jeopardy, there are also those who see the discipline's current troubles as temporary and minor.

"There are always fashions, fads and pendular swings," says Dr. Leo Rangell, a former president of the American Psychoanalytic Association. "But psychoanalysts are as much in demand as ever in key facilities, and no explanatory system of human behavior has as yet supplanted the psychoanalytic one."

Psychoanalysis is organized in America as a subspecialty of psychiatry, the medical specialty dealing with mental and emotional disorders. While other psychiatrists may use drugs, shock therapy and a wide variety of other methods, including verbal therapy, psychoanalytic therapy is entirely verbal, with reliance on free association.

In extended conversations, long-hidden infantile problems are reproduced as difficulties between the patient and the psychoanalyst (the transference neurosis). The psychoanalyst then interprets these difficulties in terms of their childhood origins and helps the patient understand and master them.

As a method of investigating the mind, psychoanalysis is almost universally accepted. But as a treatment, and as a theory of the mind, it is under heavy attack both from within and outside the discipline.

Dr. Bruno Bettelheim, one of the most prominent figures in American psychoanalysis, recently called the major theoretical structures of Sigmund Freud, the founder of psychoanalysis, "time-bound, very shaky, very dubious."

"Freud's big theoretical abstractions, thrown out in a playful, ironical way, are now taken as dogma," Dr. Bettelheim said. Comments of this nature, particularly the charge of unscientific dogmatism, once confined to bitter critics, are now commonly heard at the highest levels of psychoanalysis.

Interest Said to Decline

Many analysts agree that popular interest in psychoanalysis has declined in the last 15 years. In addition, there are several other signs that trouble many in the field:

¶Psychoanalysis is the least used of the approximately 40 recognized forms of psychiatric therapy in the United States, according to a survey by the National Institute of Mental Health. It reaches only 2 per cent of psychiatric patients and that percentage is diminishing.

¶As the mental health field expands rapidly, largely with Federal funds, psychoanalysis is losing ground to quicker, cheaper therapies that can reach slum residents and many low-income Americans who want psychological help. At $15 to $50 a session, three to six times a week for several years, psychoanalysis can often cost an individual more than $20,000.

¶Many critics charge that a lack of substantial research and theoretical development since Freud died in 1939 has resulted in an air of stagnation and lost momentum. "Almost everything we know about psychoanalysis today," said Dr. F. C. Redlich, dean of the School of Medicine at Yale University and a professor of psychiatry, "was Freud's single-handed and single-minded work."

¶Although psychoanalytic therapy is an established part of the medical order, it has not yet been proved to be effective by any scientific test.

¶The psychoanalytic world is depicted more and more as a rigidly dogmatic and defensive guild, not plugged into the major intellectual currents of the day.

Not Keeping Pace

Whatever the reasons, the growth of psychoanalysis is apparently not keeping pace with the growth of psychiatry in general, or the growth of the general population. In 1945, one out of every seven psychiatric residents (new physicians preparing to choose a specialty within psychiatry) became psychoanalysts. Now the figure is one out of 20, according to Dr. Harold Kelman, editor of The American Journal of Psychoanalysis.

Enrollment in the 20 approved training institutes of the American Psychoanalytic Association, the mainstream Freudian group in the United States, was 1,047 as of last March, an increase of 1 per cent since 1960. But in the same period the adult population of the United States has increased by 10 per cent.

"During the nineteen-thirties and nineteen-forties they had to beat the applicants away," Dr. Donald M. Kaplan, a New York psychoanalyst, recalled, speaking of the training institutes. "Now, to keep them filled at the same level as 15 years ago, they've had to drop the standards."

Association spokesmen deny Dr. Kaplan's charge, and point to records showing that the institutes are rejecting the same proportion of applicants, a little more than a half, as they did during the nineteen-fifties.

Many Escaped Hitler

Disasters provided the United States with most of its premier psychoanalysts and gave the movement particular momentum. Hitler's persecution of the Jews in the nineteen-thirties brought a distinguished generation of Middle European analysts to the United States.

Secondly, many talented doctors were attracted to psychoanalysis as a way of helping psychical victims of World War II.

During the war, for example, 2.5 million men were rejected or discharged by the United States armed forces because of emotional disorders.

Many analysts are now concluding that their field failed to capitalize on these two unexpected infusions of manpower and talent. "There's a manpower crisis," an official of the association said, "and I'm not sure we have any special idea of how to meet it."

"The crisis is reflected in the attitudes of many young psychiatric residents here at Yale," said Dr. Robert Jay Lifton, a psychiatrist at the university's School of Medicine.

"They're not choosing to be analysts, partly because psychoanalysis hasn't made any major discoveries in recent years. There's a feeling it's no longer the frontier."

For many, the frontiers are now neuropharmacology, genetics, dream research and studies of brain function. The excitement generated by these "hard," or empirically testable, studies has sharpened criticism of psychoanalysis as a body of unproven theories.

Another frontier is the community psychiatry movement, which offers relatively rapid, Federally financed help on the local level by aiming at quick change in a patient's behavior and generally ignoring (as psychoanalysis does not) the childhood roots of conflict.

With this system, which may involve drugs, direct suggestion, conditioning and a rapid inquiry into the immediate cause of distress, the Los Angeles County Hospital, for example, has cut hospital admissions from 95 per cent of applicants to 35 per cent in 10 years, and reduced the average stay of a mental patient from 180 to 5 days.

Many psychoanalysts consider the numbers impressive but the results superficial, and argue that a quick return of a sick person to his home often endangers the mental stability of his family.

Use Is Widespread

The community psychiatry approach, which is now used by more than a half of all the hospitals in the United States, draws guidance counselors, teachers, the clergymen, social workers and others into the rehabilitation process.

Because psychoanalysis cannot deal with the amount of mental illness that exists in this country, some of those involved in community psychiatry have attacked analysis as a cumbersome, dated treatment for the affluent few.

So have many involved in the bewildering variety of other competing treatments, which range from group therapies, some roughly based on the techniques of Alcoholics Anonymous, to conditioning therapies based on Pavlov's experiments with dogs.

"A psychiatrist should lead you back to reality by showing you how to act responsibly again," said Dr. William Glasser, whose "reality therapy" stresses that an analyst be firm and obtrusive in group therapy sessions. "When and where you got derailed may be interesting to both of you, but it's not worth four or five years [of psychoanalysis] to find out."

Changes Called Shallow

Many psychoanalysts reply, however, that changes in a patient's behavior can leave his underlying difficulties untouched.

"Look," said Dr. Kaplan, "it's possible to take a homosexual and turn him into a heterosexual Don Juan. He will be more acceptable to society, at least to the more virile segments of it, but he'll be just as sick as when he came in for treatment."

Psychoanalysts also object that many competing therapists "play God" with their patients, setting themselves up as the sole judges of what constitutes good and bad behavior. Traditionally, psychoanalysis aims at a patient's freedom to chart his own course in life, not adjustment to any social norms the analyst might favor.

Many analysts believe that the newer therapies are gaining at the expense of psychoanalysis because analysis was oversold to the public by the mass media after World War II.

"You had a situation where the hopes of the general public exceeded all reasonable expectations," said Dr. Rangell. "There were hopes that a generation of children could be brought up free of problems, that psychoanalytic insight would rid the world of crime, divorce and learning problems.

"Now there's a big letdown, particularly among the intelligentsia. But analysts never encouraged such utopian hopes."

Gold and Copper

Many psychoanalysts have welcomed the community psychiatry movement and have joined it, at least part time, pointing to Freud's statement that "the large-scale application of therapy will compel us to alloy the pure gold of analysis freely with the copper of direct suggestion."

That idea is that psychoanalysis has a mission to permeate and guide all efforts to improve mental health. More than 80 per cent of analysts in the association work at least part time outside their offices, teaching or advising at schools, social agencies, clinics and other institutions.

However, Dr. Robert S. Wallerstein, a psychoanalyst and chief of psychiatry at Mount Zion Hospital in San Francisco, said the formidable challenge of community psychiatry had produced "a natural temptation to react defensively and negatively" on the part of analysts.

Historically, defensiveness has been a problem for psychoanalysts. Dr. Burness E. Moore, a New York analyst who once headed the press committee of the association, said recently: "Experience with a good deal of resistance and hostility has led older analysts to exercise great caution in dealing with the outside world."

Traceable to Mockery

This traditional defensiveness, traceable to the mockery from Europe's leading intellectual centers when Freud was struggling to establish his field, led the movement to develop off the campuses and outside the medical schools.

It has also produced a suspicion of other fields of studies and a fear on the part of some analysts that psychoanalysis would be diluted from within.

As a partial result, psychoanalysis has been fractured again and again. Frequently, theoretical innovation has been greeted with suspicion, and major modifications have been labeled as "betrayals," with each new "betrayer" leaving one school of thought to found another.

"Each deviant tends to create his own orthodoxy and ultimately to become his own messiah," said Dr. Lawrence S. Kubie, a psychoanalyst and assistant professor of psychiatry at the University of Maryland Medical School. "Each group develops a tendency to outlaw the data and the theories from other schools and to view them with angry rejection and suspicion."

The American Psychoanalytic Association, founded by early followers of Freud in 1911, has seen many of its own dissidents split off into new groups outside its membership, and has come to place heavy emphasis on consolidating and preserving the heritage of Freud.

Freud Was Concerned

Freud himself feared that analysis would be watered down in the United States by a national preoccupation with innovation and change. But to its critics, the association's determination that the heritage not be squandered looks like rigidity, insistence on orthodoxy and resistance to research.

"Insistence upon internal conformity developed at a time when this revolutionary doctrine was attacked by ignorant and emotionally resistant psychiatrists," three prominent analysts — Sandor Rado, Roy Grinker and the late Franz Alexander—wrote in The Bulletin of the International Psychoanalytic Association.

"Today psychoanalysis does not need as much protection from detractors as from the danger of premature standardization and a rigidly enforced conformism."

In reply, traditional analysts argue that psychoanalysis is a unique instrument for understanding human behavior in depth, and that this understanding depends crucially upon a body of knowledge and techniques that has never been successfully abridged.

"That's why we're accused of conservatism," said Dr. Calvin Settlage of the Philadelphia Psychoanalytic Institute. "Either you adhere to proven insights or it's just not psychoanalysis. If you start reducing the frequency of sessions, as Franz Alexander did, or add other adaptations, you can't plumb to the same depth."

Lack of Research Charged

The contention that psychoanalysis suffers from a lack of research was made in the current issue of The Journal of the American Psychoanalytic Association.

"The failure of psychoanalysis to mount productive research programs during 15 or more years of generous support from the National Institute of Mental Health and foundations is now heading to a general reappraisal by granting agencies of their policy and support," wrote Dr. George L. Engel of Rochester. "Much of the blame will have to be laid at the doors of those who have failed to recognize the obligation to develop research psychoanalyst scientists as well as practitioners."

Disagreement with this contention comes from Dr. George Pollock, who, as head of research at the Chicago Psychoanalytic Institute, is now overseeing research on mourning, the psychological impact of the birth control pill, and the impact of the father at different periods of a child's development.

He said: "If it looks as though we're short on research, it's because our contribution rather gets lost—it's usually done in reference to some other discipline, and the other discipline gets the credit for the work. Work on group adaptation to crises, for example, might be picked up by an anthropologist and written up in his own field."

To charges that the association sponsors little research,

Dr. Moore said: "Associations don't conduct research, individuals do."

The association, however, recently set up its first committee to promote creative investigation.

Dr. Heinz Kohut of Chicago, who has been involved in the committee's work, said that if there had not been enough research, it was because "most people do not have creative minds." And in a healing profession, he added, "one is ordinarily pragmatically oriented —one's energies are taken up with the short-term wish to cure."

Another problem for psychoanalysis is that its effectiveness as a therapy is still questioned. Dr. Bernard Rimland, author of "Infantile Autism," created a stir some months ago arguing, in the magazine Science that "many doubts have been raised, both privately and publicly, concerning the ethics" of those who practice psychoanalysis and other talk therapies, since effectiveness studies have been so negative.

Freud, in his later years, had his own doubts about the usefulness of psychoanalysis as a therapy. He held that "the future will probably attribute far greater importance to psychoanalysis as a science of the unconscious than as a therapeutic procedure."

Yet thousands of patients, particularly those afflicted by neuroses, testify to considerable improvement through analysis. "People who have been helped know very well how effective psychoanalysis can be," said Dr. Charles Breener, the immediate past president of the association.

No Proof of Effectiveness

Dr. Breener acknowledged that no successful scientific test of effectiveness had been made. "It has not been possible," he said, "to measure in any useful way the strength of an impulse, the intensity of a fear or the severity of a conflict."

Then, too, a talk therapy is not easily measurable, nor is it easy to assign credit if a patient is improved during the course of it. Many patients get better or worse because of outside factors or normal maturation.

Many analysts work with the "one-third" rule of thumb, which is based on a number of studies that are not universally accepted. According to the rule, a third of all patients in psychotherapy will be cured, a third will be improved, and a third not helped at all.

Many of the arguments for change within psychoanalysis are bound up with the question of "lay analysis," whether the association should train and certify nonphysicians to practice analysis.

Some critics say that the ban on lay analysts helps portray the field as a carefully controlled guild, and argue that psychoanalysts are more conservative, less open to broader cultural values as a result of long preliminary training as physicians.

Ban Called Chauvinism

Dr. Robert L. Seidenberg of Syracuse, after an unsuccessful struggle to gain the admission of a few nonphysicians, said last December: "This is the kind of chauvinism that is killing psychoanalysis. This rule would have kept out Anna Freud and Erik Erikson, who have probably done more for psychoanalysis than anybody else alive. It's a failure to come to grips with diversity and nonmedical studies."

Dr. Pollock, however defended the physicians-only rule, contending as do many psychoanalysts, that the tradition is valuable because it provides a holistic approach to the patient: treatment by an analyst who knows the science of the mind as well as the science of the body.

Early in its history, over Freud's objections, the association decided that all psychoanalysts had to be physicians as a way of partly guarding against quackery and of partly gaining quickly the kind of prestige that organized medicine had long enjoyed.

In America, the word "psychoanalyst" is loosely used. ("Everybody from tea-leaf readers to psychologists can call themselves psychoanalysts," one association official said.) The association argues, however, that only its 1,255 full-fledged members, all physicians, are actually entitled to call themselves psychoanalysts. There are perhaps between 800 and 2,000 lay analysts, clinical psychologists, doctors trained outside association institutes and other personnel not recognized by the association.

Some Are Dubious

Their numbers include some of the most creative as well as some of the most dubious therapists in the field. The latter probably could not meet association standards; many of the former consider these standards too rigid and narrow.

"Medical training," said Dr. Kaplan, "turns out physicians who are preponderantly pragmatic, scarcely versed in the experimental method and the philosophy of science, and practically illiterate about the broad issues of the Western cultural tradition."

Psychoanalysis, he argued, is in trouble because it requires wisdom, sensitivity and personal virtues that cannot be reduced to a technique and passed on in training institutes.

"That's why psychoanalysis as a professional movement has either ground to a halt or is pretty much over," he said.

"It's based on virtues that are disappearing among applicants to the training institutes."

This kind of criticism has been coming steadily from the arts, a field that was one of the earliest to be enthusiastic about psychoanalysis after the war.

Norman Mailer said recently that the disenchantment set in about 15 years ago because "people in analysis began to be subjected to men who were no longer cultivated, poetic, deep and engaged in intellectual activity, but to men who were technicians, essentially interested in dominating the material before them, treating them as a commodity, as a machine to be successfully redesigned."

A most serious criticism of the psychoanalytic field is that the young and uncertain science may have lost its capacity to grow.

Freud's daughter, Anna, said in New York recently that psychoanalysis was in danger of losing the interest and sympathy of a younger generation that viewed it as an instrument to reconcile men with a society they deplored.

In a speech at the New York Medical College, Dr. Redlich of Yale charged, in effect, that psychoanalysis is systematically excluding candidates with the most creative minds.

Analysts, particularly those in the association, he said, "have created a tightly controlled shop through a careful systym of educational supervision and control. One could almost speak of censorship. The boundaries are tight. There is little room for the doubter, the critic, the maverick."

"We feel that any innovation and departure should come only after thorough training in fundamentals and an institute," Dr. Settlage commented in reply.

Psychoanalysis would develop more freely and creatively. Dr. Redlich suggested, and would learn more from other disciplines, if it were placed within the university context as a graduate school. Varations of this idea, are gaining currency.

Part of the "crisis of psychoanalysis" can be linked to its age and success.

It has been accepted long enough for the original messianic fervor to yield to a generation that sees it as part of the established order: just one available therapy among many. If it was a fad after World War II, it must now compete with newer, more highly publicized fads.

August 4, 1968

The Divided Self

*By R. D. Laing.
237 pp. New York:
Pantheon Books. $5.95.
218 pp. Baltimore:
Penguin Books. Paper, $1.25.*

Self and Others

*By R. D. Laing.
169 pp. New York:
Pantheon Books. $5.95.*

Must man first go mad in order to be sane?

By MARSHALL BERMAN

For a great many Americans, particularly young Americans, the 1960's were a time in which two of the deepest streams of consciousness—self-consciousness and social consciousness—converged. The radical vision and energy of the sixties aimed at a fusion of ideas and experiences which the fifties had found either unrelated or incompatible: political freedom and personal ecstasy, activism and mysticism, voter-registration drives and mind-expanding drugs, sit-ins and love-ins.

This fusion animated much of the most powerful literature of the decade: in the work of Allen Ginsberg, Bob Dylan, Norman Mailer, Eldridge Cleaver, for example, Americans learned to look harder and deeper at once into themselves and into the institutions and environment they lived in. They sought both to expand the self and open it up, and to create a society in which the self could survive.

As self-consciousness and social consciousness flowed together, the critical and speculative thought of the "Freudian Left" suddenly found itself in the mainstream of American culture. The term "Freudian Left" denotes a family of thinkers—Wilhelm Reich, Erich Fromm, Herbert Marcuse, Paul Goodman, Norman O. Brown are among the most prominent—who have tried to synthesize the insights of Marxist historical sociology and those of Freudian psychology, in order to give us a fuller and richer idea of what we are doing and who we are. Although some of these men began their project of synthesis as early as the 1920's, and though much of their work has been brilliantly imaginative, it was only in the sixties that they got the widespread attention and recognition they deserved.

Their theoretical perspectives opened up a whole new dimension in American social thought, a dimension of psychological depth. Their impact on American radicalism was especially striking: they provided a new direction and a new vocabulary for the emerging New Left. The essential trouble with our society, radicals began to say, is that it forces us all to play roles and fulfill functions that cut us off from our deepest feelings and needs: it alienates us from ourselves.

Once the problem was perceived in this way, two crucial questions emerged: How and why does this alienation occur? And what can we do about it? In the last few years an increasing number of people, especially young and radical people, have been turning to the British psychoanalyst R. D. Laing as a man who can answer these questions. The appearance in uniform cloth-bound editions of "The Divided Self" and the new, extensively revised "Self and Others" should be welcomed.

Although Laing's work has been known in America for only a few years, and known only in limited circles—in mental hospitals and medical schools, among students and artists and intellectuals—it has shaken just about everyone and everything it has touched. It has forced people to decide where they stand—and, implicitly, who they want to be. To a new generation of psychiatrists his

Mr. Berman, an assistant professor of political science at City College, is the author of "The Politics of Authenticity," to be published in September.

Theory

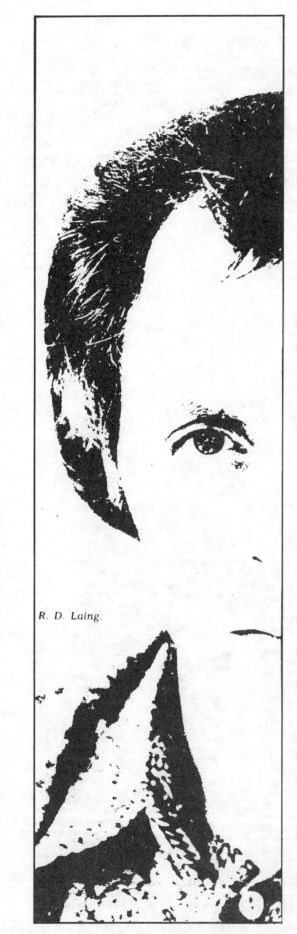

R. D. Laing.

work is inspiring, liberating; to their supervisors it is irresponsible and mind-destroying. The Living Theatre chants the gnomic last words of Laing's "The Politics of Experience" (1967; Pantheon, cloth, $4.95; Ballantine, paper, 95 cents): "If I could turn you on, if I could only drive you out of your wretched mind, if I could tell you I would let you know"; audiences are unhinged, enraged, they shout out obscenities and shake their fists.

The intensity of response which Laing evokes—both favorable and unfavorable—suggests that he really *is* turning people on, he really *is* driving people out of their minds, and he is letting more and more people know.

Laing's own radicalism has developed only as he has approached and entered middle age. The facts of the first 30 years of his life sound conventional and bland. He was born in Glasgow in 1927, educated at a grammar (i.e., state, rather than private) school and at Glasgow University (M.D., 1951), worked as a psychiatrist in the British Army, taught and practiced in Glasgow again for awhile. In the late 1950's he went to London, and got psychoanalytic training at the Tavistock Institute, the British center of Freudian orthodoxy.

It was only gradually, in the course of the 1960's, that he emerged from the protective warmth of that orthodoxy. He became an outspoken and trenchant critic of traditional approaches and methods in psychiatry. He began to experiment with the therapeutic use of mescaline and L.S.D. He established in London a therapeutic community, Kingsley Hall, where patients, doctors and staff live and work together democratically, without hierarchy, free of distinctions of rank or role.

Quite early in his career, Laing focused on a human condition which has been acutely embarrassing to psychiatry since Freud's time: the state of mind called schizophrenia. Few have ever broken through into the schizophrenic's closed world, fewer still have been able to make this world even remotely intelligible to the rest of us outside. Laing is one of the few who have got through: he has penetrated and explored this underworld, both in his patients and, increasingly, in himself; and he has come back to tell the tale. This is the source of his charismatic power. Since his first book, "The Divided Self: An Existential Study in Sanity and Madness" (1960; written mostly in 1957), he has been telling us that there is treasure buried there, and showing us maps. We can find this treasure for ourselves, he says, if we only let ourselves take this trip with him, if we follow him down and in.

In "The Divided Self," the trip begins with one of the classical accounts of schizophrenic behavior. Laing quotes E. Kraeplin's 1905 description of a catatonic 18-year-old boy, who is carried into a medical lecture room, but seemingly pays no attention to his surroundings. He does not answer or even look up when he is spoken to, but talks animatedly to himself in a long monologue which Kraeplin conveys vividly. Kraeplin finds this patient "inaccessible": "His talk was . . . only a series of disconnected sentences having no relation to the general situation." Laing is not so sure. Maybe, he suggests, the patient's talk has all too close a "relation to the general situation," but a relation that the doctor does not want to see.

Laing invites us to look more closely into this supposedly incoherent talk. For example, the patient says: "You want to know that too? I tell you who is being measured and is measured and shall be measured. I know all that, and I could tell you, but I do not want to." With a little empathy and sensitivity, Laing says, we can see that the patient is talking very plainly, and that "he deeply resents this form of interrogation, which is being carried out before a lecture-room of students." This becomes clear if we approach the schizophrenic not as a specimen, but as "a tortured and desperate human being"; if we interpret his weird and frightening behavior not as "signs of a disease," but as "expressive of his existence." Consider the boy: "What is he 'about' in speaking and acting this way? He is objecting to being measured and tested. He wants to be heard."

Laing has listened closely, more closely than anyone before him. He has "decoded" the language of schizophrenics, and transmitted some of what they are trying to tell us. Much of what they are saying, he makes clear, is "existential truth"; and very often it is a truth that we do not want to hear.

How do schizophrenics get that way? In recent years there has been much evidence that it may be essentially genetic and hereditary. Laing neither accepts nor rejects this hypothesis. He believes, however, that if schizophrenia did not biologically exist, our culture would invent it. So many people seem inexorably driven to it, trapped in environments which destroy their sense of identity before it has any chance to develop.

Laing brings to life a great variety of these insulted and injured people. Here we have space enough for only one: Julie, a 26-year-old psychotic girl. In her story Laing's enormous literary gifts unfold; his feeling for a patient's language and imagery, his ability to bring an individual human being concretely to life, the clarity and intensity of his style, pull us irresistibly into her world.

Julie feels "crushed," "smothered," "flooded," "burned up," every moment of her life, by terrible forces that never leave her in peace. The most ordinary circumstances of life constitute a mortal threat to her being. She feels that she is not a real person; she "has nobody because she is nobody." She is empty inside, and yet, somehow, innately destructive: she had better not touch anything, lest she damage it; other people must not touch her, lest they be destroyed. Terrifying images explode inside her: she was "born under a black sun"; she is a "prairie," "a ruined city," a "broken pitcher," a "well run dry"; she is "the ghost of the weed garden." The one thread that runs through everything she says is that somewhere "a child has been murdered"— a child wearing Julie's own clothes.

Laing's attempt to get at the "existential truth" of what his patients are saying leads him to investigate the context in which they are saying it. In "The Divided Self," and further in "Sanity, Madness and the Family, Volume One: Families of Schizophrenics" (with A. Esterson, 1965; Basic Books, $6), he focuses on family structures, and analyzes brilliantly the psychic pressures they generate. Thus Julie's family is perplexed: "Julie was always such a good child" until she suddenly, inexplicably went mad. Her goodness, they explain, was manifest virtually from her birth: "she never was a demanding baby." Unlike her older sister, who was always a "bad" child, Julie "never really cried for her feeds. She never sucked vigorously. She never finished a bottle." Her sister was "selfish," "greedy," "voracious," always crying, wanting, demanding. But Julie "was never a trouble." Her mother "had no bother with her. She always did what she was told." The whole family—except for her bad sister—all recall nostalgically those good old days, "before she got sick."

What is going on here? The crucial thing about Julie's family, Laing says, is that "none of the adults in her world know the difference between existential life and death." Any assertion of feelings or needs, any instinctive energy, any expression of life—from the very beginning of life—is condemned. The basic norm of this system is clear: the only good child is a dead one. Julie has picked up the signals: it is only by playing dead that she can preserve herself; if she tries to live, she will be killed.

Under such pressure, out of total insecurity, the individual constructs a network of defenses, which Laing calls a *false-self system*. The purpose of a false-self system, he explains, is to split the self off from all its activities. Thus the self is "uncoupled" from the body: the body becomes merely one object among other objects in the world, the core of a "false" self; the "true" self is felt as something detached, disembodied, hidden within.

Thus the true self is protected from participation in the life of a world that is set up to destroy it. From now on the self will be purely a spectator; it will observe, judge and criticize whatever the body, that alien object, happens to be experiencing or doing, but it will not get involved. It will leave no fingerprints or footprints in the world. It will be a stranger in a strange land. Divided, the self may be able to stand; united, it will surely fall.

"But the tragic paradox," writes Laing, "is that the more the self is defended in this way, the more it is destroyed. The apparent eventual destruction and dissolution of the self in schizophrenic conditions is accomplished not by external attacks from the enemy (actual or supposed), from without, but by the devastation caused by the inner defensive manoeuvers themselves." If the shut-up self cannot be enriched by outer experience, its whole inner world will become more and more impoverished; it will find even less living space within its citadel than it had outside. Inner life will be felt as empty, cold, dry, impotent, desolate, worthless, dead; the self will suffocate within its own walls. Worse: the false-self system will be felt as a fifth column, a base for the enemy; every move, every breath comes to be

controlled and directed by hostile, destructive forces—by a mother or father, by the authorities, by "Them" —that are continually closing in. The self grows desperate to break out. But outside it sees only the malignant power structure that drove it inward in the first place. There is nowhere for the individual to go. So he goes mad.

"The Divided Self" vibrates with the excitement of discovery, a discovery that resonates far beyond the hospital gates. Laing is steeped in modern literature and existentialist philosophy. He is aware, and he makes us aware, how much of our whole modern sensibility and awareness is rooted in the radical doubt and anxiety that permeates schizophrenics' whole lives; he evokes the alienation they feel with a vividness that strikes a sympathetic chord in all of us. Their dread of nameless threats embedded in everyday life, their sense of aloneness and emptiness, of the precariousness of a person's being— all this is fundamental to our culture. Laing points it out in Baudelaire and Kierkegaard and Dostoevsky, in Kafka and Eliot and Yeats, in Beckett and Genet. (He explores Dostoevsky and Genet lengthily and brilliantly in "Self and Others.")

Laing knew from the first, then, that he was on to something big. But he did not know at first, in 1957, how big it was. He spent the 1960's trying to discover the meaning of his discovery. The trip which at first led him into schizophrenia and away from "reality" has more recently led him through schizophrenia and back to reality, deeper into it than ever before, with a new vision—a more radical and more political vision—of how schizophrenic our reality really is.

Laing's new perspective is foreshadowed in some of the darkest passages of "The Divided Self." He intimates, uneasily, tentatively, that perhaps Julie's family is not so "deviant" after all, not so different from all other families. Is not their model of the "good child" a model that we have all grown up with—and still carry around in our heads? In growing up to be good and dead, Julie was fulfilling an ideal that was (and is) quite typical in her society —fulfilling it with a vengeance. Laing's insight into closed family systems gradually opened outward, into the larger systems in which all families are enclosed.

By 1964, in the preface to the Penguin edition of "The Divided Self" (inexcusably left out of the new Pantheon edition), his new radical vision is clearly defined. He asserts boldly that, from its deepest roots, our whole society is mad. Indeed, he suggests, the only difference between his schizophrenic patients and "normal" men is that his patients know that they are mad, while normal men deceive themselves into thinking that they are sane:

"A man who says that men are machines may be a great scientist. A man who says that he is a machine is 'depersonalized' in psychiatric jargon . . . . A little girl of seventeen in a mental hospital told me she

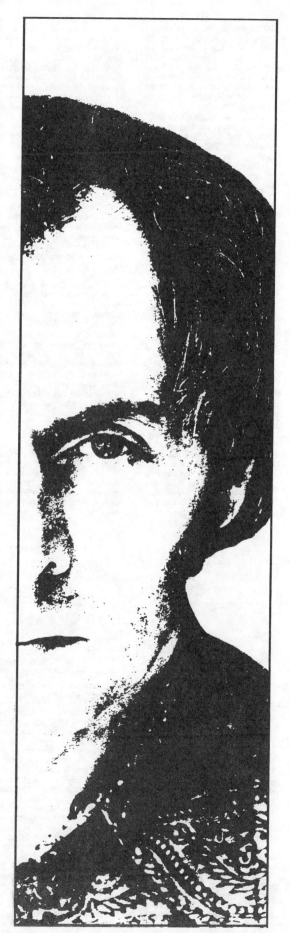

was terrified because the Atom Bomb was inside her. That is a delusion. The statesmen of the world who boast and threaten that they have Doomsday weapons are far more dangerous, and far more estranged from 'reality', than many of the people on whom the label 'psychotic' is fixed."

Laing's most recent writing, "The Politics of Experience" (1967) and the new, revised edition of "Self and Others" (1970), focus on the dilemma of psychiatry in a sick society. In "Self and Others," Laing generalizes the conceptual scheme he developed in "The Families of Schizophrenics": all social relationships, it appears, are closed "fantasy systems" whose members are alienated from themselves. Some members of these systems (few? most? all? Laing is very abstract here, and the reader is left to infer the worst) are placed in "untenable positions," in which "it is impossible to leave and impossible to stay." They are psychically up against the wall.

The members of any social fantasy system are taught by "Them," the authorities, to believe that "the box," the system, "is the whole world." It follows from this premise that the only way to get out of the box is to "step off the end of the world"—to go mad; and Laing has shown us how fearful going mad can be. Hopefully, the authorities are wrong. If they are wrong, then there are (in principle) ways for the self to get out of the box and to live sanely and happily in the world. But what if the authorities are right? What if the box *really is* the whole world? Then

madness, terrifying as it may be, is the only way for the self to survive. And Laing seems to suggest that everyone should indeed go mad.

Is the self really so totally boxed in? Laing does not make a very good case to back up his drastic indictment: his discussion of our social system is disappointingly abstract, moralistic, derivative, unconvincing; his feeling for ambiguity and contradiction, his sense of tragedy, seem to disappear. Our common sense tells us to dismiss Laing's indictment out of hand, and probably our common sense is right. And yet, having once said this, it is hard not to feel uneasy. Laing's view of society may strike us as paranoid, even schizophrenic; but it is a paranoia that strikes deep, and it creeps imperceptibly into our minds.

"She was such a good child. . . . She always did what she was told." For "child" substitute "student," "worker," "neighbor," "citizen"—any role you like. In all our institutions don't we depend on false-self systems to get us through the day? How else could we adjust ourselves to people and activities that would tear us to pieces if we cared about them? Knowing how to manipulate false-self systems: isn't this the secret of success?

"The observable behavior that is the expression of the false self is often perfectly normal. We see a model child, an ideal husband, an industrious clerk." Or a "liberated" girl who can be so refreshingly casual about her body because, as it turns out, her body has

nothing to do with *her*. Or a kept intellectual who, for the same reason, can be equally casual about his mind. It is so much easier to fulfill other people's needs and expectations, we all know, if we have no (possibly conflicting) needs or expectations of our own. It should be clear to us by now that our schizoid character structure, as much as any other power, is what makes our world go round.

Can madness really be a way back into ourselves? We must take very seriously Laing's argument that it can. It can, he says, if we go mad only for awhile, and only under very carefully controlled conditions. Then madness can propel us out of the box, and can liberate all the feelings that the box has kept locked up. Thus "the cracked mind of the schizophrenic may let in light which does not enter the intact minds of many sane people whose minds are closed." Madness may bring to the surface all our repressed fear, rage, hatred, violence and despair; but this opening up can also release all our repressed hope and love and creativity, all our buried feeling for life. We must let go, Laing believes, because only if we lose ourselves can we authentically find ourselves.

The prophetic, evangelical (some would say messianic) tone of Laing's later writings—particularly "The Politics of Experience"—is deliberate. In recent years he has moved from merely interpreting the world to trying actively, in his own way, to change it. His way has been to try to create new kinds of inner space in the

interstices of our society. He sees Kingsley Hall as only a beginning, a nuclear community from which others can grow. In these communities, he hopes, doctors, patients, friends, lovers, others, will be able to live and work together for their common health and liberation. Here men will be free to go mad, but free also to go *through* their madness, and to return to the world restored to themselves. As each one of us descends deeper and deeper into the nightmare of his own aloneness, we will be surrounded by friends who have taken such trips into themselves, and who, because they genuinely know the terror we are undergoing, will be able to help us come through.

Laing knows that these projects, even if they are realized, will be small and fragmentary at best. Kingsley Hall will share the fate of many other utopian communities: it may, if it is lucky, insulate itself from society; it will never change society. Still, it already has the distinctive value that utopias have always had.

The life and energy of Laing's vision—in his practice as well as his books—creates a little more open space for the self in the world. It is this that so many respond to. In a time when the open spaces are being closed off fast, Laing can at least give us a start in the direction we need to go. To have made such a start may be, in the end, the best thing the 1960's can leave to the hard times ahead.

February 22, 1970

The Divided Self

To the Editor:

May I comment on Marshall Berman's review of two books by the British psychoanalyst R. D. Laing in your Feb. 22 issue, "The Divided Self" and "Self and Others"?

Assigning a political scientist to review the works of a psychiatrist implies that psychiatry is not a science, or even a methodical discipline which needs any special training to master. A political scientist could not possibly know enough about psychological mechanisms or method to adequately evaluate the theories of Dr. Laing. Therefore, he could

not see what is misleading and destructive in Laing's thesis.

Berman presents Laing as a messianic figure who, at long last, has discovered the nature and cure of all our personal ills. . . . What Laing really does is blur the distinction between reality and fantasy, rationality and irrationality — and, finally, sanity and madness. He claims that insanity is desirable and necessary to understand the truly schizophrenic world; and that disorganization and disintegration are prerequisites for thinking and perceiving clearly and profoundly.

Schizophrenia actually distorts the perceptual and thought processes. It is a frightening and painful illness precisely because it is a failure of the integrative functions of the mind. . . . It is precisely because one

is disoriented that one tries to escape, through drugs or mysticism, from the necessity of adapting to his environment when he does not have the ability to do so.

The human infant is unable to cope with his world. Therefore, he is confused, dependent and self-absorbed. Only when he begins to comprehend and master his environment and to develop a sense of self can he relate to others. If he does not grow beyond the primitive level of development, he will not have the necessary emotional potential to fulfill himself and become an effective, cooperative member of a cohesive society.

We can see evidence of this disorientation and emotional crippling in many of the major trends today. We see the sub-

stitution of sensation for feeling; the demand for immediate gratification; the inability to identify or empathize with others; the sense of inner emptiness and the copping out to drugs, astrology, mysticism and magic. These and many others are the problems of our time—and Dr. Laing's alleged cure merely aggravates the disease.

Unfortunately, unless we deal realistically with these issues, we will face social disaster. No society can survive when too many people are narcissistic or unable to function adequately in the "reality" of the society, however unpleasant. In chaotic times like today, when reality is war, poverty, pollution and too-rapid social change, we need people who can accurately diagnose these problems and solve them rationally and pragmatically.

It is dangerous for society to encourage flights from reality and to sell madness as a panacea for all psychological and social disorders.

Dr. Abram Kardiner
New York City.

To the Editor:

Mr. Berman would have us believe that Laing's insights into schizophrenia are new ideas. . . . The interpretations of the case histories are exactly the same as many in psychiatric literature since the 1920's. They can be read in Freud, Sullivan, Fromm and Horney, among others.

There is considerable truth to be found in literature *and* Laing as to the meaning and psychogenesis of schizophrenia.

But nothing new . . . for a long, long time. . . .

Dr. Paul A. Barenberg
West Chester, Pa.

Mr. Berman replies:

Aristotle assumed, and never thought to doubt, that the polis, or political association, was the ideal medium for man's fullest and deepest self-expression. That was a long time ago. Now Dr. Kardiner assumes, as a matter of course, that a political scientist cannot possibly know anything about the depths of the self. We really have come a long way!

There is a lot in what Dr. Kardiner says; more, I suspect, than he thinks. I agree that the study of our political and social institutions, and the roles we play in them, yields very

little knowledge of who we really are; wherever our nature is expressed, it is certainly not there. But think of the human waste, misery and disease that spring from this gulf between our roles and ourselves! It is precisely this fatal split that leads Laing to describe our social life as schizophrenic.

Dr. Kardiner wants everyone "to fulfill himself and become an effective, cooperative member of a cohesive society." So do I. So, I am sure, does Laing. But if Dr. Kardiner were a more political scientist, he would see that, between membership in *this* society, and genuine self-fulfillment, falls a very large shadow.

Laing knows that he lives, as much as we live, in the shadow. He claims no brighter light for himself; instead, he

forces us to see how deeply we are all in the dark, because we have turned off, or never turned on, our deepest sources of power. I present him not as the Messiah, but as a prophet. (Note to Dr. Barenberg: there have been many great prophets, and there will be more, if we survive; every culture, every generation, needs it own; there are never enough.) Laing himself is not, and does not claim to be, the Way; he knows we must find our own ways into ourselves. He is trying to point out, as prophets always have done, how our institutions have become stumbling-blocks that stand in the way of us all.

We should listen to him. If we want to be and to fulfill ourselves, here and now, we need all the help we can get.

April 26, 1970

TREATMENT

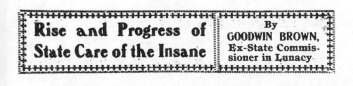

Rise and Progress of State Care of the Insane
By GOODWIN BROWN, Ex-State Commissioner in Lunacy

IT is consonant with its destiny and greatness that the Empire State should have, of all States and countries in the world, the most complete, humane, and comprehensive system of caring for this most unfortunate class.

This system, complete and harmonious as it is, like all successful organizations, was not the development of a day—practically it was the growth of half a century. It began in 1843 and was completed in 1890.

From 1843 to 1890 the care of the insane was regarded, not as a necessity required by the highest considerations of an enlightened economy, but rather as a form of charity grudgingly and often ignorantly bestowed at the caprice of unenlightened public authorities. It was not until the absolute safety and welfare of the State was dangerously threatened that the fruition of a method humane and economical was adopted. So long as "charity" was the watchword all efforts toward the proper and humane care of this class were largely misdirected, with the inevitable result of cruelty and barbarism—which, by the way, were fearfully excessive—intermixed sometimes with something akin to humanity.

When public sentiment had become sufficiently enlightened on the subject it was seen that ultimate economy as well as humanity demanded a change which charity could not effect. It was seen that it would be actually cheaper to make adequate and suitable provision for the proper care and treatment of the insane than to permit them to be at large, committing acts of violence, destroying property, and breaking up families, thereby producing widespread misery and loss of productive energy.

Prior to 1843, when the first considerable effort to properly care for the insane by the opening of the New York State Lunatic Asylum at Utica was made, little had been done to alleviate the condition of the insane in New York State. It was the almost universal practice, so far as public care was provided, to place them in jails and poorhouses. Toward the end of the first quarter of the last century the Hospital of the City of New York made a commendable beginning by the establishment of the institution which is now known as Bloomingdale, located at White Plains. For many years, however, the number which could be

cared for was limited and the accommodations were inadequate. Obviously no private corporation, no matter how charitably disposed, could cope with what was even then a tremendous problem. During the next quarter of the century, through the efforts of various philanthropists—for as yet the question was one of philanthropy and charity only—Miss Dorothea L. Dix being the most notable, the subject began to receive wider consideration.

About 1836 the first statute was enacted providing for the erection by the State of what became popularly known as the Utica Insane Asylum, which was opened for the reception of a small number of patients in 1843. The establishment of this institution by the State was the beginning of what eventually became known as "State care of the insane." For many long and weary years, however, the great mass of the insane remained in the poorhouses, for the Utica asylum was only intended for a small number of supposedly curable cases. When a patient failed to recover after the lapse of a few months, or a year or two at most, if a public charge, he was returned to the poorhouse of the county whence he came, there to remain until his tormented spirit took its flight.

The success of the Utica asylum and similar institutions in other States was such as to stimulate those who, still actuated by motives of philanthropy only, desired to extend the system thus instituted by the State so as to include all the insane. In the meantime, with the great growth of population and consequent increasing numbers of insane in the poorhouses, an agitation was begun which culminated during the civil war in the passage by the Legislature of the second great act for the care of the insane by providing for the erection of the Willard Asylum for the Chronic Insane, which was opened in 1868—an interval of a quarter of a century from the opening of the first institution at Utica.

The agitation which brought about the establishment of the Willard Asylum was a memorable one. The Legislature authorized the New York State Medical Society to investigate and report upon the question of the dependent insane, and this work devolved upon its Secretary, a young Southern physician lately located in Albany, under most romantic circumstances—Dr. Sylvester D. Willard. Dr. Willard proved himself both intelligent and humane. He entered into the work in a truly scientific spirit and with untiring zeal. His report produced a profound sensation—it revealed conditions which shocked the entire State. Among other things, he said:

"In some of these buildings the insane are kept in cages and cells, dark and prison-like, as if they were convicts instead of the life-weary, deprived of reason. They are in numerous instances left to lie on straw, like animals, without other bedding, and there are scores who endure the piercing cold and frost of Winter without either shoes or stockings being provided for them; they are pauper lunatics and shut out from the charity of the world where they could at least beg shoes. Insane, in a narrow cell, perhaps without clothing, sleeping on straw or in a bunk, receiving air and light and warmth only through a diamond hole through a rough prison-like door, bereft of sympathy and of social life, except it be with a fellow-lunatic, without a cheering influence or a bright hope of the future * * * The violent have only to rave and become more violent, and pace in madness their miserable apartments. These institutions afford no possible means for the various grades of the insane; the old and the young; the timid and the brazen; the sick, the feeble, and the violent are herded together without distinction to the character or degree of their madness and the natural tendency is for all to become irretrievably worse. * * * In some violent cases the clothing is torn and strewed about the apartments and the lunatics continue to exist in wretched nakedness, having no clothing, and sleeping upon straw, wet and filthy, and unchanged for several days. * * * Can any picture be more dismal? and yet it is not overdrawn."

Unfortunately, while the step gained was exceedingly important, the act of incorporation of the Willard Asylum provided that it was to care only for the chronic insane. This institution was designed to care for all the insane in the county poorhouses, except in the counties of New York and Kings.

Dr. John P. Gray of the Utica Asylum, with a wisdom and foresight far in advance of his time, opposed the establishment of the Willard Asylum in the lines proposed and finally adopted; namely, to care for the chronic insane. He insisted that the institution ought to care for both the acute as well as the chronic insane. From various causes, principally the opposition of the county officials, who were loath to give up the patronage and profit of caring for their chronic insane—the institution was not enlarged sufficiently to provide for all the insane remaining in the poorhouses. The Superintendents of the Poor argued—and their argument had a certain plausibility—that inasmuch as custodial care was to be provided at Willard without reference to the curative treatment of its inmates, they, the Superintendents of the Poor, might, as well be intrusted with the care of the chronic insane. This argument to some extent prevailed, and the Legislature was induced to grant exemption from the operation of the Willard act to certain counties—the number ultimately reached twenty—under conditions which contemplated humane custodial care.

Experience soon showed that the conditions could not be enforced, and thus the old inhumanities and barbarities were restored. Renewed agitation to at once and forever blot out this one of the greatest disgraces which ever sullied the fair fame of a State, was begun by the State Charities Aid Association, a voluntary society which, in its visitation of county poorhouses by local committees, because thoroughly convinced of the unfitness of these institutions as receptacles for the insane. This reform movement was uncompromisingly pursued by the Association under the able leadership of the Chairman of its Committee on Legislation for the Insane, Miss Louisa Lee Schuyler, eminent as a philanthropist and friend of the insane, and to whose unremitting efforts the successful outcome of this final effort in behalf of State care for the insane was largely due.

The principal difficulty encountered in previous agitations to improve the conditions of the insane lay in the fact that the State had no adequate machinery to enforce its statutes—there were statutes in plenty but no adequate executive power was given to any one. In 1889 the condition of the insane in the poorhouses had become intolerable. The conditions, while perhaps not as bad as those so vividly and truthfully described by Dr. Willard a quarter of a century before, were such as to call for immediate action. The number of the insane in the poorhouses had by this time reached more than two thousand—a number twice as large as existed there at the time the Willard Asylum was created. It was already seen that if the evil were to be completely abated heroic measures must be adopted.

The efforts of the State Charities Aid Association in 1888 and 1889 to secure the enactment of a law to wipe out the disgraceful blot had been threatened by a combinaion of greed and patronage which had rarely been witnessed in the halls of the Legislature. The officials having supervision of the dependent poor and insane were marshaled in solid array against a movement which threatened to destroy their immense power and to take from them the sources of great and constantly increasing revenue. In the preceding twenty-five years the number of State institutions had greatly increased, but the accommodations for the insane had not nearly kept pace with the demand for space. Each institution was separately governed by a local board responsible to no adequate central authority. So far as unity of action was concerned, they might as well have been located in so many separate States. These institutions had largely been built and were managed on the plan of "doing something for the district." In consequence, scandals and gross inefficiency were frequently charged, with results of many acrimonious Legislative investigations. No doubt many of these charges were not sustained, nevertheless they gave occasion to the enemies of State care to point to undeniable extravagances and frequent mismanagement. Millions had already been expended with inadequate accommodations, and it was said that the assumption by the State of the care of all of the insane would be followed by State bankruptcy. These arguments found many attentive listeners in the Legislature and elsewhere. In conformity with the suggestions and recommendations of many Legislative investigating committees, the Legislature of 1889, after a prolonged struggle lasting more than three months, and at the very end of the session, passed a bill creating a State Commission in Lunacy with far more extensive powers and duties than had been devolved upon any executive body theretofor having jurisdiction over the insane. Governor Hill appointed as members of the Commission Dr. Carlos F. MacDonald, Goodwin Brown, and Henry Reeves. Dr. MacDonald had for years been regarded as one of the leading alienists in the country, and his practical knowledge of the management of institutions for the insane had covered a period of more than twenty years, as he had been superintendent of three hospitals for the insane in succession. Moreover, his ideas in regard to the treatment and care of the insane were known to be of the most advanced order. He was a most pronounced believer in State care for all the dependent insane and opposed to the Willard system of caring for the chronic insane in separate institutions. The wisdom of this appointment was at once universally recognized, and there is little doubt that to his genius and energy is largely due the magnificent system of State care that prevails today in the State of New York.

Dr. MacDonald's associate Commissioners, while having had no experience in the care and treatment of the insane, had long been in the public service and had the opportunities of learning much about the management of public institutions. Mr. Reeves had served with ability and fidelity both in Congress and the Legislature and enjoyed the very highest reputation as a public officer and a public spirited citizen.

The Commission was required to visit periodically all institutions and places where the insane were in custody and to report to the Legislature and suggest such changes as might in their judgment be necessary. During the first year of its existence the Commission visited all the institutions where the insane were in custody, including twenty poorhouses, which had received special permission to care for the insane. Its report, which was submitted to the Legislature at the beginning of the session of

1890, revealed a condition of things in these so-called county asylums even worse than the State Charities Aid Association had previously reported. It was unanimous in recommending the immediate abolition of the poorhouse system, the enlargement of the present State hospitals so as to provide for the insane in the poorhouses, and the placing of all the State institutions on a curative basis by the wiping out of the statutory classification of the insane. The Legislature of that year, in conformity with the recommendations of the Commission, after a severe struggle, passed the so-called State Care Act, providing for State care of all the insane—being practically the third and last in the series of acts passed at the end of half a century—the first in 1843, the second in 1865, and the third in 1890. The following year the Commission requested an appropriation of approximately half a million of dollars, which was granted without opposition, to provide additional buildings for housing the insane then in the poorhouses. The State Care Act provided that when sufficient accommodations had been provided, the Commission should so declare, and from that time all of the dependent insane should be a State charge and the counties relieved of all charges whatsoever. The act provided that the counties of New York, Monroe, and Kings should be exempted from the provision of the act on the ground that they had provided suitable institutions for the purpose, but that they might avail themselves of the privilege of coming into the State system. In 1891 Monroe, in 1895 Kings, and in 1896 New York came into the State Hospital system. The poorhouse system ceased to exist Oct. 1, 1893, when the State care system proper went into effect. From that date no insane person has been an inmate in any poorhouse in the State, and thus ended, after an agitation of more than fifty years, one of the greatest evils that has ever disgraced the State.

All of the public insane in New York are now supported in institutions owned and absolutely controlled by the State with moneys appropriated by the Legislature. All are given that medical care and attention which their condition requires—the food, clothing, and general care do not in the least depend on anything but their physical necessity.

In 1891 the Commission in Lunacy secured the application of the competitive system of civil service examinations for the medical service, and in 1895 it adopted a uniform rate of

officers' salaries and employes' wages for all the hospitals in the State. It also established a training school for nurses in each of the State Hospitals, and the graduates of these schools obtain increased wages. An allowance is especially made for amusements and diversion, and from this fund a band of music is provided for concerts and dances. In fact, everything consistent with proper care and treatment is provided for by the State in the discretion of the Commission, which has the power to pass upon all items of expenditure. The element of charity is altogether eliminated in dealing with this class—the sole question is what amount of money will restore the greatest number of relatives and friends recovered or improved sufficiently to live at home. It is now a matter of the highest ultimate economy. A low diet, insufficient clothing, insufficient medical attendance and nursing would reduce the recovery and thus prolong the time of detention, and consequently increased expense to the State. A proper standard of care and treatment is consonant with humanity and economy.

On Oct. 1, 1896, the Commission was given supervision over expenditures. By the use of this power and unification of the system of management, a great saving was not only effected, but the standard of care and treatment was greatly improved. The average expenditure per patient was in round numbers previous to 1893 $222; the Commission reduced this to $184—a saving of hundreds of thousands of dollars. The power of revision of expenses was extended in 1896 to cover expenditures for buildings and extraordinary improvements.

The State hospitals are now operated as a unit—one charter covers all. A change in the statute which would affect one institution would affect all, and, therefore, the lawmaking power is not likely to make a change for the benefit of a locality which might injuriously affect the whole system. There are twelve State hospitals containing a total population of 24,000. One hundred and twenty-five physicians and nearly 4,500 employes are required. The fixed charges or yearly running expenses amount to about $4,000,000. There are approximately 4,500 commitments of insane each year—in some instances the same individual may be discharged and readmitted

more than once. One thousand are discharged as recovered each year, while the actual annual increase in numbers over discharges and deaths averages about 600.

Apparently there is an increase in the number of the insane greater than the increase in population. It is doubtful, however, if there is an actual increase in the ratio of insanity to the same population, for friends and relatives are less likely to care for patients at home than formerly, owing to the better management of institutions. This view is held by the Lunacy Commissioners of Great Britain. There is nothing to indicate from a careful study of the statistics that people are more subject to mental disease than formerly—in fact, the contrary would seem to be true, as the general health of the people is improving owing to the great advance in medical and sanitary science.

With the assumption by the State of the care of all the dependent insane, the following are some of the great and lasting advantages that were secured:

Absolute security against abuse and neglect.

A proper standard of care and medical treatment, including sufficient food and clothing, good nursing, amusements, and diversion.

Providing for the appointment and promotion of officers and employes in accordance with civil service rules, thus minimizing the danger of partisan influences in the State hospital service.

Economy in management and the adoption of the best methods resulting from unity of action.

Giving all the insane proper care and treatment, and giving all a chance for recovery so long as life lasts.

A higher recovery rate, which must inevitably result from the application of the methods outlined.

November 10, 1901

WATER AS INSANITY CURE.

Massachusetts Hospitals Find Baths Subdue Bad Patients.

Special to The New York Times.

BOSTON, Nov. 17.—The water cure, the most advanced method of treating mental ills, has been adopted in the insane hospitals of Massachusetts as a humane and scientific substitute for the old-time straitjackets, straps, and similar means of restraint in the case of violent or, as the hospital phrase goes, "highly disturbed," patients

Dr. H. S Frost, Superintendent of the Boston Insane Hospital, said to-night:

" We find that there is no longer any need of physical restraint, even in the most violent cases for the patient does not fear the treatment. On the contrary, he is glad to enter the bath, where he may remain for hours under the soothing influence of the warm water in which he is submerged.

" Nurses are in constant attendance to regulate the temperature of the water, to take the pulse and temperature of the sufferer, and to minister to his needs. Meals are served to the bathers. The long baths have no debilitating effect, for additional nourishment renders this impossible. Moreover, the relief of nerve depression, which the uniformly increased temperature of the water accomplishes, is of itself stimulating.

" We do not mean to say that all forms of insanity are curable by this means, but the general success has been so great that thousands of patients who were formerly tied hand and foot are now able to do sufficient work to support themselves and to help in the support of others."

November 18, 1912

State Hospital Patients.

To the Editor of The New York Times:

May I plead by your favor for a softening of the term used in your reports of the investigation of the State hospitals, when you refer to patients under State care? The word " lunatic " is a cruel and opprobrious barbarism, bound to hurt not only the feelings of patients upon whom it is thrust, but perhaps to wound still more the sensibilities of their friends.

Many years ago the State Legislature in its wisdom changed the title of the New York State Lunatic Asylum at Utica to Utica State Hospital, whereupon other State institutions in New York and elsewhere quickly followed suit. More recently, in deference to humane sentiment, the State Lunacy Commission is become the State Hospital Commission. I am well aware of the tyranny of the headline, and know that " asylum " has only six letters, while " hospital " has eight, but " patients " and " lunatics " have exactly the same number of letters. Let us, in heaven's name, do what we can to mitigate the misfortune of the sick wards of the State. G. ALDER BLUMER.

Providence, R. I., May 5, 1914.

May 11, 1914

Snug Harbor for Shell-Shocked

THE opening of the new hospital at Perryville, Md., for the special care and treatment of shell-shocked soldiers calls attention anew to the efforts which the United States Public Health Service is making to cure these men. At the present time this service has under treatment more than 12,000 discharged soldiers and sailors suffering from shell-shock and other mental disorders. Of these, 5,578 are in hospitals operated by the service. The rest are in institutions where proper care and treatment are provided under contract.

Naturally, extreme interest has been evinced in the psychology of shell-shock ever since that now familiar word came into notice through the World War. The effect upon the soldier, and the treatment for his recovery, are engaging the attention of scientific men all over the world.

"The term 'shell-shock,'" said Dr. Hugh S. Cumming, Surgeon General of the United States Public Health Service, "is a misnomer. It was coined by the British early in the war when it was thought by medical men that the undue prevalence of nervous disorder in this as compared with other wars was due to physical injury to the central nervous system, caused by exposure to bombardment—with the new high explosive shells.

"Later observations showed this view to be incorrect. Although injury to the nervous system without physical injury did sometimes occur and cause nervous symptoms, it was found that this happened in only a small proportion of cases. Medical men are now generally agreed that the predominating cause of shell-shock was a mental mechanism by which the wish, in most cases an unconscious one, to escape from the horrors and hardships of war, found expression in some form of disabling symptom, which removed the soldier to a place of safety and comfort.

"The exploding shell and its attendant horrors acted only as the last straw in a long chain of trying events which had lowered his resistance to a point where only a slight stunning or emotional disturbance was needed to give his instinct for self-preservation the ascendency over the higher ideals of the mind, of which patriotism and the sense of duty for the common good are an expression. During the period of momentary unconsciousness some chance occurrence or predisposition would determine the development of a bodily or mental state which would be perpetuated as a symptom and give the war-weary veteran his release from a situation which honor prompted him to endure and instinct impelled him to avoid. The mental conflict having been settled this way, the development of shell-shock may be considered as a triumph of the instincts over the superimposed civilization.

"As with shell-shock, so in every true case of neurosis the symptoms have no organic cause for existence. Instead, they arise in the patient's mind on the basis of an unconscious motive, and are usually caused by the inability of the patient to adjust himself to some difficult situation. When this unconscious motive (the mental origin of his disease) is revealed to the patient, the most important step in his cure has been made. It was with this understanding of the situation and by appropriate psycho-therapeutic treatment that such brilliant results in the treatment of shell-shock were obtained during the war, and every method of treatment used in the new hospital, whether work, exercise, play or mental analysis, has as its object a mental readjustment of the patient.

"The problem is to aid in restoring to usefulness that large body of men who, through failure of adaptation to military life, have had a nervous breakdown, and the basis for whose symptoms is often an emotional factor buried in their unconscious mind. Their symptoms are mostly mental and emotional rather than physical. They have lost confidence. They suffer with strange, unaccountable fears. Sensations formerly disregarded are now magnified and regarded as pathological. Perfectly natural lapses of memory are seized upon as evidences of approaching insanity. Insomnia, anxiety, fatigability, feelings of incompetency, sensitiveness to noise and hosts of other symptoms make them miserable.

"The old method of treatment of nervous disorders by absolute rest and seclusion from all forms of activity is illogical and irrational. A few persons, chiefly men who have worked to the point of exhaustion, receive benefit by a short period of such treatment. These cases, however, are not really nervous but exhausted.

"The real psychoneurotic is never cured by this method. As his troubles are a compromise with himself over his inability to meet a difficult situation, the proper environment for him during treatment is one of activity and not seclusion. Just as a child cannot be adequately educated away from the rest of the world, so a nervous case cannot be adjusted to meet the complexities of life by withdrawing himself from all activities. If apparently cured in a forest, he is likely, upon returning to civilization, to find that his old trouble is still with him.

"Patients are, therefore, encouraged not to sit around idly but to indulge in the various forms of activity that are provided for them. There is an occupational therapy department in which the man who thinks he quickly tires, mentally or physically, is encouraged to busy himself either at some handicraft or in learning stenography and typewriting. Some do useful work around the building or grounds, while others are persuaded to seek employment and work for pay while their treatment is being carried out. The timid and shy are induced to attend the entertainments and dances which are given weekly at the hospital under the auspices of the Red Cross. Skating, sledding, skiing, tennis and outdoor sports are provided, while indoors there are a swimming pool and a billiard room.

"The physiotherapy department is equipped with facilities for giving every form of bath, massage and electrical treatment that might improve the physical condition and aid suggestion. Care is taken, however, in the purely nervous cases to avoid imparting to the patient's minds the idea that they have anything of an organic nature, because if this idea becomes fixed a complete cure is impossible.

"The methods of treatment outlined above are merely aids to more important mental analysis. This has for its object the discovery of the emotional cause which underlies every nervous disorder and to uncover this it is necessary to delve into the deepest recesses of the mind. The symptoms of nervous disorders as a rule resemble or are connected by association with those experienced in some forgotten incident. This incident is discovered and its relation to the symptoms made known to the patient. He is also given a simple explanation as to the mental mechanisms concerned in producing nervous disorders in general. Persuasion and suggestion follow. The patient is encouraged to look at things in a more natural way and to help in his own cure. Numerous therapeutic talks may be required in order to arrive at a correct understanding of the case and restore the patient's confidence, hence, the necessity for a large number of medical officers.

"When a patient's symptoms are removed in this way and he finds by the numerous activities in which he has engaged that he can do many things of which he thought himself incapable, his confidence is in a large measure restored and he is ready to return to normal activities again; but with discharge from the hospital, treatment does not necessarily end. Certain cases that seem to need it are kept in touch with by direct correspondence or through their local Red Cross. By this means advice and encouragement are given when they are needed to tide over some new difficulty.

"At some time during his hospital residence each patient is brought before the entire staff of doctors to be examined, questioned and encouraged. By this means a better understanding of cases is arrived at, but aside from this the staff meeting has often been found to exert a distinct beneficial influence upon the course of symptoms.

"In a hospital treating nervous, irritable patients, some of whom have a grudge against the Government for causing their trouble and all of whom have just been released from an irksome military restraint, some restlessness, discontent and dis-

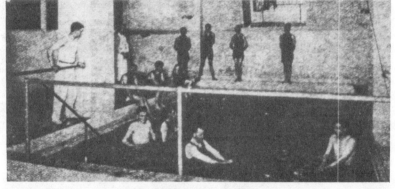

Patients in the Swimming Pool.

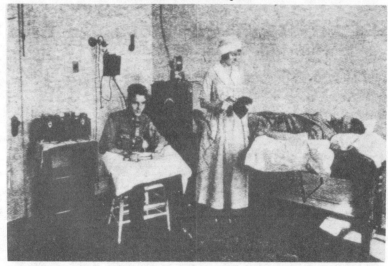

Patients Under Electrical Treatment.

order was expected. The results obtained in meeting this spirit have ur-passed our fondest expectation, and it may now be safely assumed that the institutions are free from strife and disorder as any of the general hospitals where discharged soldiers are treated.

" The officers understand that the patients are in the hospital because they are sick and are irritable because they are nervous. Every complaint, whether reasonable or unreasonable, is listened to patiently and explained away or adjusted. The nurses do much in infusing the proper spirit into the institution."

The special diseases affecting the mental and nervous system which are treated by the service are divided into six large groups, but the term " neuro-psychiatric " disorder is now quite generally used to include all of them.

It is considered imperative to recognize promptly the type of mental disorder existing in the patient. Those dealing with medical facts now recognize that certain types of unusual behavior or conduct are often the forerunner of a grave mental disorder, which, if recognized early and appropriately

treated, may be successfully dealt with in order to prevent chronic invalidism. As in all departments of preventive medicine such early recognition and treatment of the incipient case is of the greatest economy.

Of the 600,000 American disabled of the World War 200,000 have applied for compensation under the War Risk Insurance act. Of the latter number 38 per cent. come within the group of nervous and mental diseases, the largest single group of patients to be dealt with by the Public Health Service. The Public Health Service is cognizant of more than 76,000 such patients who came under the observation of the military forces. Judging by previous surveys of the Public Health Service, an additional group of patients will come to be recognized as time goes on, cases which have developed either by an unstable nervous constitution or as the result of latent injury or disease received under the stress of military service.

In order to recognize and afford appropriate treatment for this class of patients as promptly as possible, certain wards in general hospitals, or special hospitals, have been set

aside in the larger metropolitan areas to be used as clearing stations or diagnostic centres. Such centres at present are located at Boston, Mass.; New York, N. Y.; Baltimore, Md.; Greenville, S. C.; Atlanta, Ga.; New Orleans, La.; St. Louis, Mo.; Chicago, Ill.; Cincinnati, Ohio; Palo Alto, Cal.; Boise City, Idaho; Tacoma, Wash. Others are being established as rapidly as circumstances will permit.

At each of these special clearing stations or " diagnostic centres " an out-patient department is established where patients who have recovered or improved from a nervous or mental disease may come for advice and treatment and continue their occupation in' the community. Such out-patient care is afforded by men who are especially trained in this branch of medicine. Before a patient returns to his home from a hospital, however, that home is investigated to determine the suitability of the environment so as to guard against a reactivation or reaggravation of his disease. Each of these clearing stations is provided with modern apparatus for diagnostic purposes and for emergency treatment.

In its work the Public Health Service has enlisted the co-operation

and the assistance of the very best talent available in this special field. These physicians are employed as full time men, as attending specialists and as advisory consultants. The men who are performing this duty have had long years of experience and have first-hand knowledge of the occurrence of these diseases under military conditions. Among the consultants are men of national reputation and leaders of that specialty in the district in which they reside. For example, Dr. George M. Kline, Commissioner, Department of Mental Diseases, Boston, Mass.; Dr. George H. Kirby, Director State Psychopathic Institute, Wards Island, N. Y.; Dr. Roy McLean Van Wart of New Orleans, La.; Dr. John S. Turner of Dallas, Texas; Dr. Andrew C. Gillis of Baltimore, Md.; Dr. Frank P. Norbury of Springfield, Ill.; Dr. H. Douglas Singer of the State Psychopathic Institute, Dunning, Ill.; Dr. Albert M. Barrett, Ann Arbor, Mich.; Dr. William A. White, Government Hospital for the Insane, Washington, D. C.; Dr. Owen Copp, Philadelphia, Pa.; Dr. Hubert Work, Pueblo, Col.; Dr. Robert L. Richards, Ukiah, Cal.

January 2, 1921

WOULD PUT TO DEATH INCURABLY INSANE

Suggestion Made at State Asylum Viewed Favorably by Some Connecticut Legislators.

MANIAC CHAINED TO BED

Violent and Dangerous Inmate in Padded Cell Exhibited as Case for Merciful Extinction.

Special to The New York Times.

HARTFORD, Conn., Feb. 6.—A suggestion made at the State Hospital for the Insane at Norwich that hopelessly insane persons be mercifully put to death has

found favor with certain members of the joint Committee on Appropriations of the Connecticut Legislature which reconvenes in this city Tuesday.

Whether or not the plan of officially and deliberately putting chronic maniacs out of misery will come before the General Assembly in the form of a bill is problematical, for Jan. 28 was the time limit for introducing bills for such innovations and it is generally felt the idea would get short shrift from the legislators and the public of this " Land of Steady Habits " which has not yet ratified the Woman Suffrage Amendment and is still asking when does prohibition go into effect.

On an official visit to the Norwich Asylum yesterday, Superintendent Franklin S. Wilcox showed the members of the Appropriations Committee an inmate, about 50 years old and a veritable giant in stature, manacled to an iron bed placed in a padded cell some distance from other inmates. So violent and dangerous is the maniac that he has not been unshackled in five years except occasionally when three of the most

powerful guards have unchained him to give him a bath.

Superintendent Wilcox told Senator Hall of New Britain and his colleagues on the Appropriations Committee that the patient could never recover his reason and would have to remain fettered to the iron cot until death freed him. It was at this point that several members of the committee agreed that the man would be better dead than alive in the asylum, and suggested a law that would provide that persons found to be hopelessly insane after observation and examination by experts should be put to death as mercifully as possible, presumably by poison.

The advocates of this radical departure from Connecticut custom and viewpoint admitted the objection of the difficulty of selecting and authorizing the proper tribunal, even if it were possible to find any one who would be willing to issue a death warrant for a maniac.

Superintendent Wilcox reported that, whereas when he went to Norwich in 1918 there were only 1,177 patients, there are now 1,807, of whom 657 are women, but he attributes the increase to a wider understanding and acceptance of the benefits of insane hospitals rather than to any material increment of insanity in the State.

February 7, 1921

30 INSANE PARETICS CURED BY MALARIA

Long Island College Hospital Reports Marked Success With New Treatment.

HOW IT WORKS, A MYSTERY

Method of Arresting the Disease Was First Discovered in Vienna— Used on Ward's Island.

Thirty patients regarded as hopelessly insane are back at work and leading normal lives after being artificially inoculated with malaria, allowed to suffer chills and fever for two weeks or so and then treated with drugs, according

to an announcement yesterday by the Long Island College Hospital.

The thirty patients belonged to a group of sixty sufferers from paresis who have received the malaria and drug treatment at the Long Island College Hospital. Of the thirty who have not recovered sufficiently to return to work, several have shown marked benefit. Some of the patients failed to respond to the treatment. The percentage of successes, however, is considered remarkable because of the fact that paresis was regarded as incurable up to the time that the malaria treatment was discovered in Austria. St. Elizabeth's Hospital in Washington, D. C., the largest hospital in the world for mental cases; the State Hospital for the Insane on Ward's Island and the Brooklyn State Hospital for the Insane have been employing the malaria treatment with results equal to those achieved at Long Island College Hospital.

The treatment was worked out by Drs. Wagner von Jauregg of the Psychiatric Institute of Vienna and J. Kyrle of the University of Vienna during the war. The experimentation was started to test the truth of reports which had been frequently made of sudden and remarkable improvement by sufferers from paresis after they had had attacks of malaria. A number of paresis patients were deliberately inoculated with malaria. Some died, some remained unbenefited, others were helped to some extent and still others were so improved that they were

able to leave the hospital and return to their old occupations.

Investigated in Vienna.

In order to introduce the treatment at the Long Island City College, the authorities of that institution sent Dr. H. H. Morton to Vienna for three months, where he studied the methods of the Austrian originators of the treatment. On his return considerable difficulty was encountered in starting the treatment because malaria is practically non-existent in New York City, according to the statement of the hospital, which said:

"An odd fact that developed following the determination of the professors of this hospital to infect paresis patients with malaria is that they spent several months seeking a person in this city suffering from malaria. A generation ago malaria was not an uncommon disease. As a result of the progress in science, it is virtually extinct in this city today. The parasite of benign tertian malaria was found finally in a patient in the United States Public Health Hospital for Marines on Staten Island, who had contracted malaria in the tropics and was brought here for treatment."

Patients treated at the State Hospital at Ward's Island showed marked improvement on treatment with malaria only, but drug treatment by mercurial and arsenical compounds also was used at Long Island College Hospital. There is some difference of opinion among students of this treatment whether the combined malaria and drug treatment is better than the simple malaria treatment.

"The long search for the malaria patient was made necessary by the fact that it was necessary to have malaria of a mild type," said a Long Island College Hospital doctor who has been treating malaria patients. "Some of the severe types are very hard to handle and might exhaust the paresis patients very badly. It is possible to control malaria of this mild type very satisfactorily. We can stop it whenever we think that the time has come to stop it by dosing with quinine sulphate and salvarsan. Generally speaking, the procedure is to give the paresis patient all the chills and fever that he can stand. If he seems fairly sturdy, we prolong the malarial treatment, and if he is weak, give him as little of it as possible.

"After that we give him salvarsan and mercury treatment. Gradual recovery follows in many cases. Some of the patients do not respond. Generally speaking, those who have not suffered for a long time from paresis respond better than the others, but that is not always true.

"Paresis accounts for a tremendous lot of insanity and a very great number of deaths each year, so that the success of this treatment is a thing of the utmost importance to the world. Paresis usually sets in at middle age with symptoms which are hard to recognize. We suspect it when marked queerness of behavior develops at middle age in a man who has theretofore been normal. A typical picture of the disease is that of an industrious,

conservative man who stands well in every way, but who suddenly forgets careful business habits and begins to invest in wildcat stocks, to dissipate and go to pieces generally. The disease is always the result of a long-standing condition, but many patients appear to be absolutely ignorant of the fact that such a condition had ever existed. Various remedies have been tested heretofore, but the disease has previously been quite hopeless to treat.

"Just what the effect of the malaria may be is not understood, but it seems to prepare the central nervous system in some way for the beneficial action of the drugs. The drugs fail to produce benefit unless the patient is prepared for them by the malarial treatment."

Dr. George H. Kirby, who introduced the malaria treatment into the State Hospital for the Insane at Ward's Island, said yesterday that the malaria treatment was continuing there with gratifying results, and that some patients who had been treated as long as two years ago with malaria and returned to their normal occupations were still at work and showed no signs of the recurrence of the disease.

"About 15 per cent. of the admissions to the insane hospitals are due to paresis, so that this treatment is a matter of the greatest importance," he said. "The average life of the paresis patient after he reaches the hospital is one year. A few years ago all of these cases would have seemed quite hopeless.

"The action of the malaria is very obscure. It may produce resistance in the body which destroys the disease, or it may attack the disease directly. It is not correct to say that it prepares the central nervous system for the action of drugs. It has been used successfully without drugs, and there is nothing to show that the malaria itself is not quite

as effective without the help of drugs.

"The only useful drug that we have found is the arsenical combination which was produced by the Rockefeller Institute for the treatment of African sleeping sickness. That has had a good effect in many cases of paresis. We have been able to discharge a number of patients who have received this treatment. On the other hand, some patients who were not benefited at all by the Rockefeller product have been greatly improved by the malaria treatment.

"We do not speak of the malaria treatment as a cure in any case. It is too early to say that. It does, however, bring about a remission of symptoms in many cases. It is too soon to tell whether the remission of symptoms is permanent or not."

Dr. Kirby said it had been suggested that the high body heat caused by the malarial fever destroyed the germs and helped the patient, but that this was a mere guess, without evidence to support it. He said efforts had been made to treat other diseases of the nervous system by malaria, but without any success.

"We have tried it in sleeping sickness—not the African kind," he said, "but it does not work. There has been a good deal of experimenting elsewhere, but I don't know that it has been successful in any other disease."

One of the patients at the Long Island College Hospital was rapidly going blind. He had almost completely lost the sight in one eye and the other was becoming progressively impaired. The induced malarial attack stopped the progress of the eye trouble immediately. The sight did not improve, but the patient still retains a fair amount of vision with one eye.

July 5, 1925

INSANITY TREATMENT IMPROVES
Recognition of Mental Disorders as Major Health Problem Hailed as Encouraging

To the Editor of The New York Times:

The New York State Department of Mental Hygiene recently made public the results of a study of mental disease expectancy according to which approximately 4½ per cent of the persons born in New York State under existing conditions "may be expected to succumb to mental disease of one form or another" and become patients in hospitals for the mentally afflicted. This means that one person out of each twenty-two of the population is a patient in a mental hospital some time during his or her lifetime.

May I point out a significant aspect or two of these figures with regard to the national problem of mental morbidity? Approximately 75,000 new patients are admitted to the mental hospitals of the country every year. At this rate we may expect, with all the assurance of a life insurance mortality table, that 1,000,000 men and women now going about life's business will have become mental cases of more or less institutional severity in the next fifteen years.

A Major Problem.

These figures impress us all the more when we learn that there are as many patients in the mental hospitals of the country as in all other

hospitals combined. It is not the question whether mental disease is actually on the increase but the fact that there are so many persons requiring treatment for mental conditions that is significant; the fact that mental disease is now recognized as a major health problem that should be dealt with as vigorously as tuberculosis, cancer or any other widespread disease. This is a victory for the mental-hygiene movement, which sensed the importance of the problem of mental disease twenty years ago and has labored ever since to bring it to the surface.

The overcrowding of our State hospitals for mental disease is a distressing concern of State Governments throughout the nation, an index of the seriousness of the problem, but it is also a hopeful sign. It is an indication that people are beginning to think about insanity in terms of disease amenable to treatment and in many cases just as curable as bodily disorders. We are adopting a more rational attitude toward the subject, with the result that there are now more known cases of mental morbidity than before.

A More Beneficial View.

The rapid multiplication of outpatient mental clinics, the develop-

ment of psychiatric social service, and the extension of community organization and extra-institutional facilities for the treatment of mental disorders at home, all reflect a healthy change in the public point of view toward a subject that used to be discussed in whispers. There is less disposition to keep secret the fact that there has been a mental breakdown in the family, and more of an inclination to seek advice and treatment in the early stages of mental disease. This is all to the good, even with mounting hospital admission rates, because we are bringing the problem out into the open where better provision can be made for dealing with it.

The campaign of education is beginning to tell, and it is confidently hoped that in time we may bring mental diseases under control to a point comparable with the control of, say, tuberculosis, thanks to improved economic conditions and the work of the public health movement. The warfare against disease is being extended to include all the enemies of mankind, and it is the hope of the American Foundation for Mental Hygiene, which was recently organized to secure greater resources for the support of those who are fighting the battle against mental disease, that this last spectre will some day take its place among those that have lost forever their power to darken human lives.

PAUL O. KOMORA.
New York, Nov. 27, 1928.

December 2, 1928

BELLEVUE TO BUILD A $3,500,000 UNIT

Old Psychopathic Wards to Be Replaced by a Hospital for Mental Cases.

CRIMINALS' CLINIC PLANNED

Institution at 29th Street and East River Will Open for 600 Patients in Two Years.

The psychopathic wards of Bellevue Hospital, relics of an age more heedless of mental cases, are finally to pass on. A new psychiatric hospital, one of the first municipal institutions devoted solely to illnesses of the mind or nerves, is to rise on the block bounded by the East River, First Avenue, Twenty-ninth and Thirtieth Streets, it was announced yesterday by Dr. William Schroeder Jr., Commissioner of Hospitals.

The new unit of Bellevue will cost $3,500,000. It will be thoroughly modern, have new features for treatment of patients, and will be designed in the modern Italian Renaissance. The walls will be of brick, with a granite base and embellished with limestone and terra cotta. The hospital will be ready in two years and will open with 600 beds.

Clinic to Study Crime Planned.

Plans are being considered for the establishment of a special research clinic in which to carry on investigation of crime and of criminals from a psychiatric point of view. The clinical studies will be in cooperation with the Department of Correction. About 100 beds will be devoted to the investigation and treatment of nervous and "problem" children, this research to be undertaken with the Department of Education.

Dr. Menas S. Gregory will be in charge of the psychiatric hospital. The work of building and equipment will be supervised by Deputy Commissioner Louis Cohen. The architects are Charles B. Meyers and Thompson, Holmes & Converse.

"Upon the completion of the hospital," said Dr. Schroeder, "the old psychopathic wards will be discontinued and all mental or nervous cases will be removed from the Bellevue grounds. I feel that this will be to the ultimate advantage not alone of the mental and nervous cases but also to those in Bellevue Hospital receiving medical and surgical treatment.

"A large number of the more important hospitals for mental and nervous cases in this country and abroad were visited and exhaustively studied and observed."

Mr. Meyer said that in his plans special effort had been made to plan the building to coordinate, at maximum, means for interpreting symptoms, treatment and rehabilitation of patients.

Radical differences between the old wards and the new building were stressed by Dr. Gregory.

Cases Will Be Segregated.

"It has been planned to have two separate and distinct buildings," he said, "connected only by a chain of medical offices and laboratories. The greatest care has been taken to plan these buildings so as to provide every facility of caring for patients according to their individual needs and conditions. Much thought has been given to the very important problem of segregation and to the classification of the patients according to the nature of their ailments.

"To carry out this idea it has been planned to have many rooms for one, two and for three patients and several small wards. Large wards have been discarded as being obviously unsuitable for the treatment of mental illness. In planning the hospital, every feature, even the decorations, has been considered from the standpoint of the curative effect upon the patient."

Patients whose illness is of brief duration will be kept apart from those suffering from more serious disorders, Dr. Gregory said, adding that one building will house alcoholics, drug addicts, delinquents and potential criminals. The building will be in two wings, each eight stories high, connected to a third wing, ten stories in height, where will be located kitchens, supplies, living quarters for the staff and the administrative offices.

September 9, 1929

TWENTY YEARS OF WORK FOR MENTAL HYGIENE

The Movement Founded by Clifford W. Beers, Who Was Once A Patient in a Connecticut Institution, Has Grown To Activity in Many Foreign Countries

By R. L. DUFFUS.

ONE person out of every twenty-two in New York State is, or will be at some time in his life, a patient in a hospital for the care of the insane. In the country at large more than 300,000 mental patients are under treatment and this number is increasing at the rate of about 10,000 a year.

The cost of this vast total of mental ailments, measured by the expenditures necessary for the care of patients in public institutions, is $80,000,000 a year. The economic loss, due to impaired or destroyed earning power, is estimated at $143,000,000 a year in New York State alone, and its national total is at least ten times as much. Yet it is conservatively believed that half of all cases of mental or nervous disorder could be prevented if knowledge now available were applied in time, largely early in life. By the same means the lot of those who are destined to suffer from such disorders could be greatly improved.

These are some of the facts

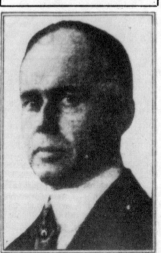

CLIFFORD W. BEERS

Founder of the Mental Hygiene Movement.

brought out at the dinner held in New York City last Thursday in honor of the twentieth anniversary of the founding of the mental hygiene movement, now international in scope. Clifford W. Beers, author of the autobiographical classic, "A Mind That Found Itself," and founder of the movement, completed at the same time nearly a quarter of a century of work for the mentally crippled and insane. From a State society formed in Connecticut in 1908 the crusade for mental hygiene has grown until it covers the United States and is active in twenty-three foreign countries.

Changed Attitude in America.

As a result, according to Dr. C-E. A. Winslow of the Yale School of Medicine, "the last two decades have done more to change the attitude of America toward mental disease and defect than all the centuries that preceded them." The hearty response to the invitations sent out for the First International Congress on Mental Hygiene, to be held at Washington next May under the honorary presidency of Mr. Hoover, indicates that the same may be said in respect of the attitude of other nations.

Mr. Beers's story has been made familiar to thousands of readers by the successive editions of his book, of which the fifteenth appeared this year. It is a vigorous, straightforward and poignant narrative of the indignities and cruelties which were practiced in public and private institutions in the beginning years of the present century against helpless patients.

Attendants were underpaid and incompetent and the inmates, as they were then called, were almost entirely at their mercy. Even some of the physicians in charge, as Mr. Beers found to his cost, were often ignorant as well as brutal. Suffering from a milder form of insanity than many of his fellows, he early made up his mind to find out the worst features of the institutions in which he was confined in order that he might later do something to reform them.

His crusade began when he was still subject to delusions and incapable of leading a normal life. Fortunately he suffered from a form of mental disorder which is highly curable. Not long after his recovery in 1903 he determined at the age of 30 to give up the business career on which he had embarked and devote the rest of his life to the cause of mental hygiene. His first step was the writing of the book, which William James, who introduced the first edition, described as "fit to remain in literature as a classic account 'from within' of an insane person's psychology."

His next step was the formation, on May 6, 1908, of the Connecticut Society for Mental Hygiene. On Feb. 19, 1909, the National Committee for Mental Hygiene, though partially organized earlier, was formally founded, with Dr. Henry B. Favill of Chicago as president and Mr. Beers as secretary.

"An Agency for Education."

The national committee, like the organization which had preceded it, was to be "a permanent agency for education and reform in the field of nervous and mental diseases; an agency for education always, for reform as long as radical changes may be needed." It was determined, however, not to become sensational. Public sentiment was to be enlisted, the cooperation of hospital officials was to be obtained, the quiet work of experts was to take the place of dramatic legislative investigations, the legal rights of patients were to be protected, information and help were to be given to those threatened with mental disease or recovering from it, and model institutions were to be established. This program, as Mr. Beers drew it up, was a veritable Magna Carta of the insane.

Mr. Beers was able to obtain the cooperation of some of the most distinguished men and women of the day. William James, Dr. Adolf Meyer, Joseph H. Choate, President Arthur T. Hadley of Yale University, President Jacob Gould Schurman of Cornell University, Dean Russell H. Chittenden of the Sheffield Scientific

School, President W. H. P. Faunce of Brown University, Jacob Riis, Dr. William H. Welch of Johns Hopkins, Henry Phipps, Cardinal Gibbons, Charles W. Eliot, Miss Julia C. Lathrop, one-time head of the Children's Bureau, all gave active encouragement, and some of them played a conspicuous part in the new enterprise.

Its first few years were rendered difficult by lack of money, and it has never yet been financed in proportion to the importance of its work. However, the initial gift of $50,000 from Henry Phipps in 1911, and subsequent gifts from Mrs. E. H. Harriman, Mrs. William K. Vanderbilt, Mrs. Elizabeth Milbank Anderson, V. Everit Macy, Payne Whitney and others, and from the Rockefeller Foundation, the Commonwealth Fund and the Milbank Memorial Fund have made it possible to begin and continue the task of education and reform. Remarkable progress has been made, though much remains to be done.

"Through the general propaganda that it has sponsored and the specific surveys that it has conducted with the financial aid of the Rockefeller Foundation, under the direction at first of the late Dr. Thomas W. Salmon," says Dr. Winslow in speaking of the national committee's labors, "the grosser evils of jail and almshouse care of mental cases have been largely eliminated, institutional facilities of a proper type have been vastly expanded and in considerable measure removed from political influence and placed under competent psychiatric direction, methods of diagnosing, classifying and treating mental disease have been revolutionized, and through provision for temporary care and observation, emergency commitments and voluntary admissions, a medical point of view has begun to replace the legal attitude that so long dominated the admission of patients to mental hospitals."

Under the direction of Dr. Bernard Glueck the national committee made the pioneer study of the mental factors in crime at Sing Sing Prison upon which the mental clinics of modern prisons have been based. Surveys of the care of the mentally ill and feeble-minded have been made in more than thirty States. When the United States entered the World War the committee assisted the government in mobilizing doctors, nurses and attendants experienced in handling mental cases.

Army Cases.

So successful was the work done that more than 70,000 mentally unstable recruits were weeded out of the national army and more than 90 per cent of the cases of shell-shock were returned to duty. Furthermore, cases of suicide and serious crime were fewer than those recorded in any army in history. Subsequently the national committee, through Dr. Salmon, played a large part in the care and rehabilitation of ex-service men suffering from mental ills.

In 1921 the committee, in cooperation with the Commonwealth Fund, undertook a study of juvenile delinquency. It was soon realized that many children who were not delinquent were in need of psychiatric guidance. To meet this need the

committee, under liberal grants from the Commonwealth Fund, helped to establish child guidance clinics, to which courts, social agencies, physicians and parents might bring problem children.

These clinics enable many children who might otherwise break down mentally in later life, or even become criminals, to become normal and useful citizens. The committee's surveys and studies indicate that two-thirds of the population of our prisons and jails are mentally deficient or abnormal. By caring for the problem child it hopes to save many individuals and to prevent others from harming themselves or the community. There are also clinics to which adults who are in need of psychiatric treatment or examination may go or be sent. Twenty years ago very few such clinics existed. Though the number now is in the neighborhood of 500, the committee believes that many hundred more should be established. A later development is mental hygiene work in colleges and universities.

One of the primary objects of the national committee's campaign of enlightenment, as explained by Mr. Beers, is to remove the superstitious horror with which disorders of the mind have long been regarded. It is pointed out that mental diseases, like other diseases, have their discoverable causes, that many of these causes can be removed, that many forms of insanity can be relieved or entirely cured, and that the "insane" person is still human. He responds to genuine sympathy and friendship even more quickly than those who are normal. It is generally recognized that the boundary line between sanity and insanity is often hard to draw, and that even supposedly sane persons can often increase their happiness and efficiency by proper psychiatric guidance.

Mental Hygiene as a Cure.

"Mental hygiene," says Dr. Charles P. Emerson, dean of the Medical School of Indiana University, "is an efficient means of preventing mental break-downs. It renders more efficient the many mental misfits of life, including the neurasthenic, psychasthenic and hysterical groups, but it presents many still wider aspects. Industrial unrest to a large degree means bad mental hygiene and is to be corrected by good mental hygiene. The various anti-social attitudes that lead to crime are problems for the mental hygienist. Dependency, in so far as it is social parasitism not due to mental or physical defect, belongs to mental hygiene. Indeed, the movement which Mr. Beers inaugurated would seem to be in large measure the solution for many social problems which might seem unrelated to psychiatry. But mental hygiene has a message also for those who consider themselves quite normal, for by its aid the man who is 50 per cent efficient can make himself 70 per cent efficient; and so on."

The National Committee for Mental Hygiene in a recent single year included, among other activities, the promotion of uniform statistical systems for use in mental hospitals; the encouragement of State mental hygiene surveys so that the needs of the population could be adequately met; a survey of psychiatric facilities in connection with courts and penal institutions; a survey of mental hygiene resources in New York City; cooperation with school authorities in giving teachers brief courses in mental hygiene for children; and the encouragement of the study of psychiatry in medical schools.

The absence of an adequate and permanent source of support led, in 1928, to the establishment of the American Foundation for Mental Hygiene. This organization is a financing body, whereas the national committee is an operating body. Its aims are "to give financial aid to work, including research, which will help to conserve mental health, reduce and prevent nervous and mental disorders and mental defects and improve the care and treatment of those suffering from these disorders."

Despite the vital importance of the subject, mental hygiene has as yet received comparatively little assistance from philanthropists. Since its organization the foundation has received several unconditional gifts, and an energetic effort is now being made to complete the first $1,000,000 of the larger fund to be raised. Dr. William H. Welch is honorary president; Dr. Arthur H. Ruggles, president; President James R. Angell of Yale, Bishop William Lawrence of Boston and Dr. William L. Russell of White Plains, vice presidents, and Mr. Beers is secretary. The board of trustees includes nationally known physicians, educators and financiers.

World-wide attention will be attracted to the movement when the mental hygiene congress convenes in Washington next May. Committees from twenty-eight countries are already organizing to assure a full representation, and workers in mental hygiene and related fields the world over will be able to compare notes, exchange information and agree upon a basis of common action.

The congress will be preceded by a survey of the status of mental hygiene work in the different countries of the world. This is already in progress under the direction of national committees. Thus the movement which started with an obscure patient in a Connecticut hospital for the insane a quarter of a century ago has grown until it girdles the earth and is already contributing to the welfare of millions of people.

November 17, 1929

SAYS INSANITY YIELDS TO CHEMICAL OFFSET

Dr. W. D. Bancroft of Cornell Reports Neutralizing Brain and Nerve Conditions.

ANN ARBOR, Mich., Oct. 4 (AP).—Insanity may now be yielding to the assaults of science, directed by physical chemists.

Dr. Wilder D. Bancroft, a chemist, of Cornell University has presented evidence to show that some forms of insanity may be caused by either one of two chemical conditions affecting the brain and nerves and that these forms of insanity likewise have responded to neutralizing chemical treatment.

Dr. Bancroft, who is editor of The Journal of Physical Chemistry, told of his researches at the eighth annual meeting of the American Chemical Society, which ended last night at the University of Michigan. He outlined evidence which indicated that insanity could be produced in normal persons by administration of chemical compounds and that some insane persons could be relieved and made at least temporarily sane by administering the same compounds.

Sodium thiocyanate has been known to produce hallucinations and ideas of oppression in normal individuals, Dr. Bancroft said. Likewise, the form of insanity known as involutional melancholia might be produced by this compound. On the other hand, he said, patients suffering from catatonic stupor have been cured by administration of sodium amatol, while others appeared to have been relieved when sodium thiocyanate was given.

Dr. Bancroft has come to the conclusion that in some form of insanity a coagulation of brain and nerve protein occurs, while in others a dispersion of protein takes place. In dementia praecox, paranoid, maniac depression and epilepsy a slight coagulation of protein has taken place in the brain, or parts of it, he said, therefore a chemical agent which has the opposite or dispersing effect on proteins should work toward a cure.

He believes narcotic addiction may be cured by judicious use of sodium thiocyanate and that developments may come soon in its use as a treatment for hay fever.

October 5, 1931

NEW DRUG IS FOUND TO COMBAT SUICIDE

Benzedrine Is Also Stimulant for Depressed and Exhausted, Psychologists Are Told.

Special to THE NEW YORK TIMES.

HANOVER, N. H., Sept. 2.—Development of a medicine which relieves mental depression and has demonstrated a tendency toward prevention of suicide was reported to the American Psychological Association today by Dr. Abraham Myerson of the Division of Psychiatric Research at the Massachusetts State Hospital in Mattapan.

The new medicine is benzedrine, a member of the adrenalin group of drugs. Dr. Myerson cited several cases when it had a "very remarkable influence" upon persons meditating suicide, in a state of extreme depression, and in the anhedonic state.

In addition, it acted as a stimulent for persons in a state of exhaustion or suffering from "morning after" depression.

September 3, 1936

'SUGAR SHOCK' IS USED TO TREAT THE INSANE

Dr. Bernard Glueck Says Insulin Injections Have Succeeded in Schizophrenia Cases.

CHICAGO, Sept. 23 (AP).—A "sugar shock" treatment for schizophrenia, one of the most common forms of insanity, was described today in The Journal of the American Medical Association.

It consists simply of injections of insulin, the standard treatment for diabetes, which lower the amount of sugar in the blood until shock is produced.

No one knows definitely just how it works, but it is based on the knowledge that various types of sudden shock literally knock an insane person back into sanity, according to the article.

The "sugar shock" treatment was explained in the journal by Dr. Bernard Glueck of Ossining, N. Y., who reported that he had "assisted in the application" of it in a number of successful cases in Switzerland during a recent European visit.

In one group of 104 cases, he asserted, the treatment—known technically as "deliberate induc-tion of the hypoglemic state"—re-sulted in "good recovery" 88 per cent of the time, enabling these patients to resume their former oc-cupations in the community. "Com-plete recovery" was reported in 70.7 per cent of the cases.

Acknowledging the difficulty of estimating the validity of therapeu-tic results in psychiatry, Dr. Glueck said that "time alone will tell how permanent the alleged cures are," but "one patient has remained en-tirely well for two years after ter-mination of the treatment and there were several whose recovery has lasted for about a year."

He credited the development of the treatment to Dr. Manfred Sakel of Vienna.

September 24, 1936

INSANITY TREATED BY ELECTRIC SHOCK

Physicians at the New York State Psychiatric Institute and Hospital of the Columbia-Presbyterian Med-ical Center are experimenting with a new method, introduced in Italy, of treating certain types of mental disorders by sending an electric shock through the brain, Dr. S. Eu-gene Barrera, principal research psychiatrist at the institute, report-ed yesterday.

Although Dr. Barrera emphasized that hope for any "miracle cure" must not be pinned on the new method, as the experiments have been in progress only a few months and findings are inconclusive, it was reported that "considerable success" had resulted in treatment of certain types of insanity.

Primarily, the treatment, if ex-periments prove it sound, is intend-ed to produce the same results as are being ob-tained through injections of metra-zol, a chemical that produces con-vulsions with beneficial effects in certain cases of insanity.

Insulin Also Used

Insulin and camphor also are used by some physicians to produce therapeutic "shock" in treatment of some types of insanity, but the new electric method, it was ex-plained, so far has been used in the treatment of "certain selected men-tal disease for which metrazol has been beneficial." It is hoped that experiments will prove the electric method to be safer, less disagree-able to the patient and less expen-sive for mass use in public clinics.

The electric shock is produced by a small portable electric box which was invented in Italy by Professor Ugo Cerletti of the Rome University Clinic. Dr. Lothar Kalinowsky, a Berlin scientist, now associated with the New York State Psychi-atric Institute here, worked with Professor Cerletti and obtained his permission to introduce the treat-ment in other world centers. He used it in Paris and London and then brought it here, where he and Dr. Barrera have been using the machine at the institute.

As far as is known these are the first experiments with electric shock for insanity to be made at a public institution in New York, al-though physicians expresesd the be-lief that some private psychiatrists might be interested in the method. Similar experiments also are said to be in progress at Johns Hopkins Hospital in Baltimore.

Although physicians were reluc-tant to earmark the new treatment as particularly beneficial for any specific type of insanity, it was said that it had been used successfully in treatment of schilzophrenia, the "split-personality" type of mental disease.

Electrodes Attached to Head

Attached to the electric box is an instrument resembling a large pair of calipers or forceps, to which elec-trodes are connected. This device is clamped to the patient's head above the ears. The patient is tested for electric resistance to de-termine how much voltage may be used. Then the current is turned on for one-tenth of a second, send-ing 70 to 100 volts—rarely more—through the brain.

The patient immediately becomes unconscious, and the shock pro-duces a convulsion somewhat re-sembling a mild epileptic fit. Upon recovering consciousness within a few minutes, the patient is unable to remember what has happened from the time the treatment was administered.

The treatment is repeated three times a week until definite results are noted.

Adherents of the electric-shock method contend that metrazol some-times is an uncertain treatment, and that the process of injection of the chemical into the veins has dis-agreeable features that sometimes instill fear in the patient The elec-tric treatment, they say, at least is not unpleasant, so the patient may be more inclined to cooperate with the physician in future treatments.

Statistics were not available on the number of patients treated and the results of the experiments here. A full report will be made through medical channels when the experi-ment is more advanced. However, it was said that "several hundred" cases wherein the electric-shock method has been used successfully have been reported in European centers.

July 6, 1940

MEN WHO 'CRACK' IN BATTLE HELPED

ALLIED HEADQUARTERS IN NORTH AFRICA, Aug. 23 (U.P.)—Swift and highly skilled psychi-atric treatment almost on the scene of battle has restored to combat fitness in record time American soldiers who "cracked" in the Sicilian battle lines under the shock of fear and horror, the Army Medical Corps reported to-day.

Front-line diagnosis and treat-ment of "battle nerves" and skilled care in rear hospitals rapidly is lowering the percentage of neurosis cases among American troops, which was moderately high during the Tunisian campaign. About 25 per cent of the men treated now are returned to limited service in a shorter time than was possible before.

Battlefield neurosis in World War I was labeled "shell shock," although the condition was not necessarily a result of the blast of a bomb or shell. It now is known to be an emotional disturb-ance resulting from terrific mental conflicts against a background of ear-splitting explosions, wounded or killed comrades, exhaustion and poor nutrition.

Few Cases Now Permanent

Capt. Lawrence P. Roberts of Orangeburg, N. Y., a psychiatrist with the United States forces in North Africa, said "the horrible mistake of the last war was in thinking a so-called shell-shocked patient was permanently ill."

"This thinking resulted in per-manent cases," Captain Roberts said. "But today we find few men who are permanently injured."

The leading exponent of on-the-spot psychiatric treatment is Major Frederick R. Hanson, a na-tive of Omaha, Neb., who prac-ticed psychiatry at Montreal.

Major Hanson devised his treat-ment from personal observation of nervous cases in the Dieppe raid and on two other similar attacks. "The longer a soldier broods on his emotional ills," he said, "the more deeply impressed the symp-toms become. We try to rid him of his fears and illusions at once."

One of the principles of the treatment, besides complete rest and relaxation, is to get the patient to talk of his battle-front experi-ences. In this manner the soldier releases his excitement in recount-ing the sights and effects that had overwhelmed him, is able to see his fears honestly and conquer them.

Mild Drug Hypnosis an Aid

Another treatment is the hypnot-ic trance, usually induced by means of a mild drug, in which the patient is led to tell his story. The soldier thus lets down the wall of inhibi-tion that had prevented him from releasing his battlefield emotions.

His physical and mental reac-tions are bared to the psychiatrist. The doctor can then work with a knowledge of the worries and fear that have been in the soldier's mind and methodically bring the man back to mental peace and stability.

The hospital in this area, with its 450 patients, is under the direction of Lieut. Col. J. E. Cox of Waynes-boro, Va. His staff of psychiatrists includes Captain Roberts, Capt. John Spiegel of Chicago, Capt. A. L. Hudson of New Philadelphia, Ohio; Lieut. Albert Glass of Balti-more and Capt. Calvin S. Drayer of Philadelphia.

August 24, 1943

GROUP AID IS URGED FOR MENTAL ILLS

Special to THE NEW YORK TIMES.

CHICAGO, May 27—The effectiveness of group psychotherapy in the treatment of men who broke under the strains of combat was sufficient to warrant carrying the technique over into out-patient work in the Veterans Administration, Dr. Martin Grotjahn of the Institute of Psychoanalysis, Chicago, declared today.

In a paper he read before the annual meeting of the American Psychiatric Association, which opened here today, Dr. Grotjahn advocated also that the method be adopted eventually by practicing psychiatrists in general.

"Soldiers live in a group, wait, feel, hope, fear and fight in groups," he observed. "Only when they are wounded or break down do they become individualized again. The moment they get better. . . . they form a group again. Their improvement is an improvement in a group."

The physician recounted the results of twelve group sessions with twenty-five enlisted men at a general hospital, where they were awaiting disability discharge. The sessions covered two months.

An advantage of the group technique, which was adopted because of disproportion between the number of patients and physicians, but has proved valuable in its own right, is that it gives the individual patient more confidence and begins his "socialization."

Describing the series as "glorified bull session," Dr. Grotjahn said his main goal as a psychiatrist was to get the emotional participation of the men, as distinguished from their purely intellectual participation. The patients' concern shifted from their afflictions in early sessions to ways and means of adjustment in later ones.

Dr. J. Louise Despert of the New York Hospital declared that chances of adjustment in schizophrenic children are greater when therapy is carried on in the psychiatrist's office than in a mental institution.

Describing seven cases of children aged from 3 to 7 years, the woman physician said the method has the advantage of not separating children from home. Results were encouraging, but the prospects of complete recovery remained doubtful.

Dr. Frederick W. Dershimer, director of psychiatry for E. I. du Pont de Nemours & Co., asserted that "industrial management is open minded about the application of psychiatry in industry, provided the psychiatrist is willing to learn enough about industry and its problems to make sense."

He added that industry employs and uses individuals who fit into eveery known psychiatric category. The inventor of nylon, he revealed, "was a known psychiatric case for years."

May 28, 1946

KNIFE AIDS MENTALLY ILL

Committee Praises Pre-frontal Lobotomies in Connecticut

HARTFORD, Conn., March 21 (AP)—The pre-frontal lobotomy, a comparatively new type of brain surgery, helped more than 80 per cent of the 125 mentally ill patients in Connecticut who underwent the operation during the past eight months, the Joint Committee of State Mental Hospital said today in a report.

Termed "a major contribution to psychiatry in Connecticut" by Dr. Burness E. Moore, one of the members of the committee, the operations are continuing at the rate of ten to fifteen each week at three State hospitals and two private institutions in Connecticut.

The report disclosed that 40 per cent of the 125 patients who underwent the operation were "much improved," and many are now leading normal lives at home; 42 per cent showed "improvement" and 11.8 per cent were "unimproved." Six of the patients died, but the report said this was below the national average for the operation.

About half the patients operated on were suffering from schizophrenia (commonly called "split personality") and had been confined five years or more.

March 22, 1947

SURGERY OF BRAIN STUDIED IN REPORT

By LUCY FREEMAN
Special to The New York Times.

DENVER, Sept. 8—Persons who undergo brain surgery for mental illness lose their emotional tensions but also lose a feeling of "self-continuity" and do not seem to care very much what happens to themselves or to other people, it was revealed today by Dr. Walter Freeman and Dr. James W. Watts, the two surgeons who have pioneered in America in psychosurgery.

This is believed to be the first public report on the effect of the operation on the personality of the patient to be made by these two men, who have performed hundreds of brain operations on the mentally ill in the past twelve years.

The report was also the work of Dr. Mary Frances Robinson, psychologist, who is working with Dr. Freeman and Dr. Watts at George Washington University, Washington, where the study was conducted. She read the report, titled "Personality Changes After Psychosurgery," at the annual convention of the American Psychological Association.

The conclusions are based on a study of sixty-eight prefrontal lobotomy patients who were seen for routine visits between February and June, 1948. The patients were described as "probably representative of the 500 or more who have made fair-to-good recoveries under the Freeman and Watts techniques."

In evaluating what has happened to the personality of these patients the authors declared, "they are freed from the tyranny of their own past and are indifferent to future problems and to the opinion of other people."

Goals Become Immediate

The patients also show "some lack of depth of personality," they reported.

"Their statements regarding themselves are objective and unconcerned and they seldom give voice to defense mechanisms," they said. "Their goals are immediate, not remote. They can recall the past as well as ever, but it has diminished interpretive value for them, and they are no more interested in their own past emotional crises than if they had happened to someone else."

These patients also "seem incapable of being humiliated now over blunders they have made in the past," the authors report.

Though they may differ individually, the behavior of each patient is in considerable measure predictable, they also revealed.

"By degrees we came to feel that there is a characteristic conspicuous by its absence in these people that is common to the rest of us and thus has gone largely unremarked by psychologists," they declared. "We have come to realize that in our own growing consciousness of the self there develops a feeling of our own duration, of our self-continuity, of being in some sense the persons we were yesterday and will be tomorrow with responsibility for both.

"And, as in living organisms duration always involves change, so we, in thinking about our past selves, are aware of change; we speak about our adjustment to circumstances. Hence, self-continuity implies self-adjustability, the effort to avoid now and in the future the mistakes we are painfully aware we made yesterday."

They asserted that "an overdeveloped awareness of self-continuity may underlie mental illness; some degree of it must be essential for successful psychotherapy."

New Tensions Barred

They concluded that psychosurgery relieves emotional tension through the severing of the fronto-thalamic tract, preventing the development of many future tensions (which make for maladjustment, but also for depth of personality) through reducing the individual's awareness of his own "self-continuity" which, they said, appeared to be a function of the frontal lobes and their connections.

All psychosurgery, if successful, checks "the terrific emotional tension characteristic of many pre-operative patients," they declared.

"If the operation is minimal, the chief effects seem to be loss of fantasy, of creative drive, of sensitivity, of sympathetic understanding of others," they explained. "If the operation is radical, patients are likely to be somewhat gross in their appetites for food and sex, careless and slovenly in appearance and largely impervious to criticism. Between these extremes lies a wide range of individual differences."

Of the sixty-eight patients studied, nineteen were men; ages ranged from 20 to 72, with 42 the most frequent; education varied from two years of rural school to a Master of Arts degree, and the illnesses lasted from one to forty years.

"Reliable differences" were noted between these patients and a control group of individuals of similar age and diagnosis who recovered without operations, it was stated.

Ronald Lippitt, president of the Society for the Psychological Study of Social Issues of the association, told the 1,800 psychologists at the meeting that he believed scientific research and social therapy would be benefited by the basic training of social psychologists in both of these fields, rather than developing highly differentiated specializations.

Most of the jobs in which social psychologists will find themselves call for the use of the skills of both researcher and therapist, he held.

September 9, 1949

PSYCHIATRIC STUDY CITES ·RECOVERIES

By LUCY FREEMAN
Special to THE NEW YORK TIMES.

CINCINNATI, May 7—A study telling what has happened thirty years after to 141 patients in a mental hospital shows that 24 per cent recovered and maintained recovery until their deaths or up to the present. The investigation is one of the few long-term studies on the outcome of serious mental illness.

The recovery figures, called "surprisingly good for a group of patients considered to have a very poor prognosis," were reported today in a paper at the opening meeting of the 107th annual convention of the American Psychiatric Association, attended by 2,500 of the country's leading psychiatrists.

Dr. William L. Holt Jr., chief medical officer of the Boston Psychopathic Hospital. and Winifred M. Holt, his research associate, presented a paper based on a study of the patients, admitted in 1921 to the Westboro State Hospital.

The authors pointed out that what they considered successful results were "obtained with a program of hospital care in which modern shock therapies played no part." They held that present-day treatment involving shock needs to be evaluated in terms of reports like the one they offered.

41% Left Hospital

Where the community accepted a former patient as mentally normal, the authors recorded the condition as recovered. Improvement, as recorded in the study meant the patient was "productively occupied within physical capacity and residing in an unlocked hospital ward or in the community."

Forty-one per cent of the 141 left the hospital. Seven per cent of the group could not be found. Thirty of the ninety patients who died had returned to their communities.

Of the twenty-three patients still remaining in mental hospitals, four were improved, the authors said, while of the eighteen still living at home, twelve had recovered. Of the thirty who died at home, twenty-two were considered to have recovered prior to their final physical illness.

Dr. John C. Whitehorn, head of the psychiatric services at Johns Hopkins Hospital and Medical School, declared in his presidential address, which opened the convention, that the present condition of psychiatry in America, in certain respects, was "significantly different" than in most countries.

Much of this difference has come about, he added, "because a number of American psychiatrists have been intensively preoccupied with the social implication of psychiatry."

May 8, 1951

MENTAL HOSPITALS FAVOR FREE ENTRY

By LUCY FREEMAN

Voluntary entering of mental hospitals marks a relatively new development nationally in the field of emotional health. There is a growing trend toward the use of voluntary commitments as the stigma attached to going to a mental hospital is gradually decreasing and more people realize that prevention may save much personal anguish.

In the last twelve years ten states have enacted laws for voluntary admissions. Forty states have laws providing for such commitments although the actual use of such a law is limited in most states, according to the recent comprehensive report, "The Mental Health Programs of the Forty-Eight States," prepared by Brevard E. Crihfield, director of research for the Council of State Governments. This report says:

"Voluntary hospitalization saves time and money for the states and embarrassment for the patient and it tends to reduce length of stay in the hospital. Voluntary admission procedures should be provided in all states and should be used more extensively."

New Jersey, California, Illinois and Ohio are among the states where voluntary commitments are high, the report showed. In New Jersey voluntary commitments were 23.8 per cent of the total mental hospital population in 1945-49.

Last year 7.4 per cent of New York State's patients entered mental hospitals of their own will. New York encourages voluntary commitments.

Preserving of Self-Respect

"It is much better for the person's self-respect to be voluntarily committed," says Dr. Newton Bigelow, the state's mental hygiene commissioner. "He then feels, 'I decided I was ill and went in the hospital on my own. I wasn't put in.' Also, his chances of being helped are better the earlier he enters a hospital."

"There is no question about the desirability of voluntary commitments," says Dr. George S. Stevenson, medical director of the National Association for Mental Health. "If one thinks of the mental hospital as a kind of safeguarding of the public, then one depends entirely on court commitments, but if one thinks of it as a hospital to help ill people, one advocates voluntary commitments."

The idea of a person voluntarily entering a hospital presents a considerable change from the popular concept of some one being "railroaded" into a mental hospital. Actually, mental hospitals across the country are so overcrowded that they are more interested in getting patients out than in keeping in those who may be less ill than others.

Extent of Overcrowding

Overcrowding is the most serious detriment to patient comfort and well-being, according to the Council of State Governments' report. About 43 per cent of the mental hospitals replying to a questionnaire (and they represented 94 per cent of the nation's mental hospitals) reported overcrowding in excess of 20 per cent. Fourteen were 50 per cent or more overcrowded.

In New York State persons are scrupulously screened by physicians after they arrive at the hospital, so that there will be no doubt about whether the patient is ill.

"Our hospitals are judged by the number of persons they get out feeling better, not by the number they keep in," said Dr. Bigelow.

Under his leadership, in the last year the state has made important strides in increasing guidance clinics, accenting prevention, using volunteers in hospitals and advancing such new psycho-therapeutic techniques as group therapy in the hospitals.

This was a year, too, when the state took care of the largest mental health population in its history. On March 31, 107,164 patients were in hospitals and 11,365 convalescing in communities. The budget for 1951-52 is reaching a peak of $143,000,000.

August 3, 1951

LAW HELD TO ABET MANY MENTAL ILLS

By LUCY FREEMAN

Emotionally ill persons committed to mental hospitals are subject to unpleasant and even harmful experiences in many states today, according to authorities in the field of mental health.

In some states they are herded into jails while awaiting disposition, made to endure trial by jury and generally treated as criminals, not as ill persons in need of medical treatment. Even the word "commit" carries the connotation of criminality and the courtroom procedure is likely to be one in which the person is "accused" rather than understood as ill, the experts maintain.

One reason for the condition is that each state has its own commitment law and these vary widely from state to state. The states that have the most satisfactory laws, according to a recent report on commitment procedures issued by the Group for the Advancement of Psychiatry, are those empowering commitment by certificate of two physicians. These include Louisiana, Vermont, Rhode Island, Pennsylvania, Maryland and New Hampshire.

The states with the most unsatisfactory laws are Texas and Mississippi which require trial by jury, the report charges, adding, "and to an extent less obnoxious are those states which utilize the permissive trial by jury on petition of patients."

Thirty-five states, according to a recent report on "The Mental Health Programs of the Forty-Eight States" issued by the Council of State Governments, provide that the mentally ill may be held in jails.

Jail Detention Scored

"Hospital authorities are strongly opposed to jail detention and to the transportation of patients by police conveyances," the report states. "They feel that the patient should be taken into custody in such a way as to show clearly that he is a sick person in need of kindly attention and assistance. If mental illness is to be recognized as a medical problem, the stigma of criminality must be removed from all procedures designed to bring the patient under care and treatment."

The Council of State Governments recommends that states review and improve their laws governing hospitalization of the mentally ill "so as to meet standards essential for safeguarding the patient's rights, promoting early recovery, and protecting the welfare of the community."

It recommends adoption of the draft act prepared in the Federal Security Agency by psychiatrists of the National Institute of Mental Health in consultation with Dr. Winfred Overholser, superintendent of St. Elizabeth's Hospital in Washington, and other medical and legal authorities.

One objection to the draft act has been raised by the National Association for Mental Health. Dr. George Stevenson, medical director, explained that two sections, one pertaining to voluntary commitment, the other to involuntary commitment, state that: "The head of a private hospital may, and subject to the availability of suitable accommodations, the head of a public hospital shall receive therein for observation, diagnosis, care and treatment any individual, etc." The words "may" and "shall" are objected to.

Wording Offers Way Out

"The present wording makes it possible for overburdened hospital superintendents to fall back on overcrowding as a reason for denying prospective patients admission to the hospital," Dr. Stevenson explained. "To turn these people back into the community without help is not only inhumane but contrary to the code of medical ethics. Too, such a procedure tends to delay the time when the community must face the problem of overcrowded mental hospitals."

States vary, too, in the administration of the laws. New York, for instance, has a strong central mental hygiene department that coordinates the activities of the state's mental hospitals and is responsible for the appointment of superintendents. While in Connecticut, for instance, each hospital has a board of trustees that appoints the superintendent.

August 4, 1951

New 'Mood-Lifting' Pill Drives the Blues Away

ST. LOUIS, May 3 (AP) — A new "mood-lifter" pill pulls people out of the "blues and woes," three physicians said today.

It helped 90 per cent of persons with mild depressions, Drs. Howard D. Fabing, J. Robert Hawkins and James A. L. Moulton of Cincinnati told the American Psychiatric Association.

One young woman was bored, fearful of meeting friends, troubled by insomnia and various aches after her engagement was broken. Six weeks of treatment with the pills had her feeling self-confident, buoyant, free of headaches and tremulous feelings, they said.

The drug, alpha (2-piper-idyl) benzhydrol hydrochloride, stimulates the central nervous system without robbing the appetite or interfering with sleep as other mood-lifter drugs do.

It also helped 65 per cent of persons with fairly severe depressions. It had little or no effect against severe mental illnesses, the physicians said.

May 4, 1954

CARE INADEQUATE FOR THE SICK AGED

By EDITH EVANS ASBURY

Thousands of New York's aged already are mentally or physically ill and live in institutions. More than half of these ailing aged are supported at public expense.

Two city infirmaries, a city nursing home, eleven state mental hospitals and 100 commercially run nursing homes house and care for the aging ill from this area. Additional hundreds are being cared for in ninety-one homes for the aged operated by religious and philanthropic organizations. Nobody, including the city's Commissioner of Hospitals, knows how many chronically ill aged men and women languish in general and voluntary hospital beds, not because they need expensive care but because there is no place to send them.

Most of the havens in which these men and women have found refuge for their declining years were not designed to handle their problems.

Bird S. Coler Infirmary, a 1,920 bed institution on Welfare Island, is an exception. One of the most modern and best-equipped facilities in the nation, it was planned to meet today's needs of the infirm aged. It was completed two and a half years ago, and already is filled nearly to capacity.

Creedmoor Hospital for the mentally ill, on the other hand, was designed to accommodate a higher proportion of younger and ambulatory patients than it now has. When it opened as a separate institution in 1935, only 28 per cent of the patients in New York State mental hospitals were senile. Today this group constitutes 36 per cent of the inmates of state hospitals.

Because most of Creedmoor's aging patients are bedfast or have limited mobility, they cannot, for instance, go to centrally located dining rooms in other buildings.

Replanning of food service for patients who cannot climb stairs, or even leave their beds—and some of the very old have to be spoon-fed like babies—is just one example of the adaption required at Creedmoor.

Homes for Aged Evolving

Similar changes, usually at great expense, have become necessary in homes for the aged. Originally planned as rest and retirement places for ambulatory, and sometimes healthy, oldsters, many of these homes are gradually evolving into infirmaries or hospitals.

There are two major reasons for the evolution. First, their original inhabitants lived for many years after entering, became chronically ill, and continued to survive for many more years. Secondly, men and women enter homes for the aged now at the age of 75 or 80, usually for health reasons.

A generation ago, the average age at admission to a home for the aged was 60 or 65, and the reason was usually a need for shelter and food.

Nowadays, men and women in their sixties have the wherewithal to buy food and shelter in their own communities, thanks to Social Security, Old Age Assistance, pensions and the like. And they show an overwhelming preference for remaining independent, and outside an institution, as long as possible.

The old idea that retired men

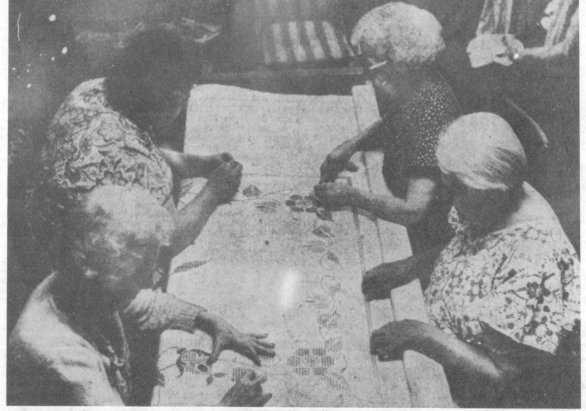

These women live at Creedmore Hospital for mentally ill, designed to handle a higher proportion of younger and more active patients than it does. Many of the ill aged languish in such institutions for lack of other facilities.

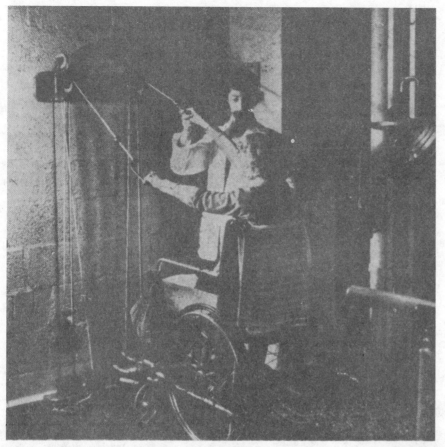

Bird S. Coler Infirmary on Welfare Island, however, was planned to handle the problems of the infirm aged. It has been completed for only two and a half years, but already its capacity has been nearly reached. Here Nurse Blanche Perry is administering physical therapy.

and women romp joyously into homes for aged, or sunny colonies in Florida to rest and relax after years of happy anticipation, has been disproved by recent surveys. They want to stay in their own homes in their own neighborhoods, near friends and relatives, regardless of the rigors of climate or penury.

Eventually, because of the increased life span, illness and enfeeblement overtake many of the aging, and they have to enter some kind of institution when they can no longer take care of themselves.

When aging men and women begin to deteriorate they are prey to a variety of diseases, and sometimes suffer from more than one at the same time.

The Disease of Senility

One of the most distressing illnesses to befall the aged and their families is senility. Medical science has not found its cause or cure. It can last for many years, during which the patient gradually grows increasingly feeble physically and mentally, requiring more and more care. The cost, over a period of years, of providing for a severely senile relative is utterly beyond the means of the average family.

Mildly senile persons can remain with relatives if there is someone to keep an eye on them. They cannot be left alone for long. They are forgetful, may wander away, may turn on the gas to make coffee and forget

to put a match to the gas. At this stage their medical needs are likely to be few.

New York's small families, usually living in small apartments, often with husband and wife both working, face a problem not to be underestimated even with mild senility. The situation is the more critical if teen-agers in the family feel shamed by grandmother's behavior, or a daughter-in-law resents the burden of caring for her.

As the disease progresses, the senile person grows more forgetful, more vague, more childish. Physical and sanitation needs, as well as personality disturbances, become extremely difficult for the average family to cope with. At this point, some kind of custodial care elsewhere is usually necessary to keep the rest of the family from being blown apart.

Senility, while it affects the mind, has physical, not mental causes. In non-technical language, it is the result of hardening of the arteries. The aging, thickening arteries permit less and less blood to flow to the brain, which becomes undernourished, starves and fails.

The disease can occur in any person, regardless of how satisfying his occupation, physical health, mental and emotional stability were during his active, mature years.

All Groups Affected

All income groups are struck. Wealthy families can hire companions or nurses, and keep the patient at home when the disease becomes severe, or they can obtain suitable institutionalization—at great expense.

If the family is supported by welfare funds, or demonstrably unable to pay for the care of the senile relative outside the home, public agencies will assume all or part of the burden.

The average, self-supporting, middle-income family, however, finds it virtually impossible in New York City to solve the problem of long-term custodial care for a senile relative in a way commensurate with its pride and self-respect.

In a nursing home—if one can be found that is willing to take a senile patient—fees will be at least $150 a month, for bed, board and nursing care alone. Medical treatment, when needed, will be billed separately.

Homes for the aged are extremely reluctant to accept senile patients, because of the more intensive, therefore more expensive, attention they require. Their financial resources are already strained to the breaking point by the unanticipated greater number of years their present population has survived, and by the resultant increase in chronic illness among them.

Another reason for the reluc-

tance to accept a senile is that his childish behavior sometimes disturbs other patients.

By reducing their own standard of living some middle-income families, at great financial hardship, manage to maintain a senile parent or grandparent. But the senile can survive for years. Usually, as things are now, the senile from the middle and lower income family eventually goes to a tax-supported institution, despite his family's financial sacrifices and pride.

Usually that institution is a mental hospital, to the further demoralization of the family and drain on the taxpayer.

State Hospitals Opposed

Many students of the problems of the aged believe that the majority of the senile do not belong in state hospitals for the mentally ill. They believe the care there is more expensive than need be for this type of patient.

According to state law, senile psychotics must be committed to a hospital for the mentally ill. Many welfare workers believe the law is sometimes loosely interpreted in order to commit nonpsychotic senile men and women because there is no place else to put them.

In the opinion of this group, the law should be rephrased to distinguish between psychotic and nonpsychotic senility. They advocate separate institutions, more like nursing homes than hospitals, for the senile.

If this were done, they argue, the senile's care would be less of a burden on the taxpayer, his last years could be spent more comfortably, and his descendants would be spared the stigma of mental illness.

Administrators of the State Department of Mental Hygiene are outraged by the latter argument. They declare that no more stigma is attached to illness of the brain than to bodily illness.

Dr. James A. Brussel, assistant commissioner, insists that "no patient is in a state hospital for the mentally ill who is not mentally ill."

"Our mental hospitals are so overcrowded now that we are hard pressed for space," Dr. Brussel declares.

"Don't you think we would be delighted to empty our beds of older people if they were not mentally ill?" Dr. Brussel demands. "Then we could reduce overcrowding and concentrate our efforts and facilities on the younger person who would receive more benefit from treatment and perhaps be cured."

A spotlight was thrown on the situation last December, when Supreme Court Justice Benjamin Brenner declared that he was sick and tired of sending old people to mental institutions simply because there is no place else to put them.

Referring to four elderly persons appearing before him for commitment, Justice Brenner said: "Since denial of custodial care and hospitalization to these people would probably result in their death, I find myself compelled to certify them as mentally ill."

Miss Ollie Randall, national president of the Gerontology Society, applauded the jurist's outburst as a "welcome shock." It underscored a problem that deserves a high, if not the highest, priority in the community—planning for old age, Miss Randall said.

Commissioner Brussel's retort is that after a thorough clinical study—"and you can be sure it was thorough"—all four of the persons to whom the jurist referred were found to be "definitely very psychotic."

Miss Randall and scores of others, including physicians and psychiatrists as well as welfare workers, believe there is merit in drawing a sharper distinction between psychotic and nonpsychotic senility, and in providing separate facilities for them.

Even a distinct wing of a mental hospital, with a different name, which would appear on the death record handed down to

his decendants, would be a humane step in the right direction, declares Justice Brenner. He also proposes that a new term "helpless aged," be used in commitment proceedings.

No layman is qualified to diagnose psychosis. Qualified psychiatrists themselves may vary in their judgment as to when the border line has been crossed from emotional disturbance and neurosis into psychosis.

To the untrained observer, mere erratic behavior may be deemed psychotic, or outward calm of a true psychotic may be mistaken as proof of normality.

Psychosis Is Defined

Dr. S. Bernard Wortis, Professor of Psychiatry and Neurology at New York University College of Medicine and director of psychiatric and neurological services at University Hospital, New York University-Bellevue Medi-

cal Center, says there is no dispute about the exact definition of psychosis.

A psychotic, Dr. Wortis says, is an individual of normal intelligence in such a state of mind as to be unable to care for his own needs, unable to deal with the ordinary requirements of his normal environment, and devoid of insight into the consequences of his actions.

The city's psychiatrists base their decision on committal recommendations on whether the senile person has reached this state, Dr. Wortis says. He denies that they take into consideration any lack of other facilities for the patients' care outside a mental hospital.

The same definition, incidentally, almost applies to a baby. And indeed, senile men and women revert to childishness as their disease progresses. As their memory fails, they forget acquired habits of self control.

This means diapering, constant change of clothing and bed linen, and sometimes resistance to being bathed and fed.

One of the most tragic sights imaginable is the wasted, feeble 90-year-old, a great-grandmother, crying piteously in her bed for, "Mamma, I want my Mamma."

Not all the aged become senile. The percentage is small. However, the numbers are large, and are bound to increase as our aged population increases. Unless some answer is found to the problems posed by their need for specialized care, its expense will continue to engulf an ever-growing number of families, and the taxpayer.

Some answers have been found to the question of how to care humanely and economically for the aged who develop other kinds of chronic illness. They will be discussed in tomorrow's article.

February 22, 1955

NEW DRUGS QUIET TROUBLED MINDS

Chemists Told of Treatment for Early Schizophrenia— Quest for Others Urged

By ROBERT K. PLUMB
Special to The New York Times.

CINCINNATI, March 31—Chemists here today were urged to press the search for new drugs that can give peace of mind to upset people.

Three important new drugs that can "tranquillize" disturbed people were described by Dr. Howard D. Fabing, a University of Cincinnati psychiatrist and neurologist. He addressed a meeting of the Division of Me-

dicinal Chemistry of the American Chemical Society's 127th national meeting here.

The three new compounds are: Alpha (4 piperidyl benzhydrol hydrochloride), sold to physicians under the trade name frenquel.

Chlorpromazine, sold under the trade name thorazine.

Reserpine, an extract of the ancient Indian snakeroot rauwolfia serpentina, sold under many trade names.

To Treat Schizophrenia

With the use of these materials, Dr. Fabing said, about six out of ten early cases of schizophrenia can be treated. The compounds have other striking effects, he noted. Post-operative hallucinations, for instance, which afflict particularly older patients, can be relieved.

The materials appear to have a specific effect on early schizophrenia, he said, apart from their ability to make the patient tranquil. Further studies of the

"peace of mind" drugs are being made through volunteers who acquire psychosis, including a schizophrenia-like condition after their intake of some of the long-known animal and plant drugs.

One of these is a chemical called lysergic acid diethyl amide, a slightly altered chemical extract of rye rust or ergot. Volunteers who took only one-tenth of a milligram of this compound, a quantity equivalent to about ten grains of salt, had violent attacks simulating schizophrenia. They lasted up to fifteen hours.

When the same volunteers were pre-treated with one of the new tranquilizing drugs, Dr. Fabing reported, they were spared the violent and terrible mental confusion characteristic of the disease. And the drug cleared up schizophrenia-like confusion after psychosis had been started artificially with lysergic acid diethyl amide.

Chemical Changes Seen

The lysergic acid compound is one of a class of chemical compounds called indoles, Dr. Fabing said. Other indoles include mescaline, used by American Indians to induce a dream-like state, bufotenin (from toads) ibogaine, tryptamine, yohimbine, cannabis and possibly marihuana. Another indole, adrenochrome, is a biological material from the adrenal gland.

All these materials have profound effects on mental processes, Dr. Fabing pointed out. The effects similar to artificial psychoses, suggest that some mental afflictions, particularly schizophrenia, might be caused by bodily chemical processes. If so, chemical treatment might succeed, he said. Dr. Fabing urged chemists to press for possibilities of treating the disturbed by chemicals.

April 1, 1955

NEW DRUG FOR ANXIETY
Wyeth Says Equanil Brings Safe and Quick Relief

Special to The New York Times.

PHILADELPHIA, Aug. 22—The development of a new drug, equanil, said to bring quick and safe relief to those who suffer from tenseness and anxiety, was announced today by Wyeth Laboratories.

The pharmaceutical concern said that the drug, a derivative of propanediol, acts as a central nervous system depressant, "lessening tension, reducing irritability and restlessness, restoring equanimity, assuring more restful sleep and generalized muscle relaxation."

In clinical studies involving more than 300 persons, Wyeth added, the drug had proved to be non-habit forming, practical and safe. It neither dulls nor dead-

ens the senses.

"Investigators working with equanil," Wyeth said, "reported that dramatic results were achieved in the treatment of tension-produced pain. * * *

"Equanil is also useful in keeping alcoholics sober after withdrawal has been completed, and has much value in accomplishing withdrawal with a minimum of discomfort."

August 23, 1955

Drop Noted in Total Of Mental Patients

By EMMA HARRISON

The first nation-wide decrease in state mental hospital patients occurred last year, the National Mental Health Committee has reported. The decline was attributed to intensive therapy.

The number of state mental hospital patients in 1956 was about 7,000 under the 1955 count. The committee noted that the decrease was even more remarkable since 1956 also was a record year for admissions. A total of 186,000 persons was admitted last year, compared with 178,000 in 1955 and 115,000 in 1945, when statistics on state mental hospital populations were first collected on a national scale.

On the basis of these figures, obtained from a report published by the Interstate Clearing House on Mental Health of the Council of State Governments, the committee queried all the states on how new appropriations were being used for patient care and how future funds could best be used.

Most states reported agreement on the need for a balanced treatment program, the committee found. The following areas of agreement also emerged in answers to the questionnaires:

¶Patients are now being treated rather than just maintained.

¶Impact of the so-called tranquilizer drugs has created the need for more medical personnel and recreational and occupational facilities.

¶Research has to be accelerated.

¶Children's and out-patient units must be increased.

Reflecting on "what turned the tide" in the mental hospital population, the committee summary found that one answer lay in increased yearly appropriations by State Legislatures, with the cumulative effect finally reversing the "seemingly inevitable rise."

It noted that, in 1945, average daily expenditure on each mental patient was $1.06. In 1956, it rose to $3.26. The committee considered this a good increase, despite higher living costs. It also observed that this figure was low as compared with the Veterans Administration's 1955 expenditure of $8.99.

Whereas in 1945 there was one full-time employe for every 6.8 patients, last year the ratio rose to one for every 3.6 patients. Increases in trained psychiatric personnel found 2,659 superintendents and physicians in state hospitals in 1956, compared with 1,458 in 1945.

Even more dramatic increases were shown in other professional personnel. Psychologists and psychometrists increased 574 per cent; social and field workers, 221 per cent; graduate nurses, 153 per cent, and other nurses and attendants, 133 per cent.

Improvement in the discharge rate also was reported. It increased from 123 patients for each 1,000 in 1945 to 175 for each 1,000 in 1954. In 1956, some of the "top state mental hospitals" were discharging from 65 to 80 per cent of first admissions, the report showed.

Summarizing state reports, the committee predicted the following trends would continue in the next two years:

¶Increased state appropriations for psychiatric research, with emphasis on physiological research.

¶Continuance of a major trend toward construction of large state institutes for psychiatric research.

¶More attention and legislative support to programs for training psychiatric personnel, with a growing trend toward state-supported stipends for residents and trainees, and the subsidizing of medical schools for expanded psychiatric training programs.

¶Development of more specific drugs for the treatment of certain kinds of mental illness, spurred by a 1956 Congressional appropriation of $2,000,000 for drug therapy evaluation.

¶More support of psychiatric services in the community.

¶More regional cooperation, especially in the fields of research and training.

January 20, 1957

HELP FOR MENTAL ILLS

Reports on Tests of Synthetic Drug Say the Results Are Promising

By WILLIAM L. LAURENCE

From more than a dozen leading institutions devoted to the study of mental and nervous diseases there are encouraging reports on the preliminary trials of a new synthetic psychotherapeutic drug. The experts say it may be "one of the major developments in the field to date." The reports are published in a special March supplement of the journal "Diseases of the Nervous System," to be issued this week when the new drug is released for prescription use by the medical profession.

The drug was synthesized in the research laboratories of Hoffmann-LaRoche, Inc., by Dr. Leo Sternbach, a group leader in the chemical research department, in what was described as "a lucky accident." Its generic chemical name is methaminodiazepoxide. It will be marketed under the trade name Librium, from the final syllables of the word equilibrium.

Librium is described as "chemically and clinically different from any of the tranquilizers, psychic energizers or other psychotherapeutic drugs now available." Nor is it related to any drug now used in medicine. It has so far been used by more than 2,000 physicians on more than 20,000 patients during the past year.

Reducing Anxiety

Dr. H. Angus Bowes of the Northwestern South Dakota Mental Health Center, at Aberdeen, states in his report that "observations on over 200 patients have convinced me that Librium represents the most significant advance to date in the psychopharmaceutical treatment of anxiety states." Other reports state that it appears to be "superior, safer and faster than any currently available agent in the treatment of common emotional disturbances." It also appears to be "remarkably effective in lessening anxiety and tension without the loss of acuity, interest or drive."

The pharmacological activity of Librium has been extensively investigated in a variety of animal species. In these studies, Librium induced muscle relaxation and a quieting effect in the usual laboratory animals (mice, rats, cats and dogs), and also showed an unprecedented "taming" action in wild, vicious monkeys, tigers, dingo dogs and other animals. In all species, it was found, fear and aggression were eliminated by the drug at doses far below those required to produce hypnosis. In addition, Librium appears to have anticonvulsant properties similar to those of phenobarbital, but lacks the hypnotic effects of the barbiturates. The animal tests were carried out in the Boston and San Diego zoos.

A report on the use of Librium as a quieting drug for hyperactive alcoholic and psychotic patients was made by Drs. Howard E. Ticktin and John D. Schultz, of the District of Columbia General Hospital and the George Washington University Medical Division, Washington, D. C. Forty-two hospital patients admitted for acute and chronic alcoholism, with or without medical complications, various psychoses and neuroses, and some with severe pain from cancer, were treated with Librium, with the following results: Anxiety and tension, as well as excessive motor excitement, were "effectively reduced in a majority of the patients"; the "best results were achieved in the alcoholic group." The result suggests that those alcoholics who drink to escape nervous tension may be helped by the drug to get relief from their tension and thereby reduce their need for alcohol.

Drs. John Kinross-Wright, Irvin M. Cohen and James A. Knight of the department of psychiatry, Baylor University College of Medicine, and the Houston State Psychiatric Institute, report on the drug's ability to modify anti-social behavior after its use on hardcore disciplinary problems in the Texas correctional system.

Prisoners Improved

In the prison group sixteen out of nineteen showed improvement. Neither barbiturates nor other tranquilizers have produced satisfactory results with these patients, "classical psychopathic personalities with lifelong histories of anti-social behavior." With Librium, "it has been possible to maintain most of them in a placid but alert state despite their tension-provoking environment."

"From these results," the report adds, "it might be predicted that the compound would be of use in conduct disturbances in children and adolescents."

By relieving anxiety and tension, the drug has also been found to induce beneficial effects on diseases in which emotional factors are involved, several of the reports point out. These include ulcers and dermatologic problems.

February 28, 1960

REFORM IS URGED FOR MENTAL CARE

Study Asks Federal Funds for Patient Treatment

By EMMA HARRISON

A national mental health program designed to change drastically the public care of mentally ill persons will be presented to Congress today. It includes a proposal to use Federal funds for treatment.

The blueprint for changes in Federal, state and local programs of care and research is a result of more than five years of study by The Joint Commission on Mental Illness and Health, commissioned by Congress on July 28, 1955.

Senator Lister Hill, Democrat of Alabama, who introduced the resolution authorizing the study in the Senate, said earlier this week in a press briefing in Washington that he was prepared to join with the commission in urging adoption of its recommendations including Federal grants for treatment. He called these grants "not only needed, but warranted."

Among the study's startling findings was that 80 per cent of the nation's 277 state mental hospitals had not kept in step with modern advances in treatment and still provided custodial care rather than treatment for their patients.

The recommendations based on studies of the financial problems, the manpower situation, the extent of mental illness, general resources and public attitudes and opinions on mental illness and health, include the following:

¶Doubling of Federal, state and local spending for public mental health services in the next five years; tripling in the next ten, with the three levels of government sharing the costs of services to the mentally ill.

¶Ending as soon as possible the present state mental hospitals program, to be replaced by specialized intensive treatment hospitals, community clinics, general hospital care and emergency clinics. All mental hospitals with more than 1,000 beds would be converted to hospitals for all long-term chronic diseases, including psychiatric disorders.

¶Encouraging in form of loans, scholarships and income-tax relief, the entrance of more qualified people into mental health fields.

¶Increasing funds for basic research and more varied and long-term research to predict and prevent various forms of mental illness.

Mental Hospitals Scored

¶Redefining of what treatment is and who may do it within various contexts—hospitals, clinics, agencies and the like. The program should include psychologists, social workers and professional and nonprofessional workers without medical training, as well as psychiatrists and other physicians.

Under the commission's proposal for changes in state mental institutions, only three of New York State's twenty-seven civil institutions have fewer than 1,000 beds. These are the model research unit, New York Psychiatric Institute in New York City with 141 selected patients, Syracuse Psychiatric Hospital with fifty-seven resident patients, and Syracuse State School for Mental Defectives with 501 patients.

The other institutions all have populations of 2,000 or more. Pilgrim State at West Brentwood had a population of 11,960 in the 1959-60 census and was overcrowded to the extent of 27.8 per cent. Altogether the twenty-seven hospitals had a total capacity of 92,326 patients, but had a population of 111,344 patients. They were 21.5 per cent overcrowded.

Dr. Jack R. Ewalt, director of the study, told a news conference held at the offices of the American Psychiatric Association in Washington, one of the thirty-six organizations participating in the study, that the mentally ill were not yet a part of the New Frontier.

However, he said, with present knowledge put to use, the nation could more than double the number of chronically ill mental patients returned to the community.

The mental hospital must be integrated into the community, the report said. A major goal should be to end its isolation—where backward, custodial systems still thrive—and bring it out into the community where it may be observed and criticized. The report asserted:

"The state hospital must cease to be treated as a target for political exploitation. Patronage must end. These hospitals and their logical community extensions — clinics and after-care programs—must be manned in all cases by properly motivated career workers and not by hacks, professional or lay. These workers need to be well trained and well paid; they need the opportunity to do a good job and hence to demonstrate to the public what they can do."

In the study, the commission found that no more than 20 per cent of the 277 state hospitals had embraced new methods to make them therapeutic rather than custodial institutions.

Patients Not Treated

More than half of the patients in most state hospitals, the report noted, "receive no active treatment of any kind designed to improve their mental conditions." It said:

"This is the core problem and unfinished business of mental health. Eight of every ten mental hospital patients are in state institutions. These hospitals carry a daily load of more than 540,000 patients and look after nearly a million in a year's time."

The quality of care may readily be judged, the report continued, by comparing the average $4.44 spent for a patient a day by state hospitals with the $31.16 for community general hospitals and $12 for tuberculosis and Veterans Administration psychiatric hospitals. State hospitals have the lowest ratio of hospital personnel to patients, 0.32 for a patient compared with 2.1 in general hospitals.

One of the ten monographs of the commission, summarized in the commission's report, observed that "the lag in the treatment of the mentally ill reflects a fundamental pattern of social rejection" that is "nowhere better evidenced than by the continued existence of 'these' [custodial and punitive state hospitals] hospitals that seem to have no defenders but endure despite attacks."

"Too many persons who are alcoholics, addicts, social misfits, or otherwise mentally ill themselves have been given mental hospital positions ranging all the way from attendant to superintendent," it charged.

But, a trend toward greater competence has lately been observed, it was added.

The report listed as "preconditions of adequate patient care" funds for personnel, training, and research; replacement of political by professional control of mental health programs and agencies and the development of a "community atmosphere that is receptive to new ideas for the treatment of mental patients."

Summarizing an unpublished report, the commission cited a monograph, "Research Resources in Mental Health."

"The enormous patient-care task the mental health professions face today is matched only by the enormous research lag in the study of human behavior," the commission found.

The research report observed that "by comparison with polio we are not even in the 1908 stage in the sense of having discovered causes . . . In the area of mental illness and health we face not only biological problems, but psychological and social ones . . . The key to much of what we need to know lies buried in bits and fragments in the area of inquiry being investigated by a dozen scientific disciplines. . . ."

The commission found it a "false assumption that basic research should be done in universities; applied research in hospitals."

Studies have shown that the mental health research tends to be concentrated in small numbers of major universities and their medical centers. There should be wider support for flexible and experimental programs in many different areas and settings, it said.

Also, it said, efforts should be made to increase communications between researchers and practitioners as well as radically to increase long-term research support and to expand and intensify basic research.

The final report written by the joint commission staff drew on the findings of the ten basic studies in cost, manpower, community resources, the roles and effect of schools and the church in mental health, research, epidemiology and public attitudes, as well as other studies in the field of mental illness and health.

The study commission, which was originated by Dr. Kenneth E. Appel of Philadelphia, a former president of the American Psychiatric Association and president of the commission, has the following officers: Dr. Leo H. Bartemeier of Baltimore, chairman of the Council on Mental Health of the American Medical Association, chairman of the board of trustees; Dr. M. Brewster Smith of Berkeley, Calif., of the American Psychological Association, vice president; Charles Schlaifer of New York, of the National Association for Mental Health, secretary-treasurer; Dr. Nicholas Hobbs of Nashville, Tenn., of the American Psychological Association, vice chairman of the board of trustees.

The Federal grants for the study, under the National Institute of Mental Health, totaled $1,410,600. Private contributions, including the cost of publishing the final report given by the American Legion, totaled $132,427, for a grand total of $1,543,027. The ten monographs of the commission, six of which have been issued, have been published by Basic Books. The final report, "Action for Mental Health" is to be published April 3.

March 24, 1961

Punishing Treatment

LAW, LIBERTY AND PSYCHIATRY: An Inquiry Into the Social Uses of Mental Health Practices. By Thomas S. Szasz, M.D. 281 pp. New York: The Macmillan Company. $7.50.

By EDWARD de GRAZIA

ARISTOTLE noticed how punishment was a sort of medicine. Dr. Thomas S. Szasz shows how the medicine administered in psychiatric institutions is a sort of punishment, and punishment of the worst sort. Here is a documented thesis that the 250,000 human beings, who each year enter our mental hospitals, are systematically shorn of most of their Constitutional rights and treated in ways to strike dread into hardened criminals.

The author, himself a psychoanalyst and professor of psychiatry at State University of New York Medical Center, declares psychiatry to be a new form of social engineering—gravely dangerous where coercive. None of the criticism Dr. Szasz levels at institutional psychiatry has to do with Freud.

This bold and iconoclastic work takes up most of the faults committed in the name of mental illness, and lays down short-run and long-run solutions. In the process, not even the famed Durham insanity ruling* is left standing—the author seeing small gain for anyone in tossing a culprit into a looney bin instead of in the jug. What emerges is an informed, inspired credo of fair treatment for all persons charged with being mentally ill.

No such person should ever be involuntarily confined (not for pseudo-criminal behavior; not for being only "dangerous" to himself or others; not for otherwise deviating from ethical, political, social or sexual norms), but if ever, *never* without a prior court hearing with right to legal counsel, access to psychiatric experts, and a jury. No person should ever be led to incriminate himself through divulgence of his communications to psychiatrists in the hire of the state.

No person should ever be "punished" under the guise of being "treated." All persons should be humanely treated while imprisoned for their crimes—whether done by reason of insanity, mental illness, spite, anger, or the wish to deny, circumvent or overthrow the system. Thus to state what is

*The Durham ruling is that an accused is not criminally responsible if his unlawful act was the product of mental disease or mental defect.

A Washington attorney, Mr. de Grazia is author of "The Distinction of Being Mad."

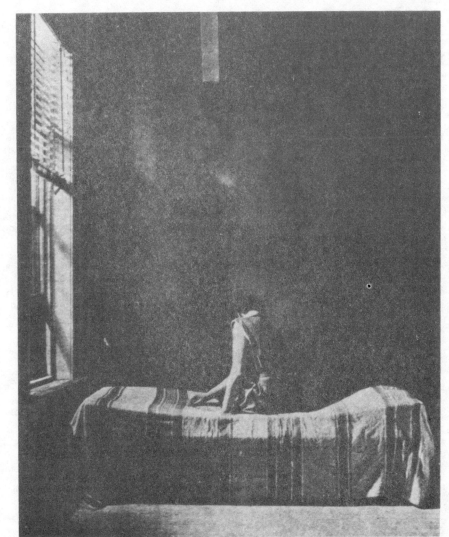

"No person should ever be 'punished' under the guise of being 'treated.'"   Photograph by David Linton.

wanted is pitiably far from what obtains.

It needs reminding that until recently neither our (liberal) criminal-law tradition nor our (backward) prison-administration philosophy ever had good excuse to invent and program such this-is-going-to-hurt-me-more-than-it-hurts-you "treatments" as electric shock, lobotomy and indeterminate (i.e., until dead or "cured") sentences for persons found involved in "potentially" criminal, deviant or otherwise obnoxious behavior. As the author points out, the Devil was the excuse for our witch-hunting forebears.

The excuse for institutional psychiatry has been that it is really the best medicine available, really in the best interests of the "patient," and really in another and high (i.e., therapeutic and scientific) league altogether than barbaric old vindictive criminal punishment. Dr. Szasz is even more alarmed over the Orwellian (even Buchenwaldian) dimensions of this psychiatric double-think, than over the many concrete wrongs he uncovers in this country's treat-

Supralegal

CERTAIN so-called therapeutic ventures have gradually assumed a supralegal existence in our society. Many public acts in the mental health field are accepted as legal, and constitutionally valid, solely because they are regarded as therapeutic. Laws sanctioning involuntary mental hospitalization and the control of so-called sexual psychopaths are two examples. However, these measures and others like them, should raise this question: When do ostensibly remedial social actions serve the purpose of moral reform, and when those of medical therapy?—"Law, Liberty and Psychiatry."

ment of the confined "mentally ill."

Dr. Szasz warns of psychiatric authoritarianism concealed in the spreading fear that we

are plagued by mental illness. From that fear stems the danger that we may be half-wittingly sowing the seeds for a bumper crop of new "inferior" beings—demi-criminals who may in reasonably good conscience be stripped of their human rights and mowed down into a sort of sub-group: they cannot be harmed (or blamed!) because they have no recognizable will, no mind to speak of, and need be put somewhere under the "best" possible care.

Although most patients, adults and children alike, are institutionalized by their loved ones, there are cases too where war, politics and religion have sent individuals to institutions. As Dr. Szasz suggests, it's a marvelous way of getting rid of trouble-makers. It can be speedier and surer than criminal prosecutions in a land where judges keep vigil over due process for accused criminals, but only nod or stare unseeing when men in white escort persons "certified" mentally ill behind tall walls.

January 26, 1964

MENTAL PATIENTS GET WIDER RIGHTS

By ROBERT E. TOMASSON

The authority to hospitalize mentally ill persons will pass tomorrow from judges to doctors when a major reform of the state's mental hygiene law goes into effect.

The new law will also end the indefinite hospitalization of non-criminal patients without legal review. This will be accomplished by the formation of a new arm of the state courts. The new agency will guarantee court hearings at specific intervals after admission.

The courts will continue, under the new law, to handle the cases of involuntary commitment of persons suspected of having committed crimes and who "do not act in the manner of a sane person." Essentially, these are persons who have been taken into custody by the police.

Described by its drafters as the country's most revolutionary mental health legislation in a century, the law seeks to encourage early voluntary treatment of the mentally disturbed before hospitalization becomes mandatory.

The state's Department of Mental Hygiene hopes this can be accomplished by making all civil admissions a medical concern removing the possibility of indefinite confinement and by a legal obligation imposed on all state and local officials concerned to encourage voluntary treatment.

In both language and theory, the new law attempts to remove the stigma often attached to court - ordered commitments, which account for about 60 per cent of the 90,000 hospital patients now being treated for mental illness in the state.

"Mental hospitals are not prisons. . . . When a person must be sent to a mental hospital against his will, he should not be treated like a criminal and be tried and convicted of being sick. Procedures for his admission are only *stepping-stones to treatment."

That statement is in the opening chapter of "Mental Illness and Due Process," a Cornell Law School Study that formed the basis for the new law.

A special committee of the Association of the Bar of the City of New York and the state Mental Hygiene Department cooperated in the four-year study. Several other private, governmental and judicial organizations offered suggestions.

The title of the new law, Hospitalization of the Mentally Ill, replaces Commitment, Custody, Maintenance and Discharge of the Insane. Certain terms will be dropped, including "insane inmate" and "custody." They are reminiscent of the era nearly 125 years ago when New York's first state hospital for "the insane" was established in Utica.

The new law is not retroactive and will affect only persons admitted (the word "committed" is not in the new measure) starting tomorrow.

The law also does not apply to mental defectives—persons with congenital defects or those who have suffered irreparable brain damage as a result of injuries or severe physical illness.

Under the old law the involuntary civil commitment of a person was initiated by the petition of a friend or relative to a judge, accompanied by a certificate of two doctors.

The petition, if granted, resulted in a certification order committing the person to 60 days of examination and treatment.

If during the 60-day period the hospital director, on the recommendations of his staff psychiatrists, felt that the patient should be retained beyond the two-month period, he filed a certificate in the County Clerk's office.

The judge's original certification then became final and no further legal step was required of the hospital in order to keep the patient for an indefinite period against his will.

The basic method for admission of involuntary patients under the new law will also involve an initial petition and a two-doctor certificate. But instead of submission of these forms to a judge, the admission will be completed if a hospital staff psychiatrist examines the person and agrees he should be hospitalized.

The old law excluded state hospital psychiatrists from this initial decision-making process.

At the time patients are admitted, starting tomorrow, an elaborate series of new legal safeguards will start to function to insure against any violations of civil liberties.

One of the most striking legal features of the new hospitalization program is the establishment of a new arm of the state courts called the Mental Health Information Service. This will periodically inform patients of their legal rights, with additional notices going to a relative and as many as three other persons.

The service, believed to be the only one of its kind in the United States, will also function as an investigative and reporting service for the courts. It will have no decision-making power.

Written notice must be given to the patient not later than five days after he is admitted, informing him of his rights. Copies must go to the information service, the patient's nearest relative and up to three others named by the patient.

Any of the recipients, including the patient, may then request a court hearing within 60 days after admission. The hospital will then send the court a copy of the request, together with the patient's file, and a date for hearing must be set within five days.

If the court decides that the patient should be retained it will issue an order authorizing continued hospitalization for a maximum six-month period.

If, however, no application is made for a hearing and the hospital director believes hospitalization beyond 60 days is needed, he must still apply for a court certification for permission to keep the patient an additional six months after the initial 60-day period.

And if treatment beyond eight months is sought, an additional order must be obtained for a maximum period of one year. Subsequent orders are for two-year periods.

At every step in this procedure the patient, a relative, up to three others and the information service are served with written notices.

Court certifications are not required however if, during his treatment, the patient agrees to remain on a voluntary basis.

The effect of the new law thus will be to abolish the indefinite, involuntary hospitalization of the mentally ill and replace it with a system that provides for periodic reviews, after a 60-day medical admission, occurring at intervals of six months, one year and then two-year periods.

A system of informal and voluntary admissions has been in effect in the state for two years, but with what is considered limited success.

In an informal admission the patient, on recommendation of a doctor, submits himself for treatment. If a hospital staff psychiatrist agrees he is suitable for treatment he is admitted and thereafter can demand his release at any time. No written application for admission is required.

A voluntary admission is one in which a person makes a written application and is accepted for hospitalization. He must stay for at least 15 days. If he then wishes to leave he must notify the head of the hospital, who must then release him within 10 after receipt of the request for discharge.

Hyman M. Forstenzer, Assistant Commissioner for Policy Planning in the Mental Hygiene Department, has noted that "many hospital directors were less than enthusiastic" about such admissions.

Mr. Forstenzer said: "They felt that their acceptance of a voluntary admission carried with it implication that they had judged the patient to have the capacity to make a decision about his need for hospitalization."

The new law prohibits any requirement that the admission or retention of patients be based on their legal capacity to make a contract.

E. David Wiley, chief counsel of the Mental Hygiene Department, has declared:

"The fact that a patient would not be considered competent to enter into a contract would not disqualify him from making application as a voluntary or informal patient or to prevent his involuntary status being changed to voluntary or informal.

"This is one of the core provisions of this law and could very well mean that most, if not all, open-ward patients in mental hospitals who are willing would become voluntary or informal patients by operation of the law. They would therefore effectively be removed from any legalistic procedures that apply to involuntary patients."

In what another spokesman for the department has called a "compromise between the legal and medical professions," the new system strengthens standby legal safeguards while emphasizing that treatment of mental illness should be a voluntary relationship between patient and doctor.

August 31, 1965

Chemical Test Used to Detect Extent of Serious Mental Ills

By RICHARD D. LYONS

A chemical test has been developed that can determine the extent and severity of serious mental illness, two brain specialists reported yesterday.

They said the test, involving the detection of a protein in the cerebrospinal fluid, has been up to 90 per cent accurate in calculating the degree of psychosis in 338 persons given the examination.

The test, the development of which started at Harvard Medical School about 10 years ago, most recently was applied to 131 patients at St. Vincent's Hospital in New York.

The developer of the test is Dr. Samuel Bogoch, director of the Foundation for Research on the Nervous System, who is associate research professor at the Boston University Medical School.

Dr. Bogoch said in an interview that the test involved tapping a small amount of cerebrospinal fluid from the lumbar region of the lower back. Cerebrospinal fluid is a clear, colorless substance surrounding the brain and the spinal cord.

The level of glycoprotein neuraminic acid, one component of the brain's gray matter, is then determined. The amount of glycoprotein neuraminic acid, Dr. Bogoch said, indicates the severity of psychosis—the lower the level, the more serious the illness. Dr. Bogoch said the test was accurate in about 90 per cent of those tested. Most of these persons were schizophrenics, but they also included persons who were depressed or manic, he said.

"There is also a correlation with treatment," Dr. Bogoch said. "If the patients improve, regardless of the treatment, the glycoprotein neuraminic acid levels increase in about 85 per cent."

In about 70 per cent of the cases in which mental patients become worse, the glycoprotein neuraminic acid levels decrease, he said. The reason for the fluctuation, as well as the reason for its link between the chemical and mental illness, is not known.

Dr. Bogoch, a psychiatrist and biochemist, first reported the relationship between glycoprotein neuraminic acid levels and schizophrenia 10 years ago. Since then, he said, its relationship with other forms of mental illness has been discovered.

He was interviewed during the final meeting of the conference on the Future of the Brain Sciences at the New York Academy of Medicine. The conference was sponsored by the Manfred Sakel Institute and the Foundation for Research on the Nervous System.

At the conference, Dr. Robert Campbell, the director of the out-patient section of the department of psychiatry at St. Vincent's Hospital, reported confirmation of the test's accuracy.

Tried on 131 Persons

Dr. Campbell said the test had been successfully tried on 131 schizophrenics at the hospital for periods of from three months to two years. He said he did not attempt to use the test on persons with other forms of mental illness. Schizophrenia is a form of mental illness marked by a withdrawal from reality. It is believed to be caused by both genetic and environment factors.

The test indicates that perhaps this is a measure of the maturation of the central nervous system, which includes the brain, Dr. Campbell said in an interview.

Dr. Bogoch said the levels of glycoprotein neuraminic acid in adult schizophrenics is comparable to the levels in normal children. This might indicate a form of chemical immaturity of the central nervous system, which would correlate with evidence of psychological immaturity in schizophrenics.

Dr. Bogoch said no attempt had been made to apply the test to children with mental difficulties in an effort to distinguish if the trouble was either retardation or psychosis.

Dr. Bogoch said the test had not been more widely employed because "most psychiatrists are not interested in chemistry and don't want to bother performing lumbar punctures" to tap the spinal fluid.

"The current mode of the practice of psychiatry is talking, not touching, so most of the laboratory procedures that general medicine uses are only employed if there is concern for gross neurological disorders, such as brain damage," he said.

"We only know that the fluctuation of the glycoprotein neuraminic acid is a reliable index of the course of mental illness," he said. "The next step might be the use of the test as a means of evaluating methods of treatment for serious psychotic disorders."

May 5, 1968

Personal Finance: When Mental Illness Hits

By ROBERT J. COLE

When Johnny came marching home after World War II, almost a quarter of a century ago, he brought back a chestful of medals, a pocketful of souvenirs, an occasional war bride—and, all too often, a certain strangeness his family and friends couldn't help but notice.

Phrases like service-connected disability, psychosomatic condition, Section 8 and psycho ward came into common usage. Top comedians such as Jack Benny and Bob Hope found that jokes about analysts and their couches were always good for a few laughs. The public finally had become aware of a problem that has always been with us.

•

Some now-forgotten comedian went so far as to remark: "Anyone who goes to a psychiatrist ought to have his head examined."

Today, psychiatry is no laughing matter.

The latest figures of the National Institute for Mental Health, compiled two years ago, would suggest that well over two and a half million people a year—18 per cent of them under 18 years old — get treatment for some form of mental illness in clinics and hospitals across the country.

Not included in these figures are the thousands of patients treated by private psychiatrists, community mental health centers now developing under a new Federal program, day and night care centers, half-way houses and residential treatment centers for children.

Fortunately, labor and management generally agree today that when an employe gets sick it does not necessarily mean a touch of arthritis or an infected finger. Very often it can also mean alcoholism or anxiety.

And, too, industry in many instances has moved quickly to provide the facilities to help mend sick employes and to hold down the heavy burden of medical bills. The list of companies with strong medical departments runs into the hundreds. Typical are those of United States Steel, Continental Insurance, Eastman Kodak, Consolidated Edison and International Business Machines.

Thousands of companies now have provisions for psychiatric care under group insurance medical plans. Most plans, such as Blue Cross and many major medical programs, provide in-hospital care. A few plans also cover in-office treatment by psychiatrists.

Unions have taken an active role in providing mental care for their members. Prominent among them are the Retail Clerks, Local 770, Los Angeles; the Teamsters union in St. Louis; the Amalgamated Clothing Workers in New York and the United Automobile Workers around the nation at plants of Chrysler, Ford and General Motors.

Some companies, when working directly with employes, even dip into emergency funds and contribute to the cost of special treatment that many employes need but can't afford.

Nevertheless, when mental illness strikes, thousands of people still find they can't afford the luxury of treatment.

•

Psychiatrists now get an average of $30 an hour. Some charge much more; a few charge less. Free treatment is a rarity Private hospital costs vary widely but $35 a day is one estimate. Total costs vary very widely but can run into the thousands for extended treatment.

If money is a key factor in obtaining treatment, low-cost (or when warranted, no-cost) mental care can be found—but it won't be quick. There are exceptions, of course, in crisis situations.

At the Manhattan Society for Mental Health, Bertram Weinert, executive director, says he can on occasion find a psychiatrist who will work for as little as $15 an hour when the patient can't afford more.

Similar organizations are available across the country. They can be found in the Yellow Pages under "clinics," through clergyman, service and welfare agencies and through the family doctor or local medical society.

Mr. Weinert notes that the Manhattan Society, when the situation warrants, will recommend an out-patient clinic, many of which across the country charge according to ability to pay. Some may have set fees, say from $3 a visit to $10 or $12 a visit.

Also available, he points out, are the psychiatric clinics of public and voluntary hospitals. One major problem, however, he notes, is that most psychiatric clinics have long waiting lists, with treatment often as much as seven or eight months away.

In summer, too, many clinics close and treatment is not available except for acute problem cases. Moreover, clinics, except for a few, like St. Vincent's Hospital in New York, are not open at night when workers are generally free.

"It's not easy to say to your employer, 'I'm leaving to go to my psychiatric clinic,'" Mr. Weinert explains.

•

In addition to psychia-trists, organizations like the Manhattan Society often can recommend other professionals such as psychologists or psychiatric social workers, who in many cases charge less than psychiatrists. In this connection, the society recommends only psychiatrists but is considering changing its policy to recommend other professionals. It also makes referrals to out-patient clinics.

Patients also might consider conferring with such agencies as Catholic Charities, the Federation of Jewish Philanthropies or Federation of Protestant Welfare Agencies.

Many people often turn to the family physician, general practioner, internist or, in the case of women, to the gynecologist. The generalist, one nationally known psychiatrist says, can, if properly trained, do "a great deal" in the treatment of all kinds of mental disorders—from ulcers to serious psychotic reaction.

Then, if the patient's job is shown to be responsible for the medical condition, the employe may be eligible under workmen's compensation regulations for outpatient or hospital treatment for whatever may be required.

August 1, 1968

Mental Health Centers Bring Psychiatry Close to Home

By NANCY HICKS

Special to The New York Times

PHILADELPHIA—A short, plump community worker excused herself from a staff meeting in a church office here the other day and walked over to a large wooden desk to make a telephone call.

"Hello, Mrs. Jones," she said. "I have the money for you to buy your furniture, so all you have to do is go pick it out."

"What do you mean you don't know what store to go to? Take the telephone book and look for one. Or go to the shopping district and look for one.

"Okay, let me know how you make out.'"

As the conversation ended, the community worker sighed. "I know it's hard," she said. "Many people are just frightened and don't know how to begin to approach this system to solve their problems. But we just have to help them help themselves as much as possible."

Mental Health Worker

The woman was not another social worker trying to help a poor family with welfare and consumer problems. Rather, she was a worker at the Temple University Community Mental Health Center here, and she was taking part in a new approach to mental health care.

The Temple University center is one of 185 such facilities that have opened around the country — in outlying areas like Sheridan, Wyo., and Nephi, Utah, as well as major cities—since the Federal Government appropriated $364-million matched funds to finance the Community Mental Health Acts of 1963 and 1965.

In 1968 the centers provided 9 per cent of all mental health care in the nation. One hundred-eighty more have been funded and are scheduled to open over the next few years.

Community mental health programs seek to decentralize psychology from large state institutions to local communities. The direction is much the same as that of medicine in general.

The programs established are drawn up according to local needs. One rural Midwestern center has a "worry clinic" for housewives. One in the Southwest works with Mexican-Americans. One in New York City has special programs for the deaf and the elderly. Often the programs make psychiatric care available near the home for the first time.

'Preventive' Effort Made

All of the centers must provide traditional services— inpatient and outpatient facilities, partial hospitalization (day or night hospitals), emergency facilities — but they also must provide "education and consultation" as part of "preventive psychiatry."

It is this factor that constitutes the "bold new approach" called for by President Kennedy six years ago when the community mental health program was first proposed.

In the years since then many of the centers have been caught up in turmoil.

Local financial support has lagged. The original law assumed that local authorities would take over financial responsibility for the centers within 51 months, but money has proved scarce on the local level.

Some leaders in the field now think that the Government was mistaken in making the local funding stipulation in the first place. In any case, legislation increasing aid to the program has passed both houses of Congress and at present is waiting action in a conference committee.

Critics say that the program waters down psychiatry by taking it out of the usual office setting, sometimes into the streets. Some groups in poorer areas are also skeptical about the program, fearing that it will try to make them "cool it," or settle for their poverty.

The defenders say, however, that the program offers a new answer to some of the larger problems affecting many people's lives. They say the program is successful because it has helped the poor and the scared mobilize inner strengths to work out the problems of daily living.

The effectiveness of the program, however, is difficult to assess, if for no other reason because mental health itself is difficult to assess.

"The centers are having an

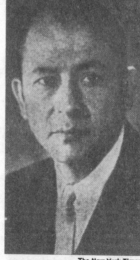

The New York Times

Dr. Saul Feldman, associate director for Community Mental Health Services of National Institute of Mental Health in Bethesda, Md.

impact on the utilization of state hospitals," said Dr. Saul Feldman, community mental health official with the National Institute of Mental Health in Bethesda, Md.

"Sixteen per cent of all patients seen in community mental health centers in 1968 were formerly hospitalized in state institutions," he said. "But many of the patients had never used mental health services before."

A System of Services

A community mental health center is not a place; it is a service-delivering system, sometimes situated in several locations. Some centers are housed in new buildings; others are in renovated structures. Many have satellite units.

Since the program is decentralized, there are many types of centers and results are mixed. In untroubled areas of the country, the programs tend to follow the traditional psychiatric approach.

In areas where many social problems exist — New York, Houston, Chicago, Philadelphia, San Francisco — the centers have become involved in community action programs aimed at eradicating the larger environmental problems in which emotional illness breeds.

There is general agreement that the program here at Temple, one of 10 in the city, is a good one. Its administrators and staff think so. Officials in Washington think so. Community mental health workers, who generally feel that their lives are overanalyzed, think so too.

The program, under the direction of Dr. Elmer A. Gardner, has built its reputation on its size and the "modern thinking" that goes into its projects.

Patients Set Own Rules

Patients at the day hospital set their own rules. They decide when a member of the group is ready to leave. The emergency unit, or Crisis Center, accepts all patients except those under arrest. (Many centers elsewhere reject actively suicidal or homocidal patients.) The police here often bring people to the center instead of putting them under arrest.

An example of preventive psychiatry as practiced under this approach was given by John B. Dunham. director of the day hospital of the Temple University Center.

He told of a woman who went to a center with her rent receipts, which showed that she had paid her rent, and a dispossess order from her landlord, which contended that she had not.

"She had all the symptoms of psychotic depression but she did not have that condition," Dr. Dunham said. "But with her housing problem, why shouldn't she be depressed?"

The center interceded with the courts, and she was able to keep her apartment.

A 16-year-old girl at a New York center was helped in a more traditional way. She had been hospitalized at a state mental institution with a severe disorder that kept her from taking care of herself. She had slept most of the time, dressed very sloppily, never combed her hair.

With drug treatment and psychotherapy in a relaxed center hospital, she has greatly improved, primping, now, as much as any other teen-age girl and preparing to return home.

While walking along North Philadelphia's Tioga Street in front of one of the three-story attached houses that make up the center, Mrs. Barbara Hodges, a mental health worker at Temple and mother of four, talked about the mental health movement.

New Concept Suggested

Maybe, she suggested, as have many nonprofessional workers, there should just be neighborhood centers that offer a range of services of which psychiatry would be only one. A newly formed community advisory board, which is making policy decisions, is working with that is mind. Its members' goal is to de-emphasize the pathology of their lives and stress other programs, such as schools and self-help efforts.

The relationship of a center to its community and especially to its nonprofessional workers — who are often part of the target population—is a pivotal factor in the smooth and effective operation of a center.

The Community Mental Health Center of the West Side Medical Center in Chicago has alleviated some of its problems in community relations by subcontracting basic field work to two black activist groups. One includes former convicts, the other students.

New York's boldest experiment, the center of Lincoln Hospital in the Bronx, was crippled by nonprofessionals who struck for several weeks last year, contendeding that they did not have enough control over operations and that the hospital had not lived up to its promise to upgrade workers, with accompanying educational programs, into professional positions. The program has never recovered its original drive.

In Brooklyn, however, the Maimonides Center is hailed as one of the best in the country. It is one of five in the city and serves a population of 110,000, the majority of whom are white working class families. It also has a large Puerto Rican population and a disproportionately large number of elderly citizens. The programs reflect all these facts.

A visit to the inpatient facility on the top floor of the four-story, modern structure showed no uniforms, pajamas, bars or locked doors, although several young girls—some former state hospital patients—were banging unharmoniously on a piano.

"If you don't lock people in, they don't feel as though they have to get out," Mark Tarail, a PhD in social work and administrative director of the program explained.

January 11, 1970

Long-Studied Drug Is Licensed For Treatment of Mental Illness

By HAROLD M. SCHMECK Jr.
Special to The New York Times

WASHINGTON, April 6— The Food and Drug Administration has licensed the much-discussed drug lithium carbonate for treatment of a common form of mental illness, the manic phase of manic-depressive psychosis.

Some experts consider the drug to be far the most effective treatment for the condition. Lithium is widely used for that purpose elsewhere in the world, but has not previously been licensed in the United States because of concern over its potential dangers.

The action by the drug agency indicates that its officers have decided the drug is too useful to be barred any longer, although it must be used with caution. It has been under study in the United States for at least five years but has been in use much longer than that elsewhere. Indeed, the study that is generally considered definitive was completed in 1954 by Dr. Mogens Schou of Denmark. The drug was first reported useful against mental illness in 1949 by Dr. J. F. J. Cade of Australia.

Manic-depressive illness is considered one of the two most common forms of serious mental illness in the United States. The other is schizophrenia.

In a telephone conversation today Dr. Frederick Goodwin of the National Institute of Mental Health said the treatment of the manic-depressive patient had been particularly discouraging in the past. Two main avenues of treatment for the manic state have beeen electroshock and heavy doses of tranquilizers. Neither has been entirely satisfactory.

Dr. Goodwin, who is chief investigator in the institute's studies of lithium treatment, said lithium seemed to treat the manic symptoms. In contrast, tranquilizers have only a sedative effect, leaving the patients subdued but still manic, he said, and electroshock treatment is usually temporary and sometimes results in severe side-effects.

The person in the manic state is usually overactive, talks too loudly and too rapidly, has grandiose ideas of his own abilities and is likely to undertake entirely impractical schemes often with the foolish spending of large sums of money. The other side of the coin is the depressive state, in which the same person may be suicidal.

The Food and Drug Administration sent out letters to manufacturers Friday announcing that lithium carbonate could be sold as a prescription drug for treating acute manic episodes of manic-depressive psychosis. One manufacturer, Smith Kline & French Laboratories of Philadelphia, announced the availability of Eskalith, its brand of the drug, today. Others are expected to follow. Since the drug is simply the carbonate salt of the metallic element lithium, it is not patentable.

The fact that it cannot be patented is considered one probable reason for the long delay in licensing it in the United States. Many drug companies have presumably not considered the effort and expense of preparing the case for it to be economically worthwhile.

Another probable reason, according to one specialist, was the bad experience doctors had many years ago with the use of lithium salts as replacements for ordinary table salt—sodium chloride—for persons who required low salt diets.

The lithium produced severe effects on the central nervous system. Study showed that the ill effects of lithium were when a person was taking too little salt. In fact, the F.D.A., in licensing the use of lithium carbonate for treatment of manic-depressives, is requiring that the drug be labeled to include the warning that it should be used only when the patient is on a normal diet.

The dose range at which toxic effects may occur is only three times the normal treatment range. That gives substantially less margin of safety than most tranquilizers.

The early symptoms of toxicity from lithium include diarrhea, vomiting, muscular weakness and lack of coordination and drowsiness, according to the required labeling. It is not recommended for use in children nor in women of childbearing age unless the alternative methods of treatment have been tried without success.

Dr. Goodwin, whose group has studied about 50 patients over a five-year period, said a great potential value of the drug is in prevention of both maniac and depressive episodes in patients subject to them.

April 7, 1970

203

Nader Report Scores U.S. Unit On Mental Health Center Plan

WASHINGTON, July 22 (UPI)—A report by a Ralph Nader group charged today that the Federally financed community mental health center system designed to replace state hospitals had been "vastly oversold" and "quickly perverted" into a new bureaucracy largely unresponsive to local needs.

"That community mental health centers are largely irrelevant to significant numbers of people and to the societal problems that certain of their advocates would 'cure' has become almost a cliche in psychiatric circles," said part I of a Nader's Raiders report that will later examine child mental health and suicide prevention.

The authors, Franklin D. Chu, a 1971 Harvard graduate, and Sharland Trotter, a 1965 Goucher College graduate, also asserted the following:

¶The National Institute of Mental Health has been a full partner in the dumping of mental patients by state hospitals into nursing or foster homes where conditions are even worse.

¶Community mental health centers routinely exclude drug addicts, alcoholics, old people, children of ethnic and racial minorities and the poor.

¶Citizens have no legitimate voice in fiscal or program policy for the centers where community boards generally include charity-minded housewives, businessmen, lawyers, ministers, judges and professional persons whose main function is to raise money.

"The centers offer mostly a collection of traditional clinical services that provide more jobs and office space for mental health professionals, but which remain inaccessible or irrelevant to large segments of the community," concluded a summary of the report by Mr.

Nader's Center for Study of Responsive Law.

The national institute has provided $529.8-million for building and staffing 476 centers in 50 states, Puerto Rico, Guam and the District of Columbia since the community center law was passed in 1963. However, only 325 centers were operating as a June 1, with the largest numbers in California, 42; Pennsylvania, 37; Kentucky, 23, and New York and Texas, 22 each.

The institute's director, Bertram S. Brown, said: "The community mental health centers program is in the process of effective and productive change. The Nader report will help that process."

July 23, 1972

8 Feign Insanity in Test And Are Termed Insane

By SANDRA BLAKESLEE
Special to The New York Times

STANFORD, Calif., Jan. 20—Can the sane be distinguished from the insane in psychiatric hospitals?

Eight individuals decided to find out. Each feigned symptoms of mental instability and was admitted to a mental hospital. The result: doctors labeled them as schizophrenics despite their best efforts to convince the hospital staff of their sanity.

Results of this three-year experiment appear in the latest issue of Science, the journal of the American Association for the Advancement of Science. The article was written by Dr. David L. Rosenhan, professor of psychology and law at Stanford University, who led the experimental group, which included, besides Dr. Rosenhan, three psychologists, a pediatrician, a psychiatrist, a painter and a housewife. They were not named in the article.

Conflicting Views Common

It is commonplace, Dr. Rosenhan said, to read of conflicting views among psychiatrists as to whether the defendant in a murder case is sane or insane. In fact, he said, "we know we cannot distinguish sanity from insanity." This is depressing and frightening, he said.

How many people are sane but not recognized as such in our psychiatric institutions? How many have been stripped of their rights as citizens? How many have feigned insanity to avoid the criminal consequences of their behavior?

In the traditional view of psychiatry, Dr. Rosenhan wrote, patients present symptoms that can be categorized, which implies a distinction can be drawn between the sane and insane.

Another view, Dr. Rosenhan said, holds that diagnoses are almost always influenced by the environment and context in which the psychiatrist examines the patient. In other words, a hospital setting prejudices the doctor to assume that a patient is mentally ill.

To test which view is correct the pseudopatients had themselves admitted to mental hospitals under assumed names and occupations. They all told the same story. They said that they heard strange voices that said "empty," "hollow" and "thud."

Otherwise, they told the truth about themselves, including relationships with family and friends, their frustrations and upsets, and their joys and satisfactions.

Some of the eight got into more than one hospital—a total of 12 hospitals were involved in the test. The hospitals were in five states on the East and West Coasts. Neither the hospitals nor the states were named in the article. Some of the hospitals were old, some quite new. Some were research-oriented. All were supported by state or Federal funds or, in one case, by university funds.

Once in the ward the pseudopatients stopped faking their symptoms. At first they were nervous — surprised they had been admitted so easily, knowing they had to get out on their own devices. But soon they settled into the hospital routine.

Nearly 2,100 Pills Given

They spoke to patients and staff members as they normally would to anyone. They accepted medication but flushed it down a toilet — as they saw some other patients do also. All told, they were given nearly 2,100 pills, primarily tranquilizers.

When asked how they felt, they said "fine," their symptoms had disappeared.

Since there was little to do in the wards all the pseudopatients took copious notes of what was happening. At first they hid their note-taking but soon saw that no one cared and they did it openly.

Some patients began to voice suspicions about them. "You're not crazy. You're a journalist or a professor. You're checking up on the hospital."

But the hospital staffs never questioned the regular note-taking. One nurse saw it as a symptom of a crazy compulsion. "Patient engages in writing behavior," she wrote on his chart day after day.

The hospital staffs often misinterpreted their feelings, the pseudopatients reported. Once a friendly nurse found a pseudopatient pacing the long hospital corridors. "Nervous, Mr.——?" she asked. "No bored," he replied.

Patients and staffs saw little of one another in all the hospitals, they found. Staff members emerged primarily for caretaker purposes, the experimenters said, and kept to themselves as if the disorders they treated were contagious.

One pseudopatient stopped a doctor. "Excuse me, Dr.——. Could you tell me when I am eligible for ground privileges?" Physician: "Good morning, Dave. How are you today?" The doctor moved on without waiting for an answer.

In one instance a patient was beaten by an attendant in front of other patients for having approached the attendant and saying, "I like you." Powerlessness was evident everywhere.

All Termed Schizophrenic

The pseudopatients' experiment was not detected at any of the 12 hospitals. Each pseudopatient was discharged with a diagnosis of schizophrenia "in remission." The length of hospital stays ranged from seven to

52 days with an average of 19 days.

The tragedy, Dr. Rosenhan said, is that labels do not go away. "A diagnosis of cancer that has been found in error is a cause of celebration," he said; "but psychiatric diagnoses are rarely found in error. The label sticks."

The physicians' failure to detect sanity, he said, may lie in their inclination to look for illness rather than health; it is better to err on the side of caution and suspect illness even among the healthy. The trouble with this approach in psychiatry, he said, is that there are such terrible stigmas attached to mental illness.

Pseudopatients Expected

To see if the tendency towards diagnosing the sane as insane could be reversed, Dr. Rosenhan arranged a second experiment. The staff at a research and teaching hospital who had heard and disbelieved the results of the first experiment were told that at some time during the next three months one or more pseudopatients would seek admittance to their hospital. Each staff member was therefore on his guard to detect any pseudopatient.

The staff members recorded their opinions about 193 patients who were admitted during the trial period. Forty-one were said to be pseudopatients by at least one staff member. Twenty-three patients were considered suspect by at least one psychiatrist.

But Dr. Rosenhan had sent no pseudopatients to the hospital. Were the patients sane or not?

"We will never know," Dr. Rosenhan said. "But of one thing we may be certain: any diagnostic process that yields so readily to massive errors of this sort cannot be a very reliable one."

January 21, 1973

Brain Surgery to Alter Behavior Stirs a Major Medical Debate

By HAROLD M. SCHMECK Jr.
Special to The New York Times

WASHINGTON, Jan. 21 — Man's brain is his last citadel of freedom and individuality, but even this is now under assault, according to critics of a practice called psychosurgery.

The word is usually defined to mean surgery on the brain for the purpose of modifying human behavior, or electrical stimulation of parts of the brain for the same purpose.

Only a few teams of doctors are known to be practicing psychosurgery, but medical experts are concerned about the lack of information on the subject and fearful about possible proliferation of the practice without adequate safeguards.

Defenders and critics of the operations spoke last week at a symposium at the National Institutes of Health in Bethesda, Md.

Concern Expressed

An audience of several hundred heard psychosurgery denounced as achieving a partial death of the patient and defended as a means of returning to manageable behavior some patients who have been wildly self-destructive and totally beyond cure through psychiatry or the use of drugs.

The symposium was organized by employes of the N.I.H. and the National Institute of Mental Health who are concerned over a proposal to appropriate $1-million in Federal funds for research on diagnosis and treatment, including psychosurgery, of behavior disorders.

"A number of employes at the National Institutes of Health have constituted themselves as an ad hoc committee having severe reservations over the use and abuse of neurosurgical techniques in the modification of human behavior," said Dr. George Ellsworth, a staff psychiatrist at the N.I.M.H. He was moderator of the Bethesda discussion.

Mutilation Charged

He said many scientists questioned the scientific basis for the procedures and were concerned over the "likelihood that they are employed principally on the traditionally powerless segment of our society—namely women, children and blacks."

Concern over the choice of patients for such operations was also expressed by the Rev. David Eaton, senior minister of All Souls Unitarian Church in Washington.

Dr. Peter R. Breggin, a psychiatrist of the Washington School of Psychiatry, said psychosurgery did make the patient more tractable and docile, but only through a generalized blunting action achieved by what he termed mutilation of parts of the brain. He described this as a partial death of the individual.

Speaking in favor of neurosurgery for extreme behavioral disorders, Dr. O. J. Andy, the chairman of the Department of Neurosurgery at the University of Mississippi at Jackson, said the procedure was done only on persons for whom all other forms of treatment were clearly hopeless; and then only with the consent of patient and family.

He described the typical psychosurgery patient as erratic, hyperactive, uncontrollably violent, given to attacks on others and unresponsive to psychiatric and psychological treatment.

He said neurosurgery could also be useful in brain damaged children and adolescents who exhibit that kind of behavior. It would allow their developing brains to mature with as normal a reaction to the environment as possible.

Dr. Andy said he had operated on somewhat more than 30 patients. In answer to a question, he said that the majority of them had been white.

Clampdown Expected

Dr. Paul D. MacLean of the N.I.M.H., internationally known for brain research in animals, said he believed the medical profession would call an end to psychosurgery. He emphasized, however, that he was not including in the definition of psychosurgery operations for obvious brain damage, as is sometimes the case in epilepsy.

Dr. A. K. Ommaya, a neurosurgeon of the N.I.H., said surgery for behavioral problems must be undertaken only with great caution, but he added that there were extreme cases in which it was warranted. He cited some grave behavioral disorders and some cases of intense and intractable pain in patients approaching death from conditions such as cancer.

Of patients for whom he considers the operations justifiable, he said: "Nobody knows the hell and misery that they live in unless you actually face such a problem."

January 22, 1973

HIGH COURT CURBS POWER TO CONFINE THE MENTALLY ILL

If Not Dangerous, a Patient Cannot Be Held Against Will Without Treatment

By WARREN WEAVER Jr.
Special to The New York Times

WASHINGTON, June 26— The Supreme Court ruled unanimously today that mental patients cannot be confined in institutions against their will and without treatment if they are dangerous to no one and are capable of surviving on the outside.

The ruling appeared likely to force the ultimate release from mental institutions of thousands of the estimated total of 250,000 patients regarded as untreated, harmless and not likely to become community charges.

"May the state fence in the harmless mentally ill solely to save its citizens from exposure to those whose ways are different?" Associate Justice Potter Stewart inquired rhetorically in the opinion.

"One might as well ask if the state, to avoid public unease, could incarcerate all who are physically unattractive or socially eccentric. Mere public intolerance or animosity cannot constitutionally justify the deprivation of a person's physical liberty."

Two Key Questions Left

The high court refused, however, to answer two related constitutional questions: whether the dangerous mentally ill have a right to treatment when involuntarily confined and whether the state can confine the nondangerous mentally ill against their will to give them treatment.

Bruce Ennis of the New York Civil Liberties Union, who argued the case in the Supreme Court, said the decision meant that "mental hospitals as we have known them can no longer exist in this country as dumping grounds for the old, the poor and the friendless." Such institutions, he said, "will have to re-evaluate the status of each patient."

Kenneth Donaldson, whose suit for damages took the case to the high court, said at a news conference here that the ruling was "a victory for common sense."

The Role of Treatment

Mr. Donaldson spent nearly 15 years in a Florida mental hospital before his release in 1971.

Chief Justice Warren E. Burger, in a concurring opinion, made it clear that he did not feel, on the one hand, that all legally confined persons had a right to treatment or, on the other, that providing treatment might justify confining an otherwise functional citizen.

Throughout the Court's opinion, Justice Stewart suggested that Mr. Donaldson, now 67 years old, might not have been entitled to discharge if he had been receiving some sort of treatment beyond custodial care, but he left the question unresolved.

A finding of mental illness "alone," Mr. Stewart wrote, cannot justify locking up a patient against his will and keeping him indefinitely in "simple custodial" confinement. Later the Justice said that a state cannot confine a harmless patient constitutionally without more than a finding of mental illness if the patient could survive safely in the outside world.

The New York Civil Liberties Union called the ruling "a landmark legal victory in the effort to oppose involuntary commitment of mental patients." Mr. Ennis estimated that it would establish a new right to freedom for "many thousands" of harmless mental hospital inmates.

Mr. Donaldson was committed to a state hospital in Chattahoochee in 1957 at the age of 50 by his father, who said the son suffered from delusions. Before he was finally released voluntarily, Mr. Donaldson brought 15 fruitless court actions; on four occasions the Supreme Court refused to hear his argument that he had a right to treatment or discharge.

In the case the high court finally accepted last fall, Mr. Donaldson sued two supervising doctors at the Florida hospital for damages for allegedly denying him his constitutional rights and failing to provide him treatment. A jury awarded him $38,500.

Right to Treatment

The United States Court of Appeals for the Fifth Circuit affirmed, formally holding that an involuntary inmate has a constitutional right to treatment that will help cure him or at least improve his mental condition.

With its decision today (No. 74-8, O'Connor V. Donaldson), the Supreme Court sent the case back to Federal District Court to determine whether Dr. J. B. O'Connor, one of the state hospital supervisors, was entitled to have the trial jury instructed that he could not reasonably have known that the Florida law supporting custodial care was invalid and thus he could not be personally liable.

In his concurring opinion, Chief Justice Burger said that government power may not be exercised "to confine a mentally ill person only if the purpose of the confinement is treatment."

"Despite many recent advances in medical knowledge," he continued, "it remains a stubborn fact that there are many forms of mental illness which are not understood, some of which are untreatable in the sense that no effective therapy has yet been discovered for them and that rates of 'cure' are generally low."

In another decision (No. 74-214, Weinberger v. Salfi) the high court upheld the constitutionality of a Social Security law that denies survivors' benefits to wives who become widows less than nine months after marriage. The vote was 6 to 3 with Associate Justices William O. Douglas, William J. Brennan Jr. and Thurgood Marshall dissenting.

His 'Friends Died There'

WASHINGTON, June 26 (UPI) —Mr. Donaldson, at a news conference in Washington after the decision came down, said he insisted throughout his confinement that he was not mentally ill and thus needed no treatment.

"I'm so angry I'll go anywhere to talk about this," he said. "I'm angry because it took 15 years out of my life without any legitimate reason. I made hundreds of friends [who] died there. They weren't any crazier than I was."

June 27, 1975

Ruling on Confining Mentally Ill Argued

By BOYCE RENSBERGER

In the seven weeks since the United States Supreme Court ruled that certain mentally ill persons may not be confined against their will, the decision has not, apparently, led to the release of a single mental patient other than Kenneth Donaldson, the original plaintiff.

Despite some early suggestions that thousands of people would soon be released from psychiatric hospitals, the decision has produced little more than controversies about its narrow and sometimes vague language and efforts to decide how, or even whether, it may be immediately applied.

In a unanimous decision announced on June 26, the Court ruled—in much more convoluted language—that a mentally ill person could not be held against his will if the following criteria were met:

¶The hospital was not offering treatment.

¶The person was not dangerous to himself or others.

¶The person was capable of living in the community with the help of friends or relatives.

Although the decision is regarded by many doctors and lawyers as a significant step forward in judicial recognition of the constitutional rights of people who suffer mental illness, medical and legal experts say each of the three conditions in the ruling is stated imprecisely enough to need further clarification.

Some of that clarification, it is held, may come through conferences between legal and mental health experts that are scheduled for the next few months, and some may have to await further Supreme Court decisions that may not come for years.

In early November, the state comissioners of mental health are scheduled to discuss the ruling at their regular annual meeting.

Each of the three conditions given in the ruling is subject to interpretations so wide that some observers have said it would be easy for most mental health agencies to say the ruling does not apply to its patients.

For example, the ruling does not say what constitutes treatment. Must it be intensive psychoanalysis, or can it be group therapy or just a tranquilizer pill, or will simply living in a "therapeutic community" suffice? There are, of course, many other possible forms of treatment.

Neither does the ruling define dangerousness. Must the person already have established a pattern of violent behavior, or is it enough that a doctor only suspects the person may commit a dangerous act? If a patient neglects his nutrition, can it be said that he is dangerous to himself?

The third condition—being capable of living in the community with help—begs another interpretation. The ruling says friends or relatives may help, but some lawyers and doctors have asked whether the help might not also legitimately come from social and welfare agencies. If a person has no immediate family or friends outside the hospital, as is the case with many who have been confined for many years, is he excluded from the ruling?

The various ambiguities and interpretations are proving such a complex matter that the National Institute of Mental Health, which has informally applauded the ruling as giving strong impetus to expansion of out-patient mental health services, has not yet issued a formal statement on what the ruling means for mental health institutions.

"We're still working on a statement that does justice to the narrowness of the decision and still takes cognizance of

206

the broader implications," said Dr. Thomas Plaut, deputy director of the National Institute of Mental Health.

No Wholesale Releases

A check with knowledgeable persons in various large states and national mental health organizations indicates that there have been no wholesale releases of mental patients. Several states say they are reviewing the status of their patients to see whether any fit the Donaldson criteria.

Paul R. Friedman, a lawyer with the Mental Health Law Project, who helped prepare Mr. Donaldson's case, said that any additional releases from confinement in the near future would probably have to be won one at a time by patients who secured their own lawyers and argued in local courts that the Donaldson decision applied to them.

At present many states have, at least as an initial reaction, said that the decision does not apply to them for one reason or another. One of the more common reasons is that all of their involuntary patients are considered dangerous. Indeed, several states have laws limiting involuntary commitments to persons deemed dangerous.

"You know what that means," one psychiatrist in a state mental health department said. "You're dangerous if they say you are and if they want to put you away, they say you're dangerous."

'A Lot of Donaldsons'

"My own opinion," said Dr. Plaut, "is that there are a lot of Donaldsons out there."

While the decision does not go as far as many advocates of the "right to treatment" had hoped, it is regarded as significant because it represents the first time the Supreme Court has approached the issue of the rights of the mentally ill.

The "right - to - treatment" concept generally holds that no person should be kept in a mental hospital unless he is receiving adequate and appropriate treatment.

Some lawyers specializing in psychiatric matters said it was significant that, in a concurring opinion, only Chief Justice Warren E. Burger said he did not believe there was such a thing as a right to treatment. None of the other Justices signed that opinion, and that is taken as meaning that the Court as a whole may be expected to broaden its mental health rulings in future cases.

The Court did say that it regarded the judgment of the adequacy of treatment to be a proper matter for courts to decide. That statement has already set lawyers to work looking for appropriate test cases to further expand the rights of mentally ill citizens.

August 17, 1975

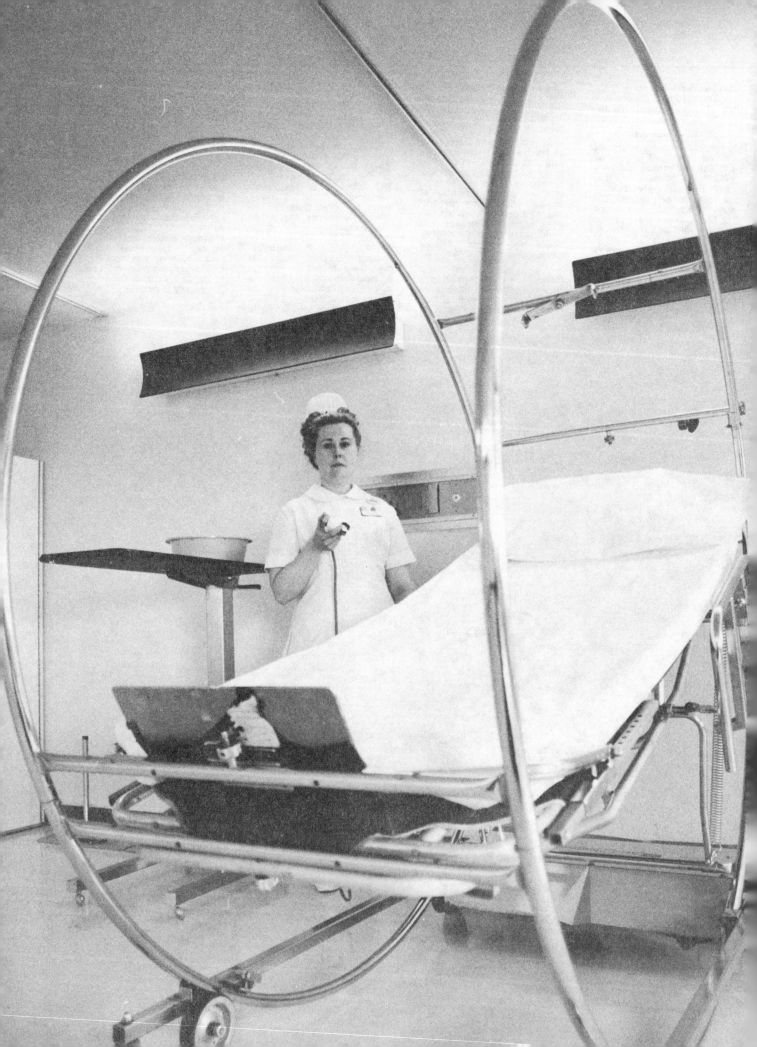

CHAPTER **3**
Health Care

A circular electric bed at New York City's Bellevue
Hospital. It is used in the treatment of paralysis,
burns and pressure sores.

Manning/NYT Pictures

A Great Doctor Who Shaped a Great Age of Medicine

WILLIAM HENRY WELCH AND THE HEROIC AGE OF AMERICAN MEDICINE. By Simon Flexner and James Thomas Flexner. 539 pp. New York: The Viking Press. $3.75.

By SAUL JARCHO, M. D.

IN the Spring of 1934 as the aged Dr. William Welch lay on his deathbed, his thoughts often turned to retrospect. Dean and archon of American medicine, he could look back over sixty important years that had elapsed since his graduation from the College of Physicians and Surgeons in New York. In these sixty years American medicine had emerged from the slough of poorly enlightened provincialism and had pursued a difficult course in the direction of world leadership. In these same sixty years —appropriately designated as a heroic age—Welch and his colleagues had transplanted to America a vigorous growth of German science. They had created laboratories, assembled libraries, constructed colleges, and trained an army of physicians and medical scientists. They had erected an entire educational system, built solidly and honored by the growing esteem of the nations.

The story of this achievement is set forth in a delectable volume by Doctor Simon Flexner and his son James. The senior author was Welch's pupil in the early days at Hopkins and subsequently directed The Rockefeller Institute; he is thus a well accredited eyewitness. The junior author has previously written on American medicine, and also on American painting. The collaboration of father and son has yielded an admirable, well-documented book in which an important special part of our national history is narrated with accuracy and interest.

Dr. William Henry Welch was descended from one Philip Welch, who in the year 1654 was kidnapped from Ireland by the soldiers of Cromwell and was later sold in Boston harbor as an indentured servant. Philip Welch subsequently gained his freedom, fought through King Philip's war, and lived to become the founder of a large and long-lived family. Philip Welch's great-grandson Hopestill Welch, a Connecticut blacksmith, fought under Israel Putnam in the French and Indian War and during the Revolution accompanied Benedict Arnold on the famous march to Quebec. This Hopestill Welch had among his descendants at least eleven physicians in three generations. The background is portrayed in Harvey Cushing's graceful essay "The Doctors Welch of Norfolk."

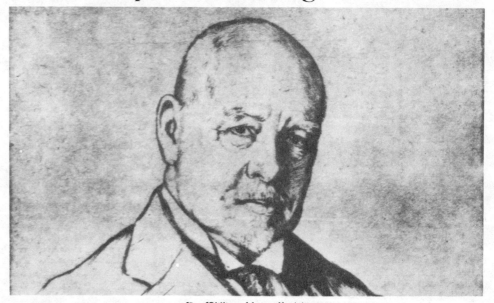

Dr. William Henry Welch.

Dr. William Henry Welch was born in 1850. Although a member of a medical family—or perhaps because of this—he seems at first to have entertained no desire to become a physician. In 1870 he was graduated from Yale College. He hoped to become a professor of Greek, but could not obtain an instructorship. For a few months he taught at a preparatory school. The teaching venture proved ephemeral. Ultimately, in the Autumn of 1872, he entered the College of Physicians and Surgeons in New York.

In those days the College was situated on East Twenty-third Street. It had not yet moved uptown to the dismal mausoleum on West Fifty-ninth Street, and the present palatial Medical Center on Washington Heights was far in the future. The required course of study lasted only three years, of which two years were spent in lectures and the third might be devoted to practical apprenticeship. The courses were not arranged in graded sequence; hence the student might buy tickets for as many series of lectures as he wished. There were no requirements for admission. Indeed, most young men went from high school directly into medical school. Except for anatomical dissections the students did no laboratory work of any kind, instruction being transmitted by means of lectures. The faculty was composed of distinguished practitioners, many of whom were also skilled in oratory. It was a principal duty of the student to prepare accurate lecture-notes and memorize them.

It must not be assumed that the older methods of instruction were completely inept. Thus Welch himself testified as follows:

One can decry the system in those days * * * but the results were better than the system. The College of Physicians and Surgeons stood then, as it has always stood, in the front rank of American medical schools. Our teachers were men of fine character, devoted to the duties of their chairs, they inspired us with enthusiasm, interest in our studies and hard work, and they imparted to us sound traditions of our professions; nor did they send us forth so utterly ignorant and unfitted for professional work as those born of the present, greatly improved methods of training and opportunities for practical study are sometimes wont to suppose.

In 1875 Welch was graduated from medical school and entered upon a brief internship at Bellevue Hospital. He now became acquainted with the great Abraham Jacobi. This proved to be a very important formative influence on Welch and on American medicine, because it was Jacobi who made Welch aware of the huge importance of Germany in scientific medicine. At this same time the Johns Hopkins University was being organized.

In 1876 Welch went to Germany. There he studied under Waldeyer, Hoppe-Seyler, and the great physiologist Carl Ludwig, and under Julius Cohnheim, a brilliant investigator who had distinguished himself by research in pathological physiology and especially by studies of the mechanisms of inflammation. In Cohnheim's laboratory Welch found himself among such outstanding young scientists as Ehrlich, Weigert and Salomonsen. In the short space of three months Welch performed a fundamental and successful research on heart failure. In 1878 he returned to New York, one of very few Americans trained to carry out scientific investigation in medicine.

The techniques and the outlook acquired in this way soon found expression at Bellevue and later at the Johns Hopkins Hospital and Medical School, where Welch occupied the chair of pathology. The professorship at Hopkins was bestowed in accordance with the advice of Cohnheim, who must be considered a lineal ancestor of American scientific medicine.

From this time forth Welch's career was one of increasing progress in bacteriologic and other research, and of ever-growing influence and responsibility in education, public health, and public affairs. As professor he not only taught but also acted as a stimulus and intellectual ferment for younger men. He was a founder and the first editor of the Journal of Experimental Medicine; for years he read the proof, checked the bibliographies and conducted all the correspondence in longhand. He had an important part in the work of the Rockefeller Foundation, greatest of medical philanthropies.

The personal and human side of Welch's character—his activities as gourmet, gourmand, baseball fan, and practical joker—should not be omitted from the record, and will be found in minute detail in the Flexners' attractive offering. The entire story is one which will be studied with pleasure by physicians, scientists, historians and by the intelligent general reader.

November 2, 1941

PHYSICIANS' ETHICAL GUIDE

AT the annual meeting of the House of Delegates, the governing body of the American Medical Association, which closed in New Orleans a week ago yesterday, the following statement of ethical principles of the profession was framed and submitted by a committee appointed for the purpose, and unanimously adopted by the delegates:

The American Medical Association promulgates, as a suggestion and advisory document, the following:

CHAPTER I.—THE DUTIES OF PHYSICIANS TO THEIR PATIENTS.

Section 1. Physicians should not only be ever ready to obey the calls of the sick and injured, but should be mindful of the high character of their mission and of the responsibilities they must incur in the discharge of momentous duties. In their ministration they should never forget that the comfort, the health, and the lives of those intrusted to their care depend on skill, attention, and fidelity. In deportment they should unite tenderness, cheerfulness, and firmness, and thus inspire all sufferers with gratitude, respect, and confidence. These observances are the more sacred because, generally, the only tribunal to adjudge penalties for unkindness, carelessness, or neglect is their own conscience.

Sec. 2. Every patient committed to the charge of a physician should be treated with attention and humanity, and reasonable indulgence should be granted to the caprices of the sick. Secrecy and delicacy should be strictly observed; and the familiar and confidential intercourse to which physicians are admitted, in their professional visits, should be guarded with the most scrupulous fidelity and honor.

Sec. 3. The obligation of secrecy extends beyond the period of professional services; none of the privacies of individual or domestic life, no infirmity of disposition or flaw of character observed during medical attendance, should ever be divulged by physicians, except when imperatively required by the laws of the State. The force of the obligation of secrecy is so great that physicians have been protected in its observance by courts of justice.

Sec. 4. Frequent visits to the sick are often requisite, since they enable the physician to arrive at a more perfect knowledge of the disease, and to meet promptly every change which may occur. Unnecessary visits are to be avoided, as they give undue anxiety to the patient; but to secure the patient against irritating suspense and disappointment, the regular and periodical visits of the physician should be made as nearly as possible at the hour when they may be reasonably expected by the patient.

Sec. 5. Ordinarily, the physician should not be forward to make gloomy prognostications, but should not fail, on proper occasions, to give timely notice of dangerous manifestations to the friends of the patient; and even to the patient, if absolutely necessary. This notice, however, is at times so peculiarly alarming when given by the physician that its deliverance may often be preferably assigned to another person of good judgment.

Sec. 6. The physician should be a minister of hope and comfort to the sick, since life may be lengthened or shortened, not only by the acts, but by the words or manner of the physician, whose solemn duty is to avoid all utterances and actions having a tendency to discourage and depress the patient.

Sec. 7. The medical attendant ought not to abandon a patient because deemed incurable; for continued attention may be highly useful to the sufferer, and comforting to the relatives, even in the last period of the fatal malady, by alleviating pain and by soothing mental anguish.

Sec. 8. The opportunity which a physician has of promoting and strengthening the good resolutions of patients suffering under the consequences of evil conduct ought never to be neglected. Good counsels, or even remonstrances, will give satisfaction, not offense; if they be tactfully proffered and evince a genuine love of virtue, accompanied by a sincere interest in the welfare of the person to whom they are addressed.

CHAPTER II.—THE DUTIES OF PHYSICIANS TO EACH OTHER AND TO THE PROFESSION AT LARGE.

Article I.—Duties for the support of professional character.

Section 1. Every one on entering the profession, and thereby becoming entitled to full professional fellowship, incurs an obligation to uphold its dignity and honor, to exalt its standing and to extend the bounds of its usefulness. It is inconsistent with the principles of medical science and it is incompatible with honorable standing in the profession for physicians to designate their practice as based upon an exclusive dogma or a sectarian system of medicine.

Sec. 2. The physician should observe strictly such laws as are instituted for the government of the members of the profession; should honor the fraternity as a body, should endeavor to promote the science and art of medicine and should entertain a due respect for those seniors who, by their labors, have contributed to its advancement.

Sec. 3. Every physician should identify himself with the organized body of his profession as represented in the community in which he resides. The organization of local or county medical societies where they do not exist, should be effected, so far as practicable. Such county societies, constituting as they do the chief element of strength in the organization of the profession, should have the active support of their members and should be made instruments for the cultivation of fellowship, for the exchange of professional experience, for the advancement of medical knowledge, for the maintenance of ethical standards, and for the promotion in general of the interests of the profession and the welfare of the public.

Sec. 4. All county medical societies thus organized ought to place themselves in affiliation with their respective State associations, and these, in turn, with the American Medical Association.

Sec. 5. There is no profession from the members of which greater purity of character and a higher standard of moral excellence are required than the medical; and to attain such eminence is a duty every physician owes alike to the profession and to patients. It is due to the patients, as without it their respect and confidence cannot be commanded; and to the profession because no scientific attainments can compensate for the want of correct moral principles.

Sec. 6. It is incumbent on physicians to be temperate in all things, for the practice of medicine requires the unremitting exercise of a clear and vigorous understanding, and in emergencies—for which no physician should be unprepared—a steady hand, an acute eye, and an unclouded mind are essential to the welfare, and even to the life, of a human being.

Sec. 7. It is incompatible with honorable standing in the profession to resort to public advertisements or private cards inviting the attention of persons affected with particular diseases; to promise radical cures; to publish cases or operations in the daily prints, or to suffer such publications to be made; to invite laymen (other than relatives who may desire to be at hand) to be present at operations; to boast of cures and remedies; to adduce certificates of skill and success; or to employ any of the other methods of charlatans.

Sec. 8. It is equally derogatory to professional character for physicians to hold patients for any surgical instruments or medicines; to accept rebates on prescriptions or surgical appliances; to assist unqualified persons to evade legal restrictions governing the practice of medicine; to dispense, or promote the use of, secret medicines, for if such nostrums are of real efficacy, any concealment regarding them is inconsistent with beneficence and professional liberality, and if mystery alone give them public notoriety, such craft implies either disgraceful ignorance or fraudulent avarice. It is highly reprehensible for physicians to give certificates attesting the efficacy of secret medicines or other substances used therapeutically.

ARTICLE II.—PROFESSIONAL SERVICES OF PHYSICIANS TO EACH OTHER.

Section 1. Physicians should not, as a general rule, undertake the treatment of themselves, nor of members of their family. In such circumstances they are peculiarly dependent on each other; therefore, kind offices and professional aid should always be cheerfully and gratuitously afforded. These visits ought not, however, to be obtrusively made, as they may give rise to embarrassment or interfere with that free choice on which such confidence depends.

Sec. 2. All practicing physicians and their immediate family dependents are entitled to the gratuitous services of any one or more of the physicians residing near them.

Sec. 3. When a physician is summoned from a distance to the bedside of a colleague in easy financial circumstances a compensation proportionate to traveling expenses and to the pecuniary loss entailed by absence from the accustomed field of professional labor should be made by the patient or relatives.

Sec. 4. When more than one physician is attending another, one of the number should take charge of the case, otherwise the concert of thought and action so essential to wise treatment cannot be assured.

Sec. 5. The affairs of life, the pursuit of health, and the various accidents and contingencies to which a physician is peculiarly exposed, sometimes require the temporary withdrawal of this physician from daily professional labor and the appointment of a colleague to act for a specified time. The colleague's compliance is an act of courtesy which should always be performed with the utmost consideration for the interest and character of the family physician.

ARTICLE III.—THE DUTIES OF PHYSICIANS IN REGARD TO CONSULTATIONS.

Section 1. The broadest dictates of humanity should be obeyed by physicians whenever and wherever their services are needed to meet the emergencies of disease or accident.

Sec. 2. Consultations should be promoted in difficult cases, as they contribute to confidence and more enlarged views of practice.

Sec. 3. The utmost punctuality should be observed in the visits of physicians when they are to hold consultations, and this is generally practicable, for society has been so considerate as to allow the plea of a professional engagement to take precedence over all others.

Sec. 4. As professional engagements may sometimes cause delay in attendance, the physician who first arrives should wait for a reasonable time, after which the consultation should be considered as postponed to a new appointment.

Sec. 5. In consultations no insincerity, rivalry, or envy should be indulged; candor, probity, and all due respect should be observed toward the physician in charge of the case.

Sec. 6. No statement or discussion of the case should take place before the patient or friends, except in the presence of all the physicians attending, or by their common consent; and no opinions or prognostications should be delivered which are not the result of previous deliberation and concurrence.

Sec. 7. No decision should restrain the attending physician from making such subsequent variations in the mode of treatment as any unexpected change in the character of the case may demand. But at the next consultation reasons for the variations should be stated. The same privilege, with its obligation, belongs to the consultant when sent for in an emergency during the absence of the family physician.

Sec. 8. The attending physician, at any time, may prescribe for the patient; not so the consultant, when alone, except in a case of emergency or when called from a considerable distance. In the first instance the consultant should do no more than make an examination of the patient and leave a written opinion, under seal, to be delivered to the attending physician.

Sec. 9. All discussions in consultation should be held as confidential. Neither by words nor by manner should any of the participants in a consultation assert or intimate that any part of the treatment pursued did not receive his assent.

Sec. 10. It may happen that two physicians cannot agree in their views of the nature of a case and of the treatment to be pursued. In the event of such disagreement, a third physician should, if practicable, be called in. None but the rarest and most exceptional circumstances would justify the consultant in taking charge of the case. He should not do so merely upon the solicitation of the patient or friends.

Sec. 11. A physician who is called in consultation should observe the most honorable and scrupulous regard for the character and standing of the attending physician, whose conduct of the case should be justified, as far as can be, consistently with a conscientious regard for truth, and no hint or insinuation should be thrown out which could impair the confidence reposed in the attending physician.

ARTICLE IV.—DUTIES OF PHYSICIANS IN CASES OF INTERFERENCE.

Section 1. Medicine being a liberal profession, those admitted to its ranks should found their expectations of practice especially on the character and the extent of their medical education.

Sec. 2. The physician, in his intercourse with a patient, under the care of another physician, should observe the strictest caution and reserve; should give no disingenuous hints relative to the nature and treatment of the patient's disorder, nor should the course of conduct of the physician directly or indirectly tend to diminish the trust reposed in the attending physician.

Sec. 3. The same circumspection should be observed when, from motives of business or friendship, a physician is prompted to visit a person who is under the direction of another physician. Indeed, such visits should be avoided, except under peculiar circumstances; and when they are made no inquiries should be instituted relative to the nature of the disease, or the remedies employed, but the topics of conversation should be as foreign to the case as circumstances will admit.

Sec. 4. A physician ought not to take charge of or prescribe for a patient who has recently been under the care of another physician, in the same illness, except in case of a sudden emergency or in consultation with the physician previously in attendance, or when that physician has relinquished the case or has been dismissed in due form.

Sec. 5. The physician acting in conformity with the preceding section should not make damaging insinuations regarding the practice previously adopted, and, indeed, should justify it if consistent with truth and probity; for it often happens that patients become dissatisfied when they are not immediately relieved, and, as many diseases are naturally protracted, the seeming want of success in the first stage of treatment affords no evidence of a lack of professional knowledge or skill.

Sec. 6. When a physician is called to an urgent case, because the family attendant is not at hand, unless assistance in consultation is desired, the former should resign the care of the patient immediately on the arrival of the family physician.

Sec. 7.—It often happens in cases of sudden illness and of accidents and injuries, owing to the alarm and anxiety of friends, that several physicians are simultaneously summoned. Under these circumstances courtesy should assign the patient to the first who arrives, and who, if necessary, may invoke the aid of some of those present. In such a case, however, the acting physician should request that the family physician be called, and should withdraw unless requested to continue in attendance.

Sec. 8.—Whenever a physician is called to the patient of another physician during the enforced absence of that physician, the case should be relinquished on the return of the other.

Sec. 9.—A physician while visiting a sick person in the country may be asked to see another physician's patient because of a sudden aggravation of the disease. On such an occasion the immediate needs of the patient should be attended to, and the case relinquished on the arrival of the attending physician.

Sec. 10.—When a physician who has been engaged to attend an obstetric case is absent and another is sent for, delivery being accomplished during the vicarious attendance, the acting physician is entitled to the professional fee, but must resign the case on the arrival of the physician first engaged.

ARTICLE V.—DIFFERENCES BETWEEN PHYSICIANS.

Section 1.—Diversity of opinion and opposition of interest may, in the medical as in other professions, sometimes occasion controversy and even contention. Whenever such unfortunate cases occur and cannot be immediately adjusted, they should be referred to the arbitration of a sufficent number of impartial physicians.

Sec. 2.—A peculiar reserve must be maintained by physicians toward the public in regard to some professional questions, and as there exist many points in medical ethics and etiquette through which the feelings of physicians may be painfully assailed in their intercourse, and which cannot be understood or appreciated by general society, neither the subject matter of their differences nor the adjudication of the arbitrators should be made public.

ARTICLE VI.—COMPENSATION.

Section 1. By the members of no profession are eleemosynary services more freely dispensed than by the medical, but justice requires that some limits should be placed to their performance. Poverty, mutual professional obligations, and certain of the public duties named in Sections 1 and 2 of Chapter III. should always be recognized as presenting valid claims for gratuitous services, but neither institutions endowed by the public or by the rich, or by societies for mutual benefit, for life insurance, or for analogous purposes, nor any profession or occupation can be admitted to possess such privilege.

Sec. 2. It cannot be justly expected of physicians to furnish certificates of inability to serve on juries or to perform militia duty, or to testify to the state of health of persons wishing to insure their lives, obtain pensions, or the like, without a pecuniary acknowledgment. But to persons in indigent circumstances such services should always be cheerfully and freely accorded.

Sec. 3. Some general rules should be adopted by the physicians in every town or district relative to the minimum pecuniary acknowledgment from their patients, and it should be deemed a point of honor to adhere to these rules with as much uniformity as varying circumstances will admit.

Sec. 4. It is derogatory to professional character for physicians to pay or offer to pay commissions to any person whatsoever who may recommend to them patients requiring general or special treatment or surgical operations. It is equally derogatory to professional character for physicians to solicit or to receive such commissions.

CHAPTER III.—THE DUTIES OF THE PROFESSION TO THE PUBLIC.

Section 1. As good citizens it is the duty of physicians to be very vigilant for the welfare of the community, and to bear their part in sustaining its laws, institutions, and burdens; especially should they be ready to co-operate with the proper authorities in the administration and the observance of sanitary laws and regulations, and they should also be ever ready to give counsel to the public in relation to subjects especially appertaining to their profession, as on questions of sanitary police, public hygiene, and legal medicine.

Sec. 2. It is the province of physicians to enlighten the public in regard to quarantine regulations; to the location, arrangement, and dietaries of hospitals, asylums, schools, prisons, and similar institutions; in regard to measures for the prevention of epidemic and contagious diseases, and when pestilence prevails it is their duty to face the danger, and to continue their labors for the alleviation of the suffering people, even at the risk of their own lives.

Sec. 3. Physicians, when called on by legally constituted authorities, should always be ready to enlighten inquests and courts of justice on subjects, strictly medical, such as involve questions relating to sanity, legitimacy, murder by poison, or other violent means, and various other subjects embraced in the science of medical jurisprudence. It is but just, however, for them to expect due compensation for their services.

Sec. 4. It is the duty of physicians, who are frequent witnesses of the great wrongs committed by charlatans, and of the injury to health and even destruction of life caused by the use of their treatment, to enlighten the public on these subjects, and to make known the injuries sustained by the unwary from the devices and pretensions of artful impostors.

Sec. 5. It is the duty of physicians to recognize and by legitimate patronage to promote the profession of pharmacy, upon the skill and efficiency of which depends the reliability of remedies, but any pharmacist who, although educated in his own profession is not a qualified physician, and who assumes to prescribe for the sick, ought not to receive such countenance and support. Any druggist or pharmacist who dispenses deteriorated or sophisticated drugs, or who substitutes one remedy for another designated in a prescription, ought thereby to forfeit the recognition and influence of physicians.

Following is the text of the report of the committee, which accompanied the document:

"To the President and Members of the House of Delegates: Your committee has given extended and careful thought to the proposed revision of the Code of Medical Ethics referred to it for consideration. As you will note on caption of report, the word 'code' has been eliminated, and the expression 'The Principles of Medical Ethics of the American Medical Association' adopted as adequately descriptive. In reference to this change it is proper to say that such action on its part is based on the idea that the American Medical Association may be conceived to occupy some such relation to the constituent State associations as the United States, through its Constitution, holds to the several States. The committee, for this reason, regards it as wiser to formulate the principles of medical ethics without definite reference to code or penalties, thus leaving the respective States, &c., to form such code and establish such penalties as they may regard to be fitting and proper for regulating the professional conduct of their members; provided, of course, that in so doing there be no infringement of the established ethical principles of the association. The committee regards as wise and well intended to facilitate the business of the parent organization and promote its harmony this course, which leaves to the State Association large discretional powers concerning membership and other admittedly State affairs.

"Your committee has retained to a large extent the phraseology of the existing code, while aiming at condensation of expression and a better understanding of some of its statements.

"The report of the committee has been reached unanimously without discussion or distrust on the part of its members, each aiming to formulate a result based on principle alone, and without regard to any past or present disagreement or misunderstandings whatsoever.

"Such being the case, the committee invites your candid and unprejudiced attention and action to the results of its labors, feeling that at least some good has been accomplished. Respectfully submitted,

"E. ELIOT HARRIS, Chairman.
"T. J. HAPPEL,
"W. H. WELCH,
"JOSEPH D. BRYANT,
"NICHOLAS SENN."

May 17, 1903

MEDICAL SCHOOLS THAT NEED CLOSING

A feature of the session yesterday of the American Hospital Association at the Murray Hill Hotel was the renewal by Abraham Flexner of the Carnegie Foundation of his fight on small and inefficient medical colleges.

According to Mr. Flexner, there are many small colleges turning out medical students who obtain their admission to these particular colleges on a flimsy grammar school education, and leave the school of medicine with an equally insecure footing in the profession

Mr. Flexner pointed with pride to the fact that twenty of the medical colleges of this class were put out of business in the last year, mainly, he asserted, as a result of a campaign among the hospitals that permitted them to flourish. He said that the main supporters of such medical schools are the hospitals in their respective towns, which permit the students to glean what knowledge they may from the institutions. In many instances, Mr. Flexner said, this assistance is given grudgingly. If withdrawn altogether, he said, the result would be for the betterment of the profession.

"Hospitals cannot subserve the purposes for which they are established," Mr. Flexner said, "unless well-trained doctors can be found to man them. Well-trained doctors must be educated largely in hospital wards. If hospitals do not afford medical schools abundant facilities for clinical instruction the hospitals must find themselves unable to discharge the function for which they exist."

He pointed out that hospitals are local institutions and that "it is as much the business of the community to look after its own wear and tear in human life as it is the business of the same community to keep its own streets in repair."

"Before the hospital opens its wards to educational uses," the speaker said, "it not only may, but must satisfy itself that the medical school applying for its privileges has in the first place enrolled a competent student body, that it has provided adequate facilities for instruction in the underlying medical sciences, both in the way of laboratories and teaching staff, and that it is prepared to take upon itself whatsoever financial obligation is incurred by introducing teaching and research into hospital wards."

Mr. Flexner named several medical colleges which, he said, ought to be closed. In the discussion which followed Mr. Flexner's address, Mrs. Margaret Engelhart, President of the Association of the Frances E. Willard Hospital of Chicago, rose at the end of the discourse and said:

"I think Mr. Flexner must be mistaken in his opinion of some of the colleges he has spoken about. At least one, to my knowledge, produces as fine a student body as could be desired, and any graduate of that school is welcome on our staff if there is a vacancy."

September 22, 1911

MEDICAL EDUCATION SCANDALS EXIST IN AMERICA ONLY

A BRAHAM FLEXNER, acting for the Carnegie Foundation for the Advancement of Teaching, has completed an elaborate report on "Medical Education in Europe," as the result of painstaking investigations carried out under his direction.

Henry S. Pritchett, President of the Foundation, has written an introductory chapter constituting a drastic arraignment of the medical institutions in this country. His conclusions, of course, are based on Mr. Flexner's report, which indicates a startling contrast between the fundamental principles underlying the educational systems of Europe and the United States. These contrasts are nearly all to our disadvantage.

It will be recalled that in July, 1910, Mr. Flexner made a report to the Carnegie Foundation on medical education in the United States and Canada, which not only dealt with the conditions of the medical schools in the two countries, but also attempted an analysis of the problem of medical education. The revelations of institutional inefficiency in that report created a tremendous sensation, not only in educational centres throughout the world, but among the general public.

At that time a reduction in the number of medical schools was recommended by both Mr. Pritchett and Mr. Flexner, with a correspondingly elevation of the standards of the remaining institutions. Other wide reforms were urged. In this connection, Mr. Pritchett made this statement at the time:

If these fundamental principles can be made clear to the people of the United States and Canada, and to those who govern the colleges and the universities, we may confidently expect that the next ten years will see a very much smaller number of medical schools in this country, but a greatly increased efficiency in medical education, and that during the same period medical education will become rightly articulated with, and rightly related to, the general educational system of the whole country.

Wide publicity of a summary of the report of 1910 evidently did make these fundamental principles clear to the people of the United States and to those who govern the colleges and universities, for in the last two years a comparatively large number of cheap institutions calling themselves "medical colleges" have gone out of business. In other instances, several small institutions have merged their interests and, as a unit, furnished the basis of sounder medical teaching.

But the present conditions in general are not satisfactory, and are condemned in the severest terms in the present report. For instance, the declaration is made by Mr. Pritchett that three-fourths of the medical schools in America would be driven out of existence if the lowest terms upon which

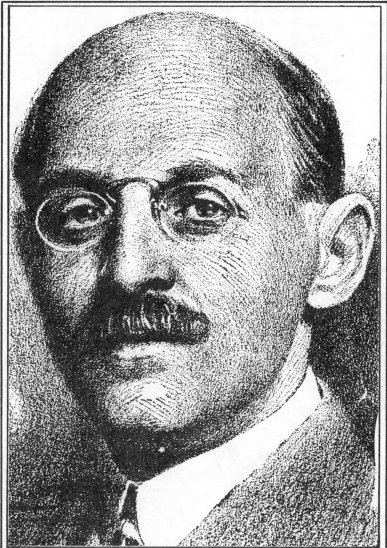

Abraham Flexner

medical schools can exist abroad were applied to this country.

While Mr. Flexner's detailed report will be read with great profit by educators and the Trustees of all institutions of learning, the deductions drawn by Mr. Pritchett are of equal, if not greater, interest to the general public. For this reason extracts from his introductory summary will take precedence in the present consideration of this vital subject. This significant avowal stands out in Mr. Pritchett's statement:

But scandals in medical education exist in America alone. In no foreign country is a medical school to be found whose students do not learn anatomy in the dissecting room and disease by the study of sick people. It has remained for the United States and Canada to confer annually the degree of Doctor of Medicine upon, and to admit to practice, hundreds who have learned anatomy from quiz-compends, and whose acquaintance with disease is derived not from the study of the sick, but from the study of textbooks.

These scandalous conditions are, it is true, less widespread to-day than they were a decade ago; yet they are still to be found in almost all sections of the country, even in the most cultivated. The State of Massachusetts tolerates in the City of Boston, the State of New York tolerates in the City of New York, the State of Illinois tolerates in the City of Chicago, the State of Missouri tolerates in St. Louis, the State of California tolerates in San Francisco, so-called medical schools that pretend to train doctors, despite the fact that they are almost totally without clinical facilities.

In no European country is it possible to find an educational farce of this description. There every school has adequate clinical resources under complete control. If the lowest terms upon which a medical school can exist abroad were applied to America, three-fourths of our existing schools would be closed at once. And, let me add, the remaining fourth would be easily and entirely adequate to our need.

Managers of feeble medical enterprises in our country pretend that they are making great sacrifices for the public good. This hypocritical pretense ought not to be permitted longer to damage the public interest. No medical school that lacks proper facilities has any other motive than the selfish advantage of those that carry it on; and no civilized country except America at this day allows such enterprises to impose upon the public.

Mr. Pritchett explains that the present report is intended to give not a detailed account of the separate schools existing in Germany, France, and England, but rather a picture of contemporary medical education in these countries. The study, therefore, is based upon an examination of representative medical schools and institutions in each country, not upon the examination of every medical establishment. For this reason no attempt is made to include a separate inventory of every school in the several countries discussed. The writer continues:

It may be added that while the primary object of this study is the benefit of medical education in America and in Canada, it is, nevertheless, impossible to treat matters of universal interest from a local and National standpoint. That which makes for the highest interest of medical science and for the true advancement of humanity through this science is common to the whole world. While the work was undertaken in the desire to improve the conditions that now exist in the United States and in Canada, it has been written from the standpoint of the advancement of medical science throughout the world. As the detailed chapters will show, there is to be found in the teaching and in the practice of the older European countries much that these newer transatlantic nations may study to their advantage, and perhaps even imitate. It is equally clear from such a careful examination as has here been made that newer countries may profit by the mistakes that have been made, or by unexpected developments that have occurred, in the experience of older nations. To-day in medicine, as in all other large human interests, the world is in reality one, and it is a backward and narrowed national view which fails to take to heart both the successes and the failures of other nations.

Mr. Pritchett insists that whether medical education is dealt with by the layman, by the medical teacher, or by the practising physician, it still remains true that it is at bottom an educational, not a medical, matter. Here is his explanation:

Considering, therefore, the medical schools in the countries under discussion from this point of view, the most striking fact that emerges from this study is the absolute dependence of professional teaching in medicine upon the general educational system of the country itself. If one admits that professional education is primarily a question of education, this result must necessarily follow; but that admission has not generally been made. One nation after another has undertaken to erect its professional schools upon the frailest foundations of general education. It is not too much to say that the result has been in every such instance a failure. This does not mean that such a system may not bring forth from time to time great practitioners.

It happens in the United States and Canada now and again that a brilliant practitioner emerges from a most inefficient and even disreputable medical school. The genius will under almost any conditions work out his salvation, but a system of education is to be judged not by its occasional brilliant successes, but by the general level of performance of those whom it undertakes to train. No one who faces the evidence brought together in these two reports can doubt the conclusion that in those countries in which the elementary and secondary school system is weak, the general level of professional education is low. Under such conditions brilliant practitioners of one profession or another occasionally arise—they will arise under any system; but the average of training will be low, and the professions will be overcrowded with a large proportion of ill-prepared men, who drag down ideals and gain their livelihood at the public expense.

Of the soundness of this conclusion there can be no more striking example than is furnished by a comparison between Germany on the one hand and the United States and England on the other. For the general high level of German professional training the German secondary school is mainly responsible. A sound and well-conceived system of elementary and secondary schools is a necessary precondition to generally good professional training; one may go even further and affirm unreservedly that any nation that undertakes to prepare men for the professions upon any other basis will, in the long run, impose upon its citizens great and unnecessary hardships.

A comparison of the conditions in the countries here studied throws light upon the precise kind of secondary education which should be provided for intending physicians. The medical curriculum, extended as it is in Europe over five years, has reached the limits of its capacity: it can contain no more. Exactly the same process has gone on in medicine as has taken place in the training of engineers. In fact, experience in these two kinds of technical education during the last fifty years has been strikingly similar. Most naturally the medical school and the engineering school have endeavored to include in their teaching some knowledge of the new sciences developed in the last half century and of their application. As a result, the burden devolved upon students of medicine and of engineering has grown enormously.

Their respective curricula have been formed almost altogether by accretion, something more being constantly put in, little or nothing taken out. As a result, both the medical student and the engineering student are called upon to carry not only a heavier load, but a load made up of more parts. Each now flies from one task to another at such a pace that little time is left for thorough preparation or for serious consideration. Consequently, there is a growing disposition to neglect the great underlying fundamental studies.

Twenty-five years ago, the medical student could even include in his curriculum a certain number of literary studies. These have been omitted, to be sure, but he is still expected in most schools to find time for elementary chemistry, elementary physics, and elementary biology. It is clear that educationally we have come almost to an impasse, that the load not only cannot be increased, but that for the sake of good teaching it must be lightened and simplified.

The medical student and the engineering student must each have a timely opportunity to ground himself in fundamental studies and to learn how to think, how to observe, how to apply. Every pedagogical consideration, therefore, points to the conclusion that the elementary underlying sciences must be learned by the student of medicine and of engineering before he enrolls himself in the professional school. A youth of twenty, in America of twenty-two, who has spent fourteen years or more in preparation, ought surely to find the time for chemistry, physics, and biology in so long a preparatory period.

A wide variation of attitude toward this question in the countries under consideration is clearly set forth in the report. Strong as is the system of secondary schools in Germany, and the even development of German medical education is mainly due to this, it still remains true that the German boy may enter the medical school, if he so desires, almost entirely without knowledge of the fundamental sciences and with the expectation of gaining that knowledge in the medical school itself. How unsatisfactory this is from the point of view of sound teaching has already been alluded to. The practical disadvantages entailed are set forth fully in the chapter dealing with this topic.

This question is warmly discussed in the United States to-day. Should the boy who undertakes the study of medicine be expected before entering the medical school to have obtained an elementary knowledge of chemistry, physics, and biology? Very intresting statements have recently appeared in American educational journals, calling attention to the fact that students who lack this preparation appear to have made quite as good showing in certain medical schools as those who have it. Without going too far into an analysis of the facts that are advanced in support of this contention, it needs to be said that even were this true it is beside the mark.

It still remains true that the youth who has not pursued these fundamental sciences does in the medical school an entirely different thing from the one who has been properly trained in them. Teachers of medicine readily admit that for students who have really mastered their elementary physics and chemistry and biology, medical education becomes a wholly different thing from what it is for those who have not gained that foundation, not only because the man so trained can begin at a different point, but also because he is familar with scientific concepts, scientific nomenclature, and scientific methods of reasoning.

Even if we may assume that students enter the study of medicine properly trained in the fundamental sciences, the problem of the curriculum is a serious one. The report shows a general tendency toward overburdening. The question naturally arises, What ought the course of study of a technical or professional school to accomplish? The medical school cannot turn out finished doctors; it cannot teach all that it is important for the practitioner to know. Under these circumstances, it does best to accept frankly certain limitations, and so to train its students that they will be disposed subsequently to remedy their own deficiencies.

Inclination of this kind appears most likely to result from a training that prescribes only the indispensable minimum, requiring in addition more thorough performance in a few directions and leaving opportunity for still further effort to those of greater energy, interest, or ability. The attitude of the German university on this point is thoroughly to be commended. Every medical faculty in Germany offers more in every department than the undergraduate student can achieve; every student is encouraged to exert himself beyond the average or the minimum in some direction or other. It is therefore not surprising that active progress beyond the point to which his education brought him is generally characteristic of the German physician.

Those interested in the development

of right educational methods will read with interest the discussion of the function of the clinical teacher. It has come to be generally conceded that not only must the basic sciences of chemistry, physics, and biology be taught by those who are primarily teachers and who give their whole time to teaching and research, but also that the more definitely medical sciences of anatomy, physiology, pathology, and bacteriology must be represented by specialists. It has not been so generally granted that the clinical teacher must also be primarily a men who devotes his life to teaching and to research.

This reform is the next great step to be taken in the improvement of medical education in the United States and Great Britain. In Germany only has it heretofore found recognition, and to this fact, next to the development of an orderly and efficient system of secondary schools, is to be attributed the high level of German medical science and medical teaching. With the more general acceptance of the view that medical education is education, not a professional incident. the conception of the clinical teacher must undergo the change here alluded to. The teaching of clinical medicine and surgery will then cease to be a side issue in the life of a busy practitioner; it will propose to itself the same objects and conform to the same standards and ideals as the teaching of any other subject of equal importance.

Turning aside from the consideration of the explicitly educational aspects of the report, Mr. Pritchett calls attention to certain lessons which it carries for those dealing with medical education in its humanitarian and social relations. Not only is the whole world to-day bound together in the discussion of all questions of scientific, educational, and social progress, the writer says, but also the people of a given nation are bound together by their common interest in such questions. Education, in any nation, he asserts, is one thing, not a series of separate and unrelated things. Under modern social conditions a nation will, therefore, inevitably lack not only industrial power, but also social contentment and efficiency, if it fails to conceive its various educational difficulties as fundamentally a single problem to be worked out by institutions related in the most vital way to each other, and representing together a national conception of progress and betterment.

The writer refers to the fact that the physician enters more intimately into individual and family life than any one, not excepting the priest, and adds:

While the average intelligent man appreciates this fact in a dim way, as a practical rule of conduct he entirely ignores it. He chooses his physician with very little more care than he chooses his coachman. It seldom occurs to him to inquire what was his previous training and what have been his opportunities. He does not concern himself with the question as to whether he is an educated man. He takes his physician on the recommendation of a friend, or on the basis of accidental acquaintance, and the notion that he should inquire in advance as to the fitness of the physician and as to the quality of his training rarely enters his mind. Moreover, the ordinary citizen fails to appreciate his individual responsibility for the betterment of the profession itself.

The future improvement of the profession in such countries as the United States depends to a large extent upon the awakening of the mass of citizens to the importance of their own attitude toward this great profession; for while the progress of medical science will continue to depend primarily on those who are connected with the profession, the elevation of the level of medical practice depends in very large measure upon the intelligence of the average citizen with respect to professional training and upon his willingness to assume some responsibility in the matter.

The following general considerations, suggested by the two reports that have been issued by this Foundation, are, in my judgment, of enormous importance to all classes of citizens. First of all, these studies have served to emphasize, particularly in the United States and Canada, the fact that medicine is a profession, not a trade. Not only is it a profession, but it is one of such enormous importance to society, carrying with it such opportunities for good or ill, that modern society is compelled to regard it as a quasi-public profession. It is not possible to allow complete freedom of choice to any who may choose to enter it. Society is compelled to insist that those who enter it shall qualify themselves for its quasi-public responsibilities and opportunities.

The difficulty experienced by young and struggling physicians in this country in attaching themselves to hospitals calls forth this criticism:

There is another point which I desire to commend to the attention of hospital trustees. This report establishes the fact that well-trained young physicians find no difficulty in attaching themselves to the retinue of hospital staff physicians and surgeons in Germany, and thus procuring for themselves the opportunity to carry on active scientific work. In America, this is practically impossible. Members of the hospital staff retain for themselves all the opportunities that the institution affords, if they are too busy with practice or too indifferent to science to use the material, clinical and other, it is wasted.

We witness, then, this strange anomaly—an American graduate in medicine can, for the asking, obtain the entrée to the clinics of Berlin, Vienna, or Munich; but in his own country, the doors of the hospital are closed in his face! It is not a pleasant task to disclose the reason back of this unwise policy. To some extent, at least, it is due to the fact that hospital physicians engrossed in practice are unwilling that their prestige should be lessened by the scientific achievements of younger men working in their wards . The laymen in control of hospitals could easily break up this selfish and unprogressive attitude, by insisting that hospital opportunities do not exist for the professional benefit of the visiting staff.

The unwillingness of the hospital trustee in America to permit the resources of the hospital to be used for medical education arises partly out of the fact that he has not yet outgrown the idea that the hospital is intended only to help the man who happens at the moment to be ill. A hundred years ago this was the case, but to-day all disease is approached from an entirely different standpoint. Every physician, every medical school, every hospital, must deal with disease not only with the idea of assisting and bringing back to health the patient who is stricken, but also in the interest of all other individuals and of the community itself.

The patient must be used, with all due regard to his own interest, to resolve the problem of disease, and to prevent the recurrence in the community of the illness with which he has been stricken. This attitude toward medicine has not yet become common among hospital trustees of the United States. They are still disposed to consider that they have done their full duty when they have given to the patients within their wards skillful medical attention and careful nursing. As a matter of fact, this is only the beginning of their duties, and no hospital can serve either its own patients or its own community more efficiently than by opening its facilities in the fullest way to a rightly conducted medical school. In order that their facilities may be thus used, the staff of the hospital must be chosen by the university on the ground of ability to teach and to investigate, as well as to practice, not by the Board of Trustees upon other grounds.

No hospital can suffer by giving this privilege to a rightly conducted university medical school. The prosperity of German medicine and the eminence of the German hospital are, as the report demonstrates, due to the acceptance of this point of view and all that it implies.

Throughout his report, Mr. Flexner emphasizes the fact that clinical teaching is the backbone of medical education in Europe. In Germany, this teaching is in the form of the demonstrative lecture; in Great Britain the clinical education is the actual and continuous participation of the student in the care of the sick. In both countries, of course, the students are armed with an introductory knowledge of the underlying sciences.

June 16, 1912

ROCKEFELLER GIVES $20,000,000 FOR MEDICAL SCHOOLS

John D. Rockefeller has given to the General Education Board, funded by him in 1902, $20,000,000, to be used for the improvement of medical education in the United States. This brief announcement was made of the gift yesterday:

"The General Education Board announces the gift from John D. Rockefeller of twenty millions of dollars, the income to be currently used and the entire principal to be distributed within fifty years for the improvement of medical education in the United States."

The working capital previous to this accretion amounted to between $35,000,000 and $40,000,000. Since the present sum is to be devoted exclusively to medical education, whereas the board's previous resources, under the terms of the charter granted it by Congress, have been devoted to "promoting education within the United States, without distinction of race, creed, or sex," the activities of the organization with respect to medical teaching will be vastly increased.

Abraham Flexner, Secretary of the board, of which Wallace Buttrick is President, said last night that the entire sum, principal and interest, would be devoted to the upbuilding of medical schools, since such was the desire of the donor. In other words, none of the money will go to educational propaganda, but all of it will be expended directly and practically.

Gift Came as a Surprise.

Mr. Flexner said that the great addition to the board's resources had been practically a surprise, those at the head of the organization having been apprised of Mr. Rockefeller's intention only a few days ago. For that reason, he explained, there has not been time to elaborate a detailed plan for the expenditure of the money. The board does not meet again until December, at which time a detailed program with respect to medical education will be mapped out.

Meantime, Mr. Flexner was able to say in a general way that just as the board in the past out of its general funds has made considerable donations to the treasuries of medical schools of such universities as Yale, Johns Hopkins, Chicago and Washington in St. Louis, it will, as soon as its plans are worked out, spend large sums for the improvement of the hospital facilities, the teaching staffs and the laboratory facilities of such schools as are decided to be worthy of help. He pointed out that under the terms of the gift while the entire principal must be distributed within fifty years, there is nothing to prevent the concurrent distribution of both principal and interest and this, he said, undoubtedly would be done.

"So far as I know," the Secretary said, "this is the first gift of its kind there ever has been. There have been large donations by wealthy men for the enrichment of designated medical schools from time to time, but I do not recall any previous instance of a big sum like this being set aside for the improvement of medical schools in general so that it can be devoted to worthy schools which

need it and so that in such schools such financial needs as that of bettering the salaries of the teaching staff, increasing clinical resources and the like, may be met."

Asked what preliminary work would be undertaken before the distribution of the $20,000,000 was started, Mr. Flexner said there would be a general survey of the schools of the country which would determine not only which ones could be improved to the general good of the country, but also what were the specific needs in each instance. In advance of the board having formulated its plans, he was unable to say how long this would take. He did say, however, that the needs of all parts of the country would be taken into consideration in apportioning such sums as it is decided to disburse from the fund.

Preference to Larger Schools.

The policy which Mr. Flexner has pursued during his long connection with the improvement of medical education in this country has been to favor the upbuilding of the larger and stronger schools, those notably which are so located that they have access to a wealth of clinical material, and it is expected that in a general way this will be the policy of the board in disbursing Mr. Rockefeller's $20,000,000.

Dr. Flexner made an attack on many of the medical schools of this country in 1910, when he was connected with the Carnegie Foundation for the Advancement of Teaching. Though he was bitterly assailed at the time, agitation which grew out of the report resulted in legislation in

many States raising the requirements for beginning the study of the medical profession and improving the educational conditions of the schools themselves. Many of the weaker schools, some of them mere "diploma mills," were driven from existence. Two years later, after a survey of German medical schools for the same organization, Dr. Flexner returned to the attack, asserting that standards of medical education in this country were below those of most of Europe.

The other officers of the General Education Board, the offices of which are at 61 Broadway, are Wallace Buttrick, President; E.C. Sage, Assistant Secretary; L.G. Myers, Treasurer; L.M. Dashiel, Assistant Treasurer.

September 27, 1919

NEW MEDICAL CENTRE

ONE of the most important new moves in medical education is just being launched at the University of Pennsylvania Graduate School of Medicine. If it succeeds, it will mean that physicians and surgeons who wish to keep in touch with the latest medical discoveries need not travel to the great universities in Europe, but can take a course of intensive study in a special branch under the acknowledged masters of that branch in America.

Heretofore, the practicioner who has been out of college for ten years, and who wants to bring himself up to date, has had to pursue his studies, as a general thing, in classes where the majority of students are lacking in practical experience, as they have but recently graduated from medical schools. Necessarily, he wastes many precious hours seeing things demonstrated that he can do almost with his eyes shut. Under the new move of the Pennsylvania Graduate School of Medicine, he can join a class of skilled physicians under the direct supervision of the acknowledged expert in a certain branch, and learn from him the final degree of perfection to which that branch has been brought. Beginning in October, 1920, the Graduate School of Medicine offers regular courses, varying in length from four months to a year, in special subjects of medical science, leading to special certificates, which give him the very latest development in the work to which he has devoted himself.

It is peculiarly fitting that the University of Pennsylvania should be the pioneer in the work. The Medical School there is the oldest in the country, founded as it was in 1765, and Philadelphia itself has a world-wide reputation as a medical centre. Now it has the opportunity to eclipse the great colleges of Vienna, Berlin, Munich and Heidelberg and make of America the recognized centre of medical advancement.

To accomplish the high aims of this new Pennsylvania institution a teaching staff of 250 men has been organized. Of this number, approximately 150 are at the head of their profession and the others are only a trifle less well known. These men, for the cause of humanity, are willing to share with their professional brothers the secrets of their success. There is no other school just like it in the country.

A Vast Project.

The reason given for the establishment of this new Graduate School of Medicine, quoting from the prospectus, is as follows:

"The prime object of the university is so to train the acceptable graduate in medicine that he shall be properly qualified to begin special medical practice or teaching and be stimulated to productive medical research. Secondarily, the university desires to perform the public service of affording reputable physicians opportunities to keep in touch with medical advances by coming into contact with the newer things in medicine as exemplified by the practice of masters in the various fields of medical endeavor.

"Realizing that the project is a vast one, the university has no thought that from the very beginning of the work of the school it will be able to cover the entire domain. Moreover, graduate medical education as here intended is new and its development must be to a considerable extent evolutionary. But the need for such education is obvious and pressing and it is within the power of the university to make a considerable beginning.

"To limited groups of suitably qualified physicians, there will be furnished opportunities for graduate study in special branches of medical and surgical practice and research in the following departments: Internal medicine, pediatrics, neurology, dermatology-syphilology, roentgenology, surgery, gynecology-obstetrics, orthopedics, urology, proctology, opthalmology, otolaryngology and medical sciences.

"The educational work of the Graduate School of Medicine is made possible by the facts that there exist in Philadelphia the factors essential to such a project, and that the university has been enabled to utilize enough of these factors in effective combination with its old and prominent medical school.

"These Philadelphia factors are: The university, which initiates, fosters and guides this additional school; with the university, the large central organization of the Graduate School of Medicine which has graduate medical education as its sole business and domain; a great American metropolis with fine medical traditions, numerous hospitals, laboratories, libraries, clinics and clinicians, and active medical specialization, education and research.

"The central organization consists of a large group of leading Philadelphia clinicians and medical educators, constituting the faculty of the Graduate School of Medicine, and of the former Medico-Chirurgical and Polyclinic institutions, which have abandoned their earlier types of medical education, and are now devoted wholly to the work of the Graduate School of Medicine. The relationships between this central organization and the other factors above mentioned arise

mainly through the members of the Faculty of the Graduate School of Medicine in their further capacities as members of the staffs of the various medical organizations of the city hospitals, clinics, laboratories, &c.

One Hundred and Fifty Enrolled.

"Students in the Graduate School of Medicine are suitably qualified physicians who become, substantially, clinical or research assistants and understudies of the members of the Faculty in medical activities throughout the city."

About one hundred and fifty physicians are enrolled for the 1920-21 course. They are from practically every State in the Union, and, what is even more significant, from many foreign countries. Scotland, Spain, Belgium, Japan, Syria, Cuba, Porto Rico, the Philippine Islands, China and Canada all have sent physicians to this new school to perfect themselves. It was stated at the school that the Faculty realizes it is hardly possible to furnish all conceivable needs or demands of the pupils enrolling in the graduate medical school, and they have not attempted to do so. The first aim is to receive only small groups of students and to have the efforts of each group devoted continuously during a reasonably long period of time exclusively to the practical and scientific study of a single well-defined department of medicine. It was also stated that it is the fixed policy of the university to form, as far as possible, an indefinite number of hospital affiliations for graduate teaching purposes only. At present affiliations have been made with twenty-two hospitals, six clinical laboratories and five medical institutions of other types.

The prospectus says: "No thought of ownership, management or control of these hospitals is entertained by the university. This university appreciates, however, the immense benefit which its graduate medical educational program may render to the public; it realizes fully how essential to it are unlimited clinical opportunities and it is firm in the belief that Hospital Boards generally will join with it in the altruistic movement and not permit the useless waste of one of their most potent opportunities for public service.

"No fixed method can be formulated for the establishment of such extramural hospital teaching affiliations. The following plan is likely to govern most cases. In general, the affiliation will only concern a small portion of the work of the hospital. A member of the medical staff of the hospital becomes, if not so already, by election of the university trustees, a teacher with appropriate title and corresponding rights as a member of the Faculty of the Graduate School of Medicine. His hospital board and the university trustees then join in validating a teaching arrangement, involving the right of said staff member, under such restrictions as are deemed necessary, to introduce his graduate medical students into his hospital work. Or the same arrangement may be made directly between the Faculty member and his hospital board. The university, will, as necessary, defray any laboratory or other expenses incidental to the aforesaid arrangements.

To See Masters at Work.

Above all things the Faculty of the school wish it understood that this is not merely a school where young doctors will be taken immediately after graduation from their medical universities, but it is an institution where physicians of standing in their communities may enroll to become medical specialists or to attain further skill in special medical practice and research. This is the primary purpose and function of the college.

The Dean of the Graduate School is Dr. George H. Meeker, who has been an active worker in the establishment of the Graduate School of Medicine.

Dr. Meeker believes that few laymen realize how vast a field of medical knowledge and skill is the daily demand.

"No one person can possibly be well qualified to serve all of the important medical needs," he said. "The standard medical licentiate, excellent though he be, is only well qualified to engage in 'general practice,' and there is a startling lack of medical establishments competent to train physicians to become medical specialists. The scope of the new school will be more readily understood when these facts are borne in mind. There is a great need for specialists, those physicians who are equipped by special training and long general experience to treat successfully many of the more serious maladies. The ordinary physician just out of college, or the practitioner without special experience, is not equipped to give this kind of service.

"The opportunities for a physician becoming a specialist are very limited. His only chance consists in attaching himself to some master as an assistant and imitating within the narrow scope allowed him the ideas and methods of this single man. Then again, while he reads his medical journals and thus keeps in touch as best he can with the medical progress of the day, he does not have the advantage of seeing those masters at work on the living case."

"Under the present plan the physician student has the advantage of the broad general experience to be got from studying under and observing the work of one hundred and fifty of the city's most eminent specialists who are giving, at a great financial loss, their extremely valuable time. He learns not one man's methods, but one hundred and fifty.

"The outcome of this venture should mean that the city will be radiating a great army of specialists, who will not only help to make it the medical centre of the world, but will reach the various provincial centres where specialists are virtually an unknown thing and raise the science of healing to immeasurably greater heights."

New School Expensive.

With a much greater number of specialists in the field the average patient will find expert treatment within his reach at prices that he can afford to pay. And while there are now great clinics in the cities where those who cannot pay anything may be treated, after the growth of the graduate school these clinics will extend to provincial centres, where the poor of a community may receive the advantage of the services of medical experts without a cent of cost to them.

Dr. Meeker said it was largely up to Pennsylvanians whether this new school was a success or not. "The school which enlists the services of 250 of Philadelphia's most eminent specialists will be run at a loss of a half a million dollars this year, and the figures will probably be the same for the following year. We can stand it that long, but after that we must have secured substantial support or we shall have failed." he said.

"Minnesota is one of the greatest States in the country in the field of medical progress. The State gives to the University of Minnesota financial support which is equivalent to the income from an endowment of $50,000,000.

"The support and development of this new Graduate School of the University of Pennsylvania is a public duty. The school is very expensive to conduct and upbuild; and the university is compelled to ask for aid. The project is primarily for the benefit of humanity; but it is also to the honor of Pennsylvanians, and we have proceeded in the faith that the humanitarian and progressive citizens of the State will not withhold the financial support without which the whole splendid project must fail."

Some idea of the extent of medical specialization may be gained from a list of specialties found in the prospectus, with the foregoing remark:

"There is no rigid list of medical specialists. However, neglecting secondary branches, variants and compounds, the following list is fairly

representative. It indicates the score and more of main pathways for medical men and the numerous departments necessary to the complete graduate school of medicine.

Practical (clinical) Medical specialists:

MEDICAL.

Internist—General.
Gastroenterologist—Digestion, &c.
Pediatrist—Children.
Neurologist—Nerves.
Psychiatrist—Mind.
Dermatologist—Skin.
Syphilogist—Lues.
Radiologist—X-Rays, &c.
Electrotheropeutist—General.

SURGICAL, &C.

Surgeon—General.
Gynecologist—Women.
Obstetrician—Midwifery.
Orthopedist—Deformities.
Proctologist—Rectum.
Otolaryngologist—Ear, nose and throat.
Ophthalmologist—Eye.
Urologist—Urogenitals.
Clinical Laboratorian—Clinical pathologist, bacteriologist, immunologist, serologist, &c.
Specialists in Medical Sciences (usually teachers and investigators)—Anatomist, physiologist, pathologist, bacteriologist, biochemist, &c.

The Administrative Board of the Graduate School of Medicine is composed of representatives of professional, social and civic activities and of the various educational agencies of the school. The present membership of the board is: Josiah H. Penniman, Acting Provost, ex-officio; C. F. C. Stout, Chairman; J. Somers Smith, Secretary, and the following:

James M. Anders, John C. Bell, James Crosby Brown, Herbert L. Clark, William J. Clothier, L. Webster Fox, F. C. Morgan, William H. Hutt, Murdock Kendrick, William A. Law, Louis C. Madeira, George H. Meeker, David Milne, and Charles Scott Jr.

The University Committee on Graduate Medical Education is at present composed of the Acting Provost, C. F. C. Stout, John C. Bell, Dr. George H. Meeker, Secretary and Dr. J. M. Anders, Dr. Ralph Butler, Dr. G. E. de Schweinitz, Dr. B. C. Hirst, Dr. J. A. Kolmer, Dr. Ernest Laplace, Dr. William Pepper, Dr. John B. Roberts, Dr. Alfred Stengel, Dr. A. J. Smith, Dr. T. H. Weisenburg.

February 13, 1921

TEACHING HOSPITALS YIELD FINE RESULTS TO MEDICINE

THE method of teaching at least one profession is taking a page from the last century. The family doctor who treated our grandparents acquired his knowledge of medicine by becoming more or less an apprentice to a practicing physician. He accompanied the physician on his rounds, read medical books in the office between calls and made himself generally useful.

In large cities there were lecture courses on medical science, lasting from twenty-six to thirty weeks a year. The student usually attended these for one or two years, depending upon the size of his income, and this was considered sufficient finishing. He had virtually no laboratory, dispensary or hospital experience up to the time he started to practice. In spite of such inadequacies the young doctor of that era acquired practical experience which those of later decades frequently missed.

In the '80s medical colleges began to spring up in all parts of the United States. The apprentice method in medicine became discredited. The student's days were filled with recitations and

laboratory experiments. He was usually so occupied in keeping up with his classes that he had no time to see the actual application of what he was studying. The theory of medicine was likely to fill his mind to the exclusion of the practical. Too often the patient was regarded not as a suffering human being but as an object of scientific curiosity. Not until after four years of theory did the medical student begin his practical observation as an interne in a hospital. By that time details of his course of preparation had lost their freshness.

Teaching Hospitals.

Leaders of the profession began to realize that while the medical school was giving the novice a wider knowledge it often slighted the first-hand contact with disease. To overcome this the teaching hospital was organized for affiliation with the medical school. The one at Johns Hopkins University, established twenty-five years ago, was among the first. Other colleges adopted

the plan, and now several teaching hospitals are in operation.

The student's position in a teaching hospital is that of an observer. His instructors constitute the staff of the hospital. Occasionally he is permitted to take histories of ward patients, but even in such clerical matters his work is closely supervised. Small groups of students accompany the ward surgeons on their tour of the wards, learning methods and practice first-hand, as did their predecessors fifty years ago. The growth of the teaching hospital has contributed more, it is said, than any other factor to America's ascendance in medicine.

Dr. George Gray Ward, chief surgeon of the Woman's Hospital in New York, says: "The recent supremacy of Germany in the world of medicine was undoubtedly largely due to the fact that all her hospitals were teaching centres. A teaching hospital or clinic will set the standard of medical practice for the profession in its vicinity, as it is an exponent of modern science in its par-

ticular field, and its educational value can hardly be exaggerated."

New Institution Here.

Hospital patients do not resent the presence of student observers in the wards. On the contrary, they are usually pleased, feeling that the attendance of a group of interested persons gives the case added importance.

There is being organized in New York a teaching centre to rank with the other great centres of the world. The nucleus of this centre is Presbyterian Hospital and the medical college of Columbia University. Twenty acres of land have been acquired at 165th Street and Broadway for the group of buildings. It is assured that several special hospitals will move their plants to this site and become part of the centre at an early date. Hospital wards, laboratories and classrooms will be combined under one roof, opening to the student an almost limitless storehouse of scientific treasures. Similar medical centres are being built in Chicago, Cleveland and Rochester.

January 11, 1925

GROUP PRACTICE OF MEDICINE.

Though Dr. WILLIAM J. MAYO is one of the world's foremost exponents of the group practice of medicine, he does not look forward to the disappearance of the general practitioner. In his address before the National Education Association he said that the physician is no longer an individual practitioner, however general, but must turn to one or another specialist for the information which in the nature of things a single individual cannot have of all that medicine has learned. He would need several lives to attain that competency, and even then collective knowledge would surpass his own.

Dr. JOSEPH COLLINS has in the current Harper's set forth in a clear and convincing article the need of such organization of specialized skill in the field of medicine as will insure to patients the advice of the highest diagnostic service and most approved treatment, whatever their ailments may be, at a cost which they are able to meet. Great progress has been made in the training of physicians. They are as well taught in America as in any country of the world, but when they persist in practicing medicine individually they fail of their maximum possible service. As it is, the poor, or very poor, do in most communities enjoy the advantages of group practice through the clinic or hospital in which specialists are associated. Those of ample means may also have such advantages, but, except in such institutions as the Mayo Clinic and the medical centres now developing, only by going from one specialist to another. The man who is neither rich nor poor is " often denied the medi-"cal service to which he is entitled "because he cannot afford it," but could have within his means if group practice were organized in some such way as Dr. COLLINS suggests:

He would go to the consulting rooms and laboratories. Here he would be received by a discerning, affable person who would seek to get enough information about his symptoms to lead him to the appropriate hopper of the medical mill. Before he is taken there it should be ascertained whether he is a wage-earner or a wage-payer. If he is a wage-earner, the firm should then and there collect the equivalent of one week's salary. If he is a wage-payer, $100 should be collected with similar dispatch, and he should be told that he may anticipate supplementary charges should his case require extensive investigation. Then the patient should be given an appointment with a member of the firm in whose province the symptoms would seem to be, who would examine and pass him on to as many others as are necessary to get a complete report. The patient is now ready for the verdict. The man who gives it to him should know not only the disease but the diseased and he should always have in mind that man's fears are magnified by illness, his hopes minimized.

The ideal way would be for the physician to have his own laboratories and assistants in such number as to cover the field of his practice, but this is impracticable. It must be constantly kept in mind, however, that, with all the organization, the service must not be impersonalized. There will ever be need of those who have skill in caring for the sick—who have the qualities of those general practitioners who have ennobled and endeared the profession. Organization has, as Dr. COLLINS has said, made medical education more efficient. The next step is to do the same for medical practice.

July 7, 1928

THE DOCTORS DIAGNOSE THEIR CASE

They Find the Medical Profession Is Now Suffering From a Number of Ills

The American Foundation recently asked leading doctors and surgeons throughout the country—especially men who have been in practice for twenty years or more—whether their experience had led them to believe that a radical change is indicated in the present organization of medical care and, if so, in what directions. The report of the inquiry will be published next week under the title "American Medicine—Expert Testimony Out of Court." This article is written by the director of the inquiry and the editor of the report.

By ESTHER EVERETT LAPE

A MAN who in the midst of a gracious, familiar room suddenly sees the walls lengthen and foreshorten, the floor and ceiling meet, would not be more puzzled than is many a medical man of today trying to keep his accustomed foothold in a world changing its dimensions under his very nose.

Thousands of doctors who in their individual lives find insufficient hours

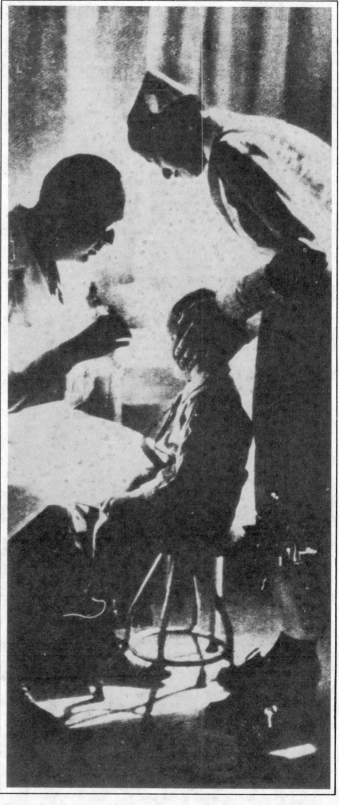

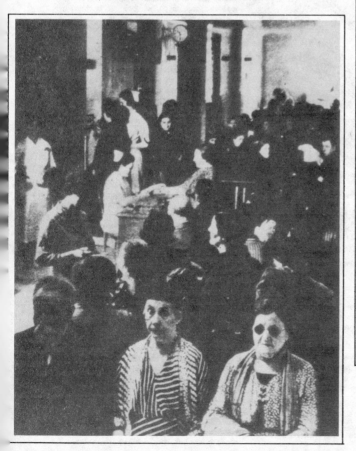

"Doctors freely admit that lack of adequate medical care is indeed an urgent national problem"—Above, doctor and patient. Left, a hospital clinic.

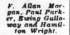

F. Allan Morgan, Paul Parker, Ewing Galloway and Hamilton Wright.

219

in any given day to get through their tasks as healer, priest, public servant, good neighbor, suddenly find themselves on the defendant's stand, under indictment because a large part of the population does not get adequate medical care. The only group (not excepting priest and pastor) with whom it is a tradition to give service without regard to whether it is paid for or not is under reproach because one-third (or one-half or some other fraction, according to the school of thought) of the country lacks the medical care it needs.

This is not another sentimentalization of the dear old doctor. The reader need not fear that we shall now throw on the screen "The Doctor" that adorns the walls of a million sitting rooms—stricken child stretched on a bed of chairs, frantic mother, tilted lamp and the benignant, saving healer. As the inquiry of the American Foundation shows, no one resents the sentimentalization of the "noblest" profession more than the modern medical scientist himself. Of the debunking of the profession in recent years, some of it quite healthy, a good part has been offered by doctors.

The net impression from the inquiry is that the doctors freely admit with the concern of those who understand that lack of adequate medical care is indeed an urgent national problem. And if the "adequate" care under discussion means modern scientific medical care at its best, doctors would be first to point out that perhaps not 1 per cent of the population now receives it. Little of it exists; and, as one contributor puts it, "The best is not yet good enough."

What the doctors—and some others—see is that the problem of inadequate medical care for millions is, in part, the problem of inadequate everything for those millions—lack of employment, lack of a living wage, lack of such conditions of health as housing, food and fuel. The doctors see that these fundamental needs impinge on their work and responsibilities, and they have made some effort to understand how. They have set up "medical economics" (curious term) committees in county medical societies to "study" the problem. But most of the best medical men in each crowded driving day are so busy meeting the problems that they have no time to study them—and no particular gift for social and economic abstractions. Daily meeting of social problems in the concrete often makes people unable to deal with them in the abstract.

The truth is that it is pretty hard to get a real doctor to look at anything but medicine. The outstanding thing about the recent inquiry is that when doctors were asked whether the present system of medical care should be changed —a question which they might have been expected to answer in terms of social and economic theorizing—they answered in terms of medicine. Their replies cover the whole field of medicine, and what they would change in that. That is their contribution to the answer the nation is seeking. They recognize the need of better distribution and lower costs, but they also know that the greatest need of all is better medicine. It is of that they write.

And the better medicine of the future

means, they realize, the end of a system in which the individual practitioner sets his own standards. This is by no means to say that the individual practice of medicine is over; it is to say that the day of individual interpretation of scientific standards has gone by. In this sense only, the day of medicine as a highly individualistic liberal profession is past and ought to be. The old form no longer fits either the social pattern or the development of medical science.

SOME of the doctors see clearly that the influence and forces that have revolutionized their calling are chiefly these two:

First, the American "industrial revolution" which swiftly changed the face of many a neighborhood and the doctor's position with it. One of the older doctors sketches the change with a few simple strokes, and thousands of his colleagues could present a similar picture:

I started my work here as a country practitioner in 1903. This city was then a village of from fifty to seventy-five houses. For many years I made my calls in the saddle within an area of from twelve to fifteen miles. Then the factories came and a new type of people swarmed in until the city and adjacent settlements had approximately 40,000 souls.
With this metamorphosis the factory and the hospital also became agents of med-

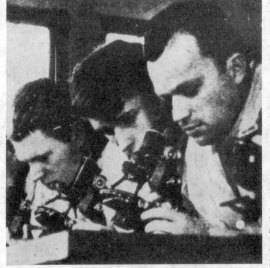

Medical students—"Many doctors are dubious of the young 'super-scientists.' "

ical care, modifying the doctor's function and changing his status.

The second and more positive influence that has operated to change the medical man's world and his own place in it is the rapid and phenomenal development of medical science itself. Many a man now living has realized the experience described as follows by a general practitioner in an Eastern State:

My practice of medicine at the beginning of my professional life and the methods now in use may be compared to the difference between a ricksha pulled by a coolie and Lindbergh's transatlantic flight.

Thirty years ago we were practicing an art with very little science and much witchcraft as its foundation. Today the scientific medicine we practice requires a great amount of art in its application and an entire omission of witchcraft.
I remember that my practice consisted of relieving patients of their pain, when possible, and very little else. Sound and correct diagnosis was not expected and was hardly ever obtained. I have delivered hundreds and hundreds of mothers of their babies (for some, an overcoat served as bed and mattress) with no boiled water anywhere in the house. I have curetted women in their kitchen, with the kitchen table serving the purpose of the operating table. I have opened abscesses under the most unsterile conditions imaginable.
Cupping in pneumonia, closing windows and pulling down shades in measles, prohibiting bathing in scarlet fever, starvation in typhoid, starvation of the diabetic, an ice-bag for an appendix, a douche after delivery, no meat in hypertension of nephritis—all of these were part of the practice of medicine, and most of my patients actually survived.

He balances the above against the procedures which he himself uses today:
Thorough urinalysis, complete blood counts and blood chemistries, Wassermanns, X-rays, basal metabolism, &c.

A GRAPHIC index of the development of medical science, as reminiscent contributors point out, is to be found in the contrast between the medical education of today and the medical education of fifty years ago. Some of the exponents, or victims, of the medical education of fifty years ago became good doctors rather in spite of than because of their "courses." Diploma mills, proprietary schools, preceptorships—these were in large degree the sources of medical training. All a man had to do was to sign up with preceptors, pay for two courses of lectures, usually of four months' duration, and pass a cursory examination given by a medical faculty or committee. Most of the medical schools were proprietary; they contained no laboratories except the chemical and had no pathological or bacteriological departments. There was almost no attempt at clinical or "bedside" instruction.

A man in those days had to fight as an individual for what he learned; since his clinical observation was his only source of competence he simply had to develop it or fail dismally in his work. Those first to admit that the training of physicians fifty years ago is a pathetic picture, from our present scientific point of view, often add that the older tradition was more efficient than the modern "spoon-feeding" system in developing sturdy, reliant practitioners.

Few medical men would want to return to the old-time medical education. Many, however, are dubious of the young "superscientist" which the modern system tends, they think, to turn out. It is not, certainly, that the young graduate of the present has too much science—but rather that he has not acquired enough science to give him the integrating power that will make his sectional information effective. Too often, some medical critics feel, the younger men have accumulated bits of information bearing on methods rather than a power to sense clinical problems as a whole. An ear, nose and throat consultant in a New York City hospital, coming from an hour of instruction in his hospital a few weeks ago, told of the "brilliant" young student who, presented with a case for diagnosis, stressed this and that scientific indication, but failed entirely to arrive at the fact that the man before him had—mumps.

ONE of the great clinicians of this age illustrates the technolistic trend of the modern student by recalling one of his rounds, as physician in chief, through the hospital ward:

We came to a man propped up in bed, gasping and heaving for breath, his chest bare, with a visible pulsation all over an enormous cardiac area that could be seen half across the room. I asked a student what he would say about the size of the man's heart, wanting of course to hear him say that the enormously enlarged heart was the so-called "cor bovinum" or "beef heart."

The youngster's reply was a commentary on present-day medical training: "I'm very sorry, sir, but the teleroentgenographic report has not yet come up from the X-ray laboratory. Shall I send for it, sir?"

Shades of Hippocrates and Sydenham! What were the boy's eyes for?

Perhaps the difficulty lies less in overemphasis on science and more in failure to get the right young men to train men capable of succeeding not only in the test-tube school but also in the school of experience and of clinical competence. There is solid support among doctors for the view that the main road to better medicine is better medical education (the notable advances of the last two decades are duly recognized) and that getting the right men into medical schools is an even sharper problem than balancing the curriculum.

IF in medical education and practice the pendulum has swung too far in the direction of overemphasis on the laboratory technique, most medical scientists seem to feel that it will safely swing back again—and that the backward swing has already begun. They think it is highly dangerous to suggest less emphasis on science. As one man puts it:

I have never in my experience in the practice of medicine seen a gross error which could be attributed to a superior knowledge in the basic principles and sciences of medicine, but I have seen hundreds of gross and pathetic mistakes which were directly attributable to a lack of appreciation of those principles of the medical sciences which have as their foundation a thorough basic knowledge.

It is not the "super-science" of the young specialist that is troubling medical critics most at the moment. It is the fact that too often specialists are not specialists. The doctor, looking at medicine—with a side glance into the crystal ball of the future—ponders the effect of this kind of "specialization" on the status and function and training of the general practitioner of the future, the diagnostician and the broad clinician. It is true enough that the rapidly expanding field of medicine, a field too large for the individual to compass, produces a bona fide specialization. But "specialists" have also been created by the public's insistence upon specialists and the doctor's inclination to profit by the greater prestige and the larger fees the specialist can command.

One of the older men ruefully observes:

Yesterday I was informed that 20 per cent of the new college graduates nominate themselves specialists after no more polish to their brains than that afforded by the tiled floors of an internship. It makes for a new definition of the specialist—the man in medicine afraid to be a complete doctor and to attack a total job.

Another raises the percentage:

From 40 per cent to 80 per cent of recent graduates are entering upon specialties, many without sufficient training and without valuable clinical experience derived from general practice.

The respectable general practitioner in a community, unable to maintain his prestige against the popular acclaiming of the specialist, turns himself into a "specialist" also—and so the ranks thicken. The president of one of the certifying boards (established by the profession in the various fields of special practice to

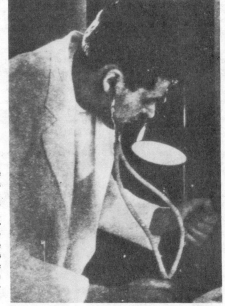

"Most of the best doctors are so busy meeting problems that they have no time to study them."

"certify" competence in the given division of medicine) points out that in 1934, roughly, a third of the physicians in active practice in the United States were listed as specialists.

Self-election in one of the specialities, surgery, has been of particular moment. There is animated comment by physicians on the free functioning of self-trained surgeons achieving their competence—when they do achieve it—by experimentation and "filling graveyards in the process." A surgeon illustrates the point by picturing two types of his colleagues:

When you go into one operating room to observe an operation for appendicitis, goiter or the removal of a carcinomatous breast or other equally grave condition, you may observe that the surgeon is using instruments few enough to be easily carried in your vest pocket; two, three or four small gauze pads or sponges; not so much loss of blood as there would be in the simplest nose bleed; practically no shock and little, if any, mortality.

In the room of another operator you will see a table covered with enough instruments to suggest a hardware display, a basket full of sponges, floor covered with bloody rags and blood, nurses excited, patient in shock and the undertaker pleased.

The first is a surgeon, scientifically trained, with his conscience saving his patient.

The second is, at best, without knowledge of his own lack of skill; at worst, in surgery for revenue only.

THIS kind of "specialization" narrows the general practice of medicine and greatly limits and lowers its quality. Men not broadly trained, perhaps not capable of broad training, unable to deal with the human entity as a whole, tend to apply persistently the particular procedures in which they have "specialized."

It is so spectacular to point an accusing finger at a curly appendix tip in an X-ray picture and tell an emaciated, overworked, high-strung little school teacher that her trouble lies there and that its removal will cause her to become strong, rosy-cheeked and placid.

Throughout the correspondence turned up by the recent inquiry there is the recurring view that a too prevalent surgical impulse is a dominant error in present-day therapy. One of the leading surgeons of the country confesses to a feeling that the

rather high maternity death rate in this country compared with that of certain foreign countries is to be ascribed to our tendency to surgical interference in obstetrics, the "craze for Caesarian sections" and for "meddlesome procedures generally." We are used to hearing the midwife blamed for poor obstetrics, but a sardonically different note is struck when the most modern of procedures is indicted.

To this whole question of facile specialization, incompetent and excessive surgery, leading doctors and surgeons are very much alive. It is recognized that the qualified specialist is an index of progress; and that the increase in the self-nominated is an index of decadence. The profession itself has set up, in twelve divisions of medicine, including surgery, certifying boards (the surgical board has just been organized) requiring demonstrated preparation and experience for certification of candidates by the board as competent in the specialty. While certification is voluntary, and the boards have no legal sanction, many medical men believe they will either control the situation entirely or guide whatever legislation may eventually be needed.

BUT will the public take the trouble to find out who is certified and who is not?

Even when special practice is limited to the qualified, and when this factor of the situation has been brought into focus, it will still be necessary to work out the answer to the question uppermost in medical minds today: What is the fate or the future of the general practitioner?

Has he a valid place, or is the medicine of the future to be practiced by specialists in groups? (If so, asks the rural practitioner, which specialists shall be sent for when the farmer's wife breaks down from overwork and child bearing?)

Has the field of medicine indeed become too large for any individual practitioner to compass? Does competent diagnosis and treatment require, in routine, the hospital, the laboratory and "the sixteen kinds of lay technicians we have summoned and trained to help us practice scientific medicine"?

Is the "doctor-patient relation," so long the sign and symbol of the individual practice of medicine, already obsolete?

THERE are those who believe it is, that the doctor-patient relation has too long served as a substitute for diagnosis, and that, as a recent graduate puts it,

the sooner it is jettisoned the better medicine in practice will be. A kindly smile, a gentle pat and a benevolent disposition hardly take the place of careful examination, thorough study and a scientific skepticism of the value of some drugs. I can't see that the argument of personal relationship is anything more than an effort of the haves to maintain the status quo.

There is another school, however, including young and old medical men alike, who believe that the personal relation will always be a part of medical therapy, whether practiced by individual or group. They admit that the individual practice of medicine has too long stressed the art of medicine at the expense of the science. But when all the false sentimental values have been stripped from the doctor-patient relation, they maintain that there remains a solid value, essential in medical therapy.

Lord Horder, when he was in this country last Spring, said of the tendency to submerge the general practitioner:

The spread of specialism and the increased knowledge-ability —if I may use such a word—of the public in medical matters have both of them combined to narrow the function of the general practitioner, who is, or who should be, the clinician par excellence, almost to the vanishing point.

I regard this as being no less dangerous to the public than it would be for the passengers if the captain left the bridge of the ship and the chief engineer, or the chief steward or the radio operator took his place.

A distinct group of "G. P.'s" defenders make no plea for his "retention" on the ground of his honorable past. He must be born again. For him, in his new incarnation, they outline a central, dominant and essential place in the medicine of the future—a medicine in which preventive as well as curative medicine will be practiced as much in the doctor's office as in the public health department and laboratory.

In this conception specialization, far from being the "down-

fall" of the family doctor, will simply enable him to practice a better quality of medicine. The reincarnated family doctor will be not the resistant rival of specialists but the employer of specialists. Far from being a secondary figure relegated to rural regions and chiefly useful in routing medical traffic to the city specialist, this "general practitioner" of the future will be the man that invokes the laboratory and calls the specialist.

THIS kind of general practitioner will be a competent person indeed. As diagnostician he will have to know enough of every specialty to know when not to rely upon his own judgment.

He will have to know how to evaluate (and therefore in a degree at least how to conduct) laboratory procedures. It is not going to be easy to produce such a man or to produce him in the number the needs of the nation will call for.

Perhaps the means of evolving this diagnostician par excellence is the most urgent problem now facing the organizers of medical education. By the same token, it must be a primary consideration in any national "planning" that aims, whether in the name of health or security, at providing the population with "adequate" medical care.

April 4, 1937

NATIONAL POLICY ON HEALTH ASKED BY 430 DOCTORS

Many Noted Physicians Join 'Revolt' Against American Medical Association

FAVOR STATE SUBSIDIES

Advocate Aid in Prevention, in Education and in Care of the Indigent Sick

A committee of internationally known physicians, including one Nobel Prize winner and several professors from the Harvard and Yale Medical Schools, made public yesterday a "medical declaration of independence," subscribed to by 430 outstanding medical men from all parts of the country, advocating a set of principles and proposals which had been overwhelmingly rejected last June by the House of Delegates of the American Medical Association, ruling body of organized medicine in America.

These principles and proposals call for the recognition by the medical profession of the principle that "the health of the people is a direct concern of the government"

and that a "national health policy directed toward all groups of the population should be formulated."

The endorsement is regarded in medical circles as the first open revolt against the hitherto unquestioned authority of the ruling body of America's organized medical profession, coming as it does in defiance of the action of the House of Delegates of the American Medical Association at its annual convention last Summer in Atlantic City.

Spread of Movement Seen

There are indications that the open defiance of the authority of the association is spreading among many of the rank and file of American physicians who had been silently opposing the attitude of their leaders and had been waiting for prominent members in their ranks to take the initiative. There are some who regard the present move as likely to result in a split in the ranks of American medicine similar to the split in the ranks of American labor.

While the announcement of the action taken by the 430 "insurgents" came only yesterday, news of its coming had reached the authorities of the American Medical Association last month, and without waiting for the official announcement the move was bitterly assailed in an editorial in the Oct. 16 issue of The Journal of the American Medical Association, official organ of that body, of which Dr. Morris Fishbein is the editor.

"A cursory analysis of the list," the editorial declared, "actually reveals the names of some physicians whose names are associated at the same time with views and actions opposed to those which they are here said to hold. Obviously some of these men must have signed merely after seeing the names of

those who signed previously and because it looked like a 'good' list.

"There appear also the names of some members of the House of Delegates which voted against some of the very propositions which these members here support. Most conspicuous on the list are the names of those deans and heads of departments in medical schools who may have signed because they saw a possibility of getting government money for clinics and dispensaries. Such careless participation in propaganda as has here occurred is lamentable, to say the least. Certainly the unthinking endorsers of the American Foundation's principles and proposals owe to the medical profession some prompt disclaimers."

In spite of this official challenge, however, the 430 physicians and surgeons have refused to make the "prompt disclaimers" suggested to them by the official organ of the American Medical Association. The list of signatures, it was announced, "is being extended."

The physicians' committee, in suggesting "changes needed for the provision of medical care to the American people," announced that they had sent the set of principles and proposals for consideration to medical organizations.

These principles and proposals, they declared, "should govern needed efforts to improve medical care, whether made by voluntary or governmental agencies, local, State or Federal." The "formulation of the principles and proposals," they added, was made "in the hope that they may receive the consideration of the National Government and of medical organizations."

Members of the Committee

The committee of physicians is composed of the following:

Russell L. Cecil, New York, chairman, Associate Attending Physician, New York Hospital; John P. Peters, New Haven, Conn., secretary, Professor of Medicine, Yale Univer-

sity School of Medicine; Milton C. Winternitz, New Haven, vice chairman, Professor of Pathology, formerly dean, Yale University School of Medicine; Hugh Cabot, Rochester, Minn., vice chairman, Consulting Surgeon, Mayo Clinic.

Also George Blumer, New Haven, Professor of Clinical Medicine, formerly dean, Yale University School of Medicine; Allan M. Butler, Boston, Assistant Professor of Pediatrics, Harvard Medical School; J. Rosslyn Earp, Albany, Medical Editor, health education division, New York State Department of Health; Channing Frothingham, Boston, Chief of the Medical Service, Faulkner Hospital; William S. McCann, Rochester, N. Y., Physician in Chief, Strong Memorial and Rochester Municipal Hospitals; George R. Minot, Boston, Professor of Medicine, Harvard Medical School, director Thorndike Memorial Laboratory; Robert B. Osgood, Boston, Professor Emeritus of Orthopedic Surgery, Harvard Medical School; Richard M. Smith, Boston, Assistant Professor of Pediatrics and Child Hygiene, Harvard Medical School and School of Public Health; John H. Stokes, Philadelphia, Professor of Dermatology and Syphilology, University of Pennsylvania School of Medicine; Soma Weiss, Boston, Associate Professor of Medicine, Harvard Medical School.

Professor Minot was one of three winners of the Nobel Prize in Medicine for the discovery of the use of liver in the treatment of pernicious anemia.

In making public the draft, together with the signatories, Dr. Peters also made public the committee's statement explaining how the draft came to be made. The statement reads as follows:

"A large number of medical men believe that the report of the American Foundation Studies in Government, entitled 'American Medicine: Expert Testimony Out of Court,' deserves the thoughtful attention of all physicians.

"As a contribution to the discussion of the subject of medical care in the United States, this self-appointed group of medical men, finding themselves in agreement, has formulated certain principles and proposals anent such care. These physicians, who have been trying to purvey medical care for many years, speak only for themselves and not for the foundation or for any other organization. They hope that these principles and proposals may suggest the lines along which effort may be made by voluntary, local, State and Federal agencies to improve medical care.

"It is recognized that the medical profession is only one of several groups to which 'medical care' is of vital concern. Close cooperation between physicians, economists and sociologists is essential. Nevertheless the medical profession should initiate any proposed changes, because physicians are the experts upon whom communities must depend. Unless the medical profession is ready to cooperate with these other groups, they cannot expect to play successfully the part which they should play, nor can they expect to enlist the sympathetic understanding of legislative bodies.

"It seems to us probable that certain alterations in our present system of preventing illness and providing medical care may become necessary; indeed, certain changes have already occurred. Medical knowledge is increasing rapidly and is becoming more complex. Changes in economic and social conditions are taking place at home and abroad. Medicine must be mobile and not static if medical men are to act as the expert advisers of those who convert public opinion into action.

"The conviction is general that action should be taken only upon the basis of demonstrated need and as experience accumulates to indicate that such action is likely to attain its ends in a nation comprising forty-eight States in which climatic, economic and social conditions vary greatly.

"Comments on these principles and proposals are invited and should be sent to Dr. John P. Peters, secretary committee of physicians, 789 Howard Avenue, New Haven, Conn."

Principles and Proposals Listed

The principles and proposals signed by the 430 medical men and now presented to the medical organizations for consideration are:

Principles

"1. That the health of the people is a direct concern of the government.

"2. That a national public health policy directed toward all groups of the population should be formulated.

"3. That the problem of economic need and the problem of providing adequate medical care are not identical and may require different approaches to their solution.

"4. That in the provision of adequate medical care for the population four agencies are concerned; voluntary agencies, local, State and Federal Governments.

Proposals

"1. That the first necessary step toward the realization of the above principles is to minimize the risk of illness by prevention.

"2. That an immediate problem is provision of adequate medical care for the medically indigent, the cost to be met from public funds (local and/or State and/or Federal).

"3. That public funds should be made available for the support of medical education and for studies, investigations and procedures for raising the standards of medical practice. If this is not provided for, the provision of adequate medical care may prove impossible.

"4. That public funds should be available for medical research as essential for high standards of practice in both preventive and curative medicine.

"5. That public funds should be made available to hospitals that render service to the medically indigent and for laboratory and diagnostic and consultative services.

"6. That in allocation of public funds existing private institutions should be utilized to the largest possible extent and that they may receive support so long as their service is in consonance with the above principles.

"7. That public health services, Federal, State and local, should be extended by evolutionary process.

"8. That the investigation and planning of the measures proposed and their ultimate direction should be assigned to experts.

"9. That the adequate administration and supervision of the health functions of the government, as implied in the above proposals, necessitates, in our opinion, a functional consolidation of all Federal health and medical activities, preferably under a separate department.

"The subscribers to the above principles and proposals hold the view that health insurance alone does not offer a satisfactory solution on the basis of the principles and proposals enunciated above."

All Fields Are Represented

The list of those that have signed the principles and proposals includes physicians in all branches of practice, in all sections of the country. Among them are, in the field of internal medicine, Francis G. Blake, physician in chief of the New Haven Hospital; Henry A. Christian, physician in chief of the Peter Bent Brigham Hospital; Eugene F. Du Bois, physician in chief of the New York Hospital; Joseph T. Wearn, Professor of Medicine at Western Reserve University and chief of medical services of the Lakeside Hospital in Cleveland; Marion A. Blankenhorn, director of the Department of Internal Medicine at the Cincinnati General Hospital; David P. Barr, physician in chief of the Barnes Hospital in St. Louis; William J. Kerr, San Francisco, physician in chief of the University of California Hospital; Ernest B. Bradley of Lexington, Ky., retiring president of the American College of Physicians; Hugh J. Morgan, Nashville, executive secretary of the Association of American Physicians, and Joseph A. Capps, senior attending physician at St. Luke's Hospital in Chicago.

The surgeons include Evarts A. Graham, chief surgeon of the Barnes Hospital in St. Louis, president of the American Surgical Association and head of the newly formed American Board of Surgery to establish and regulate standards of surgical practice in this country; Fred W. Rankin of Lexington, another member of the board; Elliott C. Cutler of Boston, chief surgeon at the Peter Bent Brigham Hospital; Frederick A. Coller, director of surgery at the University Hospital in Ann Arbor; J. Shelton Horsley of Richmond, and Samuel C. Harvey, Professor of Surgery at Yale.

The orthopedists include Frederick C. Kidner, Detroit, president of the American Orthopedic Association; Albert H. Freiberg of Cincinnati, a former president of the same association; Philip D. Wilson of New York City, a member of the American Board of Orthopedic Surgery.

The pediatricians include A. Graeme Mitchell, head of the Children's Hospital in Cincinnati and a member of the National Board of Medical Examiners; Borden S. Veeder of St. Louis, president of the American Board of Pediatrics; Philip Van Ingen of New York City, president of the American Academy of Pediatrics, and Kenneth D. Blackfan of Boston, Professor of Pediatrics at Harvard.

Among the deans of approved medical schools that have signed are Charles S. Burwell, dean of Harvard Medical School; William S. Ladd of Cornell, Loren R. Chandler of Stanford, George H. Whipple of the University of Rochester (New York), Charles W. McC. Poynter of the University of Nebraska, Earl B. McKinley of George Washington University School of Medicine, and two former deans of the College of Physicians and Surgeons of Columbia University; William Darrach, and Samuel W. Lambert.

Several men working in the field of public health have signed the draft: Dr. Thomas Parran, the Surgeon General of the United States Public Health Service; Dr. Kendall Emerson, manager of the National Tuberculosis Association; Dr. Reginald M. Atwater, executive secretary of the American Public Health Association, and, among the directors of State health departments, Henry D. Chadwick of Massachusetts, Edward S. Godfrey Jr., who directs the New York State Department; George H. Coombs, director for Maine; Clyde C. Slemons, Commissioner of Health for Michigan; J. L. Jones, State Health Commissioner of Utah; Carl V. Reynolds for North Carolina, and Frederick D. Stricker for Oregon.

Other signatories include Dr. Nathaniel W. Faxon, director of the Massachusetts General Hospital and a former president of the American Hospital Association; Dr. Louis Casamajor of New York City, member of the American Board of Psychiatry and Neurology; Dr. Fred J. Taussig of St. Louis, retiring president of the American Gynecological Society; Dr. Thomas B. Cooley of Detroit, chairman of the Council of the American Pediatric Society; Joseph B. Howland of Boston, director of the Peter Bent Brigham Hospital; J. H. Musser of New Orleans, Thomas M. Rivers, director of the Hospital of the Rockefeller Institute for Medical Research; George C. Shattuck of Boston, past president of the American Society of Tropical Medicine; A. Newton Richards, professor of pharmacology at the University of Pennsylvania; Alfred Stengel, vice president in charge of medical affairs at the University of Pennsylvania, and James H. Means, chief of medical services at the Massachusetts General Hospital.

Follows Foundation Report

The present "insurrection" on the part of the signers of the "medical declaration of independence" is the outgrowth of the report published last April by the American Foundation, established by Edward Bok, on the state of medicine in the United States. The report contained the letters of several thousand representative physicians and made no recommendations.

Shortly after the report's publication a conference of medical men and allied groups was held in New York City. Some of those present at the conference later discussed the matter with President Roosevelt.

Following these discussions with the President, a set of principles and proposals, only slightly different from those subscribed to by the 430 physicians, was adopted by the House of Delegates of the Medical Society of the State of New York. These principles were then introduced on behalf of the New York State Society before the annual meeting of the House of Delegates of the American Medical Association, which defeated the resolution after a bitter battle on the part of the New York members of the house.

Action Attacked by Journal

In its editorial attacking the action of the signers of the set of principles, The Journal of the American Medical Association published a letter which, the editorial declared, was sent by Dr. Hugh Cabot to "selected members of the association." The editorial quoted the letter as follows:

"I think it is important that a considerable group of influential and well-known physicians should assent to certain fairly general **propositions, the tendency of which will be to show that what is needed is a very broad attack along a wide front rather than more narrow attacks upon limited objectives.**

"There has, we think, been a good deal of rather just criticism of the medical profession on account of its unwillingness to advise positive rather than negative action. There seems to be some evidence that legislation looking toward compulsory health insurance has attracted a good deal of favorable attention in political bodies.

"It seems to us that compulsory insurance attacks only a very limited portion of the problem and that legislation to put this into operation might well do serious harm, not because it would not be of assistance in solving certain problems, but rather because it would help and might, therefore, tend to stop progress along a broader line."

Warns of Federal Subsidies

The editorial criticized the principles and proposals as follows:

"It should not be necessary to point out again in The Journal the danger of Federal subsidies for medical schools and the hazard of turning over to the Federal Government the control and standardization of medical schools. Such subsidies may easily involve determination of the curriculum and administration of service through the medical schools which would quite certainly interfere with the advancement of medical education and medical science and put the government right into the practice of medicine.

"Already, in some foreign countries, the government controls the number of medical students and the nature of medical education. American medicine wants no such system.

"Our government has already voted $750,000 a year for the control of cancer and suggestions have been offered that similar appropriations be made for the study of infantile paralysis, syphilis and other diseases. The danger of putting the government in the dominant position in relation to medical research is apparent.

"Still more serious is the fifth proposal, to the effect that the government subsidize private hospitals in relationship to their laboratory, diagnostic and consultative services. The nonprofit voluntary hospital is the pride of American philanthropy and a major factor in maintaining a high quality of medical service. The tender of governmental funds to such institutions for the care of an ill-defined group called the medically indigent appeals to the unthinking physicians who have endorsed these principles and proposals. Yet such an arrangement would put the hospitals promptly into the practice of medicine."

November 7, 1937

223

SPEEDED TRAINING PROVIDES DOCTORS

Medical School Step-Up Has Yielded 5,000 Above Normal Academic Production

Adoption of an accelerated program by medical schools has made possible the graduation of 5,000 more doctors than would have been supplied under a normal academic program, Dr. Willard C. Rappleye, dean of the College of Physicians and Surgeons, Columbia University, reported yesterday.

However, Dean Rappleye indicated in his annual report that the schools were not yet meeting the demands of the services and that an increase in the number of medical students might be necessary to supply, for example, 14,000 more doctors for the army by the end of this year.

Emphasizing the need for keeping up a steady supply of medical personnel for military and civilian service, the dean gave implied approval to present Army and Navy plans to draft students and then send them back to college for specialist training.

Benefit To Deserving

"Since the men for the Collegiate Training Corps will be selected because of their ability and aptitude and without regard to their ability to pay for a higher education," he said, "many promising students will be given educational opportunities which otherwise would not be available to them."

Pointing out that the problem of recognizing qualified pre-medical students under the new set-up has been considered, Dr. Rappleye declared that the choice of new medical students should not be made until the men are well into their college training.

On the question of how pre-medical students now in college should be treated, the dean expressed the hope that they "will not be inducted and given basic military training which would interrupt their preparation for medical studies." He pointed out that many of them have already completed the subjects that would be part of the proposed two-year curriculum.

Many Doctors Needed

By way of emphasizing the tremendous task facing medical schools, Dr. Rappleye estimated that the Army will need by the end of this year 48,000 doctors, an increase of 14,000 over the present staff. "The Navy's requirements," he said, "will reach close to 10,000.

Discussing the college's own contribution to the war program, he reported 174 members of the teaching staff in the armed services. Others are "called upon by various government agencies for advice in their special fields and give unstintingly of their time and talents.

"Several departments are devoting their research to war projects under government contract through the Office of Scientific Research and Development of the National Research Council," he said.

February 4, 1943

DEAN REPORTS GAIN IN GROUP MEDICINE

Dr. Rappleye of Columbia Says Trend Over the Nation Means Adequate Care, Lower Cost

POSSIBLE AS COMPROMISE

Joint Practice System Is Held of Use in Tax-Supported or Voluntary Health Systems

Medical practice in New York City and over the country is rapidly being streamlined by increasing acceptance of the principle of group practice, in which a panel of specialists combine their skills to arrive at a diagnosis and begin treatment, Dr. Willard C. Rappleye reported here yesterday.

The dean of the College of Physicians and Surgeons of Columbia University said group practice clinics were springing up everywhere. Here in the tradition-bound city, where county and state medical societies have always officially opposed group practice, the idea has taken a firm hold and more groups and fewer individual doctors are meeting the demand for medical attention.

In some professional circles it is held that group practice, if widely extended, might be the best way to meet increasing public demand for more efficient and cheaper medical care. The Federal Administration has called for passage of a payroll-tax supported national health insurance program. Opposing it, the American Medical Association has advocated extension of existing voluntary health insurance programs.

The group practice principle, which might be viewed as a compromise or might be utilized under either tax-supported or voluntary insurance plans, has been thoroughly tested and is strongly approved by the Columbia University medical college.

Integration of Specialties

"It is ridiculous to assume that any one doctor can be familiar with the great amount of knowledge that is available to medical scientists today," Dr. Rappleye said. "Specialization in medicine has been the result. Recently, it has been overemphasized.

"Now, the medical branches, the specialties, must be integrated to provide complete medical care. This is leading inevitably to the development of group practice as the modern way to practice medicine and the only way of providing up-to-date scientific medical care for any population group.

"There will always be doctors practicing 'solo,' of course, many in rural regions. Modern medical education teaches these men when to call in a specialist when it is necessary, however."

Dr. Rappleye maintained that group practice was the only way to provide the advantages of modern medical science for large population groups at a reasonable cost. He cited the experience of the medical college at Vanderbilt Clinic in the Medical Center.

This group-practice clinic was started with the idea that medical students might best learn from their professional instructors if each case examined was later considered in a group discussion with several participating specialists, each of whom had examined the patient.

Students spent their mornings seeing patients under the supervision of professional specialists and then met in the afternoon to discuss what they had separately observed. In this discussion they synthesized a diagnosis and ultimately agreed on the therapy.

Advantages in Consultation

Soon the medical center staff found that a large number of cases could be seen in a day. More important, Dr. Rappleye said, the specialists found that in many cases they could correct, amend or confirm each other's observations.

"Instead of going at examinations in a piecemeal fashion, as medicine had always been practiced," he continued, "we found that with the specialists all on hand while the patient was being seen a quick and thoroughly effective consultation could be attained.

"Everyone benefited: the patients, staff men and students. Now we keep our group practice clinic open twelve months a year with a half a dozen men always present. All new admissions go through the group panel with the exception of cases—such as a broken leg or pregnancy—where it is obviously unnecessary.

"The hospital cares for more patients than any voluntary organization in the nation. We have found we can see patients at an average cost of a little over $3 a visit, giving them the very best of scientific medical care.

"In a private office, overhead may amount to 40 per cent of a doctor's gross income. Ours is much lower. If a 'solo' doctor must call one or more specialists to see his patient, the cost goes way up. We are providing specialist services routinely when the nature of the complaint makes it necessary."

Dr. Rappleye emphasized that about 60 per cent of the work of examining new cases was done by practitioners of internal medicine, who, in a sense, are general practitioners. So doctors capable of working "solo" from their own offices in small towns are being trained at the college.

If the group practice principle is widely accepted, the dean declared, the nation now has plenty of doctors.

"In a number of situations where satisfactory standards of medical care are provided it has been shown that such services can be rendered on a basis of one doctor to 1,000 or 1,200 individuals," he reported.

June 3, 1950

MEDICAL COLLEGES IN VAST EXPANSION

By BENJAMIN FINE

The greatest expansion program in the history of medical education, to cost $250,000,000, is now under way in this country.

Almost every college of medicine in the United States is planning to increase its physical facilities. New laboratories, additional classrooms, modern dormitories and special research clinics are on the drawing board or actually under construction.

At present the country maintains seventy-three four-year institutions of medicine, and seven two-year colleges. Commissions or fact-finding committees have been set up in at least ten states to map plans for the development of new medical colleges. Some of the existing two-year schools will be expanded into regular four-year, degree-granting colleges of medicine.

These findings are based on a nation-wide survey conducted by THE NEW YORK TIMES, in which the eighty medical colleges and the forty-eight state commissioners of education were reached through questionnaires.

In the current academic year—1951-52—the medical colleges admitted the largest freshman classes in recent history, a total of 7,381 students. The total enrollment has been growing steadily since the end of World War II. Now it is slightly above 26,000, compared with 23,000 five years ago.

Despite the expansions now taking place, large numbers of qualified applicants are unable to gain admittance to any medical college in this country. Many of them seek places in foreign institutions. The records indicate that 20,000 individuals applied for admission to American medical schools for the current college year. As many of them applied to more than one institution, the total number of applications was more than 70,000, or an average of 3.5 a student.

More state and municipally owned medical colleges keep out non-residents than ever before. One-fourth of the schools exclude all students who do not reside in the state, while more than 50 per cent give preference to residents. Some of the medical colleges admit only two or three out-of-state applicants in any entering class. The Council on Medical Education of the American Medical Association reports that seventeen public colleges do not admit non-residents this year, compared with nine in 1948, seven in 1947 and none in 1946.

Of the total freshman class admitted last year by state and municipal schools, less than 7 per cent were non-residents, compared with 17 per cent ten years ago.

As a result of these geographical restrictions, some of the medical colleges have few students from which to choose. In some instances a medical school is forced to take nearly every one who applies, while other colleges can accept only one out of every twenty or thirty applicants. This makes for uneven scholarship. Whereas A or B students may be turned away in the big-name Eastern private colleges, low B or even C students are accepted in the states that enforce non-resident regulations.

Contrasts in Admissions

These figures, prepared by Dr. John M. Stalnaker, director of studies, Association of American Medical Colleges, suggest the wide variations that exist among institutions:

Medical School	Size of Freshman Class	Total Number of Applications Acted On
Alabama	80	251
Arkansas	90	185
Colorado	80	188
Georgia	89	249
Iowa	120	158
North Dakota	36	83
South Carolina	70	148

By contrast, here is the size of entering class and total number of applications acted on by institutions that have no geographical restrictions:

Albany	50	1,410
Boston	72	1,353
Chicago Medical	72	1,538
Columbia	120	2,034
Cornell	86	1,831
George Washington	95	1,824
Harvard	114	1,374
Jefferson	166	2,592
New York Medical	128	2,879
New York University	140	2,072
Pennsylvania	135	2,180
Syracuse	76	2,284

Commenting on this wide discrepancy in the number of applications received by various colleges, the Council on Medical Education observes:

"Those schools that restrict admissions to residents of a single state will probably have the greatest difficulty in finding suitable students to fill all their available places."

According to Dr. Stalnaker, a few of the schools with such restrictions are at this time taking almost everyone who applies. Some of the applicants are ill-qualified for the study of medicine, have poor academic records and poor test scores but nevertheless are admitted.

"Some state schools, which require that the student be a state resident to gain admittance," declared Dr. Stalnaker, "are literally scraping the bottom of the barrel in order to fill their classes."

Almost half of the total number of applicants for medical schools come from seven states, in this order—New York, Pennsylvania, California, Illinois, Ohio, New Jersey and Texas. Twenty-nine per cent of the New York applicants were accepted, while 50 per cent of those from Texas were admitted.

Despite the financial problems that are troubling the medical colleges, a record expansion program is well under way. Nearly half of the colleges are now engaged in fund-raising campaigns. They are seeking from both public sources and private individuals or foundations approximately $200,000,000.

Eighty-four per cent of the medical schools reported that they were planning to use this money to expand their physical facilities.

$50,000,000 for New Schools

According to THE TIMES' survey, the medical colleges will spend, within the next few years, $50,000,000 for laboratories, $30,000,000 for classrooms and $20,000,000 for dormitories. Another $100,000,000 is earmarked for research and special projects. In addition, the immediate cost for establishing new medical institutions will run above $50,000,000, making an over-all expansion program of a quarter of a billion dollars.

The University of Rochester Medical School is planning a $750,000 new wing to give added space for operating facilities and surgical supplies. The Medical College of the State of South Carolina plans to spend $800,000 for laboratories, $1,000,000 for dormitories and $8,250,000 for special and research projects, including a teaching hospital.

Vast improvements are planned at the University of Michigan Medical School. A $3,600,000 outpatient clinic will be ready for occupancy this fall, while a $3,000,000 research institute is also under construction. The college is also seeking $15,000,000 from the Legislature for a medical science building and $4,500,000 for a general children's hospital.

New Schools Being Started

To meet the increasing demands for more physicians and medically trained men, at least ten states have taken steps to build new medical schools or expand their two-year basic science schools into four-year institutions. The University of California at Los Angeles completed its medical school, and admitted its first class last September.

The University of Mississippi is proceeding rapidly with its plan to make a regular four-year medical school out of its two-year basic science institution. Dean D. S. Pamkratz of the school of medicine estimates that $8,500,000 will be needed to expand the physical facilities. An entering class of twenty-eight is to be admitted each year for the next several years. Dr. Pamkratz said that the graduate work is to be expanded, with special emphasis on general practice.

"We hope to build a rehabilitation center, a new state health department, a large student dormitory, a nurses' home and other ancillary medical buildings in the near future," he added.

The states of New Jersey, Connecticut, Rhode Island, Massachusetts and Florida have appointed commissions or set machinery in motion to found medical colleges. The Legislature of West Virginia authorized the expansion of the West Virginia University School of Medicine to a four-year program. The basic science school of the University of Missouri will be expanded to a four-year porgram, according to present plans.

All of these new medical projects are planned under public auspices. The only medical college under private sponsorship is being founded in New York City.

A $25,000,000 medical center comprising colleges of medicine, dentistry, nursing and public health is being established under the guidance of Yeshiva University. The center is to be affiliated with the city $36,500,000 hospital project in the Bronx. According to Dr. Harry M. Zimmerman, director of the new college of medicine, the institution will open in 1953 with an entering class of 100, and will eventually have a total student body of 400. The college plans to spend $10,000,000 for its basic medical building. A fund-raising campaign is now under way directed by State Attorney General Nathaniel L. Goldstein.

Thirty per cent of the nation's medical schools report that they are unable to get sufficient funds to meet their operating budgets. Many are engaged in campaigns to "keep their heads above water." Forty-five per cent report that they find it difficult to get a sufficient number of qualified faculty members. However, Dr. Zimmerman reports that the college of medicine he heads is experiencing no difficulty in enlisting an adequate staff of competent instructors.

A majority of the medical deans—78 per cent—believe that there is a shortage of doctors in this country at present, and advocate further expansion of medical facilities. Many suggest, however, that the shortage could be alleviated with better disribution. They point to critical shortages in rural areas.

For example, the University of Tennessee College of Medicine notes: "There is a definite shortage of medical service in rural areas. There is also a definite shortage in public institutions, such as mental hospitals and in public health service."

Similarly, Dean R. Hugh Wood of the school of medicine at Emory University observes: "There is unquestionably an actual shortage. The effect is magnified by the additional factor of unequal distribution of physicians."

To Admit More Students

Many institutions are increasing their enrollments to meet the demands from their communities for more physicians. However, Dr. Wood warns that classes of more than 100 may weaken the present high medical standards. Rather than greatly increase the enrollment of existing schools, additional ones should be established, said Dr. Wood, adding:

"One of the present threats to the quality of medical education stems from the fact that members of state legislatures do not understand this point. There have been several instances in the last few years in which the state government has ordered the medical school of the state university to increase its enrollment without providing additional facilities and budget."

Many medical authorities believe that the existing enrollment can be increased without lowering the quality, if sufficient funds are obtained to add to the physical plant and increase the faculty. Every one reached in THE TIMES' study urged that the high standards in medical education be safeguarded.

March 2, 1952

Study of Medical School Bias Calls National Origin a Factor

By WARREN WEAVER Jr.
Special to The New York Times.

ALBANY, July 9—A student who wants to study medicine in New York State stands a better chance of getting admitted to one of the nine professional schools if he is Protestant rather than Catholic or Catholic rather than Jewish, a report to the Board of Regents indicated today.

The report, which was made after an eighteen-month study to determine whether the state's ban against racial and religious discrimination in medical school admission policies was being observed, was cautious in charging any actual bias on the basis of the statistics collected.

Dr. Howard E. Wilson, executive assistant of the Carnegie Endowment for International Peace and author of the report, warned "these general figures are not in themselves proof of discrimination," since admission policies put considerable stress on such intangible factors as personality and character.

The figures showed, however, that in both of the two years studied—1950 and 1952—seven of the nine medical schools in the state had admitted a higher proportion of Protestant applicants than of those of either the Roman Catholic or the Jewish faith.

However, Jewish students actually topped the admissions in numbers, although the proportion was smaller in relation to the total of applications from Jewish students.

Dr. Wilson emphasized the study, while limited in the number of cases surveyed, indicated the factors of national origin and degree of Americanization might actually be more important than religion in instances where the figures indicated discrimination on religious grounds.

For example, in both 1950 and 1952 the percentage of Catholic applicants who were not of Italian descent and got into medical school markedly exceeded the percentage of Italian Catholics who were admitted. The report concluded that would-be doctors of Italian extraction had "unusual difficulty" in getting an education in New York.

"The fact that non-Italian Catholics are admitted in about the same proportion as Protestants, while Italian Catholics have a very low incidence of admission, offers evidence that factors other than religious affiliation may account for what might at first seem to be a disproportion for this religious group," Dr. Wilson said.

The report also showed Jewish applicants in 1952 had been considerably more successful in getting into medical school if both their parents were American born than if only one was, and, in turn, that the latter group had a higher percentage of acceptance than those with both parents born abroad.

This finding, according to the survey, "suggests that recency of family arrival may be a significant factor, helping to explain certain data concerning general religious groupings" and may also form "a rough index as to social-personal-cultural factors having marked influence in the selection of candidates."

The figures of Dr. Wilson's report appeared to substantiate to some extent a protest made on June 21 by the American Jewish Congress, which charged the nine medical schools in the state were treating Jewish applicants less favorably than non-Jewish ones.

However, an accurate comparison was difficult, since the statistics put forward by the Jewish group dealt only with students in a high academic bracket, while Dr. Wilson's figures covered students with varying study records.

The report included eight recommendations through which the regents, the medical schools and the undergraduate colleges might achieve a broader compliance with the 1948 Quinn-Olliffe Law, which barred discrimination in admission to any educational institution on the grounds of race, religion or national origin. These included proposals that:

¶The regents and the medical schools "explore the feasibility" of setting up a single central bureau for all medical school admission applications to conduct initial screening operations and save applicants multiple fees.

¶The medical schools formally and publicly declare their position with respect to discrimination in admission and their criteria for accepting applicants.

¶The medical schools agree on a common deadline for accepting applications and a single date for announcing results and also study the possibility of lowering the fees for filing applications.

¶The colleges undertake a more careful "sifting" of pre-medical students to reduce the number of applicants for medical schools by weeding out those obviously without qualification.

¶The regents establish an advisory Council on Admissions with representatives of education, the public and civil rights groups to advise the board on problems of this type.

On the positive side, the report stated that in 1950 and 1952 "race and color had little or nothing to do with admissibility," as the percentage of Negro and other nonwhite applicants admitted was essentially the same as that of all other groups combined.

On the negative side, the survey declared that "application of the criterion of scholarship does not explain or warrant the discrepancies in proportion of admission of Catholic, Protestant and Jewish students to New York State medical schools.

"If scholastic achievement were to be regarded as the sole determinant of admissibility, evidence would be at hand of discrimination, particularly against Jewish applicants," it continued. "However, it has already been pointed out that scholastic achievement alone does not and should not guarantee admission to the study of medicine."

The Wilson report covered 948 applicants in 1950 and 633 in 1952. Of the latter group, 28.6 per cent were Catholic, 46.3 per cent Jewish and 21.3 per cent Protestant. About one-fifth of these students got into medical schools; 15.9 per cent of the Catholic applicants got in, 20.1 per cent of the Jewish and 23.4 per cent of the Protestant.

This represented an improvement, according to the report, from the 1950 figures, which showed 10 per cent of the applicants accepted. In this group, 8.1 per cent of the Catholic students were admitted, 9.3 per cent of the Jewish students and 15.4 per cent of the Protestant students.

The schools studied were the Albany Medical College, the University of Buffalo School of Medicine, Columbia University College of Physicians and Surgeons, Cornell University Medical College, New York Medical College, New York University College of Medicine, University of Rochester School of Medicine and Dentistry and the State University Colleges of Medicine at New York and Syracuse.

July 10, 1953

First New Medical School Here in 60 Years Focuses Attention on a National Need

By BENJAMIN FINE

The opening this week of the Albert Einstein College of Medicine in the Bronx marks the first time in nearly sixty years that a medical school has been started in New York State. Indeed, this is one of the few such colleges under private auspices that has been founded since the turn of the century, and its opening provides a timely opportunity for a consideration of the status of medical education in the United States today.

Almost every report in recent years dealing with manpower problems has pointed to the need for more doctors, dentists and nurses. American hospitals have 12,000 internships available and only 6,000 internes to fill them. There are 19,000 residencies and only 12,000 doctors available. Arthur S. Flemming, Director of Defense Mobilization, said recently: "One of our principal problems is a shortage of men and women who have had the benefits of adequate medical training."

We are graduating only one new doctor for each 30,000 people. By 1960, authorities agree, this country will face a shortage of about 30,000 doctors, unless we step up our training.

Many factors are involved in the problem of the doctor shortage. Medical education is expensive—too expensive for many public universities, and far above the resources of most private institutions. For example, the Albert Einstein Medical College, which is under the auspices of Yeshiva University, is now in the process of raising $12,000,000 for the construction of its basic science building. Operating expenses thereafter will range from $1,500,000 to $2,000,000 a year. The college is to be the focal point of a $100,000,000 medical center which will also include the $40,000,000 Bronx municipal hospital center and a $45,000,000 psychiatric hospital center.

In the training of doctors, expansion is slow, difficult and expensive. The American Medical Association has set high standards for medical schools. Only Grade A schools are recognized. Classes are necessarily small; an entering class of 100 is considered to be the maximum size.

The medical profession has spent many years in building its reputation. It does not want to lower its guard now, even though more doctors are urgently needed. It agrees that more doctors are needed, but insists that they should be doctors who are trained in the best traditions of the profession.

In some quarters the question has been raised: Are the standards too high? Is the A. M. A. deliberately keeping potential medical students out of the profession for reasons not of ethics but of economics?

In a recent interview Dr. Edward L. Turner, secretary of the Council on American Education and Hospitals of the A. M. A., denied this. Dr. Turner pointed out that misunderstandings had arisen in some areas concerning the role of the A. M. A. But, he emphasized, the council and the A. M. A. have always sought to encourage the growth of medical schools, provided they were of the highest quality.

The medical profession would never permit a return to the "mail order days" of the early part of the century, prior to the reforms that stemmed from the Abraham Flexner study sponsored by the Rockefeller Foundation in 1910.

High tuition fees are a factor in keeping many qualified students from entering medical schools. In 1954-55 the average tuition fee for students attending medical schools in their own states was $646; for nonresidents it was $807. The previous year it had been $633 for residents, $772 for nonresidents. The tuition fees are grouped this way: one medical school charges less than $100; four schools charge from $100 to $199; two from $200 to $299; twelve from $300 to $399;

eight from $400 to $499; seven from $500 to $599; three from $600 to $699; eight from $700 to $799; fifteen from $800 to $899; fifteen from $900 to $999; and six, more than $1,000.

Despite these high fees, the medical schools are expanding; they enroll more students than ever before. The following table gives the year, number of students enrolled in approved medical schools and total graduates:

Year	Accredited Enrollments	Graduates
1910	12,530	3,165
1915	11,314	2,619
1920	12,559	2,680
1925	17,462	3,842
1930	21,597	4,565
1935	22,888	5,101
1940	21,271	5,097
1945	24,028	5,136
1950	25,103	5,553
1955	28,583	6,977

Dr. Turner said that there has been a rapid rise in recent years in enrollments and graduations despite high costs. Some students are still going to medical college under G. I. scholarships, either from World War II or the Korean conflict.

Then, too, seventeen states offer medical scholarships. Some states will grant aid only with the understanding that the young doctor settle and practice in that state. During 1954-55 a total of $1,151,760 in scholarship grants was available in seventy medical schools. In addition, these schools offered students $2,322,170 in loans.

However, the loans and scholarships together did not begin to meet the total needs. The students paid about $18,000,000 in tuition fees to the medical colleges.

Expansion programs for medical education are under way in various parts of the country. Last year the University of California at Los Angeles graduated its first class. The University of Miami will graduate its first class next June. The University of Mississippi completed a $9,000,000 construction plan and will admit its third-year class in June. The University of Missouri is undergoing its conversion from a two-year science to a four-year

medical college. The University of Florida will admit its first medical class next June, also. Seton Hall College of Medicine in Jersey City, N. J., will open in the fall of 1956 under present plans.

This is probably a greater growth of medical school facilities than in any comparable period. Will the additional facilities be enough to meet the needs of a growing population and the military, as well as the development of new medical and health practices?

Opinion is divided on this point. Dr. Turner believes that the existing facilities, together with those being planned, will go a long way toward developing the number of doctors needed. Other authorities, however, are dubious that the growth in medical facilities is rapid enough or large enough to meet current and future needs.

One fact which will be brought out in the annual report of the Council on American Education and Hospitals, to be issued Oct. 8, is dis-

turbing. The report will show that the number of applicants for medical school admission has dropped drastically in recent years. In 1954-55 there were about 15,000 applicants for the 7,500 positions in the entering class. They made 47,000 applications (an average of about three applications for each student). Three years ago there were more than 20,000 candidates for medical schools. And, three years ago, one out of every 3.6 students was accepted. Last year, one out of every 1.97 students found a place in a medical school.

However, these figures may be somewhat misleading. More than half of the medical schools have geographic restrictions—they will only admit residents of their state, or sometimes of the region. Which means that while one medical school may have less than 200 applications for 100 openings, another, without geographic regulations, may have more than 4,000 for the same number of openings.

September 4, 1955

Doctor's Dilemma: How to Keep Up

By LEONARD ENGEL

DURING the past two decades, every year has brought a bumper crop of advances in medicine, many of lifesaving importance. One result has been a pressing new problem for the practicing physician: how to keep up-to-date.

The lives of the doctor's patients depend on his possession of the latest medical knowledge. But it is hard for the busy physician to find time to keep up with even a part of the ever-increasing discoveries in medical science.

"Many doctors do a good job of staying abreast of major new developments," says a medical school dean, "and give their patients thoroughly modern care. Unfortunately, this isn't true of all. Many have little real opportunity to keep up. Some don't even try."

In recent months, medical leaders have been discussing numerous schemes for altering this situation. The most drastic proposal has come from Dr. Gunnar Gunderson, president of the American Medical Association. Dr. Gunderson has said that, if other measures fail, he wants compulsory periodic licensing examinations for all physicians—perhaps every five years.

The doctor's task in keeping up-to-date is not only urgent, but formidably complex.

"The physician must keep up in a double sense," says Dr. Norton S. Brown, president of the New York County Medical Society and a member of a New York Academy of Medicine committee studying the problem. "During his training, the doctor was schooled to high standards of medical workmanship. He was taught to study each patient with painstaking care. He owes it to his patients to maintain these standards depite the pressures of a crowded waiting room and an end-

less round of hospital and house calls.

"Somehow, he must also find time to keep pace with what's new. New drugs, for example, come out at a dizzying rate—several hundred a year. The physician has to know something of most or all of them—even the many that are no real improvement over existing drugs. And he must learn a great deal about those that are truly new and useful—a task that can easily consume a man's full time. Yet new drugs constitute only a small part of medical advance."

No doctor, of course, can familiarize himself with the details of new developments in all areas of medicine. This is one reason why two of every five physicians in active practice in the United States choose to be specialists. But even the specialist must know at least the broad outlines of what is being accomplished in branches of medicine other than his own.

"That's the part that keeps me reading nights and week-ends," says one New York practitioner. "I couldn't do a decent job for my patients otherwise."

A few weeks ago, a symposium on heart surgery was held at Mount Sinai Hospital in New York as part of a postgraduate course sponsored by the American College of Physicians. The speakers were six cardiac surgeons with world reputations. The audience was composed entirely of internists—specialists in internal ailments who perform no surgery. I asked an internist from Texas and another from Ohio why they were there.

"To find out which of our patients the heart surgeons can help," they replied.

Internists and general practitioners must be equally well posted in many other areas of medicine. They see most patients before other physicians. They need to know about advances in psychiatry, for example, since they

may see patients in the early stages of mental illness. Moreover, psychological factors figure prominently in a number of the ailments—such as peptic ulcer—which the internist and the G. P. treat.

IT works the other way, too. Psychiatrists must be alert to advances in internal medicine and even in surgery. Thus, anti-clotting drugs and blood-vessel surgery have recently been shown to be of value in many cases of stroke. The psychiatrist may see some of these cases, for patients with incipient stroke often have vague symptoms and are sometimes sent to psychiatrists as "neurotic."

And so it goes for every branch of medicine, from allergy to radiology. There is no branch that cannot profit from advances in another.

How does the practicing physician keep up with changes in medicine today?

Let us see how one doctor who does a conscientious job of keeping up goes about it. Dr. A.—the code of medical ethics forbids use of the name of a doctor in private practice—was graduated from medical school twenty years ago and is now in his mid-forties. His office is in a big city suburb and he has a general family practice.

One afternoon and one evening each week he drives fifteen miles to the city to serve in a diagnostic clinic in a large hospital with a strong teaching program. His motive is not the nominal fee he receives ($13 per session), but contact with a teaching hospital.

Rank-and-file doctors and medical educators alike agree that the most effective device by far for keeping a doctor's standards high and his knowledge fresh is contact with a teaching hospital. Unfortunately, only several hundred of the 7,000 hospitals in the United States (chiefly medical-school hospitals) have effective medical teaching programs.

DR. A. finds three aspects of his clinic work valuable. One is the wide range of patients he encounters. Another is the opportunity to work with an alert group of residents (young doctors taking specialty training) and with specialists. The third is the informal contact afforded him with members of the hospital staff.

"I don't know which aspect of the clinic work is most helpful," Dr. A. declares. "The clinic is a constant reminder of how medicine ought to be practiced. Since this is a teaching clinic, every hospital resource is used to obtain all relevant data on each patient. Every patient is studied as a demonstration case.

"But I especially enjoy the opportunity the clinic work gives me for talking with other doctors at the hospital. This is a pretty lively hospital. Something new is always being tried. I hear about it in consultations over difficult cases, in the corridors, in the doctors' lounge, or when I go to dinner with some of the staff."

Dr. A. also goes to meetings at the hospital to hear discussions of medical journals. In addition, he goes on ward rounds every few weeks, usually when he hears of interesting patients.

Although the city hospital is the focus for Dr. A.'s "keeping up" activities, he does not leave it at that. Once or twice a month, he attends medical society lectures. Each year, he goes to a medical convention or takes a one- or two-week post-graduate course. And he subscribes to nearly a dozen medical journals, which he generally gets to look at in bed after midnight.

"Sometimes I wonder whether I ought to cut down on the journals and get a little more sleep," Dr. A. remarks. "But then something happens that makes me pleased as punch that I do stay up and read.

"THE other week, a patient came to me with a complaint of ringing in the ears, dizziness and nausea—a combination of symptoms called Menière's disease, ordinarily caused by disease of the auditory nerve. I was about to send him to an ear-nose-throat man for ear surgery—the usual treatment for Menière's disease—when I recalled an article I had read a few weeks before in a British medical journal. An English physician had eleven patients in which Menière's syndrome turned out to be due to an ulcer or other ailment of the digestive tract rather than to disease of the auditory nerve.

"I sent my patient for gastro-intestinal X-rays. Maybe it was pure coincidence. But there wasn't anything wrong with his auditory nerve. He had a gastric ulcer, possibly cancerous."

The majority of physicians do not have Dr. A's opportunity to participate in the activities of a first-class teaching hospital. However, the practicing doctor who wants to practice up-to-date medicine has a rich assortment of other educational aids to choose from.

On a volume basis, the most important is the vast array of medical journals available to him. In the United States alone, well over 1,000 journals devoted to medicine as a whole or to its various branches are published. The total is higher still if journals in fields related to medicine, such as physiology, are counted.

In fact, finding journals that can inform him of new developments is not the doctor's problem. The hard part is choosing which journals to read. A medical editor recently pointed out that if a surgeon were to devote every evening in the month to reading only the principal journals of general surgery in the English language—all containing much information not duplicated in other journals—he could not get through one month's issues before the next crop descended upon him.

THIS flood of reading matter has given rise to a host of other publications, designed to single out and summarize the most significant reports published in medical journals or given at medical meetings. These include review and abstract (digest) journals, books, monographs and pamphlets, and special bulletins issued by agencies such as the American Heart Association. In addition, pharmaceutical companies put out magazines and newspapers—many well-edited and widely read—for physicians.

Doctors may also buy digests of medical reports recorded on tape, to be played while driving about on house calls. And closed-circuit TV has been utilized both to bring information on new developments like the Salk vaccine to nation-wide medical audiences, and to demonstrate new surgical procedures at medical conventions.

But the educational activity considered most useful by physicians—especially physicians with little opportunity to work in teaching hospitals—is the post-graduate "refresher course." More than 2,000 of these are offered each year by medical schools and organizations like the American College of Surgeons. They generally last one

to two weeks and they cover an immense variety of subjects.

In 1955 the American Medical Association questioned 4,923 of 168,000 practicing physicians in the United States on what they did to keep up with new developments in medicine. The survey showed that many put in an impressive amount of time reading, attending lectures and refresher courses and holding discussions with other doctors. Conscientious specialists reported spending 750 hours (equivalent to nearly ninety-five eight-hour days) a year in such activities; general practitioners reported almost 550 hours a year.

But the survey also disclosed two weaknesses in the various programs devoted to helping the doctor keep up. For one thing, many of these activities were found to be of limited value. Thus, numerous physicians found medical society lectures much less effective than journal reading; and journal reading was described as not to be compared either with attendance at post-graduate courses or with work in a teaching hospital.

The second weakness disclosed by the A. M. A. study is the fact that 30 per cent or more of practicing physicians take little or no part in medical society programs or other formal educational activities. What information they have on new medical developments comes chiefly from occasional journal reading or from "detail men"—the pharmaceutical company salesmen who call on doctors.

"I do not mean to denigrate the detail man," says a prominent medical educator. "The detail man deserves much of the credit for the speed with which new drugs are brought into wide use today.

"However, the detail man comes to the doctor's office to sell drugs. Aside from the fact that drugs constitute a very small part of medicine, the detail man sees the physician for a few minutes only. In that time, he can pass on only the sketchiest sort of data on one or two drugs—data often so presented as to gloss over the limitations of the drug.

"I THINK the detail man, and pharmaceutical over-promotion in general, share some of the blame for drug abuses. But I think the physician who depends solely on the detail man also deserves blame. That is not the way to practice good medicine."

Medical leaders agree that some sort of external stimulus is necessary to make some physicians work harder at raising their standards and at keeping their medical knowledge fresh. But they also concede that the fault does not lie entirely with the physician.

Numerous studies have shown that more "keeping up" facilities of every kind are needed, from additional teaching hospitals to post-graduate courses better geared to the requirements of the contemporary practicing doctor. The size of the need, however, is itself a sign of medical progress. If medicine were not changing so rapidly, there would be no concern over whether doctors were keeping up.

June 7, 1959

A. M. A. DROPS BAN ON UNIT CARE PLAN

By ROBERT K. PLUMB

Special to The New York Times.

ATLANTIC CITY, June 10—The American Medical Association today ended its long-standing opposition to closed-panel medical plans, particularly those sponsored by unions.

The move came after five years of study into what had long been one of the sharpest issues among medical men.

Although many groups that provide medical care for their members through salaried physicians were formed in the nineteenth century, they have never been officially approved by the American Medical Association.

The action today was viewed by physicians for unions as an act of recognition—and a belated one—that an individual has as much right to choose the type of medical-care program he will participate in as an individual has to select and pay his own doctor.

Union physicians also were happy that they would no

228

longer be regarded by the American Medical Association as second-class medical citizens. For the association formally declared:

"There is no generally held opinion declaring that participation in closed-panel medical care plans would render a physician unethical."

About 5,500,000 people in the United States are covered by plans in which a panel of physicians contracts to provide medical care.

The services range from lim-ited diagnostic facilities to complete medical care for a family. In most of these plans, patients have a choice among the physicians on the panel. In some plans, physicians are salaried by the panel; in others they receive a fee for service. Many of the plans are sponsored by unions. Many full-time salaried physicians are paid $12,000 to $25.000 a year or more.

The change in attitude came in the approval by the American Medical Association's House of Delegates of a voluminous Larson committee report entitled "Report of the Com-mission on Medical Care Plans."

Action on the report of the fifteen-man committee headed by Dr. Leonard W. Larson of Bismarck, S. D., has been postponed at other A. M. A. meetings. Dr. Larson is chairman of the association's board of trustees.

A special reference committee headed by Dr. John S. Detar of Milan, Mich., on Tuesday ironed out some difficulties and worked out wording upon which the delegates agreed today.

In one instance, the committee suggested that reference to the sticky question of "free choice of physician" be worded this way:

"The American Medical Association believes that free choice of physician is the right of every individual and one which he should be free to exercise as he chooses.

"Each individual should be accorded the privilege to select and change his physician at will or to select his preferred system of medical care and the American Medical Association vigorously supports the right of the individual to choose between these alternatives."

June 11, 1959

STUDENT QUALITY DROPS IN MEDICINE

Schools Alarmed by Decline in Top Applicants—Lure of Other Careers Cited

CURRICULUM CRITICIZED

Educator, in Lecture, Calls Medical Instruction Too Inflexible and Too Slow

A serious decline in the caliber of medical students is beginning to worry observers in American education and medicine.

A steady drop in the number and quality of applicants has reduced the ratio of applications and acceptances to the lowest in the history of modern American medical education. Since 1950, applications have declined by one-third, according to latest reports.

A number of alarming developments can be reported in this connection:

¶In the academic year 1950-51, about 40 per cent of all students entering medical school had a college average of A; by 1957-58, the last tabulated record, the number of A students had decreased to 18 per cent, according to the Association of American Medical Colleges. As a hopeful sign that the downward trend may begin to be reversed, the association reports an improvement in the test results of the 1958-59 applicants.

¶While medicine once was able to skim the cream of each year's crop of students, with only the law and the ministry competing, the scientific and engineering careers that have been glamorized more effectively in recent years now take the top students.

¶Medical research is having an increasingly harder time getting outstanding young men. A medical researcher said that, while medical research was one of the few areas in which the United States held a substantial lead, the comparison between a lucrative private practice and low-salaried research had begun to place the American future in that field in jeopardy.

Students Discouraged

¶Some phases of the traditional medical education program are considered obsolete by experts, thus discouraging many students who think twice before investing in an educational career that requires a greater investment of time and money than any other scientific career.

¶If students' undergraduate records are an indication, the range of quality among medical schools is very wide: In 1958-59 the number of A students in first-year classes ranged from none to 57 per cent and the number of C students ranged from none to 59 per cent, according to The Journal of the American Medical Association.

¶According to conservative estimates by the Council on Medical Education and Hospitals, at least ten new medical schools with an average graduating class of 100 students will be required between now and 1975, in addition to the expansion of many existing facilities.

The critical nature of the state of medical education was confirmed in a detailed report by Robert A. Moore, president of the Downstate Medical Center, State University of New York, in Brooklyn. The report was presented in the form of the William Henry Welch Lecture at Mount Sinai Hospital last night.

Dr. Moore confirmed the report that the percentage of college graduates applying to medical school had decreased from about 11 per cent in prewar years to about 4 per cent today.

This document sounded a warning sounded earlier by Dr. John A. D. Cooper, associate dean of the Northwestern University Medical School, to the Federation of State Medical Boards, as reported in the "education number" of the A. M. A. journal:

"The increasing mass of scientific knowledge in medicine, the medical sciences, and the behavioral sciences and the deepening complexity of medical practice call out for students with even greater intellectual capacity and dedication than in the past. If students are not equal to this heavier burden, there can only be compromise with the high level of education necessary to prepare them for the profession."

"The professions open to the college graduates," Dr. Cooper went on, "are now much broader, and they provide the prestige, intellectual satisfaction, and financial rewards comparable to those offered by medicine. * * * The vast sums of money available for fellowships and research assistantships in the expanding research budgets almost guarantee the total expense of graduate education for all but a small fraction of students in the physical, biological and behavioral sciences. Medicine has no equivalent source of subsidy for its students."

Dr. Moore's lecture examined all aspects of these growing difficulties facing medical education.

Ratio Deplored

He called it a cause for concern that the relation between all applicants to medical school and the number of freshmen enrolled had sunk to a low of 1.87 to 1.

More serious, the total of those who drop out of medical school for reasons of poor academic standing has increased from 3.4 per cent in 1954-55 to 5.3 per cent in 1957-58. Thus, despite the effort to increase the total "production" of the medical schools, almost half of the increased enrollment was lost in the freshman year.

Equally as serious as the handicaps of time and money, with tuition approaching $1,400 a year, is the medical education program itself, Dr. Moore believes. He considers it "inflexible * * * lock-step education" "that is set to the slowness and intellectual activity of the least able but passable student."

Dr. Moore said: "The abler student marks time while the tail-end catches up with him.

"I was shocked two years ago when a small group of able freshmen told me that they found the first year of medical

school less stimulating intellectually than the last year of college. Education, to attract and hold the best minds, must be stimulating and challenging. If we accept college grades as at least one index of the best mind, medicine is not attracting the same quality it did just ten years ago."

Among the measures to counter-act the growing crisis he proposed:

¶Correcting the popular misconception that it is difficult for able students to get into medical school. "No able, qualified student today will, in my opinion, fail to gain admission to some medical school in the United States," he said.

¶Shortening the total period of study, without lowering quality. Dr. Moore asked that "medicine should tidy up its own house" rather than blame the colleges and high schools for an excessively long period of education. He considers the conventional internship period an obsolete remnant of the days when the last two years of medical school were "largely didactic and formal education." Today, he said, they are "clerkships with extensive supervised practice."

¶Lengthening the school year. "It is clear that four school years of time can be put into three," he said.

Other proposals included honors programs as well as a plan of early admission, after only three, or even two years of college for outstanding students.

Medical Applicants

Following is a table showing the percentages of college graduates applying to medical school in years between 1928 and 1959:

Year.	Bachelor Degrees Granted.	Applicants to Medical School.	Per-centage.
1928	111,161	12,420	11.17
1933	137,954	12,128	8.79
1938	164,943	12,131	7.35
1942	185,346	14,043	7.58
1948	272,144	24,242	8.91
1953	304,857	14,678	4.81
1954	292,880	14,534	4.96
1957	340,347	15,917	4.68
1958	365,748	15,791	4.32
1959	......	15,169	...

January 14, 1960

U. S. DOCTOR SUPPLY AND MEDICAL SCHOOL PROBLEMS

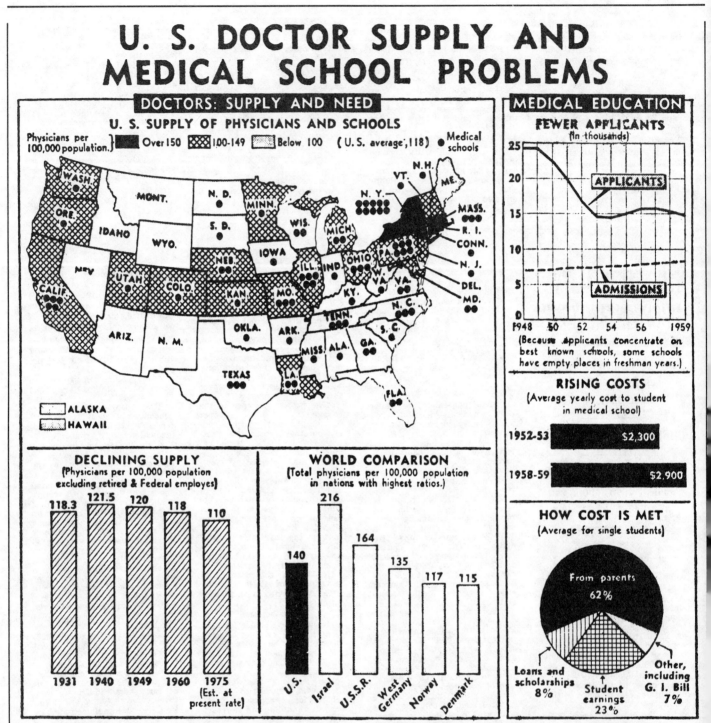

DOCTORS: SUPPLY AND NEED

U. S. SUPPLY OF PHYSICIANS AND SCHOOLS

Physicians per 100,000 population. ■ Over 150 ▨ 100-149 ░ Below 100 (U. S. average, 118) ● Medical schools

DECLINING SUPPLY
(Physicians per 100,000 population excluding retired & Federal employes)

1931	1940	1949	1960	1975 (Est. at present rate)
118.3	121.5	120	118	110

WORLD COMPARISON
(Total physicians per 100,000 population in nations with highest ratios.)

U.S.	Israel	U.S.S.R.	West Germany	Norway	Denmark
140	216	164	135	117	115

MEDICAL EDUCATION

FEWER APPLICANTS (In thousands)

APPLICANTS / ADMISSIONS

1948 · 50 · 52 · 54 · 56 · 1959

(Because applicants concentrate on best known schools, some schools have empty places in freshman years.)

RISING COSTS
(Average yearly cost to student in medical school)

1952-53	$2,300
1958-59	$2,900

HOW COST IS MET
(Average for single students)

From parents 62%
Loans and scholarships 8%
Student earnings 23%
Other, including G. I. Bill 7%

The Association of American Medical Colleges last week warned that declining medical school applications and rising costs to both students and institutions have led to a crisis stage. It estimated that at least $86,000,000 in scholarship aid alone would be needed during the next five years unless the nation's supply of doctors, already considered low, is to drop below the danger mark. The association stressed the fact that more than 80 per cent of the funds used to pay for medical students' education comes from the student and his family, while candidates for the "glamour" sciences get substantial fellowship assistance. The result was said to be that medical schools can not draw on top talent among lower income groups in the recruiting of tomorrow's physicians. Medical students pay more than twice as much toward their education as do Ph. D. students, and receive only one-fourth the financial assistance from scholarships, fellowships and assistantships, the A. A. M. C. said. At the same time, a study by The Johns Hopkins Magazine revealed that while the ratio of physicians to population has remained fairly stable for the past thirty years, it has been maintained in recent years only by the inclusion of growing numbers of foreign doctors. In 1959, a total of 8,400 doctors from ninety-one countries served in 846 American hospitals, compared with 458 foreign physicians in 1950. The current total of foreign doctors here is more than all the M.D.'s graduated from the nation's eighty-five medical schools last year. At present, 25 per cent of all residents and interns in the United States are aliens. The Hopkins estimate is that to keep up with the population growth in the United States, American medical schools will have in increase their output of physicians by 50 per cent between now and 1975, graduating 11,000 students anually instead of the present 7,400. At the present rate of growth, it says, the annual output will be 2,000 graduates short of that figure, with a subsequent drop in the ratio of doctors.

November 6, 1960

MEDICAL SCHOOLS TAKE MORE JEWS

B'nai B'rith Unit Is Told Student Ratio Doubled in 20 Years to 19%

By IRVING SPIEGEL

A marked decline in religious discrimination in medical schools was reported here yesterday by the Anti-Defamation League of B'nai B'rith.

The percentage of Jewish students in medical schools was said to be twice that of twenty years ago.

Bernard Nath of Chicago, chairman of the league's civil rights committee, made public

a four-year study at the league's forty-seventh annual meeting, held at the Savoy Hilton Hotel.

Between 1956 and 1959, Mr. Nath said, the number of Jewish students admitted to medical schools had been 18 to 19 per cent of the total enrollment whereas in 1940 they represented only 9 to 10 per cent.

This is a "heartening advance," he said, "from the days when Jews had to apply and reapply to American schools, were often turned down solely because of their religion, and then had to give up the idea of becoming doctors or else study abroad."

In 1956, the study showed, the nation's seventy-eight medical schools admitted 7,432 new students, including 1,326, or 18 per cent, who were Jewish. In 1959, out of a total enrollment of 7,675 new students, 1,485,

or 19.2 per cent, were Jewish.

Mr. Nath, noting that admission policies of many institutions were based on geographic factors, said that "since Jewish applicants are largely concentrated in Eastern metropolitan areas, geographical limitations work against them."

The speaker pointed out that when a school eased its residence requirements the situation became "more favorable for the Jewish applicant."

As an example, he cited a school in the Far West that in 1958 accepted five students from outside the state. The next year it liberalized its residence requirements and then the proportion of Jewish students in the entering class rose from 9 per cent in 1957 to 12 per cent in 1958 and 14 per cent last year.

Arnold Forster, the league's civil rights director, reporting on Ku Klux Klan activity, said

that despite losses in some areas, Klan strength "has generally risen in the last year together with an increase in violence and anti-Semitism."

He said Klan units had "participated in the race riots that shook Jacksonville, Fla., in August, 1960." He estimated Klan membership today at 35,000 to 50,000.

Mr. Forster said there were "two major competing Klan groups in the South, the United States Klans, Knights of the Ku Klux Klan, which had been dominant for six years, and the newly formed National Knights of the Ku Klux Klan."

He explained that the National Knights, formed last February, "probably as a response to the sit-in movement, is a loose confederation of splinter Klans in which each unit retains its identity and autonomy."

January 13, 1961

Negro Medical Gains

Discrimination Is Steadily Decreasing In Medical Schools Over the Nation

By HOWARD A. RUSK, M. D.

With the opening of school this month, the nation is once more plagued by isolated local outbursts against school integration.

In common with other areas of post-graduate education, integration is proceeding more rapidly and with less resistance in medical education.

Although racial discrimination in medical education does exist even outside the Deep South, it is decreasing rapidly.

In 1947, there were only ninety-three Negro students in twenty predominantly white medical schools. By 1956 there were 216 Negro students in forty-eight predominantly white schools.

Progress in South

Prior to 1948 no medical schools in the seventeen Southern states and the District of Columbia, other than Howard University and Meharry Medical College, admitted Negro students. Today, eighteen of these schools admit Negroes.

Howard University College of Medicine, Washington, D. C., and Meharry Medical College, Nashville, Tenn., are our two

predominantly Negro medical schools.

Together they graduate approximately 130 physicians annually. All of the other medical schools combined graduate about another fifty-five Negro physicians each year.

There are two particularly encouraging aspects of these changes in the last fifteen years.

First, those medical schools having Negro students would have accepted more, had more qualified Negro students applied.

Second, a number of schools have actively sought qualified Negro candidates.

Negro Physician Shortage

Our total national shortage of physicians is acute. Our shortage of Negro physicians is critical.

As compared to a total national ratio of 132 physicians to each 100,000 persons, there are but twenty Negro physicians for each 100,000 Negroes.

From 1940 to 1960 the increase in the Negro population was 46.7 per cent. In the same period the increase in Negro

physicians was but 14.2 per cent.

This sharp increase in the percentage of the Negro population is expected to continue.

The present population of the United States is 180,000,000. By 1974 it will have increased by 22 per cent to 220,000,000.

During this same period, however, the total non-white population, now 19,000,000, will increase by 37 per cent to 26,000,000.

Added to this increased demand for Negro physicians' services resulting from population growth has been an increased demand by Negroes for medical care as a result of the steady advance in the economic status of Negroes, particularly in industrial areas.

Much of the progress in improving opportunities for young Negroes in medicine has resulted from the work of the National Medical Fellowships, Inc.

Founded originally after World War II by a group of Chicago physicians concerned with local conditions, it became a national organization in 1952.

Supported by foundations and contributions, its primary activities are providing scholarships for Negro medical students and loans to Negro physicians.

Illustrative of its other activities is a publication issued last spring: "New Opportunities for Negroes in Medicine."

The booklet was written to aid high school and college guidance counselors in advising Negroes interested in the study of medicine. Copies are

available from National Medical Fellowships, Inc., 951 East Fifty-Eighth Street, Chicago 37, Ill.

Booklet Fills Gap

The publication is particularly helpful, for despite the general problem of inadequate preparation of Negroes for medical school, there is a waste of qualified Negroes desiring to go into medicine.

One reason for this is the lack in the past of proper advice and guidance, particularly in regard to selection of medical schools to which applications are made.

Just as the barriers of segregation are slowly but surely breaking down in medical schools, Negro physicians are finding it easier in most communities to get hospital staff appointments, residences and internships.

Our objective in health services as in all fields should be the eventual complete elimination of discrimination. The surest and fastest way to achieve this in medicine is to recruit more qualified young Negro men and women into medicine and then through fellowships and loans eliminate or minimize the economic barriers to medical education.

National Medical Fellowships and other groups dedicated to these objectives are making an important contribution to the over-all objective of racial integration.

September 9, 1962

The Doctors Debate Fee-Splitting

Who's responsible? As the argument continues to rage, it becomes pertinent to ask how this pernicious practice works, how prevalent it is, and why.

By LAWRENCE GALTON

AMERICAN medicine today may, on the whole, be the best in the world. It is respected for bringing to heel many once-fatal diseases and for greatly extending average life expectancy. And the curative and rehabilitative feats of American surgery grow increasingly spectacular.

But there is, it seems, an ugly, non-scientific aspect to the way some physicians and surgeons practice their calling—it involves a cold, calculating operation on their patients' dollars, a splitting of fees that amounts to buying and selling the sick with their own money.

The business of the kickback, as it can be called bluntly, or the referral fee, as it may be termed politely, has been very much in the news in recent months, leading even to bitter exchanges between august medical bodies.

When, not long ago, the American Medical Association held that it was ethical for a referring physician (usually a family doctor) to assist a surgeon in the operating room and be paid for it, the American College of Surgeons lost no time in charging that the pronouncement would only encourage fee-splitting and represented a "retreat" from organized medicine's "stanch" opposition to this practice.

Even as the A. M. A. recoiled in horror, denied the charge vehemently and deplored "the public airing of disagreements between large segments of medicine," a third party climbed into the ring—the American Academy of General Practice, representing 28,000 family doctors. Some of its top officials assailed the surgeons for having a "biased and vested" point of view and a holier-than-thou attitude, and one G. P. leader remarked bitterly:

"It takes two to tango. If there's fee-splitting going on, there must be a surgeon who is splitting the fee with the general practitioner."

As the argument within the medical profession continues to rage, the public at large may have some pertinent questions not only about the current fuss but about the nature of fee-splitting in general—how it works, how prevalent it is, and why.

FEE-SPLITTING can be as crass as this:

Called to see a patient with an abdominal pain, a physician makes his examination and announces: "Looks like appendicitis. I'll make arrangements with the hospital and with Dr. Blank. He's the best surgeon around."

The operation is done. In due course there is a bill for perhaps $5 or $10 from the family doctor and another for several hundred dollars from the surgeon. The patient pays. And the surgeon splits—handing back as much as half his fee to the family doctor.

Perhaps, in this case, the operation

LAWRENCE GALTON is a freelance writer who often deals with aspects of medicine.

is necessary and the only result of the kickback arrangement is a higher bill.

But consider another example. A woman goes to her family doctor for a check-up. Finding a small lump in the uterus, the doctor refers her to a surgeon who examines her and promptly announces: "Yes, yes. We'll operate and have you up good as new in no time."

What he doesn't announce is that he believes the lump to be a harmless fibroid that doesn't need surgery—certainly not then, perhaps never. But he has to operate and split the fee with the general practitioner or there won't be any more business forthcoming from that source.

Thus, beyond being morally reprehensible and a financial imposition, fee-splitting can lead to unnecessary surgery. And it can mean poorer-quality surgery as well—for the doctor on the lookout for a "cut" or commission may refer his patients not to the most competent surgeon but to the one who offers the most rewarding deal.

How prevalent is fee-splitting? There have been charges that it is deeply rooted and even the rule in some areas, but rare in others where it is held in the same esteem as abortion. Probably only a minority of physicians and surgeons has ever engaged in it. Still, the size of the minority has always been a mystery.

Ten years ago, a report in the Journal of the American Medical Association remarked: "Fee-splitting still goes on and will go on as long as 2 or 3 per cent of the doctors are like an equal or higher percentage of the bankers, lawyers or politicians. Human nature, being what it is, insures that the unscrupulous will always be with us."

The problem, however, is to ferret them out. As one doctor has put it, three people are involved in every case—the patient who knows nothing and the two guilty parties.

FEE-SPLITTING appears to have picked up steam about the turn of the century. It was then that aseptic techniques made operations safer. Surgery soon became frequent—and a specialty—and it was not uncommon for surgeons to bid against each other to get their patients from family doctors.

By 1903, the A. M. A. found it necessary to add to its code of ethics a ban on the "giving or receiving of commissions" as "destructive to public good and degrading to the profession." Several states legislated against the practice (and it is now against the law in twenty-three). But evidence against the guilty was difficult to obtain. Ethical doctors, even if they suspected some of their confrères, did not dare to make charges without clear proof, for fear of law suits.

In 1913, when the American College of Surgeons was organized, its purpose

was twofold: to set up standards that would restrict surgery to the able and, if possible, to the ethical. It condemned fee-splitting and required each member to pledge that "upon my honor as a gentleman, I hereby declare that I will not practice the division of fees."

But fee-splitting went on. And if, to begin with, eager surgeons had been largely responsible for instituting it in the competition to get customers, soon another influence was at work.

THE results of surgery could be dramatic. Patients often were willing to pay more for it than for the routine, less spectacular though beneficial treatment of the general practitioner. Thus, there developed a disparity between the earnings of the G. P. and the surgeon.

This situation has continued to exist. Latest figures—from a survey by Medical Economics, national business magazine for physicians—show that the typical G. P. in 1959 netted $20,000 a year before taxes while his counterpart in surgery earned $27,900.

The difference between compensation of G. P. and surgeon often is "unjust," Dr. Robert S. Myers, executive assistant director of the American College of Surgeons, remarked not long ago.

"Frequently," he said, "the general practitioner examines a patient late at night; makes the diagnosis of 'acute appendicitis'; makes arrangements to admit the patient to the hospital, and may even take him to the hospital in his own car. The surgeon comes to the hospital after the patient has been admitted and worked up, confirms the diagnosis and operates. For this he can collect from $100 to $150 with the greatest ease, but the general practitioner will frequently have considerable difficulty in collecting $5 to $10 from the patient for his necessary and time-consuming diagnostic work-up."

"RECOGNIZING this inequity," said a 1955 A. M. A. committee report on the causes of fee-splitting, "some surgeons willingly split their fees with other physicians in an effort to correct personally the resulting economic injustice. The higher surgical fee also creates intense competition for surgical patients. Some surgeons offer, or feel themselves forced to submit to demands for, a split of the surgical fee 'to meet the competition.'

"Once this practice takes hold in a community, more and more surgeons feel obliged to adopt the practice."

Further, this committee found that "the restrictions of some surgical boards work an economic hardship on the young surgeon. He has little or no referred work and is permitted to do no general practice. He sometimes feels that he is forced into fee-splitting to do enough surgery to use his training, to pay his overhead, and to support his family."

The committee recommended that a program of education be fostered by the A. M. A. to increase the public's appreciation of nonsurgical work.

BUT there is still another factor in the fee-splitting problem and the A. M. A. committee took note of it: "Arbitrary hospital restrictions on general practitioners, where they occur, create another set of economic hardships and frank hostility, particularly among those with special training in surgery that they are not permitted to utilize. As a result, some demand a split of the surgeon's fee."

The American College of Surgeons has long been against allowing surgery to be performed by any physician who has not completed a program of surgical residency. It is against giving surgical privileges on the basis of an apprenticeship kind of training and forbids its members to participate in such training of nonsurgeons. Its philosophy is that a surgeon must be capable of coping with all conditions he encounters during the course of a surgical procedure.

THE college has not been entirely successful thus far in limiting the field. A recent survey it made in cooperation with the American College of Physicians and the American Hospital Association indicates that about half of all operations in American hospitals today are performed by physicians "unqualified" to conduct surgery according to its standards.

This is not because surgeons aren't available to do them but because G. P.'s want to do them, believe they are capable and, of course, appreciate the income. Generally, the proportion of such operations is greatest in small, private, profit-making hospitals, particularly those below the 200-bed level.

Still, if the ban on G. P. operations is not complete enough to satisfy the A. C. S., it may have gone far enough to account for what Dr. Myers, in 1960, called the growth of another "pernicious, unethical practice"—that of "'feather-bedding' or 'made-work,' in which the referral of the patient to the surgeon depends upon the surgeon's reducing his fee to permit the general practitioner to charge for unnecessary [G. P.-performed] services to the patient. If the surgeon re-

fuses, he gets no more patients."

What services does the G. P. demand to do? Help provide pre-operative care, assist at surgery, and participate in post-operative care. What's wrong with this?

First, says Dr. Myers, the referring physician has no responsibility for usual "post-op" care and should not charge for it or even dabble in the area.

Such participation, he says, "usually results in divided authority, and, not infrequently, in detriment to the patient's health. To be sure, there may be a complicating condition, such as diabetes, which the referring physician is more qualified to treat than the operating surgeon, and for this he should be paid by the patient."

Second, he should not assist at an operation if the surgeon has a regular assistant, or if internes or residents are available. "The best interests of the patient are served when

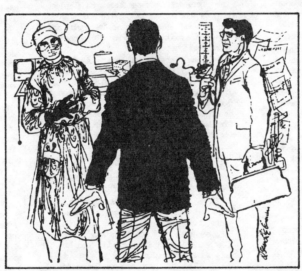

the surgeon has a regular surgical team which is familiar with his procedures and techniques. This includes a competent surgeon-assistant at surgery, and not the casual and untrained assistant."

And third, says Dr. Myers, he should not expect to take part in usual pre-operative preparation merely to gain a fee. "This does not mean that the referring physician cannot admit the patient, but the fee for this service should not be influenced—that is, raised —because surgery is performed subsequently. It should be the same as if no surgery were done."

ALL of which provides some background as to why the A. C. S. saw red when the A. M. A. resolution last year held that it was ethical for a surgeon to employ a referring physician as a paid assistant. Although the resolution made clear that if the practice was

a subterfuge to split fees or to divide an insurance benefit it would be unethical, Dr. Myers would have none of it.

Neither would Dr. Paul Hawley, director emeritus of the A. C. S., who had a comment to make about why he believed the resolution had been adopted. "The bulk of the A. M. A. is made up of referring physicians," he said.

Retorting to all this, many representatives of general practitioners maintain that family doctors are qualified to assist at surgery. They argue that for good medical care they should be with the patient before and after an operation. They also note (as has Dr. Myers, who has called the practice "unfair") that insurance companies do not pay for the extensive time spent in the hospital by the family doctor. Therefore, family doctors would just as soon assist at an operation.

At an October press conference, Dr. Carroll A. Witten, speaker of the Congress of Delegates of the American Academy of General Practice, charged that the A. C. S. wanted to prevent general practitioners from performing operations or assisting in them because "surgeons are a glut on the open market."

The primary motive of the A. C. S., Dr. Witten went on, was "to provide a livelihood for an overproduction of men in surgery. The hospital coffee shops are full of young surgeons sitting around waiting for a case."

AT this moment, there are reports that representatives of both the A. M. A. and A. C. S. are taking part in meetings aimed at reaching some agreement on how to deal with the altercation between G. P.'s and surgeons and the whole long-smoldering issue of fee-splitting.

Where does all this leave the patient?

When doctors argue among themselves, it is difficult for the layman to decide who is right. And it is to be hoped that the conferees will come up with a clear-cut solution.

Meanwhile, the patient is not entirely defenseless against fee-splitting and its danger of higher costs and poor and even unnecessary surgery.

Taking unnecessary surgery first, if an operation is to be performed in an accredited hospital, there will usually be a safeguard in the form of a tissue committee which keeps a check on operations and the justification for them. And the status of a hospital can be determined by direct questioning of the physician, the surgeon or the hospital itself.

While there are no sure-fire indications of fee-splitting, it is not out of order to suspect the possibility when a physician urges a "special" surgeon or otherwise fails to provide a choice.

Surgeons themselves have long suggested that this be regarded as a warning sign. And an A. M. A. leaflet designed for physicians to give to patients points out: "If surgery is indicated, we will discuss your choice of a properly qualified physician to perform the operation."

IF a referring physician is to act as an assistant at surgery, this in itself is not necessarily an indication of fee-splitting. For, as even the A. C. S. agrees, there are many hospitals without enough or even any specially trained assistants and the service of the family doctor may be essential.

Nor is it necessarily a sign of fee-splitting if the referring doctor participates in "pre-op" and "post-op" care—certainly not if the patient wishes it nor if there are complicating factors of a chronic nature.

In any case, it is in order —and highly desirable—for a patient or someone in the family, before an operation, to follow the suggestion implicit in a statement made many years ago by the A. C. S. Board of Regents: "The key to public education against fee-splitting is intelligent questioning of each doctor about his fee. * * * As a matter of self-protection, the patient should know who gets how much and for what."

Finally, as leaders of the medical profession try to deal with the problem, patients may make a worth-while contribution to its solution by recognizing that an honest and able family doctor who makes a correct diagnosis and a proper referral to a good surgeon can be fully as valuable as any operation, and should be rewarded accordingly, cheerfully and respectfully.

March 4, 1962

The Doctor's Image Is Sickly

By WALTER GOODMAN

NOT so long ago an editor of a popular magazine in search of his obligatory medical article would have settled contentedly for something on the order of "Should Your Doctor Tell You the Truth?" The medical feature has lost none of its popularity over the years, but today the title is more likely to be "The Truth About Your Doctor." Once portrayed for us as a scientist-humanitarian pondering the ultimate questions, the doctor is now presented in books*, magazine articles, newspaper stories and all manner of reports as a man whose main question to himself is whether he ought to pay a night call on a pneumonia case.

Young Kildares and Ben Caseys notwithstanding, the doctor's image, as reflected in what is being written about him, is in a decided state of disarray. Public opinion surveys, to be sure, show that physicians continue to be held in high esteem throughout the country. We may take these findings at face value, as the American Medical Association prefers to take them, or discount them as examples of public-opinion lag, or recognize that our attitude toward doctors is a sensitive and complex affair, not readily expressed in quantitative terms.

When it comes to prestige, for example, the doctor is at the top of the American heap, just a shade below a Supreme Court Justice and above a nuclear physicist, according to the National Opinion Research Center—but prestige is a measure of position, not of affection. That is to say, the reason a mother wants her son to be a doctor is. that she loves her son, not her doctor. A pair of sociologists writing in the January, 1963, American Journal of Sociology conjectured that resentment accompanies the deference we give to doctors partly because their high prestige sets up criteria which it is very difficult for them to meet.

Still, all polls confirm that practically everybody retains a soft spot for his own particular doctor and is well satisfied with his medical care. Our satisfaction is doubtless connected with an appreciation of the medical advances of the past 20 years, but it also owes something to sheer awe before the mysteries of medicine; we don't always know when we are getting poor treatment and are understandably anxious to give our physician the benefit of any doubt.

The reports of Dr. Ray E. Trussell, director of the Columbia University School of Public Health and Administrative Medicine, on medical care in New York's hospitals, which created something of a sensation a few years ago, showed that patients were delighted with care that the reports rated as poor. As for one's own doctor, it takes a considerable amount of courage (or perversity) to think ill of

*"The Doctor Business" by Richard Carter; "The Troubled Calling" by Selig Greenberg; "The Doctors' Dilemmas" by Louis Lasagna; "Intern" by Dr. X; "The Doctors" by Martin L. Gross; "American Medical Avarice" (not yet published) by Ruth Mulvey Harmer.

WALTER GOODMAN, an editor and author, is working on a history of the House Un-American Activities Committee, scheduled for publication next year.

the man to whom we must resort in time of trouble. As a sophisticated student of the surveys, Jacob J. Feldman of Harvard's School of Public Health, has suggested, people tend to adjust their opinions to the benefit of their physician: "Since there is evidence that many people choose their physician rather casually and only rarely leave a physician because of dissatisfaction, what apparently happens is that people are drawn to believe that they are using the 'right' doctor, the objective situation playing only a minor role in the evaluation. Clearly, it would not be very pleasant to view oneself as having the 'wrong' doctor and still keep on using him." If we begin blaming our practitioner personally, we are left with no alternative but to go out and find another —a rather arduous and uncertain undertaking.

To complicate matters further, even amid the favorable poll results we find symptoms of discontent. In a 1959 report of the National Opinion Research Center, a third of the people who were asked how much interest doctors took in their patients then as compared with 30 years before replied "a little less" or "much less." And a majority of those questioned as part of a study done for the A.M.A. in 1955 agreed with the statement, "Most doctors don't give the patient as much time as the patient would like." For all our long-standing reverence for the medical profession, it seems to have dawned upon us, bringing a sense of loss, that the doctor of today is not the doctor of the day before yesterday. He is busier, richer, colder. Especially colder.

"He's a good doctor, I suppose," runs one of those anonymous but quite believable quotations favored by magazine writers (this one from The Saturday Evening Post), "but he acts as if he couldn't care less about me." Who has not had to listen to complaints from a distraught neighbor about the doctor who is disinclined to pay house calls, the doctor who keeps one waiting in his office anteroom, the doctor whom it is impossible to reach on weekends or after 5 P.M., the doctor who keeps glancing at his watch during one's recital of ailments?

Some of these complaints, when accompanied by references to warmer times past, can be laid to the deceptive glow of memory—even during the nineteen-twenties, when the philosophic doc was still jogging along country lanes to deliver a fine baby boy in exchange for a bag of turnips, a survey-taker found physicians being described as rapacious, pompous, arrogant and inconsiderate. But the nation's personal, social and political experiences with doctors over the last 20 years provide sufficient grounds for a certain unease without resort to those fond recollections of a paternal presence during midnight hours of high temperature.

As everyone has noticed, the general practitioner of 1966 is a much busier man than his cherished counterpart of 30 years ago. The number of weekly visits from patients has more than doubled; today a typical G.P. sees about 160 patients a week, and a "good" practice may bring him 200 or even more—too many to permit the luxuries of lingering and digressing that were common in a more tranquil time. The usual office call on a G.P. lasts 10 minutes, and he makes only five house calls a week. (When, 25 years ago, our family doctor came to the house to treat my older brother, he made a point of taking a few minutes to inspect me as well, though no one asked that of him, least of all the child being inspected. Our present doctor, an excellent chap whom I have yet to dare impose on for a house visit, has never met my children; but, then, he is an internist.)

EVEN if one's family doctor is a model of patience, however, and not likely to get his name in the newspapers for refusing to tend a bloodied accident victim who stumbles into his office without an appointment, he alone cannot save the image of his profession. For he is not the only doctor a family is likely to come in contact with these days; indeed, like the bison of the plains, he is a vanishing phenomenon. In medicine, as elsewhere, it is the era of the specialist. One reason why G.P.'s are so busy is that, as demand for medical attention keeps increasing, their numbers keep diminishing. At the end of World War II, there were four G.P.'s for every specialist in the country, but only one out of five medical-school seniors interviewed in a national survey for the Surgeon General's office 10 years after the war said they planned to go into general practice. Of the 170,000 doctors in private practice today, more than half are specialists of one sort or another, and the trend is accelerating.

Whereas the relationship between a patient and his family doctor in the days when the latter treated every ailment that came up might well be rich in human resonances, the relationship between patient and specialist today is about as resonant as the relationship of a car owner with a transmission mechanic. When one is in need of a specialist, the celebrated Free Choice of Physician comes down to a combination of anxiety and ignorance. We customarily take whoever is recommended (assuming whoever is recommended will take us) and put as much faith in him as our emotional needs require and as the specialist's demeanor permits. The doctor is a stranger, the patient one gall bladder among hundreds. (No point mentioning that earache; he'll only recommend another specialist.) It is a brief acquaintance, unsatisfying except in a functional way, a few meetings of a few minutes each (which usually includes a question regarding one's medical coverage), a course of treatment, a bill.

What Ever Became Of Good Old Doc?

"Even if one's family doctor is a model of patience and not likely to get his name in the papers for refusing to tend a bloodied accident victim who stumbles into his office without an appointment, he alone cannot save the image of his profession."

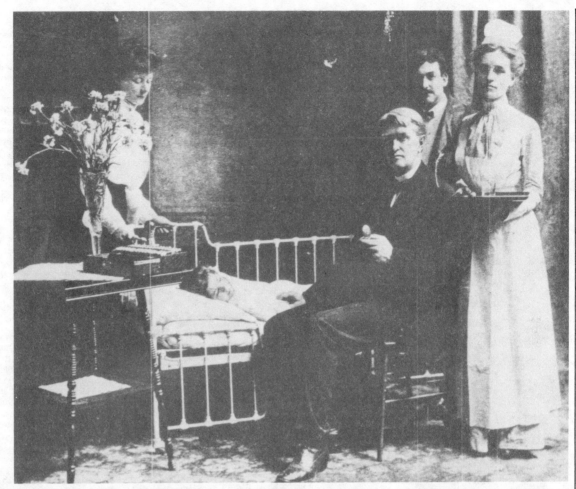

A bill. After the first flush of gratitude has died away—assuming the treatment has worked—the specialist's bill is specially unpleasant medicine. It is a high tax from a superior stranger on one's fear and helplessness, and it generally arrives after one's pain has been reduced, and one's gratitude along with it. (Sometimes, to be sure, it arrives concurrently with the pain, which doesn't help matters.)

Though doctors' fees have been rising about twice as fast as the consumer price index since 1949, they have been outpaced by services in general and left far behind by soaring hospital costs. But that is small comfort when serious illness comes and a family is barraged with expenses. The impact is not easy to forget. According to a 1963 poll of a cross section of Minnesota's adults, more than a third felt that the fees charged by most doctors are unreasonable. Insurance coverage of some sort, which much of the country now enjoys, helps, but it adds a disagreeable note of its own when the premium-payer discovers that his insurance does not quite meet the full cost of treatment. Insurance companies lay part of the blame for their ever-rising rates on doctors, and by setting up a schedule of payments for specific types of operations—say, $210 for that

gall bladder—instead of leaving the area politely hazy, the insurers have put the onus on the surgeon who thinks highly enough of himself or of his patient's savings account to charge $400. (Doctors, as we frequently hear, give time to charity cases for which they receive no pay. A 1964 study of half of Utah's physicians found that the average specialist gives his services gratis fully one hour a week.)

STILL, with all the jokes about specialists (like the definition of an internist as a fellow who specializes in being a general practitioner and the one about nobody knowing at what point the gastroenterologist is supposed to take over from the proctologist), most people seem willing to grant that there is good reason for the development of specialization, beside the fact that specialists work fewer hours and earn more money than nonspecialists. Disappointed though we may be in the seeming depersonalization of medical care, we accept it as a price of more effective treatment. Yesterday's doctor, with time on his hands and the patience of a saint, was, after all, a pretty ignorant fellow compared with today's busy M.D. with his office full of gadgets and cabinets full of miraculous drugs.

Why should he make home calls when he can handle complaints so much more efficiently in his office? As for the specialists, how else but by specializing can a physician avoid being swamped by the flood of life-saving information that has poured from the laboratories since the war? Our family doctor knows us better, but common sense grants that he doesn't know our kidneys nearly as well as the urologist.

Yet lately even this consolation has been undermined as the quality of American medical care and the skill and knowledge of America's doctors have been scrutinized and found wanting. Ten countries have a lower infant mortality rate than the United States, and the life expectancy for American men is 18th in the world. What brings these figures down to such a mediocre level in such a rich country is the inferior care available to the poor among us (the infant mortality rate among Negroes is four times that of whites), but the middle classes have their problems, too. People obliged to rely on clinics may take comfort from the spate of reports and exposés which indicate that easy access to a private physician is not always an unmitigated blessing. Doctors have proved themselves to be approximately as gullible as laymen when it comes to wonder drugs, prescribing drugs about which they know too little in quantities which turn out to be too large. The thalido-

mide episode of a few years ago was a most moving instance of the effects of misapplied medication, but it was not unique. Doctors have been charged, in headlines, with conducting experiments on patients—injecting terminal cases with live cancer cells, for example — without going through the formality of telling them about it. They continue to inflict a great many questionable operations, notably hysterectomies and tonsillectomies, and notably on persons with medical insurance—another area where the poor are in luck. They have been shown to be the frequent, if unwitting, aggravators of the ailments of those who pass through their hands. Hospitals are particularly chancy places in this regard; a few years ago staff members at the Yale Medical Service concluded after an eight-month study that 20 per cent of the service's patients had their cases complicated in some measure by the treatment they received—and this figure did not include outright errors by doctors. Every so often an instance of gross mistreatment reaches the courts in the form of a malpractice suit, and may make the daily newspaper.

PREVENTIVE care—crucial, all the experts are agreed, to any major improvement in the nation's health—appears to be practiced somewhat casually in many places. The earnest citizen succumbs to those constant exhortations to get a periodic checkup only to settle for a cursory looking-over by somebody with other things on his mind. A striking study made by the University of North Carolina in 1956 of the daily routines of 88 North Carolina practitioners, chosen at random, disclosed that about half of them "practiced from their desk chairs. Histories were almost nonexistent, and the few questions asked were often irrelevant. Patients were seldom undressed or laid down for examination. Abdominal examinations were performed with patients sitting in a chair."

Equally uncomfortable findings have been reported in New York and elsewhere, lending a certain weight to the literary tradition that warns readers off medical men of all sorts, as Petrarch warned the ailing Pope Clement VI—"I know that your bedside is beleaguered by doctors and naturally this fills me with fear." (Dickens, you may recall, attributed Oliver Twist's birth to the fact that no physicians were around to kill him with their wisdom — and Shaw, of course, commented that doctors have only triumphs to their credit since they bury their mistakes.)

LAYMEN, or at any rate those laymen who write books about doctors, are naturally concerned about the various medical deficiencies that have been coming to light recently, and their concern is edged with annoyance at the spectacle of how well America's doctors are doing despite the unkind things being said and written about them. A 1964 survey of self-employed doctors by Medical Economics found them to have a median gross income of $44,060, leaving the median doctor $28,380 after expenses.

Taking into consideration the normal rise since 1964 and the reluctance of entrepreneurs to exaggerate their earnings when it is a matter of record, you may safely assume that you will not run across many doctors who net under $30,000 a year, and if you have a run of bad luck, you are likely to encounter some who make considerably more. Doctors are in the highest 1 per cent of the nation's income-distribution list, with lifetime earnings far in excess of lawyers, not to mention dentists, and they have all the tax advantages of the self-employed to boot. (Did the $15 I handed that doctor in Chicago, whom the hotel sent up to treat my wife's virus infection, find its way onto his tax return?)

A vice president of General Motors can make $30,000 a year, or $50,000, and except for a handful of Union Square ideologues no one begrudges him. But the physician's income comes directly from his patients, not from some incorporated abstraction. (In this regard, socialized medicine can only improve the doctor's image, since people won't

have to be making out checks to him all the time.) We are prepared to accept—and even admire—in businessmen a degree of affluence that we may find unbecoming in a doctor. His prosperity serves to remind us that, as matters now stand, it is dollars rather than need that normally calls the American doctor into action, a troubling thought made more troubling by reports of kickbacks among colleagues, unsavory relationships between physicians and drug companies (spotlighted by the Kefauver hearings), and outright ownership by physicians of drugstores to which patients are directed for the filling of prescriptions. This last form of investment is currently being investigated by a Senate committee, and the Antitrust Division of the Justice Department has recently brought suit against the American College of Pathologists, representing 4,500 physicians, for price-fixing laboratory tests at an excessive level.

THE rich doctor has become a cliché of our culture, like the talkative cab driver and the dumb cop. Physicians come from far lands, as those huddled masses used to come, seeking to share in America's bounty; one Britisher not long ago exchanged a $5,900-a-year post in his own country for a job with a Michigan hospital that promises to bring him $45,000 a year. Doctors are to be found golfing at the best country clubs (Wednesday is golf day) and yachting from the docks of the best yacht clubs. They are valued clients of brokerage houses and pre-eminent consumers of luxury merchandise; a mailing list of M.D.'s is a prime tool for the seller of high-priced, low-utility items. Doctors are famous for their possession of large and tax-deductible automobiles, items which cannot be possessed without a certain degree of ostentation. To judge by the line-up of M.D. plates of a morning along the upper East Side, that part of New York City is in the grip of a terrible epidemic.

In addition to stirring up the usual emotions which displays of wealth breed in the less wealthy, particularly when the less wealthy feel that they are helping to sponsor the displays, the physicians' prosperity has enlarged what is coming to seem a veritable gulf between doctors and patients. There was a time when doctors belonged in the communities they served; this is no longer so, except in the Sutton Places and Scarsdales of the nation. (Our likable internist, by no means a show-off, lives in a neighborhood that I have small prospect of ever being able to afford. His good fortune is reassuring in a way, but it doesn't make me feel close to him.)

The great majority of medical students—nearly a fifth of them the children of doctors—come from well-to-do homes and go on to establish even better-to-do ones. Their education, beginning with their pre-med studies, through medical school and into internship and residency, is designed to narrow a man's outlook rather than broaden it, ignorance being a common side effect of expertise. Quite naturally, these promising young

fellows spend most of their free time in one another's company, a conservative company not likely to nourish empathy with lower-class patients; by the time the young men enter practice, they are well inoculated against the extra-physical troubles of the people they treat.

There is a feeling among medical students, which they do not conceal, that their years of study and the expenditure of so much of their parents' and in-laws' money entitle them to a generous allotment of creature comforts when they finally get established—usually in places where they are needed the least. (New York has about 180 doctors to 100,000 persons; South Dakota has about 70.) So propitious are the times that today a doctor has to make a special effort, like driving a Peugeot instead of a Bentley, to avoid flaunting his privileged position and leaving himself open to the envy and resentment of outsiders.

A GREAT deal of energy and money has been spent during the last 20 years in the cause of maintaining this privileged position. Observers of the activities of the American Medical Association since the war cannot help but be impressed, not to say bowled over, by the group's unflagging devotion to what it conceives to be the doctor's economic well-being. The record is familiar, but it loses nothing in the recounting.

The A.M.A., which indubitably represents the political and economic predilections of a heavy majority of its members, opposed private health-insurance plans until they proved inadequate, then championed them against Federal plans. It opposed the Kerr-Mills bill, a means-test scheme under control of the states, until the more potent King-Anderson bill came up in Congress. It has declaimed ceaselessly on the hallowed quality of the doctor-patient relationship but has fought against plans which would in no wise interfere with that relationship while extolling charity-ward arrangements in which the doctor-patient relationship becomes a matter of who happens to be on duty when the charity case arrives.

It has resisted increases in the number of medical students, out of concern for the economic position of the seller of medical care, and has succeeded in keeping the per capita doctor population constant for a generation, thereby accounting for the demand in this country for doctors from abroad. It allied itself with the drug industry against the Kefauver bill for stiffer control of the industry, and, not so openly, with the tobacco industry against efforts to bring cigarette advertising under effective control. Surveying this record, Dr. Louis Lasagna of The Johns Hopkins Medical School connects the decline in the A.M.A.'s appeal in the last two decades with the selection of A.M.A. leaders "who were less than the very best the profession had to offer." (America's medical schools harbor the most impressive critics of American medicine.)

Though the A.M.A.'s appeal seems

to have suffered a decline in the eyes of opinion makers, opinion receivers are another matter. Dr. Gallup tells us that as of December, 1965, only 7 per cent of the nation expressed unfriendly feelings for the A.M.A., and it is not realistic to expect that the organization's reputation, raised up by decades of nonpolitical works, will tumble tomorrow. Still, the A.M.A.'s incessant preachments against any changes in America's health arrangements, climaxing in its public outcries and private maneuverings against Medicare, the most popular bill of the decade, has helped spread abroad the idea that the interests of America's doctors and of America's patients are not identical.

The battle against Medicare, which the A.M.A. lost after a phenomenal expenditure of money, put the doctors in the untenable position, public-relationswise, of being against old, suffering people. Even ordinarily inattentive citizens must have been taken aback by the threats of some zealous physicians to strike against the elderly as a matter of principle and by the news that doctors are increasing their fees as much as 300 per cent in order to take full advantage of the benefits of the detested Medicare.

THERE is not a great deal that the individual physician can do about the variety of criticisms here reviewed, besides trying to be a good doctor, behaving in a civilized fashion toward his patients and perhaps garaging his Cadillac for the duration of the emergency. As Alfred McClung Lee, Brooklyn College sociologist, has observed: "Any group that has reached the intimate and trusted status achieved by the medical profession is subject to feelings both of gratitude and high expectation on the one hand and of distrust and rejection on the other." The doctor is, as far as his image goes, victim as well as beneficiary of the postwar advances in medicine. We demand more of him and he has far more to give—but time is in short supply. Without making light of the emotional needs of sick people, it appears that we must find somebody else to hold our hand through bad hours; maybe it calls for yet another specialist.

As for the more general sense that we do not know our doctor today as well as we, or our parents, used to know him, the poor man can hardly be held responsible for the disruption of neighborly feeling in a country where towns are transformed every five years and neighborhoods are destroyed overnight. We keep moving, and the doctor's clientele keeps changing. My older son has had four pediatricians so far in his 12 short years.

The medical profession, however, in the A.M.A. assembled, could do a good deal about the complaints raised against it. It could, for a start, grant that there is some justice to some of them. It could resuscitate its extensive regulatory powers, which have been allowed to lapse into a means of protecting physicians from the consequences of their errors and oversights. It could restrain its ritualistic opposition to every proposal for making medical care more accessible to more people. It could turn its remarkable energies to championing a large increase in the number of medical students and lobby for Federal scholarships for promising students from poor families. (The problem is entirely academic.)

It *could* do these things but we had better not count on it. If experience is any guide, organized medicine will treat its ailing image as one treats the complaint of a hypochondriac—by approaching it as metaphor, not reality. In all likelihood, the A.M.A. will take comfort in the public-opinion polls and lay all criticism to troublemakers and radicals. Maybe it will commission yet another public-relations firm to run an expensive campaign aimed at refurbishing the American doctor. Stories will be sent to the local press about physicians rushing to the aid of the stricken; editorial writers will be supplied with editorials on the despotism of socialized medicine in the British Isles and picture editors will receive more copies of Sir Luke Fildes's painting of the weary doctor bending over the sick child.

Images have been known to be sustained by such means, but as the doctors ought to recognize sooner than their public-relations consultants, an image is only a *symptom.* And we have all been warned by our own physician what dangers lie in wait for the patient whose symptoms are taken care of while the causes go untreated.

October 16, 1966

Shortage of Doctors Is Approaching a Crisis

Need for Physicians in U.S. Placed at 50,000—Many Areas Left With None

By RICHARD D. LYONS

The health industry of the United States, a $50-billion-a-year complex of hospitals, clinics and laboratories responsible for the well-being of every American, is suffering from a shortage of tens of thousands of doctors.

Hundreds of small towns from Wounded Knee, S. D., to Medicine Park, Okla., as well as many big city slums, are increasingly being left without family doctors as young physicians shun general practice.

The United States is losing ground to many nations in such common standards of health care as infant mortality and life expectancy at the same time that the demand for medical services is luring thousands of foreign physicians to this country.

And the nation's medical schools are facing critical financial problems while thousands of qualified applicants are being turned away for lack of places.

These are some of the findings of a six-week study of the nation's doctor shortage, including interviews with Federal officials, medical educators, hospital administrators and practicing physicians.

Most agreed that during the last decade there has been a change in public attitude toward access to medical care, that it is now regarded as a right rather than a privilege.

By enacting Medicare and Medicaid programs, the Federal and state governments have responded with the first firm steps toward underwriting and coordinating the nation's fragmented health care system. And now Federal programs tailored to meet the demand for medical services are beginning to get under way.

The most common Federal estimate of the doctor shortage is 50,000. But statistics alone, as Dr. Gerald A. Kerrigan, dean of the Marquette University School of Medicine in Milwaukee, pointed out in a recent conversation, are not necessarily a true indicator of the problem.

"The United States is relatively rich in physicians yet the national life expectancy and infant mortality rates are poor in comparison with some other nations," he said.

Dr. Robert H. Ebert, dean of the Harvard Medical School, said that "it would be a mistake to say that there is a substantial crisis but the situation

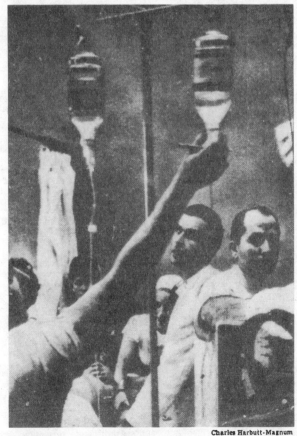

Charles Harbutt-Magnum

MEDICAL TEAM at work in St. Vincent's Hospital in New York. In hundreds of towns such services are unavailable.

is serious, especially in the central cities and rural areas."

The shortage of doctors, he said, "is being accentuated and is growing more apparent simply because more people are covered by health insurance, including Medicare and Medicaid, and they can now buy the medical care they couldn't afford in the past."

18 Operations in Two Weeks

Just after Medicare went into effect, one California ophthamologist performed in two weeks 18 cataract operations upon low-income people who had been waiting for surgical treatment for up to three years.

Before Medicare the patients were considered clinic cases and the specialist would have had to perform the operation for almost nothing. But now he can charge his "usual and customary fee," regardless of the state of the patients' finances.

According to one as yet unpublished Federal estimate, "there was an unmet need for some 20,000 practicing physicians" two years ago.

"In addition, the shortage of psychiatrists was estimated at between 10,000 and 15,000," it added. "Hospitals reported needs for some 10,000 additional interns and residents. When these and other needs are taken together, total requirements are probably about 50,000 more than the supply."

The Federal study says that the ratio of physicians in private practice who devoted themselves to family medicine, such as general practitioners, internists and pediatricians, had fallen to 50 per 100,000 persons in 1965 from 76 per 100,000 in 1950. Yet the ratio of physicians to population has remained constant over the last 20 years at about 150 per 100,000 persons, it said.

The number of nurses being trained, the report said, "has remained at essentially the same level for about 10 years" and the annual graduation rate of 35,000 a year "should be increased to between 50,000 and 60,000 by 1975."

The National League of Nursing reported 125,000 unfilled openings for registered nurses this year, while a survey by the Surgeon General's Task Force on Nursing estimated that the demand for nurses by 1970 would exceed this supply by more than 210,000.

Health Plan Staffing

The report also noted that the large prepayment medical care plans, such as the Health Insurance Plan of Greater New York and the Kaiser-Permanente medical centers on the West Coast, "provide staffing ratios of a little more than 100 physicians per 100,000 population," exclusive of psychiatrists, interns and residents.

Few medical experts have ventured to predict the extent of the growing demand for doctors' services. But Dr. Rashi

Fein, an economist on the staff of the Brookings Institution in Washington, estimated in his analysis, "The Doctor Shortage: An Economic Diagnosis," that "the total demand for physicians' visits can be expected to grow by perhaps 22 to 26 per cent by 1975 [over 1965] and by 35 to 40 per cent by 1980."

Dr. Fein's estimate took into account the expected population growth, increased personal income, a higher level of education, and the impact of Medicare, which he reckoned at between 1 and 2 per cent.

If Dr. Fein is correct, this country will need to train an additional 50,000 doctors by 1975 to meet the rising demand for medical care, even though the nation already has an estimated deficit of 50,000.

The annual number of American medical school graduates has actually risen in the last 15 years from 6,600 to about 7,600. But accompanying this increase has been a steady decline in the number of new doctors choosing to enter general practice.

The latest study of career choices of medical internes showed that only one in eight planned to become a general practitioner. At the turn of the century, in contrast, seven of eight became G.P.'s.

The situation is further complicated, according to the Federal survey, because "the number of physicians giving their time to teaching, research, administration and other activities has risen and the ratio of physicians who provide personal health services has declined."

Search for a Doctor

In Kirkland, Ill., a farm town 65 miles west of Chicago, Edwin L. Johnson, an insurance man, heads a local committee attempting to persuade a physician to settle in the community, which has been without a full-time practicing doctor for two years.

Mr. Johnson said that three persons in Kirkland had died of heart attacks this year without medical attention and several persons involved in serious accidents had been forced to "go miles to get medical aid."

Although the nearest doctor is in the town of Genoa, eight miles away, Mr. Johnson said that he was already overworked and "can hardly look after us since he has 3,000 people to take care of there."

The population of Kirkland, which has three small industrial plants employing about 225 persons, has grown from 500 to 1,000 in the last generation, Mr. Johnson said, but the lack of a physician is hampering future growth.

"Young couples are reluctant to move into town without a doctor," he said.

A medical-economic survey of Kirkland conducted by the

Sears-Roebuck Foundation showed that residents drove more than a quarter of a million miles last year making 8,000 visits to doctors in other towns. While away these persons spent almost $100,000, aside from doctors' fees, which might otherwise have gone into Kirkland's economy, the study found.

The Chicago-based foundation, which has helped more than 100 towns find doctors in the last 10 years, concluded that Kirkland could indeed support a doctor.

Backed by the foundation's survey and recommendations, the town set out to help itself two years ago. Land was donated and $40,000 raised to build a clinic containing five examination and treatment rooms, two consultation rooms, an X-ray room, a laboratory and a waiting room.

The clinic has been standing idle since it was finished 18 months ago and petunias planted in front of the building after its completion by the town's 4-H Club have long since wilted and died.

"We've been in touch with at least 125 doctors since the clinic was finished and 15 have actually come here to look over the town," Mr. Johnson said.

But none has stayed and Mr. Johnson and the other townspeople are puzzled and hurt. They cannot understand why physicians do not want to settle in communities without large department stores, libraries and theaters.

Attempts to attract doctors by other communities are apparently working no better.

Dr. George S. Palmer, director of the Florida Board of Medical Examiners, said that the state had tried and failed to draw young doctors to rural areas, offering medical students loans that did not have to be repaid if they settled in small towns of their choice for two years after graduation.

"But all the new doctors chickened out," Dr. Palmer said. "Not one student who accepted the loans settled in a doctorless town. After medical school they chose to repay the money and go into research or specialty practice in the cities while whole counties are without doctors, although I can't blame any one for not wanting to live in some parts of the state."

Wives Also Object

Occasionally it is not the doctor but his wife who balks at settling in a small community. The decision to practice in a small town has been a constant cause of argument between one Midwestern physician and his wife, who grew up in a medium-sized city.

They met and married at the state university while he was going to medical school. After internship and residency he chose to return to his hometown to practice medicine. For

him it meant a place and people he knew and loved, plus a chance to indulge his favorite sports, hunting and fishing. For his wife, however, it meant moving in among people she not only did not know but also regarded as her social and intellectual inferiors.

A study made by the New York State Medical Society has shown that the major causes of dissatisfaction among country doctors include such complaints as long, unrelieved working hours, inadequate time to study or to mingle with other doctors at medical meetings, and the lack of the educational stimuli generally found around hospitals, medical centers and clinics. Income and economic factors were not cited as causes of complaint.

A United States Public Health Service study showed that the percentage of country doctors over the age of 65 was twice as high as that of big city practitioners. In addition, the two urban areas of Nebraska, a state near the national average in the ratio of physicians to population, have twice as many physicians as the state's rural regions.

Whatever the reasons, more and more American rural communities and hamlets—in which 20 per cent of all Americans live—are without the services of resident physicians.

New Medical Materia, a trade publication, conducted two studies in an effort to locate the nation's doctorless towns. In 1959 the magazine found 1,079 such communities. Three years later the number had risen to 1,442, an increase of 33 per cent. Not included in the statistics were towns of fewer than 500 persons and those in which a doctor lived within five miles. Several experts have estimated that there are at least 5,000 doctorless communities in the nation, and that this number is rising.

'Situation Getting Worse'

"The situation in rural areas is getting steadily worse," said Norman Davis, director of medical programs for the Sears-Roebuck Foundation in Chicago. He said that "only general practitioners can offer services to rural areas and there aren't enough G.P.s."

Mr. Davis foresaw the day when rural health care might be dispensed from mobile units staffed by circuit riding physicians, pointing out that some doctors now pilot airplanes to visit patients in isolated areas.

Another alternative is already developing—the rural clinic. In such medium-sized towns as Sayre, Pa.; Temple, Tex., and Marshfield, Wis., doctors have banded together to form large group practice organizations centered on a clinic that serves not only the town but also a wide area around it. The Marshfield Clinic, with 76 physicians, serves an area of 150,000 persons.

As the family doctor has become harder to find in the country, so has his counterpart in the cities. A survey of general practitioners conducted by St. Luke's Hospital in a mixed-income section of New York City, for example, turned up almost no G.P.'s under the age of 30, showing that few recent medical graduates had chosen to start practice there.

Some cities, including New York, have telephone referral systems to provide emergency home medical service if no doctor can be found otherwise.

The nation's 6,200 general care hospitals have had to take up a larger share of the primary medical services once dispensed by the general practitioner.

The number of persons seeking treatment in the emergency room of the hospital in York, Pa., has more than quadrupled, from 7,000 to 30,000 a year, in this decade.

"The irony of the situation is that the medical profession holds sacred the right of doctors to treat patients privately rather than collectively," said one hospital official who asked that he not be named. "Yet while the average private practitioner wants to preserve 'the sacred doctor-patient relationship' he also wants hospitals to have a large staff of house physicians on call all the time so that the private practitioners won't have to get out of bed for emergencies or have their Sunday golf games disturbed."

Increases in Faculty

One Pennsylvanit physician, who gave up a full-time practice to teach, acknowledged: "I wanted some time for myself—in private practice I never had a personal life. The modern American medical school graduate has had it with solo practice because he knows that the private practitioner is the only person in the country who is expected to work 24 hours a day."

Many other physicians feel the same way. On the bulletin board of the New York Medical College was a note from a Queens pediatrician offering all his office equipment for sale because, it said, "I'm going academic full-time."

The number of full-time medical school faculty has increased to 18,000 today from 4,000 in 1952. Thus the number of faculty members increased by 350 per cent while the number of students was rising by 25 per cent.

One reason for this increase is that many faculty members are doing medical research as a sideline. A generation ago the Federal Government's support of research in medical schools was almost nothing. Today it is almost $500-million a year.

The number of medical specialists has also increased. About 5,500 doctors a year are being certified as specialists, four times the rate of 20 years ago. During that period the ratio of specialists rose from one-third to almost two-thirds of all physicians in private practice.

"Specialization has completely altered the meaning of the physician-population ratio by which manpower needs have been measured for many years," Dr. William H. Stewart, Surgeon General of the United States Public Health Service, said last year.

The trend toward specialization has been brought on by the increasing complexities of medicine, such as more sophisticated equipment and more effective though more toxic drugs.

Despite medical discoveries, better training of doctors and the rise in money being spent on health care, however, Americans do not appear to be getting any healthier.

"During the last two decades life expectancy in the United States has increased very little," Dr. Philip R. Lee, the Department of Health, Education and Welfare's Assistant Secretary for Health and Scientific Affairs, said last week.

As compared with citizens of other nations, American men and women are in 22d and 10th places, respectively, in life expectancy. The infant mortality rate in the United States is higher than that of 14 other countries. (Norway is best in life expectancy, Sweden in infant mortality.)

"So far as disease control is concerned the American health establishment is marking time—the rapid advance in saving lives has stopped," said Dr. George James, head of the new Mount Sinai School of Medicine in New York.

"Life expectancy has been practically constant for a couple of decades and so has the death rate," he said, "but hidden behind this plateau is at least one ominous fact: The spread between the level of health of whites and nonwhites is widening."

Mr. Davis of the Sears-Roebuck Foundaton, who has examined the doctor shortage in urban as well as rural areas, said "there is no motivation for a physician to practice in the inner city slums because of the uninspiring surroundings and the lack of financial rewards."

Dr. Ebert of Harvard said: "Negro areas would not get an increased share of the medical manpower even if twice as many physicians were turned out."

But the Office of Economic Opportunity is seeking to combat the effect of the flight of doctors from ghettos by setting up health clinics in central city neighborhoods, some of which contain large Negro populations, such as Watts in Los Angeles, North Lawndale in Chicago, Columbia Point in Boston, and the south Bronx.

Dr. Joseph T. English, acting assistant director for health affairs at the O.E.O., said that 41 such programs were being set up, some in rural areas, and that 10 were now in operation. He said 115 other areas had made proposals for similar clinics dispensing medical, dental and social services.

"There has been a flight to the suburbs of practicing physicians because of the tremendous frustration of trying to practice high-quality medicine in the ghettos," Dr. English said.

He pointed out that the 6,000 residents of Columbia Point were without the services of a single general practitioner before the O.E.O. had set up the clinic.

The clinics are not only starting to provide health care for more persons but also relieving pressure on municipal hospitals, on which ghetto residents have increasingly depended for medical attention.

But the hospitals themselves are having problems, including obsolescence and lack of space in some parts of the country and a shortage of internes nationwide.

Of the 14,000 openings for internes this year, only half are being filled by graduates of American medical schools. One quarter are still vacant, but one quarter have gone to foreign medical graduates, some of whom have failed tests of basic medical knowledge and are practising medicine without licenses.

September 28, 1967

Foreign Physicians, Many Unqualified, Fill Posts Left Vacant by Shortage in U.S.

By RICHARD D. LYONS

The national shortage of doctors and the rising demand for health services has led to the immigration of thousands of foreign physicians, many of doubtful ability who may arrive to practice in American medical institutions sight unseen and quality untested.

The influx of doctors from overseas has become so great in the last 20 years that as many foreign-trained physicians enter the health care system of the United States each year as are graduated from American medical schools.

About 45,000 doctors who were trained in foreign medical schools now reside in this country, and the number is increasing at the rate of 10 per cent a year.

Many of the foreign doctors, possibly as many as 5,000, have been unable to pass tests of basic medical knowledge and are practicing medicine without licenses, sometimes because of loopholes in state certification rules and sometimes with the knowledge of the hospitals in which they work.

Interviews with medical educators, hospital executives and public officials showed that some American hospitals were so short-staffed that they were advertising for doctors overseas and paying their travel expenses to come here, ostensibly for post-graduate study but often for use as cheap help.

The paradox of the migrant doctor problem is that the countries with the better medical schools and standards of health care have far fewer physicians migrating to the United States than those nations whose levels of medical education and services are poor.

England, France, Japan and the Scandinavian nations enjoy higher longevity and lower infant mortality rates than the United States, a reflection of national hystems of health care at least as good if not better, but relatively few doctors from there come to this country.

A much larger number enter from such underdeveloped nations as India, Iran and the Dominican Republic, countries with lower standards of health care and a doctor shortage of their own, and these physicians may have only the sketchiest knowledge of both English and medicine.

"This is a major national scandal and there has been no policing of foreign doctors because no central organization is responsible for them," said Dr. Harold Margulies of Washington, assistant director of the American Medical Association's

Division of Socio-Economic Activities.

Dr. Margulies, who has studied the problem for six years, estimated that from 2,000 to 5,000 foreign-trained doctors were practicing medicine in the United States without licenses.

Substandard Care Seen

"I have personally seen unlicensed foreign medical graduates working in hospitals," he said. "We have been meeting our manpower shortage in the United States with substandard people who are offering substandard care in our institutions."

While some of the foreign doctors practicing medicine without licenses do so in violation of state laws, the shortage of physicians has been so acute that many regulatory groups have not moved against them. Penalties vary widely between jurisdictions.

Some hospital officials said that the employment of foreign medical graduates was dictated through necessity as the demands increased for the staffing of emergency rooms, hospital wards and psychiatric institutions.

"Patients in many state hospitals have no hope of getting out and many doctors are uninterested in drab surroundings and uninteresting work," said one hospital executive in Chicago, who added bluntly: "So why not bring in doctors who have 'read' medicine for only six months?"

Dr. Edwin L. Crosby, director of the American Hospital Association in Chicago, attributed the influx of foreign-trained physicians to the increased demand for medical services that opened "thousands of more internship and residency posts" in American hospitals, along with the desire "of many foreign graduates for training in the United States."

He said that the association "recognizes the value of the services contributed by the participants in this foreign graduates program" and that "it is important to share our resources in medical training with other countries."

Dr. Crosby stressed, however, that the hospital association "does not believe that the presence of the vacancies and the need for physician coverage should be used to permit the employment of inadequately trained physicians or those with a substantial language barrier."

An official of the American Medical Association in Chicago said that according to association records almost 7,000 foreign doctors enter the United States every year, yet only half had passed a formal test of medical knowledge prepared by the Educational Council for Foreign Medical Graduates in Philadelphia.

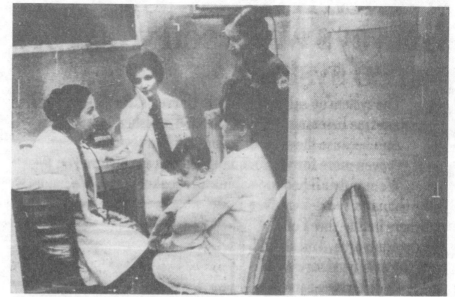

AT BELLEVUE: Early this year Dr. Sudha H. Dehejia, a specialist in child care from Bombay, was at work with young patients here. Unlike Dr. Dehejia, a number of doctors coming to the U.S. are unable to pass basic tests. Doctor drain from India has become so acute that the Indian Government this month refused to allow her doctors to come here.

The New York Times

Without certification that he has passed this test, a foreign doctor cannot enter a postgraduate training program in a good hospital, which was probably what attracted him to the United States in the first place.

May Be Listed as Orderlies

"We feel that a lot of these guys end up working in state institutions and marginal hospitals," the A. M. A. official said. "They may be on the books as broom handlers and orderlies even though they may be actually practicing medicine."

Several medical educators agreed, however, that the instruction foreign doctors receive in this country produces many fine physicians who practice high-quality medicine whether they choose to remain here or return home. But no one knows how many do eventually leave the United States.

According to A.M.A. records, there are 45,749 graduates of foreign medical schools residing in the United States. The figure includes 5,722 graduates of Canadian schools, whose standards are as high as American institutions. The countries of origin and numbers of others are: the Philippines, 5,055; Germany, 4,150; Italy, 2,811; Switzerland, 2,313; the United Kingdom, 2,110; India, 1,833; Mexico, 1,201; Korea, 1,060, and Iran, 1,000.

Federal surveys have shown that last year 2,952 foreign medical graduates entered the United States, while 4,500 more came here on exchange visas. In addition, 500 United States citizens returned home after receiving doctorates of medicine at foreign

schools. Thus, a total of 7,952 foreign medical graduates entered the United States last year while American medical schools graduated 7,574.

The drain on medical manpower has become so acute in India that this month she refused to allow physicians to take an examination that would qualify them for practice in the United States.

As one Pennsylvania medical educator said: "This country is simply stealing talent and stealing it from countries that can least afford it."

A study by the Association of American Medical Colleges seemed to bear him out. One-quarter of the positions open to interns and residents in American hospitals were being filled by foreign medical graduates, but most of the foreign doctors were not going to the best institutions.

"Most of those who do not have licenses disappear to state hospitals and some states grant special licenses to practice medicine only in that state and only in that institution," he said.

According to a list of state licensing requirements printed in the Journal of the American Medical Association, 20 states have limited licensing arrangements allowing physicians to practice medicine even though they have not been licensed to do so.

But half of the 3,000 foreign medical graduates who take state licensing examinations every year fail the tests, according to the Association of American Medical Colleges. And passing the examinations may not be a true indication of a doctor's proficiency.

None Failed in 3 States

Dr. Robert C. Derbyshire, past president of the Federation of State Medical Boards and secretary of New Mexico's Board of Medical Examiners, conducted a study of state licensing procedures between 1955 and 1965.

During that period, he said, the boards in Oklahoma, Idaho and Tennessee "did not fail a single candidate" for a license to practice medicine. In addition, Kentucky, Wyoming, Michigan, Minnesota, Alabama and South Carolina failed only 14 applicants. "The nine states with the lowest failure rates examined 10,455 candidates, with a failure rate of less than 0.14 per cent," he said.

Armand L. Bird, executive secretary of the Idaho Board of Medical Examiners, said that the failure rate was low because "applicants for licensure are screened well in advance of the test" to see if they are competent. But Mr. Bird declined to estimate how many applicants had been turned down before the formal test was given.

The Oklahoma Board of Medical Examiners reported that 20 applicants failed in the last two years, and that some failed in previous years, but that the statistics had become garbled.

The administrative assistant to the Tennessee board, Mrs. Gertrude Moore, said that 13 applicants had failed since 1964 but that they were not listed as "failures." She said that the 13 were given a second chance to pass the test and that most did.

Dr. G. Halsey Hunt, executive director of the Educational Council for Foreign Medical Graduates, said that "the licensing each year of close to 1,500 graduates of foreign schools is not a good thing for the United States."

"If these doctors stay in this country," Dr. Hunt said, "they drain something out of the economy of their homeland. They come here because it looks like greener pastures with interns making $400 a month and residents $600, even though the American graduates get the good jobs and the foreign medical graduate gets what's left."

Council statistics showed a high failure rate among those foreign doctors taking the council's test, which is given at United States embassies and consulates. About 60 per cent of those taking the test for the first time overseas fail, Dr. Hunt said, although 98 per cent of Americans would pass it.

But Dr. Hunt pointed out that many of those who failed took the examination again and that 65 per cent eventually passed. "Anyone who has passed the ECFMG is a person who has a degree of medical knowledge comparable to 98 per cent of American medical graduates," he said.

The council's test is a one-day examination containing 360 questions taken from the National Board of Medical Examiners tests that many American medical students take in place of state licensing tests. The passing score is 75. Yet only 12 per cent of foreigners score above 80, as opposed to 80 per cent of Americans.

"The ECFMG examination is a meaningless, watered down test," said Dr. Margulies of the A.M.A. He contended that while the questions were taken from the national board tests, "the most difficult questions are eliminated to allow a larger percentage to pass."

The council's annual report for 1965 says: "It must not be assumed, however, that passing the ECFMG examinations means the same as passing National Board Examinations. Questions that have been judged to be very difficult for American graduates have not been included in the ECFMG examinations."

"To use 75 as a passing grade for this exam would be okay if those who came here returned home again after specialized training," Dr. Margulies said. "But giving them patient responsibility is simply unsatisfactory."

Failure rates for graduates of foreign medical schools vary widely depending on the institution. Last year graduates of the University of Santo Tomas in Manila passed 170 state licensing examinations and failed 110. Istanbul University graduates took 158 tests and failed more than half. University of Bologna graduates passed 48 tests and failed 44. Graduates of British and Scandanavian medical schools passed 100 examinations and failed only nine.

"We are pretending that every medical degree is the same," one medical educator said. In many overseas medical schools, he added, students attend lectures for four years "and never see a patient until they come to the United States to serve as internes."

The curriculum of American medical schools devotes the first two years to instruction in the basic medical sciences, while the second two are used for clinical teaching in which the students work with patients under the tutelage of experienced physicians.

Most foreign-trained doctors entering this country are tested to determine minimum competence, but there has apparently been only one attempt to rate their over-all performance as doctors.

Dr. Erwin Hirsch, director of medical education at the Princeton (N. J.) Hospital, has been giving the same test of basic medical knowledge to American-trained doctors and physicians trained overseas for more than a year.

"The test does not pretend to prove that a man is a good doctor because you can't rate a doctor by an exam alone," Dr. Hirsch said. "But it is a devilishly clever test and the best gauge we have of measuring clinical competence. The test

takes a full day and comes pretty close to judging the art of being a doctor. Actual cases and their management are presented, including motion pictures of patients."

Thus far 60 Americans and 129 foreign doctors have taken the test, which has been given at the beginning and end of their internships. Dr. Hirsch said that there was only one American failure both times. One-third of the foreign graduates passed the test the first time, he said, but after internship two-thirds of them passed.

Dr. Hirsch said that hospitals were using a variety of "recruiting drives" for foreign medical graduates. A director of medical education in a nearby state said he received monthly letters from travel agencies in New York offering to arrange delivery of foreign medical graduates. One of these agencies is the Korea Travel Service in Manhattan, directed by Peter Ohm.

"Business is booming," Mr. Ohm told a recent visitor. He estimated that in the last three years he had placed 120 graduates of South Korean medical schools in American hospitals.

Mr. Ohm said that South Korean doctors who want to come to the United States get in touch with his office in Seoul "and we contact the hospitals here." The American hospitals advance the money for tickets to his travel agency, he said, and the Seoul office gives the tickets to the Korean doctors.

"Today if I call a hospital and say I have a doctor for them they would pay me immediately," Mr. Ohm said.

Mr. Ohm said that internship "used to be slavery, but it's not any more." He explained that some small hospitals give the air fare to the doctor as a bonus, as well as furnishing him with an apartment and a salary of $600 a month. He said that the Korean doctors seemed to be satisfied with their new jobs. "Most don't go back home once they get here," he said.

South Korea has been writing them to return to help ease her own doctor shortage.

Attempts to limit the influx of foreign doctors have failed in part because of changes in the immigration regulations.

At one time ECFMG certification was almost mandatory. Then the regulations were relaxed to let foreign doctors enter the country without certification if they had a medical degree and had practiced for at least two years in their own countries. This year the law was changed again to allow in any graduate of a medical school.

"Something should be done about it," Dr. Hunt of the educational council said.

Something is being done about it—in Canada. Medical licensure boards there are studying means of developing uniform requirements for medical licenses that would apply in all 10 provinces, said Dr. J. C. C. Dawson, registrar of the Ontario College of Physicians and Surgeons.

Dr. Dawson said that Canada's foreign doctor problem was more acute than America's because "when your immigration people tell them [the foreign doctors] to move on they come here."

But Dr. Dawson, like his American colleagues, did not envision any quick solution because of the difficulties of getting 10 provincial or 50 state boards to agree on uniform standards.

Many American private health groups are seeking to involve the Federal Government, not only in the foreign doctor problem but also in the whole range of troubles of the American system of health care.

One panel of leading medical educators estimated in a report to the Federal Government that the cost of expanding medical schools to the point that they could start to produce as many new American doctors each year as are entering from overseas could be as high as $1-billion. Yet many American medical schools are on the verge of bankruptcy.

September 29, 1967

Medical Students Plan to Return Gift Instruments

By RICHARD D. LYONS

Forty-five students at the Harvard Medical School, who said they believed that "an unhealthy relationship exists between the drug industry and the medical profession," decided yesterday to return a $40 bag of diagnostic instruments that each had been given by a pharmaceutical company.

The second-year students, who conceded that they had invited the offer last year, said in a statement that "we now feel that we made a mistake and think it proper to return the instruments" to Eli Lilly & Co. of Indianapolis.

In a letter to the company, the students said that such gifts undermined the "objectiv-

ity" of doctors and medical students because such gifts "engender a sense of familiarity and gratitude" toward those companies that dispense them.

"In a subtle but real way these attitudes can undermine the critical objectivity which must underly both the medical and economic decisions of prescription writing," the letter continued.

"In an analogous situation, it is universally recognized that an official who awards contracts should not accept gifts from bidders.

"Our aim is to establish good habits for ourselves early in our training and to promote discussion of the relationship between the drug industry, the medical profession and the patient," the letter said.

Priced at $40

Richard Pohl, 23 years old, of Lynbrook, L. I., who acted as a spokesman for the group, said the instrument package consisted of a black bag, a stethoscope, a tuning fork, a percussion hammer and a tape measure that, together, retail for about $40.

Mr. Pohl said there were about 125 students in his class, some of whom did not chose to accept the instruments when they were distributed last year.

"We want to make this a national issue if possible," Mr. Pohl said, adding that the Harvard group was talking to medical students at Tufts and Boston University in an attempt to have more instruments returned.

Last November, 36 students at the Case Western Reserve University School of Medicine in Cleveland returned similar gifts from a drug company whose name was not announced at the time.

In a letter to the New England Journal of Medicine, the Cleveland students said: "We are returning these gifts because we feel they are not gifts but rather are inappropriate advertisements. Although many of these gifts are useful, all but the most naive realize that your motivation in giving them to us is to influence our future choice of drugs."

Mr. Pohl said in a telephone interview that he and his fellow students had attempted to return the instruments to a Boston branch office of the Indianapolis company yesterday but that "no one in a position of authority was there to accept them." He added that another attempt would be made on Monday.

Attempts by The New York Times to telephone officials of Lilly in Indianapolis for comment were unavailing.

The company is but one of many pharmaceutical corporations that give medical instruments and other materials such as textbooks and sample drugs to doctors and medical students.

Some of the companies also distribute scholarships and grants to medical schools.

Dr. Richard Burack, a specialist in pharmacology at the Harvard Medical School who has been a critic of the prices and quality of drugs, applauded the students' actions.

He said in a telephone interview that "it was about time that something was done to widen the link between the drug industry and the medical profession."

February 1, 1969

Family Medicine Is Made a Specialty

By DONALD JANSON
Special to The New York Times

CHICAGO, Feb. 10 — The medical profession announced today establishment of the new specialty of family medicine.

The step is aimed at halting a quarter-century decline in general practitioners. It seeks to provide continuous personal health care for more families.

The new specialty, the first since preventive medicine achieved this status in 1948, was approved in meetings here over the weekend by the Council on Medical Education of the American Medical Association and the Advisory Board for Medical Specialties, on which all 19 existing specialties are represented. Approval came after two years of consideration.

At a news conference this morning in the Palmer House, Dr. Maynard I. Shapiro, president of the American Academy of General Practice, called the action a milestone in medical history.

He said it would end "the country's nonsystem of delivery of health care" by making available again family doctors who will know intimately the medical history of an entire family. They will minister to 85 per cent of their patients' needs and offer counsel about where to go for the rest.

Beyond restoring old-time general practice, he said, the new family doctor will be trained in psychology, sociology and other behavioral sciences "to a level never attempted before" to recognize and treat "the emotional overlay" that often accompanies disease and family strain.

Recognition of family practice as a specialty, he said, will give it the status, privileges and pay to induce medical students to enter it in both urban and rural areas.

Of more than 300,000 physicians in the country, only 72,000 now are general practitioners. The number has been declining about 2 per cent a year since World War II. Most are elderly and serve rural areas.

Fewer than 2 per cent of all 1967 medical school graduates selected general practice over specialties. Nearly half the doctors entering general practice in the United States in recent years were trained abroad, often not to the best American standards.

Dr. Shapiro, clinical associate professor at the Chicago Medical School, said he hoped creation of the new specialty would eventually reverse present figures of 21 per cent general practitioners and 79 per cent specialists.

He said that making family medicine a specialty in its own right would restore entree to hospital staffs for general practitioners increasingly shunned in recent years by medical centers and teaching hospitals.

Will Become Diplomates

Physicians passing new certification board examinations will become diplomates in family medicine, with the same specialty rank and status of diplomates in surgery, psychiatry, internal medicine and the other specialties.

The examination, devised by the National Board of Medical Examiners in Philadelphia, is to be offered for the first time by the end of this year. The examinations will be conducted by a new Board of Family Practice.

Study and residency requirements will be comparable to those for most other specialties, with three years of graduate work following four years in medical school.

Residency training programs are in operation or under development for the new specialty at 32 medical schools and hospitals, including Hunterdon Medical Center in Flemington, N. J., and West Jersey Hospital in Camden.

Dr. Shapiro said the new specialty would mean significant changes in medical school curriculums.

"The next step will be to establish departments of family practice at the schools," he said. "General practitioners will return to teaching. Students must be exposed to real practicing physicians. Now most students just don't believe we exist."

The major changes in curriculum, he said, will be to increase exposure of students to the behavioral sciences.

"Many old-time family doctors dealt in environmental and interpersonal relationships without even realizing it," he said. "Today we can teach it, and this is what the new specialty is about—teaching young doctors to practice in a scientific context those things that made the best of the old-time general practitioners great."

Doctors now in general practice may take the examination upon completing 300 hours of accredited postgraduate study in medicine. There is no clause in the qualifications document for the new specialty that permits automatic certification.

"The American public has a right to expect the highest degree of technical ability and full comprehension of the latest advances in medical science from all its doctors," Dr. Shapiro said. "We can give them proof of this for first-line physicians through this new board."

Unlike any other specialty, the family practice board will require periodic recertifications, also by examination.

Dr. Shapiro said establishment of the new specialty was a demonstration of the medical profession's "recognition of its responsibility to devise a practical response to the nation's rising health care needs."

The shortage of general practitioners has become so severe, he noted, that thousands of patients must go to internists or other specialists for periodic checkups and referral.

The principal gainer with creation of the new specialty, Dr. Shapiro said, will be the patient, who once again may have "a personal doctor" who is closely acquainted with all his health problems and consequently can offer preventive as well as emergency care.

The periodic checkups many people now get, at clinics or elsewhere, he said, are too limited and impersonal to constitute preventive medicine or to look to emotional problems. Because they do not know where to turn, he said, many people now do not go to a doctor soon enough.

"It should not be necessary to wait till you get sick to see a doctor," he said.

Dr. Shapiro said the new specialty would help close the gap between the best care available and what many citizens actually get.

In line with the name for the new specialty, the American Academy of General Practice, with headquarters in Kansas City, Mo., may change its name to the American Academy of Family Physicians, said Mac P. Cahal, executive director. He said the academy's journal, GP, also might be in for a name change. •

February 11, 1969

Protesters Disrupt Meeting of A.M.A.

By SANDRA BLAKESLEE

The American Medical Association's annual meeting opened here yesterday with a 30-minute tribute to the flag and a 25-minute invasion by liberals shouting protest at the organization's views.

The patriotic ceremony, led by a bewigged Marine Corps drum and bugle contingent, produced some moist eyes among the doctors as the 244 members of the A.M.A.'s House of Delegates assembled in the Imperial Ballroom of the Americana Hotel.

But shortly thereafter the meeting was thrown into pandemonium as a group of about 75 doctors, nurses, medical students and their supporters took over the podium to assail the organization's "conservative" leadership.

Egeberg Gives Talk

Dr. Roger O. Egeberg, recently appointed as Assistant Secretary for Health and Scientific Affairs of the Health, Education and Welfare Department, counseled the red-faced and visibly angry doctors to have tolerance toward the protestors when the session resumed later after a short recess.

"Students represent the gamut from conservative to ultra-radical," he said in his talk before the group, "and I think many of them are Maoists. But they do not represent the majority of students. I hope you will have faith in most of the students."

Generally, the demonstrators were protesting against what they say is the reactionary attitude of the American Medical Association to the total health needs of the country.

The colorful, patriotic pageant, complete with costumes, wigs and exuberant fanfare, certainly created a patriotic response among the doctors.

The display grew to a peak with the playing of "The Star Spangled Banner." The band, flag-bearers and honor guard quick-stepped out of the ballroom as the doctors stood at attention.

But before the meeting could resume, the group of young demonstrators swept down the center aisle which had just been vacated by the Marines, and seized the microphone from the A.M.A. president, Dr. Dwight L. Wilbur.

Shouting ensued until one of the protestors was given permission to speak for two minutes.

The speaker, Dr. Richard Kunnes, represented a coalition of the Student Health Organization, the Medical Committee for Human Rights, the Movement for a Democratic Society, the Health Policy Advisory Center and other liberal organizations of health professionals. Dr. Kunnes, who is 27 years old, is a senior resident in psychiatry at Alebert Einstein Hospital.

"Let's get one thing straight," Dr. Kunnes said, straining to be heard above the boos of the doctors still in the audience, "The American Medical Association is really the American Murder Association."

"You're the criminals, who rather than developing a preventive health program have prevented health programs. You're the criminals, who through your monopolistic, exclusionary and racist practices have created a vast shortage of health manpower, resulting in the needless death of countless millions."

Cries of "Shut up!" "Get out of here! and "Go to hell!" rose from the audience. Several doctors, however, sat calmly with arms folded or lit up pipes or cigars to wait out the verbal storm.

Dr. Kunne's talk lasted five minutes, rather than two, until Dr. Wilbur managed to edge up to the podium and call a recess for five minutes.

But the demonstration was not over. About 50 protestors proceeded down the aisle to join Dr. Kunnes.

They occupied the podium, causing the visitors seated on the stage behind the podium to scatter. The protestors chanted: "Hip, Hip, Hippocrates . . . Up with service, down with fees."

Dr. Kunnes, who was shouting to be heard above the din, declared that he was going to burn his membership card in the A.M.A. He proceeded to burn a card. Association officials standing next to the psychiatrist said later, however, that the card was a Blue Cross membership. Dr. Kunnes insisted it was his A.M.A. card.

Some doctors in the audience threw ashtrays at the demonstrators but no one was injured.

After 15 minutes of continued shouting and milling about by doctors and demonstrators, the protesters retired to the nearby Princess Suite to plan their strategy of disruption during the next four days of the convention, which ends on Thursday.

Dr. Egeberg, who told the A.M.A. that he had not always supported their policy positions, gave a friendly speech in which he repeated the health department's recent warning to the medical profession that health care in the nation was in a state of crisis and that the Government must have cooperation from doctors in order to solve the problems.

July 14, 1969

Internes Joining Social Activists

It is 6:15 in the evening and, for the moment at least, a fitful quiet has settled over the babies lying in the green metal cribs in Jacobi Hospital. The anxious mothers are home now, preparing dinner for their husbands and their other children; the nurses are at their stations, checking the temperature charts and the lists of medicine they are to administer.

For Peter West, the interne who has been on duty for nearly 10 hours, who will be on duty through the night and well into tomorrow, there is time for a cigarette and time to reflect on why he came to Jacobi in the northeast Bronx.

Dr. West is one of a small, but growing number of internes and residents in hospitals throughout the city who are picketing, protesting, petitioning and bringing their medical skills into the neighborhoods in an effort to make their profession more socially conscious.

"On one hand," Dr. West says, his spare frame slumped into a metal chair, "I'd hear my father — a doctor — say anyone could get medical care. Then I went to the coastal valley of California, to the migrant workers, and I saw a child die because he went to a private hospital and they sent him away to a county hospital. He died —the county hospital was 70 miles away, and he died on the way.

Care and Its Meanings

"You see all this first hand, and you see doctors oblivious to it. It's just become blatantly obvious that something is wrong."

The internship, the year between medical school and residency, is traditionally a time of staying within the confines of the hospital, of learning from senior doctors, of applying techniques studied in school, of having one's own patients. It is also a time of working 90 to 125 hours a week.

Most of the young doctors interning in New York City today, following the pattern set by generations of physicians before them, devote themselves totally to their work in the wards and in the emergency rooms.

"It's my one chance to learn from some of the best doctors in the country," an interne at Presbyterian Hospital explains.

Many young physicians believe the community benefits from such concentration. Dr. Gordon Noel, a resident at Presbyterian Hospital, says: "Unlike the students, we don't stand back in anger, wishing we could do more. Often, we think we are doing more than enough."

Some of New York's internes are looking beyond the wards and are agitating for new concepts and techniques of health care.

In their efforts to forge a more socially active brand of medicine, some of these doctors are teaching first aid to youthful activists who may become involved in violent demonstrations. Others are demanding that the city hire more nurses. And some are refusing to serve in Vietnam.

The young doctors still develop what Sinclair Lewis called "the Interne's Walk, that quick corridor step with the stethoscope conspicuous in the pocket." But they also make time to shut down clinics and picket City Hall to protest budget cuts.

"This is a different breed," said Dr. Lewis Fraad, director of pediatric services at Jacobi and one of the few senior physicians who encourage the activists.

"In the early sixties, the kids were dull—bright, but very much intent on their own careers," he said. "These kids are much more down to earth. They're interested in local problems. This is a minority, but it's a significant minority, and it's growing."

The interest in social activism is still too new to have many members or even a central organization. It manifests itself in such activities as seminars on the politics of health, held Thurs-

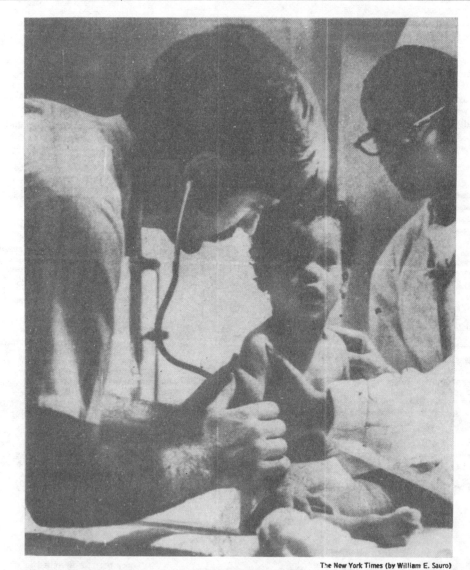

The New York Times (by William E. Sauro)

Peter West, interne at Jacobi Hospital, Northeast Bronx, examining baby in pediatrics

day nights at Judson Church in Greenwich Village, and in the demonstrations last July at the American Medical Association's convention.

Belong to New Groups

It is evident, too, in interne . membership in such groups as the Medical Committee for Human Rights, the Health Policy Advisory Center, and the Medical Resistance Union. These groups, founded within the last few years, reflect what one young physician called "the New Left of the medical profession." Their leaders say membership is increasing, but no one knows the size of their membership.

Seven years ago the municipal hospitals attracted fewer than half the internes they sought (217 out of 482) and had to seek out internes from abroad. This year, the city hospitals attracted 458 internes for 627 openings, and for the second year in a row their percentage of suc-

cess was higher than that of the private hospitals.

One of the reasons for the increase, city officials say, is the improved quality of facilities and medical instruction at the municipal hospitals. Another is the specialized training available at some of these hospitals that is unavailable elsewhere. A young interne, for example, could learn more about trauma while at Harlem Hospital than perhaps anywhere else.

But internes give other reasons for coming to municipal hospitals. "There's a kind of sorting-out process," one interne said. "A lot of people with questions about their relationship to traditional medicine go to city hospitals."

Dr. Herbert Freilich, deputy commissioner for operations in the Department of Hospitals, put it this way: "We feel that there's more of a social commitment, an attraction to big city hospitals in disadvantaged areas."

Nowhere is this feeling

more apparent than at Harlem Hospital. In 1966, Harlem sought 50 internes through the National Interne Matching Program and attracted none. This year it filled each of the 52 available staff places.

One reason is Harlem's sharply improved standards. Columbia University's College of Physicians and Surgeons became affiliated with Harlem in 1964 and a modern, 880-bed hospital has just been opened at 135th Street and Lenox Avenue, replacing the dingy building next door. Many of the house staff say they came to Harlem mainly because the hospital provides a chance to contribute to a needy community.

"Just being on the streets around here, in your whites, people come up to you and say they're sick," Dr. Marvin Anderson, a resident, said.

Some need only reassurance, but others require treatment, and to those Dr. Anderson gives the appointment slips he always carries in his pocket.

Mostly, he said, he tries to "extend the idea of good compassionate care." For, as he continued, "there's an element in the community that doesn't feel Columbia should be here; they think we're just interested in experimentation." So Dr. Anderson goes to community meetings and talks about the hospital. And he lives, eats, and shops in Harlem.

Free Examinations

Another Harlem staff doctor, Reynard McDonald, who plans to practice in the small, largely black, towns in the South, gives free physical examinations to local children.

But even for the internes who come to such hospitals as Jacobi with no plans for social action, the first few months. of internship are often enough to turn them into activists.

"In medical school everyone had his idea of a specialty, no one was interested in social problems," said Dr. William Epstein, a resident. But now, he said, he is determined to "bring to the public eye what the inadequacies are."

He said he had found "one nurse for 40 people."

Many of the internes, aware that they are what one termed "a pitiful minority," are going into the neighborhoods they serve to find support for changes they feel their profession will not make of its own accord. Two such physicians are Arthur Kaufman and Willy Shull of St. Vincent's Hospital, who plan to work with community groups to set up a treatment center for narcotics addicts.

The conflict between the majority and the minority views is reflected in dissension within the Committee of Internes and Residents, the collective-bargaining agent between the city and the house staff of the municipal hospitals,

Increase in Salary

The committee won the approval of most young doctors last year when it obtained a substantial pay raise—the interne's salary, for instance, jumped from $5,400 in 1967 to $9,000 in 1968. This year, however, when the committee decided to ask that the 1969 level of $9,250 be raised to $14,000, a dissident group objected. The power of the committee, the dissidents argued, should be used to get more meaningful benefits, such as more nurses and laboratory technicians.

Sam Rosenthal, a resident at Kings County and president of the committee, maintains that "the group as a whole is progressive," and notes that its list of bargaining demands includes such activist-favored measures as the hiring of more hospital workers.

The dissidents concede that they have little chance of "radicalizing" the city's senior doctors.

"No one objects to criticism," said Dr. Robert Elliott, an attending surgeon at Presbyterian. "But one of the hard things for the older group to accept is what seems to be a complete lack of respect for the older generation by younger students."

Dr. Elliott did not criticize the motives of the activists. But what he and other physicians do object to is the activists' methods—the picketing, the closing down of clinics, the demonstrations—and the time spent by young doctors on these activities.

Sheldon King, the administrator of Jacobi, offered this explanation of why many older doctors object to the new social involvement of the young:

"The physician enjoys a certain amount of charisma —he saves lives. I think some of them fear that when physicians get involved in the community, they lose this charisma."

September 15, 1969

Malpractice Suits Are Soaring, Doctors on the Defensive

By LAWRENCE K. ALTMAN

Witnesses at a State Senate public hearing testified here yesterday that a steep rise in medical malpractice suits was forcing physicians to practice "defensive medicine," shirk hazardous modes of treatment that could be of benefit to patients, and pass along the costs of skyrocketing insurance premiums to patients.

"One physician of every six has been sued for malpractice," State Senator Norman F. Lent told the hearing. And more than 10,000 Americans will initiate medical malpractice suits this year, Senator Lent, who is chairman of the Senate Committee on Health, added.

Because some insurance companies find medical malpractice insurance unprofitable, witnesses said, carriers are dropping out of this field and denying many physicians in some states coverage.

"Malpractice litigation is a hidden cost factor often forgotten in private and government efforts to constrain spiraling costs," said Dr. Mary C. McLaughlin, New York City Health Commissioner.

The testimony was given at the start of two days of hearings called by the Senate Health Committee to determine whether changs are needed in laws governing malpractice suits in the state. The hearings are being held in the auditorium of the City Health Department at 125 Worth Street.

Most of the 31 witnesses agreed that the boom in malpractice suits did not reflect a deterioration of the quality of medical practice in this country.

Rather, they attributed it to the following:

¶The hazards in more complex medical and surgical procedures that doctors are undertaking to explore hitherto inaccessible areas of the body and thereby extend lives.

¶The impersonal character of medicine practiced by some overworked physicians.

¶A breakdown in the relationship between doctor and patient.

¶A society that is more conscious about suing many people—not just doctors.

Because "patients often do not appreciate the complexities — and hazards of modern medical practice," said Eli P. Bernzweig, a malpractice expert for the Department of Health, Education and Welfare, they "are much more prone to blame the treating physician whenever the final outcome is not what was expected."

None of the witnesses had a specific solution to the problem. Among their recommendations were medical accident insurance programs, governmental malpractice insurance and requirements to make doctors keep up with medicine. All agreed more study of the problem was needed.

"Physicians are beginning to view each patient as a potential malpractice claimant and, as a result, practice defensive medicine," Dr. McLaughlin said.

This, witnesses said, may lead to excessive diagnostic procedures, such as unnecessary blood and urine tests, X-rays and medical specialist referrals, overutilization of hospital and nursing services, and reluctance to write facts that might suggest errors into patients' medical records.

Some doctors, Mr. Bernzweig said, even refuse emergency-room duty at local hospitals.

The doctors most prone to malpractice suits, Dr. McLaughlin said, are those practicing surgical sub-specialties, such as orthopedists, neurosurgeons, obstetricians and gynecologists, and ophthalmologists.

The reasons for suits, she said, include the leaving of foreign bodies in patients after surgery, untoward results of tight casts, technical surgical errors, adverse reactions to such drugs as penicillin and failure to obtain the informed consent of patients.

Dr. McLaughlin defined malpractice as "conduct below the standard of care for physicians practicing in the same or similar areas."

But R. Crawford Morris, a Cleveland legal expert on malpractice, said that courts used the concept of "ordinary care," not the standard of practice in a community, in deciding malpractice cases.

"It is not true that a physician's duty is to do what is accepted practice in a community but rather what is ordinary care under the circumstances," Mr. Morris said in an interview.

Though one may infer that "ordinary care" is what physicians practice in a community, Mr. Morris said that this was not necessarily so. As a far-fetched example, he said that if all physicians in a community decided not to wash their hands before treating patients and one physician continued to wash his hands, the doctor practicing good hygiene would not be guilty of malpractice.

The rates physicians pay for malpractice insurance vary with their specialties and where they practice. Everywhere they have been climbing in recent years. One doctor in New Mexico reportedly is paying more than $10,000 a year in an unusual example.

"Premiums in New York State are now above $2,000 for many physicians, with a 60 per cent increase anticipated in the near future," Dr. Max Schapira of the New York State Society of Anesthesiologists said in an interview.

Malpractice verdicts in excess of $100,000 have become common, and in three instances juries have found for the plaintiff in sums of $1-million or more, witnesses said.

Ironically, Dr. McLaughlin pointed out, "the patient's share of the ever-increasing high damage payments is less than the attorney's fees and investigation expenses."

Mr. Bernzweig said that, for the most part, the insurance industry "regards the malpractice market as totally unprofitable, and a number of carriers are withdrawing entirely from this line of business."

Dr. Raymond A. Gadowski of the American Osteopathic Association cited Hawaii, where many physicians "are suddenly finding themselves with no professional liability insurance." Some Hawaiian physicians, anesthesiologists and surgeons, he said, received as little as three days' notice of termination of their insurance when they filed renewal requests. No specific explanation for this has been advanced.

Noting that malpractice claims have been filed in this country since the last century but that they began to accelerate only about 11 years ago, Mr. Bernzweig stressed that the answer would not come from a massive Federal program "but in the collective efforts of all who have a stake in the problem." The interested parties he said, include physicians, lawyers, insurance companies, government officials and leaders of private industry.

A no-fault policy to cover the costs of unexpected complications in medical treatment was one solution proposed by several witnesses. Under such a plan, Mr. Morris said, a patient who acquired an infection after an operation, for example, would have the additional costs paid for by such insurance.

Other witnesses suggested that ways be studied for shifting claim decisions from the courts to administrative tribunals.

Commissioner McLaughlin also suggested that there be "a statutory mandate" for doctors to continue their education after completion of medical school and specialty training. Such continued education, Dr. McLaughlin said, might help reduce the number of malpractice suits and prevent avoidable deaths.

The Senate committee members said that they were surprised to learn from Elliott E. Leuallen of the New York State Education Department that except for dentists, nurses and pharmacists, the state could not, under existing laws, start disciplinary proceedings against physicians who lost malpractice suits.

September 29, 1970

Excerpts From the Carnegie Commission's Report on Medical Education in U.S.

Special to The New York Times

LOS ANGELES, Oct. 29— Following are excerpts from a report by the Carnegie Commission on Higher Education on medical education in the United States:

Americans deserve and can afford better health care. We have the highest standard of living, but not the highest standard of life—as measured by infant mortality and average life expectancy. A number of countries surpass us. In fact, in comparison with other nations, we are losing. Better health care is clearly a high national priority.

To improve health care requires:

¶More and better health manpower.

¶More and better health care facilities.

¶Better financing arrangements for the health care of the population.

¶Better planning for health manpower and health care delivery.

This report is concerned with more and better health manpower, particularly at the level of doctors and dentists.

The United States today faces only one serious manpower shortage, and that is in health care personnel. This shortage can become even more acute as health insurance expands, leading to even more unmet needs and greater cost inflation, unless corrective action is taken now. It takes a long lead time to get more doctors and dentists.

Higher education, as it trains the most skilled health personnel, has a great responsibility for the welfare of the nation. What colleges of agriculture once did for a rural society can now be done for an urban society by the health science centers— and that is to improve the quality of life for nearly all people in their areas.

Flexner Model's Flaws

The Flexner model [suggested by Dr. Abraham Flexner 60 years ago], based on Johns Hopkins, Harvard, and, before them, German medical education, called for emphasis on biological research. Science was to be at the base of medical education. The Flexner model has been the sole fully accepted model in the United States since 1910. Some schools have fulfilled its promise brilliantly; others have been pale imitations; but all have

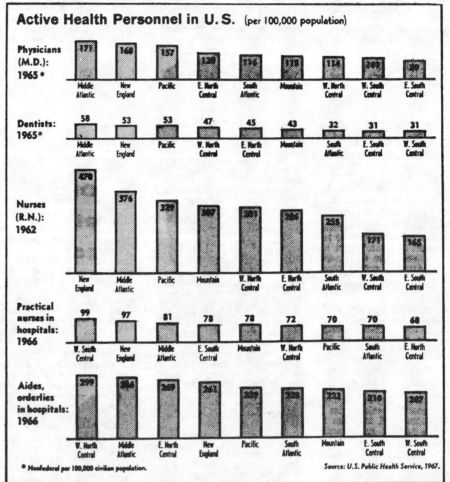

The New York Times (based on Carnegie Commission report)

tried to follow it. It has led to great strides forward in the quality of research and the quality of individual medical practitioners.

The Flexner, or *research* model, however, looked inward to science in the medical school itself. It is a self-contained approach. Consequently, it has two weaknesses in modern times: (1) it largely ignores health care delivery outside the medical school and its own hospital, and (2) it sets science in the medical school apart from science on the general campus with resulting duplication of effort.

This second weakness is now being highlighted by the extension of medical concerns beyond science into economics, sociology, engineering, and many other fields. Medical schools have had their own departments of biochemistry, but to add to their own departments of economics and sociology and engineering would accentu-

ate the problem of duplication of faculty and equipment.

Also, the better economists would rather be in a department of economics on a general campus than separated from their colleagues in a department of medical economics: members of other disciplines would have similar preferences. The self-contained Flexner model thus leads to expensive duplication and can lead to some loss in quality.

Two new models are arising: (1) the *health care delivery* model, where the medical school, in addition to training, does research in health care delivery, advises local hospitals and health authorities, works with community colleges and comprehensive colleges on the training of allied health personnel, carries on continuing education for health personnel, and generally orients itself to external service; and (2) the *integrated science* model, where most or all of

the basic science (and social science) instruction is carried on within the main campus (or other general campuses) and not duplicated in the medical school, which provides mainly clinical instruction. In this model (as in England), the medical school may be, essentially, a teaching hospital; but this is not necessary — it may, rather, carry on all its "Flexner" functions except the traditional first one or two years of science education.

Different Directions

A few schools, and many parts of schools, will, and should, stay with the Flexner model, but we believe that the nation will be better served as many schools move in different directions. A diversity of models and mixtures of models is now desirable.

Not only can the developing and new schools experiment; but as existing schools expand, they can direct their expansion in new directions

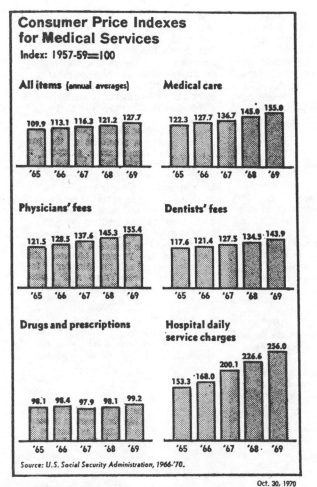

Consumer Price Indexes for Medical Services
Index: 1957-59=100

All items (annual averages)
109.9 113.1 116.3 121.2 127.7
'65 '66 '67 '68 '69

Medical care
122.3 127.7 136.7 145.0 155.0
'65 '66 '67 '68 '69

Physicians' fees
121.5 128.5 137.6 145.3 155.4
'65 '66 '67 '68 '69

Dentists' fees
117.6 121.4 127.5 134.5 143.9
'65 '66 '67 '68 '69

Drugs and prescriptions
98.1 98.4 97.9 98.1 99.2
'65 '66 '67 '68 '69

Hospital daily service charges
153.3 168.0 200.1 226.6 256.0
'65 '66 '67 '68 '69

Source: U.S. Social Security Administration, 1966-'70.

Oct. 30, 1970

so that there can be diversity *within* schools—for example, the next group of 40 additional students admitted might be asked to take their science on the main campus of the parent university. The "cluster-college" approach of changing and diversifying—rather than just duplicating on a larger scale—when expanding a general campus can be undertaken also in a health science center.

The record of the United States in prolonging life expectancy and preventing infant mortality is not impressive when compared with the experience of many other industrial countries. Although the best medical care in this country is as good as any in the world, many Americans receive inferior care, and

some health care needs go entirely untreated.

The geographic distribution of health manpower is highly uneven, and although there is no clear agreement on what ratio of, say, physicians to population is adequate, there is little question that the supply of health manpower is gravely deficient in some parts of the nation.

Health Expense Soars

Americans are spending far more on health care than ever before. In 1928-1929, total health care expenditures amounted to $3.6-billion, or less than 4 per cent of the gross national product. By 1968-1969, they had risen to $60.3 billion, or nearly 7 per cent of the GNP. Public ex-

penditures, greatly augmented after the adoption of the Medicare and Medicaid programs in 1965, were meeting 36 per cent of the total in 1968-1969, while private insurance benefits, despite the fact that about four-fifths of the population had some insurance protection, were meeting only 22 per cent.

What accounts for the sharp contrast between the high proportion of persons with some insurance coverage and the small proportion of total expenditures met by insurance benefits?

The answer lies in the weaknesses of private health insurance protection:

¶Provision for services in the hospital is much more common than for services in the physicians office or in the home.

¶There are limitations on reimbursable charges.

¶Phychiatric care is covered only on a highly restricted basis.

¶Dental care is barely beginning to be covered, although dental insurance protection is now spreading quite rapidly.

¶Charges for health services are typically made on a fee-for-service basis, and increases in costs are passed on in the form of higher premiums.

¶Hospital services are overutilized, except under prepaid comprehensive plans, partly because so many people have hospital insurance but no protection for care outside the hospital.

¶Despite much talk about the need for preventive care, insurance plans are poorly designed to encourage it.

More Students Urged

The commission believes that vigorous efforts should be made in the nineteen-seventies to induce expansion of student places for M.D. and D.D.S. candidates in university health science centers and that these centers should also develop and expand programs for the training of physician's and dentist's associates and assistants.

The commission recommends that the number of medical school entrants

should be increased to 15,300 by 1976 and to 16,400 by 1978. Toward the end of the nineteen-seventies, the question of whether the number of entrant places should continue to be increased will need to be reappraised.

The expansion in the number of medical school entrants should be accomplished through an average expansion of about 39 to 44 per cent in existing and developing schools by 1978, with nine new schools accounting for about 900 to 1,350 entrant places, adding another 8 to 13 per cent. The number of dental school entrants should be increased at least to 5,000 by 1976 and to 5,400 by 1980.

We also recommend that all university health science centers consider the development of programs for the training of physician's and dentist's associates and assistants, where they do not exist, and that, wherever feasible, such programs be initiated forthwith.

The commission recommends, also, that in developing their plans for expansion, university health science centers should adopt programs designed to recruit more women and members of minority groups as medical and dental students.

The Carnegie Commission believes that medical and dental education are critically underfunded and that greatly increased financial support is required to bring about (1) the development of a sufficient and effective supply of physicians and dentists and their associates and assistants, (2) equality of opportunity to enter these health professions, (3) effective use of educational resources, (4) regional dispersion of health manpower educational institutions, (5) equitable distribution of the cost burden, and (6) adaptation of health manpower education to changing patterns of health care delivery.

To achieve these objectives will require that the Federal Government play a major role in the financing of health manpower education.

October 30, 1970

Why More Physicians?

By VICTOR R. FUCHS

The millions of Americans who have waited long hours to see a physician or who have tried in vain to get one to make a house call will no doubt welcome the recommendation of the Carnegie Commission on Higher Education for a 50 per cent increase in

medical school enrollment. Before we swallow this medication whole, however, it would be wise to consider what it will and will not accomplish.

The recommendation is preceded by a description of the poor health status of Americans compared with the citizens of most other developed nations,

and the Commission's report implies that an increase in the number of physicians would somehow rectify the situation. This is extremely unlikely.

Consider, for instance, the most glaring and costly discrepancy, the fact that the death rate for middle-aged males in the United States is twice as high as in some other countries. Additional physicians could probably do little to reduce the heart attacks, lung cancer, alcoholism or motor accidents that destroy so many American men. Or consider the high infant mortality rates in the ghettos. Malnutrition, unwanted pregnancies, unsanitary home conditions and numerous other environmental and behavioral problems would result in unconscionably high infant death rates even if every pregnant woman received Park Avenue medical treatment.

One certain effect of an increase in the number of physicians would be to inflate the already crushingly high cost of medical care. More physicians, and especially more physicians practicing under our present system of organization and reimbursement, would mean more tests and X-rays, more drug prescriptions, more surgery and pressure for more hospital beds. The potential value of these increases should be weighed against evidence that currently points to unnecessary hospital admissions and overly long stays, overprescribing of drugs, excessive surgery and an inordinate use of tests and X-rays.

The notion that an increase in the supply of physicians would substantially reduce the price of medical care is wishful thinking, based on a misapplication of the relation between demand and supply in more conventional markets. The patient's inability to judge the quantity of care needed or the quality received means that the physician is in an excellent position to protect his earnings come what may. Furthermore, even if fees could be depressed to the point of reducing the total earnings of physicians, the effect on the cost of health care would be very small because physicians' earnings account for less than 15 per cent of the total U.S. health bill.

To reduce health-care costs we need to eliminate unnecessary or marginal utilization of hospitals, drugs and tests, and to have appropriately trained medical auxiliaries providing care for the large percentage of visits that do not require the direct intervention of a high-powered physician. The only one who can accomplish this is the physician himself. His decisions determine most of what happens in the delivery of health care. What is needed, therefore, are changes in methods of reimbursement that will give the physician a financial incentive to use the scarce resources of the system wisely. We also need a major change in the focus of medical education to prepare him for this role.

To raise health levels we need a better understanding of disease processes and control mechanisms. As research reveals more about the agents that trigger cancer or the role of diet and exercise in heart disease we can look forward to the *prevention* of illness, which is always the preferable path to better health. Beyond research, we need health and education, family planning, environmental controls and a reduction in the tensions and trauma of daily life.

The cost of turning a high school graduate into an M.D. is over $100,000 if one considers, as one should, the foregone productive services of the student as well as the direct cost of his education. Serious questions may be raised about the potential return to society, in better health, of such an investment as opposed to spending more for auxiliary personnel or research or other health-related programs. The high cost of the Commission's prescription, and of its likely side effects, should make us think twice about rushing to fill it.

Dr. Victor R. Fuchs is Professor of Economics and of Community Medicine at the Graduate Center and the Mount Sinai School of Medicine, the City University of New York.

December 19, 1970

When to Operate?

By JOHN BUNKER

The National Center for Health Statistics has recently released the first comprehensive and reliable data on operations performed in the United States. Considering the fact that more than half of hospital admissions are surgical, this kind of information is long overdue. And, of course, such data are essential if we are to begin to plan, as we must, for comprehensive medical care on a national scale.

The National Center reports that approximately 15 million operations were performed in this country in 1965, and again in 1966—the most recent years for which data have been made available—or one operation a year for every 13 persons. This might seem like a good deal of surgery, and indeed, it is twice as much as is performed in England and Wales, where the comparable rate in 1966 was one operation for every 26 persons. Not surprisingly, there are proportionately twice as many surgeons in the United States as there are in England and Wales.

Such remarkable differences in medical manpower and practices cry out for explanation, but, unfortunately, our knowledge of the indications for surgery are not sufficiently precise to determine whether American surgeons operate too often, or the British too infrequently. Probably both are true to some extent, and it seems reasonable to assume that the United States, as a wealthier country, can afford the luxury of operations that are desirable but not essential.

That wealth is a major factor in the distribution of physicians and medical care can be observed within the United States itself. Consider, for example, the discrepancy in numbers of surgeons between our poorest and our richest states: Alabama, Arkansas, Mississippi and South Carolina have proportionately half as many surgeons and half the per capita income of California, Connecticut, Massachusetts and New York. There are no published data on how many operations are performed in each state, but it seems likely that operation rates vary with the number of surgeons from state to state, as they do between the United States and Great Britain.

Detailed information on surgeons and operations for a single state, Kansas, has recently been made available by Professor Charles Lewis of U.C.L.A. Lewis compared operation rates and surgeons among 11 population regions in Kansas and made the startling observation of three to four-fold variations in rates for common operations such as appendectomy, cholecystectomy, herniorraphy, and tonsillectomy. The numbers of operations were shown to vary directly with the number of surgeons and hospital beds, and Lewis suggested that this might reflect a sort of Parkinson's Law.

Lewis suggests that as more medical services are offered, more are utilized. This extraordinary idea would appear to be totally inconsistent with the public image of medicine today as scientific and precise, each illness a discreet and identifiable entity, each calling for a specific remedy.

But the public image is not an entirely accurate one, and there are a good many factors which may help to explain the Lewis-Parkinson effect.

First, despite remarkable advances in medical practice, there are few precise yardsticks to measure the over-all medical needs of the public. In the absence of specific guidelines, doctors tend to favor active intervention. When in doubt, it is always preferable to do something rather than nothing—whether the something is operating or prescribing a drug.

Secondly, the patient himself has no way to judge either his needs or the quality of his medical care, and he generally overestimates both. More medical care is equated with better medical care, and the patient's demands tend to increase in direct proportion to affluence. Again, where there is doubt, doctors are apt to accede to their patients' demands.

Thirdly, it is now increasingly clear that our medical resources fall far short of medical potential. There are not enough doctors or dollars to bring the last word in medical care to all citizens. Therefore, when more medical care is offered, it is to be expected that more will be used.

The governments of countries where the organization of medicine is already under state control are well aware that their own medical resources are limited. Enoch Powell, the arch-conservative of British politics, says, in his new book, that the welfare state simply cannot afford an artificial kidney machine for every patient whose kidneys fail. Dr. Esther Ammundsen, Director of the Danish National Health Service, points to the widening gap between what is medically possible and what is economically feasible. She goes on to suggest that "The day is not far away—yes, it may be here already—when we simply cannot supply the personnel necessary to care for each other."

In the United States, we are only just now recognizing our own severe limitations in medical resources and in particular, medical manpower. The cry for a greater number of doctors has been raised; even more urgent is the need to examine how and where the doctors we now have spend their time and energy. More doctors in the wealthy communities mean fewer for the poor. An excess of surgeons means a shortage of pediatricians and general practitioners. More heart-lung machines means fewer medical dollars to invest in other medical needs. It is the paradox of American medicine that we can provide luxury care for the wealthy, but cannot provide basic care for the poor.

Dr. John Bunker, Professor of Anesthesia at Stanford University, is writing a book on anesthesia and surgery.

December 19, 1970

Applications to Medical Schools Up Despite a Lag in Funds and Space

By LAWRENCE K. ALTMAN

American medical schools in the last 10 years have rejected nearly 100,000 applicants—twice what Federal officials say is the current national shortage of doctors—though admissions committees considered many of those who were turned down to be "eminently qualified" to be physicians.

A record number of college seniors are seeking admission to medical schools next fall. At the same time, doctors on admissions committees are seeing an unusually high number of new faces—those of Ph.D.s and engineers displaced from other fields, socially conscious students and members of minority groups.

Because there are too few places available, medical school officials say, they are turning away more than half of all applicants at a time when competition is becoming increasingly intense for thousands of students whose grades and medical test scores are at peak levels.

In his health message to Congress Thursday, President Nixon tried to come to grips with the difficulties of adequately funding medical schools to train a sufficient number of doctors and of giving financial support to low-income students.

"The greatest barrier to admission is the lack of places available in medical schools," Dr. John M. Neff, a dean at Johns Hopkins Medical School, said in his office in Baltimore.

Dr. Neff, like other medical school officials, said that the $6,000 grant that President Nixon recommended be given each medical school for each doctor it graduated was not enough to help medical schools out of their financial plight. Further, officials pointed out, such aid would not be forthcoming for some time, even if Congress enacted the proposal.

During the last decade, the pattern of acceptance and rejection of applicants to medical schools has reversed. Whereas 10 years ago American medical schools accepted 60 per cent of those who applied to get an M.D., this year they will accept 45 per cent. Medical schools traditionally have rejected as many applicants as they have accepted.

The Association of American Medical Colleges in Washington has estimated that 75 per cent of those who apply are academically qualified by grades and test scores to get through the rigors of medical school. Thus, of the 14,200 who will be denied admission for next fall's class, perhaps 7,500 are probably qualified to enter.

In other words, just the cream of the qualified crop will get into medical school this year.

No one knows the fate of the qualified rejects, Dr. Henry Seidel of Johns Hopkins said. Upwards of 1,000 Americans each year are going to foreign medical school such as those in Guadalajara, Mexico, or Bologna, Italy, to get their M.D.s. Some transfer later to American medical schools. A few gain admission by reapplying a year later. Many go into allied health professions such as psychology. But the vast majority never become physicians.

Bids to Medical Schools

Year	Total Applicants	Avg. No. of Applications per Individ.	Accepted Applicants	Accepted % of Applicants	Total Med. School Enrollment
1949-1950...	24,434	3.6	7,150	29.3	25,103
1951-1952...	19,920	3.5	7,663	38.5	27,076
1953-1954...	14,678	3.3	7,756	52.8	28,227
1955-1956...	14,937	3.6	7,969	53.3	28,639
1957-1958...	15,791	3.9	8,302	52.6	29,473
1958-1959...	15,170	3.9	8,366	55.1	29,614
1959-1960...	14,952	3.9	8,512	56.9	30,084
1960-1961...	14,397	3.8	8,550	59.4	30,288
1961-1962...	14,381	3.7	8,682	60.4	31,078
1962-1963...	15,847	3.7	8,959	56.5	31,491
1963-1964...	17,668	4.0	9,063	51.3	32,001
1964-1965...	19,168	4.4	9,043	47.2	32,428
1965-1966...	18,703	4.7	9,012	48.2	32,835
1966-1967...	18,250	4.8	9,123	50.0	44,423
1967-1968...	18,724	5.0	9,702	51.8	34,538
1968-1969...	21,118	5.3	10,010	47.9	35,828
1969-1970...	24,465	5.6	10,547	43.1	37,756
1970-1971...	*26,000	—	*11,800	*45.3	—

Sources: Association of American Medical Colleges and American Medical Association. *Estimated.

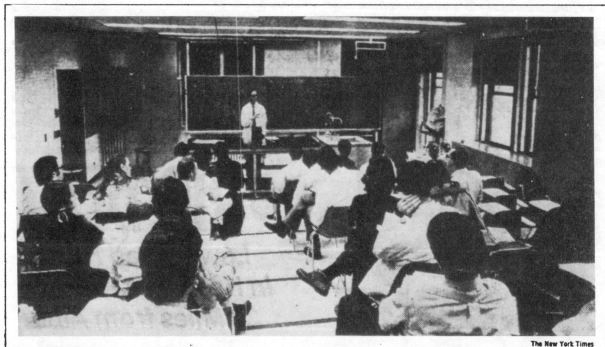

A class at Columbia Medical School. Record number of college seniors will seek admission to medical schools.

Hampered by Lack of Funds

In recent years, medical schools have made an effort to respond to demands that they develop better ways to deliver health care to the community, rather than to the individual patient. Such attempts, however, have been handicapped by declining Federal support. Federal funds to medical schools are generally given for research projects, not for teaching medicine to students.

As a result, many medical schools are in financial trouble —some nearly bankrupt and just barely able to educate those students already enrolled.

Tuition covers just a small fraction of a medical student's increasingly costlier education. Some medical educators estimate the cost to be $60,000 for each student. Tuitions amount at most to $12,000 for the four-year course.

According to officials of one-quarter of American medical schools, applications are coming from the most representative cross-section of American society ever to have sought to become physicians.

And due to fiercer competition, students are applying to more medical schools — about seven on the average — than their predecessors did.

A new computer-assisted system, which the Association of American Medical Colleges administers in Washington, allows a prospective medical student to fill out one application form and thereby petition as many as 56 participating schools for an entering place. The total cost is $600—$10 a school plus a few extra expenses.

Applications Sharply Up

This approach has sharply increased applications for next fall's classes at the participating schools. Harvard, for example, has received more than 3,000 applications for the M.D., nearly double the record 1,600 last year, according to Dr. Perry Culver. The 5,000 applications that Georgetown in Washington has received for 205 places is the most for any American medical school.

Though many students are applying to many medical schools, the total number of applicants is a record.

The medical college association estimates that 26,000 applicants, up from the record 24,465 last year, will compete for the 11,800 places available next fall in the 108 medical schools in this country. The schools are admitting about 3,000 more students each class than they did 10 years ago.

Why do so many seek to become physicians?

An increased social awareness among younger Americans and their desire for a measure of control over their destiny seem to be among the important factors. Further, medicine offers new opportunities for people with widely different educational and social backgrounds.

Specific motivations for choosing the life of a doctor are not easy to determine. Because medical schools consider applications confidential, interviews with a representative group of rejectees are difficult to obtain.

One successful applicant to the University of Indiana Medical School, Glen A. Brunk of Kokomo, for example, is taking five years to graduate from the Massachusetts Institute of Technology instead of four because he needed premedical courses. Mr. Brunk expects to receive a degree—in electrical engineering—this spring.

After spending a summer working for General Motors, where he felt he was "under-utilized," Mr. Brunk said, "I decided that medicine had quite a bit more to offer than engineering. I could make money and help people, too, and it would be a lot more personal a sort of thing."

School officials said that some reasons for the popularity of medicine could be found in the fact that medicine provides a physician with the personal autonomy to pursue a career in a wide variety of intellectually stimulating fields from pure research to pure practice without necessarily becoming part of a large impersonal organization.

"It's a chance to become their own boss," Dr. Ralph Cazort of Meharry Medical College in Nashville said.

A growing number of clergymen are also applying to medical schools. "Seminarians are saying their field isn't scientific enough for them, and the engineers say theirs isn't people-oriented enough," said Dr. W. Albert Sulivan Jr. of the University of Minnesota Medical School.

As the frontiers of medicine expand scientifically and socially, and as doctors rely more on sophisticated instruments, a variety of fields open up for individuals with different backgrounds. Electronics engineers can apply computers to medicine, for example, and social scientists can study medical problems of the ghetto.

A Lucrative Life

For some, practicing medicine can offer a lucrative, prestigious life.

"In spite of the fact kids deny it is their reason, medicine provides a very fine living," said Milton R. Geerdes of the Chicago University Medical School. "You don't see many physicians hurting these days."

Still, many physicians chose to practice, teach or do research in medical schools, where their incomes are generally one-half to one-fifth less than what they could be in private practice.

Intellectual dissatisfaction can also be a strong factor in a career change, particularly, for scientists who see Federal support for science declining and who do not feel at home in private industry.

"Jobs they have now, or the ones that are theirs for the asking, do not meet their standards for achieving their scientific or personal potential," said Dr. David Tormey of the University of Vermont Medical School in Burlington. "They want something more than the fast buck and they no longer believe it's critical to their self-importance that they rise to industrial or business heights."

In universities, too, career switching is occurring among Ph.D.'s, including those with faculty appointments.

Several medical schools such as Albert Einstein, Harvard and the University of Southern California could more than fill next year's class just with Ph.D.'s.

At the University of Southern California Medical School in Los Angeles, for example, officials said that 5 per cent of the 2,712 applicants for the 96 places there next fall were Ph.D.'s or Ph.D. candidates. Yet some schools have received no applications from Ph.D.'s.

Often Ph.D.'s, like other older students, get a cool reception from admissions committees, in part because not all Ph.D.'s have applied to medical schools with the idea of marrying their two specialties. Most schools said that they planned to accept just a few Ph.D.'s. At Columbia, for example, Dr. Frederick G. Hofmann said that less than 10 per cent of the incoming class of 137 students would consist of Ph.D.'s.

Many medical school faculty members said privately they believed that younger college students, with longer professional lives ahead of them, should not be deprived of a place in medical school to give older students a second career choice. Members of admissions committees said that they screened older applicants such as Ph.D.'s more strictly for economic motivations.

In the past, many Ph.D.'s have done poorly after entering medical school, in part because they have had difficulty in readjusting to the role of a student memorizing thousands of facts and in caring for patients through the long hours of many nights.

One Ph.D. dropped out of Chicago Medical School, Mr. Geerdes said "saying he couldn't take the amount of course work."

With the best of the highly qualified students being accepted, the drop-out rate from medical school is very low.

The cross-over of Ph.D.'s is not limited to those in science. Students with backgrounds in the humanities are also turning to medicine.

"You get very strongly the feeling that they are individuals who want to act out the helping of other people," Dr. Hofmann of Columbia said. "They want direct personal contact."

Social Concern Rises

Undergraduates are very sensitive to the difficulties that young engineers and Ph.D.'s are facing with declining Federal support and bleak job opportunities. As a result, Dr. Daniel Funkenstein, a psychiatrist at Harvard, said he had noticed that more undergraduates were changing career plans and considering medicine.

Students feel they cannot rely on Federal funds for career support, Dr. Bernard J. Fogel of the University of Miami Medical School said, and some fear that when they become scientists or engineers they will have to take any job available—not the one they would like to have.

For more and more students, doing what interests them means applying their medical knowledge to improve society.

"In the culture of today, many have discarded the old middle-class ethic of entering medicine as a means of moving upward in society," said Dr. LeRoy A. Pesch of the University of Buffalo.

"Students are making their own assessments of where the problems of today's society are," he said, "and in most cases, these problems come back to medicine. Population control, the squandering of natural resources, pollution—all of these are related to medicine. Health is involved in many social problems—poverty and malnutrition, for example."

The change in the students is widespread

At the University of Vermont, in Burlington, the contrast between the "far more liberal" freshmen and their senior class colleagues "is almost a generation gap within the student society itself," Dr. Tormey said.

"Knowing that doctors are at the top of the social heap," he said, "they [students] believe that as doctors they can have an even greater impact on changing society."

At Einstein, Dr. Bertram A. Lowy noted that "if the students who come in now for interviews stick to what they claim they will do 10 years from now, then [many of] our problems about the delivery of health services may be solved because the majority are interested in community health. They're not concerned with a private lucrative practice. They just want to go into the poor areas of the country and help people who need the help and not worry about the financial reward."

Medical schools have become socially aware of their need to increase enrollment of students from minority groups, and the student bodies are reflecting this change.

Nationally, the percentage of black students enrolled is increasing. Whereas just 2 per cent of medical students were black until about 1968, now 4 per cent of the sophomore medical class and 6 per cent of the freshman medical school class is black. In 1968-69, the nation's medical schools had 783 black students. There are now 1,509 black students enrolled.

Similarly, in recent years the number of female medical students has increased. Women made up 11 per cent of the class that entered American medical schools last fall, compared to 9 per cent two years ago.

But the lack of "adequate financial support for scholarship funds to aid needy students," Dr. Neff of Johns Hopkins said, has hampered medical schools' attempts to enroll more students from minority groups and low income families.

February 21, 1971

3,000 U.S. Medical Students at School Abroad

By RICHARD SEVERO
Special to The New York Times

GUADALAJARA, Mexico, Dec. 13—Claude D'Alberti of Fort Lee, N. J., had a solid B average when he was graduated from Queens College in June as a biology major.

He had thought about becoming a physician but had not decided. In the back of his mind was the notion that he would like to travel in Europe for a year, painting and sketching. Complicating his situation was a very low draft number.

When he finally made up his mind on medicine it was late and, with a draft call hanging over him, he did not want to risk rejection by highly competitive American schools. He had no trouble gaining admission to the Autonomous University of Guadalajara and he is busy learning that the azygous vein is the "vena acigos mayor" and that Gray's "Anatomy" is no more important than Quiroz's "Anatomía Humana."

Mr. D'Alberti is one of some 3,000 Americans who, according to American Medical Association data, are studying medicine abroad. The biggest centers are Guadalajara, with an enrollment of 1,220, and Bologna, Italy, with about 600, 80 per cent of them from New York. Americans are also studying elsewhere in Italy and in Canada, Britain—the number there is small now, only about 70, because the schools favor students from underdeveloped countries—France, Switzerland, Belgium and Spain.

Age and Religious Factors

The Americans go abroad for diverse reasons, among them these:

¶Age. Some decided to begin when they were in their thirties or even forties and were advised by medical schools at home that they were too old. One such is 46-year-old George Newell, president of the North American Students Association in Guadalajara.

¶Religion. There are many Seventh-day Adventists here; they find it more compatible with their beliefs than many schools in the States. One of them, Gwen Cheever, feels that "only six or seven colleges in the States really recognize your religious beliefs—I thought I'd just as soon come here."

Loma Linda Medical School, an Adventist institution, rejected her; she believes that prejudice against women in medicine was the reason.

¶Ethnic Background. Fifty per cent of the American group are Jewish and 15 per cent are of Italian descent (at Bologna the latter figure is 50 per cent). They sometimes say that their inability to get into schools in the United States reflects the medical profession's desire to prevent Jews and Italian-Americans from dominating the field.

¶Geography. The bulk of the students come from New York, New Jersey and California, and many complain that they suffered from having lived in areas with big populations where competition was keen. They realize that many medical schools like to have broad national representation in an effort to avert greater concentrations of physicians on the two coasts and in big cities. "I made a mistake in applying to New York schools," said Joel Albert of Oceanside, L. I. "I probably would have done better in Arizona."

¶Undergraduate Grades. Many students reported that they were at the B and C level in college and had graduated without distinction.

Uncertain and Sensitive

The Americans are uncertain of their future, sensitive about their present and embittered over what they regard as the American Medical Association's stranglehold on the profession.

"Being here makes you feel inferior when you are not," Mr. D'Alberti said. "You know what the attitude in the States is. It is in the back of your mind all the time."

Americans dominate the medical school, both in numbers—total enrollment is 3,800—and in what they pay. The annual cost, several times that of Mexicans and other Latins, is about $4,000, half of which is tuition. The assumption apparently is that because they are North Americans, they can afford it.

Although language and customs may be different at the various schools, the problems are always the same—and the biggest problem is what happens afterward.

Some foreign schools have the blessing of the A.M.A. but most do not, and it has indicated that it is not in accord with some of the teaching methods used abroad. In the case of Guadalajara and Bologna the complaint has centered on the amount of clinical experience offered, which association officials have described as insufficient.

Because of the association's hostility, graduates have found it most difficult to get interneships at home, even where there are shortages.

Six Years Instead of Four

At Guadalajara, as a result, the students spend six years instead of the usual four—four years of medical work, a year of interning in a Mexican hospital and another year of "social service," in which they work with the poor in Mexican clinics.

Before they can return home and repeat their internships in American hospitals, they must pass a special national test, developed by the Educational Council for Foreign Medical School Graduates, rather than the regular state examinations taken by graduates of American institutions.

Although no law says the students have to spend six years rather than four preparing and to take the test, they have found that good hospitals will not hire them without both

qualifications for fear of alienating the A.M.A., which supervises internships and residencies through the Joint Commission on Accreditation of Hospitals.

The students maintain that a private organization with no official status is effectively controlling who can practice medicine in the United States.

A.M.A. Fights Jersey Law

They also say that all they want is an equal chance to be tested the way students at American schools are tested, knocked down both the special test and the requirement of internship and social service outside the United States.

The American Medical Association immediately appealed. In any event, it was clear that, pending a final resolution, most hospitals were going to adhere to the A.M.A.-approved position.

The Englewood Hospital Association advised a Guadalajara graduate: "Interne applicants must be medical school graduates in possession of their final diplomas. In the case of Mexican graduates, this means you must have completed an internship and a year of social service."

On June 11 St. Michael's Medical Center in Newark informed another applicant: "Until a de-

cision has been reached between the A.M.A. and the New Jersey State Legislature, St. Michael's will be unable to accept any students into its interneship program who have not received the E.C.F.M.G. certificate. Failure to comply with the A.M.A. policy in this matter would result in our loss of accreditation."

A suit is pending in the Federal Court for the Southern District of New York, in which the Guadalajara students allege that they are being deprived of due process and that the A.M.A. is in violation of the Sherman and Clayton Antitrust Acts.

Father's School Rejected Him

The vice president of the North American Students Association at Guadalajara is Michael Ritota, who had a C average as an undergraduate at a small Roman Catholic college and who was subsequently rejected by the New Jersey College of Medicine, the St. Louis College of Medicine (Mr. Ritota's father, a New Jersey physician, went there), Georgetown and Creighton.

Under pressure from Guadalajara and Bologna students, New Jersey, California and Connecticut have passed laws that would in effect make it un-

necessary for a student to stay abroad for more than four years.

The New Jersey law, signed by Governor Cahill last April.

Mr. Ritota, who is to graduate from Guadalajara in June, and Mr. Newell have given speeches before United States medical groups in an effort to win them over. Mr. Ritota thinks he has made progress but is convinced that the A.M.A. is trying to hold the number of doctors down so that those admitted to practice can make that much more money.

Another Guadalajara student is Umberto Carnera, whose late father, Primo Carnera, was heavyweight boxing champion in 1933. Born in Udine, in northern Italy, Mr. Carnera is a naturalized American citizen and hopes to go to California after graduation and practice internal medicine.

He waited six years after college before he decided he wanted to be a physician and found that his age—he is now 31—was held against him.

"If the United States can extend itself to complete strangers," he said, "if it can help so many countries, I don't see why it can't deal with American citizens who would help to ease an American problem. I think it is going to work out."

December 28, 1971

More Doctors Defecting From A.M.A.

By EVERETT R. HOLLES
Special to The New York Times

SAN DIEGO, Calif., Sept. 3 — Dr. George Abbott is 30 years old, five years out of medical school and just starting private practice in La Jolla, an affluent and conservative suburb of San Diego. He refuses to join the American Medical Association because, to him, it is "archaic and irrelevant."

On his lapel he wears a button that says, "Caution: A.M.A. May Be Hazardous to Your Health."

The buttons have sprouted in 30 cities across the country where there are chapters of the Medical Committee for Human Rights, a militant organization of about 7,000 doctors who regard the A.M.A. as a menace to enlightened medical care.

This disaffection has already reduced the A.M.A.'s share of the nation's practicing physicians. For the first time in at least 50 years, the A.M.A.—long regarded as the nation's most powerful medical lobby—faces the prospect of having a minority of the nation's doctors as dues-paying members.

Membership Drop

In 1962, 61.5 per cent of the number of doctors of medicine

in the United States were members of the association. At the beginning of this year, 168,214 doctors—50.3 per cent of the 334,028 active physicians in the United States—were A.M.A. members, and something less than 50 per cent is expected by the end of the year.

Less apparent than the rate of defections, however, is a growing ferment within the association. Regional A.M.A officials are criticizing the organization's leadership for what they regard as its failure to appeal to the 8,000 young doctors throughout the country who enter medical practice each year.

Dr. Andrew Abernathy, a 37-year-old general practitioner in Atlanta, which the A.M.A. has long considered to be one of its strongholds, says he probably will resign from the organization next year.

"Frankly, I am sort of ashamed to admit that I belong to the A.M.A.," he said. "I don't feel that it represents the best interests of the people. It has opposed everything without offering viable alternatives."

Dr. Rufus K. Broadaway, a Florida delegate to the association's House of Delegates, is one of those who feel that

the organization's effectiveness depends on "getting into the fold more of the younger medical men and being more responsive to their views, even though this may mean changing our basic ideas."

The A.M.A.'s executive vice president, Ernest B. Howard, acknowledges that attacks from both the left and the right are "causing turmoil in the organization," particularly over the issue of national health insurance. Conservative doctors contend that the association's Medicredit proposal is a socialistic sellout; the liberals call it a weak palliative.

And the organization's equivocal stand on the Nixon Administration's Health Maintenance Organization plan for prepaid group medical care appears to satisfy neither conservatives nor liberals.

Mr. Howard insists that, except in the state of New York, where resignations from the A.M.A. are widespread, there have as yet been no significant defections — although trouble may be brewing in California.

Although the disaffection extends to almost every section of the country in varying degree, it has not assumed the semblance of an organized revolt. Essentially, the disaffection is a mood rather than a movement, at least at this point. Opposition is fragmented among a dozen other professional organizations, none of which acknowledged that they are out to wreck the A.M.A.

Although several of these other organizations report

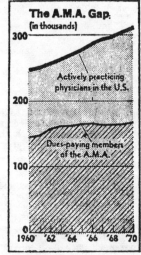

The A.M.A. Gap
(in thousands)

Actively practicing physicians in the U.S.

Dues-paying members of the A.M.A.

300

200

100

0

1960 '62 '64 '66 '68 '70

The New York Times   Sept. 4, 1971

membership gains attributed in part to the A.M.A.'s troubles, none have more than a fraction of the association's membership, or its financial resources.

Formidable Core

The core of the A.M.A.'s strength—the private practicing physician—remains formidable. Nine out of 10 doctors who belong to state medical societies were members of the association last year. The dissidents are largely younger doctors involved in public health and institutional medicine.

The erosion of the A.M.A.'s membership appears to be accelerating as a result of a boycott by younger doctors who share the opinion of Dr. Steve Halpert of Miami. He said that when he was graduated from the University of Florida Medical School a few years ago, 80 to 90 per cent of his classmates were prepared to join the association.

"Now, less than half would do so," he added. "The A.M.A. is like a closed-shop trade union. We dissidents in Florida who believe in patient-oriented medicine and not doctor-oriented health care are few, but our numbers are growing."

The association attributes many of the defections to an increase in its dues from $70 to $110, effective this year, and points to a 15 per cent increase in dues-paying members over the last 10 years. This statistic becomes less impressive, however, alongside Government figures showing that, in the same period, the number of practicing doctors increased at nearly twice that rate.

A probable loss of 10,000 to 12,000 members this year is expected by the A.M.A., principally in New York State, where members of the state medical society were released last December from an obligation to belong to the A.M.A.

California Referendum

In New York State, where the association expects to lose 7,000 to 9,000 members, 13,454 doctors had paid their current dues as of June 4—about 7,000 fewer than were maintaining membership in the State Medical Society. Last year, before the end of compulsory dual membership, the A.M.A. had nearly 27,000 New York State members.

This week, about 26,000 doctors affiliated with the California Medical Association received ballots in a referendum to decide whether they will follow New York's example and abandon compulsory membership in the A.M.A. If the association's "captive membership" hold in California is broken, it could lose another 5,000 to 9,000 members. Ohio and Colorado are considering similar referendums.

Despite the association's declining share of the nation's doctors, its strongest opponent, the American Public Health Association, which has 26,000 members and is growing at the rate of 3,000 members a year, thinks the A.M.A. is almost unassailable, "with more money, more members and more political clout than any other professional organization."

The criticism most frequently heard among younger doctors is that the A.M.A. is dominated by "old men with fixed ideas" who are out of touch with today's medical challenges and responsibilities and who look upon their affiliation with the association primarily as a protection for their economic well-being.

Not all of those who disagree with the association's policies and leadership are leaving the organization, however. There are a significant number of young doctors who intend to remain as members to work for reform from within.

One such member is Dr. Ernest Sanchez of San Diego, who has been a leader of the fight to break the A.M.A.'s

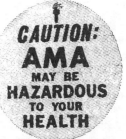

Button that is being worn by some dissident doctors who call American Medical Association a menace to enlightened medicine.

"captive membership" hold in California in the last 18 months.

But now Dr. Sanchez has had a change of heart. He is going to vote to retain the compulsory system, and is urging his anti-A.M.A. colleagues to do the same.

"I have decided that, if the California doctors should desert the A.M.A. in such numbers as have defected in New York, it might be a fatal blow to the national organization," he said.

"Without some strong organization, there would be chaos. I see no alternative. Bad as it is, the A.M.A. is better than no organization at all."

Rural Disaffection

Although the disaffection is most evident in the larger urban centers, it also extends to smaller towns and the domains of the vanishing "country doctor."

"Many of us feel that the A.M.A. is not concerned with the individual physician out in the grass roots," said Dr. William Morton of Cairo, Ga. "It tends to represent the interests of the higher-ups."

But the average small-town doctor thinks he cannot afford to sever his ties with the as-

sociation and the state medical societies, Dr. Morton said, because of his need for malpractice insurance, hospital admittance privileges, patient referrals and other fringe benefits.

Particularly antagonistic to the association are many hospital residents and interns, who represent about one-fifth of all the medical men engaged in direct patient care. They have never adhered to the association in any significant numbers and many have been denied membership.

At its recent convention in Atlantic City, the A.M.A. extended direct, low-cost memberships to residents and interns ineligible for membership in their local medical societies. The residents and interns asked for 45 seats in the A.M.A.'s House of Delegates and received one.

A group of residents and interns who call themselves the National Staff Conference are trying to form a national organization, either with the blessing of the A.M.A. or in opposition to it.

Many of the A.M.A.'s current problems spring from the discontent of older and more conservative members, such as the 400 New England doctors who have formed the Massachusetts Federation of Physicians, or the extreme rightwing, nationally organized Council of Medical Staffs.

The Massachusetts group, headed by Dr. Robert E. Kelleher of New Bedford, has been set up to deal with "economic problems ignored by the A.M.A." and specifically, to oppose most of the proposed government health plans. Dr. Kelleher says the federation's members, who represent about 5 per cent of the doctors in Massachusetts, are concerned with "the increasing government encroachment on the medical profession."

September 4, 1971

Laymen's Growing Role in Health Planning Disturbs Some Physicians Here

By NANCY HICKS

The increased involvement of lay community boards in health planning is causing new militancy and melancholy among physicians who feel they are being pushed aside and ignored in the decision-making process.

Their critics say they failed to recognize the significance of the community board movement until it became clear that public money spent for health care will, by law, be coupled with more public say in how that money will be spent.

The result is that doctors fear non-physicians interfere with patient care and "the practice of medicine."

Lay people say that is not their intention. They say they do not want to tell the doctor where to cut but they do want doctors to treat patients courteously, dispense services more to the patients' convenience, and they want to help set priorities for new services.

Similar Issues Seen

The forces involved came together last month, when the medical staff of Seaview Hos-

pital and Home on Staten Island walked out in protest over the composition of the newly formed community advisory board.

Similar issues of doctor participation and prestige underlay the decision of the Advisory Council of Medical Boards to disband last week, after the Health and Hospitals Corporation refused to let them sit in on board of directors' meetings, routinely.

"I think that we are going through a very difficult time of transition for the physician, who is trying to find his role in what is now a $70-billion enter-

prise in the United States," said Dr. Joseph T. English, president of the Health and Hospitals Corporation, which runs the city's 18 municipal hospitals. Dr. English is a primary target of criticism by the doctors.

"He has seen what he considered a highly individualistic thing — the practice of medicine — become almost overnight the third-largest employer in the United States and one of the biggest segments of the American economy," he said.

The doctors say they are not confused, but left out and they say they are hurt.

29-Member Board

It was not until December, 1971, 18 months after the formation of the corporation, that a medical and professional affairs committee was added to

253

the board of directors. The delay, Dr. English said in an interview, was a mistake. "We should have engaged the doctors in this issue of community involvement sooner," he said.

Under the guidelines set up by the Health and Hospitals Corporation, a community advisory board of 29 members was formed at Seaview, a geriatrics hospital, which in past years pioneered in tuberculosis research.

After the board was almost completely formed, and the doctors were told they had one representative, they balked. They said they had elected three members to the board. The board members said that the three names submitted to them by the doctors represented one full membership and two alternates.

The doctors then appealed to the corporation and Dr. English to disband the board. They suggested, instead, a 51-member board with "more medical input."

Dr. English refused to entertain their suggestion. He said

to intervene with a duly installed board would undermine the support the corporation sought to give community boards.

To do so would open Pandora's box for physicians to circumvent local administrators or community boards in future disputes, he said.

'Insensitive to Needs'

The doctors were told to return to the local board and ask for greater representation. Their spokesmen said, however, they should be dealing directly with the corporation.

The lack of intervention from central administration, "hurt" the doctors, one said. And they accused it of being "insensitive to the needs and fears of the doctors."

The Seaview board, which is probably the most conservative in the city, was not pleased with the doctors' attempts to circumvent it. The hospital's administrator, Joseph D.

Keeney, said the doctors were asked to join the planning committee that set up the board, but they refused to do so.

Dr. Edward H. Robitzek, the director of medical services, said that they participated by electing their three members. He said they were never asked to attend a planning meeting.

Two doctors joined a slate of 10 persons who were running in an open election for three at-large positions on the community board. Both were defeated.

"The doctors tried to come in the back door and failed," said Vincent Claffey, a Staten Island lawyer who is chairman of the board.

On March 15, a week after most submitted letters of resignation, the doctors, all of whom work on a part-time basis, failed to report for work for 11 days, until settlement was reached with the local board to expand membership to 37, including three physicians.

The Seaview situation occurred, Dr. English said, because "very early in the development of the boards, I'm not sure doctors gave them sufficient significance. Then they panicked and started moving hard and fast and caused resistance where there was none."

Advisory Role Seen

Dr. Donald C. Meyer, a dentist who is president of the Doctors Association of the City of New York, agreed in part. The association was the bargaining agent for the Seaview doctors.

"Doctors received copies of the interim guidelines, but they did not pay much attention to them," he said. "They felt the boards would be only advisory, until they were formed. Then they were sure they would be more and that medicine would not be adequately represented.

"All this dawned on doctors when they found out they would be largely excluded from the decisions the boards make. By the time they realized it at Seaview, it was too late."

April 9, 1972

Ranks of General Practitioners Growing in U.S.

By FRED FERRETTI
Special to The New York Times

FLEMINGTON, N.J., May 23 —Three years ago, Samuel Warburton graduated from the University of Pennsylvania School of Medicine with an ambition to be what was considered a vanishing species—a family doctor.

In July, after three years of family practice residency at Hunterdon Medical Center here, he will move south about 12 miles to an old gray stucco house with a mansard roof, reconditioned as a temporary "satellite" community hospital, to set up practice as a family doctor in Lambertville.

Dr. Warburton's ambition reflects a growing national trend among young doctors who want to provide primary personal care on a family level, rather than devote themselves to · research or specialization.

While the American Medical Association has not kept records on the actual number of doctors choosing family practice, an official says that "it is safe to say that it is among the primary interest of most medical students today."

In hospitals, medical centers, health cooperatives and clinics throughout the country, young medical students and residents are opting for

personal medicine. Dr. Ronald Blakenbaker, 30 years old, and director of family practice at Methodist Hospital in Indianapolis, said he chose family practice because he was touched by the queries of patients who felt that doctors were more interested in anatomy than in total personal care.

Total Care Sought

"I guess the best way to put it is that the patient felt he was just a lot of fragments and nobody really cared about his whole person," he said.

Or as Dr. Alva Baker, 28, chief resident in the family program at the University of Maryland School of Medicine, put it:

"The old G.P. [general practitioner] was forced to work at crisis medicine. People came to see him when they were sick. But we have a very strong emphasis on preventive medicine. . . . We attempt to train a man to be a specialist in breadth, not in depth."

In Denver Colo., and Cambridge, Mass., in hospitals in Illinois and Los Angeles; in Seattle, Wash., and Waco, Tex., and Jacksonville, Fla., with doctors like Samuel Warburton, Ronald Blakenbaker and Alva Baker, young men are training to be family doctors.

Dr. Warburton's choice of Hunterdon Medical Center— and its choice of him—was significant because the center, a pioneer in the training of family physicians, predated by more than a decade recent efforts by the A.M.A. to raise the prestige of family practice by bestowing on it the status of a medical specialty.

In 1969 there were 17 medical institutions offering internships or residencies in family practice. Recently, the A.M.A. and the American Association of Family Practice authorized nine more institutions to offer that training, making the total 108 nationwide.

Research Centers Shunned

According to C. H. William Ruhe, director of the medical education division of the A.M.A., in Chicago, "young medical students are more interested today in people, in getting out among people rather than staying in the medical centers, in providing personal primary care."

This attitude was "pervasive" among medical students, he said, and "we're encouraged by the trend."

In 1966, the A.M.A. recommended that family practice be raised to the specialty level following publication of a report by the Ad Hoc Committee on Education for

Family Practice. An American Board of Family Practice was created—the 20th and last specialty board—to pass on standards for teaching and practice.

While there has been a surge of interest in the number of family practice physicians, Mr. Ruhe said, it has not been at the expense of other medical specialties. What has happened, he said, has been an increase in the number of better qualified family doctors and a decrease in what he called "the old G.P., the jack of all trades, master of none."

But Hunterdon Medical Center had been training family physicians since 1953. "It was one of the pioneers," Mr. Ruhe said, "it has been one of the finest programs in the country." He added that records were imprecise, but Hunterdon might have been the first institution to offer formalized family practice internships and residencies. "It was certainly one of the first," he said.

This was done by Hunterdon because of the nature of the community in which the hospital is situated and because "we decided to work towards providing total delivery of first-line direct care for our people," said Lloyd B. Westcott, chairman of the hospital's board of trustees. "Our concept of health care delivery rested with primary physicians, backed up by sophisticated hospital-based specialists for referral."

Hunterdon County depends on the family doctor. Before the medical center was opened 19 years ago, there was no hospital for the 637-square-mile western New Jersey county. The 1970 census gives its population as 69,718.

It is primarily rural, with more than half the land devoted to farming. But with the arrival of new roads, in particular Route 78, soon to connect Clinton with New York City, the population has risen sharply.

The 25 family doctors in Hunterdon are, in the words of the medical center's director, Dr. Frederick J. Knocke, "in delivery."

When Hunterdon began its family practice training in 1953, the county had 40,000

residents and the doctors in the one-year residency program studied internal medicine, pediatrics, out-patient psychiatry, office gynecology and community medicine.

Refinement in Studies

The same studies are offered today, but there has been refinement as the one-year residency became a two-year internship and residency in 1962, and in 1969 a three-year family practice residency. Students now work not only in the hospital where, under a new agreement with the College of Medicine and Dentistry of the New Jersey-Rutgers Medical School, residents function as teachers, but also in the field, working on a family-doctor level. They will work in one of three "satellite" hospitals.

The Phillips-Barber Health Center in Lambertville, the first of these, is housed in an

old building and directed by Dr. R. Kirk Seaton. Soon it will move to a new building in Lambertville. Other satellite centers will be built in Clinton and Milford "so that we can cover the whole county," according to Dr. Knocke.

Hunterdon's director of medical education is Dr. Frank C. Snope, a graduate of New York University-Bellevue Medical Center, who had a general practice in the county for nine years before joining the Hunterdon staff.

Cooperative System

He considers the program the exemplification of "a cooperative health-care delivery system" with the family doctors providing primary care and having hospital privileges and where the specialist "does his thing" in the hospital's diagnostic center.

He pointed out that only 1 to 5 per cent of all illnesses

get to hospitals, so that "real exposure to out-of-hospital care and treatment must be a major part of the teaching." It was this philosophy, together with the lack of community facilities, that led the hospital to plan and staff its satellite centers.

The center is expected to expand from a 167-bed facility to 450 beds, while the satellite centers become full-fledged hospitals. Hunterdon will then become a thoracic and coronary center, a place for cobalt treatment, for example, while the other three centers evolve into traditional hospitals.

From a small hospital that grew out of $1.2-million of community seed money, Hunterdon has become an $11-million plant, with a $4-million annual operating and staff budget.

May 24, 1972

Unions of Doctors Are a Growing Challenge to the A.M.A.

By RICHARD D. LYONS
Special to The New York Times

SAN FRANCISCO, June 17—Faced with declining membership, a rift within its hierarchy and rising rank-and-file discontent, the 150,-000-member American Medical Association opens its week-long annual convention here tomorrow confronted with yet another challenge —the unionization of doctors.

The organizing of doctors into unions—a seeming contradiction, considering the proud individualistic traditions of the medical profession—is a rapidly spreading phenomenon abetted by a brake on physicians' incomes, in part the result of the wage-price controls program, and the intrusion of Government into the health field.

While total membership figures are difficult to determine precisely, it is probable that between 10,000 and 15,000 doctors of the 350,000 in the country are members of some type of union, although the titles of such organizations more commonly use the words association,

guild, federation or committee.

The first group of doctors banded together for collective bargaining arrangements more than 15 years ago. But the union concept has spread rapidly in the last year, with perhaps a quadrupling of membership.

This comes at a time of rising unrest among professional workers in the United States. Engineers, chemists and physicians—groups equally as individualistic as doctors—are also agitating within their ranks to organize for better salaries, perquisites and working conditions.

Still, the major move among the professions lately has involved doctors, the highest-paid group in American society with individual median incomes of more than $40,000.

"We're not just a bunch of rich doctors merely trying to get richer," insisted Dr. Sanford A. Marcus of Daly City, Calif., president of the Union of American Physicians during a recent interview. "We're trying to prevent the regimentation and nationalization stemming from socioeconomic changes in medicine from reducing the doctor to the functionary level of the postman and school teacher."

Other interviews during the last month with leaders of the doctor's union movement

throughout the country have detected a renewed sense of militancy among physicians that has not been seen since the battle against Medicare almost a decade ago. These doctors are as concerned about the manner in which medicine is practiced as they are with their incomes.

"I'm sure the A.M.A. wishes the unions would go away," said Dr. Harold A. Young of West

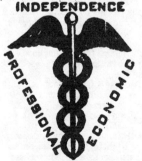

Symbol used by American Physicians Guild.

Palm Beach, Fla., the head of the 600-member American Federation of Physicians on the East Coast, "but the unions, or whatever they are called, are here to stay because the A.M.A. cannot guarantee our economic and professional independence."

As expressed by Dr. Robert Kelleher of New Bedford, head

of the 450-member Massachusetts Federation of Physicians, "We are as equally interested in affecting the climate in which medicine is practiced as the income we receive from it."

Underscoring the dissatisfaction, in this year alone doctors have taken the following steps:

¶Created the 1,000-member Union of American Physicians here in the San Francisco Bay area.

¶Set up in Las Vegas the first doctors' group to affiliate with organized labor, the Nevada Physicians Union.

¶Formed in Florida a statewide doctors' union named the Florida Physicians Association that has been given the blessing of and will operate in parallel with the state medical society.

The A.M.A. has sought to remain aloof from the union movement among its members, issuing a statement in January that "the A.M.A. is not and cannot be a union" because it would be a violation of provisions of the Sherman Antitrust Act.

Antitrust Question

Antitrust lawyers who were asked for opinions on the A.M.A. position gave differing views of this interpretation, pointing out that a clearcut decision has never been made by the Supreme Court.

The president of the A.M.A., Dr. Wesley W. Hall of Reno, Nev., whose calls for reform and redefinition of the association have met with the open opposition of other association leaders, has adopted a hands-off attitude towards unionization.

"I think this is their own business, and they are free to do what they want," he said.

Yet the unionization issue is certain to come to a boil, if not during the 121st annual convention here, certainly in the next few months as the movement grows.

Medical societies in at least half a dozen states have urged that studies be made of the benefits of unionization. The Virginia society has introduced a resolution to be debated here next week calling for the creation of a commission "to determine the most effective legal way to allow collective bargaining on behalf of the medical profession."

The collective bargaining issue involves two groups of doctors with radically different sources of income.

Most doctors now linked to unions are serving internships and residencies in hospitals that pay the physicians' salaries. A generation ago these groups worked for next to nothing in order to gain the experience and training needed for them to advance in their profession.

But over the last decade the once poorly paid internes and residents, often through the use of collection bargaining, have forced most hospitals to increase salaries markedly. A doctor in a New York hospital serving the sixth year of a surgical residency now might earn as much as $17,500 a year.

The leading group among what is collectively known as the house staff, is the Committee of Internes and Residents in New York City, which was founded in 1957.

Michael Horowitz, a lawyer for the committee, said, "There has been a quantum increase in recent years in the number of internes and residents engaged in collective bargaining."

He estimated that the committee had over 4,000 dues-paying members, while the total number of organized house staff members throughout the country was between 8,000 and 10,000.

Other organizations of house staff members have been set up in Philadelphia, Chicago, Ann Arbor, Los Angeles and Oakland.

"These doctors need the leverage that collective bargaining provides," Mr. Horowitz said. "The organizations also afford a way out between outright confrontation such as the strike and complete submission to the old way of doing things."

He said that the New York State Labor Board had opened the way for increased organization of house staffs by ruling two years ago that internes and residents were indeed employes of hospitals, rather than merely students.

Internes and residents have long been dissatisfied with low pay, overwork, the poor quality of medicine practiced in many hospitals, and their own lack of power within the medical profession. Of the 350,000 doctors in the country, about 50,000 are internes and residents.

The second group of doctors who are unionizing — totaling about 5,000 — are those who have already passed through the internship and residency phase of their training and are practicing in their communities. The largest groups are in Massachusetts, Florida, Texas and California.

The principal complaints are that their incomes are not keeping pace with the cost of practicing medicine, and that the so-called third-party payers that are now footing two-thirds of the nation's medical bills, such as Federal and state health programs and private medical insurance, are telling them how to practice their profession.

Irked With Public Image

All the doctors who were interviewed expressed annoyance with the public image of doctors as, according to one physician, "a bunch of money-hungry" people.

Doctors' incomes are rising, but the rate of the increase has tapered off. Data of the Federal Bureau of Labor Statistics in Washington show that since the wage-price freeze of last August, doctors' fees have risen about 3 per cent, while the cost of living has gone up a little over 2 per cent.

But many doctors insisted that even though the increases are about even, their costs of doing business have been rising much faster because of the complexities of medical practice.

Because of the vast amount of paper work generated by such programs as Medicare, Medicaid and the payment for professional services by private health insurance, many doctors have been forced to hire an additional secretary. Nurses' salaries and such overhead items as office rent are also on the upswing.

Dr. Kenneth G. Burton of San Antonio, head of the American Physicians Guild, which has attracted 300 members since its inception early this year, reckoned that he works between 75 and 80 hours a week and that the income from the first 43 hours of his practice goes to paying overhead.

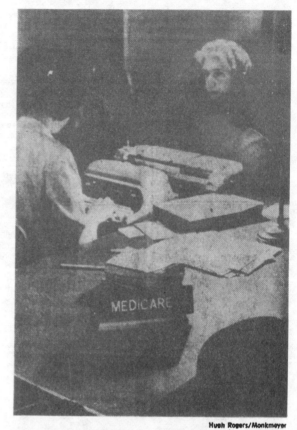

Medicare is expected to be a subject at doctors' parley

"I'm making about $13 an hour, which is less than many plumbers," he said.

Declining Incomes Cited

Dr. Burton said that during the last year five doctors in private practice in the San Antonio area were forced to give up their private offices because of declining incomes.

Without exception, those doctors interviewed vented reactions ranging from anger to disgust over reductions in fees for Medicare, Medicaid and such groups as Blue Cross and private health insurance companies.

The Social Security Administration, which runs the Medicare program for the elderly, reduced 41 per cent of all the doctors' fees that were submitted in the fiscal year 1971. In an effort to contain rising costs of the program, there have been three reductions in fee scales.

Between the fiscal years 1970 and 1971 the Medicare program increased payments for doctors only 2 per cent, although consumer prices rose 6 per cent and still more of the elderly participated in the program.

Some states, such as New York, have also reduced fees paid to doctors under the Medicaid program for the poor and the near-poor.

Dr. Kelleher of New Bedford, a plastic surgeon, said the state Medicaid program pays only $12 for the consultation of a specialist, while his normal charge is $25.

The union movement among doctors has managed to cross political and ideological lines. While membership in unions in Massachusetts, Florida and Texas might be considered to be conservative in political viewpoint, those in northern California and Las Vegas are not.

"We want to identify with the working man, to show him that we have much the same problems that he does and want to solve them the same way—through collective bargaining," said Dr. Louis L. Friedman, an organizer of the Las Vegas group.

The group, known officially as the Nevada Physicians Employes International Union, A.F.L.-C.I.O., has attracted 50 members since receiving a charter two months ago.

The local president, Dr. John L. Holmes, said the aim of the affiliation with a major labor organization, the nation's first, was "that it's the best way to make our weight felt."

"Some form of national health insurance will eventually be passed by Congress, and there has to be some group to influence the outcome of the legislation," he added. "We think a better program will result if doctors work within organized labor to offer the expertise needed."

June 18, 1972

Quaint Old Medical Practice: The House Call

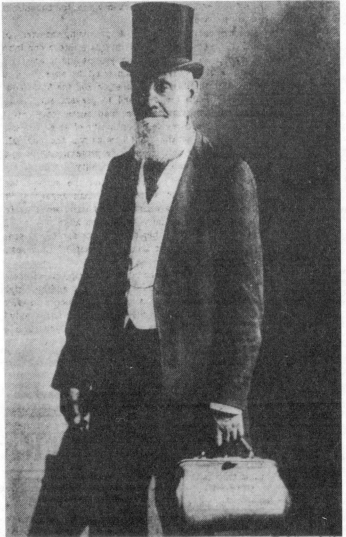

The Bettmann Archive

By William J. Welch

"Sorry, the doctor does not make house calls."

This announcement, made with cool finality to patients by a harried office nurse or by the awesome presence himself, continues to stun many doctors who have for years accepted visits to the ailing as part of their job.

To their further astonishment they discover that such a pronouncement is even considered by some patients to confer a desirable aura of splendid preoccupation on their healer, however numbed they may be when their hour of need strikes.

The time-honored expression, "send for the doctor," is no longer in fashion, but its equivalent is still a part of more doctors' lives than is remarked. In principle there are two valid reasons for making a house call: One is that the patient needs the doctor; the other—of equal weight and consequence—is that he believes he needs the doctor. Those are the two reasons for caring for the sick, in any event, at home, in the office, or at the hospital.

It is widely contended today that the house call is outmoded, that contemporary, instrumental medicine can only be instituted in a setting that corresponds to modern technology, and, if a patient really needs a doctor, he is far better served by being transported to the doctor's office or directly by ambulance to the hospital for diagnosis and treatment. This indeed is sometimes true, but by no means always.

Even a doctor who is a wizard cannot always be sure, from the message he receives, how sick the patient is. He only knows that there is trouble at the other end of the phone, a human being in distress. If it is not crystal-clear that the difficulty can be resolved or deferred—both from the human as well as the economic consideration—it can best be settled by a house call.

Even if the problem is one that requires hospitalization, much can often be done to make transportation safer and more comfortable and perhaps ward off catastrophe that might, if untended, occur en route. And even if

it turns out that only reassurance, with or without treatment, is necessary, have we become so inhuman and mechanized that we put this down as superfluous?

I have been called out of bed in the middle of the night to see an anxious patient in a panic whose painful "tumor" of chest wall turned out to be nothing but a quite normal, slightly tender, knob at the tip of the breastbone. And at 4 in the morning, I have found myself at the bedside of a frightened, breathless widow who was more under the influence of her recollections of her late husband's heart attack than in respiratory distress. But I have also treated an acute heart attack in one who might never have survived till the ambulance arrived had it not been for the emergency treatment I gave him.

The discovery of a pelvic fracture might have been dangerously delayed had I not gone to see an unsteady and irritable old alcoholic and found the tell-tale hemorrhage creeping under the skin of his inner thigh.

And there are lots of patients who are only half-well, and are going to continue indefinitely half-well, who nonetheless ought to be seen, if for nothing else than to be cheered by the presence of a doctor who is interested and cares. I am not unaware that a new generation of doctors is being trained in quite another mode by hospital-based instructors who themselves know little of the day-to-day necessity of other than the catastrophically ill.

The chief resident of a well-known teaching hospital called me the other day to say that a patient of mine who had been hospitalized for several weeks with chronic and resistant heart failure was no longer of interest to the students. They had learned all they could following his management, he said, and perhaps I could arrange to transfer the patient out of the hospital for chronic care elsewhere.

Quite apart from the fact that the patient still required hospital care, my question was, "What do you mean that they have learned all they can learn? What will they do when they are in practice and responsible for the care of such dull but resistant problems? Who will know how to care for them when those of us who are doing it now are dead and gone?"

But my question fell on deaf ears. The burning question among medical students and doctors in training today is diagnosis, and once it is made they lose interest and turn to new calamities. The real care of the sick is not part of their world, however much the sick are with us and will remain the concern of physicians.

Dr. William J. Welch, author of "What Happened In Between — A Doctor's Story," specializes in cardiology.

December 2, 1972

Self-Reform in Medical Education

By JOHN A. D. COOPER

Students entering today's medical schools are likely to find a great fement within the institutions. The medical schools are responding to society's rising expectations for better health, and the pace of change is accelerating rapidly.

Medical students are changing as well. Chances have doubled in the last four years that the entering student will be a woman. One in 10 represents a racial or ethnic minority and the percentage is rising fast. Although most entering students are from 21 to 23 years old, substantial numbers are in their late teens or early thirties.

With the competition for a medical education getting tougher, about 4 per cent of the students already have advanced degrees and many others have accumulated graduate credits. More students come from the more populous states, with New York and California supplying over 20 per cent of the applicants.

To accommodate these students and to serve the national and local communities better, the medical schools are demonstrating a remarkable ability to expand their programs and to undertake a process of self-renewal.

Traditionally, public demands for better health have brought Federal action, beginning with grants for hospital construction after World War II. Support of medical research through the National Institutes of Health followed. A Federal effort to produce more physicians began in 1963, by gradually expanding the educational capacity of medical schools. Institutional support of the schools began in 1965. That same year, the Government began partial payment for the health needs of citizens other than military veterans.

Yet the most basic problem, that of improving the quality of health care available to all Americans, has yet to be solved. It is the source of considerable controversy, involving plans for national health insurance, support of new health personnel and technology, and establishment of new systems of health care delivery.

In responding to the social need, the medical schools are reforming themselves. The greatest single change is to make the curriculums more flexible, to enable students to pursue a variety of career pathways earlier in their training.

Sixteen of the nation's 114 medical schools have abandoned the standard four-year curriculum for a new three-year program. Twenty-four other schools offer their students a three-year option. In 60 medical schools the final academic year is reserved entirely for electives, allowing students to focus their career interests before getting their degree. Fifteen schools essentially let their students take the fourth year as an internship, so that when they receive their M.D. degree, they can move directly into a residency. The internship is no longer required by any of the 22 specialty boards, although other clinical experience still is necessary.

Just what this means to students can be seen by comparing the standard curriculum of several years ago with the course of study followed in today's medical schools.

Traditionally, the medical student has spent the first two of his four years in basic science. His first year was divided between anatomy — from 600 to 700 hours of it — and biochemistry and physiology. The second year was spent between pathology, including autopsy, and microbiology and pharmacology. During these two years there was little unstructured time and little contact with patients.

In many of today's medical schools the first year is all basic science, with emphasis on cell biology and organ systems and the beginning of clinical work. The second year is required clinical experience, with students going to the wards and bedsides. Some students spend their full time studying patients.

In the traditional curriculum, the third year was mostly lectures and demonstrations with patients. But, again, students did not have much direct contact with patients. Students finally got some clinical experience in the fourth year, but they had little real responsibility for patients as they rotated through the major specialties. Such responsibilities came later, during the internship.

By contrast, the third and fourth years in many medical schools today are elected basic science or clinical activity, and the order can be interchanged. There may be no fourth year of formal schooling.

Team education is one of the innovations now catching the attention of medical schools. Since physicians will ultimately find themselves as heads of health care teams that include specially trained nurses, physician assistants and allied health professionals, medical students are working with trainees in these professions as part of their education.

Of most importance to the immediate communities they serve, schools are using facilities outside the academic health centers to teach their students. Now, students and residents may receive part of their training in rural health clinics, special out-patient clinics, community hospitals and in practicing physicians' offices.

There is a widespread belief that the supply of physicians in the United States is inadequate. This view is held in spite of our high ranking among all nations in the ratio of physicians to population.

Some of the apparent shortage can be attributed to the geographic and specialty maldistribution of physicians, and some of the needs can be met by other health personnel. Nonetheless, the medical schools have embarked on a program to educate more physicians, both by increasing the number of schools and by increasing the enrollment in established schools.

Currently, 114 United States medical schools are accepting applications. Of this total, 94 are degree-granting schools already producing M.D.'s. Another six are two-year medical schools whose students transfer to complete the degree. Fourteen other schools are in development and have not yet reached full status.

Ten years ago there were only 87 medical schools. The additional 27 have been established despite the lack of adequate financial support for construction costs and operating budgets.

The number of medical students is increasing faster. Total enrollment for the current year is 47,259. This is 3,609 more than in the previous year, an increase of 8.3 per cent. For the 1972-73 academic year, 13,570 first-year students were enrolled, 1,209 more than the previous year's freshman class, and 4,928 more than 10 years ago.

Despite these increases in both the number of schools and enrollment, applications are rising even faster. Less than 37 per cent of the individuals applying for the current year were accepted; approximately 24,000 had to be turned away. Many of those have gone to foreign medical schools, particularly in Mexico and Italy.

Just as new Federal laws and community pressures have hastened reforms in medical education, so are they changing the kind of careers today's medical students will pursue. The trend is away from the solo practitioner and toward group practice, which has been found acceptable to both patients and physicians. This approach can eventually provide one-stop medical care.

And along with this trend goes greater public acceptance of preventive health care, provided by health maintenance organizations and health service centers. We may well find that once the general public participates in such comprehensive programs the need for physicians will decline. A new division of labor among health personnel — physician assistants, nurse practitioners, behavioral scientists and family counselors— should improve health care for all patients.

January 8, 1973

Nation's Doctors Move To Police Medical Care

By NANCY HICKS

Special to The New York Times

STOCKTON, Calif. — American doctors are quietly but quickly developing a new nationwide system to police the quality and cost of the medical care they dispense.

Pushed by demands from Congress and the public for more economical use of the billions of tax dollars spent on health services, doctors throughout the country will eventually be engaging in the type of performance analysis that was started here in the northern California county of San Joaquin almost 20 years ago.

In medicine, such analysis of a doctor's work by other doctors is called peer review. Although the idea has been catching on of its own accord and is already actively practiced in dozens of locations, a new Federal law that goes into effect next Jan. 1 has put doctors on notice that they must systematically regulate themselves or face Federal regulations within two years.

"It doesn't quite have the ring of certainty now accorded death and taxes—not yet. But peer review as now mandated by Federal law is fast becoming inevitable," writes Dr. Leonard Rubin, coordinator of medical education for the Oakland-based Kaiser-Permanente Plan, which covers 1.5 million people.

The Kaiser plan has its own form of peer review, as do the Foundation for Health Care Evaluation in Minnesota, the San Joaquin Foundation for Medical Care here, and a network of federally funded experiments — widely differing organizations whose common experience is often called on to show that the peer review concept is workable.

Yet at the center of each of these diverse systems is the belief that more control must be placed on the physician, whether he is a solo practitioner, a member of a private group, or on the staff of a clinic or hospital. And this is another irritant to American doctors, many of whom are already unhappy about increasing "bureaucratic restrictions" imposed on them by publicly sponsored health programs such as Medicaid and Medicare.

Nonetheless, peer review is supported by the American Medical Association, the National Medical Association, which represents the nation's black physicians, and by many medical societies. And the new Federal legislation has made the idea something that doctors will have to deal with whether they want to or not.

The statute, a last-minute change in the massive package of Social Security amendments passed a year ago, requires that all medical cases paid for by Medicaid or Medicare — the Federal programs for the indigent and elderly, respectively —be reviewed for "appropriateness". The review is to be performed by self-designated local doctor groups that will be called Professional Standards Review Organizations, or P.S.R.O.'s.

The legislation, sponsored by Senator Wallace F. Bennett, Republican of Utah, is supposed to see that the money spent for Medicaid and Medicare — programs that accounted for $16.4-billion or about 20 per cent of the total $83.4-billion of national health expenditures for the fiscal year 1972— buys medical care of the highest quality and the lowest cost. And while the statute is

limited specifically to Medicaid and Medicare, it is seen by doctors and politicians alike as the possible framework for any future medical review system enacted as part of a national health insurance program.

Peer review is highly political.

Although the peer review organizations are supposed to be small and local, 19 states each have fewer than 3,000 doctors, making them eligible to have one state-wide P.S.R.O. under an administrative regulation passed by a special advisory peer review council to the Secretary of Health, Education and Welfare.

But because some state medical societies fear that local peer review will weaken the strength of the state organizations, Senator Lloyd M. Bentsen, Democrat of Texas, introduced a technical amendment to the peer review law that would possibly allow any state to form one state-wide Professional Standards Review Organization. That amendment has been approved by the Senate Finance Committee.

The purposes of peer review are often conflicting.

One goal of the law is for doctors who control such things as laboratory tests, hospital admissions and length of hospital stay to become just as mindful of cost as a housewife in the supermarket.

This concept of conserving basic medical resources, very much a part of medical care in developing countries such as China, is hard for American medicine to accept, given the country's high degree of medical technology.

Some practicing physicians find it absurd, for instance, to spend more than $50,000 on one kidney transplant case and then skimp on giving a blood test routinely to another patient. Yet it has been shown that unnecessary routine medical procedures push up the cost of medical care.

"Vitamin B-12 and estrogen shots alone pay the doctor's rent and put his kids through college," said Dr. George J. Williams, one of the pioneers in the San Joaquin Foundation for Medical Care.

Dr. Williams, a general practitioner in Lodi, about 10 miles from Stockton, said that the foundation's scrutiny of the need for such injections had reduced them significantly. Such injections make up only about 2 per cent of physicians' income in San Joaquin rather than the 30 per cent common in some places, Dr. Williams said.

The second goal—quality care—is more subtle, less easily defined, more difficult to achieve.

While American medical education prides itself on its heavy

scientific base, the actual practice of medicine consists of about one-third science and two-thirds "art," according to Dr. John A. Cooper, president of the Washington-based Association of American Medical Colleges. And the science is ever-changing.

Physicians are, after all, human. They make mistakes. They have differences of opinion. Their performance does not always reflect their knowledge.

The peer review system of the Kaiser-Permanente Plan of Northern California, for instance, found "significant problems" in one of every eight clinic charts it looked over and in 95 per cent of the hospital records it reviewed, according to Dr. Rubin of the Kaiser Plan.

And last year, after the United Store Workers Union in New York City, which administers its own health insurance plan, had begun requiring that members have a second doctor review each recommendation for surgery, 19 per cent fewer operations were performed than were initially recommended.

Whether this reduction of services represents quality care is still a matter of debate in the medical field. More controversial is whether cost and quality control can be reconciled in one review system.

"Many physicians doubt whether P.S.R.O.'s can obtain the two stated goals, for in many ways they are incompatible," Dr. Claude E. Welch, a nationally prominent Boston surgeon, wrote in an article in The New England Journal of Medicine.

Still, some experts feel that quality care with strong peer review will, in fact, increase health care costs.

In any case, such professional organizations as the Joint Commission on the Accreditation of Hospitals and the American Hospital Association are not counting on the review organizations to insure quality medical care. Both organizations have developed a so-called "medical audit" system for hospitals to measure their care in such terms as the rate of postoperative complications — infections, for instance — rather than the number of days a patient stays in the institution.

From the consumer's standpoint peer review may upgrade the quality of health care, but it will not provide evidence to support malpractice suits. "Malpractice suits will still be the external quality control for individual patients," said Charles M. Jacobs, a lawyer who is assistant director of the Joint Commission on Accreditation of Hospitals.

From a philosophical point of

view, some experts feel that peer reviewing will take the country one step closer to Government regulation of health services, and they wonder if direct regulation is the best route for American medicine to take.

"The Government, step by step, is being dragged into the regulation of health care and is doing so with no set policy, and P.S.R.O. is just the latest step," said Dr. Walter McClure, an astrophysicist who is also a health care specialist at Interstudy, the Minneapolis "think tank" that originated the Health Maintenance Organization scheme at the center of President Nixon's 1971 health message.

"The Government," he went on, "is drifting with just one goal in mind—cost control. But you just can't go about controlling costs. It's like trying to cure a symptom without having a diagnosis."

And politically, peer review is highly controversial.

Dr. William I. Bauer, who resigned as the first head of the P.S.R.O. office in the Department of Health, Education and Welfare, charged that the Administration had not come forth with the promised $34-million to enact the new legislation. He has been replaced by Dr. Henry E. Simmons, formerly of the Food and Drug Administration.

Some state medical societies —those in Texas and Louisiana for instance—are actively opposing the legislation, and one association of private practitioners, the Chicago-based Society of Physicians and Surgeons, has filed suit against it on the ground that it is unconstitutional.

Individual doctors, too, have protested. One Beverly Hills physician expressed his sentiments in a terse letter to Senator Bennett. "I oppose peer review. I have no peer," the doctor wrote.

Yet because of consumerism, which has brought about a general distrust of professionals, as well as the cost factors in health care, peer review is now appropriate, according to most professional medical organizations.

"Within the physician community, some still argue about whether the physician shall be accountable for his performance," said Dr. Richard E. YaDeau, a surgeon who is chairman of the board of the Minneapolis-based Foundation for Health Care Evaluation.

"As we physicians continue to debate this, the rest of the world has long since assumed that physicians are accountable—an assumption virtually unanimous throughout the non-physician community," he continued. "Actually, the issue is no longer accountability, but: by what standards shall physicians be measured and who will be their architect?"

The question of who will do the reviewing has been settled; the doctors will do it. But the question of how it will be done remains unanswered.

Most existing peer review systems are in individual hospitals—in the form of utilization review committees that check admissions to make certain they are medically justified or tissue committees that examine human tissue removed during surgery to see whether the operations were justified.

It is because these hospital-based systems have not worked in the past, politicians and physicians agree, that a new national system is being assembled. But many ask whether a new national system superimposed on the existing one will do a more responsive job. Theoretically, the national system could take over the hospital-based ones and monitor them, but the mechanism for doing this has not been worked out.

"We're moving into a totally uncharted area," Dr. Charles Edwards, Under Secretary for Health of H.E.W., conceded in an interview. "Neither the Congress nor I know where we're going or what we can achieve. We'd like to upgrade the level of health care in the country. But the question is, how do you do that?"

By Jan. 1, the country will be divided up geographically into P.S.R.O. areas in which at least 300 physicians practice.

Once this is done, local groups of doctors—not the medical societies—will petition the Department of Health, Education and Welfare to become the local reviewing agency, the P.S.R.O. This group of doctors will set standards for care for its geographic location and will check to make certain that variations from that norm are medically justified.

Physicians who are found to be chronic offenders against the locally set norms will be subject to several sanctions: They can be denied payment of claims; they can be declared ineligible to participate in the Medicaid and Medicare programs; they can be fined up to $5,000; they can have their questionable professional behavior made public. Fees will not be regulated, however.

If the system does not work to the Government's satisfaction by 1976, doctors will lose control of the program.

The peer review law is based on several models, some financed by the Federal Government. The oldest and best known, however, is the San Joaquin Foundation for Medical Care based here in Stockton.

The foundation was set up in 1954 by Dr. Donald C. Harrington, an obstetrician-gynecologist who is still its head.

As Dr. Harrington recalls, "I was going along happily practicing medicine when my brother, who was president of the boilermakers union, called to tell me that the union was negotiating with the prepaid Kaiser-Permanente Plan for care."

Kaiser employs its own physicians, and their patients pay one monthly fee for all their health needs.

Dr. Harrington's brother said that his union members were satisfied with the care they were getting from Stockton doctors, but that this new Kaiser plan was economically more attractive.

To combat this competition, Dr. Harrington set up an association of local physicians separate from the medical society. For the dues they paid, they agreed to work for a set fee for most procedures, and in some cases would also offer prepaid services to groups of subscribers.

They named their organization the San Joaquin Foundation for Medical Care. The term foundation was chosen because Kaiser was sponsored by a foundation and, Dr. Harrington said, he wanted the concepts to be parallel in peoples' minds.

Today, there are 76 medical care foundations across the country. About half of them review claims. The other half also provide medical services.

For the San Joaquin Foundation, peer review came as an afterthought.

"We set up a comprehensive program with a reasonable fee schedule for doctors. But without review, it was like writing a blank check," Dr. Harrington said.

The foundation then realized that it could not do peer review unless outpatient insurance coverage was good enough to keep doctors from hospitalizing patients to treat them. Hospital care is expensive—running to almost $200 a day in some metropolitan New York hospitals—but it is covered by health insurance. Most health insurance policies do not cover the same procedures performed in a clinic or doctor's office at a fraction of the hospital cost.

The foundation, therefore, now sets a minimum standard of insurance that can be sold in San Joaquin and the four other counties under its jurisdiction: Alameda, Amador, Calavaras and Tuolumne.

It has virtually total control of health services in the area. Ninety-seven per cent of the 330 practicing physicians in the area are members, Dr. Harrington said. Membership means the doctors are willing to accept as payment in full fee sched-

ules, set by the foundation, averaging about $8 for each 10 minutes spent with a patient. Reviewers scrutinize the number of visits, based on diagnosis, time spent with the patient, lab work and injections. About 8 per cent of all claims reach the review committee.

In addition to providing care on a prepaid basis for 47,000 MediCal (California's Medicaid program) and 37,000 Medicare patients, the foundation reviews claims for the 130,000 subscribers to other insurance programs. This means that two-thirds of the population in the area is covered in some way by the foundation, according to Boyd Thompson, executive director of this foundation and of the American Association of Foundations for Medical Care.

"We have total control of health services for the area because we control the flow of dollars," Dr. Harrington said. "We write the checks, not the insurance companies."

The foundation can and does impose strict sanctions for physicians of questionable performance. It can reduce the physician's fee, and he is not allowed to bill the patient for the extra amount.

In a few cases, doctors thought to be doing unnecessary surgery were required to have their diagnoses confirmed by other physicians before the operation could be performed. The 11 hospitals in the area know that when the foundation imposes these rules, and the hospital does not comply, the institution is not paid for the time the patient stays in the hospital.

The principle behind peer review here is the same as in any group pressure situation—the same one, for instance, that has almost every 13-year-old wearing equally faded jeans with a regulation cuff.

"There are maybe a handful of marginal doctors and being a reviewer has made me work very hard at not being considered one of them," explained Dr. Bryant B. Williams, a pediatrician who is one of 30 physician review and one of Stockton's four black doctors.

In his case, he said, peer review has not decreased his income but increased it—by making MediCal payments competitive with those paid in the community at large. As a result of this factor, about 90 per cent of the doctors in the area will take patients from MediCal and Medicare—a much higher than normal percentage.

The model in San Joaquin works, Dr. Harrington said, because the community is small enough for doctors to know one another. It would not be transferable to Boston, Baltimore or New York, he admits.

Larger scaled, less controlling models exist in other places, such as the foundation in Minnesota in which Dr. YaDeau is involved.

Unlike the San Joaquin foundation, the Foundation for Health Care Evaluation does not dispense medical care. It reviews the most expensive insurance claims—the top 15 per cent—for local companies, an activity that began in Hennepin County in 1968 and is now performed statewide.

It reviews hospital admissions for 17 of the 35 hospitals in the seven-county area. And in the Bethesda Hospital in St. Paul, of which Dr. YaDeau is medical director, the foundation is studying the records of every patient treated in the hospital in the first quarter of the year.

About 90 per cent of the 2,000 doctors in the seven-county area belong to the foundation.

"They pay $10, and for that $10 they have their fees cut if they're too high," Dr. YaDeau said.

The activities of the foundation have been felt in the area. For instance, 58 per cent of those expensive claims reviewed by the foundation in 1972 were reduced, Dr. YaDeau said. For the first nine months of 1973, the fee reduction rate was 66 per cent.

A study of hospital bed utilization has resulted in a reduction in the average length of hospital stay from 8.7 days to 6.9 days at Bethesda Hospital. When the program was started, the average length of stay had dropped to 6.1 days, then came back up.

Altogether, utilization review at Bethesda Hospital in St. Paul has reduced the cost of care for each hospitalized patient. And, the hospital no longer has a waiting list for elective surgery and it has closed down about 80 of its 300 hospital beds, turning that space into doctors' offices.

But the paradox in this—one that makes peer review unpalatable to many doctors and hospital administrators—is that the hospital is beginning to lose money by economizing.

In 1971, the hospital took in $9-million in income and realized an operating surplus of $450,000, or 5 per cent. In 1972, the first full year of utilization review, the gross income was a little higher, but the operating surplus was only $4,000, four-tenths of 1 per cent—one hospital employe's salary. This year, the hospital may run a deficit.

The way this paradox is resolved will determine whether peer review proves the strength or the bane of future health care reform.

October 28, 1973

Faulty Distribution of Doctors Linked in Part to Federal Aid

By THEODORE SHABAD

Federal medical programs are indirectly fostering a widening gap between doctor-poor inland states and doctor-rich coastal states, according to a locational analysis of American urban health care just published.

The study, issued by the Association of American Geographers of Washington, finds that a regional discrepancy in physician numbers has steadily increased over the last decade and that a Midwest center such as Chicago, for example, has been losing ground rapidly to more glamorous communities on the East and West coasts.

The migration of doctors has been explained in the past by the cosmopolitan atmosphere and the more favorable climate of the coastal areas, but the study notes that a disproportionately heavy flow of Federal dollars to these areas further accentuates the maldistribution.

The causes underlying the geographical shift of physicians are analyzed in "Misused and Misplaced Hospitals and Doctors," a so-called resource paper of the association, which is a national organization of professional geographers. Its resource papers, concerned with geographic concepts and their contemporary social relevance, are designed to supplement textbooks in college courses.

The 96-page urban health study, prepared by Pierre de Vise of the University of Illinois at Chicago Circle, is an outgrowth of a long-term project, the Chicago Regional Hospital Study, started in 1966 to improve the supply and future planning of health-care facilities.

By taking the health system of the state of Illinois as a test case, the study views the changes in physician distribution from a midcontinental vantage point. It notes, for example, that Illinois is by far the leading physician-exporting state, with 310 medical school graduates leaving in 1970.

Most of these migrants moved to California, which is described as the principal importing state of medical school graduates— 509 arrivals in 1970 — and the residence of more Illinois-trained doctors than Illinois itself.

The study, which described the United States as the "only civilized nation to have its health system controlled by private doctors and hospitals," is generally critical of the American Medical Association and in favor of national health insurance. But it contends that the Medicare program for the aged and the Medicaid system for the indigent have contributed to disparities in the distribution of physicians throughout the nation.

According to Mr. de Vise, who has written widely on the social geography of Chicago, the play of the private market should theoretically prevent the uneven distribution of physicians, assuming reciprocal licensure and free movement among states.

If physicians were dependent on only private patients for their practice, in the author's view, doctors in cities with a surplus of physicians, such as New York, Boston, San Francisco and Los Angeles, could greatly increase their income by moving to communities with a lower physician-to-population ratio.

November 3, 1973

Women in Medicine: A Dramatic Rise

By EVAN JENKINS

In a movement that could alter both the teaching and practice of medicine, American women are entering the profession in dramatically increasing numbers.

In just thee years, the number of women enrolled in the country's medical schools has more than doubled from 3,894, or 9.6 per cent of total enrollment, to 7,824, or 15.4 per cent.

Moreover, the curve is clearly rising. The percentage of first-year women students in medical schools last fall had reached 19.7, up from 11.1 per cent three years ago and only 7.8 per cent a decade ago. Further increases are expected this fall.

The increase in women has of course produced more competition for places in medical schools and some resentment from male students who feel women are taking spots that men should have. At the same time, the total number of places available has been increasing and so has the number of men enrolled in medical school, although at a slower rate in recent years than women.

Medical women—and men — foresee a number of changes as a result of the feminine influx.

In medical schools, the beginning of the end of isolation for women is already changing patterns that they have long considered discriminatory, ranging from admissions interviews to lecture-hall humor to classroom and laboratory participation. The sharp rise in women students is producing pressure for more women teachers. Finally, some observers predict much greater flexibility in medical education to permit students of both sexes to manage study and family responsibilities simultaneously.

Possible effects on practice, medical people say, include more emphasis on doctors, working in groups rather than as individuals. Again, the point would be greater personal and professional flexibility prompted by pressures on women to devote more time to family needs. A frequently-voiced expectation is that more women will be able to find members of their own sex practicing obstetrics and gynecology. And finally, there is a common feeling that women, perhaps because of social conditioning, will make medicine in general a more compassionate enterprise.

"This is really a woman's profession," said Dr. Anne Lawrence, a professor and a member of the admissions committee at the University of Chicago's Pritzker School of Medicine:

"I wouldn't be surprised if, by 1980, 50 per cent of the graduating class are women," she added. "It is suited to women's personalities, the comforting and care of the miserable."

An End of Isolation

Dr. Lawrence was one of scores of students, doctors, teachers and administrators interviewed at medical schools across the country about the rise of women in the profession. Her view that women were especially suited to medicine was widely shared by both men and women, though by no means unanimously.

In any case, the data clearly point to an end of the virtual isolation that women seeking medical careers have faced since Elizabeth Blackwell broke the profession's sex barrier in the United States by graduating from Geneva Medical College in Syracuse in 1849.

The class that entered medical school at Harvard three years ago had 11 women among its 139 students, not quite 8 per cent. This fall there will be 55 women in a class of 165—exactly a third.

Almost a third of the class that entered Columbia's school of medicine last year —47 of 147—were women and Linda Rosenthal was one of them.

"I don't feel like part of a minority group at all— there are just too many of us," she said. "My father went to medical school 25 years ago, and he keeps telling me that most of the girls were "dogs" and kept to themselves most of the time.

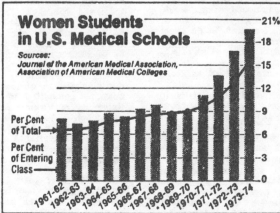

Women Students in U.S. Medical Schools

Sources: Journal of the American Medical Association, Association of American Medical Colleges

Per Cent of Total

Per Cent of Entering Class

1961-62 1962-63 1963-64 1964-65 1965-66 1966-67 1967-68 1968-69 1969-70 1970-71 1971-72 1972-73 1973-74

The New York Times/July 17, 1974

261

Things have changed comcompletely."

For some years, the percentage of women applicants accepted by medical schools has been at least equal to the percentage of men (although women have complained—and still do—that they must be extra good to make it).

What is happening now is that women are applying in greatly increased numbers, and there are two main reasons for that. One is the impact of the feminist movement.

It has changed the view, at least among women, of what is "woman's work," more women are going into law and engineering, as well as medicine. The movement has also produced direct pressure on medical schools to accept more women.

In addition, the existence of a series of antidiscrimination laws and regulations has had an appreciable effect, even though they have been enforced slowly and erratically.

There are no current data on dropouts among women medical students. A study covering the years 1948 to 1959 showed attrition for women to be 15 per cent and for men 8 per cent. More than half the women who dropped out during this period did so for nonacademic reasons; this was true for less than 40 per cent of the males.

Demand Some Changes

Medical women say they think — but can't prove — that the dropout rates may be more nearly equal these days because the pressures women faced when they were a tiny minority in medical schools are more easily handled now that they are a sizeable minority.

As their numbers increase, women in medicine are demanding an end to a lot of traditions they consider subtly or blatantly discriminatory.

A medical - school lecturer at Detroit's Wayne State University last year sought to break the ice with his students, most of them male, with this little joke:

Question: Which word doesn't belong—egg, sex, woman, rug. Answer — Sex doesn't belong, because you can beat an egg, a rug and a woman, but you can't beat sex.

It was pretty mild by comparison with some of the locker-room jibes at women that spring readily from study of the human body, but it wasn't likely to reinforce notions of women's equality. But the jokes may be changing soon, along with such practices as addressing classes as "gentlemen" and including nude girlie pictures among lecture slides, and pinup pictures in textbooks.

Beyond humor that they find insulting, medical women are attempting to combat such substantive matters as these:

¶Incidents like one that occurred not long ago at the University of Michigan, in which a woman medical student said she was not allowed to observe the complete physical examination of a male patient because his genitals would be exposed. Nearby, her medical-student husband was conducting a pelvic examination of a woman.

¶The admissions interview in which a woman, but almost never a man, is asked how a doctor can manage a career along with marriage and a family.

¶The low numbers of women on medical school faculties and admissions committies where their representation lags far behind the increase in women as students.

¶The common belief, challenged by statistics, that women, once licensed, cannot be counted on to practice medicine.

¶The virtual bar to women in some medical specialties, notably surgery.

Dr. Chandler Stetson, dean of the University of Florida College of Medicine was one who shared the view that women's capacity for "compassion" would benefit medicine. Of surgery, he declared:

"Women in general don't tend to go into surgery. They can't stand up to the operations with the blood and saws and all. It doesn't really appeal to most of them."

More Women Surgeons?

Said Dr. Nina Woodside, a faculty member at the Medical College of Pennsylvania (formerly a women's school) and head of a year-old research and reform organization called the Center for Women in Medicine:

"I guess if all the barriers were removed, women would enter surgery as often as men. Women who do select surgery do very well. But patients tend to think of surgeons as men. And surgeons certainly think of surgeons as men."

Dr. Woodside estimated in a recent interview that fewer than 10 per cent of the nation's more than 360,000 doctors were women. (The most recent date, for 1972, put the figure at 8.7 per cent.)

She and other women in medicine like to point to a study done several years ago that showed only Spain, South Vietnam and Madagascar, among 38 countries surveyed, with lower percentages of women doctors than the United States.

Given the sheer mathematics, Dr. Woodside said, it will be a long time before the sex that makes up half the population even approaches that share of the medical profession.

"But it's very clear," Dr. Woodside added, "that the idea that women don't want to become doctors just isn't true."

True or not, the idea is pervasive. It is reflected in the title of a study of women in medical schools published privately last fall and available now from the Feminist Press in Old Westbury, L. I. The title is "Why Would a Girl Go Into Medicine?" It was a question, a woman student interviewed for the survey said, that she was asked constantly.

The report's author is "Margaret A. Campbell, M.D.," reportedly a pseudonym for a woman doctor who felt that a survey alleging male bias would do nothing to help her own medical career. The question "Why would a girl?" arises in a chapter on "stereotyping."

And indeed interviews done for The New York Times at 14 medical schools suggest that stereotyping — by society, by medical school administrators and teachers, and perhaps by medical women themselves—is the norm, though perhaps an eroding one.

Calls Replies Distorted

Of the standard admissions-interview question about marriage vs. career, a woman faculty member who asked not to be identified declared:

"I seriously object to this being the issue on which women are denied access to medical school, and I know it is. Some men [interviewers] use the woman's answer either way. If she says she doesn't want children or is going to have someone take care of them, the man says, 'This is perverted, she should be home with her kids.' If she says she's going to have children, he says she's not committed to medicine."

Said Dr. William R. Sandusky, chairman of the admissions committee of the University of Virginia Medical School, "We want to know if the applicant has developed a realistic view of women in medicine. Traditionally the lady stays home to raise children."

That kind of remark incenses feminists, because it assumes that a man cannot be expected to share equally in the child-rearing and household tasks. The assumption is widely shared, and for the women professionals who share it, life can be a kind of hell. But the view is far from universal.

Still, to cope with the familiar role they are expected —and often expect themselves—to fulfill outside their careers, women in medicine have tended to enter such specialties as pediatrics, anesthesiology, and psychiatry, which offer at least the prospect of regular hours.

There is some evidence of change in that pattern — in particular, an apparent surge of interest in obstetrics and gynecology—and at the same time a hint of a kind of reverse discrimination.

"There is some social pressure from women's libbers on us not to go into pediatrics because it's sort of the 'Uncle Tom' of medicine," said Linda Rosenthal at Columbia. "But if I decide later that pediatrics is what I want, I'll do it. I'm not going to be pressured out of it."

From the view about where the "lady" stays arises the belief that women, even when they become physicians, often don't practice.

Studies cited by the pseudonymous Dr. Campbell show that women doctors practice, on average, 45 hours a week, men 50; women "drop out" of practice on average for a total of 4.8 years, men for 2.1, and women in the United States live an average of seven years longer than men, and "thus have a longer practice potential."

Although some medical women question whether women as doctors function in any way differently from men, there is a widespread feeling among both sexes that the rising feminine role will change the profession.

Balancing Roles

One common expectation is greater flexibility in both training and practice — an increase in part-time scheduling of classes and group practice arrangements that permit women, and men, to balance more easily their professional and family roles.

A lot of women think they are better suited than men to treat women patients. Patsy Parker, in her second year at Boston University's medical school, said she was considering obstetrics and gynecology because "I will treat women in a special way and hope to give them an understanding view of their bodies and the problems they may run across."

"I think we need women in ob-gyn badly," said Judy Cook who was completing her senior year at Michigan State University's College of Human Medicine. "I was pretty appalled at the attitudes of most of the doctors toward their patients. A lot of them are just not aware of the woman patient as a woman; they're so involved in her uterus."

Above all, in interview after interview, there emerged the feeling that women doctors may be more sensitive than men.

"In general, some of the

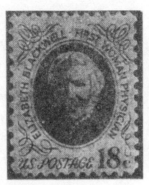

Elizabeth Blackwell, memorialized in a current stamp, broke medical profession's sex barrier in 1849. Today there are 7,824 women in medical schools.

attributes women bring to medicine are much more desirable," said Dr. Miles Hench, associate dean for admissions at the Medical College of Virginia in Richmond.

"The role-model given to women in childhood is the expectation that they be more open and feeling. This can be a positive factor in medicine. The masculine characteristic of aggressiveness can be a hindrance. But neither is absolute."

July 17, 1974

Pact Ends Doctor Strike; Staffs Return to Hospitals

By PETER KIHSS

The country's first major physicians' strike ended here last night, with an agreement to limit hours that sent internes and residents back to their regular duties at 21 hospitals. It was the fourth day of a walkout called by the young doctors in an effort to shorten drawn-out work schedules.

Leaders of the striking Committee of Internes and Residents met for nearly six hours in a caucus at the Commodore Hotel before accepting, at 6 P.M., a proposal by the League of Voluntary Hospitals.

"We are quite anxious to get back to our patients and will make every effort to get back to the hospitals forthwith," Dr. Richard A. Knutson, the president of the Committee of Internes and Residents, told newsmen shortly after the settlement was announced.

Dr. Jay Dobkin, the weary chairman of the committee's negotiating panel, who said he had been up for four nights, smiled and said, "I'm going to work as scheduled — tomorrow morning." Dr. Dobkin, who wore his white hospital trousers, is a member of the house staff at Montefiore Hospital.

The agreement, the first ever reached by hospitals in collective bargaining here to limit working hours, provides that there should not generally be more than one night's duty in a three-day period.

It also provided for a committee in each hospital to work out schedules, which would consist of an equal number of members from the house staff and the hospital medical executive board, plus an extra physician member elected by the others.

In the last hours, the union sought one addition and one clarification. The addition would have been to guarantee that no doctor would end up with longer hours under the new formula; the league refused any change in language, according to Andrew Portelli, a past president, but other sources indicated at least some hospitals would offer private assurances against increased hours for anyone.

The "clarification," understood to have been agreed to orally, was that the hospital committee members would all be physicians.

Dr. Knutson and Dr. Dobkin communicated by telephone at the end with William J. Abelow, executive director of the league, who went to the Commodore to join them in announcing the settlement.

Asked about the final vote by the 35 members of the negotiating and strike committees, Dr. Dobkin said "it was accepted by acclamation—unanimously."

Mediators Helped

Aiding the protracted negotiations were Paul Yager, regional director of the Federal Mediation and Conciliation Service, and Samuel Hacker, of his office. They were joined Wednesday night by Gayle Wineriter, special assistant to the director of mediation services, from Washington.

"We believe," Mr. Yager said, "that the two negotiating committees deserve a great deal of credit for the efforts they made to resolve this very complex problem. I believe that these negotiations represent a victory for collective bargaining."

As soon as word of the agreement was received internes and residents started returning to work, though some hospitals, including Flower and Fifth Avenue and Montefiore in the Bronx, planned to retain their emergency provisions until this morning, when most house staff shifts begin.

Those returning last night spoke of the agreement as a victory and expressed pleasure at being back at work—a sentiment that was shared by the harried attending physicians who had found themselves working virtually around the clock to take up the slack during the strike.

"We ended up with very close to what we wanted," said Shelley Kolton, a third-year medical student at Mount Sinai Hospital, who performs essentially the same duties as a first-year interne and who had joined the strike.

"The house staff in this city demonstrated the support for the union and I think that's going to be one of the most important things for the future," said Miss Kolton, who returned to work at 7:30 P.M.

At 7 A.M. yesterday the league had broken off negotiations with the union after another all-night session and had released individual hospitals to bargain separately with their own physicians. The agreement was a restated offer made by the league at 3:30 A.M.

Fifteen voluntary hospitals and six affiliated municipal hospitals for which the voluntary institutions provide some staffs had been affected. The union had said that more than 2,100 of its members participated in the walkout.

The hospitals involved have 14,000 beds, a third of the city's total. They also normally care for 10,000 outpatients a day.

How Gap Was Filled

Senior attending physicians and medical faculty members —many of them considering that rigorous work schedules were part of a physician's needed training, others sympathetic to the younger men's desire for a less demanding regimen—stretched out their own hours to handle patient problems during the strike.

The State Health Department had stepped up its watch on patient care yesterday by sending out two teams of physicians

and nurses. Andrew Krieger, assistant director of the agency's Office for New York City Affairs, said late yesterday, "so far it appears that services are being maintained very well."

Despite the break-off in talks just after dawn, Dr. Dobkin said the league's offer of 3:30 A.M. was largely one he could have recommended to the membership. He deplored a 7 A.M. deadline that he contended made it impossible to rally more than the handful of union members on hand at that time.

Even though Mr. Abelow said the 3:30 A.M. offer was withdrawn, he had also observed that an over-all agreement might still be possible. "In labor relations," he said, "we never rule anything out."

The league's first over-all limit on hours provides that "no later than July 1, 1976, no house staff officer at any hospital shall be required to perform on-call duty more frequently than one night in three, except where so provided by a majority vote of the standing committee hereinafter provided for, which majority shall include at least two house staff officers."

By May 1, the agreement goes on, the standing committee is to be established at each hospital with equal numbers of union and hospital representatives as well as a physician from the hospital medical executive board to be elected by the other members.

The committee members are to formulate guidelines by Aug. 1 for "work schedules which shall be consistent with optimum patient care, high standards of training, specialty board requirements and limitations and the health and well-being of house staff officers, including their reasonable social needs and providing for adequate rest."

The guidelines are to be "implemented by the hospital promptly, subject to budgetary limitations and existing procedures for established budgets."

No interne or resident is to be "punished, penalized or in any manner discriminated against by reason of the strike." They are to be considered as having been on "unpaid leave time for all purposes," the league proposal added.

The union has asserted that many of its members—internes who are in the first year of on-the-job training after graduating from medical school and residents who spend up to six years thereafter preparing for specialities—have worked 100 and sometimes more hours a week.

The strike had evoked a surprise statement from the two top officers of the usually conservative American Medical Association that "in important respects, it is a strike for better patient care."

The Hospitals Affected

Internes and residents of University Hospital had voted against participating in the walkout. But yesterday four of the 450 who work there and at Bellevue Hospital, which is affiliated with University Hospital, stayed out and set-up a picket line that did not affect hospital work.

The other voluntary hospitals, which had varying walkouts were Bronx-Lebanon, Brookdale, Catholic Medical Center of Brooklyn and Queens (including Holy Family, Mary Immaculate, St. John's Queens and St. Mary's), Hospital for Joint Diseases, Jewish Hospital of Brooklyn, Long Island Jewish (at New Hyde Park, Hillside and South Shore), Maimonides, Montefiore, Mount Sinai and Flower-Fifth Avenue.

Municipal hospitals affected by reason of their affiliation with teaching hospitals were Elmhurst, Coney Island, Greenpoint, Metropolitan, Morrisania and Queens Hospital Center. The municipal Health and Hospitals Corporation had agreed to start arbitration on its contract with the union on the hours issue.

March 21, 1975

Coast Doctors End Strike, Agree on Malpractice Pact

By HENRY WEINSTEIN
Special to The New York Times

SACRAMENTO, Calif., May 28—Leaders of the State Legislature and several medical organizations announced today an end of the month-long walkout by California doctors protesting great increases in malpractice insurance rates.

The legislative leaders and medical organizations said the doctors would return to work next Monday, pending the immediate activation of a Joint Underwriters Association that would provide physicians with malpractice insurance at rates acceptable to them.

They also said the legislation accepted by the physicians was only a temporary rollback of malpractice rates to the levels existing last Dec. 31.

In New York, a representatives of the state medical society said that malpractice insurance premiums for doctors would go up by only 10 to 15 per cent under rates being developed by a new doctor-owned insurance company. But some physicians still planned to curtail treatment of patients to protest the state's new malpractice law. [Page 22.]

Donald Burns, California's Secretary of Business and Transportation, said that a hearing would be held Friday in San Francisco on malpractice rates in eight California counties whose doctors had previously been insured by the Arognaut Insurance Company of Menlo Park, Calif., a major insurer than canceled its group policy for anesthesiologist on May 1.

Wesley Kinder, the state's insurance commissioner, is expected to determine at the hearing that in these areas insurance is not available at reasonable rates—defined as rates existing on Dec. 31, 1974. Then, he is expected to activate the Joint Underwriters agreement created by a new law signed by Gov. Edmund G. Brown Jr., last week.

Only a Stopgap

Leo McCarthy, speaker of the 1,700-member Society of Anesthesiologists, and the Governor stressed that the bill was a stopgap that would roll back insurance rates only until January.

A "final cure," said Mr. Brown through his press secretary, Bill Stall, "can only come through fundamental reform as set forth" in a special legislative session agenda the Governor's staff presented in mid-May, two weeks after the doctors' walkout began.

There are 14 bills now pending in the state Legislature on the malpractice question. These include measures that would limit lawyers' contingency fees; another calling for a board that would arbitrate claims and throw out frivolous ones; another requiring re-examination of surgeons convicted of malpractice, and another limiting malpractice suit awards to $300,000.

The settlement announced today was called a "good faith" gesture by both the doctors and the legislators. The doctors noted, however, that they preferred a bill passed yesterday by the state Assembly to the "stopgap" one the Governor had signed.

Introduced by Assemblyman Robert McClennan, the Legislature's only physician, the measure passed yesterday would do the following:

¶Roll back malpractice insurance rates to not more than 50 per cent above what they were on Jan. 1, before insurance companies announced increases of up to 400 per cent on some malpractice premiums.

¶Set up "pools" of all liability insurance carriers to provide malpractice policies for the next seven months in areas where they are not available or are prohibitive because of their high cost for the next seven months.

¶Impose a $100 yearly assessment for the next five years on all licensed doctors to guarantee payment of malpractice awards.

¶Require insurance companies to disclose records that would enable the state to determine if malpractice rate increases are justified.

Both bills have been opposed by the insurance industry.

The physicians prefer the McClennan bill because the earlier measure confronts doctors with a large "balloon" payment in December for future malpractice claims. The McClennan bill provides for insurance that would be initially more expensive, noted a spokesman for McCarthy, but would be cheaper in the long run.

Mr. McCarthy said he hoped legislative solutions could be given to the Governor by June 27.

The doctors made it clear today that if long-range solutions were not enacted by the end of the year they would reassess their position.

The insurance companies have come under increasing scrutiny in the controversy. Legislation has moved through an Assembly committee that would direct the Legislature's Joint Legislative Audit Committee to investigate medical malpractice insurance carriers, including Argonaut, a subsidiary of Teledyne, Inc., a Los Angeles conglomerate.

May 29, 1975

A.M.A. Liberalizes to Draw Young Doctors

By SETH KING
Special to The New York Times

CHICAGO, May 30 — The American Medical Association, faced with declining membership and struggling to emerge from several years of growing financial deficits, is slowly moving to change its image of a conservative, often stodgy champion of the medical establishment.

Perhaps the most visible aspects of an altered attitude are its espousal of a form of national health insurance legislation and its willingness to cooperate with the Federal Government in setting up panels of physicians to review treatment of Medicare and Medicaid patients.

"The American Medical Association," Dr. James H. Sammons, its new executive vice president, said in an interview, "says the Government has a proper role to play in medicine and it is the association's duty to see that it is played responsibly."

The statement represents a radical departure by the world's largest and most powerful medical society from its once unswerving opposition to any form of Government involvement in medical practice.

The change in the official A.M.A. attitude means a 'definite liberalization" as well as recognition that the association must develop a greater appeal for younger doctors, said Dr. Sammons. As of May 9, the association had lost almost 5,000 members in a year—down from 144,356 to 139,718—an erosion that took place at a time of rapid growth in the number of doctors in the United States.

Trend May Reverse

But the trend may be reversing, and younger doctors may be seeing a welcome change in the A.M.A. The association now has more interns and residents as members than it did in 1974, Dr. Sammons said.

As it has shifted attitude in an attempt to attract more support among its constituency and to become a more effective force in the Government's expanding role in medical care, the A.M.A. has simultaneously sought to deal with its extensive financial problems.

While the organization's leaders prepared for the semiannual meeting of its policymaking House of Delegates in Atlantic City next month, the A.M.A. was emerging from what Dr. Sammons called "a year of financial and psychological trauma."

The association, which operates on a yearly budget of more than $35-million, has been fighting the rising cost of its medical-education and publishing programs.

Last winter, after five years of increasing deficits, it was so short of operating funds that it had to borrow $3-million to continue these programs.

Reduced Publications

It has been forced to reduce the scope of its publications to counter a 32 per cent rise in their costs.

Earlier this month, in another move to economize, the association dismissed 77 staff members, many of them veteran employes in executive level positions.

At the House of Delegates meeting last December, the delegates refused to approve a schedule of higher dues and agreed only to a temporary $60-assessment to meet the crisis. But even this met resistance, and by mid-winter barely a fourth of the dues-paying doctors had paid the assessment. By April 30, however, more than 68 per cent had chipped in.

Dr. Sammons's selection as executive vice president by the board of trustees was in itself divisive, pitting one faction of the A.M.A.'s hierarchy against another — although this was less an ideological split than a struggle for power within the association.

"But we're beyond the trauma now and we're on the upswing," said Dr. Sammons, a Texan who spent 22 years as a general practitioner before becoming chairman of the A.M.A. board of trustees a year ago and its chief executive officer in March.

The new A.M.A. outlook, besides representing a "liberalization," is also an acknowledgement that the practice of medicine is changing in the United States, that more physicians than ever are hired employes receiving their salaries directly from hospitals or health maintenance organizations.

Another recognition by the association of the changing role of doctors is its new Department of Negotiation.

"Because of the problems with malpractice insurance carriers, with all levels of government, with the emerging hospital-physician relationships, doctors are going to have to learn to negotiate with these groups," said Dr. Sammons.

The new department will soon begin offering courses in negotiating techniques to its member doctors at county and state medical association levels.

Suggestions that the A.M.A. was being forced to become, in effect, a trade union for its doctor members or to continue losing the younger ones were a result of the lack of representation for younger members in the association, Dr. Sammons said.

"We are now saying that there is nothing a union can do for a doctor that his professional organization cannot do if it is willing," he said.

Malpractice Program

As examples of the determination of the A.M.A.'s leadership to pursue a positive, activist role, Dr. Sammons cited the board of trustees' consideration of a secondary malpractice insurance program. This would provide backup liability insurance coverage for state medical associations that negotiated malpractice liability contracts with local insurance companies.

Dr. Sammons also pointed to the A.M.A.'s changing stand on national health insurance legislation now pending in Congress.

The A.M.A. once fought stubbornly against establishment of the Federal Government's Medicare and Medicaid programs. It took a pitched battle in its House of Delegates for the association to back a national health insurance plan of its own, called Medicredit.

This plan would provide voluntary health insurance financed through private medical insurance groups, with the participants reimbursed through Federal tax credits.

The legislation the A.M.A. is now backing would require employers to offer private insurance group plans, three-quarters of which would be paid by the employers. It would also require the Federal Government to reimburse small employers who would lose money on the plan and would provide Federal funds to cover health insurance for the unemployed.

The A.M.A. has also agreed to cooperate with the Department of Health, Education and Welfare in setting up professional standard review organizations. These would be panels of physicians that would review treatment of Medicare and Medicaid patients.

But the A.M.A. won a temporary injunction last Tuesday in Federal court to block establishment of utilization review committees. These would include laymen as well as physicians and would be required to decide, within 24 hours, whether a eMdicare or Medicaid patient should continue to be treated in a hospital.

Despite the changing attitudes of the A.M.A., its new leaders do not expect a serious ideological conflict at the House of Delegates meeting.

"We've already fought our battles over whether to support national health insurance and cooperate in professional standard review groups," an A.M.A. source said. "The changes have apparently been accepted."

"If there is an argument, it will be over the proposal to increase the dues."

May 31, 1975

Soaring Malpractice Rates Are Driving Up Medical Costs

By LAWRENCE K. ALTMAN

Soaring malpractice insurance rates for doctors and hospitals have sharply driven up costs of medical diagnosis and treatment for patients and, in the view of many health officials, are threatening the quality of health care given Americans.

The sudden imposition of such drastic rate increases and the withdrawal of some insurance carriers from the medical liability field in recent weeks have dramatically focused public attention on what medical observers regard as perhaps the most important problem affecting the doctor-patient relationship in the last decade, if not longer.

And the problem has begun to extend to other health professionals. Patients going to some osteopathic physicians,

dentists and podiatrists are also paying more, largely because, these professionals say, they themselves are being charged increasingly higher rates for their liability premiums. But the rises are less than for medical doctors.

Also, the unpredictable nature of rising malpractice costs has made it much more difficult to estimate future medical care costs, thereby reducing prospects for passage of national health insurance legislation, according to some experts.

Action Taken by States

The jump in malpractice insurance rates is widely attributed to the increase in the number of malpractice suits in recent years, accompanied by a steep rise in the size of damage awards.

So important has the mal-

practice problem become that thus far this year the legislatures of at least 27 states, acting on an emergency basis, have passed malpractice bills.

The substance of such legislation has varied widely among the states. In most instances, the legislation has been described as stopgap, designed to insure the availability of malpractice coverage for doctors and hospitals, or involving the establishment of commissions to study the malpractice problem.

But a few states, such as Michigan, New York, Indiana and Nevada, have overhauled the legal tort system. Though such laws have not gone far enough to satisfy many doctors, some of the legislation, as in Indiana, has led lawyers to propose court tests of its constitutionality.

Despite the drastic nature of some legislative action, medical and legal experts and officials of organizations affected by the malpractice crisis said in interviews that they had adopted a "wait-and-see" attitude toward the results. Even radical surgery, they said, just partly solves a problem that is rooted in common law's centuries of tradition.

No single solution exists in any state, these experts said, in part because of the difficulties in reversing the effects of what has become a major industry in some states—suing doctors and hospitals.

Statistics Lacking

Statistics regarding the number and nature of malpractice suits filed are not available, because courts and medical societies do not have a system for collecting such information. Further, the insurance industry has not made data on malpractice costs publicly available.

265

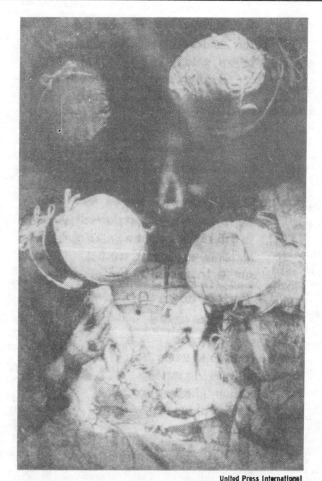

United Press International

Surgeons at work. Several U.S. doctors have stopped practicing because of the high insurance rates.

However, a few states have passed legislation requiring that basic facts about malpractice suits be reported to state officials.

In the latest development in the malpractice crisis, many hospitals have begun to raise room rates by as much as $12 a day. Later this year, other hospitals plan substantial increases in fees for X-rays, anesthesia and surgical services to help offset the costs of malpractice litigation.

In recent years, doctors have emphasized that the growing malpractice problem has led them to practice defensive medicine, that is, to order X-rays, blood and other diagnostic tests not for the patient's medical benefit but for the primary purpose of having an adequate medical-legal defense if the patient ever brought suit. In some instances, the tests represent more than an extra cost; doctors maintain that such tests pose a risk to the patient.

Now the impact of the malpractice problem is extending beyond the cost factor and defensive medicine to have a ripple effect by influencing the way Americans get medical care from their doctors.

South Dakota Problem Cited

In South Dakota, which has a number of towns without doctors, the malpractice problem has made it even more difficult for officials to attract younger physicians to serve in rural areas.

The St. Paul Fire and Marine Insurance Company, which covers most South Dakota doctors, has decided to issue new malpractice policies only to doctors who join established group practices already insured by the company.

According to the state medical society, St. Paul will not insure a new doctor who wishes to practice alone in the tradition of the old country general practitioner.

The move has made it extremely difficult for a young doctor to practice on his own. Of the 20 doctors who received licenses to practice medicine in South Dakota since mid-May, the medical society says, just one has gone into practice alone. Most such practitioners in South Dakota serve in rural areas. Their number has declined substantially in recent years.

Though malpractice has aroused doctors unlike almost any other issue in recent years,

strikes by doctors threatened this month in Hawaii and Pennsylvania have not occurred. One reason reflects the medical profession's concern about adverse publicity and the ethics of job actions that doctors in California, New York, Texas and elsewhere took earlier this year. Another reason is that doctors have agreed to judge the impact of new legislation before denying their services to more patients.

Malpractice costs are not the only reason for the rise in hospital room rates and doctors' office fees. But hospital officials predict that costs to patients can be expected to go even higher because malpractice premium bills will continue to rise.

The situation has become so bad in Alaska that may doctors there have chosen to practice without malpractice insurance because they cannot obtain coverage at what they regard as reasonable rates. Heart surgeons and other doctors have stopped practicing, forcing some Alaska patients to seek specialized care in the lower 48 states.

Elsewhere, a few doctors have retired prematurely or moved to areas where malpractice insurance rates are less costly.

To illustrate how costly malpractice insurance has become for hospitals: This year the 39 insurance companies still writing malpractice policies are charging the 5,865 non-Federal American hospitals $750-million, or $250-million more than a year ago, to protect their staffs from potential liability claims from the patients occupying their 870,000 beds.

The magnitude of the jump in malpractice rates for hospitals has varied among the states. Washington, D.C., institutions have been charged an average of 652 per cent more than last year while hospitals in Tennessee, Michigan, Iowa and Minnesota have averaged 600 per cent increases over the last year, according to the American Hospital Association in Chicago.

Yearly Cost Per Bed

According to the association's statistics, the cost to patients for malpractice hospital insurance averages $860 a bed a year. But Paul W. Earle, a hospital association vice president, said that the rates varied widely, with some hospitals paying less than $100 a bed a year.

Last week, an administrator testified in a Texas court that insurance at his Houston hospital had risen more than 20-fold, to $2,341 a bed from the $108-a-bed cost last July.

Less dramatic but still sub-

stantial premium rate increases charged the Michael Reese Hospital and Medical Center has forced that Chicago institution to announce an increase of $12 a day in room rates, to $144. Michael Reese's liability and malpractice insurance is costing $3-million this year compared with $500,000 last year. Officials have attributed the entire room rate increase to the rise in liability insurance.

Such drastic rate increases at hospitals with national reputations for quality medical care have startled some patients. But, according to Dr. Roger O. Egeberg, the Department of Health, Education and Welfare's top expert on the malpractice crisis, hospitals that tackle the toughest medical problems often have to pay the highest rates, Dr. Egeberg said in an interview:

"At a good hospital where you have experts in various fields and that possibly is affiliated with a medical school, rates are apt to be higher because doctors there treat patients in the worst condition.

"In a poor hospital when a patient turns sour and a consultant is called in, the patient might have to be transferred to the consultant's hospital because it has better facilities. If the outcome is not successful, the consultant might be included in the suit. Apparently, that's why a good hospital can have more trouble than a mediocre one."

Specialists Also Affected

The situation is similar for famous doctors such as heart surgeons whose operations demand considerable skill and pose significant risks to the patients with life-threatening diseases. Dr. Michael DeBakey, president of Baylor College of Medicine in Houston, a heart surgeon who has taught in the operating rooms of many foreign hospitals, said that he now paid $25,300 a year for the same malpractice coverage that cost $894 in 1969.

Less than two decades ago, malpractice insurance fees were so low that few hospitals considered it in figuring the cost of bed rates. Mr. Earle, the hospital association vice-president, declined to disclose specific malpractice costs per hospital bed over recent years.

However, James Ludlam, senior counsel to the California Hospital Association, said that the figures had risen from 10 cents a bed in 1953 to $4.50 now in that state. The sharpest rise came in 1970 at which time it began to jump about 40 per cent each year, Mr. Ludlam said.

But Mr. Ludlam cautioned that uniformity did not exist among hospitals in calculating the effect on bed costs of malpractice rates insurance. Some include coverage for doctors serving full-time on the hospital's staff; others do not. Some hospitals include outpatient costs; others do not. Depending on the circumstances, he said, the cost could be about $7 a day.

Medical malpractice has been considered less of a problem in rural areas than in big cities because of a reputed closer patient-doctor relationship. But even hospitals in rural areas have been hit by the soaring premium charges. A spokesman said that Blue Cross of Louisiana had received requests from several urban and rural hospitals for daily room rate increases of $7 to $12 primarily because of increased malpractice premiums.

But because of the lack of precise statistics on just who sues whom for what, it is not clear whether such rural hospitals are paying for the costs of litigation elsewhere or for problems arising within their own institutions.

Michigan Backs Arbitration

In Michigan, the Legislature passed 15 bills that among other things promote arbitration over the traditional jury system to settle malpractice cases.

Under the new Michigan law, hospitals and doctors offer a patient a voluntary arbitration form, which need not be signed as a prerequisite for care. But by signing, a patient agrees to submit to arbitration any potential malpractice dispute. The patient has 60 days after discharge from the hospital to cancel the agreement and to choose the jury trial system, under which it may take seven or more years for settlement.

By agreeing to the binding arbitration, the patient is expected to get speedier action at less cost to all parties concerned, once he institutes proceedings at the nearest office of the American Arbitration Association. A three-member board—a doctor, a lawyer and a qualified lay person—would arbitrate each malprac-

tice case. However, a court appeal would be heard by a judge, not a jury.

Michigan's experience is expected to be watched carefully because experts consider it a radical departure from traditional ways of handling malpractice.

"In the past, arbitration applied mainly to organized groups," said William Curran, an expert in legal medicine at the Harvard School of Public Health. He added, "What Michigan's law does is apply this same principle to individual patients."

2 Other Nations Contrasted

Many observers have pointed out that the United States seems to stand alone in suffering a medical malpractice crisis. England and Canada, which share the common law heritage with this country, reportedly are not seriously affected by rising malpractice insurance rates and litigation.

Officials of the American Medical Association, in pointing out that the quality of medical care is similar in these countries, have attributed the difference to the contingency fee system whereby American lawyers collect much larger percentages of settlements than is possible in Canada or England.

But others maintain that though the contingency fee is an important factor, cultural differences play an even greater role. As Mr. Ludlam, the California hospital lawyer, expressed it:

"We will always have more of a malpractice problem than other countries, even if we get national health insurance. Those other countries award practically nothing for pain and suffering whereas the United States has a tradition of compensating for these factors. The question is, how much?"

July 27, 1975

Unfit Doctors Create Worry in Profession

Revocations of Licenses, More Training Or Supervision Are Urged as Remedies

By BOYCE RENSBERGER

After long considering the incompetent or careless doctor as a rare aberration of minor consequence, the American medical profession is beginning to regard unfit physicians as a serious problem that may account for tens of thousands of needless injuries and deaths each year.

While most authorities emphasize that the majority of the country's 320,000 doctors are competent and conscientious, they estimate that as many as 16,000 licensed physicians, or 5 percent of the profession, are unfit to practice medicine. These doctors, they say, should have their licenses revoked, be required to undergo further training or practice only under close supervision.

The incompetent doctors, who treat an estimated total of 7.5 million patients a year, include some who are mentally ill or addicted to drugs as well as others who are simply ignorant of modern medical knowledge or careless in their use of it.

In recent years, evidence indicating that the problem is larger than most medical authorities had suspected has emerged from separate studies by a number of professional groups, including the American College of Surgeons, the Joint Commission on Hospital Accreditation, the Federation of State Medical Boards, the American Medical Association and the Federal Commission on Medical Malpractice, as well as the Health Research Group, a consumer-advocacy organization in Washington.

Additional evidence has been gathered by individual researchers at various hospitals and medical schools, and has been published in leading medical journals.

Among the findings are these:

¶American surgeons, a Cornell University study indicates, are performing an estimated total of nearly 2.4 million unnecessary operations each year in which 11,900 patients die as the result of complications.

¶An estimated total of 10,-

000 Americans die or suffer potentially fatal reactions following the administration of antibiotics that are not needed, according to studies at the University of Florida and Ohio State University medical schools.

¶As a result of errors in judgment it is estimated that 260,000 women undergo needless hysterectomies each year and some 500,000 children are subjected to unwarranted surgical removal of their tonsils and adenoids, studies done in several medical schools suggest.

¶Each year, according to a drug-industry marketing survey, doctors write about 161,000 prescriptions for chloramphenicol, one of the most-dangerous antibiotics, for patients whose diseases are known to be unaffected by antibiotics or who could have been treated with safer alternatives. The drug is intended for several uncommon infections such as typhoid and Rocky Mountain spotted fever. Its most serious side effect is a potentially fatal anemia.

¶About 2,200 hospitals, nearly one-third of the total in the United States, fail to meet the minimum standards of safety and adequacy of patient care required by the medical profession's Joint Commission on Hospital Accreditation. Despite this, there is no legal restriction on the medical and surgical procedures these hospitals may attempt on patients.

¶Although the Federation of State Medical Boards estimates that 16,000 doctors are un-

worthy of their licenses, state licensing agencies revoke an average of only 66 licenses a year nationwide. In most states, once a license is granted, it entitles a doctor to practice medicine for the rest of his life without any evidence that he has kept his knowledge up to date.

Pressures for Disclosure

While these and many other documented deficiencies in medical practice have existed for many years, they have remained largely hidden from public scrutiny because doctors have traditionally dealt with errant colleagues primarily within their own ranks and have rarely publicized their disciplinary actions.

These problems have lately come into public view largely as the result of two forces. One is the growing involvement of the Federal Government in paying for health services, which has focused attention, for example, on the costs, if not the hazards, of unnecessary surgery. The other is the rise of the consumer movement, which has stimulated activists, including conscientious doctors, to seek and disclose hitherto obscure information.

Perhaps the best-known example of an unfit doctor was Max Jacobson, the Manhattan general practitioner who injected hundreds of patients, including many celebrities, with amphetamines and who was himself a regular user of the drug. Dr. Jacobson's license was revoked last year, more than two years after his prac-

267

tice was described in detail in The New York Times. Many of his former patients said his injections had destroyed their lives by addicting them to the powerful mind-altering drug.

A different kind of problem was represented by Stewart and Cyril Marcus, twin brothers and gynecologists who died last summer as a result of their addiction to barbiturates. Both were once leaders in their specialty, but after becoming addicted to drugs, the quality of their work declined over a period of years.

Despite much evidence of their deterioration, officials of New York Hospital, where the Marcus brothers practiced, were slow to protect their patients or to help the doctors. Days after the hospital finally withdrew the brothers' staff privileges, they were found dead in their apartment, one of barbiturate withdrawal and the other apparently of a subsequent suicidal overdose.

Immediately after publication of The Times's investigation of Dr. Jacobson in late 1972, which revealed that several reputable doctors and hospitals knew of patients injured by his unorthodox practice yet failed to take action, many doctors and medical groups were quick to assert that the case was an isolated example of one errant doctor.

Calls for Reform

But a few physicians, including the president of the American can Medical Association, were convinced the case represented a larger problem, and seized on it in journal articles and medical society speeches to argue that the profession had to do a better job of policing itself. When the case of the Marcus brothers came up in mid-1975, it stimulated a renewal of interest in the problem. The Medical Society of the County of New York, for example, called a meeting of all local hospital leaders to discuss ways to prevent further such cases.

One of the most-outspoken critics of the way medicine polices its unfit members is Dr. Robert C. Derbyshire, a Santa Fe, N. M., surgeon who is a past president of the National Federation of State Medical Boards, the professional organization of doctors charged with disciplining their errant colleagues.

Dr. Derbyshire is one of several authorities who have independently arrived at the estimate that 5 percent, or 16,000, of the country's doctors are unfit.

The figure is based on known rates of drug addiction, alcoholism and mental illness among professional groups and on the proportion of incompe-

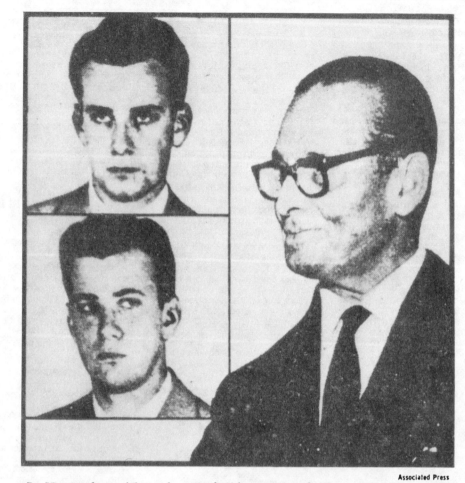

Associated Press

Dr. Max Jacobson, right, perhaps the best-known example of an unfit doctor, had his license revoked last year. At left are Cyril, top, and Stewart Marcus, gynecologists who died last summer as a result of their addiction to barbiturates.

tence uncovered through reviews of hospital case records.

Although some in organized medicine have suggested the true proportion is closer to 3 percent, the 5 percent figure has generally been accepted by the profession and is regarded by some experts as conservative.

One expert who has also suggested the 5 percent figure is Dr. Roger O. Egeberg, special assistant on health policy to the Secretary of Health, Education and Welfare.

"I've met one hell of a lot of doctors over the years and seen a lot of records and that's my feeling," Dr. Egeberg said of the estimate.

"When I first started writing and talking about this problem a few years ago, all I got was castigation from doctors and even hate mail," Dr. Derbyshire said. "Lately, however, most of the feedback is positive. I think the profession is beginning to adopt a healthier attitude toward this problem."

A Cause of Malpractice

Recent publicity over growing malpractice suits and judgments against doctors has generally attributed the problem to greedy lawyers and perfection-demanding patients. But Eli Bernzweig, a former director of the Federal Commission on Medical Malpractice, which investigated the problem for the Federal Department of Health, Education and Welfare, disagrees.

"The time has come," he said at a medical conference last year, "for all parties seeking solutions to malpractice problems to recognize that the root cause of the current malpractice problem is the substantial number of injuries and other adverse results sustained by patients during the course of hospital and medical treatment."

Another critic within the profession is Dr. Avedis Donabedian, professor of health-care organization at the University of Michigan, who has studied the quality of medical care delivered under various systems of organization.

He believes the biggest problems in medicine come not from the 5 percent of thoroughly incompetent doctors, but from the much larger body of average doctors, who, for various reasons, do not practice the best medicine they can.

"There is much evidence to indicate that the quality of care available under many cir-

cumstances falls far below acceptable standards," Dr. Donabedian said in an interview.

The American Medical Association, which represents almost half the country's doctors, has also begun to recognize the problem of unfit practitioners. Dr. Malcolm C. Todd, the association's immediate past president, devoted much of his term to campaigning for stepped-up surveillance of unfit doctors and criticized local A.M.A. affiliates for being "derelict in exercising their responsibilities" in this area.

Because medicine has been closed to outside examination for so long, popular discussion of the quality of physicians has fed on the contrast between television's superdoctor, Marcus Welby, and tales of alleged cases of missed diagnoses and botched surgery.

Evidence Hard to Get

Unquestioned evidence of medical incompetence or unprofessional conduct is hard to come by. For one thing, even the best of medicine is frequently an inexact science and, in some cases, more of an art than any science at all.

Despite remarkable advances in the last 30 years, the under-

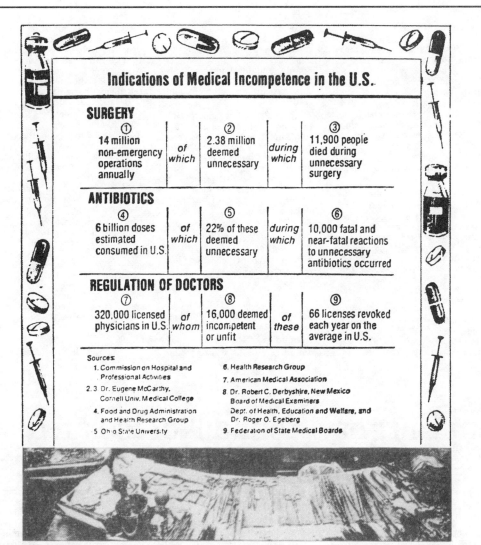

Indications of Medical Incompetence in the U.S.

SURGERY

① 14 million non-emergency operations annually	of which	② 2.38 million deemed unnecessary	during which	③ 11,900 people died during unnecessary surgery

ANTIBIOTICS

④ 6 billion doses estimated consumed in U.S.	of which	⑤ 22% of these deemed unnecessary	during which	⑥ 10,000 fatal and near-fatal reactions to unnecessary antibiotics occurred

REGULATION OF DOCTORS

⑦ 320,000 licensed physicians in U.S.	of whom	⑧ 16,000 deemed incompetent or unfit	of these	⑨ 66 licenses revoked each year on the average in U.S.

Sources:
1. Commission on Hospital and Professional Activities
2,3. Dr. Eugene McCarthy, Cornell Univ. Medical College
4. Food and Drug Administration and Health Research Group
5. Ohio State University
6. Health Research Group
7. American Medical Association
8. Dr. Robert C. Derbyshire, New Mexico Board of Medical Examiners; Dept. of Health, Education and Welfare; and Dr. Roger O. Egeberg
9. Federation of State Medical Boards

lying nature of most diseases is still not known. Even the best doctors must rely not on conclusive evidence to diagnose a disease, but on the probability that a given set of symptoms means one thing and not another.

One indication of how difficult diagnosis can be is the common experience of doctors who perform autopsies and find evidence of diseases that were never discovered before death. Dr. Michael Baden, deputy medical examiner for New York City, who performs hundreds of autopsies a year and oversees thousands, estimates that 30 to 50 percent of autopsies reveal previously undiagnosed diseases.

Most of the time the physician's diagnosis will be correct, but every doctor expects to make mistakes now and then. Judging this behavior with the advantages of hindsight and simply adding up the rare mistakes of individuals can lead to unfair conclusions.

For these reasons, the most persuasive evidence of unnecessarily bad medical practice is based not on a comparison of actual practice with a mythical ideal, but on actual practice under varying circumstances. A number of such studies have been reported in medical journals in recent years, and although the details vary, nearly all point to problems of a magnitude that, the researchers say, warrants reform.

Variations Questioned

Why, the investigators ask, should people be 5 to 10 times as likely to die during a given operation in one hospital than they are in another?

Why should the people in one region of a state be three or four times as likely to undergo the most common surgical procedures as people in another, similar region of the same state?

Why do university-affiliated doctors usually recommend against prescribing antibiotics for a cold when private practitioners do so frequently?

Why do nearly half the doctors in some places perform physical examinations with their patients fully or almost fully clothed when the accepted method is to have the patient's entire body visible?

Variations in medical practice such as these, in the opinion of many medical leaders, expose millions of patients to unnecessary risks.

Each of these problem areas represents only a small segment of medical practice that can be evaluated quantitatively. Many doctors and medical judgments cannot be directly evaluated because, for example, many doctors practice alone and their records cannot be examined, or because many diagnoses and therapies must be based on highly subjective evaluations of symptoms and other factors in the patient.

Most critics of medical incompetence say that many additional avoidable injuries and deaths must occur in these inaccessible areas.

Virtually all the studies of the adequacy of medical care reveal a great unevenness from one region to another, from one hospital to another within a region and from doctor to doctor within a single hospital.

Traditionally, organized medicine has tried to convey the belief that, except for a very few "rotten apples in the barrel," all doctors are well trained, conscientious and hard working.

But there is no evidence that the variation in quality among doctors is any different from that among lawyers, teachers, reporters or any other professional group. In virtually every occupation, there is what is known statistically as a "normal" distribution of quality. That is, there are some doctors who fall in the lowest end of the range, about as many who are in the highest end, and the vast majority near the middle, or average, part of the range.

But the problem is, some authorities note, that most patients behave as if this normal distribution of quality was not true and put unquestioning faith into whatever doctors say or do.

The 'Medical Mystique'

Dr. Marvin S. Belsky, a New York internist and author of a new book, "How to Choose and Use Your Doctor," says that the greatest problem for patients who want to assure themselves of good medical care is acquiring a willingness to judge.

"Patients in the thrall of the medical mystique," he writes, "are unwilling to examine their doctors."

The origins of the "medical mystique" are as old as the earliest witchdoctors and medicine men who jealously guarded the little genuine knowledge they had and concealed their ignorance behind pretensions of magic and authority. Then, as now, the power of suggestion played an important role in making patients feel better. The more a person believed in the medicine man, the better he was likely to feel. Practitioners of the healing arts have always known this and emphasized the need for patients to have faith in them.

"Formerly, when religion was strong and science weak, men mistook magic for medicine," says Dr. Thomas S. Szasz, professor of psychiatry at the State University of New York's Upstate Medical Center in Syracuse. "Now, when science is strong and religion weak, men mistake medicine for magic."

'Myths' Described

In his book, Dr. Belsky cites the work of Dr. Eliot Friedson, a New York University sociologist who studied the nature of the doctor-patient relationship and concluded that patients were reluctant to question their doctors' judgments because they believed several "myths of the medical mystique." These "myths," and Dr. Belsky's comments about them, include the following:

¶Doctors must make such complicated judgments fitted to each patient that no one except another doctor who has gone through the case step by step can judge the worth of the diagnosis and treatment. "Not so," Dr. Belsky says. "The diagnosing physician is often comparing symptoms to criteria that may be as basic and fixed as multiplication tables."

¶Doctors are always rational. "Doctors are human. They do get tired. Their interest does flag."

¶The quality of medicine is assured by the long and rigorous course of training a doctor must go through to get his degree and pass his licensing examination. "Actually, much of what was learned may be forgotten. Doctors' knowledge becomes stale. It requires constant replenishment through continuing education."

¶Doctors are responsible professionals, dedicated to the welfare of their patients and the public. "The truth is that dedication is variable, and doctors are no more or less dedicated than members of other professions."

According to Dr. Roger Steinhardt, chairman of the Board of Censors that investigates errant doctors for the Medical Society of the County of New York, one problem in detecting unfit doctors is the reluctance of many patients to report misconduct by their physicians. Often, he said, the relationship between doctor and patient is such that the patient is either afraid to question the doctor or is blind to obvious deficiencies.

Complaints Lacking

"Patients don't complain that their doctors are flaky or inadequate," said Gary Gatza, a spokesman for the medical society. "You would think that if patients walk into a doctor's office and it's in a mess or the doctor is obviously 'out of it,' they would turn on their heel and walk out."

Yet, the medical society says, they seldom do so. Although some 16,000 doctors are believed to be unfit to practice, state licensing agencies re-

volse only about 66 licences a year in the entire country. A common reason, according to the Federation of State Medical Boards, and local licensing officials, is the difficulty of getting patients to complain and testify.

An additional reason for the low level of disciplinary action, in the view of experts such as Dr. Derbyshire, is the fact that most medical mistakes are neither apparent to the patient nor revealed to him if a doctor discovers the fact.

The real cause of a death during surgery or following drug therapy may be evident only to a physician. But even if a doctor reports such errors to a hospital board or medical society, he is unlikely to inform the patient's survivors.

"It's just not something many doctors feel they should do," said Dr. Baden of the Medical Examiner's office. He said that autopsies there revealed the

fatal results of medical incompetence "dozens of times a year, maybe hundreds of times," but that the survivors were never told voluntarily. "If the family asks, however, we'll tell them," he said.

Because all deaths during surgery are automatically Medical Examiner cases in New York, Dr. Baden said this represented an existing way of discovering possible medical incompetence. He said he would welcome a law requiring that such discoveries be reported routinely to the proper regulatory agencies.

"Too often, these out-and-out mistakes are said to be just 'honest differences of opinion,' " Dr. Baden said. "This gives everybody the excuse not to be judgmental. We've got to start becoming a little more judgmental, and develop better means of quality control. Otherwise, we're always going to have incompetent doctors in business."

January 26, 1976

Incompetent Surgery Found Not Isolated

By JANE E. BRODY

A middle-aged man entered a leading New York hospital for the replacement of a heart valve that had been damaged by rheumatic fever. When he was taken off the heart-lung machine after his operation, his circulation failed and he died minutes later. An autopsy revealed that the surgeon had put the artificial valve in backward, preventing blood from flowing through the heart.

A young New York woman was given a local anesthetic prior to a tonsillectomy. Suddenly she got very sleepy and her blood pressure dropped rapidly. Despite various emergency measures, she died. The autopsy showed that the anesthetic, instead of entering the bed of the tonsils, had been injected into the carotid artery leading directly to her brain.

A woman with severe abdominal pain was diagnosed as needing gall bladder surgery. During the operation at a New York municipal hospital the surgeon noticed a tumor on her kidney, and without ordering a biopsy, he removed the kidney. Ordinarily, a sample of tissue would be sent to the pathologist to check for malignancy while the woman was still on the operating table.

The woman did poorly after the operation and she died before anyone could determine why. The Medical Examiner's autopsy revealed that the woman had had only one kidney to begin with, a fact the surgeon missed because no X-ray had been taken. Moreover, the removal of the kidney was unnecessary, since the postoperative laboratory report showed that the tumor was benign.

These three cases are not isolated examples. Although these incidents occurred in New York, similar cases can be found all over the country. These cases illustrate a pervasive, but usually hidden, side of American surgery, which is generally held to be the safest in the world.

The evidence is that even the safest surgery is never without some risk to the patient's life and that the American surgical profession, which is probably the best trained in the world, contains a number of unethical, incompetent and careless practitioners.

There are also, according to a major new study sponsored by the nation's leading surgical groups, far more doctors doing surgery than are needed and too many new surgeons being

trained each year, with the likely result that at least some surgeons "make work" for themselves by doing operations that are unnecessary.

More than 250,000 of the approximately 18 million Americans who underwent surgery last year died during or shortly after their operations, according to figures from the National Center for Health Statistics. That represents one death for every 72 surgical procedures.

Many of these patients were critically ill before surgery and most probably would have died had they not had an operation. For other patients, however, it was the operation itself that ended their lives. Approximately 80 percent of surgery in the United States is elective. Based on figures from the National Center for Health Statistics, a Federal agency, one in 200 persons who undergoes an elective operation dies as a result.

An unknown percentage of these deaths occurs despite the best medical care, representing the risks inherent in any surgery. But many other deaths are the direct result of careless errors made by doctors or others involved in the patient's care.

A two-year study just completed by the surgical profession of 1,493 patients who suffered complications during or after surgery found that almost half the 1,451 nonfatal complications and a third of the 245

deaths that resulted were preventable.

The study was part of a massive five-year self-examination of surgery by the American College of Surgeons and the American Surgical Association. The study, which examined data about patients treated at 95 hospitals in seven states, found that 78 percent of the preventable complications were due to surgeons' errors, with one-half resulting from faulty surgical techniques.

Some Deaths Avoidable

Whether they are due to accident, ignorance or negligence, at least 11,900 surgery-related deaths that occurred in the United States last year were entirely avoidable because the surgery involved was not necessary to begin with, according to the findings of a Congressional subcommittee.

In its report on unnecessary surgery issued last week, the House Subcommittee on Oversight and Investigations of the Committee on Interstate and Foreign Commerce recommended that a second surgeon's opinion be obtained for all suggested operations that would be paid for by Medicare or Medicaid. This, the report said, could reduce the number of unnecessary operations.

Studies by researchers at such medical centers as Stanford, Cornell and Harvard, among others, have indicated that about one in five of the elective operations performed annually in the United States is unnecessary. For some procedures, such as hysterectomies and tonsillectomies, the studies found that as many as ·one-third to two-thirds of the operations done may not be in the patients' best medical interests.

Rather, experts who have reviewed the data maintain, these questionable operations are performed because the doctor exercises poor judgment, because the patient insists on or expects surgery, because the doctor wants to protect himself from a possible lawsuit, or simply because the doctor—on whose recommendation for surgery the patient depends—earns nothing for the operations he recommends against.

A Correlation Noted

"The surgeon's bias toward performing an operation is matched by the patient's eagerness to have one," said Dr. John Bunker, a Stanford University anesthesiologist. Dr. Bunker was one of the first medical researchers to document that the amount of surgery done is directly proportional to the number of surgeons available and to whether they receive a fee for .each operation they do. He published his initial findings in 1970 in the New England Journal of Medicine.

The rate of elective surgery in the United States—up from 70 operations per 1,000 persons in 1970 to 78 operations per 1,000 persons in 1974—is the highest in the world. The American surgeon has often been described in the American medical literature as more aggressive than those elsewhere, with some operating under the widely quoted principle, "When in doubt, take it out."

The rationale for such a principle was expressed by Dr. George B. Markle, a surgeon in Carlsbad, N. M., "I go on the theory that it's better to remove an occasional normal appendix than to be too conservative and run the risk of a rupture while you're making up your mind."

Indeed, sometimes doctors are too slow to recognize the need for surgery. In 1974 a young man with severe abdominal pain went to the emergency room of a major New York hospital. He was given Valium, a tranquilizer, and sent home. His pain unrelieved, he returned to the emergency room and was given more Valium. He went home and died of a ruptured appendix.

But according to Dr. Bunker of Stanford, the more common problem is for many doctors and patients to rush into surgery, even if they are not sure it will help the problem. This approach is dangerous, he said,

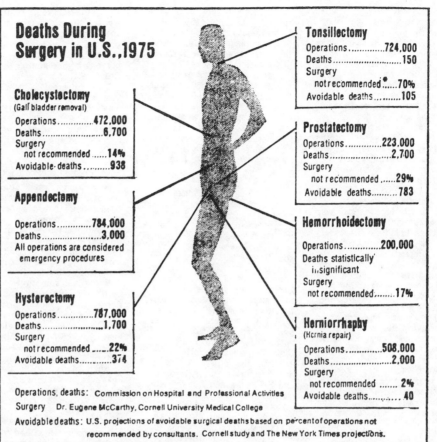

Deaths During Surgery in U.S.,1975

Cholecystectomy
(Gall bladder removal)

Operations 472,000
Deaths 6,700
Surgery
   not recommended 14%
Avoidable· deaths 938

Appendectomy

Operations 784,000
Deaths 3,000
All operations are considered emergency procedures

Hysterectomy

Operations 787,000
Deaths 1,700
Surgery
   not recommended 22%
Avoidable deaths 374

Tonsillectomy

Operations 724,000
Deaths 150
Surgery
   not recommended * 70%
Avoidable deaths 105

Prostatectomy

Operations 223,000
Deaths 2,700
Surgery
   not recommended 29%
Avoidable deaths 783

Hemorrhoidectomy

Operations 200,000
Deaths statistically insignificant
Surgery
   not recommended 17%

Herniorrhaphy
(Hernia repair)

Operations 508,000
Deaths 2,000
Surgery
   not recommended 2%
Avoidable deaths 40

Operations, deaths: Commission on Hospital and Professional Activities

Surgery   Dr. Eugene McCarthy, Cornell University Medical College

Avoidable deaths: U.S. projections of avoidable surgical deaths based on percent of operations not recommended by consultants. Cornell study and The New York Times projections.

* Estimate of various experts, not reflected in Cornell study.

The New York Times/Jan. 27, 1976

because "all treatments—drugs as well as surgery—have substantial risks and should be used only for definite indications."

Unlike drugs, whose manufacturers are required by law to state precisely when, how and for whom they should be used and what possible complications may result, there are no similarly precise guidelines for surgeons prepared by either government or medical organizations.

Except for life-threatening conditions, such as cancer, there are few clearly defined reasons for doing most operations. And even for cancer, there is sometimes debate among medical practitioners as to what kind of surgery—or whether any surgery—is the best treatment.

Under Congressionally mandated peer review, the American College of Surgeons has developed guidelines for 20 surgical procedures. The guidelines describe how an operation should be done, but not when or whether.

"Not more than 20 percent of surgery is done to prevent death or prolong life," Dr. Bunker said in an interview. "The rest is done to improve the quality of life, and we have no systematic data on the value of the results."

The riskiness of surgery is also imprecisely known. An operation that may present a one in 100 risk of death for a young, healthy patient may risk the life of one in 10 older patients whose health is already compromised.

The Odds Go Up

Because so many operations are done in this country, even a very small risk can add up to a substantial number of deaths and other mishaps. For example, tonsillectomy is one of the safest operations, with only two in 10,000 patients dying as a result of such an operation. But since 724,000 tonsillectomies are done in a year, nearly 150 patients—mostly children—die annually as a result.

Some experts maintain that 70 percent of these operations are of little or no value to the patient. It could mean, if this estimate is correct, that the lives of perhaps 100 people are lost unnecessarily each year because they are subjected to needless tonsillectomies.

The risks of surgery are manifold. They include such postoperative complications as pneumonia, blood clots, shock, infection and hemorrhage. Most of these complications are preventable or treatable, but some cannot be forestalled, and some

cause serious illness or death. The blood transfusions that are often given to ward off or reverse complications themselves cause 2,500 deaths a year, mainly because of mismatched blood and transfusion-transmitted hepatitis.

During an operation, even a highly skilled surgeon may slip and cut or burn the wrong tissue, but such a mishap is more likely to occur if the doctor is careless or ill-trained. The instances in which foreign objects have been left in surgical patients have been well-documented in malpractice cases —pieces of tubing, clamps, sponges, forceps, even a 30-inch-long towel stamped "U.S. Army."

But perhaps the most serious surgical risks are those associated with anesthesia. "No anesthesia is minor," said Dr. Marcelle Willock, director of obstetrical anesthesia at Roosevelt Hospital here and a special investigator of anesthesia-related deaths for the New York City Office of the Medical Examiner.

"In any group of perfectly healthy surgical patients, there's a one in 5,000 to one in 10,000 chance of dying from the anesthesia," Dr. Willock said. For other patients, she added, an adverse anesthesia reaction may mean permanent brain damage, leaving the person crippled for life or doomed to a vegetative existence.

"Yet if you tell a patient that, he thinks, 'That's like my winning the lottery; that will never happen to me,'" Dr. Willock noted. For all surgical patients, healthy and sick, anesthesia causes or contributes to death in one in 3,000 cases, she said.

General anesthesia — being put to sleep—is considered especially hazardous, since the very potent drugs used can interfere with the functions of the respiratory system, the heart and blood vessels, the brain and the kidneys.

But local anesthetics also can be associated with severe reactions, including anaphylactic shock (a sudden life-threatening allergic response), convulsion, choking on vomit and cardiac arrest. Dr. Willock recalled the case of a young New York girl who died a few years ago from a reaction to the local anesthetic she received while having her nose fixed.

Carelessness may also cause anesthesia-related deaths. Two patients died during surgery at a leading hospital here some years ago because workmen erred in constructing the hospital's anesthesia lines and the patients were fed the wrong gas.

In California in 1967, a 45-year-old member of the Baja Marimba Band died following plastic surgery on his ear because the oxygen tank ran out and no one noticed it until the man's brain and heart were irreparably damaged. Many hospitals now have warning beeps when the oxygen level gets low, but doctors say the systems are far from perfect.

Despite the hazards of anesthesia, Dr. Bunker points out that less than half of anesthetic administrations are handled by anesthesiologists or physicians in specialty training — those considered most qualified to give anesthesia properly and to cope with related emergencies. The majority of anesthesia is administered by nurse anesthetists or nurses with no special training.

Circumcision Hazards

Last October the American Academy of Pediatrics recommended that parents be told that circumcision of the newborn—the nation's most common surgical procedure—is not medically necessary and that its potential complications are not always trivial.

Immediate hazards, the academy said after a three-year study of circumcision, "include local infection which may progress to septicemia (an infection throughout the body), significant hemorrhage and mutilation."

Last year an estimated 1,700 of the 787,000 women who

had hysterectomies died as a result, according to figures from the Commission on Professional and Hospital Activities, a nonprofit research organization sponsored by professional medical groups.

Yet, studies have indicated, this operation is often done when more conservative and less dangerous treatments could have produced the desired result. Most doctors recommend surgery only if more conservative treatment fails.

Cost of a Backache

In 1963 a young Florida woman suffering from severe backaches was advised to undergo an operation to have her "misplaced" uterus moved. When the operation was over, she discovered that her uterus and one ovary had been removed and that, in the process, her bladder had been injured, necessitating a second operation to correct the damage.

Still, the woman's backaches persisted and she finally visited an orthopedist, who discovered that one leg was slightly shorter than the other. A lift in her shoe corrected the disparity and the backaches, but the woman, meanwhile, had had an unnecessary hysterectomy with a serious complication.

Some doctors have been accused by others in the profession of performing "hip-pocket hysterectomies," where the only beneficiary is the doctor's wallet. In England and Wales, where doctors are salaried, the rate of hysterectomies is only 40 percent that of the United States, where most surgeons are paid by the operation.

In general, compared with Britain, there are twice as many surgeons and twice as many operations done per person in the United States. How much of this surgery is unnecessary? Some American surgeons maintain the British are getting too few operations rather than the Americans too many.

Dr. Markle of New Mexico maintained, for example, that in Britain there is "a shortage of hospital beds, and over there, my patient's hemorrhoids would probably have been treated the prolonged but conservative way instead of with surgery."

Other doctors, however, dispute this view. They point to studies in the United States showing that the rate of surgery varies according to how the surgeon gets paid.

For example, in studies sponsored by the United States Department of Health, Education and Welfare, comparisons between Federal employees who are covered by Blue Cross (where doctors receive a fee for service) and those enrolled

in a prepaid group health plan (where the physicians are paid the same amount whether they operate or not) showed that surgery rates were 44 to 54 percent higher among the Blue Cross participants.

The difference in surgery rates between the two groups may suggest that patients under the Blue Cross fee-for-service system are undergoing more operations than they really need.

Prepaid vs. Fee Care

A just-completed study by the Social Security Administration found that Medicaid patients who are members of prepaid plans underwent half the number of operations performed on patients who were cared for by independent, fee-for-service physicians.

While it is sometimes argued by physicians that perhaps participants in prepaid plans do not undergo as much surgery as they should, a national study headed by Dr. Paul Ellwood, a Minneapolis medical administrator, suggested that members of such plans, where the emphasis is on preventing illness, may, in fact, be healthier.

Dr. Ellwood's study found that they were hospitalized one-third as often and spent more time at work than comparable Americans receiving regular fee-for-service, illness-oriented medical care.

Another measure of how much surgery is really needed is suggested by how many operations are recommended against when patients see a second surgeon for a consultation.

In an ongoing study conducted by Dr. Eugene G. McCarthy and Geraldine W. Widmer of the Cornell University Medical College, 1,356 members of two New York labor unions who were advised to have surgery sought a consultation.

One In 5 Discouraged

For one group in the study, for whom consultation was compulsory before surgery could be performed, nearly one in five operations recommended by the first surgeon was discouraged by the consulting surgeon.

The House subcommittee took the lowest surgical nonconfirmation rate—17.6 percent—from the Cornell study and applied it nationally to approximately 14 million elective operations done in acute-care hospitals in 1974. It then estimated that nearly 2.4 million of these operations were unnecessary.

The cost of this unnecessary surgery, the subcommittee said, was $3.9 million and 11,900 lives, using a conservative estimate of a 0.5 percent mortality rate associated with elective surgery.

Experts in the field stress, however, that there have been no adequate followup studies to determine the fate of patients not operated on because a consultant said surgery was not needed. Did their condition clear up? Did they require extensive medical care? Was their quality of life compromised? Did they eventually need surgery anyway? Dr. McCarthy of Cornell is about to conduct a study to answer those questions.

Surgery rates in the United States also are directly related to the number of surgical practitioners. For example, in different parts of Kansas, a 1969 study showed, the rate of performance of six common operations varied threefold to fourfold in accordance with the number of surgeons and hospitals beds per person.

Dr. Charles E. Lewis, who was a Harvard health-care expert when he did the Kansas study, concluded that there exists "a medical variation of Parkinson's Law: Patient admissions for surgery expand to fill beds, operating suites and surgeons' time."

The study by the American College of Surgeons and the American Surgical Association called the "Study of Surgical Services for the United States," showed there was an excess of physicians who regularly perform surgery. The study involved a questionnaire survey of a random sample of practitioners—5,880 physicians and 196 osteopaths — who listed themselves in medical directories as performing surgery, and a review of all operations performed in four regions of the country in 1970.

The report did not discuss the issue of how much surgery may be unnecessary. But the main findings of the report are that there are significant regional differences in surgery rates and that there are at least 22,000 too many doctors doing surgery now. In addition, the report said, the 12,000 to 16,000 new surgeons now in training are eight times more than are really needed.

All told, the study showed, 94,000 physicians—30.4 percent of all actively practicing doctors—do surgery full or part-time. Only 52,000 of these practitioners are specially trained and fully qualified surgeons certified by an American specialty board, such as the American Board of Surgery. Another 12,000 are internes and residents in surgical training programs who, when they operate, are closely supervised by fully qualified surgeons.

But the rest—30,000 physicians—are just doctors who have chosen to specialize in surgery, although some have had specialty training without taking or passing the examination for board certification.

'Closed Shop' Surgery?

Dr. George Zuidema, chief of surgery at the Johns Hopkins School of Medicine who served as coordinator of the study, said it found that "uncertified surgeons tend to do most of the operations that are controversial—hernias, tonsillectomies, hysterectomies and so forth."

The report also concluded that board-certified surgeons were underemployed. Distributing 18 million operations among those doing surgery, the average surgical practitioner does about 3.5 operations a week and, the study showed, board-certified surgeons average less than four operations a week.

Some experts say that to maintain a high level of skill, a surgeon should average about 10 operations a week (depending, of course, on such factors as his age and specialty.)

The report recommended that hospitals restrict the practice of surgery to qualified surgical specialists. While a few doctors have charged this would create a lucrative "closed shop" for board-certified surgeons. Dr. McCarthy believes that such a move "would enhance the over-all quality of surgery and give surgeons so much legitimate work to do that there would be neither time nor temptation to do unnecessary surgery."

January 27, 1976

Prescriptions Killing Thousands

By BOYCE RENSBERGER

Every year perhaps 30,000 Americans accept the drugs their doctors prescribe for them and die as a direct result. Perhaps 10 times as many patients suffer life-threatening and sometimes permanent side effects, such as kidney failure, mental depression, internal bleeding and loss of hearing or vision.

These figures are among the more conservative to be found in studies of the prescription drug problem by the medical profession itself. Although most medical authorities agree that some of these deaths and near-deaths could have been prevented if the doctors involved had exercised better judgment in prescribing drugs for their patients, no one knows how many.

"That a problem of preventable adverse drug reactions exists cannot be denied," says Dr. John C. Ballin, director of the American Medical Association's Department of Drugs. "The literature abounds with references to the prescription of the wrong drug or dose, to unforeseen drug reactions, or simply to the administration of a drug when none was indicated."

"You have to realize," adds a New York doctor who requested anonymity "that the whole idea of studying adverse reactions as a general problem of medicine rather than as a feature of an isolated case is pretty new."

Traditionally the nature and success of a given medical therapy has been a matter confined to the individual doctor-patient relationship. Now, with growing consumerism and Federal involvement in health care, deficiences in medical practice are coming to be studied by the medical profession as a national problem.

Dr. Sidney Wolfe of the Health Research Group, a consumer advocacy organization affiliated with Ralph Nader, estimates, on the basis of published data, that in 22 percent of cases, antibiotics prescribed in hospitals are unnecessary. Given the annual rate at which potentially fatal reactions occur with such drugs, he has calculated that more than 10,000 patients would have been spared an ordeal if the drugs were not given when not needed.

An international study, which found that American doctors write twice as many prescriptions per patient as Scottish doctors do, also found that the rate of side effects was twice as high in the United States. Because the standard health figures show the Scots to be at least as healthy as Americans, the director of the study has asked whether half the drugs prescribed by American doctors might be unnecessary.

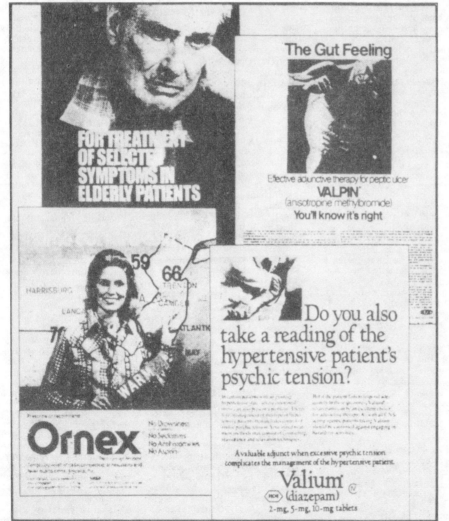

The drug industry spends $1 billion a year to encourage doctors to prescribe one brand over another. Much of this money goes for advertisements, such as these randomly chosen from medical journals. The drug makers try to influence the doctor's decision by using many of the same techniques used to sell consumer products.

273

300,00 Are Hospitalized

The international study, called the Boston Collaborative Drug Surveillance Program, is directed by Dr. Herschel Jick of the Boston University Medical Center. Dr. Jick has estimated that about 300,000 people are hospitalized in the United States annually because of a drug reaction, making this one of the 10 leading causes of hospitalization.

Dr. Jick's study found that for every 18 prescriptions written in a hospital, one adverse reaction occurs. Ten percent of the reactions are major and 1.2 percent are fatal.

Part of the adverse drug reaction problem can be traced to the bewildering variety of drugs available to doctors. About 1,200 different drugs are on the market, many more than any doctor can possibly know well. No drug is completely safe: all have potential side effects, some minor and some major. Each drug is intended for a specific use and many are not supposed to be given except under very carefully controlled conditions.

Yet any licensed doctor is free to use any drug in any way he cares to, regardless of how well or how long ago he has been trained or how diligently or poorly he keeps his knowledge up to date.

Majority Are Helped

In the vast majority of cases, patients are helped by the drugs prescribed for them. Prescription drugs are undeniably responsible for many millions of lives saved, pains relieved and miseries banished. But experts contend that in a small and possibly growing share of cases, something goes wrong.

Not long ago, for example, a 50-year-old New York woman went to her doctor, complaining of a sore throat. He gave her an injection of penicillin and within minutes she lay dead in his office, the victim of penicillin sensitivity that triggers a shutdown of breathing and circulation.

The city's Medical Examiner's Office found that the doctor had failed to make a standard test for such sensitivity, which afflicts one in every hundred persons. The doctor had not even asked whether she had a history of sensitivity.

Warning Not Heeded

In another case, a 48-year-old New Jersey man was hospitalized by his doctor because of a kidney infection. The doctor chose to combat the infection with neomycin despite the manufacturer's warning that the antibiotic was to be avoided in kidney disease cases.

If neomycin builds up to high levels in the blood, it can permanently damage hearing nerves. Because the kidneys are needed to remove foreign chemicals from the blood, any disease reducing their efficiency could allow a dangerous build-up of neomycin.

The New Jersey doctor did not know this, and his patient gradually lost his hearing and became totally deaf. His condition is permanent.

"Although the occasional horror story becomes known, usually through a sensational malpractice trial, there are literally thousands of others that the public doesn't hear about," said a New York doctor who sought anonymity. "Some adverse reactions send people into the hospital and they're treated as medical problems like any other. But a lot of them never go beyond the private physician's office.

"Look," the doctor continued, "some of these guys who practice all by themselves don't keep up with the scientific literature and don't even recognize an adverse reaction. They treat it like just another symptom and prescribe another drug for it."

Efforts to determine the total number of deaths caused by adverse reactions have been few. One of the most widely cited studies was made in 1971 by Dr. Samuel Shapiro and his associates at the Lemuel Shattuck Hospital and the Tufts University Medical School, both in Boston.

Dr. Shapiro studied 6,199 consecutive drug cases in several hospitals and found 27 fatal reactions, 22 of which killed patients not already terminally ill.

Dr. Wolfe has projected this rate to the 10 million patients admitted to hospital medical wards and calculated that about 30,000 hospital patients are killed annually by prescribed drugs. No one knows how many patients die from prescription drugs taken outside hospitals.

Antibiotics Misused

Other studies have suggested there may be as many as 160,000 deaths due to drug reactions. Such studies are hotly disputed by the drug industry, which generally contends that many of the deaths were among patients already seriously ill or that national projections are invalid, or both.

The single most widely prescribed class of drugs and the one that causes the major share of adverse reactions is antibiotics. The American Medical Association's Department of Drugs concluded that "this group of agents may be the most improperly used class of drugs in all medicine."

From 1967 to 1971 the population in the United States grew by

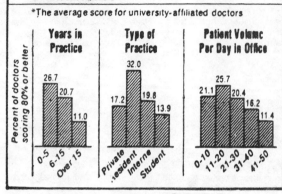

Percent of Doctors Scoring 80%* or better on Test of Their Knowledge of Antibiotics

*The average score for university-affiliated doctors

Years in Practice			Type of Practice				Patient Volume Per Day in Office				
26.7	20.7	11.0	17.2	32.0	19.8	13.9	21.1	25.7	20.4	16.2	11.4
0-5	6-15	Over 15	Private Resident	Interne	Student		0-10	11-20	21-30	31-40	41-50

Percent of doctors scoring 80% or better

The New York Times/Jan. 28, 1976

The doctors who are most up-to-date on how to prescribe antibiotics are those most recently graduated from medical school and those who see only a modest number of patients a day, according to a study of 4,513 doctors. The study, a 50-question test, was given by the Network for Continuing Medical Education. Results were in the New England Journal of Medicine.

about 5 percent. Over the same interval the number of antibiotic prescriptions filled in drugstores grew six times faster, according to drug-industry marketing surveys. In 1967 Americans were put on antibiotics once every two years, on the average. By 1971 the rate had climbed to nearly once a year. By 1972 antibiotic factories were turning out eight billion doses a year, of which two billion were exported.

Experts on infectious diseases say there has been no appreciable change during the same period in the incidences of diseases warranting antibiotic therapy or in the types of antibiotics available. This rate, they say, suggests the average adult has a bacterial infection requiring antibiotics only once every five years.

Increase in Prescriptions

The rise in antibiotic prescribing is often attributed by practioners to growing patient demand. Whenever a patient goes to a doctor with an infection, they say, the patient expects and sometimes demands an antibiotic. Many private practitioners have remarked that it is easier to accede to such demands and keep patients satisfied than to withhold the drug and risk alienating them.

"The gap between the actual antibiotic prescribing practices and the ideal practices recommended by infectious-disease specialists appears to be widening," said Dr. Henry E. Simmons, then United States deputy assistant secretary for health, and Dr. Paul D. Stolley of the Johns Hopkins School of Hygiene and Health in a 1974 article in the Journal of the American Medical Association

One suggestion that doctors may not know as much as they should about antibiotics is the generally poor showing of physicians participating in the National Antibiotic Therapy Test, a voluntary exercise devised by the private Network for Continuing Medical Education. Of the first 4,513 doctors to take the 50-question, multiple-choice test, half scored 68 percent or worse.

Dr. Harold C. Neu, head of the division of infectious diseases at Columbia University's medical school, who devised the test, said the results "brought home to me that many physicians are not as conversant with antibiotics as they ought to be."

Superinfection a Hazard

The test was designed to be difficult enough to challenge the best doctors. Thus, even university-affiliated physicians, who are presumed to be the most up-to-date practitioners, averaged only 80 percent correct. Of the private practitioners, the family doctors for most Americans, only 17.2 percent scored 80 percent or better.

In addition to adverse reactions, one of the most feared hazards of antibiotic therapy is superinfection. The effect of combating an infection can be to encourage a worse infection by a microorganism resistant to the antibiotic. Superinfections, once started, are fatal in 30 to 50 percent of cases.

Ordinarily, many species of bacteria live in the human gut and various other parts of the body. Some can be harmful, but because they compete and keep one another in low numbers, none becomes a threat to health.

When a broad-spectrum antibiotic is given for some infection, it may kill not only the target bacteria, but also many others in the body's normal flora, leaving one or two resistant species to proliferate without competition.

Thus, a bacterial species may suddenly explode in numbers and toxicity, overwhelming the body. Experts agree that some risk of superinfection occurs every time any patient is put on broad-spectrum or medium-spectrum antibiotics, those capable of killing a wide range of organisms.

Upsurge in Patients

In recent years doctors have noticed an upsurge in the number of patients developing infections from the body's normal bacteria, known as Gram negative, and some have linked this rise to the growing use of antibiotics. Other doctors contend, however, that the rise in Gram negative infections is due to the larger proportions of elderly and severely debilitated patients in hospitals today.

Dr. William R. McCabe, an infectious-disease expert at the Boston University medical school, reported in the New England Journal of Medicine, that the incidence of such infections may now be as high as 1 percent of all patients admitted to hospitals. Thus, given the 30-million annual hospital admissions, there may be as many as 300,000 cases of superinfection. If a third are fatal, Dr. McCabe said, superinfection alone may account each year for 100,000 deaths.

"We are dealing not with a scattering of local institutional problems, but with a full-blown national epidemic," said an editorial in the Journal of Infectious Diseases, which independently calculated "a minimum of some 50,000 deaths" related to superinfection.

Various medical experts have estimated that between one-fifth and one-half the antibiotics given are not really necessary and that, therefore, the same proportion of deaths due to Gram-negative superinfection could have been prevented by more intelligent prescribing of antibiotics.

Antibiotics also account for another potential hazard—an adverse reaction to the drug itself. One study conducted at the University of Florida of 7,765 hospitalized patients found that 341 suffered adverse side effects of the drugs they had received. Most victims recovered soon, but 48 patients died or almost died. If the same proportion holds nationally, then 55,000 people a year die or almost die from antibiotic reactions.

Because most of those people needed an antibiotic in the first place, the risk of an adverse reaction had to be taken. But, if 20 percent of the antibiotics given in hospitals are unnecessary, as experts such as Dr. Wolfe of the Health Research Group estimate, then perhaps 20 percent of those potentially fatal reactions need never have happened.

"Prudent non-use of antibiotics could have prevented over 10,000 life-threatening adverse drug reactions," Dr. Wolfe told a 1974 Congressional hearing on overprescribed drugs.

One of the most controversial uses of antibiotics is in treating viral infections because, with rare exceptions, known antibiotics do not affect viruses.

In 1973, for example, about 7.5 million Americans suffering from runny noses and coughs went to the doctors and were diagnosed as suffering nothing more than the common cold. About 95 percent came away with a prescription, more than half for antibiotics that cannot kill cold viruses. Some of the antibiotics were among the more hazardous available.

These figures are from confidential market-research studies conducted for the drug industry by International Marketing Services in Ambler, Pa. The numbers are projected from a sample of about 10,000 doctors who are paid to report all their diagnoses and drug prescriptions. Annual compilations of the statistics are printed and sold chiefly to drug manufacturers. The New York Times has obtained copies of the statistics pertaining to certain diseases and drugs.

Drug-industry figures show that about 277,000 patients were given the closely related and potent antibiotics Lincocin and Cleocin, both of which are known to have a high rate (up to 33 percent) of harmful side effects such as colitis, an intestinal ailment that can be fatal. The drugs are intended for serious infections of "strep" and "staph" bacteria that are resistant to safer antibiotics.

Perhaps the antibiotic best known for causing serious side effects is chloramphenicol, commonly prescribed for typhoid, Rocky Mountain spotted fever and other uncommon infections. A potential side effect of the antibiotic, however, is a fatal anemia.

Chloramphenicol's lethal properties have been well known and publicized for over a decade. Yet Dr. Wolfe estimates from the drug-industry surveys that one in every four prescriptions for the drug are for diseases in which it is known to be useless or for which there are safer alternatives.

For example, if the drug industry's own figures are correct, doctors prescribed chloramphenicol for the common cold 12,000 times in 1972. Another 24,000 prescriptions of the drug were written for "acute upper respiratory infections," which, like colds, are almost invariably viral. In all, 161,000 prescriptions for chloramphenicol were written for, in Dr. Wolfe's words, "diseases for which no competent physician could reasonably argue chloramphenicol is indicated."

Although some physicians argue that no antibiotics should ever be given for a common cold, others maintain that if a "cold" is bad enough to send a person to a doctor, more serious bacterial complications may well have set in. In such cases, antibiotics could be useful.

In any event, the appropriate antibiotic, most experts would agree, would be something other than chloramphenicol. Similar reasoning applies to several other diseases for which the drug was used. Yet 161,000 times a year physicians apparently choose one of the most dangerous antibiotics known when a safer drug was available or no drug at all should have been used.

Parke, Davis and Company, the drug's developer and largest supplier, has long recognized chloramphenicol's hazards and now routinely includes in its labeling the warning, "Chloramphenicol must not be used when less potentially dangerous agents will be effective. It must not be used in the treatment of trivial infections or where it is not indicated, as in colds, influenza, infections of the throat, or as a prophylactic agent to prevent bacterial infections."

Because doctors are legally free to prescribe drugs as they see fit, however, such warnings are only advisory.

While the vast majority of ailments treated by doctors receive appropriate medication, if any is necessary, at least one ailment may be receiving the wrong medication in the vast majority of cases.

Of the 2.4 million women who went to their doctors for nausea and vomiting due to pregnancy, 98 percent, according to the drug-industry survey, were put on a drug. Of these, three-quarters were given Bendectin, a brand name for a combination of three drugs in one pill.

This drug, which accounts for $27-million a year in sales, was evaluated by the National Academy of Sciences and found to lack substantial evidence of effectiveness. The American Medical Association's Council on Drugs studied the product because of its overwhelming popularity and called it an "irrational mixture" with "no evidence that [the ingredients] are effective either alone or in combination." The council's verdict on Bendectin was, "Not recommended." If a drug is needed to reduce vomiting, it said, another class of drugs, which cost about one-fourth as much, would be a better choice.

In addition to high price and low efficiency, doctors who incorrectly prescribe Bendectin can expose their patients to the risk of a variety of adverse reactions. According to information supplied by the manufacturer, Merrell-National Laboratories, the following may occur: Dry mouth, dizziness, blurring of vision, thirst, drowsiness, vertigo, nervousness, epigastric pain, headache, palpitation, diarrhea, disorientation and irritability.

Merrell-National says that additional reactions may occur on rare occasions, including fatigue, sedation, rash, constipation, loss of appetite, painful urination and, ironically, nausea and vomiting.

Dr. John Chewning, a spokesman for Merrell-National, said in an interview that the drug company still considers Bendectin to be an effective drug and is conducting studies that it expects will demonstrate the drug's efficacy.

When these studies are completed they will be submitted to the Food and Drug Administration. If the new evidence is not sufficiently persuasive, the Federal agency says it will ban the drug from the market.

Side Effects Listed

The list of Bendectin's side effects is not an unusually long one for a prescription drug. Similar lists are issued by the manufacturers of most of the drugs on the market today.

They are all given on a piece of paper, called the package insert, which Federal law requires manufacturers to include with every package of a prescription drug sold to a pharmacist. The insert must also include chemical descriptions of the drug, its proper uses and types of patients for whom the drug could be especially hazardous.

Because doctors seldom see the package insert, the same information is available to them in a book called the Physicians' Desk Reference. Because much of the information is written in technical language beyond the vocabulary of most laymen, pharmacists have traditionally removed the insert before selling the drug to the patient.

Patients who wish to see the information can consult the Physicians' Desk Reference in a library or request the insert from the druggist. Contrary to what some pharmacists have told patients, there is no law prohibiting the patient from having the insert.

Ads Promote Drugs

How does the average doctor learn what drugs are good for

275

the treatment of a disease or what hazards the drug poses?

For many doctors, who left medical school before most of the current drugs were developed, their knowledge is gained in about the same way that ordinary consumers learn

of a new detergent or of the nicotine content of a cigarette brand.

Advertisements in medical journals, free samples, door-to-door salesmen and direct-mail promotions are widely used by drug manufacturers to build

brand recognition and acceptance by doctors.

Some medical experts say that doctors are not swayed, that most regard drug companies as biased sources of information and, instead, read scientific articles in journals

and go to scientific meetings to keep up.

Drug companies, on the other hand, say most doctors do rely on their advertising and they spend more than a billion dollars a year to maintain their efforts.   January 28, 1976

A.M.A. Disputes, but Others Praise, Series About Incompetent Physicians

By JOHN NOBLE WILFORD

The top executive of the American Medical Association said yesterday that the five-part series on incompetent doctors and inept medical practices published in The New York Times last week "stated many things that need stating," but that some of the conclusions were "unjustified" by the evidence on which they relied.

In addition, the Pharmaceutical Manufacturers Association described the article in the series concerning the misprescription of drugs as "dangerously negative and misleading."

These comments were among more than 100 responses received to date from physicians, nurses, dentists, professional organizations and patients, many of whom said they had suffered as a result of medical practices such as those described in the series.

A large majority of respondents, including some physicians and many professionals in the health-care field, praised the series and said that it performed a long-needed public service.

On the other hand, others contended that the series had performed a disservice by undermining patients' confidence in their physicians. Among these respondents were some physicians who challenged the accuracy of estimates published by The Times of deaths and life-threatening reactions caused by incompetent and unnecessary surgery and drug prescriptions. It was these estimates that formed the basis for much of the A.M.A.'s criticisms. The association's official position was stated by Dr. James H. Sammons, in a letter to Arthur Ochs Sulzberger, publisher of The Times. As executive vice president, Dr. Sammons is the A.M.A.'s chief operating officer.

The Times's series said that an estimated total of 11,900

people died each year as a result of unnecessary surgery, that perhaps 10,000 fatal and near-fatal reactions occurred annually after the use of unneeded antibiotics and that perhaps 30,000 deaths a year were caused by adverse drug reactions generally.

The estimates reported in The Times by health-care experts were derived as projections from studies published in the Journal of the American Medical Association and the New England Journal of Medicine.

Dr. Sammons' letter said:

"In arriving at national estimates of deaths from 'unnecessary' surgery and wrongly prescribed drugs, The Times, in some cases, relies on studies that are not statistically projectible. In others, the national estimates are built on studies whose methodology has been questioned, both in the medical literature and by experts in the field."

Dr. Sammons said that consequently the conclusions of The Times's articles were "open to serious question." His letter continued:

"It should be stated for the record that Eugene G. McCarthy, M.D., author of the study on which the projection of 11,900 deaths from 'unnecessary' surgery ultimately rests, qualifies his own findings. 'As a result of a number of factors,' he writes in his original article, 'the findings presented here cannot be applied to the general population undergoing elective operations.'"

Dr. McCarthy's study, in which this quotation appears, was published in The New England Journal of Medicine on Dec. 19, 1974. The New York-based study found that when the opinion of a second surgeon was mandatory prior to an elective, or non-emergency, operation, 17.6 percent of the operations were not recommended by the consulting surgeon.

Other Programs Cited

Dr. McCarthy is a member of the department of public health of the Cornell University

Medical College in New York City.

In an interview last month with The Times, Dr. McCarthy said that since the publication of his report, other surgical consultation programs had been established elsewhere in the country and that the preliminary results of all of them were similar to the findings of his own study.

In addition, during the preparation of the series Dr. McCarthy helped The Times to arrive at the number of operations nationwide on which an estimate of unnecessary surgery could be protected. The number Dr. McCarthy suggested is essentially the same as that used by a Congressional subcommittee, whose projections The Times used. The American Medical Association objected to the subcommittee's figures as being "intellectually dishonest."

Dr. Sammons also asked why The Times failed to take into account the "authoritative, contrary assertion" of Dr. George D. Zuidema, chief of surgery at the Johns Hopkins Medical Center, who in testifying before a Congressional subcommittee last summer, said:

"A total of approximately 18 million operations is carried out annually in the United States, and it has been alleged by some that as many as two million of these operations, or one-ninth of the total, are 'unnecessary.' These allegations, however, are totally unsupported by data."

Dr. Zuidema was coordinator of a just-completed five-year survey of surgical practices in the United States, which was sponsored by the country's leading surgical organizations. Some health-care experts have asserted that there are no accurate national data on unnecessary surgery because the surgical profession itself has never addressed the question and has failed to take the opportunity to study it in the profession's huge survey.

Dr. Sammons also said that he had "difficulty accepting The Time's statements on death by prescription drugs." He noted that The Times had said that "the figure of 'perhaps' 30,000

deaths a year is characterized as 'conservative.' "

Dr. Sammons said that this "glibly quoted" figure was analyzed by Dr. Michael Halberstam, an internist in private practice in Washington, who concluded that it was based on a study whose findings had been misinterpreted.

Some Terminally Ill

The study in question was done by Dr. Samuel Shapiro, a clinical pharmacologist, and his colleagues in Boston and published on April 19, 1971, in the Journal of the American Medical Association. The study found that 27 deaths had resulted from adverse drug reactions among 6,199 consecutive medical patients entering a hospital. He reported that five of the 27 patients had been terminally ill to begin with and he discounted their deaths in his conclusions.

The Times reported that Dr. Sidney Wolfe of the Health Research Group, a consumer organization in Washington, had taken the 22 deaths among initially nonterminal patients called drug-caused in the Shapiro study and arrived at a rate of 3.5 fatal drug reactions per 1,000 patients.

Dr. Wolfe estimated that 30,000 hospitalized patients died annually from adverse drug reactions. Others in the field used the same statistics to project a death rate several times higher.

Quoting Dr. Halberstam, Dr. Sammons wrote:

"Any physician who read Dr. Shapiro's case histories would have to conclude that all but two of the 22 patients already had a fatal disease and were mortally ill."

This was not the conclusion reached by Dr. Shapiro and his colleagues and published in the A.M.A.'s journal. They said that of the 27 patients who died, five "were considered terminally ill immediately prior to the onset of their reactions, and though drug therapy was judged responsible for their death, life was probably not appreciably shortened as a result. The majority, 15 patients, were severely ill, but it was believed that their lives, at the time of their reactions, were not otherwise in immediate danger. The remaining seven patients were moderately ill."

Similarly, the Pharmaceutical Manufacturers Association, in a letter to The Times, took issue with the estimates of adverse drug reactions quoted in the series of articles. The pharmaceutical group cited the conclusions reached by "a group of distinguished pharmacologists under the sponsorship of Medicine in the Public Interest [a nonprofit corporation studying issues in medicine and science]," which included the following:

¶"Current estimates of the magnitude and cost of the adverse reaction problem are completely unreliable because they are derived from a data base that is incomplete, unrepresentative and uncontrolled."

¶"The majority of reported adverse drug reactions are minor functional gastrointestinal disturbances."

¶"Many - fatalities allegedly attributed to adverse reactions occur in gravely ill patients."

The pharmaceutical association suggested that The Times consider the findings of a University of Florida study, published in the Journal of the American Medical Association on Oct. 7, 1974, which found that 5 percent of patients admitted to a hospital suffered adverse reactions to antibiotics and 17 of the 6,063 patients studied had severe reactions. One patient died.

This was, in fact, one of the studies that formed the basis for the projection of 10,000 fatal and near-fatal reactions to antibiotics published by The Times in its series of articles. Although he objected to the precise projections used by The Times, Dr. Sammons of the A.M.A. said that "physicians would agree with The Times that some percentage of surgery is unnecessary" and that "to some extent drugs are prescribed or administered incor-

rectly or unnecessarily and sometimes with adverse patient reaction.

Dr. Sammons added: "We would further agree that there are physicians in practice who are impaired physically or mentally, and other physicians whose efforts to continue their own education leave something to be desired."

The Times series was also criticized by Modern Medicine Publications, based in Minneapolis, an affiliate of The New York Times Company, in a memorandum reproduced in an advertisement on Page 26. There is no editorial connection between Modern Medicine Publications and The Times newspaper.

Jersey Group's Comment

Others who wrote or telephoned to The Times were forthright in their favorable comments about the series. A

spokesman for the New Jersey Hospital Association said, for example: "Your articles were absolutely right on about the way these doctors are handling incompetence."

A nurse from Newtown, Pa., said: "I would like to see this series required reading for all consumers of health care. The premise that 'the doctor knows best' and will function in the best interest of his client is no longer a valid one."

Two doctors from Woodcliff Lake, N. J., said the articles in the series were "generally well executed and points reasonably stated."

A New York woman wrote: "My husband, who is a surgeon in community medicine, often has lectured medical societies on such issues, and we both feel that the series is what journalistic enterprise and responsibility are all about."

February 6, 1976

DRUG ADS DROPPED OVER TIMES SERIES
By MARTIN ARNOLD

Because of a five-part series on medical incompetence that was published in The New York Times last month, pharmaceutical concerns have canceled advertising worth $500,000 from Modern Medicine, a magazine owned by The New York Times Company.

An official for the magazine, who wished to remain anonymous, said yesterday that the drug concerns had canceled 200 pages of advertisements in the magazine. A one-page advertisement in the magazine costs $2,500. The magazine usually carries about $3.5 million worth of ads a year.

The magazine is operated wholly independently from The New York Times. On Feb. 6 the magazine took an advertisement in The Times in which

it criticized The Times's five-part series.

That advertisement, in the form of a memorandum to the editors of The Times, not only dissociated the magazine from the conclusions of the series, but also sought to show advertisers that the magazine had not been consulted by The Times when the series was being prepared.

An officer of the magazine said that those advertisers who canceled their advertisements felt that "you don't feed people who beat you up."

The magazine, which has a circulation of 160,000, is published twice monthly nine months of the year and once a month in July, August and December. Its office is in Minneapolis. It is one of 260 medical publications in the country; in advertising income it is second.

Burton C. Cohen, president of the magazine, said, "We are confident that whatever advertising may be scheduled to be withdrawn will be rescheduled for Modern Medicine in the near future." February 6, 1976

Medical Series: The Contrary Views

To the Editor:

Before the record closes on your five-part medical series, [Jan. 26-30], one important point should be made: The A.M.A. is not alone in disputing many of your facts, assumptions and conclusions.

Samples of authoritative, contrary views:

●New England Journal of Medicine: ". . . data used were at times inaccurate, at times manipulated and at times subjected to inappropriate extrapolation." Its calculation of "unnecessary" deaths because of gallbladder removal: one-tenth of The Times'.

●U.S. Assistant Secretary for Health, Theodore Cooper, M.D.: "One would easily conclude . . . that doctors and health industries spend most of their time in unnecessary activities, i.e., intricate, complex, self-satisfying, technical exercises for profit alone. It is not necessary for me to challenge the inappropriate calculations and extrapolations in these articles."

●Ralph S. Emerson, M.D., head of a recent New York State surgical study: ". . . . the Brooklyn-Long Island Chapter of the American College of Surgeons sponsored a study of the surgical procedures in twelve hospitals . . . The incidence of unjustified surgery in the 833 consecutive cases was less than 1 percent." This varies considerably from The Times' 17 percent figure.

Excerpts from letters to The Times that were not published:

●The Commission of Professional and Hospital Activities, a source of data for the series, cites eight "mistakes or problems. . . . Your total should have shown only 300,000 appendectomies and 1,000 deaths." The Times reported 784,000 emergency appendectomies, 3,000 deaths. No mention of these factual errors has been made.

●Leighton D. Cluff, M.D., former chairman, Department of Medicine, University of Florida College of Medicine, whose figures were cited: "The incidents of drug reactions in a state referral hospital . . . where persons with complicated or rare medical prob-

lems are often cared for may not be representative of the average community hospital. Therefore, it is invalid to use these figures to project nationwide incidents."

●Francis D. Moore, M.D., chief-in-surgery, Peter Bent Brigham Hospital, Boston: ". . . the sample of operations upon which the articles are based is much smaller than the authors indicate; the incidence of unnecessary operations has not been determined at all, merely the number of operations in which opinions differ, and, finally, the mortality in these operations is not provided in the critical incident study and is far less than 12,000 a year."

Few if any authorities have endorsed your statistical projections. And I do not see how The Times can defend the promotional banner—"Should You Trust Your Doctor?"—under which the series appeared.

JAMES H. SAMMONS, M.D.
Executive Vice President
American Medical Association
Chicago, April 20, 1976

May 6, 1976

WHY THE QUACK FLOURISHES-- DIFFICULTIES OF SUPPRESSING HIM

PUBLIC attention has recently been focused on the subject of medical quackery by the statement made at a meeting of the Medical Society of the County of New York by its counsel Champe S. Andrews, that during the convictions for this particularly mean and heinous offence. There has been much criticism of the work of the society, because of the smallness of this number, when considered in connection with the fact that it is estimated that there are 20,000 illegal practitioners regularly doing business in New York.

The medical quack is divided by Mr. Andrews into five great classes. They are those who prey on the consumptive poor, the charlatans who advertise that they treat men only and who prey on the fear and ignorance of their victims, the occultists, the midwife in illegal practice, and those who make unwarranted use of the title "Doctor," in which class is included the proprietor of the diploma mill, and the druggist who prescribes. The convictions which have been obtained have been distributed among all these classes, and they have undoubtedly had the effect at least of making those who remain in the business more careful than they were before.

"I consider the consumption fakir one of the most dangerous in the lot," said Mr. Andrews, " and he is one of the most difficult to convict. He preys on those who have practically abandoned hope of recovery in the regular way, and often his treatment hastens the end. Usually it prevents the patient from seeking proper treatment. The trouble about convicting these men is the same as that which attends the conviction of the ' men only ' fakirs. The principal is very seldom in evidence himself. Some of the worst advertising quacks are men of wealth, who have their yachts, and at this season are probably cruising off the Bermudas. Their offices are placed in charge of a broken-down physician, or often of a student who has failed to pass his examination and has no diploma at all.

" Most of them operate a chain of offices, and they pass their men along from one to another, so that one man is not long in one place. All this adds to the difficulty of conviction. An amusing feature of the business is the evidence which we have obtained of the extent of their advertising, from the Mayor and the Postmaster. These officials receive literally hundreds of letters a month from persons scattered all over the country inquiring as to the standing of Dr. So and So. They are all turned over to the County Medical Society, and at the last meeting of the society ninety such letters were read. Some of them came from as far away as California.

" The occultists are a comparatively futile and harmless lot. As a rule their treatment consists of incantations and the administration of some harmless drug, or perhaps of bread pills. As long as they confine themselves to palmistry and fortune telling we do not bother them, but very few of them seem to be able to abstain from invading the field of medicine. As a rule, however, they only get a few superstitious and sentimental women. It is to meet this condition that the law declaring palmists and fortune tellers to be disorderly persons was passed.

" With the midwife we have no quarrel as long as she confines herself to her legitimate field, but there are a great many who do not. Take up any one of half a dozen newspapers, and you will find in them scores of advertisements of midwives who conduct an illegitimate practice, worded so that the nature of their business is perfectly apparent. I consider these people the most dangerous class of malpractitioners in New York, and in addition to their illegal practice they are almost always blackmailers when the opportunity offers itself.

" The men who use the title of ' Doctor ' without warrant and the fake diploma sellers are as bad as any. Druggists are often offenders in this respect. They seem to think very often that their business gives them a right to the title. The fake diploma men do a flourishing business. One of them, whom I convicted twice, Joseph Rohrer, has issued hundreds of diplomas. He issued a sixty-five-page catalogue alleging offices in eight of the capitals of Europe and styled himself ' President of the International Massage and Movement Cure Institute.'

" Somewhat in line with this is the traffic in genuine physicians' diplomas. A short time ago an advertisement appeared in one of the newspapers offering diamonds valued at $5,000 for the diploma of a physician who had been dead not more than two years. The man who gets a diploma like that is almost beyond detection, unless he is given away by an enemy. We did convict in one such case a little while ago. A valet to a distinguished physician in London stole his master's diploma after his death and moved to another part of London, where he practised for a time. Finally he came to this country and tried to do the same thing here, but we learned about him and put a stop to his career.

" Some of the minor forms of medical charlatanism are the exploitation of particular cures, such as the water cure, the air cure, the sunlight cure. All of them have merit if properly used and are used by regular practitioners. The quacks, however, exploit them as a cure for every known disease. In this class are the patent medicine cure alls, but they cannot be reached unless the fakir prescribes them in particular cases. There is no law to prevent a man from diagnosing his own ailment and prescribing any poison that he likes for himself.

" Now, why is it that with all these quacks constantly operating so few convictions have been obtained? The answer is the inherent difficulty in getting evidence. In the very nature of these cases the victim is loath to come forward and expose his or her frailty or weakness by testifying against them. Many of them come to us with information given on the express condition that their names shall not be exposed. Such information is, of course, of no use in securing a conviction. The result is that all our cases have to be made with detective evidence, and it is extremely difficult to secure the right sort of detectives. Many of them must be women, and we are never able to use them more than once.

" As soon as an arrest is made the whole crew of malpractitioners in the same line is advised. When the day comes for the examination the courtroom is filled with them, and every one in the business has a good look at our detectives. If they try to do any work for us again they are asked to leave as soon as they appear in the quack's office.

" The nature of the work to be done in obtaining the evidence also makes it very expensive. We must have the evidence of two detectives, and each one must make several calls on the persons we are after. Their fees are heavy, and they must be paid in advance. To convict Blinn and Conrad, two of the most notorious malpractitioners whom he have succeeded in getting recently, cost us $1,000. One of them got a fee of $500 from our detective. I think it is safe to say that of the 500 convictions which we have obtained 475 were obtained on the evidence of detectives."

November 20, 1904

DOCTORS ASSAIL PATENT MEDICINE ADVERTISING

At the twenty-second annual dinner of the New York State Medical Association, held last night in the big ballroom of the Hotel Astor, that part of the public press which makes a practice of printing objectionable patent medicine advertisements was roundly denounced.

Dr. William J. Mayo of Minnesota, President of the American Medical Association, the first speaker introduced by Dr. J. Riddle Goffe, President of the New York body, who acted as toastmaster, sounded the keynote of all the speeches when he said that the nostrum evil was the gravest confronting the medical profession at the present time.

He declared that the 30,000 members of the National association should work as a unit to discountenance the promiscuous publication of patent medicine advertisements and to bring into disrepute the papers that printed them.

Dr. Goffe said that the association had as a guest Samuel Hopkins Adams, who is engaged, as a member of the editorial staff of a weekly, in conducting a campaign against the booming of proprietary medicines that are either of doubtful value or positively harmful. Although Mr. Adams was not on the list of speakers he was invited to tell what he knew of the situation.

" I am sorry to say that the investigation that I have made into the matter of the publication of patent medicine advertisements has revealed very discouraging conditions," said Mr. Adams. " A large part of the American press is really held in slavery by proprietary medicine interests, and this is to be explained by the fact that for the $250,000,000 of capital invested proprietary medicine men spend a larger proportion for advertising than any other class on earth.

" The papers, be they daily or weekly or monthly, that accept and print advertisements of so-called medicines that are.

in reality harmful preparations are willfully injuring the health of the public.

"Take one medicine, which has received the public indorsement of statesmen, ministers, soldiers, and sailors. It is a great advertiser, and I tell you in all seriousness that you can manufacture it for yourself if you have an alcohol stove. Just put the alcohol in a bottle, add three times as much water as you have alcohol and put in a dash of red ink. There you are. And you can get drunk on it, too. [Laughter.]

"The religious press is worse than the lay press. It will boom worthless nostrums in its editorial columns for a price and throw in a few Biblical quotations for good measure."

The Rev. Dr. George R. Van de Water denied the sponsorship of the Church for many "religious publications," as they had been termed.

"The churches have nothing to do with these papers," Dr. Van de Water said. "They are simply individual undertakings for profit, organized by men who have space to sell to all comers.

"It's an evidence of the prevalence of graft. It is graft in one shape or another that is responsible for very nearly all the evils on earth. It is a question of graft when a hansom cab drives up to a minister's home at midnight and a man jumps out and offers a large sum of money to the minister if he will perform a marriage ceremony which may be off color.

"It is graft when you are asked as physicians to perform operations and prescribe medicines which you know you should not. It is graft when a newspaper or periodical sells its columns to quack doctors and fake medicines, knowing that by so doing they are imperiling the health of their readers."

Other speakers were Dr. Sucuki, Surgeon General of the Japanese Navy, Martin W. Littleton, Borough President of Brooklyn, and Louis E. Bomeisler.

"The Protection of the Water and Milk Supply" was discussed by Health Commissioner Darlington, ex-Commissioner Lederle, and others yesterday.

"What we want," Dr. Darlington said, "is chemicalized water filtration. Four years ago the land about the Croton watersheds could be bought for about $25 to $100 an acre, but to-day the price has been raised from $500 to $1,000 an acre.

At this high price it is impossible for the city to buy it. One acre of a filtration plant would cleanse 3,000,000 gallons of water a day.

"The enormous consumption of bottled spring, artificial and mineral water is largely an indirect tax upon the people. Poor people cannot afford it. They should have filtered water. A filtration plant, when the public expense of caring for sick and burying the dead is considered, would pay interest on the investment.

"It is an old idea that flowing water purifies itself. Within half a mile of its impure source, the impurity which may be discovered by chemical methods may be entirely lost. Bacteriologically, however, the impurity does not change perceptibly. Where we have human contamination we may look for human diseases to follow."

Dr. Darlington denounced an act of the last Legislature regarding water rights in Putnam County, which gives the residents of the county the right, after the city has constructed the reservoirs, to fish and row in them as well as the lakes.

October 19, 1905

MONAGHAN HASTENS TO TRIM QUACK LIST

Christian Scientist practitioners were classified inadvertently in the same category as patent medicine makers and hypnotists in the latest bulletin of the Department of Health, issued yesterday from the office of Health Commissioner Dr. Frank J. Monaghan, and as a result Dr. Monaghan said last night that some of his subordinates "will have to do some tall explaining."

The bulletin, listing forty-four "quack" cures and warning the public against their exorbitant claims of effecting cures, scarcely had been made public before a storm of protest was raised. Included in the list were Christian Scientists, Couéists, psycho-analysts and physical culturists.

The inclusion of these four was due to an error. Dr. Monaghan hastened to say last night, and he declared that orders for its correction would be issued at once.

"Other than these four, the list stands as printed," he said. "The object of enumerating these quacks is to guide the public mind in the right direction and warn them of the outrageous claims they make. Particularly do these claims appeal to the illiterate and unintelligent.

"Naturally medical men refute all their claims. Many complaints have been received by the department from medical men, and it was to inform the public of these complaints that the list was issued.

"Couéism may be all right in its way, and undoubtedly it has helped some people; so also, perhaps, have psychoanalysis and physical culture. And, of course, Christian Science is not to be regarded in the same light as drugless healing or beautifying establishments."

The bulletin in its present form reads:

"The Bureau of Public Health Education of the Department of Health, through the Weekly Bulletin, some time ago, requested physicians and other citizens to send in complaints relative to irregular medical practice.

"In consequence a large number of complaints were received by letter, telephone and in person. A tabulation of the different classes to which the individuals complained about belonged was made for office information.

"As it is thought that the information is interesting as indicating the wide realm from which quacks are drawn, and the serio-comic titles assumed by some, we publish the occupational classification of the individuals in question in the following list:

"Aero-therapy."	"Electronapro-
"Astral" healers.	therapy."
"Autothermy."	"Geo-therapy."
Beautifier Establish-	Hypnotist.
ments.	Hydro-therapy.
"Biodynamo-chro-	Herbalist.
matic" therapy.	Helio-therapy.
"Blood" specialists.	"Irido-therapy" diag-
Bone setters.	nosticians.
Cancer "cures."	Kneipp cure.
"Chromo-therapy."	"Leonic" healers.
"Christos" (blood	Mental and spiritual
washers)	healing.
Christian Science.	Medical gymnast.
"Chromopathy."	Mechano-therapy.
Coueists.	"Naturologist."
Diet-therapy.	"Naturopath."
Diathermy.	"Neuro-therapy."
"Drugless healers."	"Naprapath."
Electro-therapy.	Optical Institutes.
Electrotonic methods.	Obesity curers.
Electric light diag-	"Psycho-analyst."
nosis.	Patent Medicine Men.
"Electryonic" meth-	"Photo-therapy."
ods.	Physical culture.
"Electro-homeo-	"Physio-therapy."
pathy."	

Four Arrested as Fake Doctors.

Charged with practicing medicine without a license, Otorine Menmoli, 30 years old, who described himself as a student, of 211 Avenue A, was arraigned yesterday in Essex Market Court before Magistrate James M. Barrett, following his arrest on a warrant issued by Chief Magistrate William McAdoo. He was held in $500 bail for examination next Wednesday.

According to an affidavit which Albert Angelini of 26 Humbolt Street, Hoboken, signed, Menmoli was summoned to attend Angelini's sister, Mrs. Ida Heidelburger, at 211 Mott Street, in June, 1923, and, after many visits, at each of which Menmoli diagnosed her case differently, she was removed to Columbus Hospital, where she died.

While the affidavit states that Mrs. Heidelburger died after June, 1923, it was said at Columbus Hospital that the records there showed that Mrs. Heidelburger was admitted to that institution on April 17, 1923, and died there on April 25, or nearly two months before Menmoli is accused of having attended her.

It was announced by Assistant District Attorney Michael Ford in charge of the prosecution of fake doctors, that Adele Fluth, 2,010 Seventh Avenue, known as a "naturopath," was arrested by Policewomen Isabel Goodwin and Adele Pries, who allege she treated the latter, although not registered. B. C. Friedrich, 8,424 Twenty-third Street, Brooklyn, is accused of treating Mrs. Mildred Smaldon, 329 Third Avenue, and of borrowing $500 from her, as well. Raoul Pareant, 505 West 134th Street, is charged with treating Mrs. Carmelia Vuto, 311 East 112th Street, for dog bite.

The arrests are the first in the District Attorney's campaign against quacks.

February 15, 1924

U. S. WARNS PUBLIC ON URANIUM 'CURES'

WASHINGTON, March 17 (UP) —The United States Food and Drug Administration has warned that fraudulent uranium "cures" were sweeping the country.

In testimony before an Appropriations subcommittee of the House of Representatives, made public today, the agency also said deaths from cancer and other serious diseases were increasing because of "false cures."

The information came from George P Larrick, Food and Drug Commissioner. He urged approval of his agency's request for a 7½ per cent fund increase for the twelve months to start July 1. That would give it $5,-484,000 for the next fiscal year.

Mr. Larrick said lack of adequate money had made it impossible for his agency to keep up with a boom in quacks of all kinds. These, he said, included "health-food faddists catering to the ill, gullible and misinformed."

He said his agents also had been unable to keep pace with the growing use of "bootlegged" sleeping pills and other drugs, and use of "insect-infested • • • and decomposed foods."

But the newest problem for his agency, he said, was the growth of fake uranium "cures" that have "sprung up by leaps and bounds all over the country."

March 18, 1955

U. S. and A. M. A. Pledge Drive To End Billion-a-Year Quackery

By MARJORIE HUNTER
Special to The New York Times.

WASHINGTON, Oct. 6 — Americans were pictured today as spending more than a billion dollars a year in false hopes of getting well, getting slim or regaining lost youth.

That was the consensus of speeches made by medical and Government officials, including two members of President Kennedy's Cabinet. They spoke at the first annual National Congress on Medical Quackery.

The two-day congress is sponsored by the American Medical Association and the Food and Drug Administration. More than 600 persons attended today's opening session and heard thirteen speeches.

The Government officials and medical leaders pledged a full-scale fight on quackery—the practice of fraudulently offering cure-alls for such things as pains, bald heads and wrinkled skin.

Speakers attacked the three main forms of quackery:

Device quackery, including machines to cure assorted diseases or cause loss of weight; nutritional quackery, including health fads and vitamin supplements; and drug and cosmetic quackery.

Gone are the loud-talking medicine men of the past, only to be supplanted by sophisticated hucksters, the congress was told.

Too often the public thinks that quackery "went out with river boats, sideburns and the snake-oil hawker," said Dr. Leonard W. Larson, president of the American Medical Association.

"Quackery of today is commercial, it is almost respectable, it is cosmopolitan, it is modern," Dr. Larson said. "To me, one of the most difficult challenges facing us is to strip off this mask of respectability and to show the public the vicious, scheming villainy beneath."

Dr. Larson asserted that quackery "often operates under a pseudo-medical guise."

In this way, he said, "quackery draws patients into its fleece-lined spider's net of fraud and heartbreak."

Witch Doctor Gone, Too

Abraham A. Ribbicoff, Secretary of Health, Education and Welfare, said that the "witch doctor's tom-tom has given way to the illustrated brochure; the medicine show extravaganza to the television commercial."

He said that it was well known that he and the American Medical Association did not always agree on every subject.

"Today, we do not want to talk about giving each other trouble," he continued. "We want to talk about how to bring trouble—bad trouble—to a common foe: the charlatan and the quack who prey upon the innocent in search of better health."

The possibility of intensifying the battle against quacks was suggested by Postmaster General J. Edward Day and Paul Rand Dixon, chairman of the Federal Trade Commission.

Mr. Day said he was considering using a law, designed primarily to combat obscene matter, to impound fraudulent medical products pending outcome of court cases.

Will Seek Congress' Aid

Mr. Dixon said he would seek to persuade Congress to pass a pending bill giving his commission the authority to issue temporary cease-and-desist orders in food, drug and cosmetic cases.

Othre pledges of Government support in seeking to stamp out quackery came from Assistant Attorney General Herbert J. Miller Jr., speaking on behalf of Attorney General Robert F. Kennedy; and Commissioner George P. Larrick of the Food and Drug Administration.

Mr. Larrick said the most widespread and expensive type of quackery was the "promotion of vitamin products, special dietary foods and food supplements."

"Millions of consumers," he said," are being misled concerning their need for such products."

The annual cost of vitamin and health food quackery, he went on, is estimated at half a billion dollars a year.

Dr. R. W. Lamont-Havers of the Arthritis and Rheumatism Foundation said that about $250,000,000 was spent annually by arthritic victims in a vain attempt to relieve suffering.

He said the cause and cure of arthritis had not been found, but that sufferers still turned to anything that offers hope. He suggested that physicians try to inform patients better.

A program to discourage young men and women from enrolling in chiropractic schools was urged by Oliver Field, director of the American Medical Association's Department of Investigation.

"As the sage has observed, all the tribes of the earth love to have their backs rubbed, but it remained for the Americans to make a profession out of it," Mr. Field said.

He complained that the Government had given war veterans money to attend chiropractic schools.

October 7, 1961

HOSPITALS

THE NEW JOHNS HOPKINS HOSPITAL.
BALTIMORE, May 8.—The Johns Hopkins Hospital, which was formally opened yesterday, is thought to be the most richly-endowed, largest, and best institution of the kind in the world. It is open to the poor as well as to the rich. It cost $2,000,000, and the 17 buildings, with one or two exceptions, are connected by covered passages. Telephones connect the different apartments, and everything about the institution is wonderfully complete. There are buildings for physicians, nurses, and students as well as for patients and contagious diseases. The lecture room for clinical instruction will accommodate 250 students.

An emergency fund of $100,000 for the benefit of Johns Hopkins University has been contributed by a number of persons. Mr. and Mrs. Lawrence Turnbull of Baltimore have endowed a memorial lectureship of poetry with $20,000.

May 9, 1889

HOSPITAL BABIES TAGGED

"Pinafore" is not repeating itself in the maternity hospitals of New York. There are no mixed babies, and the "upper crust" baby has no chance to become exchanged with the "plebeian," as in the sad tale of Little Buttercup in the classic opera of long ago.

It is a marvel to an outsider how in a hospital where there are half a hundred, more or less, of exactly the same carmine complexioned infants, t'other is told from which. There might be some uncertainty as to whether a distinction was always made if in most of the hospitals, as soon as the little morsel of humanity arrived in the world, it was not immediately tagged for identification. There is some method of doing this in most of the maternity hospitals in the city, where little mortals are ushered into life.

There was published not long ago an account of the way the tagging of new born infants was done in the Johns Hopkins Maternity Hospital of Baltimore. There, it seems, as soon as the baby arrives a rubber adhesive plaster is clapped on its innocent little back, and on this is written in indelible ink the name, number, and any necessary details. The plaster will remain for an indefinite period, does not come off in the bath, and is always in place to surely and positively tell who the baby is. As far as investigations have gone, this precise method of tagging is not in use in New York, though a nurse, who has seen the tagged babies at the Johns Hopkins, says it is an excellent method, and a doctor familiar with it also agrees that it is one of the best methods of marking known.

As for babies being mixed, quite a thorough search only revealed one story, and that case was only known by hearsay, and occurred nobody knows how many years ago, in the Dublin Lying-in Hospital. One of the principals of the mixing was the professor of obstetrics, who was the instructor in that line of medical work of a physician now in New York. The story was one which the doctor related at intervals as an illustration of possibilities in handling small babies.

One day, the story goes, several babies entered this world of woe at almost exactly the same time at the Dublin Hospital. The reception room for new babies at this hospital was under a big rotunda, where a big open fire was kept burning. There was a fender to keep the sparks from flying, and as the babies arrived they were laid on a slab in front of this fire wrapped carefully in blankets to keep them warm, until their wardrobes should be prepared, or there was a lady's maid or valet ready to attend to their first toilets. That was where all the trouble came in. When the doctors were ready to take up the mites by the fire the truth gradually dawned upon them that they had not the slightest idea which of those babies was which. There was no means of telling, but a baby was given to each mother and they never knew the difference, for the doctors never told.

There has been sometimes, they say, a slight confusion of names in the little foundlings who go to Randall's Island by way of the Department of Outdoor Poor. They are named by the Commissioner in the city, properly tagged, and started on their journey. But in some way the tags get mixed. It does not make so much difference when Mary is tagged Susan, but when Elizabeth is tagged William and William tagged Elizabeth, what a humiliation to William's manly spirit, until the nurses have straightened out the babies, and William wears his own individual tag and is himself again.

The only other case of mistaken identity that can be found is where the mother does not know her own baby and insists that the baby given her afterward is not the one she has taken to the hospital. This is usually in cases of older babies, which come from the poorer homes in the city. When they are taken to the hospital they are frequently dirty, frowsled, and dressed in shabby, dirty clothes. The first thing done to the child is to wash and dress it, and this simple process often makes a genuine transformation in the appearance of the child. Then frequently the mother will not see her baby for two or three weeks, and in that time it changes from a sickly, emaciated little creature to a healthy, plump baby, and with the change in its complexion, caused by a rational system of bathing, it is altered so greatly that she will declare that it does not belong to her.

As for the method of identification of the babies at the different hospitals, at Bellevue there is a strip of adhesive rubber plaster put around the baby's wrist, marked with an indelible pencil with the baby's name and number, or only the number if it has not a name, and any necessary details. At the Nursery and Child's Hospital the marking is about the same. A little bracelet, as they call it there, is put on each baby's wrist. It is made of the plaster, a narrow strip doubled together so that the two sticky sides are together, fastened carefully at one end, and the bracelet is made large enough to move a little on the wrist, but not large enough to slip over the hand. On this the baby's name and number is written as soon as it is dressed in its first gown.

Incidentally it is interesting to know that of babies born in the hospital it is very seldom that there is one who has not a name waiting for it, and by which it is marked as soon as it is dressed. Twin babies came to one mother the other day, and for even this double number there were names enough to go around, and the mother announced them immediately.

Nurses all say that there is as much individuality in a little baby as in an older one, and once seen there is no danger of confusing identity. At the New York Infirmary for Women and Children they have a particularly attractive room for the small babies. They have it to themselves, and their little beds are in the shape of baskets of iron, dainty little affairs, which are hung from the wall. The maternity ward in the hospital is not large, and there are not under a dozen little babies in the hospital usually at a time. They are all tended separately, and in each little basket are the baby's name and number.

As soon as a mother has seen her baby there is no danger of her forgetting it, if the nurses should. There was a good illustration of that the other day. One poor little baby was not getting enough to eat to keep him in a healthy condition, while another had enough and to spare. So without remark the baby who needed food was taken to the mother of the baby who had too much. No one told her that it was not her baby, but she knew it immediately, and said so.

At the Sloane Maternity Hospital, where they probably have more little babies at a time than in any hospital in the city, often not far from a hundred, they tag them by the wrists. At the New York Foundling Asylum the babies are marked with little cards tied to the waists of the little gowns. Two babies sleep together in a crib, and when the children are undressed for the night the cards stay with the little frocks, ready to be put on in the morning. When a baby is sent out to board, or wherever it goes, it wears this card marked with all necessary particulars and its number. These numbers at the asylum date from the first child received there, and include all of the children—those born there and the mites of a few hours old taken in—and the numbers put on the cards now are in the thirty-first thousand.

At the Mothers' and Babies' Hospital they tag the babies at the waist with a regular business tag, such as is used to mark mercantile goods, and at the Hahnemann Hospital they are not tagged at all. They have only a small number of babies, half a dozen or so at a time, and it is never found difficult to identify them. They are put to sleep by themselves in little beds made for the purpose, high at the head against the wall and low at the foot and broad, so that three or four babies will only comfortably fill a bed.

All nurses say without hesitation that, no matter how small a baby is, it has its individual characteristics and there is not the slightest difficulty in distinguishing it from any number of other babies. The doctors are some of them less certain.

Dr. L. L. Seaman, for a number of years chief of staff of the maternity department at the Charity Hospital, says the babies there were marked in a way similar to those at other hospitals, with tags fastened around the neck. He has never known of a case of mixed babies.

May 20, 1900

THE NEW YORK HOSPITALS

The general relation of the people at large to the hospital has greatly changed within recent years. The hospital is now considered a beneficent institution, not only for the poor, but for the people of moderate means and even for the wealthy. Going to a hospital does not mean, either, that the case is practically hopeless. It means better care for the patient, with a great relief to the family from physical as well as mental strain, and it may mean a lessening of expense. Investigation in different hospitals shows a marked increase in the number of private patients. This is appreciated by the hospital authorities, for the bulk of their work being purely benevolent and conducted with a large outlay, the private patients, who pay for their comforts and the attention they receive, help to support the other work.

"There is an increase of at least 75 per cent. in the number of private patients we receive at this hospital," the Superintendent of the Roosevelt Hospital said, speaking of the private patients the other day, "within a comparatively few years. There were six rooms for private patients when I came here, seventeen years ago, and we have at the present time twenty-eight of our thirty-nine private rooms occupied. Private patients were not encouraged at that time.

"We do not emphasize the point of economy to a patient who comes to the hospital. In the private rooms there is paid something more than the cost, and in this way we obtain a certain income for the benevolent work in the wards where the patients may or may not pay a cent. There is no doubt but there is a great advantage in many cases for the patient who comes to a hospital. In the ordinary dwelling, where there are many draperies and much upholstered furniture, there is no chance for the antiseptic conditions that are so essential in case of sickness. In the hospital there is everything that is required for any emergency, and there are always members of the house staff at hand when the visiting physician is away. Then take a case of typhoid fever, the special treatment is with cold baths, into which the patient is placed to reduce the temperature. We have here portable bathtubs, which are used for this purpose, and which would not be found in a private house, and the work is greatly simplified.

"The rooms range in price from $25 to $75, the greater number being $25 and $30 rooms. If the case is not serious there need be no extra expense for a special nurse, and the patient is attended by one of the regular nurses of the hospital. If it is necessary to have special treatment, we have always on our list a number of graduate nurses, sometimes as many as twenty-five, who can be called upon at short notice to do the work. For each twelve hours the nurse is paid $4. Of this she receives $3, the remainder paying her board. The nurse is necessary in serious cases, and often the presence of a special nurse is a great comfort to a nervous patient.

"In case of friends who desire to enter the hospital with the patient, they can take a room at the regular price and remain in the hospital until the recovery of the patient. A wife sometimes comes with her husband, or a mother with her daughter. We have a wealthy Fifth Avenue woman, who has taken one of the best suites in the hospital, here now, and who has brought with her her husband and her companion. They probably will have been here six weeks before they leave. The woman and her companion have one room, and the husband another, and he comes and goes as he pleases. It is a great convenience. A person of wealth can of course create proper conditions in a case of illness if there is time, but it means a great amount of effort, and by coming to the hospital they can go home comfortably when they are convalescent and not find it necessary to disinfect the house.

SOLVES A PROBLEM FOR MANY.

"The possibility of going to the hospital solved a problem for people living in hotels. I have in mind one case of a young man above his majority who was living with his parents at a hotel when he was taken sick. The three came to this hospital, the father and mother staying the entire time that the son was ill."

There is a special pavilion for the private patients at the Roosevelt Hospital, and the rooms are fitted up with every convenience. There is the little metal bedstead in each room, pretty furniture of either birch or mahogany, with a wardrobe, bureau, a big easy chair and couch, and pretty rugs on the floor. The two pieces of upholstered furniture are covered with denim and have over this pretty slips of figured chintz which can be removed and laundered. In some cases of fever, like typhoid, these pieces are removed from the room.

There is a diet kitchen and serving room on each floor from which meals are served after being sent from the kitchen and where the pretty china and silver tea and coffee services are kept. There is an attractive reception parlor in which the visitors are received.

At St. Luke's Hospital they tell the same story of the increasing demand for private rooms. The figures of their last report show the increase in the past year.

"I do not see why treatment in a hospital should not be an economy as well as a benefit in other ways," said the Superintendent of St. Luke's Hospital. "Take a surgical operation for instance. In an ordinary household there is not the complement of effects required for the work. When an operation is performed there is not only the surgeon to pay but the etherizer, and the assistant as well as the nurse. In other cases, such as pneumonia and typhoid fever, and where baths are required, treatment can be given in a hospital that it is very difficult to give in a private house.

"Our charges here are from $3 to $6 a day. Take a medium price, $4 a day, and estimate what the patient will receive for it. In a serious case the physician would feel it necessary to call at the house several times a day, while in a hospital he can leave the patient in charge of the members of the house staff, and they are always ready in case of an emergency. One nurse has charge of four patients where there is no special attendant, and in cases where the illness is not very serious or does not require constant attention it may not be necessary to have a special attendant, perhaps only a night nurse. After the most serious part of the illness is over, the special nurse can be discharged and one of the regular nurses take the case. Medicines and dressings in a surgical case are included, and there are the delicacies for the sick which are given the patient which would add materially to the cost of caring for a patient at home. The patient is better off and the house is not upset.

"Friends coming with the patient is discouraged here. When patients are very ill temporary accommodations can be arranged for them. It can be put down as one of the advantages of a hospital that the relatives and friends do not take care of the patients. It is much better for them not to be under the care of any one who is overconcerned for them. We have no special pavilion for private patients, and no accommodations for their friends. Possibly they would be admitted more freely if we had greater accommodations. The income from the rooms benefits the general work. The charitable work is the chief work of the hospital. The big work done at the Roosevelt and the New York Hospital for the poorer people is the primary work, and it is growing more and more expensive every year.

"It cost us last year 1.82 per capita for our ward patients, that is $12 plus per week. The largest sum taken from any patient is $10.50. We do not turn any one away who cannot pay; all are treated alike, and nurses and doctors do not know one from the other. Modern surgery, modern medicine, and modern sanitary conditions are expensive, and even the method of building makes an additional first cost. This building is put up in the pavilion form, and in every one of our wards the sun shines some part of the day on every pleasant day."

AT THE NEW YORK HOSPITAL.

At the New York Hospital the new private patient pavilion opened a couple of weeks ago speaks for itself as to the demand for rooms for private patients. It is a large building, facing Sixteenth Street, and will accommodate sixty patients. Half of the rooms were engaged within the first week after the opening, and it is expected that there will be another influx of patients after New Year's, as people, when it is possible, put off leaving home until the holidays are past.

The new building has everything that modern sanitary knowledge can suggest and is like a great hotel, with its rooms prettily furnished with brass bedsteads, couches, Morris chairs, writing desks, open fireplaces, double doors to each room, diet kitchen, and serving rooms, lavatories and bathrooms on each floor. There is pretty china for the service of meals, with every convenience for keeping the stores and cooking. A cold-storage plant will be put in soon.

In addition to the private rooms there are semi-private wards, four of them with eight beds, and ten in the remainder. Patients pay $14 a week for beds in these rooms, and this includes the attendance, with only the additional expense of the surgeon's fee. These semi-private wards are to be found in other hospitals in the city.

In the maternity as well as the general hospitals there is noticed an increased tendency among people of means or in comfortable circumstances to take advantage of the opportunities offered them in such places. There are private rooms in the Sloane Maternity Hospital, and in some cases the wives of physicians have been treated there. At the Mothers and Babies' Hospital, Lexington Avenue, they say that the demand for private rooms is increasing, and noticeably so within the last year. The increased tendency of people to live in a limited space in the city makes hospital treatment desirable. Many of the patients have been women living in flats, boarding houses, or hotels.

Women can have rooms for $10, $20, and $30 a week, and there is one suite of rooms for which there is a charge of $50. There are two patients in the $10 room, which is off one of the wards, and there is a more elaborate bill of fare for the patients in the more expensive rooms, and special attendants. In the $50 suite there are separate rooms for tending the mother and baby.

Many people who have had the experience of being ill in and out of the hospital are greatly in favor of the former, especially where, as in many cases, the breaking down of some member of the family from overwork and anxiety follows, where the patient has been ill at home, although the trained nurse may also have been in attendance.

December 31, 1900

BELLEVUE OF THE PAST AND PRESENT

THERE is a great deal of curiosity about the "new Bellevue," as it is called, on which work is now in progress, and which is intended to make Bellevue one of the greatest, as well as one of the most interesting, municipal hospitals in the world.

Other big hospitals have a consecutive history of their foundation and progress. Bellevue has not. Very little is known about old Bellevue. A book called "Contemporary Biography of Eminent Men in the State of New York," published in 1878, gives a number of facts concerning men connected with Bellevue's early days, but beyond occasional fragmentary newspaper articles nothing has been written of the human side of this great institution. There are still men in Bellevue who remember the effort of one old pensioner to do it. He turned in his "copy" at the end of one year's hard labor, and in 32,000 words had just reached the description of the breaking of the ground for the foundations of the first hospital building. His story was never finished.

The foundation of what is now a portion of the main building of the famous old charity hospital, and which will be incorporated in the new one, was laid in 1811. At that time the City Almshouse, close by the present City Hall, was very much overcrowded. Before the Revolutionary war New York had few poor persons to take care of. After the war immigrants from Europe, most of them penniless and without friends, began to pour in so rapidly that in 1795 the corporation was obliged to look around for a larger almshouse. Bellevue was decided upon. The now populous tenement neighborhood was then a beautiful woodland, varied in surface, with a bold shore and a wide sweep of the river, unconfined by wharves and bulkheads. Blackwell's Island was still covered with trees.

PRISONERS AS NURSES.

In the early days of Bellevue no trained nurses smoothed the pillows of the sick. They were cared for, after a fashion, by male and female prisoners from the penitentiary, rough and rude characters, the dregs of the worst element in a rapidly growing city. The majority of the convict nurses, too, were foreigners, and did not understand what they were told to do. There was always one continuous grievance; the doses of whisky and other spirits sent from the medicine room to the patients seldom reached their bedsides.

In 1816 the almshouse and hospital had become so large as to require the services of a resident physician and surgeon. There were two visiting surgeons who went to the hospital twice a week and advised the house staff. At that time the Superintendent of the almshouse made all the appointments, even the physicians. They were removable at his will. Dr. John Van Buren was resident for thirty years at an annual salary of $500. The penitentiary was so crowded in the Spring of 1822 that a treadmill was started in the hope that it would terrify evil-doers and reduce the number of prisoners. It was worked by male and female prisoners, and could grind from forty to fifty bushels of corn a day, quite enough to supply the almshouse and the penitentiary. The formal opening of this treadmill was a public event, attended by the Mayor.

Objection was made to purchasing this site because it was too far from the city—about three miles. Finally, in 1811, the Corporation paid about $3,500 for six acres of land, a portion of the original Rose Hill Farm, extending from about Twenty-first Street to Thirtieth Street and to Third Avenue.

The stone for the new almshouse was quarried on the property. The cornerstone was laid by De Witt Clinton. The war of 1812, with England, blockaded the harbor and the work progressed very slowly. The main building was about 320 feet long, three stories high, and 50 feet wide. Two hospitals were built in the rear, a penitentiary for petty commitments, a workhouse, and a chapel. The total cost was $418,794, an extravagance at that time which called forth more criticism than the appropriation for the subway to-day. The original purchase was sold in parcels to pay for it.

WHEN TYPHOID RAGED.

In 1825 a malignant typhoid fever broke out in Bellevue, carrying off many of the patients and their convict nurses. The pestilence was beyond control for a month, and was finally made the subject of legislative investigation. It resulted in Dr. Isaac Wood, sometimes called the "Father of Bellevue," being appointed resident physician. Under his management the hospital and prison departments were permanently separated, and other sanitary reforms instituted.

Finally politics began to creep into Bellevue, and Dr. Wood retired. Positions were regarded as party prizes, and the management became lax. Licentiousness, disorder, and filth abounded. There was another epidemic of fever, more deaths, and the Common Council jumped in. An investigating committee heard testimony from all the leading physicians in the city, and finally, in 1849, the office of resident physician was abolished, and the management of the hospital was turned over to a medical board.

The first annual report of Bellevue was made by Dr. Crane, in 1848. The yearly average then was about 1,000 patients. The physician in chief was a busy man, and the care of the patients was left largely to medical students, who paid tuition fees to the chief. The mortality was about one patient in five, and some of the reports of deaths entered on the books were original. One of them reads:

"Visitation of God and also a contusion of the head."

According to the report of Warden Charles Sutton in 1851, the number of patients treated annually was 5,000. This Warden replaced the rickety wooden bedsteads with iron ones, built a kitchen and laundry away from the wards, and introduced gas and steam heat. All these improvements came gradually and covered a period of four years. The patients began to climb up to 6,000 and 7,000 a year, so that in 1857 another story was added to the main building.

The reports of the successive wardens are very much alike, thanking God and the Commissioners for favors past and favors to come. A large part of the present sanitary improvements was due to the efforts of the late Dr. James R. Wood, who was a fast friend and frequent visitor at the hospital, as well as one of its principal operating surgeons. Some of the most difficult and still remarkable operations performed by that eminent surgeon took place in Bellevue. Dr. Wood was largely instrumental in founding Bellevue Medical College, and was the founder of the anatomical and pathological museum now connected with it.

All day and all night long ambulance wagons are running in and out of Bellevue gate, answering and returning from hurry calls for the injured. Patients too poor to go anywhere else find shelter at Bellevue. Even as it stands to-day, there is no institution to compare with it in this country, and in its remodeled form it will be one of the foremost public hospitals in the world.

When an ambulance reaches the receiving ward—one of the most pitiful places to visit in New York—a bell summons the house surgeon or one of his assistants. The case is quickly diagnosed, the patient sent to a ward, and a ticket number placed over his or her bed. If the patient is a woman and she is unconscious, as most women are who are taken there, means of identification can be attended to afterward. In the ward a doctor and a nurse do all that is necessary for the present, until the house physician makes his rounds and gives further orders.

The white man and the black man, honest man and thief, in cots side by side, all undergo the same treatment. None is too poor or too abandoned to be admitted. The dirtiest tramp that walks the street can get as good, often better, treatment than persons with homes who send for the family doctor.

The Medical Board, which has exclusive control of the Medical and Surgical Departments of the hospital, is composed of some of the most eminent physicians and surgeons in the city. They make their own assignments for the year, arranging it so that eight or nine of their number visit their special divisions every day. The thirty or more young doctors who are kept at the hospitals for daily service in the wards go through the divisions with the specialists. They are absolutely under their orders in the method of treatment; they cannot leave the hospital without the permission of the warden; they must be ready promptly when wanted; their discipline is almost military.

Visitors are admitted under certain regulations, but most of the unfortunates that fill Bellevue's wards have no friends to call on them. Sometimes patients whose beds are side by side strike up an acquaintance, but oftener than not the silence in a ward with one hundred persons is unbroken except by the nurses. The colorless faces, with closed eyes, are like the faces of the dead. A man falls asleep after a brief chat with a man in the bed next him, speaking hopefully of the morrow. Before morning curtains are hurriedly drawn around the bed.

September 13, 1903

COST OF NEW BELLEVUE WILL BE $11,000,000

World's Greatest Hospital That Will Shelter 3,000 Patients.

TO COVER THREE CITY BLOCKS

New Structure Will Be Full of Windows and Fresh Air, and It Will Take Ten Years to Complete It.

For the next ten years, if the plans of the architects are approved, the City of New York will be building in installments the greatest hospital in the world. The cost of the enormous structure, containing twelve pavilions and embodying all the appropriate improvements of modern science, will be $11,000,000—something less than one-third the price paid for the underground railroad from the City Hall to the Bronx. The hospital will be the new Bellevue, of which a generation of overworked physicians have dreamed, and the plans were made public for the first time yesterday afternoon.

Dr. John W. Brannan, President of the Board of Trustees of the City Hospitals, and Messrs. McKim, Mead & White, the architects, chose the occasion of a lecture by Dr. Brannan in Havemeyer Hall for showing the plans. Not only were drawings of the new Bellevue exhibited and explained, but there were charts of the new Harlem and Fordham Hospitals, as well as of the improvements now in progress on Gouverneur Hospital. The appropriation of $75,000 made by the city for securing plans provided for remodeling all of the four institutions under the Trustees.

The cost of the new Bellevue building—$11,000,000—does not include the expense of condemning the East River block between Twenty-eighth and Twenty-ninth Streets, just north of the present Bellevue site. That block, which will make the hospital grounds cover three whole blocks, is now in process of condemnation. Most of the property is cheap, but the electric light plant alone, Dr. Brannan estimates, will cost the city about $1,000,000. Nor does the $11,000,000 include the filling in of a large strip of what is now river. The War Department, by special action, has consented to the extension of the bulkhead line so that it will include enough space to make a rectangle out of the three blocks.

The new hospital, in which nearly 3,000 patients may be treated, will cover almost all the available space from Twenty-sixth to Twenty-ninth Street. Along those two streets, extending from the river to First Avenue, will be two great wings, and they will be connected by a series of structures including the central administration section and two smaller wings. These smaller wings will be parallel with the big wings. On the four ends of the small wings will be cupolas, architecturally similar to the tall dome in the very centre of the building.

NEW GROUNDS SPACIOUS.

On the river side of the hospital and on the First Avenue side the grounds are to be about 250 feet across, and if there ever comes a time when the facilities need further stretching still other sections of the structure, now unplanned, may be erected so as to make a quadrangle with the dome in the centre and with courts under it to the east and west. The authorities, however, say they hope this never will be necessary, as the institution is intended primarily to be one distinguished for its all-light wards, its plentiful sunshine, and its clear sweep of unobstructed breezes.

In the accompanying illustration the hospital is shown as it will look from First Avenue. Its appearance from the river will be practically the same, except that on the water side there will be seven full stories instead of six, because of the slope of the ground from First Avenue.

Over the entire building will be a roof garden, to which many elevators will run. No ward will be without its elevator. At certain points on the roof will be glass-inclosed sections, where weaker patients may be sheltered and yet out of doors. In bad weather these covered areas will be capable of extension.

Fresh air, plenty of it all the time, that is what Dr. Brannan says is the main thing in a modern hospital. In no other institution anywhere has this idea been carried out as it will be in Bellevue. Besides the ample roof, there will be a multitude of balconies. To quote Dr. Brannan: "There is enough room on top, but these balconies will be useful for patients who are not able to find an attendant ready to take them up to the roof. They can't go up by themselves, but it will be easy to step out on the balcony. We want open-air places whither they can step at all times, on the moment the notion strikes them. I believe our discoveries about the advantage of outdoor air in the treatment of tuberculosis have had more than anything else to do with the realization that the same element is good for acute maladies."

Eight out of the twelve pavilions will have their windows toward the river, and in them there will be no bed from which the occupant cannot see the water at all times by a slight movement of his body, and in every ward the windows will occupy more space than the spaces between. Bellevue is to be a hospital of windows, fine views, and sunlight.

SITE OF THE NEW HOSPITAL.

The block between Twenty-eighth and Twenty-ninth Streets is now in process of condemnation. The dotted lines show the new bulkhead limit ordered by the War Department at the request of the hospital trustees.

TO BUILD BY DEGREES.

The plans of the architects are intended to be very general. Few of the details have been worked out, for the building must be done by degrees as the construction of the American Museum of Natural History is being carried on at Central Park West and Seventy-seventh Street. There will be one wing built at a time.

Up to date, the Board of Estimate and Apportionment has been asked for $702,000 for the first pavilion, and the trustees expect to get that sum before the Summer is over. Now that condemnation proceedings have been begun for the block between Twenty-eighth and Twenty-ninth Streets, the closing of the one block of Twenty-eighth Street will be taken up. This was considered a stumbling point at the start, but the matter is adjusting itself. At first the neighboring merchants complained that they could not get along without the East Twenty-eighth Street pier, but when the Dock Department agreed to make a pier at the foot of East Thirtieth Street the "kicks" ceased. The Board of Estimate will be asked within a few weeks to close the street as soon as the new pier is ready.

One of the city officials protested against the elaborate dome in the centre of the hospital, said Dr. Brannan. This dome, however, is not solely an ornament. It is

there that quarters will be prepared for 125 doctors, so that they will not be jammed into unwholesome, cramped rooms, as they are to-day. The Assistant Superintendent also will have his room there, and there will be a sitting room and a gymnasium for the internes.

The nurses, too, are to be well cared for. While in a few cases the younger physicians may sleep two in a room up in the dome, every nurse will have a separate bedchamber. Working twelve hours in a regular shift is the nurse's lot, and it has been decided that they ought to have every comfort without extravagant accommodations, however—during the "off hours." There is to be no more contracting of tuberculosis among employes because the city fails to house them like human beings.

FRESH AIR AND LOTS OF IT.

As for the other three hospitals under the Board of Trustees, Dr. Brannan told of the balconies now being added to Gouverneur, which was planned originally without regard to the need of fresh air, and about the fine buildings proposed for the Harlem and Fordham Hospitals. The Harlem, now located at One Hundred and Twentieth Street, at East River, will be at One Hundred and Thirty-sixth Street and Lenox Avenue, while the Fordham will occupy four acres of land secured out of the grounds of St. John's College, at Crotona Avenue and Southern Boulevard, opposite Bronx Park.

As the Southern Boulevard runs through the park, there can never be a trolley line running by the Fordham. The main building there is to be of simple architecture, with a fine roof garden and other improvements like those of the new Bellevue, on a smaller scale. The Harlem, too, will have its open roof, its comfortable quarters for both doctors and nurses, and its facilities for giving the patients plenty of room and light.

Dr. Brannan lectured for more than an hour before showing the new plans. He told about many things the layman does not know. When he first became a Trustee, he said, he believed that Bellevue ought to be rid of alcoholic, insane, and prison patients—classes which no other city hospital entertained.

"I have decided, though, that we should continue to care for them all," he said. "But we must have the facilities for doing so."

The recent overcrowding, he continued, was not to be called temporary. Bellevue and the other hospitals had reached their limits. Though not much had been said about it, the fact was that during the Winter the City and Metropolitan Hospitals were in just as bad a way as Bellevue.

"In the Metropolitan," he said, "there were not only patients on the floors, but they lay in the corridors as well during the season of greatest crowding."

For the first time in the history of the city, he said, as far as he knew, private hospitals sent their pneumonia patients to Bellevue this past Winter. More than 130 were sent down there. He told of serious cases made worse by transfers from hospital to hospital when beds were so scarce that even an old woman with a fractured hip had to be sent from pillar to post seeking a place to lay her head. He told of the male nurses at Bellevue—the only male nurses in any hospital—and how it finally had been decided to have a woman at the head of every ward, despite the fact that the men had objected strenuously in some cases against working under women.

"Speaking of nurses," he continued, "Bellevue has one nurse to nine patients. The private endowed hospitals have one nurse to four or five patients. Sometimes conditions at Bellevue have been worse even than this. Last week there were thirty-eight patients to two nurses in a ward. It is a physical impossibility for patients to receive anything like the proper care under such circumstances."

Of the ambulance system of the city, Dr. Brannan said he thought it haphazard to some extent, but still very efficient. He explained the district scheme, and how some hospitals had to cover more territory than they could cover thoroughly. It was not generally known, he said, that ambulance surgeons received no salaries at all, but were doing the work as part of their training.

He told of the new rule at Bellevue—that all cases of unconsciousness, from whatever cause, must be brought to the hospital for diagnosis; also all cases where the ambulance surgeon was in doubt, despite the old tradition about "roasting" the new man for a mistake, a custom not to be heard of hereabouts. Referring to the police, he said:

"And whenever the police order a patient to be carried to the hospital, that order must be obeyed. That is our rule. The police are not doctors, but they have had tremendous experience. When they say a man ought to be taken in, they are generally right. It is also a rule for the ambulance to go wherever a policeman orders, no matter how far out of a district. The police do not order outside trips without good reason. When they order the surgeon to go further, they are almost always right in doing so."

HARVARD TO BE CENTRE OF $20,000,000 MEDICAL PLANTS

FTEEN new buildings, of a total value of nearly $4,000,000, which will be parts of five hospitals, are under construction almost within a stone's throw of the Harvard Medical School in the Boston Fenway district. The five new hospitals, two of which will move into new quarters, added to the eleven medical institutions which already comprise the Harvard medical group, will make the hospital and clinical facilities of that school extraordinary.

Within a radius of half a mile from the Harvard Medical School there are built or under construction sixteen medical institutions, constituting the most wonderful medical plant in the world. When buildings now under construction are completed and in operation all the institutions will represent in value of buildings and capitalized funds about $20,000,000. Some of the sixteen will not have more than friendly relations with the others, but all are or will be engaged in medical work, and those who are acquainted with the detailed plans of the various boards of trustees say that the five new hospitals now being built will be so closely related to the Harvard School that it would be hard to tell them apart. Practically every one of the hospitals does or will specialize in certain kinds of disease.

Already the collection of medical institutions grouped in the Fenway is the largest single aggregation of buildings devoted entirely to the science of healing in the world, but its combined pre-eminence will be so great when the present projects are realized that every ailment, disability, infirmity, or physical misfortune of mankind can be treated in the narrow confines of the Fenway medical plant.

Incurables, the cancerous, consumptives, persons near insanity, women ailing from their peculiar diseases, individuals suffering from malnutrition, those afflicted with dental troubles, and children with any complicated troubles, all these could find in this radius institutions specially built for their needs, as well as others taking a more general class of patients.

The institutions already built and operating are varied in their work, but their utility will be greatly increased by the completion of the following six:

Harvard Memorial Cancer Hospital, being erected.

Thomas Morgan Rotch, Jr., building, which will house the Infants' Hospital, approaching completion.

Children's Hospital, to cost $500,000. Plans drawn and accepted and construction subject to decision of Board of Managers.

Peter Bent Brigham Hospital, fund of about $6,000,0000 for buildings and maintenance combined. Construction under way.

State Psychopathic Hospital, $600,000 appropriated for grounds and building. Construction under way.

Robert Brigham Hospital, amount of fund unstated. Foundations in, but construction halted.

Added to this there is a project to erect a Harvard dormitory and medical union clubhouse, to cost at least half a million dollars, and conducted on the same principle as the Harvard Union and dormitories, but for medical and dental students. These buildings would be open to all students and would provide facilities for dining, formal meetings, social gatherings and, as well, the best features of life in modern dormitories. The plan was put forward by Dr. J. Collins Warren about two years ago, but was halted by lack of funds to continue it.

The institutions now within easy distance of the Harvard Medical School and connected with it by reason of clinical exchanges, number nine, and are as follows:

Harvard Medical School, Longwood Avenue, extending to Van Dyck Street.

Harvard Dental School, Longwood Avenue and Wigglesworth Street.

Nutrition Laboratory of the Carnegie Institution of Washington, west side of Vila Street.

House of the Good Samaritan, Francis and Binney Streets.

New England Deaconess Hospital, 175 Bellevue Street.

Channing Home, Francis and Bellevue Streets.

Free Hospital for Women, Pond Avenue and Cumberland Road, Brookline.

Woman's Charity Club Hospital, Parker Hill, Roxbury.

New England Baptist Hospital, Parker Hill Avenue, Roxbury.

Co-operation rather than a more formal connection will mark the relations between the entire number of institutions, but the great advantages to be derived from close association are emphasized by the plans to extend the power plant of the medical school, which already serves four institutions, to meet the needs of four more. The single plant will provide light, heat, and power for about $6,000,000 worth of buildings when all the construction has been completed, and will be the largest institutional power plant in the world.

At present the medical school power station supplies the five huge marble buildings of the medical school, the dental school, the Carnegie nutrition laboratory and the House of the Good Samaritan. Plans are under way to extend it to serve the new Children's Hospital, the Thomas Morgan Rotch, Jr. memorial building, which will be the future home of the Infants' Hospital, the Harvard Memorial Cancer Hospital and

the Peter Bent Brigham Hospital, all of which possess real estate in what was originally the Harvard Medical School property of twenty-six acres.

The great significance of the work to be done by the entire series of establishments working separately and together was indicated by Dean Henry A. Christian of the Harvard Medical School.

"There were twenty-six acres in the original tract secured in the Fenway for the medical school," said Dean Christian, " and all but the eleven acres needed by the school itself have been taken by the other institutions which are centring in this district.

"This series of co-operating institutions will work together with the purpose of applying the most approved methods to the treatment of diseases, of furnishing the best facilities for the investigation of disease, and of giving medical instruction.

"Large as the medical plant as a whole will be, there will be no general director. I expect it will require close to $1,000,000 a year to maintain the plant we will have within almost a stone's throw of the administration building here. The medical school itself spends about $250,000 a year.

"Altogether the facilities for hospital treatment will amount to nearly 600 beds, and probably 2,000 people will be inmates, employes, students, and teachers or physicians in the buildings in this medical centre.

"There is little likelihood for duplication in following the well-defined purposes laid down, while together the institutions leave little in any branch of medicine untouched.

"Concentrating the purchasing power of the various institutions has been discussed, and it is probable that some scheme will be worked out.

"Doubtless the growth of this district as a medical centre will bring an increasing number of people to the vicinity."

A central information bureau for all disease discoveries is one of the great benefits foreseen by the doctors from the consolidation of the medical plants of so many institutions. It is hinted that a strenuous effort will be made to bring here permanently men who have risen to the foremost rank in their profession and to maintain them here for purposes of treatment of patients and investigations by laboratory and other means.

Another point of view was given by one of Boston's most prominent physicians, who pictured the great world benefit to be obtained by what he called the "intensive study and practice of medicine," which can be pursued with the advantages presented by the great group of medical institutions.

"Such a tremendous advantage for the public and the world will be gained that no one can estimate it," said he. "Take the case of cancer. With the facilities at command and the broad field offered for general medical work the man who has proved the value of a treatment can be secured and work here, not as an experimenter, but as a proved expert.

"There will be no tendency to make the hospitals experiment stations, but there will be a constant effort to bring here the best men obtainable, to give the best care of the sick, and to administer the best treatments that have been found valuable by testing."

December 31, 1911

URGES MORE CLINICS IN MEDICAL SCHOOLS

The current number of the Survey contains an article by William H. Welsch, M. D., LL.D., Baxley Professor of the Johns Hopkins University, favoring a wider coalition between medical schools and hospitals. In his article Dr. Welsch tells how " both at King's College in New York and at what is now the University of Pennsylvania, in the eighteenth century, the essential need of combining clinical instruction with the teaching of the medical school proper was recognized, and later the institutions furnishing these opportunities drifted apart."

Dr. Welsch said that Columbia University and the Presbyterian Hospital are fortunate in the alliance they have recently made to render the hospital more useful; enable it to serve the needs of both patients and the community more efficiently; will secure the best professional service for the hospital, and will make the hospital the centre of larger ideals by permitting education, by advancing knowledge, and by exemplifying the best in practice. And also that such an alliance will benefit the university, by enabling it to give the best clinical instruction to its students, and afford improved opportunities for advanced study.

Dr. Welsch says:

"Owing to the fact that our hospitals and schools have drifted apart, it is difficult at the present time to arrange affiliations between them. This separation

of functions did not exist at the beginning. Indeed it is curious to observe how correct were the ideals of the medical schools in this country in the eighteenth century. I feel, in solving its own problems, the Presbyterian Hospital has done a great service to medical education in America, because it has indicated how the problem can be solved elsewhere, not necessarily on precisely the same terms, but along the same general lines.

"There is practically no division of opinion among medical men as to the influence upon hospital service of these additions; but laymen are apt to conjure up in their minds conditions under which the inroads of medical students into a hospital would be disturbing to the order and quiet of the wards, and where the examination of patients for purpose of teaching might be harmful to the sick. For these alleged reasons the public may be induced to pause, at least, before accepting the idea that the use of a hospital for teaching increases its value in the treatment of patients. But those who have had experience know that nothing is further from the truth than such a conception of reduced service, for it has been demonstrated that, instead of weakening the humanitarian efficiency, the educaitonal and research functions increase the value of the service which a hospital fulfills in the care of its patients.

" As has already been stated, one of the reasons why ward patients are better served by the new arrangement is that the hospital is in a position to secure for its wards the very best professional service available; and by a permanent agreement of this kind the best professional service is secured not only for the immediate present but for the future.

"A hospital of this type will not only have the most talented men on its staff, but the men will also be of a distinctive type—not necessarily truer, better principled, but men singularly devoted, who realize that their first duty is to the allied interests of the hospital and the school, and that their life work and main enjoyment are to lie in the practice of medicine in the wards and private rooms of the hospitals, in teaching medical students, in the advancement of knowledge, and in the development of their departments of medicine.

" They are men who will not become absorbed in a large outside practice, be it even a consulting practice, which would interfere with this work. If, then, the hospital secures men of this type, who are to give their lives to the service of the patients, will not the hospital be better served, will not the ward patients be better cared for? The presence of the students in the wards will also tend to the better care and treatment of the sick and injured.

"From the method which is essential for the adequate training of medical students to-day great advantage is derived by the patients, because the latter are studied more carefully and thoroughly. The more thoroughly they are studied, the more will be known about the diseases that afflict them, and the better will be the chances of successful treatment. It is, therefore, beyond dispute that a teaching hospital connected with a university medical school makes better provision for the care of its ward patients than a charitable hospital with no other aim beyond the care of the indigent sick, important as that is.

" At the period when students are thus admitted into the wards they are not materially less fitted to work there than is the ordinary interne when he begins his work. This practical teaching begins usually in the fourth year of the medical school, when the students have already been taught the methods of physical diagnosis; they have already had opportunities of study in the out-patient department of the hospital. They come, therefore, not ignorant; and they work always under the close supervision and control of heads of departments and their associates. In the wards, students take clinical histories, make examinations of patients, and analyses of blood and other body fluids—taking charge, in fact, of a part of the routine necessary for the orderly working of the hospital."

February 19, 1912

FINEST HOSPITAL IN THE WORLD IN CINCINNATI
Elaborate Plant on the Segregated System Won After Ten Years of Hard Municipal Fighting.

THE City of Cincinnati is building what is expected to be the finest general hospital in the world. It will consist of thirty group buildings, eighteen of which have already been finished, all planned according to the latest ideas of hospital construction. The cost of the plant will approximate about $3,000,000. The buildings will be in the suburbs, but adjacent to and within a few minutes' access from the centre of the city.

Ten years ago Cincinnati was one of the worst equipped cities in the United States in the matter of hospital accommodations. Its chief municipal hospital was situated near the centre of the city, and on the banks of a foul canal. The main building was of the tumbledown variety. It was also infested with vermin, and overrun with rats and mice. The health, fire, and police authorities finally condemned the building. It was unsafe and unsanitary. It was really a fire trap, and the city officials began to dread what might happen if the place ever took fire.

The awakening of the political powers was the result of the indomitable persistency of a well-known citizen of great influence and power in civic matters, a man of the highest public and private repute, a recognized leader in all movements for municipal betterment, Dr. Christian R. Holmes. For several years Dr. Holmes had been Chairman of the Board of Hospital Commissioners. For years and years he had called attention to the deplorable condition of the city hospital. For years and years the hospital had to get along with meagre appropriations. There were few votes to be obtained in a place where scientific management and operation were demanded. Gradually the building ran down and the rats moved in. The Board of Hospital Commissioners were fighting a losing game, and they knew it. If worst came to worst, there would some day be a big smash-up when an epidemic or a fire would so arouse the people that the politicians would be swept aside. Some of the politicians also foresaw what would come. But Dr. Holmes and his colleagues were not content to await until a catastrophe should arrive. The sick had to be considered.

So Dr. Holmes and his colleagues had recourse to public agitation. They enlisted the zeal and public spirit of the people.

Finally the call for a new hospital became so masterful that the political authorities who had given Cincinnati a bad name throughout the land began to run for cover. Of course, the city ought to have a new hospital. They had been for it all along. They simply wanted to get public spirit crystalized so that the city should have the best that could be obtained. Dr. Holmes was the finest product of public spirit that they knew. They were proud of him, and to show that they meant what they said, and had always been for him, they actually tried to join in a great public dinner given to him in honor of his great effort to awaken Cincinnati. The new hospital was now assured. The fight had lasted for a decade. The city authorities voted $3,000,000 for the new hospital, and it was also voted to accept Dr. Holmes's ideas for its construction and equipment. He wanted the best there could be, and he was told to go ahead and make the institution up to date in every particular.

Accordingly, Dr. Holmes visited the best hospitals in Europe and this country, and studied their equipment and construction. He formulated his plans for segregated buildings, in accordance with the most improved ideas of hospital building. He selected a site of thirty acres away from the congested part of town, yet within easy reach, on high ground, surrounded by wooded hills.

In laying out the grounds and planning for the hospital buildings, attention was paid to the future expansion, and enough ground has been purchased to accommodate buildings for 100 years to come. An extensive study having been made of hospital construction, ideas were adopted from the Rudolph Virchow Hospital in Berlin, the Eppendorf Hospital in Hamburg, the Johns Hopkins in Baltimore, and others. The new hospital is built upon the corridor-pavilion type of the Johns Hopkins. The buildings are constructed more for utility of the interior than beauty of exterior.

This description of one of the ward buildings fits them all. The building is four stories high, with a bright and clean basement. On the fourth story is a roof garden, which connects with the top ward. Each floor is in itself a complete hospital, or what is technically known as a ward unit. It consists of a ward, containing twenty-four beds; four end rooms, treatment and lecture rooms, service kitchen, dining room for convalescent patients, bathroom, sink room, nurses' room, toilet and washrooms, linen closet, storeroom, blanket-warming closet, sun parlor, and corridor. If at any time it becomes necessary to isolate one of the floors, all the requirements for the operating of a complete hospital are there. This arrangement is repeated in all the ward buildings on the grounds.

The contagious group, devoted to scarlet fever, measles, and diphtheria, and consisting of three buildings, is a complete hospital in itself. It has been in use for nearly two years. There are few hospitals like this in the world. Here the patient is allowed to see a relative. The visitor is taken into a special room, puts on a cap, gown, and covering for shoes, and is then permitted to go to the patient's bedside. Upon leaving, the visitor is led into a disinfecting room and thoroughly disinfected. By an arrangement consisting of a wall of plate glass, the dead may be viewed by relatives without fear of contagion, an innovation in public hospitals.

Dr. H. T. Summergil of New York City, an expert in his field, will be the Superintendent of the new hospital. The new hospital group will not only have the advantage of an ideal situation, easily accessible from all parts of the city and suburbs, but the environment is such that there is no danger of encroachment of any kind. When finished it will stand as a monument to the awakened public spirit of Cincinnati.

December 1, 1912

285

Best of Care for Every Hospital Patient

By DR. JOHN G. BOWMAN,
Director of the American College of Surgeons.

WILL your treatment make a soldier of this man? Can he fight when you are through with him?

These are questions which the doctor in the United States Army today must answer as he goes about his work. In the case of a wounded soldier, who clearly cannot serve in the ranks again, the question is: Can you make this man capable to earn his living? The test of medical and surgical treatment in the army is in terms of men who can fight; or, failing the power to fight, the test is in terms of power to earn one's living. Results are what is wanted, results that mean strength to the army or happiness to the incapacitated man. Probably never before have practical results been demanded of the medical profession as they are demanded today in the army.

What does this military insistenc upon results mean? Just this: It means an effective effort to give each soldier, wounded or ill, the best service known in medicine and surgery. Every detail of that service is checked up, and for that reason unnecessary surgical operations, incompetent surgical operations, lax or lazy medical diagnoses are practically impossible to occur.

Where did the army get its medical efficiency of this character? Back of it all is a big idea, a "vision," a determination on the part of the leading surgeons of this continent which found expression four years ago. There was no world war then. But these surgeons met in Washington and with the highest seriousness that ever comes to men they asked: "Is the best surgery too good for the humblest patient? Are the standards of surgery as practiced in the great centres too good for the smaller communities? Have we no leadership in us to face these questions? Is there the slightest reason why we should not take hold with all the strength in us and force the right sort of ideals in surgery to come true all over our continent?"

That meeting in Washington was the beginning of the American College of Surgeons. It was the beginning of a great idea which today saves the life of many a soldier as well as the lives of untold thousands of laymen.

What did these surgeons do? They organized. They set for themselves the bringing about of the highest class of medicine and surgery in every community where medicine and surgery are practiced. In broad outline they proposed a continent-wide standardization of hospitals as a practical method to make their aim come true. Then they gave out of their own pockets more than $500,000 in order to set their plan into action.

Almost spontaneously that meeting set the most unselfish and idealistic project ever undertaken in any profession into action. But the very magnitude of the project inspired caution. It called for conservative leaders. Dr. John M. T. Finney of Baltimore was elected President and Dr. Franklin Martin of Chicago Secretary General. Dr. Martin was the man in whose mind the "vision" of an American College of Surgeons first took form, and it is interesting here to note that when Congress years later created the Council of National Defense the President of the United States appointed Dr. Martin as a member of that council in recognition of his ability to make big worth-while things happen.

But to come back to the story of the college. Its first task was to perfect its organization. Strong, active committees were appointed in each State in the Union and in each province in Canada, and through these committees 3,000 additional surgeons were admitted to Fellowship in the college. The college, it must be remembered, is a society of surgeons and not a teaching institution. Its members are known as Fellows, and all surgeons of worthy character and of real competence are welcome to Fellowship. The college enrolls today 3,700 Fellows.

When matters of organization were fairly accomplished, actual headway toward hospital standardization was still a long way off. An enormous inertia had to be overcome. In many a community things were "good enough as they are." Also it was difficult for doctors, hospital Superintendents, and laymen to understand that the college had no ulterior or selfish motive in its work. It was difficult to understand that the aim of the college was exactly the aim of every good hospital; that it was exactly the highest aim which the medical profession had long ago set for itself, and that that aim was simply to bring to every man, woman, or child who was sick or injured the best possible care, no matter where the patient lived or what his circumstances were.

In a tentative fashion, therefore, hospital standardization was approached. Widespread good-will was essential to success. On behalf of the Catholic hospitals, Cardinal Gibbons reviewed the proposed program and gave his verbal and written approval to all of it. Later Father Charles B. Moulinier, S. J., President of the Catholic Hospital Association, became a member of the staff of the college engaged in this work, and is in that position today. The American Hospital Association unanimously indorsed the program and appointed a committee to co-operate with the college. Practically all opposition fell away as soon as the project and the motives back of it were really understood.

Up to this time the whole plan remained in broad outline. But when expressions of heartiest co-operation streamed in from doctors, hospitals, and laymen in more abundant measure than any Fellow had dared to hope, then came the time for specific details of the plan. Just what standard was to be set up?

In order to answer this question the Fellows of the college elected a Standards Committee in each State and province of the two countries. These committees met for two days in Chicago. About 250 surgeons were present, together with a large group of hospital Superintendents, internists, hospital trustees, and laboratory workers. This body centred its attention on three questions: What do we have in hospitals? What do we want in hospitals? How do we propose to get what we want in hospitals?

Out of the conference came a plan of action, a plan definitely formulated, but essentially the same as the one proposed by the charter members of the college at the first meeting. The entire emphasis was placed upon results in the care of patients. It was standardization not of material things, not of bottles, or apparatus, or buildings, or reputation of doctors, but of principles. The patient, the patient, the patient! The beginning and the end of all medical service and of all hospital service are the welfare of the patient. As the prime factor in hospital standardization, therefore, the college asks: What was the matter with the patient? What did the doctor do for him? Was the patient relieved or cured? If not, why not?

Then came the war. The leaders in surgery, filled with the purpose of carrying scientifically sound surgery to the furthest districts of the continent, volunteered in the army, and the swift consequence was that the essential ideas of standardization, now studied for years, were put into practice in the army. But let us see, further, what that plan is.

If doctors are to know the results of their work they must have exact facts. They must know what has happened to each patient. In other words, they must keep what are known as case records. Case records tell the story of each case under such headings as these: Complaint of the patient, diagnosis on which treatment was based, laboratory analyses, physical findings, important points of operation or treatment, complications of convalescence, and post-operative or final diagnosis.

The keeping of complete case records, therefore, is the first requirement in hospital standardization. There is no debate as to whether that requirement is sound. But the second requirement is even more important. The keeping of the records is in itself not enough. The second step is to profit by these records. The college asks that all physicians and surgeons who practice in any given hospital meet at regular intervals, and that with the highest seriousness in their hearts they review the results of their work. They are to ask themselves in a fearless, calm way: What did we do for our patients? Were they relieved or cured? If not, why not? They are to analyze their own work in order to answer such questions.

By way of illustration, let us see what may happen at one of these meetings: Suppose that the doctors meet to review the work done in a given hospital during the last three months. Suppose that an analysis of the surgical cases under review shows that 6 per cent. of the patients developed infection during convalescence which reasonably were chargeable to the hospital. The facts as to the per cent. of infections may easily be determined from properly kept records; and it goes without saying that these infections are a serious indictment of the surgical service. Now let us assume that 90 per cent. of the cases developing infection were patients of a particular surgeon. Under such circumstances the position of the college is that an obligation rests upon the doctors to demand that either this surgeon discover the cause of his unsuccessful work and remove that cause, or that he discontinue practice in the hospital.

As a people we have come to look upon service from the medical profession as a right, very much as we conceive our right to hold property. If a man has his foot crushed, for example, in a street accident, he gets medical care irrespective of his ability to pay for that care. In so far now as we accept the idea that we have a right to health, it follows that the hospital is a public service corporation, and is accountable to the public for the quality of all of its work. The time has come when the hospital, as an institution, should in all fairness make to its community a true accounting of its work.

How, the college asks, can any hospital guarantee honest, competent service to its patients if it does not know the truth as to what happens to its patients? Not only should the hospital know exactly what happens to its patients, but it should make every reasonable effort to see that mistakes due to carelessness, laziness, or lack of training do not occur a second time. A hospital in which no earnest attention is given to these matters is sometimes merely a boarding house for sick people, and not a benefit to its community.

What does this plan of standardization have to do with the hospital laboratory? That is an interesting phase of the problem. As soon as a doctor who practices in a hospital realizes that his success or failure with each patient comes under the scrutiny of his fellow-practitioners, he gathers a sharpened incentive for success. He takes no chances with mere guesswork in diagnoses. He demands every laboratory facility which may help him find out what is the matter with his patient. It is only human that he should throw more intense earnestness into his work. And what has actually happened is that in many a hospital a first-class laboratory, under a competent laboratory worker, is today in operation where, until recent years, no need for such a laboratory was really expressed.

As for the cost to the hospital of putting the whole plan into action, little need be said. The real cost is one of effort on the part of the staff. Even in the smallest communities the public has responded liberally when the doctors have asked for help. The fact is that no community, however small, can afford to maintain a hospital only 50 per cent. efficient. In this connection the inspiring fact is that 90 per cent. of the hospitals of this continent has taken up the program of the college with an earnestness that means success. Further headway is an evolution. The college has no authority to enforce its program and wants no such authority. It asks co-operation only on the basis that its purposes and methods of accomplishing these purposes are right.

June 2, 1918

Hospitals No Longer Are Feared.

Among the changes of recent years is one in the feeling entertained by the public through all its strata toward hospitals. Not so long ago those institutions were regarded almost wholly as places to which the sick poor could be sent, and the sick poor for the most part thought that such a sending was a condemnation to death or not far from it.

Once there was some excuse for that belief, and while the old stories about the "black bottle" probably never had any foundation in fact, there is no doubt that before the days of antisepsis and asepsis hospitals were breeding grounds for the pathological bacteria, and those who did not carry infection to them were apt to acquire it after their arrival.

Those days, fortunately, are past, and for whatever reluctance to take hospital treatment that may now survive among the unenlightened there is no basis. More and more, the rich and the well-to-do—the people in what are called comfortable circumstances—go to hospitals when they are to have surgical operations and when they are seriously ill, for it has become widely known that even in the best of private houses the chances of recovery and of mitigating suffering are less than they are where all the conveniences and facilities of advanced medical science are at hand.

One effect of this change in sentiment and habit is not so fortunate, at least from the standpoint of those who must raise money to meet the increased expenses due to the new forms of treatment and the larger demand for beds in wards and private rooms. Hospitals always were hard pressed for money, but never, probably, did their managers realize the need so much as now, when practically all of them are obliged to make strenuous efforts to secure funds for better equipment, more trained nurses and larger buildings.

December 9, 1921

Tallest Hospital in the World To Be Erected on the East Side

The New Beth Israel Hospital, to Cost $3,000,000, Will Occupy Block Front Facing Stuyvesant Square and Have Eighteen Floors—Cornerstone to Be Laid Next Sunday.

The cornerstone of the new Beth Israel Hospital, which is to occupy the block in Livingston Place, between Sixteenth and Seventeenth Streets, opposite Stuyvesant Square, will be laid with appropriate ceremonies on Sunday, Nov. 5.

The structure, which will be the tallest hospital building in the world, will cost, according to the architect, Louis Abrahamson, about $3,000,000, exclusive of the land.

It will cover a plot 184 by 120 feet and have four floors below the street level and fourteen above.

The land was purchased several years ago at a cost of about $500,000.

Buff colored brick, with granite, limestone and terra cotta trimmings will be used, together with a tiled roof, in the Italian style of architecture. G. Richard Davis & Co. are the builders.

In the lowest level of the building will be the boiler room and oil tanks, with a capacity of 40,000 gallons. Oil will be used as fuel in heating the building instead of coal.

The sub-basement will contain the storage rooms, engine and refrigerating plant. The engine plants include electrical machinery and pumps. The laundry will occupy about 150 feet of space in length and will be the largest hospital laundry in the city. The basement also will contain kitchens and cooking laboratories.

A diagnostic clinic will occupy the Sixteenth Street end on the first floor. This will be the only clinic of this nature in New York. The emergency department, social service department and lecture auditorium, where religious ceremonies and entertainments also will take place, occupy the remainder of the floor.

The executives offices, X-Ray department and internes' quarters will be on the second floor. The third floor is given over to the children. A playroom, roof garden and infants and childrens departments occupy the entire space.

The maternity department is on the fourth floor. The fifth, sixth and seventh departments are entirely used for private rooms. On the eighth floor is the therapy department. Private rooms fill the ninth floor; convalescent rooms the tenth.

On the eleventh floor will be a laboratory for experimental work and research; on the twelfth there are seven operating rooms; on the thirteenth helio-therapy and a solarium, and on the fourteen a nurses' lecture room.

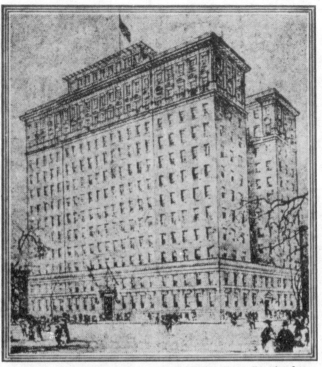

Sketch of New Hospital as It Will Appear When Completed, by the Architect, Louis Abrahamson.

October 29, 1922

The Fifth Avenue Hospital

By RUSSELL B. PORTER

To any one who has observed how many hospitals are bleak houses — dingy, smelly, unattractive buildings that inspire fear and distrust, situated in noisy, slumlike surroundings — the sight of the new Fifth Avenue Hospital, which occupies the block front between 105th and 106th Streets, must come as a pleasant surprise. Riding up the avenue between the stately mansions of the rich and fashionable on the one hand, and the natural beauties of Central Park on the other, one comes suddenly upon this great white structure opposite the horticultural gardens — a structure that one might readily imagine as a modern hotel or apartment house, or a millionaire's country club, or anything magnificent and comfortable, anything but a hospital.

It stands superbly white against the green background of the park, a towering nine-story building with the graceful lines of the North Italy Renaissance clinging to the structural design of a Manhattan skyscraper. Shaped like the letter X, with the elongated side lying upon the avenue, its straight lines modulated into curves, its row of columned loggias running up the centre of the Fifth Avenue side, and its mosque-like red roof, the edifice cannot fail to attract the attention of any one with an eye for the unique and beautiful.

This effect is calculated especially for its psychological reaction upon the prospective patient. Consider the "ambulatory case," the man who goes to the hospital, but is able to walk. If he has any esthetic sense he will be thinking of the present scene instead of the future he may dread, as he walks or rides up to an entrance back of the semicircular plot of green grass which the X-shaped design makes possible in front of the hospital. He finds an interior in harmony with the exterior. The room in which he finds himself is a high-ceilinged, circular rotunda, with an air of spaciousness and comfort and dignity that reminds one of the lobby of a modern hotel of the first class. It is decorated in soft tones of French gray, buff and tan, restful to the eye, and is further distinguished by an entire absence of hospital noises and smells, equally restful to the nerves. These features are in effect throughout the hospital. The color scheme is uniform on every floor, unobtrusive ventilating devices take away odors, and acoustic machines and sound-proof walls make the building as near sound-proof as possible.

Even on entering an anteroom to give his pedigree the patient is protected from any suggestion of the misery or suffering that one associates with life in a hospital. The only persons he sees are office employes, visitors and walking patients. If a patient is unable to walk, he is admitted by a separate driveway at the rear of the hospital, and is taken upstairs to his room by a special elevator.

Formalities of registration completed, our ambulatory patient is escorted upstairs to his floor. Here, as before, the absence of hospital sounds, sights, smells, gives him confidence and comfort. Stepping out of the elevator, he discovers himself in a spacious landing of the same size and shape as the first floor rotunda, with a floor supervisor opposite the elevator, as in a modern hotel; at the left a well-furnished visitors' room and, further on, an open-air loggia. Radiating like spokes from the hub, four corridors proceed from this centre—four long corridors flanked by private rooms.

For this is the wardless hospital. Except for the children's floor, where wards are desirable, every patient has a private room. Every room is an outside room, with a maximum of light and air. There are no inside rooms, no courts. In this respect, the hospital is the only one of its kind in the world. The X-like design, which is responsible for this, also makes it possible for the floor supervisors and nurses, standing at the hub, to command a view along all four corridors. If a patient wants something, he presses a button in his room, and a red light flashes on in the corridor outside his door. The red light remains "on" until a nurse comes inside the room and puts it out by pressing another button.

The rooms themselves give almost all the space and comfort and luxury of rooms in a big hotel, and, like such rooms, they have been furnished with the idea of providing a homelike atmosphere. A typical floor has fifty-four single rooms for patients, each 8½ to 9 feet wide by 16 feet long. There is a window in every room. Those on the Fifth Avenue side command a beautiful view of the northern end of the park, with Harlem Mere, the horticultural gardens, and the meadows. The rooms are furnished with wooden bureaus, tables and chairs, designed for comfort and painted in accordance with the general decorative scheme. The beds are comfortable, and are fitted with a mechanical device that enables the nurses to elevate the head and knees with a simple motion like cranking a Ford. The walls are painted gray. The absence of the stereotyped white enamel furniture and white walls is a relief to the eye and soul.

One need not fear, however, that too much emphasis has been placed upon the esthetic side, to the disadvantage of the material. Here beauty is combined with efficiency. In building this hospital, with accommodations for 300 to 350 patients, at a cost of $3,500,000, no expense has been spared to provide every scientific equipment for the best possible care and treatment of the patient. Many of the rooms have private bathrooms. All have private lavatories and are equipped with everything that the patient needs. This insures prompt bedside service, and makes it unnecessary for nurses to go flying back and forth in the halls for extra equipment.

Automatic telephones and telautograph machines enable the nurses and doctors to summon others and order equipment from any part of the hospital without making a sound to annoy the patients. By these methods, orders are sent for food, surgical dressings, linen, &c., to the central service department in the basement, which has control of orders for every department in the hospital. The cooking is done by white-robed chefs in large, sanitary kitchens, equipped with one set of ventilators to bring down fresh air, and another set to take up the cooking odors and dissipate them in the air outside the hospital.

The hospital has its own refrigerating plant, and it makes ice cream in large quantities in a mammoth freezer run by electricity, without ice. In the basement are a laundry with the largest mangle in the world and enough other equipment to wash the clothes of a whole neighborhood; a storeroom for dressings and instruments as well stocked as the average drug store, if not better, a special room for sterilizing dressings, and a cafeteria restaurant for nurses and doctors, to mention only a few of the features.

Electric dumbwaiters carry the food and supplies for the patients upstairs from the basement. Each floor has a service room, which is located to the right of the landing as one gets off the elevators. The nurses operate the dumbwaiters by pressing buttons, and take the trays off for their patients. These service rooms also contain diet kitchens where skilled dietitians prepare special food for those who need it.

Such is the ordinary life of the patient. Now, suppose that he must submit to an operation. The entire eighth floor is then his province. There is a series of seven operating rooms in one wing, while the other wings are devoted to various highly developed scientific departments. The patient about to undergo an operation is taken first to one of a series of anesthetizing rooms, which have nothing at all of the operating room atmosphere about them. They are like little parlors, and are furnished with curtains, rugs and wooden furniture, all in harmony with the general scheme. The operating rooms themselves are equipped with the latest scientific and hygienic methods. There is a lighting system of such power and variety that it has been found possible to discard the traditional whitewashed walls. As in the room for patients, the walls are painted a restful shade of gray.

The concentration of the X-ray, pathological, bacteriological and other laboratories and other scientific departments on the same floor as the operating rooms enables the operating surgeons to have all the facilities of diagnosis and research at their fingers' ends for whatever emergency may arise. There is an X-ray library, for instance, with pictures of the interiors of patients' bodies always ready for study. A man can be taken into a specially equipped room and his physician can look right through his body to find what troubles him.

The invaluable effect of proper and complete diagnosis of patients' conditions is realized in the laboratories. The hospital staff can carefully estimate and record the chemistry of the blood, the secretions and excretions of the body. They can register graphically and record permanently the heart functions by means of the electrocardiogram. The medical staff is able to use a new and highly important test in the estimation of the basal metabolic rate, which not only registers the most fundamental process of the body, but differentiates groups of diseases and materially assists in the diagnosis of some very complex conditions. The importance of such examinations is self-evident, as certain diseased conditions and surgical complications have shown no material decrease during the past ten years, solely because of the lack

of a complete diagnosis at an early stage of the illness.

Simply as an example of the emphasis placed upon the psychological condition of the patients, it may be mentioned that the instruments with which the basal metabolic tests are made are very terrifying for a patient to look at, but are harmless and painless and easy to operate in the hands of a skilled physician. But to save the patient from fear that might break down his resistance to disease, the hospital authorities have arranged things so that he is in a separate room from the awesome machinery while the test is made, so that he does not see it at all.

The entire sixth floor is used for maternity cases and is arranged with the most modern equipment available for the care of mothers and new-born babes. The second floor is the children's floor, and is known as the Laura Franklin-Delano Foundation, as the Fifth Avenue Hospital was organized by the combination of the old Hahnemann Hospital and the Laura Franklin Free Hospital for Children. It has a capacity of 75 to 100 youngsters. Among its features are glass cubicles, without roofs, for children just admitted and under observation for infectious and contagious diseases, so that they are separated from one another, but are still able to play and talk back and forth, and see each other. When they leave the cubicles they go into wards. They have indoor and outdoor playrooms and a classroom for lessons. The period of convalescence must be a delightful one in this hospital. First there are the open air loggias. Here one takes the air and diverts himself with a view of the park. Here also is the only place in the hospital where one may smoke. This is where modern woman puffs her cigarette in a modern hospital. Yes, the nurses say that even the maternity cases do it. Then there are indoor sun parlors, and, finally, the magnificent roof tops, four of them, where the patient can find any variety of sun or shade, or warmth or coolth or change of scene.

To the west he sees the park, with its lake and trees and gardens. Northwest, Morningside Park and Morningside Drive, the Cathedral of St. John the Divine, Columbia University, a glimpse of Riverside Drive, the Hudson and the Palisades. Due north, a fascinating labyrinth of apartment and tenement house rooftops, covering a life teeming with secret emotions, passions, tragedies, comedies, successes, failure, that the roof-top observer can only imagine. Rooftops bound together by ribbons—ribbons of elevated lines. Flung eastward more housetops, more ribbons, then the

East River, Hell Gate, Hell Gate Bridge, Queensboro Bridge. One can feel the diversified life and commerce of the great city pulsing all around him. It puts new blood into the convalescent's veins merely to think of it. Southward the heart of the city — the marts of trade and commerce, the centres of art and culture, everything that makes life worth while. Down in the street, on all sides, men and women walking or riding or doing business or making love—like Lilliputians to a Gulliver who is recovering from his weakness and about to burst his thongs.

This beauty and efficiency which have been described are not, as one might have imagined, the exclusive property of the rich. The hospital is for all. The purpose behind it has been to make available the ideal type of hospital service for everybody, regardless of class, creed or color. In planning it, its sponsors found that the hospital problem had been solved for the rich, who could pay for what they wished, and for the poor, who get a free modern ward service in city hospitals and privately endowed institutions. But the problem remained unsolved for the great in-between class — men and women of moderate means who do not wish luxury, who will not accept charity, and yet need as careful attention as the rich or poor.

It is to the man-in-between that the Fifth Avenue Hospital caters. Its aim is to give him all the necessary privacies and comforts of the private room, all the most modern scientific equipment, all the peace and contentment of mind necessary to recovery. He pays what he can afford. The rates are "from nothing up." The very poor, who can pay nothing, are provided for. One-third of the cases are to be free. The entire children's floor is free. There will be special accommodations, also, for those who can and wish to pay for them, but these will be luxuries. Every one will get the same attention, outside of luxuries, no matter what he pays. In fact, the nurses and doctors attending a patient will not know how much he pays unless he tells them himself.

The hospital has recently been opened and put into operation. Its sponsors say that it is already proving that it meets a great need. They say it will demonstrate that the ward system is a relic of the Dark Ages. Wards were once thought necessary for the sake of economy; they say, but the Fifth Avenue Hospital proves that the single-room system is justified by its economy. There is no waste of heat or light, as rooms not in use can be shut off, while a ward must be kept open and lighted if only half occupied. Elimination of sex and disease classifica-

tions allows the maximum use of floor space. While sometimes a man's ward is overcrowded, at the same time a woman's ward is almost empty. Moreover, single rooms can be redecorated and renovated one at a time, without closing a whole ward.

Newly admitted patients, it is pointed out, are spared the vicarious suffering caused by the pains and moans of the old patients, and the old patients are spared the disturbance caused by the admission of new patients to a ward. Isolation in private rooms decreases the danger of infection and contagion. Visitors can be admitted to private rooms at all hours, in the discretion of the attending physician, thus giving the patient intercourse with his family and friends, and giving his room a homelike atmosphere, in contrast to the restricted visiting hours and cheerless air of wards. The temperature of private rooms can be altered to suit the needs of individual patients, and their beds can be placed near the windows to get the most possible air and light.

In addition, it is pointed out, the man in moderate circumstances gets the advantage, in this sort of hospital, of the most modern idea in medicine—that of preventing disease, prolonging life, and increasing efficiency, by frequent examinations and overhauling of the human machine. Examina is and diagnoses of this kind require delicate and costly apparatus and specialty skilled diagnosticians. In the past the rich have profited most by this kind of preventive treatment. Now, however, any patient who enters the Fifth Avenue Hospital is entitled to it. He will get a complete physical examination. It will take a few days to give him this, so that the single room system, allowing the examinations to go on undisturbed, is considered ideal for the purpose.

Those who are responsible for the Fifth Avenue Hospital regard preventive medicine as a great service which they can perform, not only for the individual, but also for the community. To keep the human producing unit in efficient working order is a duty to the community, as they see it. Therefore, they intend to embark upon a campaign of public education to show the advantages of such treatment, and to enable the general public to avail itself of the most modern methods. With such aims, and with such equipment, is it any wonder that the people of the Fifth Avenue Hospital are convinced that their kind of a hospital will be the hospital of the future?

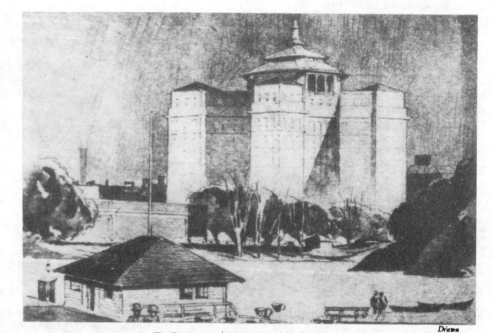

The Fifth Avenue Hospital, Seen From 110th Street.

Drawn by H. R. Shurtleff.

MEDICAL CENTRE PLANS ANNOUNCED

The greatest medical centre in the world, which is to cost approximately $20,000,000 and is to embody the latest developments in coöperation between hospitals, medical colleges and research institutions, is assured for New York City with the announcement last night by the Board of Managers of the Presbyterian Hospital of its decision to erect a building jointly with the College of Physicians and Surgeons of Columbia University at Broadway and 168th Street.

The structure, which will be the core of the centre to be erected around it, will cost $10,000,000, exclusive of the land. That section to be occupied by the College of Physicians and Surgeons will cost $3,000,000, which already has been subscribed. The Presbyterian Hospital section will cost $7,000,000, of which $2,500,000 is available, leaving $4,500,000 still to be raised.

The announcement of the plans was made by Dean Sage, President of the Presbyterian Hospital. The joint administrative board representing the hospital and the school is headed by William Barclay Parsons, with Dr. C. C. Burlingame as executive officer.

When the medical centre is completed there will be available in one place the services of leading specialists in every branch of medicine, commanding the finest equipment that money can buy. The institution will surpass Berlin, Vienna or any other centre in Europe.

It will be the first complete adaptation of the medical centre idea to the needs of New York City. It is planned to include, in a well coordinated form, every type of special hospital and institution necessary for the treatment of any patient and the training of any specialist who has to do with the protection and promotion of health.

Study of Medical Centres.

The tentative plan was first announced three years ago. Since that time careful study of the medical centres now in operation at Johns Hopkins, Harvard, Yale and other institutions, has been made by the joint administrative board.

In addition to all the facilities for the care of patients, the new building will provide a place for scientists to collaborate in research work, and will have the equipment for training practitioners of the highest type. Thus the centre in itself will, according to President Sage, embody the three principal branches of the science—care, research and teaching. It also will contain a nucleus for a medical group of wider scope, and it is expected that around it will be drawn such institutions as a dental school, a maternity hospital, a children's hospital and a neurological institute.

The announcement says that the site, which is the old American League Baseball Park, offers ideal advantages for a medical centre. The park, which is twenty acres in extent, is a residential district overlooking the Hudson. There are good transportation facilities to any part of the city and ample room for expansion.

The arrangements at the new hospital will be designed to the last detail for the comfort and welfare of patients. James Gamble Rogers is the architect. In the general hospital section there will be ten ward floors with sixty-four beds on each. Each floor will be divided into small wards with from one to twelve beds. Efforts will be made to make the patient feel that he is not merely one of many, but that he will receive all the personal attention that a small hospital would give, together with the great resources and the skill of the large hospital. Each floor also will have two diet kitchens, three sun parlors, a treatment room and a laboratory.

Time Saved for Faculty.

The hospital section of the building will be directly connected with the medical college. Faculty members, who will also be on the staff of the hospital, and students observing, will thus no longer lose the time they now must spend in going between classrooms, hospitals and laboratories scattered in various parts of the city.

The private pavilion, with 125 rooms, will also be attached to the building, and the income from these rooms will be devoted to meet the cost of free work in the wards. One of the features will be private rooms to be rented to relatives and friends who wish to stay near patients.

The Presbyterian Hospital was founded in 1872 by James Lenox and has cared for thousands "without regard to race, creed or color." On the average, over 65 per cent. of its ward service is free. Last year 27,000 persons were served in the hospital and outpatient department. It was among the first hospitals to introduce the Lister method of aseptic treatment in operations and to introduce medical social service for patients, and visiting nurse work.

The hospital has had no new buildings since 1892, when the present structure on Seventieth Street and Madison Avenue was erected following a disastrous fire. This building is now antiquated and it is impossible for the hospital to carry on its work there longer, according to the Board of Managers. The hospital for several years has been affiliated with the College of Physicians and Surgeons and the new building will make possible closer coördination of effort.

Within a short time the Presbyterian Hospital will launch a campaign—the first public appeal it has ever made—for gifts in order to raise the $4,500,000 necessary to complete the building fund. Members of the Building Fund Committee are Thatcher M. Brown, Cornelius R. Agnew, the Rev. Dr. George Alexander, Robert W. Carle, Henry W. de Forest, W. E. S. Griswold, Dean Sage, Johnston de Forest, Samuel H. Fisher and William Sloane Coffin.

In commenting on the new medical centre yesterday Dr. Samuel W. Lambert said: "Such an affiliation of school and hospital, developed through the close physical contacts of adjoining buildings, makes possible the only solution of the proper development of scientific medical laboratories of the school and of practical medicine in the wards of a hospital.

"The intimate work in scientific research and in clinical medicine of the combined staff of such a medical centre gives the patients the best opportunity for the accurate diagnosis and for the cure and relief of their diseases. It gives to the students of the school proper balance between a foundation in science and an experience in the clinical art of medicine."

October 5, 1924

HOSPITAL EXPANSION PLANNED BY U. OF P.

Special to The New York Times.

PHILADELPHIA, Dec. 19.—Plans for the expansion of the medical school and hospital of the University of Pennsylvania into what is expected to be the largest and most perfectly equipped medical centre in the world were given out tonight by Dr. Alfred Stengel, Professor of Medicine at the University.

A program involving millions of dollars will be discussed by university officers and prominent medical men and educators at a dinner and conference here on Jan. 10, to which 1,200 invitations have been issued. Dr. Henry S. Pritchett, President of the Carnegie Foundation; Dr. Hubert Work, Secretary of the Interior, and Josiah H. Penniman, President of the university, will speak at the conference.

Dr. Stengel said the program involved the erection of new buildings, establishment of numerous foundations, clinics and hospitals for research and observation of every type of disease, and the introduction of revolutionary methods in hospital isolation.

Dr. Stengel made no estimate of the exact sum required to carry out the program, but it is agreed that it will run into many millions of dollars. Fulfillment of the complete plan will be a matter of years, but it is hoped to begin immediate work toward four goals partly made possible through gifts already received. Efforts will be made, it is understood, to bring to the university recognized leaders in every branch of medicine and surgery as Faculty members and lecturers.

A new departure in hospital methods on a large scale will be introduced with the establishment of an "out patient" department, in which persons may receive treatment for certain periods every day and continue at their work, instead of entering the hospital for long stays.

Another objective is the erection of suitable buildings to house clinics of every type, each separate medical and surgical specialty to be presided over by its chief, who will be the senior professor that subject in the medical school.

Plans call for a fireproof hospital with 1,000 beds, a staff of 100 internes and 500 nurses. This, it was said, would do away with most of the present buildings of the University Hospital, except the maternity building an the J. William White surgical pavilion. An administratino building of twelve stories, also to contain 400 beds, is to be the central unit of the proposed new group.

Dr. Stengel said the institution planned to establish a "medical press" to issue pamphlets on the latest developments in medicine and surgery, to pass upon the authenticity or falsity of medical discoveries, and to offer general medical information to the public.

No "medical trust" would be involved in the hospital scheme, it was emphasized. Although the central idea is the treatment of the "middle man" who does not wish to go to a charity ward and feels he cannot afford other hospital treatment, most of the patients will be sent to the University Hospital direct by their family physicians.

December 20, 1926

TRAINED NURSES SEEK NEW TRAINING SYSTEM

By EUNICE FULLER BARNARD.

THE nursing profession is taking stock of itself. Its responsible leaders are convinced that, from an economic and educational viewpoint, something is radically wrong with the profession. The nurse complains that under the present system of nurse distribution she receives little more than a living wage; the patient complains of the high cost of nursing. The leaders of the profession hold that the present hospital method of training nurses has led to many defects that must be corrected if the American standard of nursing is to be raised.

Facts about the profession were laid before three national nursing organizations in convention at Louisville a few weeks ago. The report was made after an eighteen months' survey of the nursing field by the Committee on the Grading of Nursing Schools, cooperatively maintained by the three national nurses' organizations, and by the American Medical Association, the American College of Surgeons, the American Hospital Association and the American Public Health Association. The Chairman of the committee, which has embarked on a five-year program, is Dr. William Darrach, Dean of the College of Physicians and Surgeons of Columbia University. The director of the survey and author of the 600-page report is May Ayres Burgess, an educational statistician.

The Unemployment Problem.

It is estimated that the hospital training schools turn out graduate nurses at the rate of 20,000 a year, and it is contended that these schools, with their large crop of graduates, are at the root of the trouble today. There are, it is said, too many free-lance nurses, and as a consequence there is much unemployment among them, the typical private-duty nurse having only seven months of work out of the year.

The report makes these points:

Hospitals not only train their students. They use them as a working staff, because they believe it is cheaper, and the young recruits can be kept under a more rigid discipline. Therefore the phenomenal increase of nurses is due not to the public's need of them but to the hospital's need of more students. The first duty of the training school is to keep the hospital staffed with a constantly renewed corps of vigorous, often unpaid, students. To do this it cannot always choose them too nicely or provide for them after graduation. The hospital in effect has economized at the expense of the future welfare of nurses, patients and physicians.

The committee recommended to the convention that hospitals be staffed with graduate instead of student nurses, and that the training of students be put on a more disinterested basis. "The decision as to whether or not a school of nursing should be conducted in cooperation with a given hospital," reads the committee's resolution, "should be based solely on the kinds and amounts of educational experience which that hospital is prepared to offer."

Hospitals should not be expected to be responsible for nursing education, or to pay for it out of funds collected for the care of the sick, according to the committee. "The education of nurses," it is asserted, "is as much a public responsibility as is the education of physicians, public school teachers, librarians, ministers, lawyers and other students planning to engage in professional public service, and the cost of such education should come, not out of the hospital budget but from private or public funds."

The Surpluses of Nurses.

How the present situation has arisen and its unhappy effects on nurses, patients and medical practice is a story extending over the last quarter century. The training of nurses is less than seventy years old in this country. Up to 1890 we had but thirty-five nursing schools, and the number of graduates was negligible. By 1900 there were several hundred schools, but trained nurses were still at a premium. Today there are more than 2,000 schools and hospitals, eager for student labor, and new ones constantly are opening.

In the same period, since 1900, the history of medical schools has been the exact opposite. Their number has been deliberately cut in half, from 160 to 79, due to a concerted effort of the physicians to limit and improve the quality of their profession. Today four nurses are graduated annually for every doctor.

What this means in human terms is that hospitals often accept students, who are not suitable in education, ability or character to satisfy patients or physicians after graduation, or even to make a financial success of their profession. In the three years of hospital training every act of the students' waking life is known, checked and controlled. Thus, says the report, "it becomes possible for the school to admit as students many young women who will be useful hands and feet in the hospital wards, but who are not at all safe prospects to go out into the completely unsupervised activity of graduate nursing after the hospital is through with them."

Of the nurses graduated within the last five years, one-sixth, the survey finds, have never been beyond the first year of high school. "If the proportion still holds for 1928, it will mean that something like 3,000 of this year's graduates will be so poorly educated that they would have difficulty in getting positions in a good department store."

The use of student labor by hospitals is sharply criticized by Dr. Burgess.

"Who can imagine," she says, "a bank, for example, openly preferring to staff its offices with utterly untrained students, teach them all it can in three years, and, as soon as they have learned the rudiments of banking, discharge them all and seek a new supply of untrained students to take their places? Or who can imagine a public school system placing all its schools in the hands of normal school students, letting them teach as long as they remain in normal school, but the moment they receive their diplomas, telling them:

THE VISITING NURSE

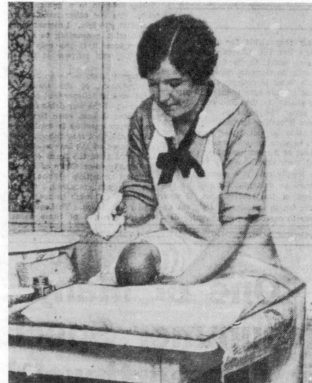

She Is the Friend of the Tenement Baby.

'There is no place for you in the public school system. We run our public schools on student labor. You go out now and support yourselves by being governesses!'' Yet that is very nearly what most of the best hospitals in this country are saying to their own graduate nurses.

"There would seem to be something radically wrong with the educational methods of these hospitals if, after they had the educating of a student for three years, they would honestly prefer to start the training process all over again with raw material, rather than to avail themselves of the services of their own product.''

In view of the situation, it is time, in Dr. Burgess's opinion, for some large hospital to try the experiment of providing full graduate nursing on a self-supporting basis. "Is it,'' she asks, "an unreasonable thing to suggest that the famous hospital ought seriously to consider placing at least part of its nursing service in the hands of skilled nurses?''

According to Miss Marion Rottman, superintendent of nurses at Bellevue Hospital, which now maintains a large training school, such a plan as Dr. Burgess suggests is not only reasonable, but feasible. "Every hospital,'' she said, "should depend on graduate nurse service, supplemented by student service part time. It would largely eliminate the present system, in which the hospital patient who can afford it feels it necessary to employ a special graduate nurse in addition to the student nurses supplied by the hospital.''

At present the nurse's lot is not a happy one. In the pleasant mythology of the popular poster and advertisement, the nurse is always a stalwart young goddess. In the composite photograph provided by the committee's report she is shown to be often a lonely and aging woman, now working long hours under heavy strain and again waiting in enforced idleness with no work at all.

The private-duty nurse today, it is found, earns on an average but seven months' wages in the year. Four months each year on the average she is out of work, resting or waiting the hoped-for "call." And one month a year, the astonishing figures show, she is giving her services free—nurs-

ing relatives, friends or patients who cannot or do not pay.

While patients and physicians complain of the nurse's high wages, and often of her inadequate service, the nurse herself is caught in a treadmill of long hours, precarious income, lack of leadership and of stimulus to professional growth. Her fee of six or seven dollars a day, which under her present uncertain employment conditions she must charge, works a real hardship on the average wage earner who needs her services. Such a charge is in many cases of protracted illness sufficient to sweep away a family's savings, and to force the butcher and the grocer to wait months for their money. Physicians, indeed, have reported that a third of their patients who needed special nurses did not have them, usually because they could not afford the price.

So the whole system of private-duty nursing seemingly needs to be put on a new basis that will fit the patient's purse as well as the nurse's need of a more assured income, shorter hours, leadership and professional growth. To meet all these needs the report urges the system usually spoken of as hourly nursing.''

The returns from physicians and patients, according to the report, show that with the present method of twelve and twenty-four hour service the call for nurses has about reached the saturation point. "There is reason to believe, however,'' it states, "that many people who are now entirely without any nursing service would be glad to pay for it on an hourly basis. Everywhere there are probably many mothers of sick children who do not feel that they can pay $7 a day to a twelve-hour nurse, but who would gladly pay $2 a day to have a nurse come in and give certain of the more difficult treatments. Probably there are large numbers of chronic cases in every community for which some service is needed daily and for which the relatives or the patients would be glad to pay a $2 or $3 fee for a a short period of daily care and yet would feel wholly unable to employ a full-time nurse.''

The nurses who would come to

such cases should, it is held, be sent out from a central responsible and supervising agency. They would be on regular salaries paid monthly by the organization. They would belong to a regular staff on eight-hour shifts. The registry administering the service would be open night and day, and assignments to night duty or holiday duty would be taken in rotation by the different members of the staff.

A New Incentive.

"It would seem entirely feasible,'' states the report, "to establish some system by which the nurses enrolled would be classified according to experience and ability. It would seem fair for registries to establish a scale of charges according to the degree of skill of the nurse.

"When patients and physicians called the registry for a nurse, they could be given a choice so that they could secure a low-priced semi-skilled nurse or a high-priced highly skilled nurse, according to what they felt was needed and what they were willing to pay for. Such a scheme of graded service and graded charges, with ample opportunity for the nurse to rise from group to group as she demonstrated her value, would seem to offer professional stimulation to the nurse, and at the same time to meet a real need on the part of physician and patient.''

Nurses would then be working under conditions which most people take for granted. "They would work together in a professional atmosphere,'' points out the report. "They could discuss the problems of their cases with their group leaders. When they did especially good jobs of nursing, there would be some intelligent person who knew what that work implied and who could give the professional appreciation which every one needs.''

Hourly nursing, more or less of this sort, is already being tried out in a number of cities. In some cases it is an extension of the work of the visiting nurse association. In other places it is arranged by a nurses' registry, and in a few instances it is under the joint control of both types of organization.

July 29, 1928

Dr. Mayo Criticizes Hospital 'Salesmanship'; Finds Human Treatment of Patient Lacking

CHICAGO, Oct. 14 (P).—Dr. W. J. Mayo, surgeon and chief of staff of the Mayo Clinic at Rochester, Minn., adversely criticized hospitals today in addressing the annual hospital standardization conference, which prefaces the clinical congress of the American College of Surgeons. Dr. Mayo charged the hospitals with too much salesmanship and too little humanity.

Super-salesmanship in management of some hospitals often resulted, he said, in the patient being placed in surroundings which, however, they might appeal to his esthetic sense, were above his means.

"My own experience has been that patients in a well-planned ward, even with a moderate degree of privacy, on the whole will make a quicker recovery than in a private room with

two attentive nurses who unobtrusively, in caring for the physical needs and increasing the happiness of the patient, may suggest a mental state in which the diseased condition is exaggerated sympathetically,'' he said.

Dr. Mayo defended the trained nurse, asserting that at present, her fine training was wasted in scrubbing floors, making beds, giving patients baths and other tasks a hospital maid could be trained to do in six months.

Dr. Franklin H. Martin, president of the congress, came to the defense of hospitals. He said the average cost of hospital bed and board, which included general nursing, was lower than the cost of similar room and board at a respectable hotel.

Dr. Martin suggested it would be fair to give the patients in advance

a probable estimate of the cost, which would include hospital nursing and laboratory and operating room expenses.

The average income of physicians was low in comparison to the incomes of those in other professions, Dr. Martin said.

"Twenty-five years ago an average income of an independent doctor in this country was less than $1,000. Today it is about $2,000,'' he stated.

Dr. Malcolm T. MacEachern, associate director of the College of Surgeons, reported that greater skill and better equipment have so greatly increased the efficiency of plants devoted to restoring human health that the average stay of patients in hospitals today has been cut to half what it was ten years ago.

"The stay of most hospital patients today ranges from eight to fifteen days,'' Dr. MacEachern said.

The mortality rate in hospitals has been cut in half in the past decade, he added.

October 15, 1929

NEW HOSPITAL PLAN AIDS MIDDLE CLASS

The "Middlerate Plan" of the Massachusetts General Hospital in Boston, through which 2,500 persons were able to get hospital care for serious illnesses at a cost within the reach of middle class incomes, is discussed in a report of C. Rufus Rorem, made public yesterday by the Julius Rosenwald Foundation.

The hospital's Baker Memorial Pavilion, opened in the Spring of 1930, was built for persons of moderate means, the report explains. Semi-private and private rooms are provided at rates of from $4 to $6.50 a day, including all usual drugs and all the nursing required by any but gravely ill patients. A schedule of moderate fees in this service has been arranged by the hospital staff, which has agreed that no patient be asked to pay a doctor's bill of more than $150 in all.

Before admission, the patient, or some member of his family, discusses financial arrangements with the hospital's admitting officer. The probable cost of the illness is estimated and the method of payment is arranged. It may be in instalments if necessary. The entire amount is collected by the hospital which turns the doctor's share over to him, thus relieving him of the possible uncertainty and difficulty of making collection. It is expected that the service will become self-supporting after it has been established long enough to be fully in use. The Julius Rosenwald Fund has agreed to meet half of the deficit during the initial period of experiment up to a total amount of $150,000.

The 2,500 patients cared for during the first year of the Baker Memorial Pavilion's operation include white collar workers, skilled artisans and lower salaried professional people. The average income of the patients has been $4,000 for a family of four. The average cost of the illnesses of the patients, including hospital room, nursing and X-rays, if needed, any extras and the doctor's fee, has been approximately $100. In many cases, the report says, it was less than that and, in a few, much higher.

The plan is designed to provide care for persons who cannot afford the hospital rates and professional fees in the hospital's regular private room service but who can, and should, pay more than ward rates which give the hospital only half of its actual cost of care and provide no payment at all for the physician. An analysis of the record, the report declares, shows that these patients would have had to use the ward service if there had been no such plan. Under it they receive medical care of the highest standard at rates they can afford, without profit and without charity.

Mr. Rorem says that the use of the Baker Memorial Pavilion, as of the other services in the institution, is limited to 200 members of the hospital's staff. During the year 183 staff members cared for patients under the "Middlerate Plan" and payments by patients to physicians reached an aggregate of $147,000. Mr. Rorem says that in contrast to some similar experiments in smaller cities, the medical staff of the hospital has been cordial and cooperative in its reception of the plan.

In a foreword to the report Dr. Michael M. Davis, director for medical services of the Julius Rosenwald Fund, says:

"Amid the widespread discussion among the trustees, physicians and superintendents of hospitals as to how to provide for the much advertised 'person of moderate means,' an attempt to raise money to meet his needs has been more prominent than the effort to devise a service the cost of which he could pay. The Baker Memorial plan was inaugurated to accomplish the latter—to provide services to the hospital patients at moderate rates, rather than to help them pay for their care.

"Persons of moderate means number many millions souls. A plan to support to them out of the income of endowment funds would require that this country invest for this purpose, and take out of production, use in business or educational enterprises, an immense amount of capital."

Dr. Davis believes that further experience will show how much hospital costs can be lowered by administrative economy, while still covering the cost and a fair return to the physician, and may indicate some plan of annual payments that families could make in advance as a form of insurance against hospital sickness so that they would have the funds to meet the costs at need.

September 13, 1931

A SCHOOL FOR THE NURSE

By CAROLYN C. VAN BLARCOM.

THE announcement last week that the Presbyterian Hospital School of Nursing has become the Department of Nursing in the Columbia University College of Physicians and Surgeons marks a significant advance in nurse training. It indicates great progress toward replacing the time-honored apprenticeship system with true education.

Until recently nurse-training schools in general have been integral parts of hospital organizations. Students have been enrolled primarily to do the work of the hospital. Training and education have been inevitably subordinated to hospital chores. During the boom years, when hospitals increased rapidly in number, exploitation of student nurses also increased.

Added to the yearly output of carefully trained nurses from good schools was a flood of graduates from schools that were often little more than diploma mills. While the population of the United States increased 62 per cent from 1900 to 1930, the number of graduate nurses increased 2,374 per cent. They are still being turned out, good, bad and indifferent, at the rate of 25,000 a year. The result, as might be expected, is too few good nurses and too many poor ones ranging over the country.

Unhappily, it is not always easy for the average lay person to cull the good from the bad, for any one who will may call herself a "trained nurse." The title of registered nurse, abbreviated to R. N., is a safer guarantee. It may be used only by a nurse who has graduated from a school that meets the requirements of the official educational body in the State of registry and who has passed the State board examinations.

Wide Survey Made.

Leaders of the nursing profession have been greatly disturbed by the lack of proper training. Accordingly, in 1926, the profession initiated an exhaustive study of nursing conditions. The investigating body, the Committee on the Grading of Nursing Schools, was headed by Dr. William Darrach, dean emeritus of the College of Physicians and Surgeons, and included in its membership representatives of the American Medical Association, American College of Surgeons, American Hospital Association and American Public Health Association, as well as various nursing organizations.

The kernel of the committee's conclusions after eight years of careful study is: "Fundamental improvement in nursing education is a vital necessity for the health of the American people and presents perhaps the most important opportunity in the whole field of American education. We have great need of nurses with better training than that which is given by the typical hospital school. We need schools for professional training on a par with the schools of other professions."

Other professions have passed along the road of evolution that nursing is traveling today. Once young men prepared themselves for the bar by "reading law" and doing add jobs around a lawyer's office, would-be doctors prepared themselves by assisting some physician in his practice. But those days are past. Medical students are now trained in a medical school, attached to a university, on the one hand, and on the other, to a hospital of widely inclusive services. Medical students receive much of their training in hospital wards. But every detail of their work has a place in their education and none of it is done to save money for the hospital. Nursing remains the only profession in which the apprenticeship system still prevails.

Hospital Training Essential.

Nurses, like doctors, must be trained in schools attached to hospitals. Nothing can replace the educational value of bedside care, given under instructive supervision. But this training, it is held, must literally be training, and not merely hospital work. And always the nurse's theoretical training must go hand in hand with the practical. The more she understands of the whys and wherefores, the more efficient will be her ministrations.

With the progress steadily being made in all branches of medical practice—diagnostic, preventive and curative—there is an increase in the responsibilities of nursing and in its opportunities. It is no longer enough for a nurse merely to carry out specific orders. There is always a "nursing program," which is an entity in itself, and the doctor takes it for granted that the nurse is capable of carrying out this program without detailed instruction.

The intelligent, better trained nurse has already been so influential in improving individual and community health that steady progress is being made toward broadening her opportunities so that her value to society may be further increased. Schools for nursing are now integral parts of such universities as Yale, Western Reserve, Vanderbilt, University of California, Washington University, University of Minnesota and University of Wisconsin. Many other schools, although not parts of universities, are assuming more and more the character of professional schools.

Stiff Training Prescribed.

Such a school is the one at the Presbyterian Hospital. It has long functioned as a real school, with a definite three-year course of practical and theoretical instruction. In order to be graduated a student must be on hospital duty for three calendar years—less three weeks for vacation—must complete the prescribed academic course exactly as she would at high school or college. The practical instruction includes specified periods spent in the care of various classes of patients—medical, surgical, obstetrical, psychiatric, children and those with special disorders.

The theoretical instruction includes not only the principles of nursing but the study of anatomy, physiology, chemistry, materia medica, bacteriology, dietetics and many aspects of public health and community problems. The student nurse's day in such a well-conducted school is eight hours.

In sharp distinction to this orderly and comprehensive curriculum is the haphazard career of a student in the diploma-mill type of school. Her hours of duty are irregular and often cruelly long. She goes to lectures when she has the time and inclination. She may hear the same lecture each year for three years or she may not hear it at all.

The Patient Suffers.

She may be graduated without ever having seen the inside of the operating room and may never have had any contact with obstetrics, treatment of children or other branches of nursing. Such a nurse is not eligible for examination and registration by State authority and may not call her self an R. N. But she may don a crisp white cap, call herself a trained nurse and

take into her care a patient whose life literally depends upon that knowledge and experience which may be obtained only in the course of such thoughtful training as is now given in schools that function as educational institutions.

Perhaps therein lies the significance of the Columbia announcement. The Presbyterian Hospital School of Nursing remains unchanged in its new affiliation. The same courses of practical and theorectical instruction will be given by the same doctors and nurses. The field work will continue to be done in the hospital wards, laboratories and diet kitchens as heretofore. But the entire emphasis on nurse training is changed as the school becomes a department of a university medical school and ceases to be a department of a hospital.

Individuals, as well as entire communities, it is contended, will benefit increasingly as nurse training schools in general outgrow the old apprenticeship system and evolve into modern, scientific educational institutions.

November 24, 1935

PWA PROVIDES HOSPITAL AID

Special Correspondence, THE NEW YORK TIMES.

WASHINGTON, May 15.—More than 40,000 beds will be added to the facilities of American hospitals under the current PWA program. Both Federal and other hospitals will be the beneficiaries. PWA has refused aid to over-hospitalized towns and cities, but has approved many projects for communities that hitherto have lacked adequate hospital facilities, and has undertaken more than 500 hospital projects, including both new construction and the improvement of existing hospitals.

New facilities have been provided for Eskimos in Alaska, for lepers

in the Virgin Islands and for many of the Indian reservations in the West. The Marine Hospital at New York City and the Naval Hospital at Philadelphia, each costing above $2,000,000, are two of the largest projects. All told, WPA operations will add about 8,000 beds to Federal hospitals.

About 400 communities will now find it possible to modernize the surgical departments in their hospitals, to add new and more efficient X-ray and other scientific laboratories and to increase their medical equipment and enlarge their clinics. Federal aid is also being extended, through PWA

loans, to many institutions specializing in mental or other diseases.

PWA has come to the assistance of several communities with half completed hospitals. The Alleghany General Hospital in Pittsburgh is an example. This was an $8,000,-000 enterprise, started in 1929. Lack of funds, caused by the depression, made necessary a suspension of work in 1931. The PWA then assisted the enterprise with a loan and the hospital will soon be completed.

WPA has allocated $50,000,000 or more for hospital construction and improvement. States, towns and cities have contributed about $75,-000,000 to supplement the Federal grants.

May 17, 1936

HOSPITALS HELD BEST FOR MATERNITY CASES

American Hospital Group Replies to Dr. DeLee, but Emphasizes Need for Efficiency

Special to THE NEW YORK TIMES.

ATLANTIC CITY, Sept. 14.—A modern hospital with a properly planned and intelligently supervised maternity department is the best place in the world for a maternity patient, although babies are better off born at home than in a poorly equipped and carelessly managed hospital, it was stated here today in a report submitted to the American Hospital Association by its committee on public education. The association is holding its thirty-

ninth annual convention here.

The report came as an answer to Dr. Joseph B. De Lee, Chicago obstetrician, who last year contended that babies were better born at home than in hospitals. The committee, headed by Dr. A. J. Hockett of New Orleans, made its report on the basis of a compilation of information obtained from the "most eminent specialists in obstetrical practice" in the country.

Mrs. Franklin D. Roosevelt visited the convention this afternoon and viewed its exhibits with Dr. C. W. Munger of New York, retiring president of the association. She spoke tonight at the dinner of the American Occupational Therapy Association at the Hotel Chelsea. She stressed the value of cooperation in professional service.

September 15, 1937

HOSPITALS CURBING 'FRILLS' FOR SICK

The shortage of nurses and the reduction in the number of physicians on hospital staffs are leading to subtle changes in hospital procedure in which the patient still gets the best of care but with the gradual elimination of all "frills," it was learned yesterday.

The new conditions, it was revealed, are leading to a type of rationing in which the time of the doctors and nurses is the factor rationed. The critically ill are given priority and the period of convalescence is being curtailed as much as is deemed compatible with the patient's health.

While the hospitals are still doing their best to provide private nurses to patients who want them, such private nursing is becoming more and more difficult to obtain. In such cases, it was learned, the situation is explained to the patient and he generally adjusts himself to the idea of being cared for by the general duty nurse.

Miss Grace Warman, vice chairman of the New York State Nursing Council for War Service and also principal of the School of Nursing and Superintendent of Nurses at Mount Sinai Hospital, explained the development as a result of the emergency of what she described as "nursing time economy."

Many duties previously performed by registered nurses, such as bathing patients, making beds and similar duties, are now being taken over as much as possible by volunteer nurses' aids, who are given special courses at the hospital. In this manner the nurse is left free to perform other duties.

"We are trying to get people to realize," she said, "that unless they absolutely need private nurses it is their patriotic duty to get along without one. It is the doctor who decides whether a patient needs a private nurse, and even then it may not be possible to obtain one. The private duty nurse has to be conserved for those who absolutely need one."

Patients are also appealed to not to stay in the hospital any longer than is absolutely necessary in the convalescent period, it was learned. Here, too, the doctor decides when the patient is sufficiently recovered to be sent home.

Prior to the emergency the determining factor in admitting a patient to a hospital was the availability of a bed. Today, however, the determining factor is whether the patient can be properly cared for. This means that priority is given to those who need immediate hospitalization. Here, too, the physician decides whether the patient must be admitted to the hospital at once or whether the admission can be postponed with safety to a later date.

Dr. Charles F. Wilinsky, Deputy Commissioner of Health, Boston, in an article in the current issue of the New England Journal of Medicine on "Hospitals and the War," says that the hospitals face the challenge of adjusting themselves to curtailed personnel and rising cost and scarcity of supplies while at the same time maintaining the high standards which are important for the preservation of life.

"Judgment in its keenest form," he states, "will have to be exercised. The use of substitutes and relatively simple methods and procedures will be justified. The critically ill must have priority, and there must be a rationing, so to speak, of doctors, patients and hospital beds when that appears necessary."

February 6, 1943

HOSPITAL SETS PACE IN SOLDIER SALVAGE

By SIDNEY SHALETT

Special to THE NEW YORK TIMES.

WASHINGTON, April 14—Brig. Gen. Shelley U. Marietta, commanding general of the Army Medical Center in Washington, known as Walter Reed Hospital, has a simple formula for the tremendous job that is being done. They work for two things—to save lives and salvage human bodies.

That simplified formula is entirely accurate, but it covers a multitude of activities so vast and so important that cataloguing them constitutes a Roll of Honor for the Army Medical Center in which the entire nation can take pride.

A visit authorized by the War Department to this center, which includes, in addition to the famous Walter Reed General Hospital, schools for Army doctors, dentists, veterinarians and technicians, and a special division where vaccines and viruses for men and animals are developed and manufactured, revealed something of the scope of these activities. There were insights into the miracles of plasma, X-ray and radium; explanations of scientific work that is being done to prevent tooth decay; demonstrations of the wonders that plastic surgeons can perform for men wounded or burned in modern war, such as a hint that X-ray might be used to cure the age-old curse of the infantryman—foot calluses.

Yet there was something else revealed that was not written down on the bare list of clinics and laboratories which the tour was to encompass. That something was the magnificence of the human spirit.

Spirit of Youth Unquenched

At Walter Reed a glimpse of the stark, brutal side of war was

THE ARMY 'SAVES LIVES AND SALVAGES HUMAN BODIES'

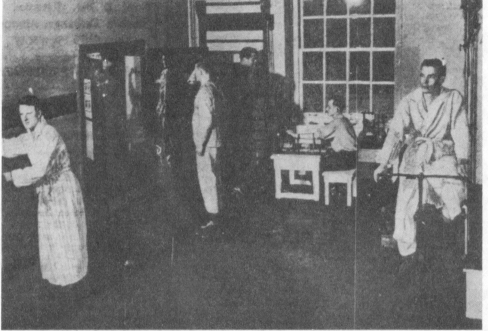

A section of the physical therapy gymnasium in Walter Reed Hospital, Washington, D. C., where soldier patients returned from action in the field recover the use of their limbs through exercises.

The New York Times (U. S. Army)

gained. It was not so vivid a glimpse, perhaps, as that which might be seen on the battlefields. Yet it was the sort of stuff that helped make men and women pacifists in the Twenties: boys—fine boys, the cream of American youth —with faces twisted and burned from plane crashes; men with arms and legs maimed from the tearing impact of enemy steel; others with minds vague and bruised from what they have seen.

Yet—and this is the magnificence of it—these men are neither afraid nor sorry. They know that the game is dangerous, but they tell you they think the stake, which is freedom, is worth it. They also tell you they are ready to go back and fight some more, as soon as they are able.

The young officer with the hideously scarred features is ready to return to Africa and fly again when they finish giving him a new face; the gray-haired sergeant would take the next boat back to Africa if his shell-torn leg would let him.

These are the lives they are saving and the bodies they are salvaging at Walter Reed, and the Army doctors (most of whom were recruited recently from civilian life) are inspired by the work they are doing.

One-Third of Cases Mental

Nearly one-third of the casualties now being shipped back from war zones, Army doctors have estimated, are mental or nervous cases. Some come from North Africa and the South Pacific, but many are from places where they have not seen actual combat yet. It is the job of the neuro-psychiatric section of the hospital to straighten out their minds.

As Army psychiatrists explained it, these men are not insane. Many of them are constitutional psychopathic cases who, occupying "obscure little grooves" in civil life, got by quite nicely. It was only when thrown up against the routines and rigors of Army life that their minds slipped. In many cases their minds are stronger, in fact, than they were before their mental crack-ups.

Occupational therapy is one of the methods used. The men work under supervision at activities specially prescribed by their physicians. Here a soldier in the maroon-colored fatigue uniform of the hospital works at making a yellow hook rug, with "Waac" worked into it in large brown letters. Another works skillfully at a jigsaw, cutting out a large American eagle. Some make belts, ship models, chessmen; others embroider.

One—and he has empty, faraway eyes—stands in a corner, painting a rather weird picture in oils on a board. It is a picture of a woman with a strange coiffure; the swirling lines are oddly reminiscent of Van Gogh.

There is another room where occupational therapy is used, but this room is for soldiers whose bodies, not their minds, were hurt. Movement is wonderful for loosening up injured members. Over in a corner a big Negro, his legs in braces, works diligently at a loom. Elsewhere a tough-looking soldier, his foot in a cast, is making a colonial rug.

"Thirty-two months ago," he tells you, "a ten-wheel truck ran over my leg. They were going to amputate, but they decided there was a chance to save it. They did. Hell, I'll be better in a couple of months, and maybe I can get over there and do something."

On a table is a skillful, if rather satirical, clay bust of Hitler.

"The boy who did that is back in the Army now," a nurse says. "Don't be surprised that he made Hitler look like that. He was a Polish boy, Radzinski, I think his name was."

The hospital has a device called The electroencephalograph that enables its brain surgeons to locate tumors and disturbances inside a man's head, even though he cannot see inside the skull. By placing the patient inside an insulated cage which keeps out extraneous electrical impulses, and by "pasting" (not inserting) electrodes on his head, the surgeon gets a graphic record of the brain impulses, which write their own reactions in wavy lines on a recording machine. It is invaluable for weeding out men psychiatrically unfit for service.

The plastic surgeons of Walter Reed are doing a brilliant job. You have to have a strong system to watch even movies and pictures of the work they do, much less look

at the men on whom they perform their merciful operations. Men, come in whose faces, hands and legs look hopeless; yet, when the Walter Reed plastic surgeons get through with them, they can go out among their fellow-men again, secure in the knowledge that their appearance will not shock those who see them.

Some of these operations used to require years; now, through improved methods, some patients may be restored in a few months. Skin grafting in burn cases has been aided greatly by the Padgett dermatone method, doctors said. This "slices" off skin grafts of a uniform thickness, replacing the old method of removing skin sections for grafting purposes by a razor.

Plastic surgeons pointed out an interesting fact about skin grafting: only in the case of identical twins, they said, may one person's skin be successfully grafted to the body of another person. They said it is as yet one of the "inexplicable wonders of nature."

The Maxillo-Facial research department is another branch of the plastic surgery department. Here they make ingenious duplicates for missing parts of faces, which the victims don as an actor would put on his make-up. Latex rubber is largely used, but the technicians are searching for an equally mobile, yet more durable, material.

The physical therapy section is another department where the starkness of war and the courage of the men who fight them are equally hammered home. Strapping soldiers lie under heat lamps, or grope in gymnasiums to exercise paralyzed muscles. One big fellow with a useless leg sits patiently attempting to pick up pebbles with his toes. Another—"I caught a bullet in North Africa, and I'd like to go back and return it to 'em," he explains—laboriously turns a wheel with his braced arm.

New X-Ray Exhibited

In the X-ray department, Major Aubrey O. Hampton exhibited one of the new developments of the war. It is a field unit X-ray machine, small enough to be transported and operated by emergency power in the field. There is one model especially adapted for transport by plane. It can be used for both plate and fluoreoscopic work, and has helped save many lives by locating bullets that have twisted

their way into men's bodies.

Major Milton Friedman showed a 200,000-volt machine adaptable for either X-ray or radium treatment, that has "arrested"—medical men use that term rather than "cured" — many cases of cancer among soldiers. Major Friedman told of men who have been flown back to the United States from points as far away as India for radium, X-ray and surgical treatment for malignant tumors; apparently cured, they returned to their posts. Reflectively, he added that a number of officers, who knew they could not be cured and that they were going to die in a short time, insisted on being allowed to go back to battle, rather than end their lives in the easier surroundings of home.

Major Friedman demonstrated how radium — a few powder-like specks inserted into a gold or platinum cell, then put into a needle or capsule and inserted into the spot to be treated—is used. He said radium is "cheap" now since new sources have been discovered —only $30 a milligram, or $120,-000 a teaspoonful, compared with the old price of $125 a milligram, or $500,000 a teaspoonful.

"In attacking malignant tumors," he explained, "radium is the high-explosive bomb, while X-ray is the long-range shell."

Major Friedman also revealed that it has been discovered that X-ray is valuable for eliminating certain types of foot callouses. It actually has been used on some foot sores where feet have become crippled, he stated. The infantryman of the last World War had no comforts like this.

In another section of the hospital doctors demonstrated the use of something that is even more precious than radium, though it runs through every one's veins and every one can give it—blood plasma.

Men used to die on battlefields because they could not get blood transfusions when they needed them. With plasma, both liquid and dried, available, lives of fighting men are being saved. It is a comparatively simple process to prepare the plasma, which, in its liquid state, resembles an amber-colored shampoo and in its dried state a lightish brown sugar, yet doctors consider it, along with de-

velopment of the sulfa drugs, one of the great life-savers of this war.

In this connection Colonel George R. Callender, Assistant Commandant of the Army Medical Schools, commented that the American soldier in this war, because of plasma, sulfa and other scientific developments, has an infinitely greater chance to survive than his father did in 1917-18. Other Army doctors added that the kits of sulfa powder which soldiers take on the battlefield with them to sprinkle over their wounds if they are hurt are proving an immense aid to morale.

Back in the days when the draft was young, you used to read in the newspapers of how Joe Doakes, who wanted to get in the Army but couldn't because of bad teeth, spent six days and $600 in the dentist's chair getting new teeth made. Those days are gone forever, a visit to the dental school disclosed.

Now, as Major R. M. Appelman put it, "if a man has two opposing jaws," they take him in the Army, and Uncle Sam provides the teeth. The Army Medical Center has a veritable assembly line for turning out dentures and is sending out more than 2,000 plates and partial plates a month now. There is a "bank" for instance, perpetually kept stocked with 70,000 spare teeth to fit the jobs that are being sent out. Ingenious substitutes for critical materials, such as rubber, also have been developed.

In the research department of the Dental School Captain Ned B. Williams exhibited his work on a vaccine which, it is hoped, will attack the lactobacillus believed to cause tooth decay and thus prevent the disease that makes many of these 2,000 dentures a month necessary. It will be a great boon to humanity if the vaccine is perfected; right now it has passed the stage of experimentation on guinea pigs, and Captain Williams and fourteen others are taking the vaccine themselves to see what happens. In six months he hopes to have at least an indication of whether it will work; in a year perhaps "some conclusion."

The medical schools also add to the strengt hof the Army. Walter Reed is giving 1,200 doctors a year special training in tropical medicine and other peculiar Army problems.

April 15, 1943

---

37 HOSPITAL SHIPS SERVE ARMY, NAVY

By ARTHUR H. RICHTER

Declaring that the supplying of the necessary tonnage to furnish our armed forces with hospital ships was one more way in which the American merchant marine has proved its worth as a military

auxiliary, Frank J. Taylor, president of the American Merchant Marine Institute, said yesterday that it was fortunate that the United States had a merchant marine from which vessels could be drawn for this purpose.

Mr. Taylor said that in 1939 the Army had no hospital ships and the Navy only one. Today our armed services possess a fleet of thirty-six new hospital ships, with a capacity for approximately

22,000 patients, which is considered by many to be the equal of, or better, than that of any other nation, he added.

Many of these gleaming white ships are converted American luxury liners, while the others have been drawn from the ranks of the Liberty ships and ex-cargo type troop transports, he said. The merchant marine has made available thirteen former passenger liners, twelve Maritime Commission C-type freighters, six Liberty ships

and two other cargo vessels. Three troop carriers, formerly merchant ships, also have been converted to fit into our "mercy" fleet.

Maximum Safety Assured

"These conversions," Mr. Taylor said, "were designed to insure maximum stability and safety. On board, facilities include operating rooms, dispensaries, a pharmacy, laboratories, refrigerating rooms, sterilizing units, wards and dressing stations for all types of war illnesses, physical and mental.

"Electrically operated 'mechanical cows' provide milk and ice cream. Dining halls, lounges and a variety of recreation equipment make the vessels examples of unsurpassed service. They are air-conditioned throughout and as fireproof as is possible in ship construction.

"Averaging 600 beds, these ships have a total capacity of about 22,-000 casualties. Perhaps the best land comparison for one of America's ultra-modern hospital ships is to say that it is the floating equivalent of a seven to nine-story hospital covering a small city block."

Mr. Taylor explained that the operation of hospital ships was unique among wartime sailings because, unlike other vessels, they operate in the open, without secrecy. As each hospital ship is completed, he pointed out, official notification of her commissioning is given to the governments of Germany and Japan, in accordance with the terms of the 1907 Hague Convention.

Hospitals ships travel fully lighted at night over routes not commonly used by convoys and give frequent wireless identification and position locations. They are easy to identify by day or night as they are painted white from smokestack to waterline, with the hull encircled by a broad green band and with giant red crosses painted on either side amidships, on deck and on the funnel. Many of the funnel crosses are electrically lighted for night identification.

According to institute statistics, the "leaders" of the fleet are three former world-cruise ships, the American President Lines' Presidents Madison, Buchanan and Fillmore. Two of the Grace Line's Santa ships, later known as the Irwin and the Kent, also are members of the fleet.

Other ex-passenger ships include a number of popular coastwise liners, well known in this port, such as the Iroquois, Algonquin and Seminole of the Clyde-Mallory Line, the Acadia of the Eastern Steamship Company, the United Fruit's Munargo and New York & Cuba Mail liners Siboney and Yucatan.

The Relief, only hospital ship in service before the war, was built in 1920, and has served with the Navy since. The Larkspur has had an interesting career, starting out as an auxiliary of the Imperial German Navy in 1901 as the Breslau. She was taken over by the United States in the last war and served for many years as the Navy destroyer tender Bridgeport before being converted into a hospital ship.　　November 12, 1944

VETERAN HOSPITALS WIDELY CRITICIZED
By LEO EGAN

Whatever decision Congress makes with respect to the scope of medical and hospital services to be provided for war veterans through the Veterans Administration, a complete overhauling is needed to improve medical and nursing standards, in the interest of veterans, medical science and public health. Such is the opinion of many impartial and distinguished physicians and scientists familiar with Veterans Administration hospitals and medicine.

Underlying a great mass of medical criticism of veterans hospitals in the last year and a half is a feeling that medicine and hospitalization have been treated as stepchildren by General Frank T. Hines, the Administrator of Veterans Affairs and the Veterans Administration. The primary concern of the Veterans Administration has been pensions, bonuses and disability claims, according to some critics. It also is charged by some doctors that more attention has been devoted to the construction of monumental hospital buildings than to the standards of care within them.

In support of this criticism, physicians usually point to the fact that some of the Veterans Administration's facilities, as its hospitals are officially known, are headed by managers who are not doctors, and that the Deputy Veterans Administrator in charge of hospitals, construction and supplies is Col. George E. Ijams, who is not a doctor. Before the last war he was in the insurance business in Baltimore and achieved distinction in World War I by selling $200,-000,000 worth of Government life insurance to American soldiers in France. The medical director of veterans hospitals is Dr. Charles M. Griffiths, one of many subordinates serving under Colonel Ijams.

While many physicians, especially men of reputation who have visited veterans' hospitals as consultants, dispute the allegation that veterans receive third-rate treatment, there is an unusual unanimity among medical men, including these consultants, that the quality of Veterans Administration medicine could be vastly improved. There is also wide agreement that a tremendous waste of research and clinical material takes place in veterans' hospitals.

Unlike most civilian hospitals, whether supported by voluntary contributions and fees or by public monies, Veterans Administration hospitals obtain their medical and nursing staffs through civil service. These full-time, salaried physicians and nurses are supplemented from time to time, as special cases require, by part-time consultants and specialists from civilian hospitals and private practice.

Under the usual civil service procedure, promotions in the medical and nursing staffs are based on length of service and an "efficiency" rating, based on reports from the head of the institution in which the doctor or nurse is serving.

Including pay and allowances, Veterans Administration physicians receive from $3,200 to $9,000 a year, plus, for the present, a $648 war service overtime bonus. But these salaries fail to attract many of the most promising young doctors or the more capable older ones, even in normal times, according to many medical authorities.

Among the reasons for this, it is said, is the fact that until recently, the Veterans Administration never has encouraged teaching within its institutions and therefore these were not approved for residencies or internships by the American Medical Association or the American College of Surgeons. Young doctors in Veterans Administration service have not, therefore, been able to use their experience to qualify for any of the "boards" that give recognition from organized medicine to specialists.

Failure of the American Medical Association or the College of Surgeons to approve Veterans Administration hospitals in itself implies no criticism of them. Hospitals are rated by these two agencies only when they provide teaching facilities. Those that provide no teaching, as has been the case in VA facilities, are not rated at all. Recently a few veterans' hospitals, among them the Kingsbridge facility in the Bronx, have decided to encourage residencies and are having no difficulty getting the necessary approvals from organized medicine.

Another factor discouraging applications for service in veterans' hospitals is the lack of prestige of their medical staffs. In the years they have been in existence the veterans' hospitals have failed to build up such a tradition as attracts doctors, particularly new graduates, to the United States Public Health Service, Columbia-Presbyterian Medical Center, the Army and Navy Medical Corps and other institutions of wide reputation.

Despite these conditions, the Veterans Administration is able, in the opinion of most impartial medical men, to attract a large number of capable physicians, but all too frequently discourages them from keeping abreast of the latest developments in their profession, from putting into effect new techniques and new therapies or making any substantial contribution to the advancement of medical science.

With few notable exceptions, veterans' hospitals are located at places distant from large medical centers. The architecturally imposing structures generally constitute a small community of their own, with the result that the medical and nursing staffs are insulated from contemporary medicine and from outside social contacts. In such atmospheres the social and professional jealousies and intrigues so typical of peacetime Army camps flourish, discouraging initiative and dulling ambition. Frequently the medical libraries of such hospitals are poorly stocked.

There are other discouragements, too. Physicians are assigned on the basis of hospital needs, at the moment rather than their special aptitudes. Practice is regulated rigidly by a thick volume known as Rules and Procedures, which specifies in great detail what a doctor shall do, while new techniques, therapies and medicines can be prescribed only after they have been tested and approved by the VA research center in Washington. Social workers assigned to institutions are not available to the medical staff to help clear up home or environmental problems that may be preventing a patient from obtaining maximum benefits from hospitalization because they are used to investigate disability claims.

But none of these restrictions, irksome as they are to many VA physicians, is as annoying as the volume of paper work they must perform. Reports, notes, observations and memoranda that are dictated to stenographers in most hospitals are written first in longhand in the Veterans Administration by the physicians themselves. Actually the volume of work is heavier than civilian physicians ever have to carry. This is because every patient in a veterans' hospital, regardless of his ailment or infirmity, is regarded officially as a "compensable," i. e. if he is not yet drawing a disability allowance from the Veterans Administration he may soon apply for one. And allowances to disabled veterans account—and will continue for many years to account—for the great bulk of the VA budget.

Indicative of the resistance to medical innovations in the Veterans Administration hospitals is the matter of occupational therapy for tubercular patients. Some years ago physicians in civilian tuberculosis hospitals became convinced that the diversionary type of occupational therapy was inadequate and insufficient. It consisted of such occupations as basket weaving, handiwork, needlecraft or leather working. While it served to divert the patient's attention from his ailment and gave him something to occupy his mind and hands, it did not provide him with any useful skill that could be used to earn a living later.

As an improvement, a start was made in civilian hospitals with purposeful occupational therapy, consisting of such things as typewriting, stenography, printing. Patients whose physical condition permits now receive in many hospitals aptitude tests and counsel in choosing a new occupation—where one is needed—that will enable them to become useful members of the community with a minimum of risk of recurrence of their ailment.

Where introduced, purposeful occupational therapy has proved a great success. By giving the patient a goal to work for and new hope, it has brought about enormous reductions in the twin problems of TB sanatoria—absences without leaves and discharges against medical advice.

The use of purposeful occupational therapy was started in 1939 at the New York City Sanitarium at Otisville, N. Y., and has been greatly expanded and improved since then with results that are completely satisfying to hospital and health authorities.

But despite this record, the Veterans Administration only now is considering the introduction of such treatment. A group of its occupational therapies have been receiving instruction in its use from the National Tuberculosis Association. When they have finished they will organize a demonstration to prove to the Veterans Administration that it should be introduced generally and will then give instruction to other VA therapists.

In justification of their attitude, Veterans Administration facilities contend that the World War I veterans who until recently constituted the bulk of their TB cases, were not interested in learning new vocational skills and were above the age bracket at which the best results were obtained in civilian institutions with purposeful therapy. Most World War I veterans are in the 45 to 55 age group. Most of those receiving purposeful therapy at the New York City Sanitarium in Otisville are under 30.

The new shift to purposeful activity is being explained by the influx of World War II cases in the lower age limits.

May 16, 1945

DISEASES OF AGED HOSPITAL PROBLEM

A shift in the emphasis of hospital care from acute illnesses to degenerative and long-term ailments is noted in the August issue of The Bulletin of the Hospital Council of Greater New York, to be issued today.

"The great advances in medicine within the last fifty years have either eliminated or brought under control the acute diseases and infections which formerly took so great a toll in the lives of young people," the publication says.

"Improved surgical techniques, new drugs, equipment and methods of practice and the solution of so many environmental health problems, have largely been centered around the acute diseases and have resulted in increasing numbers of people continuing to live longer lives.

"This extension of the average life span, plus the gradual decline in the birth rate and the drop in immigration, has caused a shift in the population distribution. Today, even though half the population is under 30 years of age, society is faced with the growing problem created by the increase in the number and percentage of people living beyond the middle years of life and into old age."

As the population ages, the report continues, problems of serious consequence to the community arise as a result of the increasing need for services and facilities for patients with such diseases as arterio-sclerosis, high blood pressure, rheumatism, nephritis, diabetes, and other illnesses of long duration.

To help restore the hope and usefulness of these patients and reduce the "staggering cost" to the community, the council recommends the establishment of facilities for long-term care in connection with general hospitals, an increase of rehabilitation and home services and more facilities for teaching, training and research.

Referring to its "Master Plan for Hospitals and Related Facilities for New York City," the council estimated that 16,000 beds would be needed in eighty general hospitals by 1950 to care for 86,-400 residents, who by then will be disabled for a year or more. The 16,000 beds, nearly one-eighth of all the beds, are exceeded only by the number required for general care and the mental diseases.

September 17, 1947

ONE OF 10 IN NATION HOSPITALIZED IN '47

Yet City After City Warns That Rising Deficits May Deprive Many Persons of Care

DEMAND FOR BEDS UP 50%

Nonprofit Institutions, Hard Hit by Debts, Serve More Than Half of U. S. Patients

By LUCY FREEMAN

City after city throughout the country reports that its voluntary hospitals are confronted with mounting deficits. The tragic effect may be to deprive many persons of adequate hospital care, according to a survey just completed by THE NEW YORK TIMES.

One out of every ten persons in the nation entered a hospital as a patient last year and the majority went to the voluntary hospitals.

The 2,921 voluntary nonprofit hospitals took care of 9,198,159 of the 15,153,452 persons admitted to hospitals in 1946, according to the latest figures available from the annual census of hospitals registered with the American Hospital Association. Of 38,000,000 visits reported by out-patient departments in 1946, almost half were attributed to the voluntary hospitals.

The demand for hospital care has increased 50 per cent since 1940, as reported by the American Hospital Association. In 1936 there were 8,646,885 admissions to the nation's hospitals. This rose to 10,087,548 in 1940 and to 15,153,-452 in 1946.

First Hospital in 1751

The first voluntary hospital, the Pennsylvania Hospital in Philadelphia, opened its doors in 1751 to the sick poor. Since then the nongovernmental hospitals have become indispensable to the country's health services. In recent years it is estimated that voluntary hospitals took care of 60 per cent of all patients, 70 per cent of all free cases and 76 per cent of all births in hospitals.

Two factors have combined to increase the importance of the voluntary hospitals in the life of this country—the changing concept of the hospital and the changing concept of medicine.

Historically speaking, the voluntary hospital came into existence largely for the care of the sick poor who could not be nursed adequately in their own homes. Most of New York's hospitals were established between 1840 and 1880, voluntarily supported by churches, fraternal and racial groups or philanthropic individuals on behalf of the community's needy. In those days the man of means who became ill was nursed at home.

The great increase in hospital facilities in the present century has been due in large part to the development of anesthesia, aseptic surgery and scientific medicine, the authorities explain. The new techniques, both diagnostic and therapeutic, required elaborate and costly equipment as well as trained personnel that only a large institution such as a hospital could provide. Medical men were quick to see the advantages of treatment in institutions where conditions could be controlled.

Become Medical Centers

As the quality of medical care, nursing, surgery and therapy increased, the man who could afford care turned to the voluntary hospital. Now the modern hospital has become a medical center providing the latest methods of treatment. Years ago only the sickest patient received a thorough examination; today every patient gets a routine physical examination, a laboratory check-up and, at many hospitals, the benefits of a therapeutic service.

This has been accompanied by a changing concept of hospital care.

"We believe hospitals should prevent as well as heal illness," says one hospital administrator.

Thus more attention is paid to diagnosis in the belief that an ounce of diagnostic cure is worth a pound of post-operative care. Medicine now studies the "total patient," considering body and mind as inter-related, discussing the patient not only from the physical point of view but the psychological as well.

The creation of social service departments has helped in the solution of personal problems that often retard recovery. Services for convalescent care have prevented recurrence of illnesses and have shortened the periods of recovery. Home service has provided a check on discharged patients; one hospital estimated this saved three times what it would have cost in readmissions.

Hospitals, therefore, have become social as well as medical institutions. They are now community health centers, places to go to get well, as opposed to the old concept of places in which to die.

Fewer Born in Homes

Several factors are responsible for the recent demand for hospital services. Where once births took place chiefly in homes, now nearly everyone in the larger communities is born in a hospital. In New York, for instance, 98 per cent of all babies were born in hospitals in 1946. Throughout the nation two out of every three babies were born in hospitals in 1946; the births in hospitals have increased 76 per cent since 1940.

As an indication of the efficient hospital care for the public, only 1.8 maternal deaths in a thousand were reported in New York in 1946. A minimum of two deaths per thousand was regarded as a goal beyond attainment only a few years ago.

The passage of workmen's compensation laws and the rapid expansion of hospital insurance, particularly the Blue Cross plan, have made it easier for persons to pay for hospitalization. Today 30,000,-000 persons are members of the Blue Cross and 20,000,000 others are covered by commercial health insurance. These plans make it simpler for the hospital to obtain prompt payment of bills for patients who otherwise may be unable to meet the full costs, including doctors bills.

The facts that people are living longer and diseases of old age are increasing have multiplied the need for care of the aged patient. Unemployment of older people since the war has brought a large demand for clinic services as they complain of recurring chronic ailments, minimized during the period of occupation.

While the number of hospital beds has increased from 1,096,721 in 1936 to 1,468,714 ten years later, the need has increased still more. The report of the Commission on Hospital Care estimates an additional 195,000 beds are needed for use in general hospitals alone. The average daily census of patients in hospitals rose from 980,516 in 1936 to 1,239,454 in 1946.

Not only is hospital care big business in terms of the number of people served but it is also big business in terms of the monetary value of the physical property needed to provide the services. It is one of the top ten major industries of the country. Hospital plants had a value of more than $4,400,000,000 in 1946.

In order to provide care for patients, expenditures have increased $462,593,000 in 1946 over 1945; from $1,500,762,000 to $1,963,355,000 in civilian hospitals. Salary needs accounted for 56.2 per cent of the total expenses of all types of hospitals.

The number of full-time hospital employes increased from 608,732 in 1945 to 829,500 in 1946. Of these, 381,258 were employed by the voluntary hospitals. Counting additional part-time and volunteer employes, hospital workers of all types numbered more than 1,000,000 in 1946.

The ratio of nurses, graduate and student, to the population has improved steadily. In 1910, it was one nurse, for 1,116 persons; in 1940, one nurse for 357, and, in 1946, one nurse for 316. Today, with the trend toward the forty-hour week and the increase in the number of patients, the need is for more nurses. An enrollment of 50,000 first-year students in schools of nursing is sought this year.

The modern voluntary hospital no more resembles the hospital of two generations ago than the streamlined automobile does the horse and buggy. Yet the public asks today's hospitals to function on financial horsepower adequate only for outmoded hospitals.

The scope of medical service has widened but the sources of income have decreased. Only a few voluntary hospitals in rural areas, serving small groups, face the future with any degree of certainty.

February 24, 1948

HOSPITAL-AID PLAN HAS 347 PROJECTS

By BESS FURMAN
Special to THE NEW YORK TIMES.

WASHINGTON, July 1—The national hospital construction program, under which the first project was approved only six months ago, now numbers 347 projects in forty-two states, the Public Health Service announced today.

Construction now in process will add 11,846 general beds to the nation's facilities, at a total cost of $160,734,258 of which the Federal Government under the Hill-Burton act pays one-third; the states and local communities two-thirds.

The Federal Government's contribution was $46,246,067 during the six months. With the opening of the new fiscal year today, an additional $75,000,000 becomes available for the fiscal year to end July 1, 1949.

The New York State hospital plan, accepted only last week, undoubtedly will get started under this new appropriation. Public health officials complimented it highly as being carefully worked out to meet the needs of the state.

Contrary to general predictions, the Public Health Service reported, the neediest areas have been able to meet the two-to-one fund-matching plan and hospitals actually are being constructed in remote rural counties. While the expectation had been that fifty-bed hospitals would be the smallest built under the program, many twenty-five-bed hospitals are being built. At the request of many states, the Public Health Service staff of hospital architects has worked out plans for a twenty-five-bed hospital and has prepared cost estimates for it.

Florida counties were reported as in the front row in requests for new hospitals. This was explained as partially due to that state's heavy taxes on race-track betting, which are equally divided among all Florida counties. The poor counties, receiving as much as the rich ones, have been earmarking their funds for hospitals. The first hospital built and dedicated was at Live Oak, Suwannee County, and Surgeon Gen. Leonard A. Scheele went there for the ceremonies.

Mississippi was also mentioned by the Public Health Service as one of the needy states in which, by great local and state effort, money is being raised to build new hospitals. Mississippi is one of eight states which have enacted legislation authorizing state funds for allotment to communities for use in matching Federal money for such construction. The other states are Alabama, California, Illinois, New York, North Carolina, Virginia and Utah. The Territory of Alaska also has this system.

Under a special $3,000,000 fund authorized under the Hill-Burton Act for inventories and surveys of the states, a nationwide system of state hospital building plans has now been drawn up. An analysis of the first 44 state plans showed that 1,361,895 hospital beds were needed.

The Public Health Service has worked out an estimated equipment costs program based on information received from more than 600 manufacturers and distributors of hospital equipment and materials.

The estimated equipment costs ranged from $58,399 up to $96,499 for a 50-bed hospital; $95,440 to $158,127 for a 100-bed hospital; $170,345 to $291,107 for a 200-bed hospital.

New Jersey now has two hospital construction projects under the Hill-Burton plan, a 29-bed new hospital at Menlo Park to cost $834,000; and a 110-bed wing to an existing hospital at Greystone Park to cost $456,000. Connecticut has three, a 110-bed addition to a hospital at Putnam to cost $650,000; a 47-bed general hospital at Willimantic to cost $463,300; and a remodeling at Sharon to add 53 beds and to cost $103,000.

July 2, 1948

Shortage of Nurses Found A Peril to Health of Nation

By HAROLD FABER

More nurses are working today than ever before in the nation's history, yet a critical shortage of nursing service exists in almost every city and rural area.

The extent of the shortage cannot be indicated in precise statistics, because nobody knows exactly how many nurses there are, but anybody who visits a hospital anywhere can see there aren't enough nurses.

Reports from over the country describe the shortage as "critical," "severe," "serious," "acute," and "pressing." What is meant is, hospitals have been forced to shut wards, new installations cannot be opened and new programs for health service cannot be started.

In Boston, for example, more patients could be admitted to hospitals if there were nurses to care for them. The shortage of hospital beds in Atlanta is masking a shortage of nurses. In Alabama, nurses are leaving the state for better jobs.

Chattanooga is following the pattern everywhere — nurses are "spread thin." The Chicago area is not graduating enough nurses to meet its needs. Even though patients are waiting for care, almost all of the thirty-nine hospitals in and around Cleveland have vacant beds because of a lack of personnel.

Only forty-two of Iowa's ninety-nine counties have public health service nurses. Detroit officials are worried about how they are going to staff four new hospitals. In Los Angeles the nurse shortage would be worse if there were enough hospital beds to meet the city's needs.

In New York, three municipal hospitals cannot operate at full capacity, a fully equipped child health center cannot open, and visiting nurse services have been cut. Philadelphia is "extraordinarily short" of public health service nurses.

Pittsburgh authorities admit that nursing service is below standard. In Salt Lake City, nursing groups are afraid to ask for a forty-hour week because of the shortage. Seattle officials estimate their nursing staffs at one-third to one-half under strength.

What is happening is that the nurse shortage is becoming a menace to national health. Moreover, there is every indication the shortage will become "more critical," "more severe" and "more acute" in the near future.

Anybody who tries to determine exactly how many nurses there are, and exactly how short the country is, will soon find himself lost in a maze of mathematical maneuvers.

Three years ago the country had 506,050 nurses, of whom 300,533 were active, according to an inventory by the American Nurses Association. Another inventory is being made by the association and figures will be available next month, but until then any calculation of how many nurses we have is a matter of "educated guessing."

These are the factors that can be used: The 300,533 active nurses early in 1949, plus the graduating classes of 21,379 in 1949, the 25,790 of 1950 and the 28,794 of 1951, less a yearly drop-out, calculated at 6.5 per cent, or about 20,000, for the profession.

From these figures, some mathematicians get results ranging from 316,500 to 330,000 as the number of nurses active today. Some think there may be more. A statistician for the Health Resources Advisory Committee puts it this way: "Use 330,000 and you won't be far wrong."

How many nurses do we need? An estimate of 381,886 to provide for "absolutely minimum" civilian requirements was made last year by representatives of nursing organizations. This is how they broke down their figures:

Non-Federal hospitals (general, allied and special) and educational programs in nursing	237,339
Public health	30,000
Industrial	18,000
Private duty	53,000
Other (including office)	27,000
Federal civilian hospitals	16,547
Total	**381,886**

If that estimate, which excludes the increased needs of veterans hospitals, is accepted, as it is by all groups studying the subject, the current shortage in numbers can be put at about 50,000 exclusive of military needs.

Why is the shortage so great, if we have more nurses than ever?

There is general agreement among nursing and other health groups that we need more nursing service because of the tremendous expansion of health and medical services, emphasized today by the mobilization program. The following factors have changed the pattern of medical and, therefore, of nursing care:

1. The rising average age of the population.
2. The growth of population and its urbanization.
3. The growth of hospitalization and group health plans.
4. The change in the techniques of medicine, such as the use of "miracle" drugs that keep alive patients who formerly would have died, and getting patients out of bed faster.
5. The spread of nurses out of hospitals into industry and public health services.
6. The large increase in the number of mothers who have their babies in hospitals.

Everyone agrees on the growth of nursing service calls, but there is a difference of opinion as to whether we need more nurses, or better trained nurses. Nursing groups in general insist both are necessary. Some medical groups, such as the American Medical Association, believe there is no actual shortage of nurses, and that the

present number would be enough, if they were used properly.

One of the key factors in the shortage is not the number of nurses, but their distribution. Nurses, like everybody else, prefer to work from 9 to 5, forty hours a week, with Saturdays and Sundays off. And jobs with these conditions are available, especially in the fast-growing field of industrial nursing.

From all parts of the country comes word that hospital nurses are leaving their low-paying jobs to take positions with the Veterans Administration, which has a starting salary of about $1,000 a year more than in most hospitals, or to accept commissions in the Army, Navy and Air Force.

In the face of all these considerations, there is a growing belief among nurses that the numerical size of the nursing shortage is an academic question. Taking a realistic approach, they hope for, but do not expect, a large growth in the number of girls who enter nursing school and, therefore, an increase in the number of graduates.

This opinion is based on the realization that there is a manpower shortage in general and that other fields are competing for the young woman high school graduate.

Why don't more girls enter nursing? The answer from all over the country is the same: Girls know they can make as much money or more with less preparation — as secretaries, saleswomen or in industry; they know that nurses are overworked and they know that nursing schools still retain some of the conventlike atmosphere that makes study distasteful.

The main reason girls enter nursing is the spirit of service, but girls today, in an expanding labor market, have a choice that perhaps their mothers did not: Nursing is not the only career that offers an opportunity to serve. For example, the armed forces are seeking to enroll 72,000 young women before July.

If the present rate of recruitment is maintained, 4 per cent of all girls, or 42,000 to 44,000, will enter nursing schools each year for the next four years. Not until 1958,

when the babies of the war years begin to reach nursing school age, can there be any significant increase expected in the number of new candidates, according to the following table prepared by the Health Resources Advisory Committee:

Estimated New Students in Schools of Nursing, 1950-59

Year of Admission	Females At Age 17½	Nursing School Enrollees*
1950	1,101,000	44,185*
1951	1,039,000	41,667*
1952	1,079,000	43,200
1953	1,085,000	43,400
1954	1,066,000	42,600
1955	1,093,000	43,700
1956	1,135,000	45,400
1957	1,124,000	45,000
1958	1,167,000	46,700
1959	1,238,000	49,500

*Actual enrollment.

Taking all these factors into consideration, nursing leaders and educators have come to the conclusion that the solution to the nursing shortage will not be found in recruiting more girls, although that is necessary, but in training them and the working nurses for today's pattern of nursing, in which the nurse is the leader of a team of nonprofessional workers caring for the sick and preventing disease.

March 3, 1952

HOSPITALS BIG BUSINESS

With an annual expenditure of $4,000,000,000, hospitals have become the fifth largest business in the country, Dr. Madison B. Brown, executive vice president of Roosevelt Hospital, told the American Surgical Trade Association

yesterday.

Dr. Brown addressed the organization of dealers in hospital supplies at their semi-annual meeting in the Waldorf-Astoria Hotel. He asked them to submit suggestions for improvements in hospitals to the administrators of of each institution where they sold equipment.

Tracing the rise of hospital costs since 1940, Dr. Brown said that patients were getting more service than they were paying for. He explained that their criticism of high hospital bills was caused by failure of hospital authorities to translate costs with mediums patients could understand.

December 17, 1952

HOSPITAL AID LAW IS TEN YEARS OLD

By BESS FURMAN

Special to The New York Times.

WASHINGTON, Aug. 11.— The tenth anniversary of the Hill-Burton Hospital Construction Act on Monday will find its "new program" rolling at last.

This act to provide Federal aid to build hospitals where they were needed most originated as bipartisan legislation. It was sponsored in the Senate by Lister Hill, Democrat of Alabama, and Harold H. Burton, Republican of Ohio, now on the Supreme Court bench.

Since the Hill-Burton legislation was signed by President Truman on August 13, 1946, it has helped to build and put in operation more than 2,000 hospitals providing more than 95,000 beds. A majority have been general hospitals.

In 1954, the Eisenhower Administration pushed through an extension of the act to provide categorical grants to four types of health facilities. Mrs. Oveta Culp Hobby, then Secretary of Health, Education and Welfare, contended that these special facilities were critically needed to relieve the loads of general hospitals.

Eligible for Federal earmarked funds are diagnostic or

treatment facilities, chronic disease institutions, rehabilitation centers and nursing homes.

As late as December 30, 1955, only fourteen of these special projects totaling only $800,000 had been approved by the Public Health Service. It began to seem that most of the first appropriation of $21,000,000 earmarked for the four categories would revert to the Treasury June 30, 1956, since the needed health facilities would not be built.

However, Dr. John W. Cronin, in charge of the hospital construction program of the Public Health Service, told the Senate Appropriations Committee in January of this year that he believed about 175 projects would be approved by June 30. This seemed so far-fetched to the committee that it injected a skeptical note in its official report to the Senate.

However, Dr. Cronin's estimate fell short. The fiscal year ended with 182 projects having been approved. They totaled $18,932,595 of the initial $21,000,000 appropriation.

Of the 182 projects approved: Sixty-four were diagnostic and treatment centers in forty states; thirty-eight were chronic disease centers in thirty-one states; thirty-eight nursing homes in thirty-one states; forty-two were rehabiltation projects in thirty-five states.

Dr. Cronin explained that the original Hill-Burton program had been similarly slow in starting because surveys and plans

had to be made in every state.

After the Hospital Extension Bill became a part of the Hill-Burton Act, it took six months for the eight member Federal hospital council to promulgate regulations as required by law. Then the states had to make surveys on which to base their plans in the four fields. The state plans came in with a rush after Jan. 1 this year. Fifty-two have now been received from states and territories. Only that of the Virgin Islands is missing.

For fiscal 1956, Congress appropriated a second $21,000,000 in the four categories; and a third $21,000,000 for 1957.

Dr. Cronin reported that the rehabilitation centers and the diagnostic and treatment centers were developing in many places as new units of university medical schools.

The first special facility project approved was the Pinal Nursing Home at Florence, Ariz., which will have fifty-three beds in a building fifty yards from the Pinal General Hospital. This, too, set a pattern being widely followed. The nursing home, in these cases, will function under the same hospital board, same physicians, same chief nurse, same dietician as the hospital. When the nurses homes are completed, ambulatory patients will move into them from the general hospital and thus free hospital beds for the acutely ill.

"About 25 per cent of general hospital beds are occupied by

chronic patients, and there is a 200,000 bed shortage in general hospitals," said Dr. Cronin.

The "old program" under the Hill-Burton Act, Dr. Cronin said, is as strong as ever, as popular as ever, with as much demand as ever. Its scope has been limited only by the size of the Federal appropriations which are matched on an elaborate formula under which the needier states get the most money.

For fiscal year, 1957, Congress appropriated $102,000,000 for the original program, an increase of $14,000,000 over the previous year.

Up to the close of the last fiscal year, the cumulative cost of all facilities approved under the act was $2,460,000,000. Of this, the Federal Government had contributed $781,000,000. This had been matched by local sponsors' funds totaling $1,696,000,000.

All the hospitals constructed under the act are nonprofit institutions.

The program has been concentrated strongly in states of low average income. Fifty-two per cent of the projects were in the Southern states, 22 per cent in the North Central states, 14 per cent in the North East states and 12 per cent in Western states.

Fifty-four per cent of the projects were situated in communities of less than 5,000 population. Only 12 per cent were in cities of more than 50,000 persons.

August 12, 1956

HOSPITAL STRIKE ENDS IN 46TH DAY AS PACT IS VOTED

1,100 Union Members Roar 'Aye' to Plan Their Chief Calls a 'Partial Victory'

7 PICKET LINES HALTED

All 81 Voluntary Institutions Asked to Ratify Terms— Wide Acceptance Seen

By HOMER BIGART

Hospital strikers roared approval yesterday to an agreement ending the bitter forty-six-day strike at voluntary institutions.

Eleven hundred nurses' aides, cooks, orderlies, porters and housekeeping workers squeezed into the ballroom of the Diplomat Hotel and shouted "Aye" when proposals described as a "partial victory" were read to them. A loud but solitary "No" was also heard.

Leon J. Davis, president of the striking union, Local 1199 of the Retail Drug Employes Union, said that the agreement provided only "backdoor recognition" for his union. But he added: "We'll be in the front door before long."

Mayor Gets Statement

The agreement, arranged by Mayor Wagner after weeks of negotiation, was embodied in a statement of policy by the hospitals. John V. Connorton, president of the Greater New York Hospital Association, handed it to the Mayor late yesterday.

Mr. Connorton denied that the agreement provided for union recognition. Neither, he said, did it provide for a union structure within the hospitals.

The policy declaration will apply to those of the association's eighty-one member hospitals that ratify the document. The seven hospitals that were struck were members of the association.

Mayor Wagner predicted that the majority would go along, since most of the association members had participated in the negotiations. He said he was "delighted" by the ending of the strike and hoped that the peace would last for years.

Decisions to Be Prompt

He said that he understood that the declaration would be considered promptly by the boards of all the voluntary hospitals. "Am I right, John?" he asked Mr. Connorton. Mr. Connorton nodded affirmatively.

The provisions for grievance machinery and wage reviews were couched in such terms that both Mr. Connorton and Mr. Davis appeared correct in their conflicting interpretations.

In the mediation of grievances, workers may be represented by anyone they designate. The union considers this "foot-in-the-door recognition" because there is nothing to prevent a worker from choosing a union official.

Wage levels would be reviewed annually by a twelve-man "permanent administrative committee" composed of six hospital trustees, to be named by the hospital association, and six public figures to be designated by the chief judge of the Court of Appeals.

The agreement calls for a minimum hourly wage of $1 an hour with a wage boost of at least $2 a week to every employe whose weekly wage is not increased by $2 through the lifting of the hourly rate. The struck hospitals put this wage rate into effect several weeks ago.

The hospitals promised not to discriminate against employes who joined or remained members of any union. They also promised to drop all legal action against the union except an appeal from a decision by Justice Henry Epstein in State Supreme Court.

Justice Epstein ruled on June 12 that the strike was a "bona fide labor dispute" and refused to punish the union's leaders for contempt of a no-strike injunction. He contended that voluntary hospitals were subject to a section of the Civil Practices Act that makes injunctions difficult to obtain.

Both sides agreed that an important matter of law was involved and that the appeal should be continued but with the understanding that no punishment would be sought by the hospitals.

Picket Lines Withdrawn

Picket lines were withdrawn from the hospitals yesterday and Mr. Davis said the strikers would start drifting back to their jobs today.

The hospitals are not obligated to take all of them back at once. But they have promised to reinstate them "as quickly as practical and feasible, unless guilty of violence."

Mount Sinai, the largest of the struck hospitals, said it would mail reinstatement cards to all workers who had not reported by 11 A. M. today except for thirty-five employes charged with violence.

The vote to end the strike came at a meeting that was relaxed and jubilant, with no more tension than a clambake.

Mr. Davis made no attempt to explain the fine points of the agreement, and other officials said that one point—the classification of nonprofessional employes—was still in dispute.

The hall was stifling. Men sat around in T-shirts, fanning themselves with newspapers. Many of the women brought their children and the din was terrific.

Cautions Strikers

Mr. Davis cautioned the strikers, most of them Negroes and Puerto Ricans with no prior union experience: "Be patient. Don't create imaginary things. Don't make it more difficult. Don't be offensive. Don't be provocative. Act like organized workers."

After the vote, the strikers met in groups to elect their representatives. Mr. Davis said these representatives were, in effect, shop stewards although the term was offensive to the hospitals.

He also said that the six public members of the wage-review committee would be selected by the chief judge of the Court of Appeals from a slate nominated by the union. This statement was challenged by a hospital association spokesman who denied that such a procedure was part of the agreement.

Mr. Davis announced that the drug union was setting up an "independent" division for the hospital workers.

Meanwhile the hospital association approved its policy declaration at a general membership meeting. Then Mr. Connorton took it to the Mayor.

At City Hall Mr. Connorton said:

"Unpleasant as the strike has been for all concerned it will have accomplished a great deal for both the hospitals and their employes if it has dramatized to the public the urgent need for hospitals funds from increased Blue Cross income, from the city and from the public."

The city's first major hospital strike began May 8 at Mount Sinai, Lenox Hill, Beth David, Beth Israel, Bronx and Brooklyn Jewish Hospitals and spread June 5 to Flower and Fifth Avenue Hospital.

Union recognition was the key issue. As private, nonprofit institutions, the hospitals contended that they were exempt from provisions of the State Labor Relations Act and were not obliged to engage in collective bargaining with any union.

Their adamant refusal to recognize Local 1199 fanned a confused and intensely bitter labor dispute. The support and prestige of the entire labor movement in the city was committed to Local 1199. The struck hospitals were strongly backed by the Greater New York Hospital Association, which represents eighty-one voluntary institutions.

There were undertones, too, of racial tension. Most of the strikers were Negroes and Puerto Ricans. The charge of racial exploitation was raised by labor leaders, who said that the hospitals were taking unfair advantage of the pool of cheap labor from the slums.

Despite this explosive element, there was only one major outbreak of violence. It came June 9 when street fighting broke out between pickets and the police near Flower and Fifth Avenue Hospital. Seven pickets were arrested in the fifteen-minute clash.

On the same day, Mayor Wagner released a peace formula devised by his special three-man mediation board. This board consisted of William Hammatt Davis, chairman; Aaron Horvitz and Joseph P. McMurray.

Neither labor nor management was entirely happy with the Davis formula. But Mayor Wagner approved it as a basis for settlement and summoned both sides to all-night meetings in City Hall.

June 23, 1959

Hospital-Bred Infection Thought More Prevalent Than Estimated

Experts' Guesses on Incidence Range From 1% to 30%—A. M. A. Finds Danger of Germs Is Exaggerated

By JOHN A. OSMUNDSEN

No one knows the real magnitude of the problem of hospital-acquired infections.

It is certain, however, that more persons are developing new infections unnecessarily while in hospital for other disorders than the best available statistics would indicate.

Most hospitals estimate that between 1 and 2 per cent of all their patients develop such infections.

Other authorities, however, say that the rate is closer to 5 per cent.

A British medical journal, The Lancet, has noted editorially that the frequency of hospital-acquired infection varies all the way from 3 to 30 per cent.

One way in which these differences of opinion might arise was suggested in a report earlier this year of an eighteen-month evaluation of hospital infections in six Government hospitals. The study was conducted by the United States Veterans Administration Cooperative Committee for Hospital Infection.

Infection Rate Higher

Before the study began, the frequency of infections was reported to be in the range of one-half of 1 per cent to 2 per cent, the committee wrote. During the study, however, the infection rate jumped to between 4 and 5 per cent.

And "in one of the large general hospitals where a compulsive and energetic assistant chief of service personally sought all infection in an effort sustained over several months, the frequency fluctuated between 13 and 15 per cent," according to the report. "On his promotion elsewhere," the report continued, "it dropped precipitously to the more comfortable pre-study level of 1 to 2 per cent."

The committee concluded that "the frequency of significant staphylococcal infections in general medical and surgical hospitals ranged between 10 and 13 per cent."

Aside from inefficiency in identifying and reporting their infections, another reason why the cases rate is probably underestimated has been cited by Dr. Reimert Ravenholt. He is director of the division of epidemiology and communicable disease control for the Seattle-King County Department of Health in the State of Washington. He said:

"Most physicians, including pathologists, ascertain only the anatomic site of infection at post-mortem; rarely is an attempt made to determine the [causative] agent."

Autopsy Findings Cited

When Dr. Ravenholt reviewed 7,837 deaths in Seattle-King County in 1956, he found from autopsy data that certainly more than 100 and possibly 200 of the deaths had involved staph infection. The original death certificates had listed only four deaths from that cause.

In a more recent study reported in The Journal of the American Medical Association, the infection rate in a group of newborn infants rose 10 per cent after autopsy figures had been carefully rechecked.

Some authorities say that such findings may overstate the case because staphylococci are extremely hardy germs, and their presence after death may in many cases be irrelevant. These experts do not deny, however, that more deaths are caused by these infections than are so designated.

The occurrence of infection long after patients have been discharged is another factor contributing to the low estimates many hospitals make of the problem.

Study of Infant Cited

A study was conducted by Dr. Valerie Hurst and Dr. Moses Grossman of the University of California Medical Center in San Francisco sixteen months after an outbreak of impetigo, a rash. It revealed that:

"Although only twelve of the infants had contracted impetigo while in the nursery, staphylococcal disease that seemed attributable to exposure in the nursery subsequently occurred among an additional thirty-one infants."

The report in the May 12 number of The New England Journal of Medicine went on to note that mastitis, boils or other skin disease had developed in sixteen mothers, twenty of the infants' brothers and sisters, and ten fathers. Most of those infections would not be considered hospital-acquired by many authorities.

Despite the growing number of scientific reports on this problem in medical journals both here and abroad, some authorities insist that the seriousness of the situation has been exaggerated.

An editorial in the July 9 number of The Journal of the American Medical Association, for example, accused the lay press of producing "a distorted echo of the medical reports." It might be argued that the editorial exaggerated the exaggerations it alleged. Nevertheless, there is little doubt among many authorities who have studied the infection problem for several years that an increasing number of hospital-acquired cases are caused by inadequate techniques and inappropriate use of antibiotics as well as by breaks in hospital aseptic procedures. The Journal's editorial tends to discount these factors.

Dr. Ravenholt, for example, has said that "only the better hospitals recognize that they have any staph problem."

Because hospital infections are frequently caused by germs resistant to most antibiotics, programs to control the menace have largely been aimed at killing the organisms before they can infect.

Three such programs concentrate on keeping certain critical areas of the hospital free from contamination by using chemical germicides, bacteriacidal radiation and other aseptic measures.

At Duke University, for example, Dr. Deryl Hart has reported reducing the rate of infection of "clean," or uncontaminated, wounds to .24 per cent by performing all surgery for the last twenty-three years under ultra-violet radiation, which is lethal to germs.

Another infection-prevention program utilizing ultra-violet radiation is being carried out by Dr. Edward Phillips and his staff at the Mount Sinai Hospital in Los Angeles.

It is called the Robbins Aseptic-Air System. It consists of seventy-two closed ultra-violet chambers installed in the basement and attached to the air-conditioning system. Although encouraging results were reported in February, the effectiveness of the system is still under study.

The frequency of clean-wound infections is reported to have been kept within the remarkably low range of one-quarter of one per cent for two-years at the Huggins Hospital in Wolfboro, N. H., with a "critical-care zone" system conceived by Dr. Ralph Adams.

Extra Precautions Taken

According to this system, special aseptic procedures are followed in the operating suite, the premature nursery and nursery, and the isolation unit. These critical zones are sterilized frequently with germicides. Hospital employes entering them must don "sexless, sizeless, sideless, quick-change, double-breasted" gowns, protective booties over their shoes, and, in certain cases, fitted filter masks.

Those environmental control systems have focused so far only on special areas of the hospital that are believed to be most infectiously hazardous to patients.

Because it is uncertain how and where infections are contracted, one system has been developed to render the entire hospital environment not only sterile but also actively lethal to bacteria over long periods. The Permachem Corporation of West Palm Beach, Fla, was the developer.

It was reported last week to have kept three hospitals in New York State, Virginia and Oklahoma free from hospital-acquired infection for more than two years.

Moreover, several large-scale bacteriological cultures of the hospitals' air, floors, walls, furniture, blankets and linens were reported to have failed to detect any bacteria. Only when vacations interfered with the housekeeping procedures in the Culpeper Hospital in Culpeper, Va., were a few bacteria found, most of them in dirt.

The Permachem system owes most of its effectiveness to the powerful, long-lasting germicides used. They consist of organo-metallic complexes, organic acids and quaternary ammonium compounds.

Used in Varied Ways

Those substances are blended into paints, floor waxes and window-cleaning preparations, sprayed on walls and furniture, added to the laundry rinse water, put into air-recirculation filters and into floor-cleaning solutions.

The system was first tested under carefully controlled conditions at the Francis Delafield Hospital, Columbia-Presbyterian Medical Center, by Dr. Perry Hudson. He is now a professor of zoology on Columbia's faculty of pure science and on the staff of Montefiore Hospital in the Bronx.

Dr. Hudson found that the system was more than 80 per cent effective in eliminating bacterial contamination from the environment over long periods. This finding was recently confirmed by Dr. Mary Barber at the Hammersmith Hospital in London.

Thus, several studies and practical applications of systems for controlling the hospital environment indicate that unnecessary infections can be prevented.

The extension of such concepts beyond the hospital environment seems clearly to be needed and is already being tried to a limited extent.

The object of all of this work is, as Governor Rockefeller said at a recent public-health meeting, to find some way of "controlling our environment and the chronic illness in it before our illnesses control us."

August 15, 1960

HOSPITALS CHIDED FOR REGIMENTING

Ounces of prevention are becoming pounds of regimentation in a growing number of hospitals throughout the country, a study finds.

It attributes the trend to an increasing tendency of hospitals to put organizational requirements ahead of the individual needs of patients.

The criticism comes from a physician and a sociologist, who term the approach inconsiderate, inflexible and inept.

Unless sweeping changes are made in the "whole concept" of hospitalization, the report warns, the hospital will become simply a "convenient place" to apply medical and nursing techniques with hardly any notice of the patient involved.

The authors of the report, titled "The Hazards of Hospitalization," are Dr. Leon Lewis and Rose Laub Coser. Their findings appear in the current issue of Hospital Administration, a professional journal.

In some cases, they said, the patient appeared to be "incarcerated" instead of hospitalized.

But they also found that rebellion against the inroads of regimentation was beneficial to the patient. The one who complains about the hospital usually gets well faster than the one who passively accepts the hospital's routine, they said.

And the patient who is allowed to be up and around, to take care of his own needs and to worry about what is going on at home or at the office usually was found to recover more rapidly than the one who lies in bed all day, heeding the hospital's advice of not to worry about anything.

One trouble, as they saw it, was that hospitals try to keep patients out of the way of daily routine for the sake of "organizational efficiency," which meant that the patient spent most of his time in bed whether it was needed or not.

Caution on Bed Rest

The bed, they advised the hospital administrators, should be looked upon as "a useful but dangerous instrument."

"Bedrest should be prescribed with the same cautious consideration as drugs," they said, otherwise the patient would be left to the "hazards" of inactivity, disinterest and enforced passivity.

What was worse, they said, was that a patient forced into the passive acceptance of supervision, relieved of the need to make decisions and isolated from the outside world may not be willing to reassume the obligations of ordinary life when released.

The call for change envisioned a more active role for the patients whenever possible and a closer link between them and the attending staff.

Much of what they found wrong with hospital methods was blamed on "intrenched" procedures. But they felt the outlook for change was favorable.

"The most expensive type of comprehensive care," they said, "is less costly in the long run than prolonged custodial hospitalization."

August 28, 1960

ELECTRONIC NURSE GUARDS PATIENTS

By ROBERT K. PLUMB

Electrical bed attachments to provide continuous monitoring of the conditions of acutely ill patients are among the devices in a new Roosevelt Hospital ward that opened yesterday.

The devices, attached to eight beds, will check on the patients' pulse and respiration rates and temperatures and will take electrocardiograms and electroencephalograms.

A nurse at a central electronic observation panel can keep these physiological processes in the eight patients under constant observation and make permanent records of them.

A new special-care unit with seventeen beds in all was opened at the hospital as a laboratory to work out ideas for the new Garrard Winstron Memorial Building. That 400-bed addition to the hospital, at 428 West Fifty-ninth Street, will be opened in 1962.

The $110,300 unit supplements the surgical recovery room at the hospital. The electrical set-up was installed by EPSCO, Inc., of Cambridge, Mass.

Electronic monitoring of physiological processes has long been used in operating rooms. But hospital spokesmen believe that the new Roosevelt unit is the first completely monitored system for patient observation to be established in New York City.

Dr. James E. Thompson, chief of surgery at the hospital, said, "At the end of our experimental period, we shall have a model acute-care unit which will not only save patients' lives but also cut medical costs, eliminate waste of personnel and equipment and serve as a model for other hospitals throughout the country."

Dr. Howard A. Patterson, president of the hospital medical board, emphasized that the new ward was a "child of the nursing shortage."

Round-the-clock nursing requires three nurses for each patient each day, he pointed out. The seventeen beds in the special-care unit will require five to eight nurses each shift, he said.

The unit will handle the seventeen sickest patients in the hospital.

Marianne Hartmann, who has been at Roosevelt since 1952, is in charge of the unit. Her assistant is Anne Skelly.

Present plans call for twelve nurses to take care of the seventeen beds. Miss Hartmann estimated that the unit would cut in half the number of nurses needed to take care of the seriously ill.

November 23, 1960

Disposable Hospital Devices Gain

By RICHARD RUTTER

A significant trend within a trend is developing in the hospital supply field.

The big or "outside" trend is one of rapid growth. Sales of hospital equipment are at an estimated rate of $500,-000,000 to $550,000,000 a year. They have been steadily increasing in recent years and they are expected to continue to rise, probably much more rapidly in the years ahead.

The "inside" trend is toward increasing the use of disposable hospital and medical equipment. The importance of this development was dramatized all too vividly recently by a tragic case in New Jersey in which more than a dozen persons died of hepatitis reportedly caused by a contaminated injection needle or infusion apparatus.

A pre-sterilized, disposable needle—and other disposable-type equipment such as syringes, gloves, tubing, matress covers, masks and waste container liners—is used only once and then discarded. Chances of cross-infection are said to be reduced drastically.

Vast Rise Foreseen

In 1960, there were about 1,628,000 hospital beds available in this country. By 1975, about 3,243,000 beds are expected to be needed. This projection is based on these factors:

¶A population growth to about 225,000,000 to 230,000,000 by 1975.

¶Increased public awareness through "education" programs and the like—of the importance of medical care coupled with an improved per capita financial ability to afford hospitalization. Some form of a Federal program of medical care for the aged, as planned by the Kennedy Administration, probably will become law sooner or later.

¶The rapid growth of urban areas. This is where hospital utilization has been greatest.

¶The growth and spread of hospitalization insurance. Today, about 74 per cent of the population has some form of hospitalization insurance, compared with 48 per cent ten years ago.

¶The number of those in the 65-and-over age group is expected to grow more rapidly over the next twenty-five years than the rest of the population. This is the age group most in need of hospital and advanced medical care.

The hospital supply field is a comparatively small one, with 150 to 200 manufacturers in the field. Of those, a handful—such as the American Hospital Supply Corporation, Evanston, Ill.; the A. S. Aloe Company, St. Louis; the Will Ross Company, Milwaukee, and the IPCO Hospital Supply Corporation, New York—do the bulk of the business. But the extent of that burgeoning business is indicated by the number of distributors, 550 to 660 or more.

As medical technology has advanced, a change has taken place in the distribution of supplies—through "education" programs plies to hospitals. In past years, salesmen made their "pitch" by talking to the hospital purchasing agent or administrator. Purchasing agents still play an important role, but the decision as to what type of equipment is to be used is often made these days by the people in the hospital who actually use the prod-

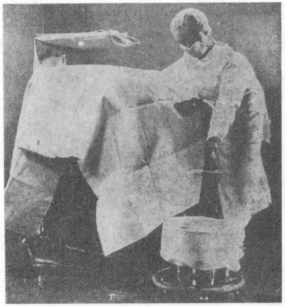

Trend toward use of disposable items in hospitals is manifest by waste liner, syringe, needle and the table drapes.

uct. Salesmen, perforce, must be able to demonstrate and create a demand for their company's line on a professional level.

The greatest part of the average hospital's expense budget goes for labor, perhaps as much as two-thirds. This creates a special problem as compared with industry—where the labor factor is, of course, a substantial one. Industry can reduce payroll costs by means of technological improvements and, eventually, automation. For a hospital to shave costs and maintain high standards of patient care without reducing personnel the main solution would appear to be in labor-saving equipment. And that is where disposable supplies come in.

Storage Space Cut

Besides the matter of built-in sterilization, disposable equipment reduces the need for storage space. It saves the many man-hours that are required for cleaning, sterilization and preparing supplies for re-use—such as sharpening injection needles.

Disposable items are now said to account for about 10 per cent of all hospital supplies and the percentage is growing.

New items are constantly being added to the variety of disposable products. Recently, for instance, IPCO Hospital Supply in cooperation with the Phillips Petroleum Company developed disposable liners for hospital containers. These liners are made of Marlex, a polyethylene plastic material. The Scott Paper Company has come up with Dura-Weve, a reinforced material made by laminating rayon with two or more layers of high wet-strength paper. This is being used in place of cloth for things such as towels, sheets, examination gowns, aprons, bibs, pillow cases and surgical packs.

The cost of medical care has been the fastest single rising item in the cost of living in recent years. Disposable equipment is probably not the answer to this serious economic problem, but it may help at least to check the trend.

February 5, 1961

New Patient Care Theories Require New Hospital Designs

By GEORGE AUERBACH

Modern theories of patient care and the myriad services involved in tending the sick are fostering changes in hospital architecture.

The numerous facilities required to afford complete care for the sick have led to the construction in suburban towns of rambling hospital complexes. In a large metropolis, where limitation of land prevents spreading, services must be placed vertically in such a manner that patients are as near as possible to all facilities.

The need to improve and expand existing hospital facilities has induced the Federation of Jewish Philanthropies of New York to earmark $60,700,000 of the $104,365,000 it hopes to realise from its current building fund drive for hospitals and medical-care agencies.

A four-year survey of the group's hospital plants has indicated that many old buildings

and makeshift quarters must be modernized or replaced. More than a dozen hospitals will be involved in the agency's program.

Large Outlay Involved

Because of the large outlay required to build and equip a hospital, it must remain serviceable for about fifty years, according to Saul Horowitz, president of the H. R. H. Construction Company and a member of the federation's building fund committee. Careful planning is needed to facilitate later expansion or renovation to meet population increases and to accommodate new medical practices.

The federation's hospital building program will include such facilities as circular pavilions, wings with outside corridors that double as patient lounges, multi-building complexes, and the construction of a surgical center between two patient-care pavilions.

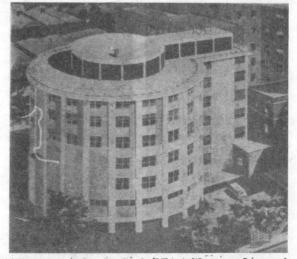

Rendering shows circular building with unusual amount of window space at Maimonides Hospital in Brooklyn.

303

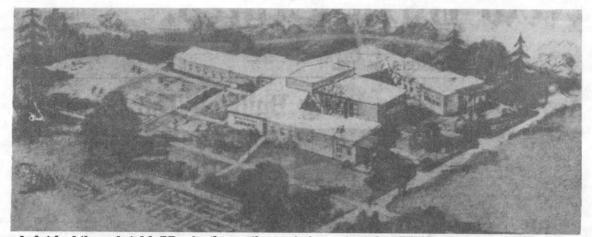

A sketch of the projected building for therapeutic care to be constructed at Hillside Hospital, Glen Oaks, Queens.

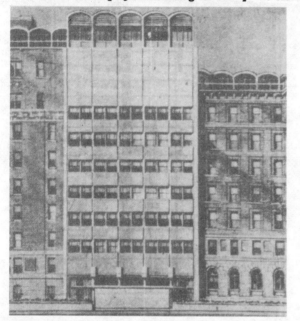

Mount Sinai Hospital, on Fifth Avenue, has received permission to close off 100th Street in order to build a surgery center between two patient-care structures.

A semi-circular addition to the Beth Israel Hospital at Stuyvesant Square and Seventeenth Street will have 300 beds. A semi-circular pavilion with 200 beds and sixty-six bassinets will be built at the Maimonides Hospital at 4802 Tenth Avenue in Brooklyn.

The circular arrangement provides more window space than does a rectangular wing. It also facilitates intensive nursing care, because all rooms are close to the nurses' station in the center of the semi-circle.

Plan Aids Surgery

This floor plan also is advantageous in surgical departments. All operating rooms can be close to the equipment in the center of the circle. This arrangement is superior to long corridors in rectangular buildings, where equipment and nurses' station may be as far as half a city block from some patients.

Ten buildings will be added to Montefiore Hospital in the Bronx. The complex will enable the hospital to expand its services and to operate more efficiently. The additions include a research center, ambulatory services building, staff apartments, emergency suites, storage facilities, central kitchen, diagnostic and treatment center, in-patient facilities, science laboratories and more rooms for patients.

The Long Island Jewish Hospital, a six-story structure opened in 1954, is too small to meet the needs of the area. The building was planned for expansion, and four additional floors will be added. The new floors will add 166 beds to the present 500, and will permit the enlarging of other facilities.

A new building for therapeutic activities will be built at Hillside Hospital in Queens, the city's only voluntary psychiatric hospital for the treatment of acute mental patients responsive to active therapy. The rambling building, when completed, will consolidate theapeutic activities scattered in several locations, will combine research facilities and will provide a sixty-six-bed patients' wing.

The Home and Hospital of the Daughters of Israel will be moved closer to the Long Island Jewish and Hillside hospitals, to create a complex of geriatric-psychiatric-medical facilities. A 300-bed structure with balconies and large glass windows will be built for patients at Daughters of Israel.

There is little room for expansion of Mount Sinai Hospital on Fifth Avenue. However, permission has been obtained from the city to close 100th Street and to build an addition over the fifty-foot-wide street, between existing structures to the north and south.

A ten-story surgery center will be built on the street level and will abut the two patient-care hospital units on either side of 100th Street. The new facilities will be readily accessible to both patient pavilions.

December 24, 1961

HOSPITALS BUILD SUBURBAN UNITS

Special to The New York Times

PITTSBURGH, April 28— Big downtown hospitals, like banks, are establishing branches for more convenient service to suburbanites.

By doing so, downtown hospitals, often surrounded by decaying city blocks, put down new roots in economically healthy communities. Suburban areas get branch hospitals with the full medical and administrative resources of long-established institutions.

Forty hospitals in the country now operate branch units, sometimes at distances of 20 miles. A two-year study financed by the Government Public Health Service describes 11 hospitals in nine states, each of which operates one or more branches with a single medical staff, management and board of trustees.

The Hospital Planning Association of Alleghany County released today what it identified as "the first description of the growing pattern of metropolitan hospitals operating branch units."

"Our downtown hospitals are the product of centralization," Philip B. Hallen, project director for the association said. "As decentralization depopulates and decays the central city, urban hospitals become less convenient to patients and staffs, but they cannot possibly relocate their physical facilities, which represent multimillion-dollar investments.

"On the other hand, new suburban communities, often serving only as dormitories for central cities, cannot initiate comprehensive hospital facilities. To establish new facilities causes a serious drain on the already short supply of professional and technical personnel."

One expedient, the report indicated, is for small hospitals to affiliate with larger medical centers to provide fuller and better service. Another is for major hospitals to establish branches.

Most multiple-unit hospitals are operated by voluntary, non-profit corporations. The oldest two-unit system in the study was the Youngstown (Ohio) Hospital, which established a branch in 1929. Grace Hospital in Detroit started a suburban unit in 1946.

Baptist Memorial in Houston, Tex., has a branch and plans three additional 100-bed hospitals. These will be on freeways that provide good motor connections with the parent hospital.

April 29, 1963

HOSPITAL DESIGNS TREAT OWN 'ILLS'

Innovations Aid Staffs and Add to Patients' Comfort

New designs in hospitals are curing some of the ills that plague buildings intended for the care of the sick.

Among the major problems confronting hospitals today are overcrowded medical wards and a shortage of staff personnel. To some degree, these conditions are being combated by innovations in the design and equipment of the buildings themselves.

Architects are designing buildings to help hospital administrators distribute their staffs more evenly throughout the building. New equipment is being stressed as a way of making more efficient use of doctors and nurses.

A shortage of funds has generally kept hospitals lagging in adapting modern building equipment to their needs. For instance, air-conditioning has been incorporated into the design of hospital buildings only during the last few years.

Operations Are Rescheduled

In addition to contributing to the comfort of patients, air-conditioning has permitted hospitals to function more efficiently. Until the advent of air-conditioning, most patients in need of operations not of an emergency nature chose to have their surgery done during the cooler months of the year, from September to May.

But during these same months hospitals have larger numbers of patients suffering from long-term illnesses—respiratory diseases, heart ailments, arthritis and the like. In warmer weather, the number of patients requiring hospitalization for chronic complaints decreases.

With air-conditioning, elective surgery can be done during the summer with as much comfort for the patient as during the winter. Moreover, many pagery done during their summer vacations, saving themselves time and expense.

From the hospital's point of view, shifting surgery from winter to summer months makes it possible to even out the patient load the year around.

According to Edwin E. Fairfield, an architect whose firm, Crow, Lewis & Wick, has designed more than 150 hospitals, medical wards today are being arranged so that patients with the same needs may be grouped together and receive specialized care.

Recovery rooms for post-operative care, minimal-care units where patients are allowed to tend to many of their own needs, and intensive care sections for patients under constant medical supervision are all becoming standard arrangements in the design of hospitals.

Instead of having a private nurse for each patient requiring close attention, one nurse in a specialized ward can keep close check on a few patients at one time.

Mr. Fairfield finds that most private hospitals are now designed without large wards. Patient rooms today are mostly semi-private, with some four-bed wards.

Having only a few patients to a room allows the hospital greater flexibility in distributing patients by illness, age and sex. Such arrangements help make patients more comfortable in their surroundings, and provide them with better care.

Other new features in hospital design are electrically-operated beds and rooms painted with soft pastel colors.

Many hospitals today, Mr. Fairfield notes, engage professional interior decorators when they plan a new building.

October 13, 1963

HOSPITALS BUILT WITH FEDERAL AID MUST INTEGRATE

Ban on Separate-but-Equal Facilities Is Left Standing by the Supreme Court

WIDE IMPACT EXPECTED

Rights Group Hails Action —Says It Will Affect 2,000 Institutions in the South

Special to The New York Times

WASHINGTON, March 2 — A decision that hospitals built with Federal aid may not segregate their patients or their staffs was left standing today by the Supreme Court.

The United States Court of Appeals for the Fourth Circuit, dividing 3 to 2, handed down the decision last November. It held unconstitutional a provision of the Federal hospital aid law authorizing separate-but-equal facilities.

Today the Supreme Court declined to review the case. As is customary in such actions, it gave no reasons. But the circumstances made it all but certain that the effect would be a new and broad assault on racial practices in the South.

The N.A.A.C.P. Legal Defense and Educational Fund, which handled the case, hailed the Supreme Court's action, saying it would "affect 2,000 hospital and medical facilities throughout the South."

Hailed as 'Entering Wedge'

Jack Greenberg, director-counsel of the fund, said the decision would "put an end to keeping Negroes out of white hospitals or segregating them within the hospitals, and requiring them to give up their Negro doctors and hire white doctors if they wanted treatment." He went on:

"It will be an entering wedge for Negro physicians into the mainstream of medical practice in the South. We wait to see whether the medical profession will voluntarily follow the law or whether a long, hard process of litigation such as we have had with schools will be necessary."

The immediate legal effect will be in the Fourth Circuit, which covers Maryland, Virginia, West Virginia and North and South Carolina. All Federal courts there are now bound by the rule against hospital segregation.

The other Southern states are in the Fifth Circuit, except for Arkansas, which is in the Eighth, and Tennessee, in the Sixth. These other circuits could differ with the Fourth, but the best guess is that they probably will not.

The case at issue today involved two hospitals at Greensboro, N. C.

The Moses H. Cone Memorial Hospital admitted only a few Negro patients and gave no staff privileges to Negro doctors or dentists when the case began, in 1962. More recently the hospital has said it will consider Negro staff applications.

The Wesley Long Community Hospital, so far as the legal record shows, is completely segregated.

Both are nonprofit hospitals operated under North Carolina law as private charitable corporations. But both have had substantial Federal aid in recent construction, Cone $1,269,-950 and Long $1,948,800.

The aid was given under the Hill-Burton Act of 1946, named for Senators Lister Hill, an Alabama Democrat, and Harold H. Burton, an Ohio Republican who later went to the Supreme Court. The act forbids discrimination in general, but with this key proviso:

"An exception shall be made in cases where separate hospital facilities are provided for separate population groups, if the plan makes equitable provision on the basis of need for facilities and services of like quality for each group."

It was this proviso that the Fourth Circuit held unconstitutional. The opinion was by Chief Judge Simon E. Sobeloff.

The key question before the Court of Appeals was whether the hospitals were so private in character that they were not covered by the Constitution. The Constitution condemns only racial discrimination by governmental action.

State's Role Noted

Judge Sobeloff found that there was deep involvement on North Carolina's part in the two hospitals. He relied heavily on the fact that the Hill-Burton Act itself required state participation in several ways, such as making an over-all state hospital plan.

Thus the Fourth Circuit concluded that these hospitals were too public in character to practice segregation. The logic of the opinion would seem to apply to any other institution receiving Hill-Burton aid.

The suit was originally brought by 11 Negro doctors, dentists and patients. The Justice Department intervened on their side, agreeing that the Hill-Burton proviso was unconstitutional and that segregation at the hospitals should be enjoined.

The decision could have some impact on the forthcoming civil rights debate in the Senate.

The bill as passed by the House declares void all segregation provisions of Federal law, such as the Hill-Burton proviso. And it orders agencies giving direct aid to end segregation in the programs.

This case could be said to accomplish part of the objective of that portion of the bill, but only part. It would have far less sweeping effects than a general Congressional command to end discrimination in Federally aided projects.

March 3, 1964

HOSPITAL COSTS FOR LABOR SOAR

By AUSTIN C. WEHRWEIN
Special to The New York Times

CHICAGO, Aug. 1—Hospital labor costs have increased 545 per cent since World War II, the American Hospital Association said today.

According to an association survey, the average daily cost to the hospital for each patient has risen from $9.39 in 1946 to $38.91 in 1963, an increase of 314 per cent.

During this same period, the total expense of an average stay in the hospital—slightly more than a week—increased from $85 to $298, the association said.

The Labor and patient costs averages are for non-Federal short-term general hospitals. These are hospitals that admit patients with all types of illnesses or injuries.

The survey of the 5,684 hospitals was published in the 1964 guide issue of Hospitals, the journal of the American Hospital Association, the survey was made in 1963.

Dr. Edwin L. Crosby, director of the association, said:

"Hospitals are working to raise salaries of their personnel to levels comparable to other fields. In addition, increased medical specialization and advanced technology have resulted in hospitals needing many more skilled, well-trained individuals who must be paid according to their abilities."

He said many hospital specialists and technicians were performing jobs that were unknown 10 years ago. The public has also turned to hospitals for more health care, he added.

The survey showed that last year 241 employees were needed to care for every 100 patients. In 1946, the ratio was 148 to 100.

The hospitals surveyed employed almost 70 per cent of all hospital personnel in the United States. They spend 69 per cent of all hospital dollars and have 64 per cent of all hospital assets.

Besides the non-Federal short-term general hospitals, the survey covered 1,454 long-term, Federal and other types of hospitals.

The total employment in all 7,138 hospitals registered by the association in 1963 was at a record high — 1,840,287, 77,330 more employes than in 1962.

Total payroll expenses of all hospitals—long term and short term—reached $7.3 billion in 1963. This represented 66.3 per cent of the total budget of $10.9 billion expended by all hospitals. In 1946, all registered hospitals spent $1.1 billion on wages out of a total budget of $1.9 billion.

Other factors in the rising costs,Dr. Crosby said, are costly equipment, new special services, and the public's demand for increased service and facilities. Nonlabor costs have increased 425 per cent for non-Federal short-term genera, hospitals since 1946 and by 328 per cent for all hospitals.

August 2, 1964

Problems in the Making of a Surgeon

By WALTER SULLIVAN

Although everyone wants a surgeon to develop the highest possible skills, no one wants to be practiced upon. While this dilemma has been brought to the fore by the new programs that enable all to pay for their treatment, its roots lie deep in history.

For centuries surgeons were frustrated in their efforts to learn anatomy by taboos denying them access to the human body. They had to resort to graverobbers to learn their trade. Furthermore little formal training was available. The most popular school was the army, where surgeons were kept busy amputating limbs and closing up wounds. Until the discovery of anesthesia in the mid-19th century surgeons spent most of their time repairing rather than removing diseased organs such as an infected appendix.

Then, during the 19th century, a number of great virtuoso surgeons appeared in Europe and students flocked to learn from them. This method of "preceptorship" teaching by one master still predominates in much of Europe and the Soviet Union, according to surgeons who discussed the situation here last week.

A New Method

However, toward the end of the century, a new method of teaching surgery began to evolve at the Johns Hopkins Hospital in Baltimore. Its innovator was William Stewart Halsted who invented the "residency" method of training in use in this country today.

He and his colleagues, while at Roosevelt Hospital in New York, introduced cocaine as a local anesthetic without realizing its addictive properties. While undergoing tests, a number of them became addicts before realizing what had happened.

Dr. Halsted also invented the rubber gloves now standard in surgery. His theater nurse was plagued with skin infections, so he had tight-fitting gloves made for her. Then, realizing that such gloves could be sterilized—giving the surgeon sterile hands—he had his hands cast in bronze so that skin-tight gloves could be made for himself. (Ultimately he married the nurse).

It was Halsted's residency method that was uppermost in the minds of surgeons as they met last week to discuss whether or not the training program is in danger. The occasion was the annual meeting of Allen O. Whipple Surgical Society whose name honors another great teacher of surgery. The headquarters of the society is at Columbia University's College of Physicians and Surgeons, associated with the Columbia-Presbyterian Medical Center at 168th Street and Broadway.

Dr. George H. Humphreys II, president of the society and head of surgery at the college, described the residency system as the foundation of American superiority in this field. Under the system, in general use for only a generation, a surgeon completes his four years of medical school, plus one year of internship, and then spends three to five years as a "resident" in a hospital.

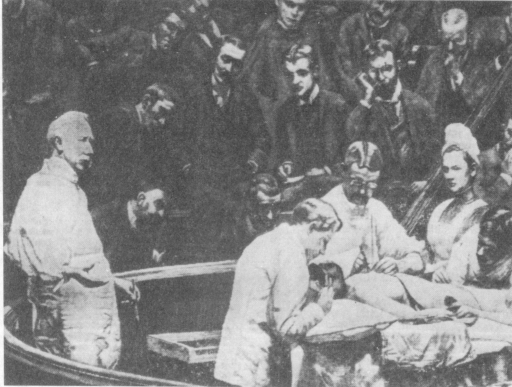

Painting by Thomas Eakins from the Bettmann Archive

VIRTUOSO: This 1889 painting typifies the "virtuoso" period of American surgery. Entitled "The Clinic of Dr. Agnew," it shows the teacher lecturing to the gallery while a junior surgeon works on the patient. This form of instruction has largely been replaced by the residency system, where surgeon trainees participate in operations conducted by many specialists.

The Problems

Instead of serving as an apprentice to one man, he works with specialists in various forms of surgery. Thus, it is argued, he obtains a far broader experience than under the old preceptorships. In gradual stages he does more and more of the surgery himself.

The advent of almost universal medical insurance, through the Medicaire and Medicaid programs as well as such private plans as Blue Shield, affects the residency program in two ways: the charity wards, where residents obtained their experience, are vanishing and the insurance programs, public and private, by and large refuse to pay for surgery performed by residents.

In the past a patient who could not pay had little choice as to who treated him. The teachers of surgery argue that this did not mean charity patients were used as guinea pigs by novices. On the contrary, they say, ward patients in teaching hospitals received more and better attention than the average hospital patient. Participants at the conference cited statistics to show that operations performed by residents in university teaching hospitals and Veterans Administration Hospitals score in the high success brackets.

But now, in effect, there are no more charity patients. It has therefore become necessary to persuade a certain number of those admitted to hospitals to enter the teaching section voluntarily. The Columbia - Presbyterian Medical Center, 10 months ago, set aside 110 semi-private beds on two floors as its teaching section.

Dr. Robert B. Hiatt, associate professor of surgery, said that the task of this unit is "to care for the patient who comes to be treated by an institution—not by an individual."

Candidates for admission to the unit are told that they will be cared for largely by medical students and residents, but under the supervision of the medical faculty. If there is surgery, a predominant part of the work will be done by a resident, but the professor may intervene if necessary.

"It has been an amazingly successful experience," Dr. Hiatt said. Most of the patients accept these terms—probably in part because they are assured of immediate admission.

What most troubled the American teachers of surgery was what Dr. David V. Habif termed the "financial penalty" imposed on residency programs by the current policies of public and private in-

surance plans. Dr. Habif is professor of surgery at the College of Physicians and Surgeons. The Federal program will not reimburse a salaried resident, i f he does the operation, nor will it pay the surgeon-teacher or "attending surgeon" unless he is present during the operation.

When a professor of surgery on full salary is present, he can collect a fee, which he customarily turns over to the hospital to support its training program. What concerns the surgery teachers is the insistence on their presence.

All of this denies badly needed funds to the teaching hospitals. Under heavy workloads the professor is often present only for the critical part of an operation. Or he may be only on call. A number of speakers argued that a trainee must operate completely on his own—with the professor merely on call—before he is fully qualified.

However, Dr. Harold Safian, medical director of United Medical Service (Blue Shield) in New York, pointed out that it would cost Blue Shield as much as $3-million a year to support the surgery done for its subscribers on a teaching basis.

The Proposals

Various solutions were dis-

cussed. One was for Federal medicare legislation to recognize the team approach to surgery, much of which is now done by groups of specialists. Payments could be made to the team. Another suggestion would allow certain institutions, such as university hospitals, to charge the surgical fee that would normally be collected by an individual. Yet another idea was that the Government should directly subsidize the residency programs as a vital stage in medical education.

A major obstacle to such plans apparently lies with the majority of surgeons who are not in the teaching business. They compete with the teaching programs for patients and are not eager to see their rivals subsidized.

The tone of the meeting was not hostile to Medicare. On the contrary, the program as a whole was generally supported. Dr. J. Engleburt Dunphy, chairman of the department of surgery at the University of California School of Medicine in San Francisco, said: "If nothing else comes out of Medicare we are going to give happier care to an awful lot of people."

March 19, 1967

Use of Commercial Blood Donors Increases

By LAWRENCE K. ALTMAN

The reluctance of most Americans to donate blood for transfusions, combined with a rising natural demand for blood, is forcing physicians to use an increasing amount from persons who sell their blood for profit. Among those who sell their blood are some drug addicts and derelicts.

The result is a sort of "transfusion roulette" on a national scale, for commercial blood has a higher risk of causing such infections as hepatitis or malaria and doctors have no way of knowing for sure which pint of blood may be contaminated.

And yet with blood in chronically short supply in many major cities—in New York this week the supply dropped at one point to less than enough for a single day—doctors and patients have little choice but to rely on commercial blood, for better or worse.

Specialists are aware of this critical aspect of health care in the United States, but relatively few studies have been made of the specific problem and its ramifications. In inter-

views with blood bank officials and doctors, however, these elements emerged.

¶Despite the higher risk of hepatitis from commercial blood, few doctors pay attention to the source of the blood they use.

¶Though the danger of hepatitis is well known, it is estimated that more than half such cases go unreported.

¶Despite recent advances in methods of fractionating blood, thus permitting its more efficient use, many doctors fail to take advantage of this and also tend to give unneeded transfusions.

¶As Americans travel more abroad, bringing diseases back with them, an increase in malarial infections resulting from blood transfusions has become a problem.

¶In some areas the blood shortage has become so acute that special requirements are made of hospital patients who may need blood. One hospital in New Jersey now has a mandatory preadmission blood donation policy.

¶Psychological studies are being made to determine the reasons why so many people are apathetic about donating blood.

Only 3 Per Cent Give Blood

According to the American Association of Blood Banks, only a small fraction—about 3 per cent—of those Americans qualified to donate blood actually do so. "There is definitely a shortage of blood donors," a spokesman for the American Medical Association says. Although no definitive statistics exist, the A.M.A. estimates that people give about 6.6 million pints a year.

Although statistics gathered by the association show a small annual increase in the numbers of units of blood donated, the increase in donations has not kept up with the growing need for blood. In 1964, for example, more than 4.2 million units of blood were transfused; by 1967, the number had grown to more than 5 million units and by 1968 to more than 6.5 million units. The number of units collected during those years went from 6.3 million to 6.6 million to 7 million.

How much of the blood used comes from commercial banks is unknown, but doctors in New Jersey have found that 35 per cent of transfusions there used commercial blood.

Doctors interviewed in New York City estimate that 60 per cent of the blood transfused here comes from commercial sources.

The fact that commercial blood carries with it a higher risk of infection has brought about a doctor's dilemma.

Closing commercial blood banks because of high transfusion-associated infection rates, many physicians say, would cause more deaths among individuals deprived of blood for emergencies than save lives from infections such as hepatatis and malaria.

"You cannot destroy a large per cent of the source," Dr. Martin Goldfield of the New Jersey State Health Department said, "unless you substitute a mechanism to get adequate voluntary blood." Dr. Goldfield, among many other physicians, said a blood insurance program, in which the "premiums" are paid in blood, might help meet the problem.

Commercial Blood Defined

Commercial blood is a term that can be defined in several ways, but doctors generally use it for the blood that individuals sell to profit-making blood banks. The term does not cover the processing and testing fees that almost all hospitals charge patients, even for voluntarily donated blood.

Some nonprofit community blood banks pay donors. A few have a list of professional donors whom the blood bank pays

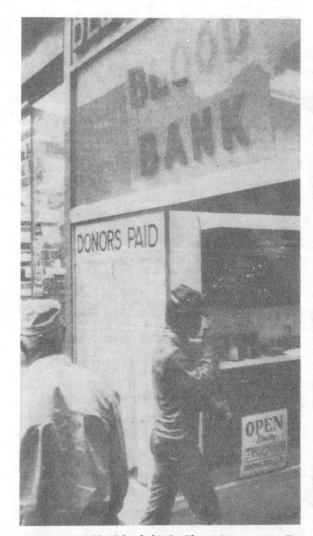

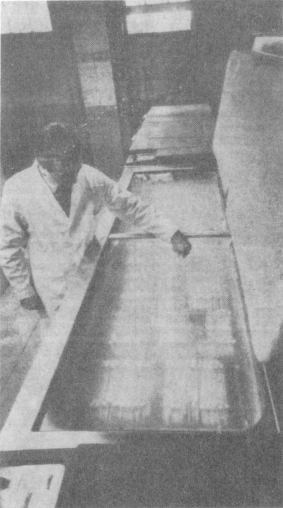

The New York Times (by Jack Manning)

A commercial blood bank in the Times Square area. Because only 3 per cent of Americans qualified to donate blood actually do so, hospitals are being forced to buy blood from commercial banks, which pay their donors.

At the Greater New York Blood Bank here, liquid nitrogen tanks such as these are used to freeze rare blood types so that they can be preserved indefinitely. This technique is more expensive than conventional storage methods.

for giving blood, often rare types, on demand. A spokesman for Blood Services, which describes itself as a nonprofit organization, said that for the inconvenience of donating it paid up to $10 for 76 per cent of the 237,350 pints it provided hospitals last year.

In some of the 24 cities its banks serve in 12 states from California to Mississippi and Arizona to North Dakota, Blood Services reportedly is the community's only blood bank.

But doctors generally do not include semi-commercial community blood banks, or professional donors, when they talk about the commercial blood problems.

Though doctors are not certain about the precise reasons why, they are certain that hepatitis is a more frequent complication — as much as 10 times — from commercial than from volunteered blood.

Patients Hospitalized Longer

Such complications hospitalize patients longer, increase their already high hospital bills,

lengthen their convalescence at home, and keep them away from work longer. Moreover, doctors note that transfusion-associated hepatitis kills at least 1,500 Americans each year.

A hepatitis blood test now exists. But doctors, while considering it worthwhile to perform this test, emphasize that it is no panacea because it detects only about one-quarter of blood contaminated with the hepatitis virus that inflames the liver.

When most people think of transplants, such organs as hearts or kidneys probably come to mind. What they may not realize is that physicians' greatest triumph in transplants has been with blood, a liquid human tissue.

Perhaps because of such success, no one knows exactly how much blood Americans sell or donate, nor how much of it is used or discarded. The American Medical Association estimates that people give 6.6 million pints of blood each year, about half to the American Red Cross.

Just one state, New Jersey, has tried to obtain accurate statistics on the acquisition, distribution and complications of bood transfusions. There, doctors have found that 35 per cent of transfusions use commercial blood.

One in 17 Gets Transfusion

About one of every 17 patients receives a transfusion during his hospital stay, the Professional Activities Study of the Commission on Professional and Hospital Activities in Ann Arbor, Mich's has found in a limited survey.

Newer techniques, such as open-heart surgery, that permit affected individuals to live more productive lives often require dozens of pints of blood for one patient. Also, doctors often need to give more transfusions as improved therapy permits patients with leukemia, chronic anemia and some forms of cancer to survive longer.

However, Dr. Hugh Chaplin of Washington University School of Medicine in St. Louis, among other physicians, has se-

riously questioned whether transfusions with whole blood, instead of fractionated units, "reflects good medical practice, or merely a thoughtless habit."

Even so, demand for blood exceeds volunteer supply.

To reduce this gap, business began profiting by buying blood from individuals and selling it to hospitals. Such commercial blood banks now exist in just about every large city in this country. Such banks can ship blood for use elsewhere, if it is not used locally.

Percentages of commercial blood used varies widely with the locality. Doctors interviewed said that almost 60 per cent of the blood transfused in New York City is commercial. About half of it is in some Chicago hospitals, one-quarter in some Virginia hospitals, and less than 5 per cent in Buffalo hospitals. In some cities, like Seattle, none is used.

Physicians use commercial blood because, in their professional judgment, the benefits of such tranfusions outweigh their risks. A patient injured in an automobile accident, bleeding from a ruptured artery or organ, such as spleen or liver, can die if he does not receive enough blood speedily. During such emergencies, remoteness of possible infection at some time in the future is of relative unimportance.

But not all transfusions are given for emergencies.

Doctors have prolonged the lives of thousands of Americans with transfusions for complications of many diseases. In such situations, the timing — not the need — of the transfusion is elective. In other words, physicians often can achieve the same results if they give the transfusion one or two days later.

Yet, in such elective situations, all of the doctors interviewed said that they did not look to see whether the blood their patients received had come from paid or volunteer sources, which officials said they do by examining labels on the plastic bags of blood. Nor, the doctors said, did they inform their patients of the increased risk of infection.

Friends Can Donate

"I never thought about doing it until you asked," one Virginia physician replied, "but from now on I will refuse commercial blood for nonemergency transfusions for my patients." Most patients, he said, can call on relatives and friends to donate.

Dr. Goldfield of the New Jersey Health Department is one physician who has not only thought about the complications of blood transfusions but has also pioneered studies on the subject as well. Four years ago, Dr. Goldfield began analyzing cases of hepatitis reported to his department at Trenton. Then with the aid of a nurse and medical students, who made it

a summer project, they surveyed patients' charts in records rooms of New Jersey hospitals.

Dr. Goldfield found that the risk of developing hepatitis was 3.4 times greater "following transfusions of blood from paid donors than from volunteers." Further, he said that preliminary analysis of his data indicated that there was no significant difference between hepatitis rates following transfusions from different commercial blood banks. Elimination of all commercial blood in New Jersey, he said, would prevent about two-thirds of that state's transfusion-associated hepatitis cases.

Dr. Goldfield's continuing study shows that even in New Jersey, whose data on communicable diseases health officials elsewhere consider among the most complete in the country, hepatitis cases are underreported.

Hepatitis Unreported

Despite a vigorous campaign to get doctors and hospitals to report hepatitis cases, Dr. Goldfield said, only 85 of the 241 cases his survey found in 1967 and 145 of the 297 found in 1968 had been reported to his health department. These totals did not count New Jersey patients hospitalized for transfusion-associated hepatitis elsewhere.

From the hepatitis blood tests that his laboratory technicians had performed, Dr. Goldfield concluded that even when commercial blood had been hepatitis-tested, the risk of hepatitis from paid blood was still 2.5 times greater than that tested from volunteers.

With an increasing number of American servicemen returning from Vietnam, where they are often exposed to malaria, and with the growing number of Americans who have traveled

in the malarious areas of the world, malaria infections resulting from blood transfusions are becoming a problem.

When Dr. Howard B. Shookhoff of the New York City Health Department diagnosed a case of transfusion-induced malaria recently, Public Health Service doctors traced the blood to a commercial bank near a Southern military base. Further investigations showed that two other individuals acquired malaria from transfused blood that had been obtained from military donors from the same commercial blood bank.

Some physicians criticize blood banks for not using Madison Avenue advertising techniques to recruit more voluntary blood donors. These physicians have also suggested that studies be undertaken to better understand the psychology of the voluntary donor so that the 3 per cent of the eligible population that gives blood might be increased.

Lagging replacement programs at hospitals aggravate the need for commercial blood. Accordingly, some doctors criticize hospitals for complacent attitudes and for not exerting more pressure on a patient's relatives and friends to donate at peak periods of psychological incentive.

Hospitals that have made concerted efforts to urge patients' families to donate before admission or at the time their relatives or friends are transfused have had impressive records.

Barnert Memorial Hospital Center in Paterson, N. J., for example, established and stuck to "a mandatory preadmission blood donation policy." Harvey Schoenfeld, the center's director, wrote in the American Hospital Association's journal that "the key, it appears, is firm administration of the policy."

As a result of Barnert's success, Mr. Schoenfeld said in an interview, other hospitals in Passic County have reinstituted or begun similar successful programs.

Elsewhere, a few doctors have reported that they withdrew one or two pints of blood from some patients about a week before the patients had elective surgery. Dr. George Milles and his associates at Augustana Hospital in Chicago reported in the hospital association's journal earlier this summer that they have been transfusing a growing number of patients with their own blood since 1961. There are physiological limitations to such "autotransfusions," however.

Autotransfusions are also used for individuals with religious convictions against receiving someone else's blood, such as Jehovah's Witnesses, and for those people with rare blood types.

Unquestionably, the safest blood is your own. Accordingly, some doctors look to the day when blood freezing techniques will enable Americans to insure themselves with their own blood.

Some blood banks, such as the Greater New York Blood Bank Program here, are using freezing techniques on a limited basis to preserve indefinitely rare blood types. But the techniques costs — about three times those for conventional 21-day storage — prohibit its greater use.

Meanwhile, until more Americans donate more often, doctors said that they must rely more frequently on commercial sources. This means, they said, that patients will spend more money and physicians more time treating cases of hepatitis and other transfusion-associated infections.

September 5, 1970

Blood Relationship

By ANTHONY LEWIS

LONDON, Jan. 24—A book on methods of collecting blood for medical purposes: It would be hard to imagine a subject less likely to interest the general reader or throw light on broad issues of social organization and values. But that book has just been published in Britain, and it is attracting the fascinated attention it deserves.

It is "The Gift Relationship" by Richard M. Titmuss, professor of social administration at the London School of Economics and one of this country's most respected social thinkers. Americans who wonder whether the economics and ethics of the marketplace

are ultimate goods would do well to become familiar with its teaching.

Blood is a commodity in growing demand the world over; in the United States roughly six million units a year are collected. The question is how to obtain the supply.

In Britain virtually all blood is given by voluntary donors. They get nothing tangible in return except a cup of tea. Most other countries rely to a substantial degree on payments or other inducements. Even the Soviet Union gives days off work, housing advantages and in half the cases money.

In the United States about a third of the total supply is bought. Most of

the rest is given with other incentives: prisoners who get time off, citizens who are given a right to draw on blood supplies in the future, and so forth. Less than 10 per cent of the blood is volunteered without any strings.

The book compares the American and British systems in terms of simple efficiency. Professor Titmuss uses four tests.

First, the adequacy of supply: In Britain there have been no significant blood shortages; the supply from voluntary donors increased 77 per cent between 1956 and 1967. The U.S. does have shortages: There are no national statistics, but Professor Titmuss estimates that the supply rose only 17 per cent between 1957 and 1967.

Then, wastage: There is almost none in Britain, less than 2 per cent. American experts have estimated that 15 to 30 per cent of all blood collected in the U.S. is wasted by becoming outdated before it is used.

Cost: A unit of blood costs 5 to 15 times as much in the United States as in Britain.

Last, purity of the product: In Britain the incidence of disease from transfused blood is near zero. In the United States there is a severe risk of hepatitis, surveys showing that it strikes 2 to 4 per cent of patients. The reason is plain: Much of the supply comes from addicts, alcoholics and others who sell their blood for money and are more likely to be diseased. Titmuss writes, "the commercialized blood market fails.

"It is highly wasteful of blood, and there are characteristic shortages. It is administratively inefficient; the so-called mixed pluralism of the American market results in avalanches of paper

and bills and greater accounting and computer overheads. The price to the consumer is greater. And the blood is more likely to be contaminated."

Professor Titmuss enjoys pricking the marketplace worship of economists. He notes wryly that, under their system of reckoning the gross national product, donated blood adds nothing to G.N.P. but sold blood does—even when it is wasted.

But his purpose and his achievement are deeper than economics. He shows us that altruism works in a modern society, indeed that it is necessary. Hobbes and his followers are wrong when they say that man can be moved by nothing but his own immediate self-interest.

The remarkable volume of blood donations in Britain must mean that man has a real need to give. The need has, if anything, increased with the complexity of modern society and the remoteness of its institutions.

A person who gives blood of his

own free will, for the benefit of patients unknown, contributes to something vital and scarce in our world: the sense of community. The donor helps to create the assurance that he and all of us live in a society where people do not act only out of Hobbesian selfishness, where one gives to a community and may receive from it.

The British are not inherently more altruistic than other people, Professor Titmuss says: They have just been wise or lucky enough to institutionalize altruism. They have done so not only with the blood supply but in medicine generally, through the National Health Service, "the most unsordid act of British social policy in the twentieth century."

"It is a good feeling to give blood," one elderly woman here said when told about Professor Titmuss's book. It is a good feeling also to participate in a system of health care that rejects commercial values. January 25, 1971

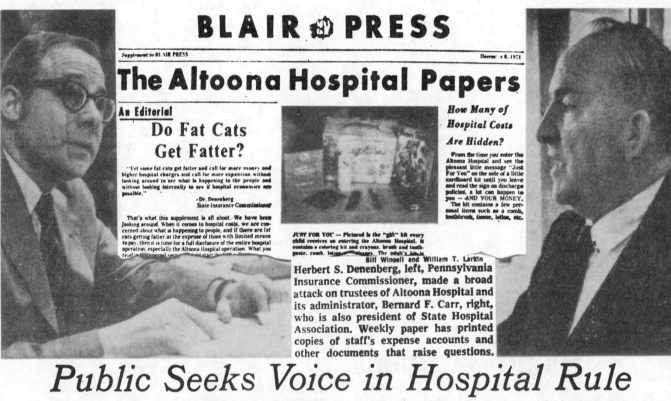

BLAIR PRESS

Supplement to BLAIR PRESS   December 8, 1971

The Altoona Hospital Papers

An Editorial
Do Fat Cats Get Fatter?

"Yet some fat cats get fatter and call for more money and higher hospital charges and call for more expansion without looking around to see what is happening to the people and without looking internally to see if hospital economies are possible."

– Dr. Denenberg
State Insurance Commissioner

That's what this supplement is all about. We have been looking around. When it comes to hospital costs, we are concerned about what is happening to people, and if there are fat cats getting fatter at the expense of those with limited means to pay, then it is time for a full disclosure of the entire hospital operation, especially the Altoona Hospital operation. What you read...

How Many of Hospital Costs Are Hidden?

From the time you enter the Altoona Hospital and see the pleasant little message "Just For You" on the side of a little cardboard kit until you leave and read the sign on discharge policies, a lot can happen to you — AND YOUR MONEY. The kit contains a few personal items such as a comb, toothbrush, tissue, lotion, etc.

JUST FOR YOU — Pictured is the "gift" kit every child receives on entering the Altoona Hospital. It contains a coloring kit and crayons, brush and toothpaste, comb, lotion...

Bill Wingeil and William T. Larkin

Herbert S. Denenberg, left, Pennsylvania Insurance Commissioner, made a broad attack on trustees of Altoona Hospital and its administrator, Bernard F. Carr, right, who is also president of State Hospital Association. Weekly paper has printed copies of staff's expense accounts and other documents that raise questions.

Public Seeks Voice in Hospital Rule

By RICHARD D. LYONS
Special to The New York Times

WASHINGTON, Jan. 3 — The administration of local hospitals, an area normally left to doctors and bankers, is coming under increasing public scrutiny as alarm over soaring health costs spreads.

New York, New Jersey, Connecticut and five other states have passed laws in the last two years that give the public a voice in the setting of the rates charged by hospitals, the planning of new institutions, or the mandating of full disclosure of the finances of medical centers. Six other states have legislation pending.

The change in attitude is being led by consumer advocates, armed with improved knowledge in health affairs.

Hospitals as a group are being increasingly criticized as being so poorly managed that their very inefficiencies are

contributing to increased medical costs.

Accountability Issue

A subtler issue is whether the local hospitals that have been built and maintained by a combination of governmental and private funds should be held legally accountable to the community of their actions.

Pennsylvania will soon become the 15th state to grapple with these issues, in part because of a relatively ob-

scure battle there during the year over the management practices and financial affairs of the Altoona Hospital.

That controversy involves, on the one side, the administrator and board of trustees of the Altoona Hospital, an expanding, 430-bed institution that is the largest in this economically depressed area of west-central Pennsylvania, and, on the other, a group of angry townspeople, plus state officials and Blue Cross. Money is the central issue, with the hospital's directors complaining that more is needed through higher rates because the institution is being short-changed by Blue Cross, Pennsylvania Medicaid, and Medicare.

Counter Charges

For their part, state officials, Blue Cross officers and some townspeople accuse the directors of administrative inefficiency, financial mismanagement, and empire building.

The two sides have flung charges and counterclaims at each other almost all year, starting with a decision by the management of Altoona and three smaller local hospitals in February to withdraw as participating Blue Cross institutions.

Since then there have been public hearings and investigations by state officials, testimony by angry citizens, rebuttals by the hospital's administration and, in the most bizarre action, the printing by a weekly newspaper of "the Altoona Hospital Papers."

This paper, The Blair (County) Press, has issued two 16-page supplements, free of advertising, containing copies of 50 hospital expense accounts, liquor bills, dinner checks, travel vouchers and other documents that raise both major and minor questions about the institution's management.

"If the leadership of the hospital isn't improved and better management practices instituted, the result in a few years is that this area won't have the hospital," said H. A. Barnhard of Roaring Springs, the newspaper's publisher.

"The situation here is just like that of the Penn Central Railroad," Mr. Barnhard went on. "The management was a mess, the board of directors didn't take action to correct the conditions, and the railroad went bankrupt just as the hospital may in a few years if its administration isn't changed."

The analogy strikes home in Altoona, a fading railroad town where the Penn Central, which is in receivership and has laid off workers, is

the biggest employer. Ninety years ago the Pennsylvania Railroad donated the land on which the hospital stands.

Mr. Barnhard said the documents proved that "the management has been playing fast and loose with the money it takes in from patients." Some of the photostats show that the hospital paid for trips to Las Vegas by doctors and their wives, rooms at Miami Beach hotels, and cocktails and dinner for as many as 120 persons at a local country club.

With less titillation but more importance, other copies offer a blurred glimpse of the hospital's management practices and aspirations, such as: an outline for a $20-million expansion program; demand notes of over $1.4-million on top of mortgages of $1.8-million; payments of $300,000 a year to a computer company that hospital officials say gives poor service, and a payment of $22,228.67 to one doctor for one month's services.

The disclosures followed an investigation by Herbert S. Denenberg, the State Insurance Commissioner, into the reasons why the hospital dropped its participation in Blue Cross. He levied a broad attack on the actions and policies of the hospital's board of trustees and its administrator, Bernard F. Carr, who also is president of the State Hospital Association.

Mr. Denenberg first charged conflict of interest in that 10 of the 20 trustees were linked to local banks, including eight members associated with the Mid-State Bank of Altoona, which has lent the hospital well over $1-million.

Mr. Denenberg pointed to a report of the hospital's auditors, Main-Lefrentz and Company of Pittsburgh, stating that rather than losing money the hospital had been making money, at least in the recent past.

According to one accounting estimate, the hospital had in a six-year period in the 1960's taken $2,250,000 out of operating revenues—that is, the money spent on their

patients—to pay for expansion.

Rating and Reimbursing

The Blue Cross issue is a complicated problem involving the accounts the insurer is willing to pay for the costs of hospital services and the amounts the hospital wants to charge patients and be reimbursed for by Blue Cross.

Blue Cross audits the books of a participating hospital, determines what the association considers to be the true cost of providing services, then negotiates a repayment contract with the hospital.

In Altoona's case, Blue Cross of Western Pennsylvania noted that it had granted steady rate increases to a point where the hospital was being reimbursed at the highest rate of any of the four institutions of its size and class in the area, about $77 a day.

Hospital officials took the position that this still did not meet the real cost of providing services which, they said, were some 20 per cent greater. Requests for an increase in reimbursement funds were denied by Blue Cross.

The hospital then dropped Blue Cross for its own employes, switched their coverage to a private health insurance company, advised area residents to do the same, and last July canceled its participation as a Blue Cross affiliated hospital.

This led to consternation among local Blue Cross beneficiaries because they were unsure as to what their medical insurance benefits were. In addition, 50 local companies switched to other insurers even though premiums were higher.

After six months of charges by both sides over the justification for the action, the four hospitals returned to participation in Blue Cross.

Mr. Carr and members of his staff insisted that many of the relatively petty complaints that had caught the public's attention were nonsense. These included a hospital charge of $1 for a popsicle for a young patient, and the payment of $3,800 for 100 ashtrays. The officials maintained that travel expenses were normal for a

business with a gross of $13-million yearly.

Mr. Carr said Blue Cross was still not paying its fair share, while Medicare and Medicaid patients were costing the hospital $20,000 a month on the amounts the programs were reimbursing the hospital.

Conceding that the hospital did indeed pay some radiologists and pathologists large amounts for services —one radiologist was paid over $200,000 in one year— Mr. Carr said the money had actually been divided by several specialists, rather than only the one to whom the check was addressed.

As to expansionism, Mr. Carr said it was necessary "to serve the people of this area."

The intent would be puzzling since Altoona, which has a population of 63,000, has lost 20,000 people in the last 40 years. As to the economy, one state assessment showed that the only increase in Altoona in the last decade has been in liquor sales.

All of the hospital's 14 interns are graduates of foreign medical schools, which have been criticized as being inferior, while autopsies are conducted on only one-third of the bodies, about half the average of a good hospital.

The problems at the hospital have led W. William Wilt of Hollidaysburg, the local Republican Representative in the state legislature, to plan to introduce legislation mandating that every Pennsylvania hospital adopt a uniform accounting, auditing and reporting system so that "everyone could know where it stands."

But Mr. Denenberg believes that such legislation, which is in effect in Connecticut, Arizona and California, does not go far enough in "making hospitals toe the line of their responsibility."

"We need comprehensive regulation of hospitals by such things as a certification that the hospital actually is needed, as well as controls over the rates charged," he said.

January 4, 1972

Health Care Base for Needy Set by U.S.

By RICHARD D. LYONS
Special to The New York Times

WASHINGTON, April 18— Elliot L. Richardson, the Secretary of Health Education and Welfare, ordered today 6,308 health care facilities, including half the nation's hospitals, to

provide a minimum level of free services to the poor.

If an institution does not comply with the order and cannot demonstrate sufficient reason for not doing so, it faces penalties up to and including the revocation of its license.

The order was in the form of a notice in today's Federal Register giving proposed regulations implementing a little-used section of the Hill-Burton Act. Under this law $3.7-billion has been dispensed in grants and loans to hospitals, rehabil-

itation institutes, public health centers and skilled nursing homes over the last 26 years.

"Reasonable Volume"

The legislation, technically Title VI, Section 622 of the Public Health Service Act, states: "There will be made available in each such hospital or addition to a hospital a reasonable volume of hospital services to persons unable to pay therefor, but an exception shall be made if such a requirement is not feasible from a financial standpoint."

The required services under today's order would be at a level not less than 5 per cent of an institution's operating cost and not less than 25 per cent of its net income.

A spokesman for the Health Services and Mental Health Administration, a branch of the Health, Education, and Welfare Department that oversees the Hill-Burton funds, said it had on file data showing that the degree of compliance ranged from a high of 8 per cent to less than one-hundredth of 1 per cent.

Mr. Richardson's order would go into effect within 30 days

but may well be challenged in the courts.

Opposed by Hospital Group

The American Hospital Association issued a statement several months ago, before the wording of the regulation had been settled, opposing its intent. The statement said the nation's community hospitals were already living up to an acknowledged responsibility of providing some degree of free health services.

Yet the issue was forced by five class action suits brought by lawyers, mostly paid for with funds from the Federal Office of Economic Opportunity, against the Health, Education, and Welfare Department in the District of Columbia, West Virginia, Florida, Louisiana and Colorado.

The nationwide effect of the order is to strengthen the legal

weapon that poor people have to force hospitals and other institutions that have accepted Federal funds to live up to the letter of the law.

"If the Legal Aid Societies get hot, the hospitals are going to have to provide a lot more health care to the poor," said one department official.

Two Categories

The wording of the regulation, however, provides an escape clause for two types of health care facilities: those in serious financial difficulties, of which there are many, and those operating in areas of affluence where there are almost no poor people, of which there are few.

The H.E.W. Department will leave it up to those state agencies regulating and licensing hospitals to enforce the new regulations.

As the rules were written, any health care institution that

has ever accepted Hill-Burton funds, no matter when or how much, has to abide by the directive. The institution must file with the appropriate state agency an annual report either showing that it has met the requirements or giving a reason why not.

According to the regulations, if the state agency is dissatisfied with an institution's justification for not providing the minimal level of benefits, penalties may be imposed "which may include, but not need be limited to, a license revocation and termination of state assistance and court action."

The hospital also has the right to appeal to the Secretary of H.E.W.

The order affects 3,608 non-profit hospitals and 2,700 other health care facilities. In 1970 there were 6,715 non-Federal hospitals in the country.

April 19, 1972

Trauma
When It's A Matter Of Life And Death

Brakes screech. Impact. Half in, half out of the car window, the driver lies unconscious, his body broken and bleeding.

This is trauma, the technical term used to describe severe injuries that threaten life or permanent disability. Millions of Americans sustain such injuries each year at home, at work and on the road; 110,000 die of them.

Trauma is the leading cause of death of Americans from age 1 to 38. Yet care in most places is poor—or worse.

"Thousands of lives are lost through lack of systematic application of established principles of emergency care," the National Academy of Sciences-National Research Council charges in a recent report. Summing up the report, a correspondent for the British

journal, The Lancet, says that 80 per cent of America's 25,000 "ambulances" are hearses, limousines, or just station wagons, "manned by attendants who are often untrained and ignorant of the very basic principles of emergency care," and "who carry the injured to the nearest hospital regardless of its equipment or staff."

But during the last year the Federal

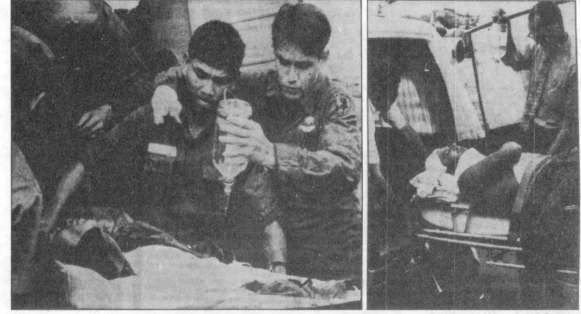

United Press International; David R. Zimmerman

The technique of speeding highly coordinated medical care to the wounded on the battlefield in Vietnam, at left, is being applied to victims of serious accidents in a statewide campaign in Illinois, at right.

Government has begun to fund research and demonstration projects designed to improve trauma care. Early results on a bellwether program covering an entire state, and one that may be a model of trauma care for the nation, were reported to the American Medical Association at its recent annual meeting. The area served by the program is virtually all of Illinois outside of Chicago. Its cost is low—a few million dollars—because for the most part existing resources have been used.

The aim of the Illinois Trauma Care System is to provide every down-state Illinoisan with the same highly coordinated trauma care that military surgeons developed during the Korean war, and refined in Vietnam, where it has yielded the lowest casualty death rate of any American war.

This care consists of: Rapid initiation of treatment, if possible before the patient is moved; rapid transportation to the trauma center; and immediate and definitive surgical and medical treatment by specially-trained trauma teams. The techniques used include kidney dialysis and assisted breathing, along with round-the-clock monitoring, instant care of complications and rapid treatment of infections.

The methods have already been introduced into civilian casualty care in city hospitals around the country. In Chicago at Cook County Hospital, the trauma unit now saves 99 per cent of its patients, many admitted with what surgeons call "knife and gun club injuries" incurred in ghetto violence.

The drive to provide comparable trauma care in the rest of the state—especially in rural areas where most fatal traffic accidents occur—was initiated by two young, dynamic surgeons, Drs. David Boyd and Bruce Flashner, who had worked in the Cook County trauma unit. In starting the system, they gained the ear of Illinois Governor Richard Ogilvie—whose life was saved by prompt, effective emergency care after he was injured in battle during World War II. Dr. Boyd says the Governor "oiled the bureaucracy for us and expedited the launching of the trauma system."

The first task was to establish a network of local, areawide and regional trauma centers. Forty of Illinois's 300 hospitals now are so designated. To concentrate resources, manpower and skills the other hospitals were urged to drop trauma care. Local trauma centers, with the most basic resources, serve areas 50 miles in diameter. Areawide and regional centers provide specialized care the local centers cannot afford.

The state's major contribution has been to hire for each center a trauma coordinator (T.C.), a new kind of civilian emergency care expert. All are former military corpsmen. They are available at all times by radio or phone. They talk to emergency workers at an injury scene; advise them how to stabilize the patient; and tell them where to take him. While the ambulance is en route, the T.C. calls in the required trauma surgeons and other specialists.

The T.C. helps decide if a patient should be kept at a local center 10 miles from an accident, or, after having first been stabilized, ought rather be moved to an areawide or regional center, hundreds of miles away perhaps, where a broken neck or other grave injury can be expertly attended. The T.C. arranges the transfer, perhaps by helicopter or plane.

All Illinois emergency vehicles are being equipped with radios to reach the trauma coordinators. Ambulance attendants are receiving special training. In fact, training for all emergency workers, including police, firemen and nurses is being provided.

In its first 16 months, Illinois's Trauma Care System handled 20,000 patients. Previously, Dr. Boyd estimates, 8 per cent of injured persons died after first aid arrived. Today the figure is 2 per cent—an improvement, he says, that brings the life saving rate among civilians injured in Illinois to the same rate as that of soldiers wounded in Vietnam.

—DAVID R. ZIMMERMAN

Mr. Zimmerman is a freelance who specializes in science and medicine.

November 5, 1972

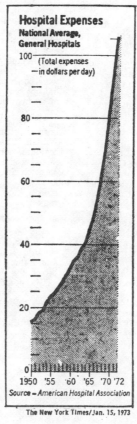

Hospital Expenses
National Average,
General Hospitals

100 — (Total expenses
— in dollars per day)

80 —

60 —

40 —

20 —

0

1950 '55 '60 '65 '70 '72

Source = American Hospital Association

The New York Times/Jan. 15, 1973

January 15, 1973

Substandard Care Is Found in the Majority of 105 Hospitals in Federal Spot Check

By DAVID BIRD

More than half of the hospitals surveyed in a nationwide Federal spot check last year were delivering substandard care because they had "significant health and safety deficiencies," according to a Government report now in preparation.

The survey was taken to determine whether the nation's hospitals were providing adequate care for their patients, whose bills are increasingly being paid by Federal funds.

Of the approximately 7,000 hospitals in the United States, 105 were included in the random samplings. Of those 69 were found deficient. Four of the hospitals surveyed were in New York City. Of those, three were found deficient.

"I was extremely surprised at the results," said Stanley Rosenfeld, section chief for hospitals of the Department of Health, Education and Welfare's Bureau of Insurance, who is working on the report. "I expected something like 10 per cent might be found deficient. These figures are astounding."

Other Deficiencies Cited

The survey covered 33 states, Mr. Rosenfeld said, and showed that many of the hospitals did not meet fire safety regulations — that they have inadequate exits, no fire detection system or sprinklers or inadequate fireproofing to prevent the spread of fire.

Other serious deficiencies, he said, included improper drug records, so that patients were in danger of being given improper medication; inadequate numbers of nurses, so that it was impossible to care for all patients; lack of control in the dietary departments, so that patients were not being given the foods prescribed for them and even in some cases were being subjected to malnutrition, and poorly kept medical records, so that proper follow-up treatment was impossible.

Although the Federal Government has poured billions of dollars into the nation's hospitals since 1965, when legislation set up Medicare to pay hospital bills for the aged and Medicaid to do the same for the poor, it was not until recently that the Government was even allowed to check directly on whether the hospitals were adequate.

Medicare is funded entirely by the Federal Government. Last year some $1-billion in Medicare funds went to New York state hospitals alone. Washington generally provides 50 per cent of the Medicaid payments. The state and local governments divide the remaining cost. Last year more than $1-billion in Medicaid funds was distributed to New York State hospitals.

While the 1965 laws committed the Federal Government to a major role in supporting the nation's hospitals, there was no provision for the Federal Government to check on whether the hospitals were adequate.

The monitoring role was given to a private group supported by the hospitals. The legislation said the hospitals were "deemed" to meet Federal requirements for health and safety if they had been accredited by the Joint Commission on the Accreditation of Hospitals.

Commission's Makeup

The joint commission derives its income from the hospitals it inspects. The board that guides the commission is made up of 20 commissioners—seven from the American Hospital Association, seven from the American Medical Association, three from the American College of Physicians, and three from the American College of Surgeons.

Under the original legislation, the Federal Government could not question the judgment of the joint commission in accrediting a hospital. If Federal officials received complaints about a hospital, they could forward the complaint to the joint commission, but there was no requirement that the joint commission act on the complaint.

"As a result," said one Federal official, "not many complaints were forwarded."

In 1972, however, the Congress passed legislation allowing the Government to spot-check the joint commission. That program just got under way last year. It is the results of the first year of the survey that are now being drawn up into a report for the Secretary of Health, Education and Welfare.

"Something is wrong with the present system, we definitely think so," said Mr. Rosenfeld.

The joint commission, which has headquarters in Chicago, has a staff of 250 persons and an annual budget of more than $7-million. Its director is Dr. John Porterfield.

'We Do the Best We Can'

"We are what you would call industry-oriented," Dr. Porterfield said in a recent interview. He said that because the accreditation program had to be supported by the hospitals, its scope was limited by how much the hospitals were willing to pay.

"We do the best we can in a marketable product," he said. "This effort has to be supported by the hospital."

He said the joint commission's surveys might not have stressed fire safety because "we're not fire inspectors, we're physicians and nurses."

But then he added that fires had been rare in hospitals and that perhaps such stringent fire safety regulations as the Federal Government requires were not really necessary.

"You don't buy hailstone insurance on your tombstone," Dr. Porterfield said.

Federal funds for both Medicare and Medicaid come through the Department of Health, Education and Welfare but they come through separate parts of the bureaucracy. Medicare funds go through the Social and Rehabilitation Service. In order to avoid duplication Medicare officials are supposed to notify their Medicaid counterparts if there are any problems in the hospitals.

"They piggyback on our findings," said a Medicare official who conceded that his bureau did not really have any findings of its own until it began checking on its own last year.

"To date we have not been notified of any problems," said William Toby Jr., the deputy regional commissioner of the Social and Rehabilitation Service, which oversees Medicaid in the New York, New Jersey, Puerto Rico and Virgin Islands region.

'We Are in the Dark'

Mr. Toby said it was impossible for his office to check on the hospitals directly because there are only eight people in the regional office.

"We don't know what's going on," he said in a recent interview. "We have to rely on another agency. It's clear to us now that we're in the dark."

The three hospitals in New York City that were found in the Federal survey to have "significant health and safety deficiencies" despite their accreditation by the joint commission were Jamaica Hospital at 89th Avenue and Van Wyck Expressway in Queens and two Brooklyn institutions, Caledonian Hospital, at 132 Parkside Avenue, and Victory Memorial Hospital at 9036 Seventh Avenue.

All three are private, nonprofit, or voluntary, hospitals.

Charles G. Marion, the executive director of the 292-bed Jamaica Hospital, said he felt the inspectors on the spot check were too tough. "I think they were trying to justify something—their jobs, maybe," he said.

According to Federal records Jamaica Hospital received $3,-948,803 in Medicare funds alone from the Federal Government in 1974.

Radar Ovens Relocated

At the 213-bed Caledonian Hospital, S. George Zingale, the executive director, said he had moved to correct the deficiencies in the hospital, which was built in 1925.

One of the deficiencies was the location of new radar ovens so that they blocked a corridor and the lack of crash bars for emergency opening of exit doors.

Mr. Zingale said the crash bars had been installed "and fortunately we had an old laundry chute where we could relocate the ovens."

Caledonian Hospital received $3,266,046 in Federal Medicare funds last year.

Miss Mildred C. Moriarty, administrator of the 254-bed Victory Memorial Hospital, said steps had been taken to correct the deficiencies found there. One of them was that the institution had an inadequate medical library. The hospital told the Federal Government it would expand the library. The hospital received $2,857,807 in Medicare funds last year.

The hospitals where the serious deficiencies were turned up in the surveys were notified that they had lost their "deemed" status. That is, they no longer were deemed to meet Federal regulations by virtue of their joint commission accreditation. There was no penalty, however, and no reduction in Federal payments to them.

"There is nothing in the law that would allow us to reduce payments," said Mr. Rosenfeld.

March 23, 1975

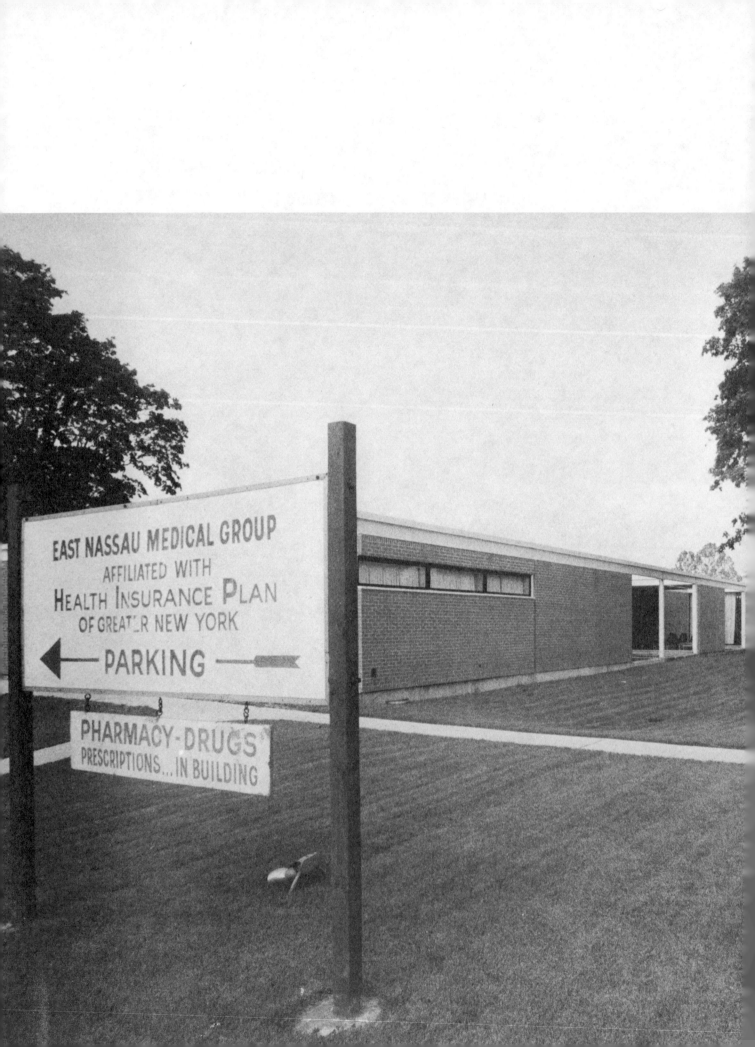

CHAPTER 4

Medicine and Society

An increasingly familiar sight: a group practice building. This one is in Hicksville, Long Island, and is affiliated with the Health Insurance Plan (H.I.P.).

Walker/NYT Pictures

JOHNS HOPKINS SETS SURGEONS' FEE LIMIT

Eminent Specialists in Hospital Dissent From Ruling Based on Economic Inquiry.

Special to The New York Times.

BALTIMORE, Md., July 28 (Copyright, 1921, by The Baltimore Sun).—The Board of Trustees of the Johns Hopkins Hospital has just issued the following dictum: The maximum fee that any surgeon ought to charge for an operation, no matter how wealthy the patient may be, is $1,000. The maximum charge that any physician ought to make for attending patients in a hospital is $35 a week.

The dictum takes on the force of an order to physicians and surgeons practicing in the hospital, limiting fees to be charged.

The effect of the ruling will be felt not only in the hospital, but, because of the standing of Johns Hopkins, in the city of Baltimore and throughout the United States.

The ruling was issued after long consideration of all the conditions surrounding physicians and surgeons, the cost of living, scale on which physicians and surgeons are required to live and the like. In it many eminent scientists at the hospital concurred.

A letter signed by the trustees of the hospital was sent to all members of the hospital staff making this announcement. Nobody was slighted, although it applies only to the part-time professors and their assistants in the Medical School and those physicians and surgeons of the Hopkins staff who practice at the hospital.

The full-time professors and members of their staffs are not affected, because all fees received by them go into the "pot," as the William H. Welch Fund

is designated, and are distributed to the various full-time departments. But it does affect such men as Dr. L. S. Barker, Dr. J. M. T. Finney, Dr. Thomas S. Cullen and many others who are not on the full-time basis. It is understood that very few, if any, of these men like it, and many of the top-notchers dislike it very much.

$5,000 Fees Not Uncommon.

The letter to the physicians and surgeons who practice in the hospital was couched in very diplomatic language. Its meaning, however, was perfectly clear and unmistakable. Baldly stated, it was that no physician practicing in the hospital could charge any patient more than $35 a week. Some of them, it is said, have been getting from $10 to $50 a visit, according to the means of the patient. Also, that no surgeon practicing in the hospital may charge a patient more than $1,000 for any operation, no matter how serious the operation may be, and no matter how much money the patient may have. Charges of $2,500 for surgical operations are said to have been common, and charges of $5,000 are said to be not uncommon.

This was the institution's answer that physicians and surgeons, especially the big specialists, were charging all that the traffic would bear. They may do it, outside, but it cannot be done, henceforth, in the Johns Hopkins Hospital.

The rule, which was promulgated a short time ago, does not, of course, affect the practice of physicians and surgeons outside the hospital. The hospital authorities do not undertake to exercise any supervision over the charges made by those members of its staff who practice in other institutions, or in their own offices, or the homes of their patients.

It was suggested that the rule might cause the most eminent of the medical and surgical men to take their very wealthy patients from out-of-town to institutions other than the Hopkins Hospital, and that the hospital would lose in this manner. No danger of this is feared, however, because it was said that any member of the medical school or hospital organization attempting to dissuade a wealthy patient from going

to the Johns Hopkins Hospital would at once convict himself of intending to make a charge greater than the hospital authorities thought fair and reasonable.

Effect in Court Cases.

The greatest effect of the new ruling, however, will not be felt in the Johns Hopkins Hospital. It will be felt in every corner of the United States, for the action of the hospital trustees sets a standard of charges for medical and surgical treatment that will have to be followed elsewhere, and those who make greater charges will be in danger of being regarded as profiteers.

It was pointed out today that the ruling would have another far-reaching effect. In case a man of wealth called in a surgeon for an important operation in any part of the country and was charged a fee of say $2,500 or $5,000, he could, if he so minded, contest the bill in the courts, and unless there were very exceptional circumstances connected with the operation, the court would be likely to abide by the declaration of the Johns Hopkins Hospital that $1,000 was all that could reasonably be charged. The ruling as to fees also would furnish grounds for the executors of estates of rich men to contest bills which might be rendered by physicians or surgeons for services.

The action of the Johns Hopkins Hospital Trustees establishes, so far as is known, a precedent. No other institution of high standing has ever before made such a ruling affecting members of its staff, and there has been no standard by which the courts could be guided as to the reasonableness of the charges for such services as physicians and surgeons render.

A forerunner of the action by the hospital Trustees was the statement made by Dr. J. Whitridge Williams, Dean of the Medical School, in an address he delivered a couple of months ago to the medical alumni of the University of Maryland. On that occasion he declared that the greatest danger confronting the medical profession was the love of money, and said the time had come when a halt would have to be called on many members of the profession who profiteer on their patients and charge all the traffic will bear.

"As a result on this tendency on the part of many physicians," he said, "I believe the doctors of the present time are not held as high in the opinion of the public as the doctors of former years. Many men regard medicine as a means of making money rather than as a means of doing good. The field of medicine is no place for the man who wants to make money."

July 29, 1921

SURGEONS CRITICISE FEE LIMIT OF $1,000

Medical Men Here and in Other Cities Say Johns Hopkins Dictum Is Unfair.

So many of the better known New York surgeons are away on vacations or were absent for week-ends yesterday that nothing like a consensus could be had, really representative of medical opinion in this city, on the action of Johns Hopkins Hospital in limiting surgeons' fees to $1,000 for an operation and attendance fees to $35 a week.

A number of those who were found were reluctant to discuss the subject for quotation, but among the few who did talk announcement that the Johns Hopkins plan had aroused some opposition. Emphasis was laid on the cost

of acquiring the technical skill, training and experience requisite to really good surgery, attention was drawn to the amount of charity work most medical men perform, and fear was expressed that the attendance fee in particular would result in relegating much of the after care to subordinates.

Some support was found for the system generally credited to the Mayo brothers' hospital at Rochester, Minn., where the surgeon's fees are based on a percentage of the patient's annual income. A similar system is in use at the Broad Street Hospital here. There also was talk of the wisdom of paying fixed salaries to hospital surgeons and it was said that the Presbyterian Hospital was in progress of instituting that system.

Dr. Lefferts A. McClelland, President of the Medical Board of the Broad Street Hospital and himself a surgeon, characterized as "ridiculous" the ruling of Johns Hopkins authorities on surgeons' fees.

"How is it possible to compute the money value of saving a life?" he asked. "Take a jurist who by his pleading in court saves his client's life —the money that his long legal training has cost him is a parallel of what it costs a surgeon to perform an operation. The vast majority of the work of eminent surgeons is done for nothing. Just the other day I myself did an op-

eration to remove a brain abscess which cost me in loss of other appointments and in railroad fare alone over $200, yet all I got in return was 'Thank you.'

"I have talked with many surgeons today who are in entire agreement with me on the Johns Hopkins ruling—among them Dr. Maximilian Stern, in charge of neurological work at the Broad Street Hospital, and Dr. W. B. Savage, President of the Medical Board of the South Side Hospital at Babylon, L. I."

Dr. McClelland predicted that surgeons in other parts of the country would pay no attention to the Johns Hopkins dictum, but would continue to charge what they thought was right and proper in relation to their patients' incomes.

A reported interview with Dr. A. J. Barker Savage, Acting Superintendent of the Broad Street Hospital, to the effect that a similar limitation of rates had obtained for over a year at that institution, was mentioned to Dr. McClelland, but he said that all that was compulsory there was the basing of fees on income by a regular percentage, without a limit on the actual amount of the charge. This was confirmed by those on duty at the hospital, who said that there had been no criticism of the system, the initiation of which is credited to the Mayo brothers.

A superintendent of one of the largest hospitals in New York City, who would not permit his name to be mentioned, had this to say of the Baltimore fee ruling:

"It is no concern of a hospital what a surgeon shall charge his patients in the institution. The patients are there not because it is one or another hospital but because the surgeon to whom they went for treatment had them brought to it, so that the matter of payment for operations and treatment should rest strictly between the patient and his surgeon."

Regrets Discussion of Fees.

One young surgeon, who is associated with one of the best known surgeons in New York, regretted that the question of fees should have been brought before the public in any way.

"It is very regrettable that any controversy over fees should be brought up at all," he said. "How are you going to determine what is a just fee? What is a large fee to one doctor is a pittance to another. Did you ever see a rich doctor? There are a few, but they have made their money by curing very wealthy people who, out of gratitude, make them large gifts of money."

"A set fee for surgical operations might be an effective method for a hospital to adopt, where the resident surgeon is paid a yearly salary by the hospital to do its surgical work and the fees from individual cases are turned into the hospital; but it hardly strikes me as a fair proposition for the ordinary surgeon," said Dr. Guilford S. Dudley, acting chief of the second surgical division at Bellevue Hospital.

"Johns Hopkins is largely run on such a basis, I think, and that is probably why the Trustees established a fixed rate. The Presbyterian Hospital here is being reorganized along the line and will soon have all of its work done by surgeons who are paid a yearly salary by the hospital.

"For the private surgeon, however, the fairest method of compensation to my mind is the Mayo Brothers' way, where a certain percentage of a patient's yearly income is charged as the bill for the operation.

"It hardly strikes me that stopping of large fees would curtail the amount of free clinical work done, as every surgeon would probably continue with his free clinical work out of regard for the ethics of the profession and from his own love of the work.

"The worst feature of the Johns Hopkins edict is the limitation of charge for attendance on a patient to $35 a week. This reduces the fee per visit to about $2. It is hardly likely that a fine surgeon would attend a patient in bad cases where the treatment required changing dressings twice a day to keep the patient in comfort for that small a fee. He probably would turn it over to the house surgeon and the patient would be deprived of the best services of the specialist who performed the operation."

Heartily Endorses Limit.

Emphatic endorsement of the limiting of surgeons' fees to $1,000 was given by Dr. James Garfield Dwyer, Consulting Surgeon of the Manhattan Eye and Ear Hospital.

"I am absolutely in favor of the action of the Johns Hopkins authorities," said Dr. Dwyer. "The limiting of fees to $1,000 is a step in the right direction, and I have been advocating such a rule for a long time. There is no reason why a surgeon should go above that sum, and he can scale down his prices for the poorer patients."

A New York surgeon who would not be quoted by name declared that the practice of gouging patients for operations has been prevalent heretofore.

"'All the traffic will bear' has been the rule," he continued, "and many surgeons have charged $1,000 and $2,000 for removing adenoids or tonsils. It is high time that this was stopped, and I hope that the Johns Hopkins decision will have a strong effect in reform."

The opposite viewpoint was expressed by the private secretary of a prominent surgeon, now on his vacation. She said that his attitude was against restricting doctors and surgeons in their charges, since they could and should be trusted to adjust their fees to the means of the individual patient.

The opinion of Dr. John W. Brannan, President of Bellevue and Allied Hospitals, was sought, but he refused to see reporters, sending word by an attendant that he had "nothing to say" on the Johns Hopkins ruling.

Chicago Criticises Dictum.

Special to The New York Times.

CHICAGO, July 29.—In years gone by a doctor's wife had to take in boarders to eke out a living, but today no physician would be able to establish a practice unless he lived in a neighborhood of the better class, owned an automobile and had an office in one of the Loop's best buildings. This is the consensus of opinion of Chicago's physicians, who were apparently of one mind in declaring that the edict of the Board of Trustees of Johns Hopkins Hospital in Baltimore that the fee for a major operation should not be more than $1,000 and the charge for hospital attendance $35 a week is all wrong.

If the wealthy man does not pay a large fee, physicians would not be able to take care of the poor, it was said at the office of the Chicago Medical Society. Even now, it is stated, one-third of the patients do not pay their doctor's bills at all, and the physicians have been forced to establish a clearing house to collect them.

"No Board of Trustees in a hospital can decide what a doctor's services are worth," said Dr. Franklin Martin, Secretary General of the American College of Surgeons. "Do you know that nine-tenths of the operations performed by the best surgeons in Chicago today are done for the poor without charge? Their livelihood must come from somewhere. If the well-to-do are not assessed reasonably high, the poor will suffer for it."

"Very well and good," said Dr. Carl B. Davis, who was reached as he emerged from an operation room at the Presbyterian Hospital, "only I think it would be fair to apply the same limit to banks, corporation lawyers and specialists in other lines of business. In other words, why put a limit on the doctor's fee alone? Each patient is charged according to his ability to pay. There are a great many charity patients who can obtain treatment only because of the fees paid by some man who is able to pay them."

Dr. Louis D. Smith, head of the special committee of the Chicago Medical Society, said: "I don't think the operating fee limit is a just one. You have to take the financial status of the patient into consideration. If life is worth no more than $1,000 to a man with a fifty-thousand-dollar a year income, why then, perhaps, the fee is a fair one."

The $35 a week limitation for hospital attendance, Dr. Smith thought, was just, as did Dr. William Franklin Harpel of the Advisory Board of Hahnemann Hospital.

"Except in special cases," said Dr. Harpel, "the limit on the fee for hospital attendance is a fair one. In many instances the charge could be made lower. On the other hand, there are patients whose condition is such that a physician has to be in attendance much of the time. Under these circumstances $35 is too low."

Dr. C. Pruyn Stringfield likewise was opposed to the $1,000 limitation for major operations.

"The way surgeons and physicians look at the subject," he said, "is that they average the fees with the patient's ability to pay. The man who has a big income certainly should be charged more than the man who is earning $1,000 a year."

Dr. Max Thorek, surgeon in chief of the American Hospital, similarly opposed the ruling of $1,000 an operation, as did a number of Chicago doctors. Dr. Thorek said the medical profession for centuries has been donating its services to the poor and turning the financial burdens over to wealthy patients. "If a wealthy magnate brings his wife to me and I save her life, I charge the limit," said Dr. Thorek. "My theory is that if he can buy a $100,000 yacht, he can pay generously for his wife's life."

For Freedom of Fees.

Special to The New York Times.

PHILADELPHIA, July 29.—Surgeons and hospital officials in this city today expressed emphatic disapproval of the action taken at Johns Hopkins limiting the fees to be charged for operations and hospital attendance. It was the consensus of opinion that the ruling will affect the scale of charges or operations and treatment very little, if any, outside of Baltimore. Furthermore, physicians had no hesitation in saying the edict is distinctly unfair and certainly unwise.

The idea of limiting the fees of some of the better known members of the staff of the Pennsylvania Hospital appealed to a resident staff surgeon of that hospital as being wholly impracticable.

"It would have the effect," he said, "of driving away from the hospital all but charity patients, for the doctors would simply remove their patients to a hospital where no such ruling was in force."

In discussing the question of fees to private patients, one of the leading surgeons in the city said:

"It very often happens that fees of $50,000 or $75,000 are paid to lawyers of high repute for an opinion. Now, supposing the man who pays such a fee has a wife or child who is seriously ill. If a surgeon, by means of careful diagnosis, skill and technique, is able to save that person's life, is it not worth more—certainly as much—as the lawyer's opinion?

"If people generally knew of the many mornings that are given by most prominent surgeons in this city to charity work for which they neither receive nor ask any remuneration whatever," he continued, "the matter of fees would be more clearly understood.

"I have no hesitation in saying there is very little 'gouging' going on in Philadelphia. Personally, I have known of very few cases. For major operations, where the skill of the surgeon has saved the life of a patient who can well afford to pay amply for the service, I feel that the bill should be commensurate with the service and the patient's ability to pay. This does not mean 'gouging,' but to limit a surgeon's fee would be clearly unfair."

Many of the leading surgeons in the city are agreed on the freedom of fees in Philadelphia.

Several of the hospitals in the city have taken the attitude that it is none of the hospital's business what members of their staffs charge private patients. The resident surgeon of one hospital said fully 70 per cent. of the operations performed there by one of Philadelphia's leading surgeons are charity operations, for which he receives no fees.

Unwarranted, Says St. Louisan.

Special to The New York Times.

ST. LOUIS, July 29.—Prominent surgeons here were loath to express an opinion concerning the action of Johns Hopkins University in limiting fees. Several who declined to be quoted, however, said they did not believe it was in the jurisdiction of any institution to say what a surgeon should charge for his services.

Dr. Harvey G. Mudd declared that such an edict was an unwarranted interference and in his opinion was a restriction which could never be effectual for the reason that the matter of fees for medical services permitted no arbitrary ruling.

"I would not like such a restriction to be placed upon any surgeon," he commented. "There are so many varying circumstances which govern the subject that a limit of $1,000 would be absurd. For many cases the surgeon receives nothing. Fees are based entirely upon the patient's ability to pay."

Dr. E. A. Babler was of the same opinion. He does not believe there is any ethical restriction upon a surgeon's fees.

"The only fair basis upon which we practice is the regulation of fees according to the wealth of the patient," he said. "A large fee means no more to a wealthy man than a moderate fee to one of less fortunate circumstances. In the sum total those who are able to carry the burden are assessed the most, and the many charity cases for which the doctor receives nothing make the balance."

QUALIFICATIONS ON LIMIT.

Johns Hopkins Authorities Must Approve Charges Exceeding $1,000.

Special to The New York Times.

BALTIMORE, Md., July 29.—"The Johns Hopkins Hospital has not said finally and without qualification that a patient may never, under any circumstances, be charged more than $35 a week for medical attention, nor more than $1,000 for an operation. But it has said that when more than these sums is charged the hospital authorities must be informed of the circumstances and must approve the charge."

This statement was made today by Judge Henry Harlan, President of the Board of Trustees of the Johns Hopkins Hospital.

The Trustees adopted those recommendations after consultation with the medical board of the hospital, Dr. Harlan continued, because it was known that some very large fees had been charged. The medical board and the Board of Trustees felt that some limit should be fixed. But they do not fail to recognize that there are some cases in which larger fees for either surgical or medical services are justifiable. When such larger fees are charged, however, the hospital authorities must approve them.

"There is no plan to fix charges for each order of operation, is there?" Judge Harlan was asked. "That is to say, that an operation for appendicitis should cost so much or an operation for another malady so much?"

"Of course not, that is not practicable," Judge Harlan answered.

It is understood that the real reason for the action, Judge Harlan was told, was that some well-to-do people had been charged large sums just because they were well-to-do, and that they resented the charges and associated Johns Hopkins Hospital with their resentment. There was some resentment of such charges and some association of the hospital with them, Judge Harlan answered.

In taking control of the fees which may be charged its patients, it is said, Johns Hopkins is blazing a new trail in hospital administration, just as Johns Hopkins Medical School blazed a new trail when it adopted the full-time professorship idea, which other medical schools are now adopting.

July 30, 1921

HOSPITAL FEES HIT THE MIDDLE CLASS HARD

Present System Favors the Rich and the Poor— Medical Men Suggest Ways to Lower the Cost of Illness

A SCALE of minimum and maximum fees for physicians and surgeons has been fixed by the Medical Society of the District of Columbia. Minimum fees range from $2 for a minor office consultation to $300 for certain major operations. Maximum fees for similar services run from $10 to $5,000. Charity work is permitted, but Washington doctors will not otherwise deviate from the scale, which, it is pointed out, will enable people of moderate means to obtain the best medical skill at a cost within their reach.

By WILLIAM L. CHENERY.

THE wife of a professional man employed in lower New York became ill on Jan. 1. Good doctors were consulted and her trouble was correctly diagnosed as cancer. Two operations were attempted, but on Easter Day she died.

The family was in moderate circumstances, the man's salary being about $125 a week. By economy they had accumulated $10,000 through the effort of a lifetime. The surgeons were considerate, and the largest fee demanded was $300. In spite of this, nursing charges, hospital expenses, payment for ambulances and the various special treatments prescribed by competent advice amounted to more than $8,000.

At least 85 per cent. of the people to-day have much smaller incomes than this man had and the families that have accumulated as much as $6,000 are still fewer. Disease, however, does not centre its attacks on the rich.

Is it possible for a family in moderate circumstances, for the average middle-class family, to sustain the burden of serious disease without impoverishment? The question is raised by the experience of this one man, who expended more than half of his entire savings in a brief period in a vain effort to combat disease. It is the problem faced by every one in moderate circumstances.

The difficulties encountered are, furthermore, increasing in complexity as medical science advances. It is not a question of profiteering or extortion, but rather of rising costs. The kind of procedure essential to diagnosis and treatment is inherently expensive. The cost of good treatment has risen out of proportion to incomes. What is the answer?

Profession Recognizes Problem.

Mutual insurance schemes offer one solution. Henry Ford has offered another in the Ford Hospital at Detroit. In that institution medical and surgical fees and the charges for special treatments are so regulated that the cost of sickness does not swiftly consume the product of the thrift of a lifetime. There is, however, just one Ford Hospital, and all middle-class Americans do not live in Detroit. What is the situation of New Yorkers?

Last week the Medical Society of the District of Columbia adopted a fixed scale of fees, establishing minimum and maximum charges for various types of service. Local doctors are also giving thought to the issue, and the Public Health Committee of the New York Academy of Medicine is making a continuing study of the hospitals in this city. The preliminary findings made have been published in a report prepared by E. H. Lewinski-Corwin and published by G. P. Putnam's Sons. In these studies hospital costs and the capacity of the public to pay are both considered. The conclusions represent the best thought of the medical profession in this city.

It is often said that the best medical treatment can now be obtained only by the poor, who must accept charity, and by the rich. The statement is measurably true, but it is not an indictment of the hospitals or of the doctors. Only a small portion of the public can be guests at the most expensive hotels or enjoy costly motor cars or play polo. The difference, however, is that the best medical treatment is often essential to life, while high-priced luxuries are non-essential.

It is desirable to make the best medical care available for every one, millionaire, charity patient and member of the middle class, while the wider distribution of the dearest luxuries is not a problem of great public concern. A man may live happily without ever once riding in a fine motor car; but if sickness befalls him he must have the medical equivalent of these few ultimate luxuries.

What are the costs of being ill in New York? All of the hospitals in New York City together spend about $35,000,000 annually. This is an average of about $6 for every resident of the city.

The Public Health Committee obtained figures from various hospitals in order to ascertain the charges actually made to private patients. In the private general hospitals the charges for private rooms vary from $3 to $15 a day. More than half the rooms cost from $5 to $8 a day. The largest numbers are priced at $7 and $8 a day. The cost of semiprivate beds—that is to say, rooms with two or more beds in them—ranges from $2.50 to $7 a day, although the greater number of rooms are valued at from $3.50 to $4.50 a day. The ward rates are from $2 to $3 a day.

Cost of Board Varies.

Thus considerable latitude exists as to the cost of board for pay patients in hospitals. By the use of ward facilities it is possible to get by cheaply. Private rooms are undoubtedly the more desirable. The problem, accordingly, is to get private rooms at prices within the means of persons moderately well to do. Hotels, which are organized for profit, have not found this difficulty insuperable. It is possible to rent rooms in good hotels for as little as $2 or $3 a day.

The room rates in the hospitals for the treatment of special diseases are higher than those in the general hospitals, and the rates in the proprietary institutions are still higher.

The X-ray fees charged by the hospitals vary widely. A skiagraph of the head may cost $5, or it may cost $30. An X-ray picture of the stomach may cost $15 or $75, depending on the number of plates taken. Charges to private patients for operating rooms vary somewhat. In many institutions the charge is from $10 to $15, but in one hospital it is $25, or even higher.

The average cost to private patients in one of the hospitals has been reckoned to be $20 a day. This includes special nursing, which constitutes about 48 per cent. of the bill. The ward patients averaged about $4.16. In another general hospital an average for private patients showed $405 for each case; semiprivate patients paid $42 each, and ward patients paid but $11 a case. Most of these were tonsil operations, however, and the stay in the hospital was brief. A third general hospital reported an average cost of $15 a day to private patients, $7 a day to semi-private and $4 a day for those who used the wards.

In view of these facts the Public Health Committee of the New York Academy of Medicine reported: "The greatest need of change in social policy lies, however, in relation to the large group referred to as 'the middle class.' Of the total number of 4,425,114 persons making individual income tax returns in 1918, 1,495,878, or 33.83 per cent., reported incomes of $2,000 to $3,000, and 932,336, or 21.06 per cent., incomes from $3,000 to $5,000; in other words, 54.89 per cent. of all tax returns were made by persons earning between $2,000 and $5,000 annually.

"The mode of living and the educational standards of this group are such that most of them dread the atmosphere and association of a public hospital ward, and the idea of charity and of free medical services is repugnant to them. This raises the question whether, in those hospitals which are not operated for profit, the scale of rates for room and board as well as all other charges should not be regulated in accordance with the income of the patients.

"The need of moderately priced hospital accommodations for people whose incomes range from $2,500 to $7,500 is one of the most crying social needs in relation to hospitals."

Analyzing Hospital Costs.

What are the possibilities of reform? Plainly the cost of caring for private patients must be sustained by some one. If the essential charges are greater than the majority of individuals can bear, who is to carry the load?

The answer to this question involves some consideration of what are the actual costs involved in maintaining hospitals. To this the Public Health Committee of the New York Academy of Medicine has given attention. As to this they say: "The reports of the United Hospital Fund for the last decade show a continually mounting cost for the maintenance of hospitals. In the group of 56 hospitals for which comparative statistics are available, the general hospitals have shown an increase from $2.46 per day per ward patient in 1912 to $4.72 in 1921, and $4.64 in 1922. The per capita costs in the special hospitals have risen from $2.09 in 1911 to $3.92 in 1921 and to $3.90 in 1922."

According to other reports made to the same authority, 45 hospitals in Manhattan and the Bronx and 11 in Brooklyn got 70 per cent. of all their income from pay patients and from contributions by the city. During the last few years, moreover, the number of pay patients has increased relatively. Some of the hospitals show surpluses at the end of the year. Thus Roosevelt Hospital reported a surplus of $239,259 in 1921 and slightly more than $200,000 the next year.

The general hospitals, however, do not earn what would be regarded as fair profits if they were operated as business concerns. It is thus apparent from their statements that, as at present organized, the service rendered is generally at cost. If lower rates are to be fixed, it is probable that fundamental reorganization must be attempted.

Typical bills rendered by the different hospitals show in detail the costs of various diseases as experienced by patients who have undergone treatment. Here are some characteristic cases: Chronic appendicitis in one hospital required a stay of twelve days. The hospital bill was $231.25. Of this, $96 was for board, $35 for operating room fee, $2 for laboratory, 25 cents for drugs and $98 for special nurses. Of course the surgeon's fee was in addition to that, but the hospital bill itself was relatively small.

The largest bill listed by this hospital was for $1,658.05 for a patient suffering from nephritis. This person stayed in the hospital sixty-five days and the charge for nursing was the largest item, being $917. At the same hospital a patient suffering from arthritis stayed in a ward for fifty-one days, and the total charge was only $204. It is worth noting what enormous proportion in the sickness bill the nursing item represents.

Hospital treatment was originally designed for the very poor. A hospital was a charitable institution; those persons who were in comfortable circumstances were treated at home. It was slowly discovered that treatment could be more effectually managed in the hospitals, and consequently all classes tended to resort to them.

The first hospital in New York was a room in the "Publick Workhouse and House of Correction," erected in 1736,
on the site of the present City Hall. One room, 25 feet by 23 feet, with six beds, constituted the hospital. Bellevue is the development of this original institution. The lingering public prejudice against going to city hospitals may doubtless be partly explained by the historical antecedents of the present capacious institutions.

For this reason, while the hospitals maintained chiefly through taxation have expanded quite as much as have the privately managed institutions, they do not meet the necessities of the middle classes. The unfortunate tradition that the hospital was designed first for prisoners and for public charges still influences those who know nothing of the origin of the institution and less of the facilities at present offered. It is none the less clear that municipal ownership at this time is not demanded as a relief from the high cost of sickness. Other remedies are preferred.

What some of the new developments may be was indicated by President George Vincent of the Rockefeller Foundation at the opening of the Vassar Brothers Hospital at Poughkeepsie.

Hospital Insurance.

Dr. Vincent said: "It has been customary to say of the hospital service in the United States that only the poor and the rich receive the best service. In the past, and to a considerable extent in the present, there is a basis of truth for this statement, but increasingly hospitals are putting good service within the reach of every member of the community.

"One of the problems is to distribute the cost of sickness in such a way as to prevent it from crippling the finances of an individual or a family. In countries like Germany and England, compulsory health insurance under State auspices has been introduced. In Cuba there has been a remarkable development of hospital associations, to which members make a monthly contribution that guarantees free hospital care in case of illness. Recently similar voluntary hospital societies have been organized in London. Many industrial corporations have introduced hospital services to which the employes and the company make equal contributions."

In the Cuban experiment 52,000 per-
sons pay $2 a month to associations that offer hospital care in case of need. All told they contribute a million and a quarter dollars a year, which provides good hospital service. In effect, what they have done is to establish a mutual health insurance society comparable with the national health insurance developed in Great Britain and in Germany.

The Cuban organization avoids State insurance, which is not popular in the United States, and at the same time provides a method by which the benefits of public health insurance are extended to classes that are very sensitive about maintaining their independence and would be inclined to refuse to use public facilities, even where the hospitals maintained by taxation were clearly superior.

Some Possible Experiments.

In this country, which, as it happens, is far richer in hospital facilities than are any of the nations of Europe, the problem of the middle class has just begun to be recognized. The Public Health Committee of the New York Academy of Medicine has gone on record as recognizing the need of accommodating rates to the thin purses of the majority of the public, but the costs of running hospitals have not shrunk.

The Ford Hospital, which has no charity patients, yet regulates all fees and charges and keeps its rates within the reach of the moderate income, is one kind of solution. It is at least conceivable that other hospitals of the Ford type will be established. An institution that renders such positive service is likely to have imitators even though, as in the case of the Ford institution, it also has its hostile critics.

Another kind of solution may be found in an American adaptation of the insurance principle. In Chicago definite progress has been made by the employers in the garment industry in providing against unemployment through mutual insurance. This is a strictly American plan, and it is not subject to the same criticisms that have been aimed at state unemployment insurance abroad. Similarly, it would be natural for some American community to explore the possibilities of the Cuban idea of hospital associations.

November 9, 1924

THE CRISIS FOR THE HOSPITALS AND THE PLAN BRITAIN EVOLVED

Hospital service for patients who cannot pay has put such a burden on privately maintained American institutions that 110 which could not get funds have had to close. Newton D. Baker, chairman of the Welfare and Relief Mobilization, recently called attention to the plight of the hospitals, and the American Hospital Association has asked that funds be appropriated from moneys raised for relief. The crisis lends interest to the following account of new schemes of hospital maintenance adopted in Great Britain. The author is secretary-treasurer of the International Hospital Association.

By E. H. LEWINSKI CORWIN.

THE economic stress of the last three years has revealed in a disquieting manner the insecure foundations on which the entire structure of our private hospitals rests. In view of the reliance which our communities have placed on the private hospital, the situation calls for measures that will do more than bridge over a temporary difficulty. There is need for constructive statesmanship to place our voluntary hospitals on a firmer financial basis.

From one end of the country to the other come reports of the sorry plight of our hospitals. Recently the cry was sounded rather alarmingly in a booklet issued by the Hospital Association of Pennsylvania. The booklet points out that "patient revenue in many instances is less than half what it was"; that income from endowments "is no longer a bulwark"; that "State aid rarely covers more than 25 to 30 per cent of free work and includes none of the cost of dispensary work"; that "there is practically no income from voluntary gifts or contributions." These statements appear the more serious as one continues to read the report, and discovers that there is no constructive or hopeful answer to the question, "What are the hospitals to do?"

Expenditures Greatly Reduced.

Managers have evidently done all they could to reduce expenditures by rigid economies and the slashing of wages of personnel; they are facing the necessity of limiting free patients; they have borrowed from banks to the limit, and now "in times like these" they find themselves powerless. They state that "management can do no more. Operating economies must find a limit on the line bordering good hospital care. Somewhere, somehow, hospitals must find new or increased support." But in view of the uncertainty of all sources of revenue they say that they do not know whence it will come.

No doubt a great many of our private hospitals are close to the brink of insolvency; but it is hardly conceivable that "management can do no more" to meet the difficult problems facing them. Further economies can and must be introduced in many instances. Certain sources of income can be increased. In New York the hospitals, by an understanding with the insurance carriers,

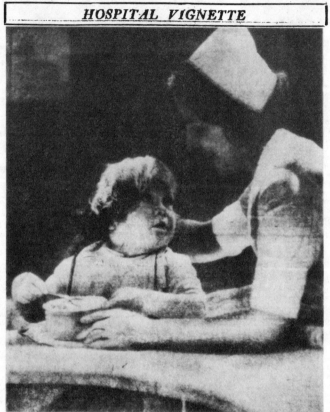

HOSPITAL VIGNETTE

Paul Parker photo, courtesy Welfare Council of New York City.

have raised the rates for workmen's compensation cases. In some States the hospitals have obtained by legislative enactment a priority lien on indemnities paid to patients treated in hospitals for injuries sustained in automobile and other accidents.

Other Sources of Revenue.

The granting by cities of either direct subsidies to hospitals or the payment for the care of public charges on an adequate basis can be made to yield a larger income. It does, however, call for a great deal of consideration as to how far this should go, as does also the question of the payment by relief agencies for the hospital care accorded to their wards—the provision of adequate hospital care for the destitute, it is considered by the advocates of this policy as being of equal moment with provision of shelter, food and clothing. There are still other possible sources of revenue. The situation, therefore, should not be regarded as desperate, but as requiring well-considered and thoughtful communal action.

The experience of Great Britain in this particular regard is worthy of close study. The hospital situation in that country became acute a decade or so ago. The burdens of taxation, the disorganized trade following the World War, and the growing difficulties of providing employment impoverished the British population, and the maintenance of social insurance placed enormous responsibilities on the government ex-

chequer. The wealthy families became less able to meet the growing demands on the part of various charitable endeavors, and the situation of the voluntary hospitals in Great Britain in the beginning of the last decade became so desperate that a special committee was appointed by the government early in 1921 to inquire into the situation. This special committee was presided over by the Viscount Cave.

A British Decision.

The government committee reported under date of May 21, 1921. To the fundamental question as to whether the voluntary hospitals should be encouraged to continue, or whether it would not be more desirable that they should be turned over to the State and be henceforth maintained by taxation, the unanimous answer of the committee was to the effect that "the money loss to the State would be a small matter compared with the injury which would be done to the welfare of the sick for whom the hospitals are provided, the training of the medical profession and the progress of medical research," if the voluntary hospital should be allowed to pass.

The committee recommended that a Parliamentary grant of £1,000,000 be made, and that the money be distributed under the direction of a specially appointed voluntary Hospitals Commission. Such a commission was appointed under the chairmanship of Lord Onslow, but the grant voted by Parliament was reduced to £500,000. The Hospitals

Commission rendered its final report in 1928.

The commission, like its predecessor, the government committee, laid stress on the need of broadening the basis of support of the hospitals through so-called contributory schemes.

In the words of the government committee report, "if the voluntary hospital is to continue to prosper, it must rely not only on the large subscriptions and gifts, but also, and to an increasing extent, on moderate and continuous contributions from all classes of the community." But it was insisted that there must be a direct quid pro quo for these contributions.

Contributory Schemes.

It may seem strange that, in a country where compulsory insurance against the contingency of illness exists, there should be need for further arrangements to provide for hospitalization. In Great Britain the treatment provided for by law in case of illness is of a kind which can be properly undertaken by a general practitioner "of ordinary professional competence and skill." The health insurance act does not provide for treatment requiring the facilities of a hospital. The government committee did not express a definite opinion as to the desirability of broadening the scope of the act to provide payment for hospital care.

There were already in existence several schemes of contributory collections, outside of individual hospitals—those of Oxford, Sussex and the several Hospital Saturday and Sunday Funds. In London the collections were made by several agencies, of which the Hospital Savings Association became most important.

There are at present at least 270 hospital contributory schemes in Great Britain, differing from one another in details of practice and privileges accorded to their contributors. They have an enrolled membership of about 6,000,000, not including dependents of contributors. They contribute annually into the treasury of the voluntary hospitals £2,500,000, or from 60 per cent to 70 per cent of the entire income of the hospitals.

A brief description of the plan evolved by the Merseyside Hospitals Council of Liverpool may suffice to bring out the essential features of the contributory hospital schemes.

In the Liverpool area there are twenty-two voluntary hospitals and all of them have agreed to pool their resources as a unit and to abstain from making individual appeals to the community for support. The city authorities, the public assistance officers, organized labor, the medical profession, the churches and the university have allied themselves with the hospitals in conducting annually a financial campaign for the maintenance of hospitals.

The industrial workers have consented to make weekly contributions toward the support of hospitals and toward their own protection in case of illness requiring hospitalization. The employers of labor have agreed to deduct the voluntary contributions of their workmen and to turn them over to the central fund under the Merseyside Hospitals Council, plus their own contributions, the size of which varies. The employers, as well as workmen, are represented on the central council as on its various committees. In other words, the Merseyside Hospitals Council serves both as a community chest for the hospitals and as a quasi hospital insurance fund.

The plan, as it has been worked out there, is only a few years old and is admittedly an experiment. The penny in the pound contribution was initiated simply because of its slogan value and the ease with which contributions could be calculated. It does not take into consideration the size of the family of the contributor. It bases the contribution in proportion to earnings of the individual rather than in proportion to the risk involved.

In return for his weekly contribution, the fund guarantees to the contributor and his dependents the payment of hospital treatment, if and when needed, as well as auxiliary services, such as ambulance service, surgical appliances, extra nourishment, convalescent care, spa treatment and so on. Although the council has practically succeeded in balancing the hospital budgets, it recognizes that the penny in a pound contribution is inadequate to meet the cost of hospitalization. For the time being the council has decided to keep the penny in the pound basis intact, but it is asking every one to give a penny for each pound and a part of a pound, the employer to add one-third of the collection in his organization.

Overcoming the Deficits.

Thus every one in the scheme will pay a penny if he earns a pound or less; he will pay two pence if he earns two pounds or less; and three pence if he earns three pounds or less and so on. With this change in the contributory scheme, the average contribution will range from 3¼ to 3½ pence a week, and this contribution is expected to meet the existing hospital deficits and to pay for all the auxiliary services.

Under an act of Parliament of 1929, the former poor law hospitals have been taken over by the municipalities and are providing for certain types of infectious and chronic maladies and for acutely ill patients who are destitute. A contributor to the Merseyside fund, sent by a physician to a municipal hospital, is, by virtue of the arrangement made, free from financial investigation. Under this plan the wife of the contributor and his bona fide dependents, that is, those who are resident with him and wholly dependent upon his earnings, are entitled to full hospital benefits.

The Merseyside contributory plan admits also clerical employes, provided their incomes do not exceed the limits agreed upon in concert with the medical profession as insufficient to obtain adequate service in any other way. Persons whose incomes exceed the minimum are not precluded from sharing in the contribution of a penny in a pound, and they may obtain admission to a voluntary hospital on the recommendation of their family doctors, but they are not entitled to free medical service while in the hospital.

The point may be raised whether the pattern of organization and function of the British contributory schemes is applicable in this country. In many of our large cities, and in some counties, we have hospitals maintained by tax funds, which offer free service to those unable to pay for hospital and medical care. Those who use these services need not be certified by the authorities as paupers. There is, therefore, less urge here on the part of wage earners to provide for the contingency of illness on an insurance basis. In this country of "rugged individualism" there is more paternalism in many avenues of life, particularly in provision for the sick, than in any European country outside of Soviet Russia.

Adapting the Plan.

For American purposes the plan would have to provide for the higher levels of our industrial population, as well as for clerks and salaried employes, small shopkeepers and the like. This may lead to the inclusion in the plan of facilities of a semiprivate character, which would raise problems of organization entirely outside of the scope of British experience and which, in a large American city, would require for their solution an extent of cooperation which hitherto has not existed among the hospitals.

Another difficulty which would have to be overcome before any such plan could be put into operation here is that of the relationship of the insured to the physicians inside and outside of the hospitals. These problems are not only of a financial nature; they relate to proper professional service and the hospital affiliations of physicians and surgeons. Whatever form the group insurance plan for hospital care may take in this country, if it be adopted at all, it will not be in the nature of a sickness insurance as understood abroad. It will be merely a voluntary distribution of the burden of cost of hospital care throughout the community for the benefit of the participants as well as for the hospitals.

American Experiments.

The experience of several American hospitals which have independently organized group insurance plans is rather encouraging from an actuarial point of view. Baylor University Hospital has demonstrated that a group insurance plan could be worked out. Two other hospitals in Texas are meeting the financial problem for themselves and their patients in this way, and the Hahnemann Hospital in Philadelphia is experimenting with a plan of similar character. An association was formed in Brattleboro, Vt., to provide a similar opportunity for the people of that city, and recently the hospital in Cooperstown, N. Y., serving a rural section, organized a method of providing medical and hospital care in the community on a rather comprehensive scale. The Cooperstown experiment, however, is more in the nature of a sickness insurance and may find application in only a limited way in rural sections.

There is a movement on foot in several communities to afford opportunity to provide against the contingency of hospital care on an insurance basis. In Essex County, N. J., the hospital council has voted in favor of proceeding with such a plan. This undertaking undoubtedly will be watched closely by other communities.

November 13, 1932

SOCIALIZED MEDICINE IS URGED IN SURVEY

Wilbur Committee Advocates Community Centres to Treat and Prevent Illness.

WEEKLY OR MONTHLY FEES

Taxes or Insurance Would Help Defray Cost—Report Based on Five-Year Study.

Socialization of medical care for the people of the United States, based on a system of group practice and group payment, with community medical centres to provide complete medical service, both preventive and therapeutic, in return for weekly or monthly fees, in the form of insurance, taxation, or both, are the basic changes in American medical practice recommended by a majority of the Committee on the Costs of Medical Care, of which Secretary of the Interior Ray Lyman Wilbur is the chairman.

The committee, consisting of forty-eight experts who were selected as representatives of private medical practice, institutions and special interests, public health service, the social sciences and the public, submitted its final report yesterday during the National Conference on the Costs of Medical Care at the New York Academy of Medicine, attended by leaders in medicine, public health, industry, labor and women's organizations, educators, economists and others.

Dr. Parran Opens Conference.

The conference was opened on behalf of Governor Roosevelt by Dr. Thomas Parran Jr., New York State Commissioner of Health, who read a message from the President-elect in which he expressed the hope that the committee had "arrived at a practical policy for the present emergency."

Dr. Parran read Governor Roosevelt's message at a luncheon, at which Secretary Wilbur presided. The speakers were Professor C. E. A. Winslow of Yale, vice chairman of the committee, who presented an interpretation of the committee's recommendations; Dr. Nathan B. Van Etten of New York City, who presented the viewpoint of the committee's dissenting minority; Dr. Lewellys F. Barker of Johns Hopkins University, Baltimore, who spoke from the physician's point of view, and President Livingston Farrand of Cornell University, who spoke from the point of view of public health.

The committee's final report, consisting of 236 printed pages, to be published this week by the University of Chicago Press, is the culmination of an exhaustive study on a nation-wide scale of all the major aspects of medical service. The report, it was stated, "will provide for the first time a scientific basis on which communities throughout the country can attack the perplexing problem of providing adequate medical care for all persons, at costs within their means.

The final recommendations were supported by thirty-five members of the committee, while the remaining thirteen dissented. Of these, eight physicians submitted a minority report, two dentists signed a second minority report, while one member of the public health group and one from the social sciences group signed separate dissenting opinions. Seven of the dissenting members among the physicians and the two dentists all come from the private practice group. One member of the institutions and special interests group joined the dissenting physicians.

The development in each city of one or more hospitals into a "community medical centre" is described as the "keystone" of the committee's recommendations. These centres would provide complete medical services in return for weekly or monthly fees, with, when necessary, some supplementary support from tax funds. Professional procedures, according to the report, would be under the control of the physicians, dentists and other practitioners, and financial responsibility would rest with a board representing the public.

The personal relations between patient and practitioner should be carefully maintained in such centres, the committee says. Such organization, it is asserted, would be fairer to practitioners than the present system because it would provide them with higher average incomes and would give the largest rewards to those with the greatest experience and ability.

The recommendations in general, the report states, provide for the development of existing machinery rather than the construction of an entirely new organization.

The Principal Minority Report.

The principal minority report recommends that (1) government competition in the practice of medicine be discontinued and its activities restricted entirely to certain types of service; (2) government care of the indigent be expanded with the ultimate object of relieving the medical profession of the burden; (3) coordination of medical service be considered an important function for local communities; (4) united attempts be made to restore the general practitioner to the central place in medical practice; (5) that the corporate (i. e., organized) practice of medicine be vigorously and persistently opposed as wasteful, inimical to high quality, or productive of unfair exploitation of the medical profession; (6) careful trial be given methods which can rightly be fitted into our present institutions and agencies without interfering with the fundamentals of medical practice, and (7) that State or county medical societies develop plans for medical care.

The Governor's Message.

Governor Roosevelt's message read as follows:

Dear Doctor Parran:

Since it is impossible for me to be in New York on Nov. 29, will you please represent me at the final meeting of the Committee on the Costs of Medical Care, express my sincere regrets that I personally cannot be present and convey the following message:

"Those of us who believe that the promotion and maintenance of the public health is a vital function of government have long been concerned with the relation of medical care to mass health. Because large groups of the population seemed unable to provide themselves with adequate medical services the problem was of major importance five years ago, when you began your studies. It is of vastly more importance now because of the changed economic situation.

"Millions of men, women and children are now in need of all the necessities of life, including medical care. Moreover, the reluctance of the self-sustaining population to spend from reduced earnings for anything except emergency service must inevitably result in the postponement of needed medical, dental, nursing and hospital service. Such continued postponements, we can anticipate, ultimately will have a profound effect upon the health of the nation as a whole.

"It is for this reason that many Americans are deeply interested in the conclusions and recommendations of your committee. I hope that you have arrived at a practical policy for the present emergency whereby more and better medical care may be made available for those in want and for those to whom the disaster of illness would mean destitution. But whatever the practical next steps you may have designated, I hope even more that you have not failed to establish the ideal we should strive for over the next span of years. If you have been able to show us how adequate medical care may be made available for the entire population, with its tragic differences in ability to pay for the costs of such care; if you have set up a goal toward which the citizen and the government, the voluntary agency and the professional group, all may coordinate their efforts in a planned progress whose only consideration is the common good—then I, as an American citizen, am honored in this occasion to thank you for it."

Sincerely yours,
FRANKLIN D. ROOSEVELT.

The concluding session of the conference, following a dinner last night, was addressed by Dr. Wilbur, Dr. John Hartwell, president of the New York Academy of Medicine, who spoke on "The New Outlook for Medicine," and President James R. Angell of Yale University, who spoke on "The Future and the People's Health." Dr. Wilbur discussed "the high points in the committee's recommendations."

Dr. Wilbur Replies to Critics.

Dr. Wilbur answered criticisms that the majority report meant "State medicine," declaring that the medical profession was on its way toward some form of community organization, whether it liked it or not, and arguing that it was in the interest of both the profession and the public to have the profession control this movement instead of leaving it entirely in the hands of legislative bodies. He cited the United State veterans hospitals as examples of "State medicine" already in existence. The majority report, he continued, was designed to keep the medical profession in control of such movements.

He declared that the cost would not be prohibitive, as existing institutions would be used. Voluntary contributions were favored at first, he said, as a gradual approach to compulsory payments through a group insurance plan. The cost of complete service, he said, should not be more than $20 to $40 per capita for everything.

President Angell urged that nothing be done to make the career of medicine unattractive to the highest type of men, to rob the doctor of his sense of personal responsibility to his patient or to frighten the public by radical-sounding phrases. Declaring that he would fear State medicine in the United States, he said he believed some development of the nature indicated in the majority report was coming, and commended the spirit of this report as likely to keep this experiment a thoughtful, controlled one, surrounded with safeguards.

Dr. Hartwell cautioned that nothing be done to destroy the relation between the private doctor and the patient who is able to afford treatment, to deter the best men from going into the practice of medicine, to place too great a tax burden upon self-supporting persons or to permit political interference with medical and hospital service.

After the dinner it was announced that the American Committee on Medical Costs had been organized to support the majority report and to answer criticisms of it. The committee includes Morris L. Cooke, engineer and director of the Germantown Hospital, Philadelphia, chairman; Dr. Livingstone Farrand, president of Cornell University; Dr. Michael Davis, director for medical service, the Julius Rosenwald Foundation; Evans Clark, director of the Twentieth Century Fund, and William J. Schieffelin, president of the Druggists' Supply Corporation.

The committee on costs of medical care has been supported by eight foundations and two other organiza-tions—the Carnegie Corporation, the Josiah Macy Jr. Foundation, the Milbank Memorial Fund, the New York Foundation, the Rockefeller Foundation, the Julius Rosenwald Fund, the Russell Sage Foundation, the Twentieth Century Fund, the Social Science Research Council and the Vermont Commission on Country Life.

Committee Spent About $1,000,000.

During its five years of research the committee expended an estimated total of about $1,000,000, while the work performed without cost by the various organizations and indi-viduals mentioned by Dr. Wilbur is estimated at about $500,000 more, thus making the total cost about $1,-500,000.

Dr. Wilbur expressed the hope that when the present committee goes out of existence Jan. 1, 1933, some other organization may be formed for the purpose of promoting further research in the field of medical economics. It is also hoped, he stated, that a continuing organization may immediately be formed to promote experimentation and demonstrations in local communities along lines proposed in the committee's recommendations.

November 30, 1932

MEDICAL JOURNAL ATTACKS REPORT

Special to THE NEW YORK TIMES.

CHICAGO, Nov. 29. — The Journal of the American Medical Association will attack the majority report of the committee on the costs of medical care, made public in New York today, in an editorial in its next issue, of Dec. 3, it was announced today. The editorial will support the first minority report, which was signed by members of the Medical Association.

"Briefly, the majority report recommends that medical practice be rendered largely by organized groups associated with hospitals, and it expresses the hope that those groups will maintain the personal relation-ship between patient and physician so essential to good medical care," the editorial will read.

"In contrast with this recommendation of the majority report, the minority bluntly recommends that 'united attempts be made to restore the general practitioner to the central place in medical practice.' Those two reports represent the difference between incitement to revolution and a desire for gradual evolution based upon analysis and study.

"The majority report urges reorganization of the medical practice, the development of centres, insurance; if necessary, taxation to provide funds; expansion of public health services. The minority is willing to test any plan that may be offered if it conforms to the medical conception of what is known to be good in medical practice."

The editorial will charge that the director of the work, Harry H. Moore, Ph. D., revealed his personal bias for insurance schemes and for governmental practice in a book he has published.

"The rendering of all medical care by groups or guilds or medical soviets has been one of the pet schemes of E. A. Filene, who probably was chiefly responsible for establishing the committee and developing funds for its promotion," it will say.

"The physicians of this country must not be misled by utopian fantasies of a form of medical practice which would equalize all physicians by placing them in groups under one administration. It is better for the American people that most of their illnesses be treated by their own doctors, rather than by industries, corporations or clinics."

November 30, 1932

QUAKER CITY BATTLE GOES TO PHYSICIANS

By LAWRENCE E. DAVIES.

Editorial Correspondence, THE NEW YORK TIMES.

PHILADELPHIA, Jan. 28.—This city has become a battleground in the spreading movement for socialization of medicine. While other States and localities are testing or planning to experiment with projects based on some of the recommendations contained in the recently published report of Dr. Ray Lyman Wilbur's Committee on the Cost of Medical Care, Philadelphia physicians have marked up two clear-cut victories over what their spokesmen regard as unwarranted layman-directed invasions of the realm of medicine, the city's third industry.

Within the last few weeks both the Hahnemann and Germantown hospitals have surrendered to the demands of the organized medical practitioners and dropped aid plans designed to furnish low-cost hospitalization to wage earners. The doctors plan to continue their fight by centring attacks upon less highly advertised projects of somewhat different character at a few other hospitals and eventually demanding the payment of physicians for dispensary work.

The Philadelphia County Medical Society's committee on medical economics, headed by Dr. Seth A. Brumm, appears now to have the whip hand. It is determined to nip in the bud any tendency toward medical socialization, which it scorns as the brain child of "men or groups with no altruistic concept." There are reputable members of the Philadelphia County Medical Society and the Homeopathic Medical Society who say privately that some form of medical socialization is inevitable, but so far they have shown no inclination to engage in a public controversy with society officials.

$150 Service For $10.

The aid plan abandoned at Hahnemann Hospital called for the payment, by any employed person, of $10 a year, for which he was guaranteed hospitalization worth up to $150 during the year should the need arise. A proposal to include doctor's fees at a total cost to the patient of $15 a year had been dropped previously upon the protest of staff physicians. Some 500 applications were accepted before the hospital trustees took final adverse action, and the hospital's agreement with this number will be fulfilled.

The Germantown Hospital planned to make available, at an annual fee of $15, complete hospitalization and physician's care in case of serious illness to workers at industrial plants provided at least 50 per cent of the employes subscribed. The experiment was to be limited to 1,000 persons during the first year and was not to be open to any unmarried person earning more than $1,500 a year, nor a married one receiving over $2,000, with $200 additional allowed for each dependent. The agent selling the plan to an industry would collect a 25 per cent commission on the first year's subscriptions and the $11.25 left to the hospital from each patient would be prorated between the institution and the physicians.

Staff doctors defeated the plan after Dr. Henry C. Munson, secretary of the county medical society, had notified Louis Neilson Clark, managing director of the hospital, that if the project, termed "unethical," were put through, the institution would be removed from the accredited list of the American Medical Association and staff physicians would lose their standing in recognized medical societies.

Chairman Brumm defends the work of his committee partly on the basis of a questionnaire sent out to medical society members. According to his figures, compiled from 1,500 replies, 90 per cent of the physicians asserted that their patients were satisfied with present methods of medical care.

Ulterior Motives Seen.

"The various experimental plans have been put forth to meet emergencies that do not exist," says Dr. Brumm. "The doctors have been scared by lay organizations. Since Bismarck started this, the politicians, insurance companies and industrial concerns backing plans for socialized medicine all have had ulterior motives. We know, for instance, that the big insurance companies are losing money every year on health insurance so they're out to unload on the taxpayer.

"In 1920 we had 175 free clinics in the United States; today we have 8,000. From 1920 to 1930 the population increase was 1.3 per cent. During that period, our ten most prosperous years, the contact visitation to out-patient service totaled 50,000,000 a year. Was it because we had no money?

"We want the poor people taken care of but that is not a medico-economic responsibility; that's a governmental responsibility. We'll supply the medicine but not the economics. We have been giving $20,-000,000 worth of free medicine in Philadelphia annually. The white-collar class must learn to budget the item of medical care. If it can budget death it can budget medical care."

In spite of the committee's vigorous stand both John M. Smith, director of Hahnemann Hospital, and Managing Director Clark of the Germantown Hospital predict that hospital aid plans of some kind are certain to gain root here and they advise the doctors to cooperate so that the plans will not get out of their control, as has been the case in various European countries with exceptions such as Denmark and Sweden.

January 29, 1933

SICKNESS INSURANCE GAINING NEW GROUND

Medical Care on an Annual-Fee Basis Is Now Urged by Numerous Organizations

New trends in medicine were discussed at the annual meeting of the American Medical Association held last week in Milwaukee. One of these trends, toward sickness insurance, is here described by the director of medical services of the Julius Rosenwald Fund.

By MICHAEL M. DAVIS.

CHANGES in medical service are proceeding with unusual rapidity these days. The depression is accelerating some of them. Others are being influenced by the reports of the recently disbanded Committee on Costs of Medical Care.

Change does not merely happen. Some changes follow the sweep of general social trends; apartment-house living, for instance, increases the number of people who go to hospitals during sickness. Other changes spring from new scientific discoveries; the practical wiping out in many communities of typhoid fever and malaria has substantially altered the kind of practice on which local doctors depend. Still other changes result from the conscious effort of individuals or organized groups. A physician in a large Southern city wrote me recently:

The local profession fully realize that an economic readjustment in medical practice is inevitable, and through a committee of fifteen which has just been appointed are now considering the various plans which have been adopted throughout this and other countries with the idea of recommending that one which to them seems best suited to give service to the patient and some remuneration to the doctor.

Subsequently I met with that committee of fifteen, the chairman of which is a distinguished surgeon and former president of the American Medical Association, to discuss their plan of action. This, tentatively, was to offer medical care to people of modest income in their community at a fixed annual fee; in other words, a plan of sickness insurance.

In California the State medical society has advanced beyond the tentative stage. Last February it published a bulletin approving a plan of voluntary sickness insurance which it encourages county medical societies to organize. For an agreed annual fee, paid into a central organization, formed not for profit but as a mutual benefit agency, subscribers would receive medical care from any member of the county medical society whom they selected as their physician.

The California Plan.

California presents, in fact as well as on paper, other significant trends. In its railroads and other large industries employes quite generally obtain medical care on an annual-payment basis. The idea of sickness insurance has become widespread enough among the people on the Pacific Coast to make it generally salable.

The energetic business promoter has not failed to grasp the opportunity. Some small insurance companies and some specially organized "medical service" or "hospital associations" are selling sickness insurance to individuals or groups and hiring doctors to furnish care. The liberal promises which are made at the time of the sale are not usually borne out by the actual contract, which the prospective patient is too likely to sign before reading. Legislative regulation of these commercial medical contracts has become an active issue in California. The plan of the California Medical Society is doubtless due in part to the desire to check commercialization, by meeting in a better way the demand which is recognized to exist among a large proportion of the people.

Action in New York.

In New York the State medical society, at its annual meeting in April, adopted a committee report which endorsed two of the plans which had been recommended by the Committee on the Costs of Medical Care: first, more adequate medical care of the unemployed and indigent and payment to physicians for such service and, second, group hospitalization—paying for hospital care by an annual fee.

Two months before that the American Hospital Association had issued departments of the local government have made arrangements for medical service on an annual-payment basis from the Ross-Loos Clinic, a well-established "private group" organization of about twenty-five physicians, who own their own buildings. For $2 per month they obtain medical service at home, clinic or hospital, complete except for nursing and dentistry, and their dependents also receive care without charge, except hospitalization and medicines, and for these they get reduced prices. In the Central and Far West, several other organized groups of physicians furnish care to organized groups of people in return for an agreed annual sum per person.

A North Carolina Plan.

In Roanoke Rapids, N. C., five mills and their employes set up a hospital and a plan of complete medical service more than ten years ago. Eight thousand of the 12,000 people of Roanoke Rapids have paid 25 cents a week, and until 1931 an equal amount was put in by the employers. During the depression the mills found it no longer possible to continue their payments; but the employes voluntarily doubled their weekly amounts, and the service continues.

Similar plans are common in the mines, lumber camps, and railroads, especially in the West. In a relatively few instances, as in the case of the Endicott-Johnson Shoe Company in Binghamton, N. Y., and the Homestake Mining Company in South Dakota, the whole cost is borne by the employer. Altogether, about two million Americans now receive medical care under voluntary sickness insurance.

During the depression, taxation or charity has had to provide medical care for thousands of persons who in prosperous days were able to pay for it themselves. New York State has set an example to the country by setting up, under the Temporary Emergency Relief Administration, a plan whereby physicians are recompensed from relief funds for authorized care given in the homes of persons who are receiving relief. Representatives of local medical societies and of local commissioners of public welfare supervise the work and deal with such questions as the reasonableness of bills, principles in allocating cases to physicians, &c. In the same State, also, a work-relief project is paying unemployed nurses, under the supervision of existing nursing agencies, for the care of clients at home.

In New York City the dental society has set up a plan, in cooperation with a voluntary public-health agency, whereby persons above the "ordinary charity level" but unable to pay for dental care can obtain it from dentists who have agreed to give service for low,

stated fees to be paid by the patients themselves. In Chicago the dental society provides free service to persons in receipt of family relief. A large central clinic is in operation, supported by relief funds. Six hundred dentists are at present giving their services free to a thousand patients a month.

In Cleveland several hundred physicians of standing have placed themselves on a voluntary panel, agreeing to provide, free or for whatever amount the patient can pay, services to persons who apply at clinics but who have previously been of the group accustomed to pay a private physician.

A Study in Michigan.

From Michigan comes a major illustration of an effort by physicians to make systematic plans both for the long-range and for the immediate demands of medical service. More than a year ago the State Medical Society appointed a committee of seven prominent physicians, with Dr. W. H. Marshall of Flint as chairman, to study medical service throughout the State. From the economic standpoint, the object of the investigation has been "to study the specific buying power of [the various districts in] Michigan and to discuss whether there is much left in the family income for insurance, medical care, &c. Population per square mile, assessed valuations, acreage in farm lands and employment of the population are variable factors in different districts of the State which definitely color the picture of medical care." From the medical standpoint, the incomes of physicians, the distribution of doctors, dentists, nurses, hospitals and health agencies have also been studied.

Michigan's plans have not yet been called to general public attention, but, declared The Michigan Journalist of April 7, "the medical societies of thirty-three States have expressed interest in it and have desired information concerning the methods used and the facts collected." This committee, it is stated, will not only report a substantial body of facts but also make recommendations for action.

The Problems of Change.

Change has brought problems as well as progress. Unprovided-for sickness, uncertain and uneven costs of care (high costs in some cases), overspecialization, shortage of doctors and hospitals in rural areas, unsatisfactory financial conditions of many physicians, nurses and hospitals are problems which existed before the depression. The depression has accentuated these problems and sharpened the sense of need for change.

These problems and needs sit upon the doorsteps of the American people and of the professions concerned with medical care. Changes in medical practice are not merely impending; they are occurring. The country is full of significant trends and experiments.

June 18, 1933

Increasing Work of Hospitals.

It is significant that the first national professional agency to set forth some constructive program in this field should be an organization of hospitals. For the number of hospitals and the scope of their work have been steadily enlarging. With our 7,000 hospitals and 6,000 clinics are now associated two-thirds of the practicing physicians of the country.

Recently a thousand hospitals have taken the step of supplying quarters wherein local physicians may carry on private office practice. This is a noteworthy measure for reducing doctors' overhead, saving patients' time, making the hospital more of a medical centre for it locality, and supplying an important incentive to coordinated work among physicians.

In Los Angeles some 9,000 employes of business establishments... Last February it published a bulletin approving a plan...

MOST DOCTORS BACK HEALTH INSURANCE

By DR. GEORGE GALLUP
Director, American Institute of Public Opinion

The attitude of American doctors toward one of the most controversial public issues in medicine today, health insurance, has been measured by the American Institute of Public Opinion in a special preliminary survey.

The issue was freshly raised two days ago at the San Francisco convention of the American Medical Association. The institute survey, which covered representative doctors in all States, shows that:

More than seven out of ten doctors polled favor the principle of health insurance, by which an individual assures medical and hospital care by regular payments to a health fund.

The chief reason why doctors approve the idea, the survey shows, is that they think it will provide a more regular income. Those opposed to the plan think it would tend to "commercialize" the medical profession. A small percentage of doctors said they favored health insurance to pay for hospital care but not for doctors' care.

More than eight doctors in ten think that the movement toward health insurance will grow in the next few years. Even doctors who oppose the movement believe it will gather strength.

There seems to be little agreement among physicians whether health insurance, if widely adopted, would decrease or increase the income of the medical profession. Twenty-seven out of every 100 in the survey said they had no opinion. Of those holding opinions, nearly half said they thought doctors' incomes would be increased, while the other half said they would be decreased.

The institute's special study of doctors' opinions on health insurance supplements a general survey of the public's attitude, which was reported last week. This survey found 53 per cent of the population willing to enroll under some group insurance plan.

The survey of doctors found no substantial difference of opinion between general practitioners and specialists. Both types voted in favor of health insurance by almost the same majority. Differences of opinion between city doctors and country doctors were also slight, both favoring health insurance by more than 70 per cent.

Another question is the development of "group" practice—the banding together of doctors into clinics. The institute asked doctors:

"Do you think the standards of medical practice are raised when physicians practice in groups, as in clinics?"

The results show an almost even division of opinion, with a slight majority (53 per cent) saying that group practice is beneficial. The chief reasons given were that "two heads are better than one," and that group practice provides greater facilities and equipment for research. Doctors opposed to group practice declared, on the other hand, that "clinics are apt to become too much of a machine."

The survey also asked doctors: "Do you believe many persons in your community go without adequate medical care because they are unable to pay doctors' fees?" Although the majority replied in the negative, nevertheless a substantial number (37 per cent) said that inability to pay prevented many persons from having adequate care. When the same question was put to the general public, the institute found that more than four out of every ten citizens had to forego medical care, at times, because of the cost.

June 15, 1938

HEALTH INSURANCE FAVORED BY MILLIONS

Survey Shows Many Would Pay $3 a Month

Millions of Americans are interested in a new system of paying the doctor and the hospital—the system of voluntary health insurance—according to a nation-wide cross-section survey by the American Institute of Public Opinion, of which George Gallup is director.

The institute's study, which comes after months of debate on the merits of health insurance by physicians, medical economists and government officials, indicates that approximately 25,000,000 persons would be interested in paying as much as $3 a month for complete medical and hospital protection.

This is a figure that many economists believe would be "the top" for guaranteed medical care. Some existing insurance plans are providing such care for as little as $2 a month:

If the cost were limited to this latter figure, the institute survey indicates that approximately 32,000,000 persons would take advantage of it.

The results of the institute survey are especially significant in view of a plan announced by Senator Robert M. Wagner of New York to introduce a major national health measure in the present session of Congress. It is expected to include voluntary health insurance.

After a year of controversy the American Medical Association has indicated it will offer no opposition to health insurance so long as it is voluntary.

The institute survey indicates that the bulk of the potential customers for medical and hospital insurance come from the upper and middle economic groups. They come, in other words, from those earning at least $20 a week.

But a large group of Americans earning less than $20 a week say the cost would still be too high; they could afford to pay only $2 to $3 a month, "if the whole family can be included for that."

January 22, 1939

FAMILY PHYSICIAN 'VANISHING' IN CITY

The family physician is disappearing among self-supporting New York families of small means, "who make numerous and varied choices among physicians, clinics and hospitals during a year and who change frequently from one medical resource to another," the Committee on Research in Medical Economics reported yesterday.

The committee called attention to the results of a survey made under its direction by Miss Gladys C. Swackhamer. The study, covering 365 families, will be published tomorrow.

In a foreword to the study, Michael M. Davis, chairman of the Committee on Research in Medical Economics, points out that the report does not claim that the families studied represent anybody but themselves and that "the reader must judge for himself as to how significant the findings are for other families in New York or elsewhere." Mr. Davis disclosed that a similar study in a much smaller city is under way and that general conclusions must await information from more families and from a number of different communities.

Income Figures Listed

The families embraced in Miss Swackhamer's study live on the lower East Side, the West Side and in Harlem. Some 32 per cent had incomes of less than $1,000; 49 per cent from $1,000 to $1,999; 14 per cent from $2,000 to $2,999, and 5 per cent more than $3,000.

"Although 47 per cent of the families used both private and agency care," Miss Swackhamer reports, "22 per cent used private care only, and 31 per cent used agency care only."

Most of the private physicians utilized were general practitioners and their fees were usually $2 for office visits and $3 for home visits.

"The families make numerous, varied and uncoordinated choices among physicians, clinics, hospitals, proprietary medicines, home remedies and other resources in time of illness," Miss Swackhamer points out.

"The family doctor is a vanished ideal among two-thirds of the families and is very imperfectly represented among the remaining third.

"Informed Choice Infrequent"

"Informed choice of physician is infrequent. The cause is not only lack of information on the part of the patient or family, but the difficulty and cost of securing information from expert sources.

"Change from one medical resource to another is frequent. The frequency of change must reduce the continuity and effectiveness of treatment and the degree and value of personal relationships between patient and physicians.

"Economic and psychological factors combine in motivating choice and change of physicians and other medical resources.

"Cost or the fear of cost is a pervasive element, commonly influencing choice, often causing delay in securing care and frequently impelling change from one medical resource to another."

In releasing the report for publication, the committee suggested that "the study puts the burden of proof on those who make shibboleths of free choice and personal relationship with physician without looking to see how far these essential principles are actually effective under existing conditions of private medical practice."

May 14, 1939

HEALTH INSURANCE WON IN UNION PACT

Special to THE NEW YORK TIMES.

PHILADELPHIA, Aug. 25—An agreement imposing on the employer the obligation to provide health insurance for his workers was adopted today by the International Ladies Garment Workers Union and the Philadelphia Waist and Dress Manufacturers Association. It was the first time such a clause had been written into a labor contract, union officials said.

Immediate and future wage increases and a reduction in weekly working hours were also embodied in the contract, which was praised by David Dubinsky, president of the union, as "a progressive step in employer-employe relations in our industry and the result of mutual understanding between our union and an association of employers ripe with the experience of many years."

The health clause will apply to 10,000 workers in Philadelphia plants making cotton dresses and blouses.

It calls for an assessment each week of 3½ per cent of the payrolls of the members of the employers' association. One per cent will go into a fund to provide vacations with pay and 2½ per cent will be used to establish a system of weekly sick benefits and a medical clinic to supervise the health of the workers.

The agreement is for twenty-nine months and becomes effective immediately to supplant an agreement scheduled to expire Feb. 1.

An immediate wage increase of 7 per cent was provided, and, in view of the increasing cost of living, a 5 per cent increase on Feb. 1. Wage benefits to the workers under the contract will be about $2,500,000 a year, Mr. Dubinsky stated.

Working hours were reduced from forty to thirty-seven and one-half hours a week for all shops producing garments wholesaling at more than $15.75 a dozen.

August 26, 1941

NEW MEDICAL PLAN STARTED IN JERSEY

Special to THE NEW YORK TIMES.

NEWARK, N. J., July 10—A non-profit plan, designed to provide medical and surgical services for its subscribers, while allowing them to choose their own physicians, went into operation today in New Jersey for the first time when contracts were distributed to 700 employes of Peter J. Schweitzer, Inc., a paper manufacturing concern of Elizabeth, N. J.

Approved by the Medical Society of New Jersey, the service is offered by the Medical-Surgical Plan of New Jersey, assisted by the Hospital Service Plan of this State. Dr. Norman M. Scott, executive vice president and medical director of the plan, said here today at his headquarters at 31 Clinton Street that the organization was concentrating for the present on enrolling groups of 100 or more employes in war-production plants, thirty of which are negotiating for the service.

The plan offers benefits, tentatively fixed on a schedule, ranging up to $150 for medical and surgical care in semi-private accommodations of any approved general hospital in the State. Only specified illnesses that require hospitalization are compensable. An individual subscriber pays 75 cents a month. Subscriptions covering all members of a family group, regardless of the number of children, cost $2 a month.

The subscriber, it was emphasized, has "free choice" of his physician and surgical benefits are available regardless of the number of required hospital admissions in the contract year. Medical benefits are allowed in cases requiring more than three days' hospitalization, provided that twenty-one days have not been used in a contract year.

Enrollment will be made available in each county where at least 51 per cent of the licensed physicians have agreed to participate. More than half of the physicians in the State already had approved the plan, it was said, but the required proportion has been met so far only in nine of the State's twenty-one counties, including Essex, Hudson, Bergen and Passaic Counties.

The plan is under supervision of the State Department of Banking and Insurance. The facilities of the Hospital Service Plan are being used for enrollment, which also places the medical-surgical arrangement under the supervision of the State Department of Institutions and Agencies.

Other officers of the plan are Dr. Thomas K. Lewis, president; Dr. Edward W. Sprague, vice president; John S. Thompson, secretary-treasurer, and Dr. William J. Carrington, Dr. Harry N. Commando, Dr. Augustus S. Knight and Dr. Elton W. Lance, trustees.

July 11, 1942

A. M. A. LOSES FIGHT IN SUPREME COURT ON A HEALTH PLAN

By LEWIS WOOD

Special to THE NEW YORK TIMES.

WASHINGTON, Jan. 18—Ruling unanimously, the Supreme Court upheld today the conviction of the American Medical Association and the District of Columbia Medical Society, local affiliate, for violating the Sherman Anti-Trust Law by conspiring to block the activities of Group Health, Inc., a government employe cooperative.

Justice Roberts wrote the opinion approved by all the present eight members of the high court except Justices Murphy and Jackson, who did not participate since the case came under their purview when Attorneys General.

The court left undecided the question whether a physician's practice is "trade," in the meaning of the Sherman law. Justice Roberts based his decision on the conclusion that the association and the society conspired to restrain Group Health, which he said was operating within "the sphere of business."

He refused to hold the medical societies immune from prosecution. They alleged that their dispute with Group Health was covered by the Clayton and Norris-La Guardia acts.

Whereas lower court decisions were filled with details of alleged unfair practices by organized medicine against Group Health, the Roberts opinion did not discuss these activities. It merely reiterated part of the testimony given in lower courts and discussed the legal procedure of those tribunals. Mr. Roberts closed his discussion with the words, "The judgments are affirmed."

Group Health Is Described

Group Health, around which the four-year dispute revolved, was described by Justice Roberts as "a nonprofit corporation organized by government employes to provide medical care and hospitalization on a risk-sharing prepayment basis." Physicians were employed on "a full-time salary basis" and hospital facilities were sought for treatment of members and their families.

"This plan was contrary to the code of ethics of the petitioners," said Justice Roberts, referring to the medical societies.

"The indictment," he went on, "charges that, to prevent Group Health from carrying out its objects, the defendants conspired to coerce practicing physicians, members of the petitioners, from accepting employment under Group Health, to restrain practicing physicians, members of the petitioners, from consulting with Group Health's doctors who might desire to consult with them, and to restrain hospitals in and about the city of Washington from affording facilities for the care of patients of Group Health's physicians."

The controversy arose in December, 1938, when the medical associations and twenty-one physicians of Washington and Chicago were indicted as participants in an unlawful combination and conspiracy to restrain trade. Also indicted were the Washington Academy of Surgery and the Harris County (Houston, Texas) Medical Society.

A Federal district court threw out the case on the ground that medical practice was not "trade" under the Sherman act. The local Circuit Court of Appeals reversed that decision and ordered trial of the suit.

Early Defendants Are Cleared

Some of the defendants were acquitted by order of the court and others were found not guilty. The association was fined $2,500 and the society $1,500.

The conviction was sustained by the Circuit Court of Appeals and has been approved by the Supreme Court. Through intervening procedure the number of defendants was stripped to the association and the society.

"Much argument has been addressed to the question whether a physician's practice of his profession constitutes trade under Section 3 of the Sherman Act," Justice Roberts said.

"In the light of what we shall say with respect to the charge laid in the indictment, we need not consider or decide this question."

In describing Group Health, he remarked:

"The fact that it is cooperative

328

and procures services and facilities on behalf of its members only does not remove its activities from the sphere of business."

Justice Roberts approved the action of the Circuit Court in holding "the calling or occupation of the individual physicians immaterial if the purpose and the effect of their conspiracy was such obstruction and restraint of the business of Group Health."

Indictment Is Summarized

Justice Roberts alluded to the conspiracy charges, as outlined in the indictment:

"Restraining Group Health from doing business; restraining members of Group Health from obtaining adequate medical care according to Group Health's plan; restraining doctors serving Group Health in the pursuit of their calling; restraining doctors not on Group Health's staff from practicing in the District of Columbia in pursuance of their calling; restrain-

ing the Washington hospitals in the business of operating their hospitals."

Whereas the medical societies argued that they were charged with five separate conspiracies and entitled to trial on each, Justice Roberts agreed with the Appellate Court that the indictment charged only a single conspiracy as follows:

"The medical societies combined and conspired to prevent the successful operation of Group Health's plan, and the steps by which this was to be effectuated were as follows: (1) to impose restraints on physicians affiliated with Group Health by threat of expulsion or actual expulsion from the societies; (2) to deny them the essential professional contacts with other physicians, and (3) to use the coercive power of the societies to deprive them of hospital facilities for their patients."

Justice Roberts added:

"We think the courts below correctly construed the indictment. We agree that the case was one for submission to a jury."

Plea of Exemption Is Denied

As to the third point, the medical societies, said Justice Roberts, contended that their controversy with Group Health over employment of doctors was covered by the Clayton and Norris-La Guardia acts, which concern disputes not prosecutable under the Sherman Act.

"They insist," he stated, "that as the petitioners and Group Health, its members and doctors, other doctors and hospitals, were either directly or indirectly interested in a controversy which concerned the terms of employment of doctors by Group Health, the case falls within the exemption of the [two] statutes and they cannot be held criminally liable for violation of the Sherman Act.

"We think, however, that petitioners' activities are not within the exemptions granted by the statutes. They [doctors] were interested in the terms and conditions of the employment only in the sense that they desired to pre-

vent Group Health from functioning by having any employes. Obviously there was no dispute between Group Health and the doctors it employed or might employ in which petitioners were either directly or indirectly interested."

Thurman Arnold, the assistant attorney general who prosecuted the case, acclaimed the Supreme Court verdict. The result, he said, was of far-reaching importance "because it holds that when defendants restrain free availability of services in the market it is immaterial whether they are professional men or whether they are a nonprofit, cooperative corporation."

Dr. A. Magruder MacDonald, president of the District Medical Society, expressed disappointment, but said that the issue was dead. He promised that the society, which he called "the representative medical organization" in Washington, would not lose sight of its 100-year-old tradition of service.

January 19, 1943

MEDICAL CENTER FOR UNION

Ladies Garment Workers Will Open It in Philadelphia

Special to THE NEW YORK TIMES.

PHILADELPHIA, Feb. 12—The International Ladies Garment Workers Union (AFL) will open here on Feb. 26 what is described as the first medical center in the country to be operated solely for union members. The center will have a staff of twenty-one physicians, in addition to nurses and technicians, according to Isidor Melamed, former business agent of the union, who will act as director, and 90 per cent of the services will be free.

The center will occupy a four-story brick building at Twenty-second and Locust Streets, which formerly housed the Italian Consulate. Costs will be defrayed jointly by the union, which has a membership of about 14,000 here, and clothing manufacturers, who have pledged 3½ per cent of their weekly payrolls.

February 13, 1944

HOSPITAL SERVICE NOW 10 YEARS OLD

The Associated Hospital Service of New York, founded ten years ago tomorrow as a nonprofit community enterprise for the prepayment of hospital bills, will mark this milestone in its history with the enrollment of its two millionth member.

Three thousand five hundred members will go to hospitals in the New York area this week for an average stay of 9.9 days and for 92 per cent of them there will be no extra hospital charges to pay. Some of them who are members also of the United Medical Service will have, in addition, no doctors' bills to worry about.

The association, now growing at a record rate of 50,000 members a month, is the largest of eighty-five cooperative hospital insurance groups, including five in Canada

and one in Puerto Rico, which are known collectively as the Blue Cross and are affiliated with the Hospital Service Commission of Chicago, which sets up standards and acts as a coordinating agency.

$75,000,000 Paid in Year

Latest figures place Blue Cross membership at 17,500,000 and it is advancing by 85,000 a week. Blue Cross affiliates last year paid 1,400,000 bills totaling $75,000,000 to 3,500 hospitals.

The current spurt in the enrollment in the New York area—the 1944 increase topped the previous year's by 218 per cent—is particularly noteworthy, association officials feel, in view of pending legislation designed to make health insurance compulsory. The voluntary method of paying hospital bills, they say, has passed the experimental stage and a decade of experience has shown indisputably that it works.

Frank Van Dyk, executive vice president, who, with a staff of six assistants, started the association

off by enlisting Fannie Hurst as its first subscriber, now directs a force of 700 at the offices at 370 Lexington Avenue. He attributes the present expansion of membership partly to the availability of ready cash, both among workers and employers, and to the recent enrollment of several large groups on an industry-wide basis, including the pocketbook, hotel and furniture workers.

Many Employers Pay Cost

A further factor is the result of a gradual process of education. "People talk more about health security today," he says. But more interesting, he observes, is a definite and fast-growing trend among employers to pay all or part of the cost of hospital insurance. A majority of the members now being enrolled for the first time are being enrolled on that basis. An employer contribution is deductible from taxes and is not considered an increase in violation of the Federal wage stabilization program.

"Such contributions," Mr. Van Dyk says, "have proved a sound personnel policy and today there are roughly 1,000 employers making contributions. We don't require this, of course, but our salesmen suggest its possibilities. I think that employers are recognizing more and more that personnel relations are as important as public relations."

As assets have mounted—they stood at $13,607,192 at the end of last year—additional benefits have been made available. Subscribers are entitled to twenty-one days a year in a semi-private room and receive without additional cost prescribed diets, use of operating room, X-rays, drugs and medicines, including penicillin, laboratory examinations, and the use of physiotherapy and other equipment. After twenty-one days, 50 per cent of charges for the next ninety days are paid. Last December, as a special dividend, twenty-one days of full benefits were made available for each different illness in the year.

May 6, 1945

TRUMAN ASKS LAW TO FORCE INSURING OF NATION'S HEALTH

By FELIX BELAIR Jr.
Special to The New York Times.

WASHINGTON, Nov. 19—President Truman told Congress in a special message today that "the health of this nation is a national concern" and asked immediate action on a five-point legislative program of preventive and curative medical aid, including a compulsory health insurance system under the present social security program.

Besides the compulsory insurance feature and a new plan for "payment of benefits to replace at least part of the earnings that are lost during sickness and long term disability," on which he proposed to say more later, the President's program called for the following things:

Broadening the present program of grants in aid to States for construction of hospitals and related facilities.

Expansion of public health, maternal and child health services.

A plan for strengthening professional education and medical research.

After the reading of the message, bills to carry out its objectives were introduced by Senator Wagner of New York and Representative Dingle, Democrat, of Michigan. The measures were referred by the Senate to its Committee on Education and Labor, and in the House to the Interstate and Foreign Commerce Committee.

Anticipating cries of "socialized medicine" which were heard from the Republican side of the Senate, the President said in his message that was precisely what his proposal was not. He called the compulsory health insurance program a system of prepaid medical costs, then added:

"The American people are the most insurance-minded people in the world. They will not be frightened off from health insurance because some people have misnamed it 'socialized medicine.'

"I am in favor of the broadest possible coverage for this insurance system. I believe that all persons who work for a living and their dependents should be covered under such an insurance plan. This would include wage and salary earners, those in business for themselves, professional persons, farmers, agricultural labor, domestic employes, Government employes and employes of non-profit institutions and their families.

"In addition, needy persons and other groups should be covered through appropriate premiums paid for them by public agencies. Increased Federal funds should also be made available by the Congress under the public assistance programs to reimburse the States for part of such premiums.

"Premiums for present social insurance benefits are calculated on the first $3,000 of earnings in a year. It might be well to have all such premiums, including those for health, calculated on a somewhat higher amount, such as $3,600.

"A broad program of prepayment for medical care would need total amounts approximately equal to 4 per cent of such earnings. The people of the United States have been spending, on the average, nearly this percentage of their incomes for sickness care. How much of the total fund should come from the insurance premiums and how much from general revenues is a matter for the Congress to decide."

Mr. Truman emphasized that his proposal was not socialization of the medical profession. People would be free to choose their own physicians, though participants in the compulsory system.

"Likewise," the President said, "physicians should remain free to accept or reject patients. They must be allowed to decide for themselves whether they wish to participate in the health-insurance system full time, part time or not at all."

The President asserted that the all-important difference between what he proposed and the present doctor-patient relationship was:

"Whether or not patients get the services they need would not depend on how much they can afford to pay at the time."

Since medical services were personal, Mr. Truman said, the compulsory-insurance system should be highly decentralized in administration with the local unit as the keystone of the program to assure its adaptation to local needs and conditions.

"Subject to national standards, methods and rates of paying doctors and hospitals should be adjusted locally," he said. "All such rates for doctors should be adequate, and should be appropriately adjusted for those who are qualified specialists."

The President recalled that nearly 5,000,000 men between the ages 18 and 37 were classified as unfit for military service, or about 30 per cent of all those examined.

November 20, 1945

Text of the President's Health Message Calling for Compulsory Medical Insurance

WASHINGTON, Nov. 19 (AP)—President Truman's message to Congress on a national health program follows:

To the Congress of the United States:

In my message to the Congress of Sept. 6, 1945, there were enumerated in a proposed Economic Bill of Rights certain rights which ought to be assured to every American citizen.

One of them was: "The right to adequate medical care and the opportunity to achieve and enjoy good health." Another was the "right to adequate protection from the economic fears of * * * sickness."

Millions of our citizens do not have a full measure of opportunity to achieve and enjoy good health. Millions do not now have protection or security against the economic effects of sickness. The time has arrived for action to help them attain that opportunity and that protection.

The people of the United States received a shock when the medical examinations conducted by the Selective Service System revealed the widespread physical and mental incapacity among the young people of our nation. We had had prior warnings from eminent medical authorities and from investigating committees. The statistics of the last war had shown the same condition. But the Selective Service System has brought it forcibly to our attention recently—in terms which all of us can understand.

30 Per Cent of Draftees Unfit

As of April 1, 1945, nearly 5,000,-000 male registrants between the ages of 18 and 37 had been examined and classified as unfit for military service. The number of those rejected for military service was about 30 per cent of all those examined. The percentage of rejection was lower in the younger age groups, and higher in the higher age groups, reaching as high as 49 per cent for registrants between the ages of 34 and 37.

In addition, after actual induction, about a million and a half men had to be discharged from the Army and Navy for physical or mental disability, exclusive of wounds; and an equal number had to be treated in the armed forces for diseases or defects which existed before induction.

Among the young women who applied for admission to the Women's Army Corps there was similiar disability. Over one-third of those examined were rejected for physical or mental reasons.

These men and women who were rejected for military service are not necessarily incapable of civilian work. It is plain, however, that they have illnesses and defects that handicap them, reduce their working capacity, or shorten their lives.

It is not so important to search the past in order to fix the blame for these conditions. It is more important to resolve now that no American child shall come to adult life with diseases or defects which can be prevented or corrected at an early age.

Medicine has made great strides in this generation—especially during the last four years. We owe much to the skill and devotion of the medical profession. In spite of great scientific progress, however, each year we lose many more persons from preventable and premature deaths than we lost in battle or from war injuries during the entire war.

We are proud of past reductions in our death rates. But these reductions have come principally from public health and other community services. We have been less effective in making available to all of our people the benefits of medical progress in the care and treatment of individuals.

Inequality in Medical Care

In the past, the benefits of modern medical science have not been enjoyed by our citizens with any degree of equality. Nor are they today. Nor will they be in the future—unless Government is bold enough to do something about it.

People with low or moderate incomes do not get the same medical attention as those with high incomes. The poor have more sickness, but they get less medical care. People who live in rural areas do not get the same amount or quality of medical attention as those who live in our cities.

Our new economic bill of rights should mean health security for all, regardless of residence, station or race—everywhere in the United States.

We should resolve now that the health of this nation is a national concern; that financial barriers in the way of attaining health shall be removed; that the health of all its citizens deserves the help of all the nation.

Lists Basic Problems

There are five basic problems which we must attack vigorously if we would reach the health objectives of our economic bill of rights.

1. The first has to do with the number and distribution of doctors and hospitals. One of the most important requirements for adequate health service is profes-

sional personnel — doctors, dentists, public health and hospital administrators, nurses and other experts.

The United States has been fortunate with respect to physicians. In proportion to population it has more than any large country in the world, and they are well trained for their calling. It is not enough, however, that we have them in sufficient numbers. They should be located where their services are needed. In this respect we are not so fortunate.

The distribution of physicians in the United States has been grossly uneven and unsatisfactory. Some communities have had enough or even too many; others have had too few. Year by year the number in our rural areas has been diminishing. Indeed, in 1940, there were thirty-one counties in the United States, each with more than a thousand inhabitants, in which there was not a single practicing physician. The situation with respect to dentists was even worse.

One important reason for this disparity is that in some communities there are no adequate facilities for the practice of medicine. Another reason—closely allied with the first—is that the earning capacity of the people in some communities makes it difficult if not impossible for doctors who practice there to make a living.

The demobilization of 60,000 doctors, and of the tens of thousands of other professional personnel in the armed forces is now proceeding on a large scale. Unfortunately, unless we act rapidly, we may expect to see them concentrate in the places with greater financial resources and avoid other places, making the inequalities even greater than before the war. Demobilized doctors cannot be assigned. They must be attracted. In order to be attracted, they must be able to see ahead of them professional opportunities and economic assurances.

Nation Short of Hospitals

Inequalities in the distribution of medical personnel are matched by inequalities in hospitals and other health facilities. Moreover, there are just too few hospitals, clinics and health centers to take proper care of the people of the United States.

About 1,200 counties, 40 per cent of the total in the country, with some 15,000,000 people, have either no local hospital, or none that meets even the minimum standards of national professional associations.

The deficiencies are especially severe in rural and semi-rural areas and in those cities where changes in population have placed great strains on community facilities.

I want to emphasize, however, that the basic problem in this field cannot be solved merely by building facilities. They have to be staffed; and the communities have to be able to pay for the services. Otherwise the new facilities will be little used.

2. The second basic problem is the need for development of public health services and maternal and child care. The Congess can be justifiably proud of its share in making recent accomplishments possible. Public health and

maternal and child health programs already have made important contributions to national health. But large needs remain. Great areas of our country are still without these services. This is especially true among our rural areas; but it is true also in far too many urban communities.

Although local public health departments are now maintained by some 18,000 counties and other local units, many of these have only skeleton organizations, and approximately 40,000,000 citizens of the United States still live in communities lacking full-time local public health service. At the recent rate of progress in developing such service, it would take more than a hundred years to cover the whole nation.

Sanitation Measures Needed

If we agree that the national health must be improved, our cities, towns and farming communities must be made healthful places in which to live through provision of safe water systems, sewage disposal plants and sanitary facilities. Our streams and rivers must be safeguarded against pollution. In addition to building a sanitary environment for ourselves and for our children, we must provide those services which prevent disease and promote health.

Services for expectant mothers and for infants, care of crippled or otherwise physically handicapped children and inoculation for the prevention of communicable diseases are accepted public health functions. So too are many kinds of personal services, such as the diagnosis and treatment of widespread infections like tuberculosis and venereal disease. A large part of the population today lacks many or all of these services.

Our success in the traditional public health sphere is made plain by the conquest over many communicable diseases. Typhoid fever, smallpox and diphtheria—diseases for which there are effective controls — have become comparatively rare. We must make the same gains in reducing our maternal and infant mortality, in controlling tuberculosis, venereal disease, malaria and other major threats to life and health. We are only beginning to realize our potentialities in achieving physical well-being for all our people.

3. The third basic problem concerns medical research and professional education.

We have long recognized that we cannot be content with what is already known about health or disease. We must learn and understand more about health and how to prevent and cure disease.

Need for Research Stressed

Research—well directed and continuously supported—can do much to develop ways to reduce those diseases of body and mind which now cause most sickness, disability and premature death—diseases of the heart, kidneys and arteries, rheumatism, cancer, diseases of childbirth, infancy and childhood, respiratory diseases and tuberculosis. And research can do much toward teaching us how to keep well and how to prolong healthy human life.

Cancer is among the leading causes of death. It is responsible for over 160,000 recorded deaths

a year, and should receive special attention. Though we already have the National Cancer Institute of the Public Health Service, we need still more coordinated research on the cause, prevention and cure of this disease. We need more financial support for research and to establish special clinics and hospitals for diagnosis and treatment of the disease especially in its early stages. We need to train more physicians for the highly specialized services so essential for effective control of cancer.

2,000,000 Mentally Ill

There is also special need for research on mental diseases and abnormalities. We have done pitifully little about mental illnesses. Accurate statistics are lacking, but there is no doubt that there are at least two million persons in the United States who are mentally ill, and that as many as ten million will probably need hospitalization for mental illness for some period in the course of their lifetime.

A great many of these persons would be helped by proper care. Mental cases occupy more than one-half of the hospital beds, at a cost of about $500,000,000 per year —practically all of it coming out of taxpayers' money. Each year there are 125,000 new mental cases admitted to institutions.

We need more mental-disease hospitals, more out-patient clinics. We need more services for early diagnosis, and especially we need much more research to learn how to prevent mental breakdown. Also, we must have many more trained and qualified doctors in this field.

It is clear that we have not done enough in peacetime for medical research and education in view of our enormous resources and our national interest in health progress. The money invested in research pays enormous dividends. If any one doubts this, let him think of Penicillin, plasma, DDT powder and new rehabilitation techniques.

The High Cost of Care

4. The fourth problem has to do with the high cost of individual medical care. The principal reason why people do not receive the care they need is that they cannot afford to pay for it on an individual basis at the time they need it. This is true not only for needy persons. It is also true for a large proportion of normally self-supporting persons.

In the aggregate, all health services—from public health agencies, physicians, hospitals, dentists, nurses and laboratories—absorb only about 4 per cent of the national income. We can afford to spend more for health.

But 4 per cent is only an average. It is cold comfort in individual cases. Individual families pay their individual costs, and not average costs. They may be hit by sickness that calls for many times the average cost—in extreme cases for more than their annual income. When this happens they may come face to face with economic disaster. Many families, fearful of expense, delay calling the doctor long beyond the time when medical care would do the most good.

For some persons with very low income or no income at all we now use taxpayers' money in the form of free services, free clinics and public hospitals. Tax-supported, free medical care for

needy persons, however, is insufficient in most of our cities and in nearly all of our rural areas. This deficiency cannot be met by private charity or the kindness of individual physicians.

Each of us knows doctors who work through endless days and nights, never expecting to be paid for their services because many of their patients are unable to pay. Often the physician spends not only his time and effort, but even part of the fees he has collected from patients able to pay, in order to buy medical supplies for those who cannot afford them. I am sure that there are thousands of such physicians throughout our country. They cannot, and should not, be expected to carry so heavy a load.

5. The fifth problem has to do with loss of earnings when sickness strikes. Sickness not only brings doctor bills; it also cuts off income.

7,000,000 Always Ill

On an average day there are about 7,000,000 persons so disabled by sickness or injury that they cannot go about their usual tasks. Of these, about 3,250,000 are persons who, if they were not disabled, would be working or seeking employment. More than one-half of these disabled workers have already been disabled for six months; many of them will continue to be disabled for years, and some for the remainder of their lives.

Every year four or five hundred million working days are lost from productive employment because of illness and accident among those working or looking for work—about forty times the number of days lost because of strikes on the average during the ten years before the war. About nine-tenths of this enormous loss is due to illness and accident that is not directly connected with employment and is therefore not covered by workmen's compensation laws.

These then are the five important problems which must be solved, if we hope to attain our objective of adequate medical care, good health, and protection from the economic fears of sickness and disability.

Offers Program to Congress

To meet these problems, I recommend that the Congress adopt a comprehensive and modern health program for the nation, consisting of five major parts—each of which contributes to all the others.

First: Construction of Hospitals and Related Facilities

The Federal Government should provide financial and other assistance for the construction of needed hospitals, health centers and other medical, health and rehabilitation facilities. With the help of Federal funds, it should be possible to meet deficiencies in hospital and health facilities so that modern services—for both prevention and cure—can be accessible to all the people. Federal financial aid should be available not only to build new facilities where needed, but also to enlarge or modernize those we now have.

In carrying out this program, there should be a clear division of responsibilities between the States and the Federal Government. The States, localities and the Federal Government should share in the financial responsibilities. The Federal Government should not construct or operate these hospitals. It should, however, lay down minimum national standards for construction and operation, and should make sure that Federal funds are allocated to those areas and projects where Federal aid is needed most. In approving State plans and individual projects, and in fixing the national standards, the Federal agency should have the help of a strictly advisory body that includes both public and professional members.

Adequate emphasis should be given to facilities that are particularly useful for prevention of diseases — mental as well as physical—and to the coordination of various kinds of facilities. It should be possible to go a long way toward knitting together facilities for prevention with facilities for cure, the large hospitals of medical centers with the smaller institutions of surrounding areas, the facilities for the civilian population with the facilities for veterans.

The general policy of Federal-State partnership which has done so much to provide the magnificent highways of the United States can be adapted to the construction of hospitals in the communities which need them.

Second: Expansion of Public Health, Maternal and Child Health Services.

Our programs for public health and related services should be enlarged and strengthened. The present Federal-State cooperative health programs deal with general public health work, tuberculosis and veneral disease control, maternal and child health services and services for crippled children.

These programs were especially developed in the ten years before the war and have been extended in some areas during the war. They have already made important contributions to national health, but they have not yet reached a large proportion of our rural areas, and, in many cities, they are only partially developed.

No area in the nation should continue to be without the services of a full-time health officer and other essential personnel. No area should be without essential public health services or sanitation facilities. No area should be without communnity health services such as maternal and child health care.

Hospitals, clinics and health centers must be built to meet the needs of the total population, and must make adequate provision for the safe birth of every baby, and for the health protection of infants and children.

Present laws relating to general public health, and to maternal and child health, have built a solid foundation of Federal cooperation with the States in administering community health services. The emergency maternity and infant care program for the wives and infants of service men —a great wartime service authorized by the Congress—has materially increased the experience of every State health agency, and has provided much-needed care. So too have other wartime programs such as venereal disease control, industrial hygiene, malaria control, tuberculosis control and other services offered in war essential communities.

Favors Larger Grants to States

The Federal Government should cooperate by more generous grants to the States than are provided under present laws for public health services and for maternal and child health care.

The program should continue to be partly financed by the States themselves, and should be administered by the States. Federal grants should be in proportion to State and local expenditures, and should also vary in accordance with the financial ability of the respective States.

The health of American children, like their education, should be recognized as a definite public responsibility.

In the conquest of many diseases, prevention is even more important than cure. A well-rounded national health program should, therefore, include systematic and widespread health and physical education and examinations, beginning with the youngest children and extending into community organizations. Medical and dental examinations of school children are now inadequate. A preventive health program, to be successful, must discover defects as early as possible. We should, therefore, see to it that our health programs are pushed most vigorously with the youngest section of the population.

Of course, Federal aid for community health services—for general public health and for mothers and children—should complement and not duplicate prepaid medical services for individuals, proposed by the fourth recommendation of this message.

Third: Medical Education and Research.

The Federal Government should undertake a broad program to strengthen professional education in medical and related fields, and to encourage and support medical research.

Professional education should be strengthened where necessary through Federal grants-in-aid to public and to non-profit private institutions. Medical research, also, should be encouraged and supported in the Federal agencies and by grants-in-aid to public and non-profit private agencies.

In my message to the Congress of Sept. 6, 1945, I made various recommendations for a general Federal research program. Medical research—dealing with the broad fields of physical and mental illnesses—should be made effective in part through that general program and in part through specific provisions within the scope of a national health program.

Federal aid to promote and support research in medicine, public health and allied fields is an essential part of a general research program to be administered by a central Federal research agency. Federal aid for medical research and education is also an essential part of any national health program, if it is to meet its responsibilities for high grade medical services and for continuing progress. Coordination of the two programs is obviously necessary to assure efficient use of Federal funds. Legislation covering medical research in a national health program should provide for such coordination.

Fourth: Prepayment of Medical Costs.

Everyone should have ready access to all necessary medical, hospital and related services.

I recommend solving the basic problem by distributing the costs through expansion of our existing compulsory social insurance system, This is not socialized medicine.

Everyone who carries fire insurance knows how the law of averages is made to work so as to spread the risk, and to benefit the insured who actually suffers the loss. If instead of the costs of sickness being paid only by those who get sick, all the people —sick and well—were required to pay premiums into an insurance fund, the pool of funds thus created would enable all who do fall sick to be adequately served without overburdening anyone. That is the principle upon which all forms of insurance are based.

During the past fifteen years, hospital insurance plans have taught many Americans this magic of averages. Voluntary health insurance plans have been expanding during recent years; but their rate of growth does not justify the belief that they will meet more than a fraction of our people's needs. Only about 3 per cent or 4 per cent of our population now have insurance providing comprehensive medical care.

A system of required prepayment would not only spread the costs of medical care, it would also prevent much serious disease. Since medical bills would be paid by the insurance fund, doctors would more often be consulted when the first signs of disease occur instead of when the disease has become serious. Modern hospital, specialist and laboratory services, as needed, would also become available to all, and would improve the quality and adequacy of care. Prepayment of medical care would go a long way toward furnishing insurance against disease itself, as well as against medical bills.

What System Would Cover

Such a system of prepayment should cover medical, hospital, nursing and laboratory services. It should also cover dental care—as fully and for as many of the population as the available professional personnel and the financial resources of the system permit.

The ability of our people to pay for adequate medical care will be increased if, while they are well, they pay regularly into a common health fund, instead of paying sporadically and unevenly when they are sick. This health fund should be built up nationally, in order to establish the broadest and most stable basis for spreading the costs of illness, and to assure adequate financial support for doctors and hospitals everywhere. If we were to rely on State-by-State action only, many years would elapse before we had any general coverage. Meanwhile health service would continue to be grossly uneven, and disease would continue to cross State boundary lines.

Medical services are personal. Therefore the nationwide system must be highly decentralized in administration. The local administrative unit must be the keystone of the system so as to provide for local services and adaptation to local needs and conditions. Locally as well as nationally, policy and administration should be guided by advisory committees in which the public and the medical professions are represented.

Fees to Be Adjusted Locally

Subject to national standards, methods and rates of paying doctors and hospitals should be adjusted locally. All such rates for doctors should be adequate, and should be appropriately adjusted upward for those who are qualified specialists.

People should remain free to choose their own physicians and hospitals. The removal of financial barriers between patient and doctor would enlarge the present freedom of choice. The legal requirement on the population to contribute involves no compulsion over the doctor's freedom to decide what services his patient needs. People will remain free to obtain any pay for medical service outside of the health insurance system if they desire, even though they are members of the system; just as they are free to send their children to private instead of to public schools, although they must pay taxes for public schools.

Freedom of Physicians

Likewise physicians should remain free to accept or reject patients. They must be allowed to decide for themselves whether they wish to participate in the health insurance system full time, part time, or not at all. A physician may have some patients who are in the system and some who are not. Physicians must be permitted to be represented through organizations of their own choosing, and to decide whether to carry on in individual practice or to join with other doctors in group practice in hospitals or in clinics.

Our voluntary hospitals and our city, county and State general hospitals, in the same way, must be free to participate in the system of whatever extent they wish. In any case they must continue to retain their administrative independence.

Voluntary organizations which provide health services that meet reasonable standards of quality should be entitled to furnish services under the insurance system and to be reimbursed for them. Voluntary cooperative organizations concerned with paying doctors, hospitals or others for health services, but not providing services directly, should be entitled to participate if they can contribute to the efficiency and economy of the system.

None of this is really new. The American people are the most insurance-minded people in the world. They will not be frightened off from health insurance because some people have misnamed it "socialized medicine."

I repeat—what I am recommending is not socialized medicine. Socialized medicine means that all doctors work as employes of government. The American people want no such system. No such system is here proposed.

Under the plan I suggest, our people would continue to get medical and hospital services just as they do now—on the basis of their own voluntary decisions and choices. Our doctors and hospitals would continue to deal with disease with the same professional freedom as now. There would, however, be this all-important difference: whether or not patients get the services they need would not depend on how much they can afford to pay at the time.

I am in favor of the broadest possible coverage for this insurance system. I believe that all persons who work for a living and their dependents should be covered under such an insurance plan. This would include wage and salary earners, those in business for themselves, professional persons, farmers, agricultural labor, domestic employes, Government employes and employes of non-profit institutions and their families.

Provision for Needy Persons

In addition, needy persons and other groups should be covered through appropriate premiums paid for them by public agencies. Increased Federal funds should also be made available by the Congress under the public assistance programs to reimburse the States for part of such premiums, as well as for direct expenditures made by the States in paying for medical services provided by doctors, hospitals and other agencies to needy persons.

Premiums for present social insurance benefits are calculated on the first $3,000 of earnings in a year. It might be well to have all such premiums, including those for health, calculated on a somewhat higher amount, such as $3,600.

A broad program of prepayment for medical care would need total amounts approximately equal to 4 per cent of such earnings. The people of the United States have been spending, on the average, nearly this percentage of their incomes for sickness care. How much of the total fund should come from the insurance premiums and how much from general revenues is a matter for the Congress to decide.

The plan which I have suggested would be sufficient to pay most doctors more than the best they have received in peace-time years. The payments of the doctors' bills would be guaranteed, and the doctors would be spared the annoyance and uncertainty of collecting fees from individual patients. The same assurance would apply to hospitals, dentists and nurses for the services they render.

Federal aid in the construction of hospitals will be futile unless there is current purchasing power so that people can use these hospitals. Doctors cannot be drawn to sections which need them without some assurance that they can make a living. Only a nation-wide spreading of sickness costs can supply such sections with sure and sufficient purchasing power to maintain enough physicians and hospitals. We are a rich nation and can afford many things. But ill-health which can be prevented or cured is one think we cannot afford.

Fifth: Protection Against Loss of Wages From Sickness and Disability.

What I have discussed heretofore has been a program for improving and spreading the health services and facilities of the nation, and providing an efficient and less burdensome system of paying for them.

But no matter what we do, sickness will of course come to many. Sickness brings with it loss of wages.

Therefore, as a fifth element of a comprehensive health program, the workers of the nation and their families should be protected against loss of earnings because of illness. A comprehensive health program must include the payment of benefits to replace at least part of the earnings that are lost during the period of sickness and long-term disability. This protection can be readily and conveniently provided through expansion of our present social insurance system, with appropriate adjustment of premiums.

Insurance for Wage Losses

Insurance against loss of wages from sickness and disability deals with cash benefits, rather than with services. It has to be coordinated with the other cash benefits under existing social insurance systems. Such coordination should be effected when other social security measures are reexamined. I shall bring this subject again to the attention of the Congress in a separate message on social security.

I strongly urge that the Congress give careful consideration to this program of health legislation now.

Many millions of our veterans, accustomed in the armed forces to the best medical and hospital care, will no longer be eligible for such care as a matter of right except for their service-connected disabilities. They deserve continued adequate and comprehensive health service. And their dependents deserve it, too.

By preventing illness, by assuring access to needed community and personal health services, by promoting medical research, and by protecting our people against the loss caused by sickness, we shall strengthen our national health, our national defense and our economic productivity. We shall increase the professional and economic opportunities of our physicians, dentists and nurses. We shall increase the effectiveness of our hospitals and public health agencies. We shall bring new security to our people.

We need to do this especially at this time because of the return to civilian life of many doctors, dentists and nurses, particularly young men and women.

Appreciation of modern achievements in medicine and public health has created widespread demand that they be fully applied and universally available. By meeting that demand we shall strengthen the nation to meet future economic and social problems; and we shall make a most important contribution toward freedom from want in our land.

November 20, 1945

A. M. A. PICTURES 'CONTROL'

Says Plan Would Put Medicine in Politics—Backs Some Points

CHICAGO, Nov. 19 (P)—The Journal of the American Medical Association approved parts of President Truman's national health program today, but said that compulsory sickness insurance provisions would submit physicians to "politically controlled medicine."

An editorial, to be published in the Nov. 24 issue, said Mr. Truman's proposal for extending medical education and research through Federal grants would put the Federal Government in control of medical education. Of the President's proposal for Federal financial aid to States and localities for building up hospitals and other health facilities, the editorial said the Hill-Burton bill for such funds had the approval of the A. M. A., "subject to safeguards which are in the text reported by the committee which conducted hearings"

Asserting that the recommendation for expanded maternal and child health service was essentially that contained in the Pepper bill, the editorial said that "the passing of a nation-wide compulsory sickness insurance bill ought to make unnecessary" the Pepper measure's proposals.

The journal expressed approval, however, of Mr. Truman's recommendation for compensation of workers during sickness and disability.

November 20, 1945

BRITAIN'S DOCTORS ASSURE NEW PLAN

Special to The New York Times.

LONDON, May 28—The British Medical Association Representative Body voted today to advise the medical profession to join the Labor Government's National Health Service.

By supporting a decision of the British Medical Association Council early in May, some 360 representatives meeting here have made it certain that the health service will be worked from its inception on July 5.

It has been a long uphill fight by the Government, led by Aneurin Bevan, Health Minister, who started out by antagonizing the doctors, dentists and specialists to such an extent that an overwhelming majority of them—as much as 90 per cent in some categories—voted against the Government measure. For a while it looked as if the health service would be gravely jeopardized but after discussions with leading doctors, Mr. Bevan made a number of concessions and another plebiscite of the profession was held in April.

This showed that while a majority was still against accepting service, a substantial minority was in favor and its members would be numerous enough to give the health service a start.

The British Medical Association Council thereupon advised the profession as a whole to cooperate, subject to ratification by the Representative Body at its meeting today.

There was a heated discussion at the meeting, with the chairman of the association, Dr. Guy Dain, arguing in favor of acceptance and Lord Horder, physician to King George VI, taking a diehard oppositionist viewpoint.

It appeared for a while that Lord Horder's school of thought would win. However, Dr. Dain argued throughout that the trend among doctors was more and more in favor of cooperating with the Government and that to recommend acceptance would be sensible, it being understood that Mr. Bevan would continue negotiations on outstanding matters.

These matters include the terms and conditions of the service of consultants and specialists and some special problems concerning dentists.

Dr. Dain pointed out that the health service was going into effect whether they liked it or not and that those who stayed out would lose compensation for the good-will of their existing practices. He asserted that a plebiscite taken today would show a majority of the profession in favor of cooperating.

The council's resolution advising the profession to cooperate was carried late in the afternoon by a large majority, while motions of no confidence in the council were similarly defeated overwhelmingly.

This removes the last possibility that the Socialist Government's comprehensive health service, which takes care of everyone from the cradle to the grave, would be blocked or get off to a crippling start.

Everyone realizes that it is going to take much patience and experiment to get it working smoothly for nothing so comprehensive as this has even been tried in the western world.

It is going to be relatively costly since each adult will be paying the equivalent of one dollar a week for the rest of his life, well or ill, and the Government knows that it must produce results or face a great storm. Today's votes mean at least that the doctors will do their best.

May 29, 1948

333

BRITAIN SOCIALIZES WIDE HEALTH FIELD

Free Medical Service Extended to Cover 27,500,000 Persons —Dentists Hesitant

By CLIFTON DANIEL
Special to THE NEW YORK TIMES.

LONDON, July 5—Britain's Socialist Government put into effect today a "cradle to grave" social security system that is declared to be the most comprehensive in the world.

With some difficulties and delays and still some resistance from physicians and dentists whose professions are being virtually nationalized, four new social-security acts extending and consolidating existing measures came into force. By far the most extensive of these is the National Health Service Act, which provides free medical attention for every man, woman and child who chooses to accept it.

During the day, two physicians practicing in partnership in a southern suburb of London found themselves with 2,700 registered public patients, but with no official forms on which to write free prescriptions.

"I gave them a few kind words, told them that perhaps medicine wasn't needed and sent them away," said Dr. A., senior member of the partnership.

As did 86 per cent of Britain's physicians, Dr. A. originally voted against serving under the National Health Scheme, but like more than 18,000 other general practitioners, he changed his mind when he saw that resistance was useless and impractical.

After Dr. A decided to join the service his telephone and doorbell rang constantly for four weeks—until he put up a sign asking applicants just to drop their registration forms in his mailbox.

Under the Government's previous health insurance scheme, Dr. A and his partner had 1,200 manual laborers and low-salaried workers registered as patients. The rest of their practice was private and they had a gross annual income of about £4,000 [$16,000].

Compensation for Losses

Nearly all private patients have now registered for free service, and today Dr. A was contemplating the prospect that the partnership income would be cut to £2,400, out of which operating expenses would have to be paid.

An additional 7,500,000 persons have put their names on physicians' lists under the new act. Added to the 20,000,000 registered for medical panel service under previous legislation, this means 27,500,000 now registered for free service. [The figures are for England and Wales, to which the act applies; Scotland has a separate Ministry of Health.]

Dr. A. and his partner are entitled to compensation for loss of private practice; the national average payment to physicians will be £3,500 [$14,000] a year.

"The only thing that is keeping me from going nuts," said Dr. A., "is the thought that some of my private patients will stick by me and continue to pay for special service."

Among dentists, early returns today from an official canvass showed that a third of the nation's total had decided to join the Health Service. [Reuters reported the number of dentists signed up as about 6,000.] Most dentists are holding out for concessions from the government.

Hospitals in Public Service

Of Britain's 2,987 hospitals, 2,751 are today automatically under Government ownership—most of the exempt hospitals are those of religious orders—and specialists connected with the hospitals are largely cooperating.

Druggists and opticians, whose services and supplies will be free to registered patients, are participating in the National Health Service.

Besides the health act other three measures taking effect today are:

(1) National Insurance Act, which provides an improved and more uniform scale of benefits for unemployment, sickness, motherhood, widows, orphans, old age and death. The act extends compulsory insurance to about 3,500,000 self-employed and unemployed persons, two-thirds of whom have not yet registered as required by law. The act will cover about 25,500,000 persons, and most men and single women of working age will pay weekly contributions, as will their employers. For men over 18 this amounts to about $1 a week.

(2) Industrial Injuries Act, which takes workmen's compensation out of the hands of private companies and places it under Government management.

(3) National Assistance Act, which creates a National Assistance Board to take over from local authorities the functions of providing relief and welfare aid to those not fully protected by insurance.

These measures were initiated by the social security report prepared by Lord Beveridge at the behest of Winston Churchill's wartime Coalition Government; they have been enacted under the Labor Government with some Socialist refinements.

It has been estimated that the Insurance Act alone will cost £511,000,000 in 1948, rising to £788,000,000 in 1978 as the number of old-age pensioners increases.

Of the totals, the British Treasury will pay £175,000,000 rising to £453,000,000. The Health Service, paid for entirely out of taxation, will cost an estimated £250,000,000.

July 6, 1948

2 Contrasting Health Plans On Trial Here and in Britain

By FRANK S. ADAMS

Two new, contrasting methods of providing medical and hospital care for large groups are on trial. One is the system of governmental health care, which is receiving its greatest test in Great Britain. The other is that of the voluntary, nonprofit agencies that are developing in this country.

Students of public health and medical economics will follow the workings of the two systems with close attention, and the public undoubtedly will observe their relative merits with interest. The verdict of public opinion almost certainly will determine the nature of future legislation in this country.

The British program is a universal, compulsory, tax-supported and government-administered program, under which every person, rich and poor alike, is entitled to free medical, dental and hospital care. It was put into effect on July 5 after protracted opposition from the British Medical Association. Official estimates place its cost for the first nine months at 180,000,000 pounds.

Several differing types of voluntary, non-profit agencies have evolved in this country in recent years. The best known is undoubtedly the Blue Cross plan, which now provides hospital insurance for 30,000,000 persons in the United States and Canada, at moderate rates that vary from place to place.

Prepayment plans for meeting part or all of the costs of medical care have come into being still more recently. In New York 1,000,000 persons are covered by such plans, and their membership is increasing at an extremely rapid rate. The national membership is more than 6,000,000.

These plans, however, have not crystallized into a single pattern. To the accompaniment of a controversy within and without organized medicine, there have developed several major types of nonprofit agencies, exemplified in New York by the United Medical Service. the Health Insurance Plan of Greater New York and Group Health Insurance, Inc.

The need for some kind of a prepayment plan, either governmental or voluntary, to meet medical costs has been demonstrated conclusively, according to the opinion expressed last week by one leading American student of the problem, Louis H. Pink, president of the Associated Hospital Service of New York and vice chairman of the Blue Cross Commission.

If the voluntary plans in this country grow fast enough to do the job, most Americans would prefer them, he said, because of the wider choice allowed individuals and organizations and the greater control they would have over the scope and quality of their medical coverage.

He acknowledged, however, that if the voluntary agencies failed to meet the test of public approval, the Government inevitably would have to step in with some kind of a national program. Several bills for that purpose have been brought forward in Congress.

Descriptions of the workings of the British plan and of the principal agencies now functioning in this city follow:

Great Britain

Some form of national health service has existed in that country since 1911, and by the outbreak of World War II in 1939 about half of the population was covered by it. On July 5, however, a new National Health Service Act, based on the principles of the Beveridge Report, went into effect in England and Wales. [Scotland has a separate Ministry of Health.]

The new plan will make available to all, free of charge, medical service, including medicines and specialist care; hospital accommodations when needed, and dental services, although there will not be enough dentists at the beginning to give service to everyone, and priority will be given to nursing and expectant mothers, and young children.

Most British hospitals were taken over by the Government under the new scheme, and are administered through a system of regional boards. The regions are planned so that the service in each one can be associated with a university medical school. Out of 2,987 hospitals 2,751 were taken over when the new act went into effect.

Patients who prefer to do so may continue on the fee-paying basis with their family physicians, but observers expected that this would be confined largely to the upper income groups. On July 5, 27,500,000 persons had been registered for medical panel service.

under the new act, and it was predicted that ultimately 90 to 95 per cent of the population would obtain their medical treatment through it.

The British Medical Association opposed the act for a long time, but at length reluctantly gave way after the Government had made some concession with regard to methods of payment, freedom of expression, and geographical restrictions on further entrance into service in "overdoctored" areas.

Physicians have the choice of taking part in the service or not. Those already in practice have the option of receiving a fixed annual payment of $1,200, with the addition of capitation fees, or of depending entirely on higher capitation fees. Doctors setting up in practice will be paid entirely by the first method for the first three years. Doctors have the right to refuse a patient.

Although 86 per cent of physicians of Great Britain originally voted against serving under the act, more than 18,000 of them eventually agreed to serve under it. Many of them, however, have continued to protest that their incomes would be halved by the workings of the act, and that they might find themselves with more patients than they would have time to care for.

Blue Cross Plans

The Blue Cross Plans for providing hospital insurance began in Dallas, Tex., in 1929 when a group of school teachers founded the first one. There are now ninety-one plans, including five in Canada and one in Puerto Rico, and they had 30,254,456 members as of March 31, 1948. The largest plan, Associated Hospital Service of New York, has 3,400,000 members in and near New York City.

The Blue Cross Plans vary slightly, but most of them provide twenty-one to thirty days or more a year of hospital care in a semi-private rom. The charges range from $10 to $14 a year for individuals, and from $24 to $26 a year for families, regardless of the number of children under the age of 18.

In most cases they cover the cost of bed, board, general nursing care, customary drugs, use of the operating room, laboratory tests, special equipment, and in some cases X-ray examinations. In New York, the maternity allowance on the family contract was increased

last year from $60 to $80. Patients who prefer a private room to the semi-private accommodations specified in the plan are allowed $6 a day toward its cost.

The Associated Hospital Service includes in its membership 25,000 employe groups, and 10,000 local employers contribute all or part of the subscription charges for their employes, and in some cases dependents as well. Like all the Blue Cross Plans, the Associated Hospital Service is a non-profit, community enterprise, under the control of a board of directors that includes representatives of organized medicine, business, industry and labor.

United Medical Service, which calls itself "The Doctors' Plan," was established with the support of the New York State Medical Society and seventeen local county medical societies in the State. It is designed along the lines approved by the American Medical Association, which emphasizes the free choice of a physician and the payment of a fee to the doctor for services.

Subscrbers may enroll under any one of three plans. Under the Surgical pian, allowances of specified amounts up to $225 are paid toward physicians' fees for surgical care. The surgical-medical plan adds to this additional payments for medical care in a hospital, up to a maximum of $200.50; and the surgical-medical plan provides additional allowances for specialist care, or home or office treatment.

These allowances will pay a participating physician's fee in full if the subscriber is single and has an annual income of not more than $1,800, or is married, with a family income not exceeding $2,500. If his income exceeds these amounts, the participating physician may ask the patient for the difference between the UMS fee and his usual charge. Subscribers, if they prefer, may consult non-participating physicians, who receive the same fees.

United Medical Service had an enrollment of 833,122 members on March 31, 1948, but it is growing so fast that officials said last week this had increased to 950,000. It is affiliated with and administered by the Associated Hospital Service of New York. It is one of fifty-two "Blue Shield" plans for prepayment of medical costs, which on March 31 had a total membership of 6,473,439.

Hospital Insurance Plan

The Hospital Insurance Plan of Greater New York, which originated wtih a committee convened by the late Mayor Fiorello H. La Guardia in 1943, began operations on March 1, 1947 and by last week had enrolled 122,000 members. Its proponents say that it offers the most comprehensive medical coverage available.

HIP enrolls only groups of employes, in which the employer agrees to pay at least half the cost of the coverage. In some cases this is extended to dependents also. It has an income ceiling making ineligible persons and families with incomes of more than $5,000 a year.

Its largest contracts are with New York City and with the United Nations, but it also has contracts with labor unions and industrial concerns. It was selected as the best available plan for city employes by a committee named by Mayor O'Dwyer, which made an exhaustive report on Aug. 15, 1946. Roughly two-thirds of its present members are city employes.

HIP operates through a group service plan. It has twenty-five groups of physicians functioning in the city and is organizing additional ones. Each consists of twenty to twenty-five physicians, including general practitioners and an appropriate variety of specialists. Its capitation fees are scheduled so that the average compensation to a doctor devoting his full time to group work should be $10,000 a year.

Each member has a choice of any group in his borough, and of any one of a number of general practitioners in each group. The average fee to HIP at the present time is $25.50 a person, and it is self-supporting, according to Dr. Dean A. Clark, its medical director. It was financed in its early stages by grants from the New York Foundation, the Albert and Mary Lasker Foundation, and the Rockefeller Foundation.

HIP has not received the approval of the New York State Medical Society, which does not approve of group practice, and which stipulates that to get its approval a majority of the governing board of a voluntary insurance plan must be made up of medical men recommended by the society.

The State Medical Society recently urged its members not to affiliate with plans that had not received its approval, but according to Dr. Clark the recommendation went unheeded by the 700 physicians who are under contract with HIP, virtually all of whom, he said, are members of the society.

The present makeup of the board of directors includes eight physicians, four labor leaders, eight representatives of business and industry and four persons selected on an individual basis. Its chairman is Dr. Willard C. Rappleye, dean of the College of Physicians and Surgeons of Columbia University. It also has a medical control board made up exclusively of physicians, which has final jurisdiction over professional questions and standards.

Group Health Service, Inc.

This organization, started in 1939, was the pioneer in the field in New York City, but it has been outstripped in numbers by UMS and HIP. It has 35,000 members and has contracts with 3,500 physicians, according to Arthur H. Harlow Jr., its president. Its membership consists largely of groups in which the employer pays the total cost.

It permits the free choice of any physician anywhere and pays cash allowances up to $225 for various kinds of medical and surgical care. Families with an income of not more than $3,000 and individuals up to $1,800 are covered in full if they go to participating physicians, but other physicians may charge their regular fees. Group Health also offers a system of double indemnities for double premiums, designed to appeal to persons in higher income levels.

Group Health began on July 1 an experiment in permitting individual enrollment under rigidly controlled conditions. This had always been considered one of the great problems that voluntary insurance plans had to face because of the danger of getting a preponderance of persons who are in imminent need of medical or surgical care, unless enrollment is by groups large enough to permit a distribution of risks. The experiment is being followed with close attention by observers in the field.

July 18, 1948

FREE MEDICAL HELP IN BRITAIN TO STAY

By CLIFTON DANIEL
Special to The New York Times.

LONDON, April 3—After a trial of nine months, Britain's universal free medical service, whose operations are being studied by those interested in a similar service in the United States, has definitely come to stay.

"If there were going to be any breakdown, we would have had it by now," an official of the Ministry of Health said as the end of the first nine months approached. "That phase has been successfully overcome."

There is no single substantial political or professional group in the country that proposes to abandon the service, fundamentally alter its character or drastically cut its costs.

"The best measure of its success," said a supporter of the Labor Government recently, "is that the Conservative party is eager to

point out that it was for the health service all the time."

A prospective Conservative candidate for Parliament acknowledged that the health service was the most popular measure enacted by the Labor administration and that one of the major problems of Conservative policy was how to make legitimate criticisms of the operations and costs of the service without seeming to attack its objectives.

Cost Troubles Economists

The only serious questions now being raised about the health service concern its administration, its

efficiency and its cost in relation to the national budget as a whole. The cost, which is admittedly higher than the Government had anticipated, has been troubling economists, who fear that the burden of social services assumed by the Socialist Government may be becoming heavier than the national economy can carry.

Forty per cent of all incomes in Britain are taken for taxes as compared with about 25 per cent in the United States, a fact that the Economist calls "fantastic" and "appalling." Roughly one-third of the entire Government budget is expended on social services.

When the Health Service Law was enacted its cost was budgeted at £150,000,000 ($600,000,000) per year. In fact, the cost for England, Wales and Scotland in the first nine months was £208,000,000 ($832,000,000). Nearly £260,000,000 ($1,040,000,000) has been budgeted for the first full fiscal year that began on Friday.

Even so the opposition obviously does not dare to propose a major cut. In its recent economic survey the Government stated that the cost of service would be stabilized at the present level and with that the Conservative party is believed to be content.

In the forthcoming general election campaign, it is expected that the Conservatives will take a new line, emphasizing that the Government by providing a minimum average of medical service for everybody has destroyed the priority once enjoyed by the most needy and that general practitioners who are the principal servants of the system are overworked and underpaid.

Not Enough Doctors

Despite its great cost, the health service budget does not include any important provision for capital improvements. A pamphlet issued by the British Medical Association said:

"Under the new service 28,000,000 more persons suddenly became entitled to medical treatment without payment of fees. But there are no more doctors than there were before.

"There can be no hope for a long time to come of providing all doctors necessary."

About 50,000 hospital beds in Britain are empty because of the shortage of staff and, according to the medical association, 30,000 patients are waiting for admission to hospitals in London alone. The country needs 45,000 more nurses, the association said, and has no immediate prospect of finding them.

The health centers that were to have been one of the principal features of the health program—several hundred of them were to have been built throughout the country—cannot be built because of the shortage of labor and materials. Housing has first priority.

"Of £260,000,000 to be spent next year not one penny is for brick and mortar," one health expert said last week. No major program of construction has yet been projected.

Despite the deficiencies of the service, however, there is no disputing that the great majority of Britons are pleased with it. They are deaf to cries of alarm about its cost to the nation.

"They are getting the same service as before—or even more—without paying for it," a medical official remarked recently. "Why shouldn't they be pleased?"

About 93 per cent of the 48,000,000 people in England, Wales and Scotland have enrolled in the service. Most of those who have not enlisted probably will do so once they require medical attention.

Even though they are overwhelmingly opposed to the terms of the service offered to them, about 20,000 of the country's 21,000 general practitioners have entered the program. Nearly all of the country's 14,000 druggists are filling prescriptions at the Government's expense. Nearly all of the 10,000 dentists are participating.

Prescriptions are being filled at the rate of about 200,000,000 a year as compared with an estimated 150,000,000 before the service started. Spectacles are being dispensed at the rate of 9,000,000 pair per year instead of an estimated 8,000,000, and 9,000,000 patients are receiving dental treatment instead of 8,000,000—all of which has run up the costs.

In examining these statistics for guidance to the United States, British experts advise Americans to take account of the fact that conditions in the two countries are not necessarily comparable.

First, Britain is a small compact country with a dense population that is served by excellent communications and can be easily reached by a community medical service.

Second, Britain did not start universal medical service from scratch. As long ago as 1911 free health service had been instituted for lower-income classes and nearly every doctor in the country had been making some contribution to it. The new service was simply an extension of the old to cover the entire population.

Third, the political atmosphere for the introduction of the new service was well prepared long in advance. When the Health Service Law was enacted the Socialist Government was in power and all political parties and the medical profession as well were agreed in principle that such a system was required.

All Entitled to Benefits

Britain's health service is more comprehensive than anything yet contemplated in the United States. It is literally both universal and free. Anyone in the country is entitled to its benefits. No one needs to pay directly for medical treatment. Each working citizen makes a small weekly contribution to the service along with his payments for other social security benefits. The remainder of the cost is paid out of ordinary taxes collected by the National Treasury.

In order to get the benefits of the service, the citizen must register with a general practitioner. He can choose his doctor. The doctor can either accept or reject him as a patient.

Once registered, a patient simply goes to the doctor or summons him whenever treatment is needed. If something more than the services of a general practitioner is required, the doctor sends the patient to a specialist or hospital.

The general practitioner receives an annual fee from the Government for each patient on his list. The patient pays nothing unless he wants and can afford more than the minimum essential attention.

In order to obtain dental or ophthalmic treatment, the citizen needs only to apply to the nearest qualified dentist or optician.

April 4, 1949

AMA Lists Health Plan Tests, With Local Units as Judges

By WILLIAM L. LAURENCE
Special to THE NEW YORK TIMES.

ATLANTIC CITY, N. J., June 9—The House of Delegates of the American Medical Association gave a nod of approval for the first time today to lay-sponsored voluntary pre-payment health plans when it voted to forward a set of twenty principles to county and state medical societies for their guidance in determining the eligibility of such plans for approval.

While this action still leaves it up to the county or state societies to approve or disapprove of any lay-sponsored medical insurance plans, the move is regarded as a distinct step forward in liberalizing the attitude of the association toward plans not fully under the control of the medical profession. Hitherto only medically sponsored voluntary prepayment plans could hope for any official approval by the AMA or its units, and it is believed that the move made today will give an impetus to the formation of lay-sponsored groups, of which there are about eighty in the United States at present, with a membership of about a million.

The twenty principles were worked out through conferences during the past year between the Council on Medical Service of the AMA and the Cooperative Health Federation of America, composed of representatives of organized labor, farm organizations, health cooperatives and other consumer groups.

Under the action taken today cooperatives and other types of lay-sponsored voluntary health plans may now expect to gain the seal of acceptance of organized medicine if their organizations are in accord with the twenty principles.

The principles had been "tentatively initialed" by the representatives of the Council on Medical Service and the Cooperative Health Federation. In approving these principles for the guidance of county and state societies the House of Delegates added the further qualification that local areas might find it necessary to add minor modifications without changing the fundamental intent involved.

Dr. Dean A. Clark, president of the Cooperative Health Federation, who is also medical director of the Health Insurance Plan of Greater New York (HIP), issued a statement expressing gratification in behalf of the Cooperative Health Federation over today's action.

"We regret, however," he added, "that by requiring such health plans, before seeking AMA approval, to be approved by the very state and local medical societies which have been bitterly opposed to them in the past, the House may well have nullified the spirit of its own action.

"In the light of the discriminatory practices against doctors taking part in such plans still carried on by some state and local medical societies, and of the many state laws sponsored by organized medicine which prohibit the formation of lay-sponsored pre payment plans for medical care, the Cooperative Health Federation of America can only take a 'wait-and-see' attitude concerning the practical results and benefits for voluntary consumer action which may be expected to flow from the House of Delegates' action.

Local Reactions Awaited

"While today's action is a considerable step toward the recognition by organized medicine of the right of consumers voluntarily to organize to provide health care for themselves, through agreements with doctors of their own choice, its real effectiveness will depend upon the spirit with which it is received and acted upon by the AMA's state and local units.

"Had the AMA been willing to assume national responsibility in forthright fashion for approving or disapproving health plans organized and sponsored by the people, as it does in the case of hospitals and medical schools throughout the country, a forward step of considerably greater significance would have been taken.

"As it is, the House of Delegates' action may constitute no more than lip service unless a marked change takes place in the attitude on certain of the state and local medical societies toward efforts of the people to solve voluntarily for themselves their economic problems connected with medical care. Only if these constituent societies accept these principles with the genuine spirit of cooperation shown by the AMA's Council on Medical Service in this year's negotiations and by the House of Delegates today, and only if these societies take action in good faith to approve consumer-sponsored plans that conform to the principles, can today's action have any important effect on consumer groups.

"The Cooperative Health Federation hopes that, following the stand taken by the AMA today, its constituent societies will show such a spirit of cooperation and will act speedily to assist consumer groups to obtain necessary enabling legislation for lay-sponsored health plans in every state and to wipe out once and for all the discrimination which has been practiced against doctors desiring to enter into agreements with consumers to provide health service for them.

"The CHFA pledges its fullest cooperation to the AMA and to every state and local medical society toward giving these principles real effectiveness."

June 10, 1949

A. M. A. Sets $1,100,000 Ad Drive To Kill Truman's Health Program

By WILLIAM L. LAURENCE
Special to THE NEW YORK TIMES.

SAN FRANCISCO, June 26 — The Board of Trustees of the American Medical Association has approved the expenditure in October of $1,100,000 in a newspaper and radio advertising campaign in an effort to deliver a knockout blow to the Administration program for compulsory health insurance.

This was announced today in a progress report of the coordinating committee for the national education campaign of the association, presented to its House of Delegates at the opening of the House's ninety-ninth annual session. The House of Delegates is the policy-making body for organized medicine in this country.

The publicity campaign will seek to reach every American through five-column advertisements in more than 11,000 daily and weekly newspapers during the week of Oct. 8.

About 300 radio stations will carry hundreds of thirty-second and one-minute announcements. Full-page advertisements will appear in thirty leading national magazines.

The campaign will aim to bring the Administration's compulsory health insurance measure to a vote on the floor of Congress as soon as possible. The association is confident that the bill will be defeated overwhelmingly. At the same time the program will seek to stimulate the growth of voluntary health insurance programs. The committee report said:

"Tens of thousands of doctors, all over America, who have carried medicine's case to the people, often at great sacrifice in time and money, will continue to be heavily burdened until this issue is resolved. We cannot afford for that reason, as well as others, to permit the delaying tactics of our opponents to turn this into a long-drawn war of attrition. It has become imperative, if we are to avert an unending, exhaustive fight for survival, that we find a way to make public sentiment on this issue unmistakably clear."

"To Crystallize Public Opinion"

The expanded program, the report said, has one specific objective—"to crystallize public opinion into a public mandate on this issue."

"We want an articulate public opinion, speaking with a voice that the socializers in Washington cannot defy nor ignore. We are confident that if given an opportunity to speak on this issue, the people in every section of America would say 'no'—and say it so emphatically that socialized medicine would become a dead issue, even in the offices of the Federal Security Agency. We intend to give them that opportunity."

The advertising budget approved by the A. M. A. Board of Trustees consists of $560,000 allocated to newspapers, $300,000 to radio and $250,000 to national magazines. About 144,500 doctors in every community in the country will share the cost of this program through the payment of annual dues of $25, inaugurated last year.

The message "will be geared to selling both a commodity and a principle," the report said.

"The commodity which the A. M. A. copy will advertise," it was stated, "is an already widely accepted, thoroughly recognized, American product — voluntary health insurance."

"The principle which the A.M.A. copy will seek to strengthen and bulwark is the basic American ideal of individual freedom, individual initiative and freedom of opportunity—under a free economy, as opposed to the alien philosophy of a government-regimented economy," the report said.

During the last six months, the report added, "more than 8,000 new organizations" have endorsed the A.M.A.'s stand, bringing the total of endorsing groups to 10,234.

Quotes U. M. W. Journal

In addition, the report continued, "doctors all over the nation, exercising their rights as individual citizens, are campaigning actively for candidates whose convictions square with sound American principles—and are just as actively opposing those men in public life who have espoused the alien philosophy of socialization."

The report quoted from a United Mine Workers Journal editorial commenting on the defeat of Senator Claude Pepper in the recent Florida primaries. "In forty years of covering political campaigns in the nation and in many states,'" the committee quoted, "'your editor has never witnessed such effective and quiet solicitation of votes as demonstrated by Florida doctors, druggists, dentists, hospital staffs, insurance companies and pharmaceutical representatives, aided and abetted by other professional men.'"

The campaigns for 1949 and 1950 will cost the American doctors $4,500,000, of which $1,500,000 was expended in 1949.

Dr. Shields Warren, director of the Division of Biology and Medicine of the Atomic Energy Commission, participated in a symposium on atomic energy in war and peace. He said that atomic energy and its products promised advances in medical research that would surpass the gains of the past.

"The use of radioactive tracers available in a multiplicity of forms has virtually revolutionized many of our techniques," he said. "It has brought some problems that seemed difficult or impossible of solution by other techniques within the possibility of solution."

Dr. Warren also said that atomic defense could not be considered apart from civil defense problems in general. He attributed the slowness in civil defense planning to "the fact that serious decisions regarding conduct in time of war are extremely delicate and difficult to make in time of peace."

"Fortunately, the American Medical Association has not been lagging and the Council on National Emergency Medical Service of the A. M. A. has planned a program of action that should be of material aid in the solution of the complexities ahead," he asserted. "This program of the council deserves reiteration:

"1. Establishment of emergency medical service committees in each state medical society.

"2. Each state must urge upon its Governor the absolute necessity for adequate state civil defense enabling legislation.

"3. Each state must urge its Governor to appoint a state director of civil defense with the necessary responsibilities and authority to act.

"4. Each state should appoint a civil defense advisory committee to advise its Governor and the civil defense director. Representatives of state medical societies should, with advantage, serve on this advisory committee.

"A defeatist attitude on civil defense will get us nowhere. The problem is not hopeless. The initial steps in the provision of knowledge as to medical aspects of atomic warfare and as to the means of monitoring a radioactive disaster have already been taken."

Dr. Evarts A. Graham, Professor of Surgery at Washington University School of Medicine and surgeon-in-chief at Barnes Hospital, St. Louis, received the American Medical Association's distinguished service award for 1950. Dr. Graham is best known in the medical field for his pioneer work in lung surgery for cancer.

June 27, 1950

A British Doctor Weighs the Health Service

Here is a report on one general practitioner's experience and reaction to five years of socialized medicine.

By CLIFTON DANIEL

LONDON

DR. GEORGE THOMAS HARPER, a general practitioner in the village of Upper Waldrop, one of the many dormitory towns on the fringes of Greater London, gives every appearance of being a happy man. After five years in the National Health Service—five years of collecting his fees from the public treasury—he is agreeably surprised to find that he has a prosperous practice, that he has kept his professional freedom, and that his relationship with his patients is still satisfying.

When the Health Service, a nationwide and comprehensive medical and hospital service, paid for mainly out of taxes and available to everybody, was inaugurated on July 5, 1948, Dr. Harper was far from happy. "We were all quite panicky," he recalled not long ago. "Every doctor with a good class of practice wondered what the hell was going to happen."

Dr. Harper (the physician's name is fictitious, and so is the name of the town) had turned over most of his afternoon's work to his young assistant and was taking a long lunch hour to talk with a visitor about his experiences in the Health Service.

Sixteen years ago Dr. Harper and his wife—she was 25 and he was 26—borrowed money from their families and from an insurance company to buy a place for him in a three-man medical partnership in Upper Waldrop. (Before the National Health Service, medical practices were bought and sold in Britain, and partnerships were common.) Dr. Harper was just beginning to get established in the town when the war started and he volunteered for the Navy. He served in ships all around the world, and he remarked in passing, "I was sunk at Dieppe."

SIX years to the day after he left home, the doctor came back and started again the slow process of building up a medical practice. Then, in less than three years, when he was beginning to hope for a larger share in the profits of the partnership, the Health Service Act was put through Parliament by the Labor Government.

"One was very apprehensive of the effect on an area like this," the doctor said. "We thought it would be disastrous. We felt that if the patients went for it in a big way we were going to suffer."

By "an area like this" Dr. Harper meant a middle-class residential suburb. Upper Waldrop stands apart from the thickly clustered satellites of London and, although it lies between two big factory towns, it is inhabited not so much by industrial workers as by owners, managers and directors and business and professional men. It has a lot of open land and still calls itself a village, although it now has 16,000 inhabitants. The managerial and professional classes live down in the town in brick and half-timbered villas behind garden walls, and they look askance at a low-cost housing development that has been built on the hill above them.

The medical partnership in which Dr. Harper was the junior member had the best practice in a highly competitive and "over-doctored" area. Its clientele numbered five to six thousand patients, only 800 of whom were "panel patients" —that is, workers receiving free treatment under the national health insurance program that preceded the National Health Service. (Some 22,000,-000 workers were entitled to use the "panel" service.)

BECAUSE of uncertainty about the future of a practice so largely composed of private patients, the three doctors decided to dissolve their partnership. Two went into the state service. One continued with private practice, seeing his patients exactly as before and charging his usual fees. Recalling the decision that he had to take, Dr. Harper said, "Basically, I felt, taking the population as a whole, that the Health Service was a good thing, but like most doctors I was rather resentful of the methods used in introducing it." The doctors as a profession first voted overwhelmingly not to accept the terms of employment proposed by the Labor Government—then they capitulated when they saw their stand was futile. Both the Labor and Conservative parties had voted for the Health Service and the British Medical Association itself was in favor of the plan in principle.

Approximately 18,500 general practitioners, Dr. Harper among them, joined the service. Only 500 elected to remain in purely private practice.

"Having accepted the service, I thought the only thing to do was go ahead and make it work," Dr. Harper continued. "I was 37 years old and still had twenty-five to thirty years of working life ahead of me. There was no use carping."

In the first year of the Health Service, between 1,500 and 1,800 patients placed themselves on Dr. Harper's list. All were free to choose. They could continue as private patients, if they wished to pay the fees, or enroll with any Health Service doctor they liked. About 47,000,000—97 per cent of the population—chose the Health Service, and Dr. Harper said, "I got far more than I thought I would." Most of those

who signed on with him were formerly his private patients. He got others from the practices of doctors who did not enter the service, including his former senior partner. Since 1948, Dr. Harper's list has grown steadily and now numbers just over 4,000. The list, when divided between him and his assistant, is just about the national average per doctor.

DR. HARPER, who lives in a house that for more than a hundred years has been occupied by doctors, left the living room and went down the corridor to his surgery (the British name for a doctor's office). He came back with several large manila envelopes containing an accountant's neat figures on the earnings of the practice.

"I don't understand these things," the doctor said. "I just look at the totals and take the rest for granted."

After several false starts and mistakes, Dr. Harper finally calculated that in the year before the Health Service the three-man partnership had a net income of £10,667, of which his share, after expenses, was £1,500.

In the first year of the service, Dr. Harper's own net taxable income was £2,112—more than he received from the partnership. As he collects seventeen shillings a year from the Government for each patient and will get an annual bonus of £500 under a new pay scale recently adopted, his income is now still larger. In 1951-52 his gross was £4,667, but the accountants have not yet calculated the net.

TWO thousand pounds is a fair middle-class income in Britain, and in the case of a doctor it is larger than it looks. As Dr. Harper uses his house as his office, he is allowed income tax deductions for a part of the rent and part of the gas, light and water bills, for the wages of a cleaning woman and part of the wages of the man who tends his large and lovely garden. He also deducts 90 per cent of the cost of operating his car and the salaries of his secretary and his assistant. He even manages to pay "a little bit" to his wife. Mrs. Harper, who always uses the pronoun "we" in speaking of the doctor's practice, is a professional as well as personal helpmeet for her husband.

"Considering the financial circumstances of the country," Dr. Harper remarked, "I think I am doing financially as well as I would have done if I had remained in private practice. Our type of high-class practice would have changed any-

CLIFTON DANIEL of The Times has watched Britain's health program from his London post.

way because of high taxes."

The doctor also has a sense of security that he did not have before. He gets his money from the Government and no longer has to worry about whether his patients can pay. The cost of the Health Service is met mainly by taxes, plus a weekly levy of ten pence (less than 12 cents) paid by employed persons and their employers, and charges to the patient for a part of the cost of prescriptions, dental treatment, surgical appliances, false teeth and spectacles. As one who "never liked the financial aspects of medical practice" or "assessing the ability of patients to pay," Dr. Harper said, "I like the feeling that the money is coming in."

Only £600 of Dr. Harper's income represents fees from private patients, of whom he still has about 150. "It's the old brigade who have remained as private patients," he said. The majority are elderly people or Conservatives who hate any form of nationalization. As many of them are chronically ill, they find it expensive to stick to their principles.

"Private patients are dying off faster than they are being replaced," the doctor added. In the past five years his fees for private patients have increased very little, Dr. Harper said. "One is afraid of killing the goose that lays the occasional golden egg," he explained.

Even so, quite a number who started out as private patients, particularly younger couples with children, have "gone on the state," Dr. Harper commented. "If I had the same income, I think I would go on a doctor's list too."

MRS. HARPER entered the room and joined the conversation. "People in an area like this would have a free doctor before they would have a free school for their children," she said.

The advantages of being a private patient are mainly those of convenience, the doc-

—————— HEALTH SERVICE FACTS ——————

Who is eligible?
Anyone in Britain, regardless of nationality, is eligible for full medical care from Health Service doctors and dentists of his own choosing. Ninety-seven per cent of Britain's population has joined the service since its inception five years ago.

How many doctors have joined?
About 18,500 general practitioners. Their net incomes average (before taxes) $6,272. They may compete for private patients with the 500 "G.P.'s" who have remained in private practice. About the same proportion of Britain's 7,000 specialists are in the Service.

Who pays for the service?
Ninety per cent of the cost is paid through taxes amounting to about $22 per capita. There are also direct payments. Public patients must

pay part of the cost, for example, of spectacles and dentures and must pay 14 cents toward the cost of each prescription.

What is the patient entitled to?
Patients are entitled to the services of a general practitioner—home and office calls—and specialist care, hospitalization, ambulances, surgery, blood tranfusions. Grievances arising over quantity or quality of service, if they cannot be settled informally, may be brought to the attention of the National Health Service.

Many Britons who still pay the higher costs of private care, on a regular or occasional basis, feel that it is worth the price—in convenience, comfort and a more satisfactory relationship between doctor and patients. And many doctors agree with them.

tor said. "I think I'm a bit soft about it," he conceded. "I don't honestly think I make any difference in the standards of treatment between public and private patients. But, while I am not prepared to give private patients better treatment, I am prepared to consider their convenience and comfort more." State patients with mild and nonconfining illnesses are expected, for example, to go to the doctor's surgery and wait their turn. Private patients with similarly mild complaints can pay to have the doctor call on them.

Some private patients, Mrs. Harper remarked, are less demanding than public patients because they are personal friends of the doctor, they know how hard he works and they lean over backward to avoid imposing on him.

THE afternoon was more than half gone, and the doctor, with his visitor, set out in his new car to make a few calls. The first was to the home of a neurotic, chronically ill, mid-

dle-aged woman. Dr. Harper obviously dreaded the visit, and he was in and out of the house before his companion, waiting in the car, had time for a cigarette.

"A woman like that is a menace to the Health Service," Dr. Harper said, half humorously. "At 17 bob [shillings] a year she's a dead loss. She'll never get well." No matter how many times a year the doctor may attend such a patient he still gets only seventeen shillings for his work. At the same time," Dr. Harper went on, now talking seriously about his patient, "I feel sorry for her. Her aches and pains are real enough to her. And I regard her as a test of my patience and understanding. I keep hoping that I will be able to do something for her."

The next call was on a small boy who had recently had his tonsils out. The doctor and the boy were obviously on friendly terms, and while they talked the visitor asked the mother, the wife of a research

chemist, how the family liked being "on the state."

She had only one complaint: "You feel you can't call on the doctor for as much as you would like." Her attitude, Dr. Harper said, was unusual—and welcome. Some patients, he said, try to get as much as they can—not so much out of the doctor as out of the system.

WHEN the Health Service first started, it produced a "vast increase" in the total amount of work, Dr. Harper recalled. People came to his surgery with trivial complaints that formerly they would have ignored or treated themselves—but both the doctor's attention and his prescription were free. (An initial charge of one shilling for each prescription has since been levied. Dr. Harper and his wife were astonished at how long some people would sit in his surgery waiting for a dozen aspirin.

The number of such visits has since declined, the doctor said. Still, he calculates that he does 30 per cent more work for the same number of patients—"a lot of it done very quickly."

The doctor stopped outside one of the new municipal houses on the hill and went in to see a child with measles. He was quick again. "One has to cut out the frills," he said. "In the old days I couldn't have got out in under fifteen minutes. It was a much more leisurely life, no doubt about that. Now one is too busy to be entirely happy that one is doing the job properly."

On the way back across town, Dr. Harper turned into the driveway of Upper Waldrop's hospital, which has thirty beds and is staffed by the doctors of the town, assisted by visiting specialists and consultants. It used to be a "voluntary hospital" supported largely by private contributions, but it now belongs to the Health Service. Even so, Dr. Harper obviously still felt possessive as he proudly showed his visitor around the wards.

HEALTH SERVICE DOCTOR AT WORK

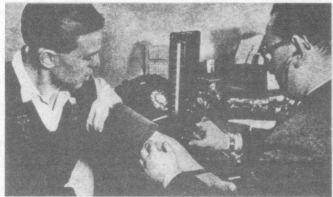

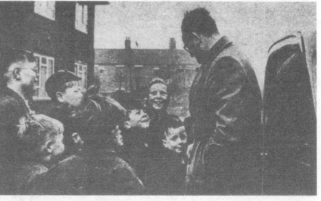

OFFICE CALL—It begins this London Dockland physician's day. The patient had an eye complaint, and is getting his blood pressure take in a general checkup.

MAKING THE ROUNDS—On his twenty to thirty calls a day, he is recognized on sight, like a country doctor. He has treated all his young greeters shown above.

The matron was hidden away, having a quiet cup of tea with another nurse. When she was found, she proved to be a middle-aged mock-tyrant, very economical with her words. "I prefer it this way," she said concisely. "I feel we are part of a unit. If we need something—say an oxygen tent—we know that we can call on the Health Service for it." Aside from their own hospital, the people of Upper Waldrop have access to two larger ones in near-by towns.

DR. HARPER'S last stop was at the home of a senior civil servant whose income is about the same as the doctor's but who is, nevertheless, a Health Service patient. By chance, the patient, who was being treated for intestinal ulcers, had a seizure that seemed suspiciously like a heart attack just before the doctor arrived. The patient's wife was agitated, but she managed to give her attention to the visitor while the doctor examined her husband.

"I hated the idea of going on the state," she said, "but my husband said he wouldn't be a private patient and our doctor wasn't going into the Health Service." The visitor surmised that the man was either one of those who thought the service socially desirable, or, as he was paying for it with his taxes, intended to have his money's worth.

"I never thought I'd be able to have another doctor," the wife said, "but we are more than satisfied with Dr. Harper. He comes to us as if we were private patients."

Dr. Harper came downstairs and gently, without using any alarming words, told the wife that her husband should have an electrocardiograph examination next day. Driving away, Dr. Harper seemed a little exasperated. The patient expected and was getting the equivalent of private service but he was reluctant to pay for a special visit from a heart specialist on the specialist's day off.

On the way back to his surgery, Dr. Harper, talking about bureaucratic interference in his work as a Health Service doctor, said that in theory there was a great deal, but in practice very little. "I think there should be more interference," he declared—a statement that certainly would astonish the leaders of the Fellowship for Freedom in Medicine.

"After all, it is public money," Dr. Harper said, explaining that he was speaking of financial, not medical, control. "So far as clinical treatment is concerned," he said, "one has complete freedom. You do whatever you feel is justified."

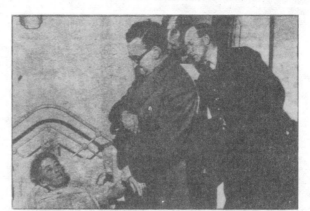

BEDSIDE—More patients than ever line his waiting room but he recognizes no change in mission to be where he is needed.

At the surgery only a few patients were waiting. It was raining steadily and it was obviously healthier to stay at home with a minor ailment than to take it to the doctor. Dr. Harper gulped a cup of tea and spent the next hour or so seeing patients. On a normal day he receives thirty to fifty in his surgery and calls on twenty to thirty more.

"Quite frankly," he commented, "I don't want to go on to the end of my days working as I have worked for the past few years." Supper was mostly cold and Mrs. Harper served it herself while their son watched television in the living room. Their daughter was away at boarding school. Over coffee the visitor remarked that Dr. Harper's opinion of the National Health Service seemed to be, on balance, more favorable than unfavorable, and he asked whether the doctor would not list his objections to the service.

"THE biggest objection," the doctor began, "is a rather indefinite one. You have the feeling there's a sort of power behind the scenes that can interfere. You feel there is a third party between you and the patient. It is not as great as you feel it is, but it is there."

Also, the patient "has the whip hand," Dr. Harper said. He can "push the doctor around" and the only recourse for the doctor is to ask that the patient be transferred to another man's list—and push him around for a while. The doctor has no contract or guaranteed working conditions. His responsibility to his patients continues 365 days a year and twenty-four hours a day. A patient who directly pays only a few shillings a year may call on the doctor as often as he likes.

The telephone rang, as if to underscore the doctor's last point. "One could sum all that up by saying that the Health Service Act was designed for the benefit of the patient rather than the doctor," said Dr. Harper when he returned from answering the phone. "It's a one-sided agreement, I think."

Still the drawbacks to the service are not nearly as great as Dr. Harper had thought they would be—"aside from the fact that one has had to work rather too hard to get the income one wanted," he said.

"You never get the income you want," interjected Mrs. Harper, who was clearing the table.

"Well," the doctor replied, "the income you think you deserve, shall we say?"

AFTER supper some friends of the Harpers came in—a dentist who is also a qualified medical doctor, the heart specialist, and their wives. The dentist, who is required by the Health Service to get the approval of a committee before he can undertake any work except emergency treatment and cleaning, was by no means as satisfied as Dr. Harper. He said the service had destroyed the old relationship between patient and doctor and had "commercialized" the practice of medicine.

The heart specialist, who said that state work took up nineteen-twentieths of his time, shared some of the dentist's dissatisfaction.

"You mean to say," the dentist said to Dr. Harper with great astonishment, "that you weren't actively against the service in the beginning?"

"No, not in theory," the doctor said, and he told of a woman who had been in his surgery that evening.

"You know, doctor," she said, "I couldn't have come to see you tonight if there hadn't been a Health Service."

Dr. Harper paused. "As a doctor," he said, "I hate the idea that people can't get the attention they need because they can't afford it."

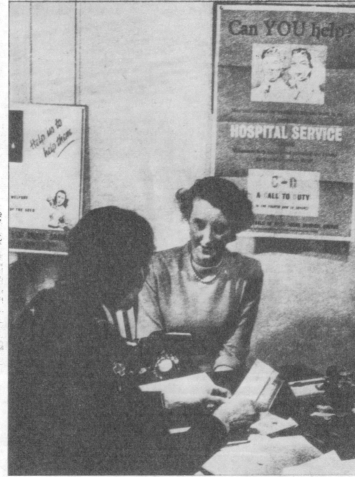

"Britain's Health Service provides broad hospital as well as medical care." The girl is being interviewed for voluntary nursing in a state hospital.

July 5, 1953

PLANS INSURE 70% ON MEDICAL BILLS

Coverage in U. S. Has Grown Swiftly Since 30's, but Problems Remain

By ROBERT K. PLUMB

Insurance to pay hospital or medical bills was first offered to the American people in the Nineteen Thirties.

By 1940 health insurance had become a major factor in the financing of health services. According to a recent estimate of the Health Insurance Council, in 1940 slightly more than 9 per cent of the population of the United States had some type of hospital insurance, 4 per cent had some type of surgical insurance and about 2 per cent had some type of medical insurance.

The growth of this type of insurance in the last fifteen years has been described by the experts as "phenomenal."

In brief, the council reports that last year 66 per cent of the people had hospital insurance, 56 per cent had surgical insurance and 35 per cent had some limited medical insurance.

Tremendous Impact

This year about 110,000,000 Americans—nearly 70 per cent of the population—have some form of voluntary health insurance. The impact of this insurance coverage on the organization of medical care—on hospitals, doctors and health service—is tremendous.

One implication of the spread of voluntary health insurance stands out. Most persons who can get it and pay for it are sold on the effectiveness of modern medical care. They like their doctors and the services that they buy in doctors' offices, clinics and in hospitals. They are largely reconciled to the fact that good medicine is expensive. They are willing to put the money aside to pay for care when they need it in the future.

If this enlightened and informed public interest can be capitalized upon by medical planners, health services may become a lot better in the future than they have been in the past.

Figures on the number enrolled in one or another of the various forms of health insurance now available are no indication, of course, of the ability of the available insurance plans to meet the health needs of the insured. There are some woeful inadequacies. Most tragic are the instances in which the insured believe, incorrectly, that their insurance will "pay all the bills."

For example, a middle-aged couple set out for a Sunday drive on the New Jersey seashore several months ago. The husband, drove at a moderate speed . He dozed. The car swerved off the road and into a tree.

The Car Is Fine

Two weeks later a mechanic finished repairing the car by jamming the automatic transmission in place.

"This guy was sure lucky he was insured," the mechanic said. "This thing was a wreck when it came in here. The bill will be about twelve hundred bucks. All but fifty paid by the insurance company."

Things were not going so smoothly in a hospital three blocks away. The motorist had been thrown into the steering wheel. His chest was crushed. His wife had fared worse. She went through the windshield. In two weeks the couple had hospital and doctor bills totaling close to $2,000. Half of this was paid by the family health insurance plan. The couple were thus only half through their treatment. And the most expensive part of their treatment—when insurance benefits begin to taper off—was yet to come.

Lucky to be insured? Yes. But too bad they were not insured as adequately as their automobile was for a common accident.

Two major directions for expansion of voluntary health insurance are pointed in a study just published, "Family Medical Costs and Voluntary Health Insurance: a Nationwide Survey." The study was sponsored by the Health Information Foundation. The two directions are:

1. Expansion in terms of the number of people covered by voluntary health insurance.
2. Expansion in terms of the benefits to be offered on an insured or a prepayment basis.

Vertical Expansion Slow

Voluntary insurance plans have expanded their horizontal coverage of the nation's population, but vertical expansion—improvement in the insurance coverage of those already enrolled—has been slower to develop.

Between 1930 and 1940 many different kinds of voluntary insurance were started. According to the study by the Health Information Foundation Blue Cross was the pioneer. This plan was organized to help pay the hospital bills of subscribers. Blue Shield was organized shortly after Blue Cross to help families pay the cost of surgery. And Blue Shield has been expanded to help pay the cost of physician's services, other than surgery, in hospitals.

In ten years the medical society-sponsored plans flourished. Consumer groups were organized to set up cooperative with salaried doctors working together in medical groups; hospital bill plans spread, and insurance companies began to write coverage for doctor and hospital bills.

The nonprofit Blue Cross and Blue Shield programs were f ahead in the number of subscribers. Blue Cross was ahead until 1950 and Blue Shield was ahead in 1939. Since those years the foundation survey indicates private insurance companies have been in the lead and they are still gaining.

Other types of insurance programs have had a slower growth, perhaps because they require substantial capital investment for modern medical

centers. These "comprehensive" prepayment medical care plans provide groups of salaried physicians who take care of the limited number of subscribers in an insurance group.

These plans—the principal one is the Health Insurance Plan of Greater New York—now cover about 4 per cent of the population. Other groups are the Group Health Association in Washington, the Kaiser Permanente Foundation in California and the Ross-Loos Clinic in California.

Enroll in Groups

About three-fourths of the families who now have some form of health insurance joined the insurance plan through enrollment in a group, usually a group of employes. The foundation study reports that 10 per cent of all families who have bought health insurance through a group have all of their premiums paid by employers; 49 per cent have part of their premiums paid by employers; 41 per cent have no contribution from employers.

Health insurance has recently become one of the important labor contract "fringe benefits" and as such is the subject of negotiations between union and management in many instances. As a result, the insurance has been studied in increasing detail by labor economists in the last few years.

The principal types of voluntary health insurance, a brief statement of advantages and disadvantages and costs follow:

Blue Cross pays part of private-room hospital bills and the costs of many drugs, tests and laboratory fees incurred in hospital treatment of certain diagnosed afflictions. Blue Cross is usually sold in combination with Blue Shield, which helps pay for medical treatment or surgery if performed in a hospital or (under limited circumstances) in a doctor's office.

The subscriber to Blue Cross or the Associated Hospital Service hospital-bill plan pays $4.36 each month. In combination with Blue Shield (United Medical Service, as it is called in New York) medical and surgical coverage is added and this insurance comes to a total of $7.76 a month for each covered family in New York.

For this premium, a family with an income of less than $4,000 a year going to a physician on a Blue Shield panel will not pay any additional fee for in-hospital medical services for the family. If the family income is above $4,000 a year, or if it uses a physician not on a Blue Shield panel the physician may charge any amount he wishes in addition to the allowances paid by Blue Shield. Some newly written Blue Shield contracts increase to $6,000 the family income limit under which insurance payments will be accepted by doctors as total payment for treatment.

Blue Cross and Blue Shield, nonprofit and sponsored by "organized medicine," are designed to pay many hospital bills as well as medical or surgical bills while in the hospital. Under Blue Cross-Blue Shield, payment is made only in case of hospital

confinement and there is usually a thirty-day limit to a hospital stay. In New York there is a twenty-one day limit for semi-private rooms. Beyond these limits subscribers must pay part of their hospital bills in most cases.

Blue Shield is designed as "fee for service" contracts in which physicians and surgeons are paid on a fixed scale for each individual service they perform. This is believed to be an advantage, for it allows doctors to operate in their traditional "free enterprise" fashion while the insurance company pays a part, at least, of the bill.

But the limitation of these plans to paying for medical treatment inside hospital walls is believed to be a serious disadvantage. For one thing, it is feared that some phyhicians may direct the admission of their patients to hospitals whether it is necessary or not.

Drawback Cited

The two plans also do not help pay the cost of diagnostic services outside the hospitals. Since diagnosis is the keystone of medical treatment—and modern scientific advances have made diagnosis costly — insurance-induced hospital admissions might rise. Recent studies suggest that such hospital admissions have increased.

A more serious drawback, in the view of critics of Blue Cross and Blue Shield, is that these plans make no attempt to provide complete medical services to their subscribers. And they do not make any real assessment of the quality of care that the subscriber receives.

The list of services that are not now paid for by Blue Cross and Blue Shield include diagnosis, preventive health services, physical examinations, home and office calls, consultations and the whole range of splendid new techniques that are available outside of the hospital.

Probably 90 per cent of all physician services are provided outside hospitals. Most Blue Shield plans limit their payments for physicians to services provided in hospitals. Most subscribers to Blue Shield are reimbursed only for part of the surgeon's fee—medical expenses other than a surgeon's fees may not be paid.

Flat Payments Made

The health insurance written by commercial companies varies widely. Generally, it is written to pay specific sums of money to the insured upon his demonstration that a specific injury or accident has occurred.

In its simplest forms commercial insurance may be written as a "dread" disease coverage. For instance, a few years ago, before the Salk vaccine was developed, commercial concerns offered to pay up to $5,000 in expenses incurred by parents of children stricken by polio during the next two years for a payment of $10. Similar policies covering other specific "dread" disease situations were written.

Other types of insurance pay flat sums of money for loss of time, limb or vital faculty. And some provide the insured with money when he is in the hospital

341

or away from work. Some plans will pay fixed surgeons' or physicians' fees for specific ailments and others will pay doctors' bills. As in other types of insurance, commercial health insurance varies widely with the company and the "fine print" in the policy.

A typical personal accident, sickness, hospital and surgical insurance sold to preferred risk individuals by commercial companies offers combined accident and sickness insurance that pays $75 a week up to 104 weeks for total disability for men at a premium of $20.50 each quarter. Hospital and surgical insurance may be added to this basic coverage for men at an additional cost of $7.50 a quarter. (Together this insurance costs $9.33 a month for the insured individual.)

The hospital and surgical coverage pays specified fees for listed operations up to a high of $255 for surgery and up to $9 a day for sixty days for hospital room for each accident or illness. It pays other fees such as $30 for operating room and laboratory fees, $36 for three or more blood transfusions, etc.

In comparison with these allowances, hospital costs in New York City average about $20 a day and surgeons are free to charge the patient as much as they wish in addition to the fee paid by the commercial insurance company.

The disadvantages of the commercial insurance, as its critics see them, are the same as the disadvantages of Blue Cross and Blue Shield. Also, critics of commercial insurance believe that companies are trying to select risks as they select for other types of coverage. This will leave uninsured a great non-preferred risk population.

A fast-growing new type of commercial insurance is the so-called "major medical expense" insurance. This insurance is written to pay the "catastrophic costs" of very long and expensive medical care in hospitals. In its usual form the holder of major medical expense insurance must pay the first $100 (or $200 or $300 or more) of his medical expenses, then the insurance pays, usually 75 to 80 per cent, of the costs of medical care, up to a maximum of $5,000 or $10,000.

Used as Supplement

Major medical expense insurance may be written to supplement Blue Cross and Blue Shield or commercial insurance. Or it may be written as the basic insurance protection of an individual or family who feels able to pay his or its own routine medical expenses, saving insurance protection and prepayment plans for the "catastrophic illness," in a financial sense.

Cost factors and other terms of major medical insurance vary widely. However, a typical policy pays 75 per cent of medical expenses over $500 up to a total of $10,000. This insurance costs $150 a year for a 48-year-old father, his wife of the same age and their 16-year-old child. The insurance is cancellable after age 65. It does not cover mental diseases, rest or pregnancy.

Supporters of major medical expense insurance hold it to be an important addition to the presently available Blue Cross-Blue Shield plans and to commercial insurance. Critics say this form of insurance must always have a "deductible" feature (to keep premiums low) and must hold the insured individual or family responsible for a fourth or so of expenses they incur even after the period of deductibility. These features, they say, will always make this form of insurance too costly to be of use to low-income families. And major medical expense insurance, they say, can in no way provide the broad range of prehospital medical services that are necessary to keep persons well, rather than paying the bills when they get sick. It is predicted that physicians' charges are likely to spiral under insurance of this type. This might lead to ever-increasing cost of medical care.

The Health Insurance Plan of Greater New York is the major example of comprehensive prepayment medical care program. Founded in 1947, H. I. P. has 500,000 subscribers, including men, women and children from more than 700 employed groups, about half the subscribers are employees of the City of New York. A family with children pays $7.60 a month for both H. I. P. and Blue Cross. The employer, city or private, pays the same. City employes are free to enter or not as they see fit, but if they do not join, the city will not pay its portion of the premium for another type of insurance.

In H. I. P., thirty-two groups of physicians in six counties—each medical group including family physicians, pediatricians, surgeons and all other types of specialists—join together to contract to provide all the medical care for the subscriber. This includes medical care at home, in a physician's office and in hospitals. It also covers diagnostic tests, visiting nurses and ambulance service—without any extra charges. H. I. P. is both an insurance plan and an organization of doctors to provide care most effectively on a prepayment basis. Each of the medical groups has a modern medical center where all X-ray, laboratory and office specialty services are provided.

Critics of H. I. P. charge that it does not provide "free choice of physician." However, proponents of the program say this is a specious argument. The reason they cite: under the fee-for-service system, a patient is always limited to a choice from among those physicans whose fees he can afford to pay.

Backers of H. I. P. say that it provides the only way for subscribers to purchase on a prepayment basis all the medical services they will need. H. I. P. service is not predicated upon hospital admission, although most H. I. P. subscribers also belong to the Blue Cross program in order to pay hospital bills if hospitalization becomes necessary. The combination of insurance and organization of medical services into H. I. P. has been going on here for a decade.

January 8, 1957

More Buying Medical Policies To Pay for 'Catastrophic' Bills

By FARNSWORTH FOWLE

Insurance against "catastrophic" medical expenses is growing rapidly.

In New York State, more than 90 per cent of the population has some form of health insurance, according to the Health Insurance Institute, an information center supported by the insurance companies. But only a fraction of these persons are protected against the kind of bills that accumulate when a major, protracted illness or accident strikes at a family's economic foundations.

The fraction with major medical protection increased by 350,000 to 1,836,000 in 1957, according to a preliminary estimate by the institute. This would mean coverage of nearly 11½ per cent of the state's population by the end of that year.

Major medical expense insurance does not pretend to cover all of a bill or every bill from a physician or hospital. As it has evolved, these policies are written to cover the bulk— usually 75 or 80 per cent—of the biggest bills, up to ceilings usually set at $5,000, $10,000 or even $15,000.

This means that the purchaser continues to carry 20 or 25 per cent of the risk. This "co-insurance" protects the insurance companies against the temptation to doctor and patient to agree on a high figure the company would have to pay in full. At best, the patient or his family will have to pay enough of the bill to feel the pinch.

Another characteristic of most major medical policies is the "deductible" feature: The purchaser knows that he will continue to have to pay the routine smaller bills himself, up to a specified limit of $25, $50, or perhaps $500, where the policy takes effect.

This deductible feature is familiar to many purchasers from their automobile insurance.

Some major medical policies are written as comprehensive policies, covering medium hospital and medical bills, as well as large ones. Others are written specifically to supplement some other type of protection, such as Blue Cross and Blue Shield.

But even in these cases, they often do not take over at the point where Blue Cross or Blue Shield coverage runs out: They may specify a deductible sum above the prepaid bill before the insurance company begins to pay the larger share.

One reason that major medical coverage is growing so rapidly now is that it got off to such a late start compared with other types of insurance, and is hurrying to catch up. It was only ten years ago that the first such policy was written for a group of General Electric Company employes.

Real Demand Cited

A decade's experience has shown that there is a real demand for such policies despite the expense, and that their administration is not too complicated from the insurer's point of view. The Health Insurance Institute recently reported that 130 insurance companies now offered such policies, and that 13,262,000 persons had this kind of protection by the end of 1957.

The cost of "major medical" varies as widely as the precise terms. Maximum benefits may be set at $5,000 or three times that amount; the deductible amount may be set at $300—or a fraction of that amount or several times it. And much depends on the age and family situation of the person buying the coverage. For a couple of 35 with two children, the annual premium for a $10,000 maximum benefit, $500 deductible policy may range from $84 to $112.50.

Another cost factor is whether a person is buying insurance for himself and his family or whether he is protecting them through a group policy which costs less because of simpler administration. Most persons with major medical protection are under group policies. Where the group works for the same company, the employer often helps to pay the bill.

State Workers Join

One of the largest of these groups in the state is made up of the state's employes. Last year, 82 per cent of them voted to join the State Employees Health Insurance Program before it came into effect on Dec. 5, 1957. Including retired employes and dependents, it now covers 197,800 persons.

The plan, drafted by the state's Temporary Health Insurance Board working through the Civil Service Department, starts with basic contracts for Blue Cross hospitalization benefits and Blue Shield medical-surgical benefits.

Then comes the supplementary major medical expense coverage. This contract is with the Metropolitan Life Insurance Company, one of nine major commercial insurance companies that bid for it. It covers 80 per cent of bills in excess of those covered by the Blue Cross-Blue Shield insurance, except for the first $50, which is deductible. The maximum benefit is $7,500 in a calendar year and $15,000 for one person in a lifetime.

The cost of this comprehensive combination for covering only the employe is just under $62 a year, of which the state pays half. If it also includes the employe's family, the cost is just over $178 a year, with the state paying 35 per cent. The "major medical" cost is less than one-fifth of the combined total.

Alternatives Listed

For state employes in certain areas there are these alternatives:

A combination of Blue Cross with Group Health Insurance, Inc., or with Health Insurance Plan of Greater New York, in the areas served by these two non-profit organizations. The state contributes the same amount of money for the employe choosing either of these combinations as it does for the state-wide combination, including the Metropolitan major medical policy.

An official of the State Department of Civil Service said last week that a large majority of employes with this choice had preferred the state-wide plan.

For the first year of the plan, he said, the number of complaints was not unreasonable.

"Nobody's dropping it," he observed.

New York is the first state to introduce such a comprehensive plan for its employes, he said, and inquiries are coming in from California and other states.

Insurance companies and medical societies have long been anxious about one feature of major medical insurance plans: Because the plans do not specify a scale of fees to be paid for particular operations or services, there has been a fear that some physicians might abuse it by asking maximum fees rather than the "reasonable" charges called for in the contracts.

Doctors Are Warned

On May 27, the New York County Medical Society heard a warning from its retiring president, Dr. Philip D. Allen, that such increasing of fees might "kill the insurance concept" and bring Government intervention in health insurance.

Metropolitan's experience with the new plan has been reassuring in this respect. A spokesman said last week that fees were working out satisfactorily, with "very few signs of abuse by the medical profession."

As the new plan approaches its first anniversary, it is opening its doors to local government authorities in the state. Under a law passed in Albany this spring, cities and counties and other local bodies (except for New York City) may decide to offer the plan to their employes, paying the same share as the state does for its workers. Including dependents, this could add roughly 225,000 to those under the plan.

September 8, 1958

42% RISE REPORTED IN MEDICAL COSTS

Average American families are paying 42 per cent more for personal health services than they did in 1953, a survey shows. The total bill is now about $294 a year, the Health Information Foundation reported yesterday.

Two major factors were cited: Increased use of services and rising costs.

The study, covering a twelve-month period in 1957-58, was made by the foundation in cooperation with the National Opinion Research Center of the University of Chicago. A similar one was made in 1953.

Most spending went for physicians' services, the survey shows. The doctor bill took 34 per cent of the health dollar. Hospitals took 23 per cent; drugs and medication, 20 per cent; dental services, 15 per cent, and other medical goods and services, such as eyeglasses and special duty nursing, 8 per cent.

Researchers found great differences in the amounts families spent. One-third spent less than $100 and another third spent from $100 to $299. The other third spent more than $300, with 16 per cent of these families spending more than $500 in the twelve-month period.

The survey also found that women spent more a year for personal health services than men. The women spent an average of $111, and the men, $77.

February 15, 1960

KENNEDY SUBMITS AGED CARE PLAN; STIFF FIGHT LIKELY

By JOHN D. MORRIS
Special to The New York Times.

WASHINGTON, Feb. 9— President Kennedy laid before a divided Congress today a broad program of Federal insurance to provide medical care for the aged.

In a special message the President also outlined other measures he said the Federal Government should take to deal with the "harsh consequences" of illness.

The message, read to the House and Senate by clerks, immediately drew manifestations of stiff opposition. Everett McKinley Dirksen, the Senate Republican leader, and Charles A. Halleck, House Republican leader, were among the first to record their opposition.

The health insurance part of the program faces especially strong resistance despite the backing of the Democratic leaders of Congress.

Aid to 14.2 Million

It calls for hospital, nursing home and other care for about 14,200,000 persons 65 years or more of age who are eligible for Social Security benefits under the Old Age, Survivors and Disability Insurance System.

The new benefits would be financed by higher Social Security payroll deductions. Employers and employes would pay about $1,500,000,000 a year in additional taxes to finance the program.

The President's other recommendations supplement the health-insurance keystone of his program. They are somewhat less controversial but are likely to meet considerable opposition from opponents of Federal spending for social-welfare projects.

They would be financed from general treasury revenues, presumably without a tax increase.

They include:

¶Federal scholarships for medical and dental students.

¶Grants for construction, expansion and restoration of medical and dental schools.

¶Funds for construction of nursing homes and for improvement of nursing-home services.

¶Broader programs of research and rehabilitation, including increased appropriations for maternal and child health and welfare. A National Institute of Child Health and Human Development and a center for research in child health would be established.

In proposing a health insurance system under social security, President Kennedy redeemed a campaign pledge. But aside from the open hostility of Republican leaders, the plan received a cool reception from some key Democrats.

Representative Wilbur D. Mills, Democrat of Arkansas, had no immediate comment as chairman of the House Ways and Means Committee, which has initial jurisdiction. He opposed similar plans last year. The committee is closely divided on the issue.

It was understood that Administration officials had failed to persuade him to introduce its health-insurance bill, even as a routin gesture without committing himself to support it. The probable sponsor, it was reported, is Representative Cecil R. King of California, the next ranking Democratic member of the committee.

To finance the new insurance system, President Kennedy recommended a two-part tax rise. Present Social Security rates are 3 per cent each for employers and employes and 4½ per cent for the self-employed. They apply to the first $4,800 of a person's annual pay.

Under the Kennedy proposal, the first increase would take effect Jan. 1, 1962, when the tax would become applicable to the first $5,000 instead of $4,800 of earnings. Then, on Jan. 1, 1963, an additional levy of one-quarter of 1 per cent each would be imposed on employers and employes and an additional three-eighths of 1 per cent on the self-employed.

Automatic Increase, Too

The rate increased would be added to an automatic rise— scheduled for 1963 under present law—of one-half of 1 per cent each for employers and employes and three-fourths of 1 per cent for the self-employed.

Thus, the 1963 rates would be 3¾ per cent each for employers and employes and 5⅝ per cent for the self-employed.

An employe who earns as much as $5,000 a year now pays $144 in Social Security taxes and his employer matches it. He would pay $150 in 1962 and $187.50 in 1963 as a combined result of the higher base, the proposed rate increase and the automatic rate increase already scheduled.

Benefits for all specified services except nursing home care would start July 1, 1962, with the nursing-home provisions taking effect six months later. The specified benefits are:

343

¶Up to ninety days of hospitalization in a single attack of illness. The patient would pay $10 of the daily costs for the first nine days. The insurance plan would pay the full costs after that.

¶Skilled nursing home services up to 180 days immediately after discharge from a hospital. Combined hospital and nursing home care would be limited to 150 units, with each day of hospitalization counting as one unit and each two days of nursing home care as one.

¶Clinic diagnostic services for hospital outpatients, or those who visit hospitals for services without being admitted

as inpatients. Costs in excess of $20 would be covered.

¶Community visiting nurse services and "related home health services" for a limited time. Officials said the limit would probably be 240 days.

Medical and surgical costs are not covered by the Administration plan. It differs in that major respect from a much-disputed bill that Representative Aime J. Forand, Democrat of Rhode Island, unsuccessfully sponsored in the last Congress.

The proposed new system adheres to the basic framework, however, of both the Forand bill and a measure by Mr. Kennedy in the Senate last year.

Various versions of the Forand bill were rejected by the House Ways and Means Committee. The Kennedy bill was defeated on the Senate floor, 51 to 44.

In his urging Congress to pass his health program, Mr. Kennedy said:

"As long as people are stricken by a disease which we have the ability to prevent, as long as people are chained by a disability which can be reversed, as long as needless death takes its toll, then American health will be unfinished business."

'Not Specialized Medicine'

Mr. Kennedy declared that

his program was not "socialized medicine."

"It is a program of prepayment of health costs with absolute freedom of choice guaranteed," he said. "Every person will choose his own doctor and hospital."

Administration officials estimated the cost of benefits under the new insurance plan at about $1,100,000,000 in the first year of full operation.

They said no figures were available on total costs of the various supplementary proposals to be financed from general revenues.

February 10, 1961

A. M. A. MAPS FIGHT ON AGED-CARE BILL
By DONALD JANSON
Special to The New York Times.

CHICAGO, Feb. 14 — The American Medical Association announced today an "all-out effort" to prevent passage of President Kennedy's medical-care program.

It described the program as the most "deadly challenge" ever faced by the medical profession.

The association will provide all member doctors with posters entitled "Socialized Medicine and You" for display in their offices. Physicians were urged to discuss the points made in the posters with their patients.

The drive, to be aimed at the public through a broad advertising program as well as through chats with doctors, was described in a special issue of The A. M. A. News.

The association supports the existing program, passed by Congress last August. It provides Federal-state aid only to

elderly citizens who lack the means to pay for medical care themselves.

The Administration plan, introduced yesterday, would provide medical aid to 14,200,000 persons over 65 years of age without a means test. It would be financed by increasing Social Security taxes.

Fears Federal Controls

The medical association, to which 80 per cent of the nation's practicing physicians belong, considers this "socialized medicine" that would lead to Government controls over hos-

pitals and medical practice.

The drive against the Administration bill may be conducted by radio and television spot announcements as well as by national and local advertisements in newspapers and magazines.

The "Socialized Medicine and You" posters were designed, the article said, so each doctor could "discuss frankly with his patients the impact Government medicine would have on both the patient and the physician."

February 15, 1961

MEDICAL AID IN BRITAIN

By SETH S. KING
Special to The New York Times.

LONDON, July 7—Fourteen years ago this week Britain's National Health Service came into being, bringing with it womb-to-tomb medical and dental care for everyone.

In the days since its inception it has had its confusions and difficulties. It has been praised and damned, with equal fervor, by both doctor and patient.

But fourteen years after its birth, two unchallengeable conclusions can be drawn: The British people want it and would not hear of any radical changes in what they have; British doctors are still skeptical of some of its methods, but 98 per cent of them participate voluntarily in some phase of the National Health Service.

From the system's beginning in Britain there have been no rebellions by doctors such as Saskatchewan is now experiencing.

Today, out of the 42,000 qualifying physicians practicing or administering hospitals, the British Medical Association estimates that barely 500 are engaged exclusively in private practice.

Changes Tried

This virtually universal ac-

ceptance does not mean that the British medical profession has made no attempts to amend the system the Labor Government imposed on them in 1948.

There have been constant efforts by the medical societies to improve the lot of the doctor, and, in their opinion, to make the service more attractive to the patient.

Some of these efforts have succeeded. Others are still being pursued.

The National Health Service functions with relative simplicity. A new patient begins by getting from local authorities a list of doctors practicing in his neighborhood. He chooses one and presents himself at this doctor's surgery (as his office is called). He is given a small card to fill out and on it he writes his name and address, his age, and his national insurance number. If he is a non-resident foreigner, he does not need to have a number.

He takes his turn in the usually crowded waiting room. The doctor examines him and prescribes a remedy. If he needs additional treatment, such as surgery, physiotherapy, special appliances, or whatever, he is referred to one of the hospitals in the neighborhood. There he is treated, or makes application to be treated when his turn

comes, by a resident specialist.

House Calls

A National Health patient may ask his doctor to make a house call on him. The response to this is considered no more reluctant than for most general practitioners in the United States.

For virtually all the medicine the patient requires he pays a fee of two shillings (twenty-eight cents) for each prescription. If he needs special appliances, he may be asked to pay part of the cost of these.

For all this the head of each family pays 10 shillings 7 pence ($1.48) a week. Three-quarters of this goes to unemployment and other relief and only one-quarter for the National Health Service.

If he is not satisfied with his doctor, he may change to another in his neighborhood.

The general practitioner in the National Health Service is paid on the basis of a "capitation fee." He receives a set amount annually for each patient who registers with him, regardless of whether he treats that patient once or daily. There are other added fees paid to him for certain services. Rural doctors get special allowances as compensation for the generally fewer patients they treat.

An individual doctor may handle a maximum of 3,500 patients. The average city general practitioner has about 2,000 patients on his list. For this, plus his extras, he earns about £2,425 ($6,790).

A specialist, beginning at the age of 34, gets a base annual salary of £2,550 ($7,100). As he grows older and becomes more skillful, this may rise to £3,900 ($10,920). In addition, if he becomes an outstanding man in his specialty, he will be given merit awards, decided by the local medical board where he practices. These may run as high as £4,000 ($11,200) a year. So the handful of top specialists may earn as much as £7,900 ($22,120).

In addition, both specialist and general practitioner may legally have as many private patients as he chooses to handle. In the case of the specialist, private patients are referred to him by other doctors when these patients choose to get their treatment in the specialist's private clinic or nursing home. Private patients come to general practitioners during the hours when the surgery is not maintained for National Health patients.

Under these conditions, it is obvious that the specialist has the best of both worlds, with his fees for public patients guaranteed through a Government salary while he may also be paid by as many private patients as he attracts.

The general practitioner has less to cheer about and it is here that the greatest discontent with the system is voiced.

'Glorified Attendants'

With the rise of personal incomes in Britain, more people are indulging in the extra attention they get as private patients, and the incomes of many general practitioners are rising.

For the patients themselves, there are certainly annoyances in the system. Britain is shockingly short of hospital bed space. A child who needs a tonsillectomy may wait, under National Health, as long as nine months before his turn comes.

It is genera'iy conceded that

a general practitioner often cannot give enough time to routine examinations that might catch some diseases earlier.

But the British public has embraced the security that National Health gives them, and they would not be without it. The poorest dust-bin man has access to Britain's greatest surgeons and her best hospital care and he has no worry of how to pay for it.

"It's true that we may not get as much personal attention and sympathy from a doctor under the National Health as we might in private systems," a British business man explained not long ago. "But we know we are going to get treatment when we need it, and no matter how much we need, we aren't going

to mortgage our future to pay for it."

The discontent of some British doctors over the system is getting more attention of late in the British press. A spirited debate is going on over how many British doctors are migrating and whether Britain is training enough medical students.

Doctors Leaving

Some private studies have produced claims that as many as 600 doctors are leaving Bitain each year to work elsewhere. The Government has challenged these assertions. It argues that the National Health System is actually increasing by 500 doctors a year after retirements and deaths have been replaced.

It has been estimated in the

last week that about one-third of the doctors who are now protesting so bitterly in Saskatchewan are British doctors who migrated there because they refused to practice under the National Health Service.

But however an individual doctor or patient may feel about the National Health scheme, there is no British politician bold enough to attack it outright.

Even Enoch Powell, the current Minister of Health, who is a paragon of modern Toryism, took the trouble recently to point out that the National Health Service has carried the support of all major political parties in Parliament and that therefore it could not properly be called "socialized medicine."

July 8, 1962

AGED SAID TO LACK HEALTH COVERAGE

By AUSTIN C. WEHRWEIN
Special to The New York Times.

CHICAGO.

The Hospital Research and Educational Trust, closely allied to the American Hospital Association, has published a study that says the elderly and poor are without adequate health insurance coverage.

The research for the report preceded the height of the controversy on the Administration's plan for medical care for the elderly under Social Security, and the study takes no stand on that program.

However, in general, it deals with many aspects of the hotly debated proposal.

On Oct. 14, the American Medical Association published a study that said statistics led to the "irresistible conclusion" that the Administration's proposals

were "built on a monstrous fraud."

The association concluded that "the aged as a group are substantially better off on the average than younger Americans."

A summary of the trust's two-volume report, just issued, said:

"Less than half the aged (65 and over) have any health insurance at all, and one-third of all low-income persons have no coverage."

For the population as a whole, it said, only a fifth lack coverage.

The three-year study, running to 1,500 pages and offering 537 statistical tables, was made in Michigan, beginning in 1957.

"While Michigan is the subject of the study, its implications are national rather than simply local," Dr. Joseph H. McNinch, a medical doctor and director of the trust, said this week. "In addition to providing a sample of national problems, the study produced

methodology for further study that is applicable across the country."

The study was directed by Walter J. McNerney, formerly director of the program in hospital administration at the University of Michigan School of Business Administration. He is at present president of the Blue Cross Association.

The study said that the health insurance of the elderly and of low-income groups usually paid a smaller proportion of the expenses than that of other groups.

"Low-income families tend to have greater total medical expenses than all but very high income families," the summary said.

It said that the use of health care services increased steadily as family income fell below $6,000 a year.

Cases Called Unpredictable

Mr. McNerney noted that, in general, medical and hospital costs were unpredictable, unrelated to income and that by

the "irony of events," low-income groups paid a higher percentage and a higher actual money sum for such care than those better off financially.

It said one problem group, which it called "relatively small," was at the bottom of the income scale and included a larger-than-average proportion of Negroes and other nonwhites, farm laborers and nonfarm service workers.

Another problem group is made up of those who lose insurance because of irregular employment. The study urged unions and management to do something about this, because laid off workers tended to drop coverage.

Coverage for retired persons, the survey said, is largely limited to nongroup policies at higher rates.

"The aged are peculiarly and unpredictably vulnerable to medical expenses, and uniquely low in resources to meet these expenses," the summary said.

December 18, 1962

PRESIDENT SIGNS MEDICARE BILL; PRAISES TRUMAN

By JOHN D. MORRIS
Special to The New York Times

INDEPENDENCE, Mo., July 30 — President Johnson flew to Independence today and signed the medicare - Social Security bill in a moving tribute to former President Harry S. Truman.

Mr. Truman, beaming, sat beside Mr. Johnson on the stage of the Harry S. Truman Library auditorium. More than 200 persons, including Vice President Humphrey, Congressional lead-

ers and Administration officials, witnessed the ceremony.

President Johnson chose Independence for the signing because Mr. Truman was the first President who proposed a Federal program of health insurance under Social Security.

It was in a special message Nov. 19, 1945, that Mr. Truman asked Congress to enact such legislation.

'A Reality for Millions'

"The people of the United States love and voted for Harry Truman," the President said, "not because he gave them hell but because he gave them hope.

"I believe today that all America shares my joy that he is present now when the hope he offered becomes a reality for millions of our fellow citizens."

The 81-year-old former President, opening the ceremonies with a brief talk, found himself uncharacteristically at a loss for words at one point.

"I am glad to have lived this long and to witness today the signing of the medicare bill," he said.

Then, welcoming those who came to Independence, he groped briefly for a phrase to express his feelings.

Johnson Hails Program

"I thank you all most highly for coming here," he said. "It's an honor that I haven't had done to me—well, quite a while, I'll say that to you."

In his address at the signing ceremonies, Mr. Johnson said:

"No longer will older Ameri-

cans be denied the healing miracle of modern medicine. No longer will illness crush and destroy the savings that they have so carefully put away over a lifetime so that they might enjoy dignity in their later years."

The Senate completed Congressional action on the bill Wednesday, capping a 20-year effort to steer such legislation to final passage.

The bill expands the 30-year-old Social Security insurance program to provide hospital care, nursing home care, home nursing services and out-patient diagnostic service for all Americans over 65 years old.

It also sets up a supplementary program of Federal insurance covering most of the doctors' bills and some other health costs of persons over 65. The supplementary insurance will be available on a voluntary basis with participants paying $3 a month in premiums.

Other provisions include a 7 per cent increase in cash benefits under the present old age, survivors and disability insurance program.

To finance the basic hospital and nursing care insurance and the new cash benefits, Social Security taxes will be increased in steps over the next 22 years starting next Jan. 1.

Both the basic and supplementary insurance programs start next July 1. The 7 per cent rise in cash benefits is retroactive to last Jan. 1. Checks for nearly $1 billion, covering eight months of retroactive payments for 20 million beneficiaries, will be mailed in September.

The medical care programs will not go into operation until almost a year after the bill was enacted. The delay was intended to allow time for drafting administrative rules.

The bill does not specify how doctors and hospitals will be paid for their services. But it is expected that the rules, to be set forth by the Department of Health, Education and Welfare, will funnel much administrative activity through such established organizations as Blue Cross, Blue Shield and possibly some private insurance companies.

The medical care program covers all persons who have reached 65, with some minor exceptions.

Coverage for Doctors

It covers 17 million persons eligible for Social Security and 2 million others who do not fall under Social Security's present old-age, survivors and disability insurance program. Medical benefits to the latter group will be paid for by appropriations from general revenues, not from Social Security funds.

Of the 2 million persons, only 350,000—persons in their seventies who under previous laws did not have enough wage credits to qualify—will be entitled to cash benefits. They will receive payments of $35 a month. Those still not covered by Social Security are people who did not meet the requirements for coverage at the time

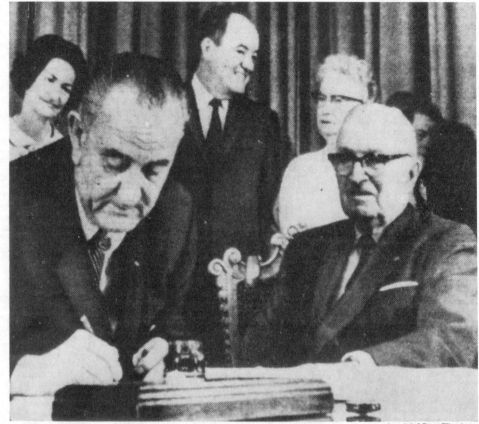

Associated Press Wirephoto

MEDICARE BILL SIGNED: President Johnson signing bill, with former President Harry S. Truman at his side, in Truman Library at Independence, Mo. Behind them are Mrs. Johnson, Vice President Humphrey and Mrs. Truman.

they retired, many of them self-employed persons or domestics, and their widows.

The new law extends Social Security coverage to self-employed physicians and to hospital internes, the last major group that had been exempt from coverage.

President Johnson used 72 pens to sign the measure and passed them out to members of Congress, labor leaders, Administration officials and others who filed across the stage and shook his hand.

He gave the first one to Mr. Truman and the second to Mrs. Truman.

Wilbur J. Cohen, Under Secretary of Health, Education and Welfare, got two pens. So did Andrew Biemiller, chief lobbyist for the American Federation of Labor and Congress of Industrial Organizations, and Lawrence F. O'Brien, the White House Congressional liaison officer.

Forand Receives Pen

Mr. Cohen was an early advocate of medicare legislation. He and Mr. Biemiller and Mr. O'Brien did much to lobby the present bill through Congress.

Others receiving pens included Representative Wilbur D. Mills, Democrat of Arkansas,

and Senator Russell B. Long, Democrat of Louisiana, the House and Senate managers of the bill; Representative Cecil R. King, Democrat of California, and Senator Clinton P. Anderson, Democrat of New Mexico, co-sponsors of the measure, and former Representative Aime J. Forand, Democrat of Rhode Island, who sponsored a much discussed medicare bill as 1957.

Mr. Johnson and Mr. Truman chatted privately for a few minutes before and after the ceremony. The President later flew to his Texas ranch for the weekend.

July 31, 1965

Digest of the New Social Security Law

Special to The New York Times
WASHINGTON, July 30 — Following is a digest of major provisions of the medicare-Social Security law.

HEALTH INSURANCE

Insurance for persons over 65 years old is provided under two plans, one designated as "basic" and the other as "supplementary," starting July 1, 1966. The basic plan automatically covers everyone who is 65 except aliens with less than five years of residence

in the United States, aliens without status as permanent residents and Federal employes eligible for Government health insurance under another law. Participation in the supplementary plan is optional, subject to the same eligibility requirements.

Basic Plan

This insurance will be financed by increases in the Social Security payroll tax. The cost of benefits for about 2 million aged persons not covered by the present Social Security or Railroad Retire-

ment Insurance programs will be met by appropriations from general tax revenues.

Benefits under the basic plan include:

HOSPITALIZATION

Up to 90 days in each spell of illness. The patient pays the first $40 of hospital costs. If he stays more than 60 days, he pays $10 for each additional day up to the 90-day limit. A spell of illness starts with the first day of hospitalization and ends when the patient has spent 60 consecutive days without hospital or nursing care.

The insurance covers room and board, prescribed drugs while hospitalized and other services and supplies except private duty nursing and services of physicians other than internes or residents in training. Christian Science sanatoriums and psychiatric hospitals are included. But there is a lifetime limit of 190 days in a psychiatric hospital.

NURSING HOME CARE

Up to 100 days in an extended care facility in each spell of illness after a stay of at least three days in a hospital. There is no charge to the patient for the first 20 days. The patient pays $5 for each day above 20, up to the 100-day limit.

HOME NURSING

Up to 100 visits by nurses or technicians in a one-year period following the patient's discharge from a hospital or extended care facility. The insurance covers the full cost. The services furnished must be in accordance with a plan set up and periodically reviewed by a physician.

DIAGNOSTIC SERVICES

Tests and related diagnostic services, other than those performed by physicians, that are normally provided by hospitals to out-patients. The patient pays $20 of the charge for each diagnostic study— that is, for diagnostic services provided by the same hospital in a 20-day period. The patient also pays 20 per cent of the charges above $20, and the insurance covers the remaining 80 per cent.

Supplementary Plan

Persons enrolling in this plan will pay $3 a month in premiums. The Federal Government will match this with a payment of $3 a month for each participant. The Federal share, about $600 million a year, will come from general tax revenues. The insurance supplements the basic plan by covering most other major medical expenses except those for dental services, medicines and drugs.

The coverage includes:

¶Physicians' services, including surgery, whether performed in a hospital, clinic, office or home.

¶Up to 100 home nursing visits each year in addition to those allowed under the basic plan and without any requirement for prior hospitalization.

¶Various services and supplies, whether provided in or out of a medical institution, such as X-ray and other diagnostic tests, radiological treatments, surgical dressings, splints, casts, iron lungs and other specified prosthetic devices, artificial arms, legs and eyes and ambulance service.

A participant in the plan pays $50 of his annual costs for the services and supplies covered. He also pays 20 per cent of the annual costs above $50 while the plan pays 80 per cent.

CASH BENEFITS

A 7 per cent increase in all cash benefits under the present Social Security program of old age, survivors and disability insurance is retroactive to last Jan. 1, with all recipients entitled to at least $4 in additional monthly payments.

The minimum monthly benefit rises immediately from $40 to $44. The maximum for a single retired or disabled worker is increased from $127 to $135.90. Maximum family benefits are raised from $254 to $309.20.

For most persons going on the benefit rolls in future years, monthly benefits will be further increased as they acquire higher wage credits under provisions for payment of Social Security taxes on $6,600 of annual earnings instead of the present $4,800. Maximum benefits will be $168 for a single worker and $368 for a family.

Retirement Test

The bill increases to $1,500 the amount that a retired worker may earn in a year without losing part of his Social Security pension. The old exemption was $1,200. There will be a reduction of $1 in benefits for each $2 of earnings from $1,500 to $2,700 and a dollar-for-dollar reduction on earnings above $2,700. This replaces a $1 for $2 reduction on earnings from $1,200 to $1,700 and a dollar-for-dollar reduction above $1,700.

About 750,000 persons will be entitled to a total increase of nearly $300 million in annual cash benefits under the provision.

Widows' Benefits

The bill gives widows of workers covered by Social Security the option of drawing benefits at the age of 60 on a reduced scale. Full widows' benefits will still be payable at the age of 62

For a widow who exercises the new option, the monthly benefit will be 71½ per cent of what her husband, if living, would have received at age 65. If a widow does not start drawing benefits until she is 62, she is paid 82½ per cent of the husband's benefit.

About 185,000 widows are eligible for the new option.

Child Benefits

Children of retired, disabled or deceased workers will be eligible under the bill for Social Security dependency benefits through the age of 21 if they are attending school or college. Only those under 18 are now eligible. About 295,-000 children will qualify.

New Payments

The bill adds to the benefit rolls about 355,000 retired workers and widows by reducing coverage requirements for persons in their seventies. The minimum requirement of six quarters of employment in jobs covered by Social Security is reduced to three quarters. Payments of $35 a month are provided for women at the age of 72 and men at the age of 76.

Cash Tips

Employers will be required to withhold Social Security taxes and also income taxes on tips reported to them by their employes. The employer, in passing the taxes along to the Government, will not have to match the employe's Social Security contribution on income from tips, as he does on other pay. However, workers will earn the same increase in retirement benefits as they would have earned if both the employer and employe shares of the tax were paid on the tips.

Doctors' Coverage

Self-employed physicians and hospital internes, numbering about 175,000, are brought under the old age, survivors and disability insurance program. They constituted the last major group exempt from coverage. Salaried physicians were already covered.

Disability Payments

The bill relaxes the present rigid requirement for payment of disability benifits under the Social Security insurance program. About 60,000 disabled workers and dependents are expected to qualify for new benifts.

TAXES

A series of increases in Social Security taxes will start next Jan. 1 to finance costs of the basic health insurance plan and liberalization of the old age, survivors and disability program. The tax, shared equally by employers and employes, is now 7¼ per cent. Under previous legislation, it was scheduled to rise in two steps to a maximum of 9¼ per cent in 1968.

Under the bill, the first $6.600 of a worker's annual pay will be subject to the tax after Jan. 1. The present base is $4,800. The combined employer-employe rate will rise in seven steps to 11.3 per cent in 1987.

Income Tax Deduction

Taxpayers no longer will be allowed full deductions for medical and drug expenses of persons over 65. The rule now applicable to younger persons is extended to all by the bill. It limits the deduction to medical expenses that exceed 3 per cent of the taxpayer's income and to costs of prescribed medicines that exceed 1 per cent of his income.

However, the bill also provides a new allowance for all taxpayers, regardless of age, on health insurance costs. The taxpayer will be permitted to deduct from his income half the premiums paid each year without regard to the 3 per cent rule on medical expenses. The maximum deduction under this provision is $150. Additional expenses, including insurance premiums, will still be deductible to the extent that they exceed 3 per cent of the taxpayer's income.

WELFARE AID

The bill authorizes increases of about $400 million in annual Federal grants to states for public assistance (relief of the needy) and other welfare programs. It consolidates the Kerr-Mills medical assistance program with five related programs and sets Federal standards for the scope of benefits and eligibility of beneficiaries.

A new program of health care for children in impoverished families is established, with $185 million in grants authorized for the first five years. Grants for maternal and child health services and aid to crippled children are raised in four steps from the present level of $80 million to $120 million in 1970.

By revising the general formula for public assistance grants, the bill raises annual Federal authorizations by $150 million.

July 31, 1965

Medicare Law in Brief
Special to The New York Times

WASHINGTON, July 30—*Following in brief is what the medicare-Social Security bill signed by President Johnson today will mean to persons over 65:*

Hospitalization—Up to 90 days for each illness. The patient pays the first $40 of hospital costs. After 60 days, he pays $10 a day up to the 90-day limit.

Nursing Home Care—Up to 100 days in an extended care facility in each illness after a stay of at least three days in a hospital. The patient pays nothing for the first 20 days. He pays $5 daily thereafter.

Home Nursing—Up to 100 visits by nurses or technicians in a one-year period after a patient's discharge from a hospital or extended care facility.

Medical Benefits—Those who pay $3 a month in premiums will receive, among other benefits, physicians' and surgeons' services and other services and supplies.

Social Security Benefits—The minimum monthly benefit rises immediately from $40 to $44. The maximum for a single retired or disabled worker goes from $127 to $135.90. Maximum family benefits rise from $254 to $309.20.

Widows—Widows of workers covered by Social Security may either start drawing benefits at the age of 60 on a reduced scale or wait for full benefits at 62.

July 31, 1965

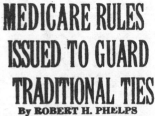

MEDICARE RULES ISSUED TO GUARD TRADITIONAL TIES

By ROBERT H. PHELPS
Special to The New York Times

WASHINGTON, May 30 — The Government is issuing rules for Medicare that it says preserve the traditional doctor-patient relationship.

The instructions, which the Social Security Administration is sending to the 230,000 medical doctors and 4,000 osteopaths in the country, set guidelines for determining "reasonable" fees and outline two methods of receiving payments.

On the sensitive subject of fees the guidelines permit a doctor to vary his fee for a medical service and allow some doctors to charge more than others for the same service.

Doctors who fought the adoption of Medicare have expressed fear that the Federal Government would insist on regulations that would interpose bureaucrats between the physician and his patients.

But Dr. Philip R. Lee, Assistant Secretary for Health and Scientific Affairs of the Department of Health, Education and Welfare, said in an interview that he saw nothing in the rules that would "alter a doctor's relationship with his patients."

The two principal benefits of the Medicare program, payment of hospital and doctor bills, begin July 1. Hospital coverage is automatically given to almost all of the 19.1 million persons 65 years of age or older, but coverage for physicians' services is voluntary.

Last Day to Register

Tomorrow is the last day to sign up for the doctor-bill insurance before the next enrollment period, which begins on Oct. 1, 1967. Social Security offices remained open today to give the elderly an 11th-hour chance to sign up for this insurance. More than 17 million have decided to pay $3 a month for the medical insurance.

Dr. Lee noted that there had been "rumors" that some doctors were raising fees in anticipation of Medicare, but he emphasized that there had been no "documentary" evidence to support such reports.

He said some increases in fees could be expected because "it is clear that the cost of medical care is rising."

Under the regulations, which Dr. Lee helped draft, neither the doctors nor the patients will deal directly with the Government.

Seventy intermediaries — many of them Blue Cross and Blue Shield plans—will set regional scales of fees on which payments to doctors will be based.

If the doctor wants to, he can submit his bills for Medicare patients directly to the intermediary, which will send him a check. If the doctor does not want to deal with an intermediary he can send the bill to the patient, who then pays the doctor and is reimbursed when he submits the bill to the intermediary.

In either case a one-page form must be submitted to the intermediary. The patient fills in part of the form. The part to be filled in by the doctor asks fewer questions than forms for some Blue Shield plans.

Dr. Lee predicted that most doctors would work with the intermediaries because of the ease of collecting bills. Doctors who choose this plan must agree, however, to charge no more than the "reasonable" fees set by the intermediaries.

The doctor who bills the patient directly can charge whatever he wants, but the patient will be reimbursed only on the basis of the "reasonable" fee.

Under the Government's guidelines, intermediaries must consider two factors in establishing "reasonable" fees. One factor is the customary charge that the doctor makes for the particular medical service.

The other factor is the prevailing range of charges in the locality—the charges most frequently used by doctors. The reasonable fee cannot exceed either the customary or prevailing charges.

Medicare will pay for 80 per cent of the reasonable charges, except for the first $50, which the patient must pay.

The regulations permit a wide variety of prevailing—and thus reasonable—charges for the same medical service.

Specialists are permitted a higher range of charges than are general practitioners offering the same treatment. Thus a bone specialist could charge a higher fee than a family doctor for setting a broken arm.

Doctors in big cities can charge more than those in small towns, on the basis of the fact that their costs are higher. Medical complications and extensive travel time by doctors can also cause fees to rise.

May 31, 1966

Doctors' Fees Up As Much as 300% Under Medicare

By MARTIN TOLCHIN

Physicians have raised their fees for patients 65 and over by as much as 300 per cent since Medicare began July 1.

The widespread increases were confirmed yesterday by leading physicians and health insurance officials in the city.

However, officials of medical societies in Westchester and Nassau Counties said that although physicians' fees had risen gradually in the last two years, there had been no sharp increase since Medicare went into effect.

The city physicians contended that they had raised the fees of only those patients whom they had carried at lower fees than prevailed in the rest of their practice. Many were long-standing patients who were retired or financially dependent, they said.

'Eliminating a Discount'

A Medicare spokesman commented, however: "This is a situation in which the professional takes advantage of the plan."

He added that only a small percentage of physicians' bills had been received by the Social Security Administration and that it was too early to discern a trend.

The Government pays 80 per cent of a physician's fees after the first $50 annually under Part B of Medicare. It costs subscribers $3 a month in premiums.

Some physicians said that they had raised their fees so that they could accept the Government fee as full payment and not attempt to collect the 20 per cent from the patients.

A professor of internal medicine who said that he had raised the office-visit fees of some older patients from $10 to $15 to conform to his regular fees, explained:

"I'm not raising fees but eliminating a discount."

Dr. George Himler, a Manhattan surgeon who is chairman of the coordinating council of the city's five county medical societies, said that he had tripled the fees of some older patients.

"A lot of these people were of substandard means," he said. "Many of them I've been carrying at $3 and $5 office visits for years, because there was nothing to raise them with. Now they're being raised."

Dr. Himler said that $10 was his customary fee for an office visit.

Patients Pay Less

He noted that physicians customarily had adjusted their fees to take into account the patients' ability to pay. Consequently the rich have paid more and the poor less, he said.

"This Robin Hood idea is going out the window," Dr. Himler said. "These [poorer] patients are not going to be second-class patients the way they used to be."

An internist who said that he was raising fees for office visits for many older patients from $5 to $10, to conform to his general practice, pointed out that under Medicare the doctor would get more although the patient would pay less.

In his case a patient who formerly paid $5 will pay only $2, or 20 per cent of the new fee of $10, he said.

A surgeon on a university faculty said:

"Like every major medical policy, you put down what you'd like to get and hope for the best. If I get a reasonable fee from the Government, I won't even try to collect the rest."

He said that he had charged $600 for a hip nailing, for which Blue Shield presently provides an allowance of $300. The Blue Shield subscriber is supposed to pay the balance of the bill, but this is often waived with older, poorer patients, he said.

'Subsidizing' Resented

A leading Blue Cross official said: "I've heard doctor after doctor say, 'Why should I continue to subsidize something that is no longer paid for by the patients?'"

Physicians' fees mounted steadily in the year that ended last June, according to an official of the Bureau of Labor Statistics of the United States Department of Labor.

Fees for family physicians rose from an index figure of 121.1 in June, 1965, to 128, based on an average of the period 1957-9, which is indexed at 100.

Fees for office visits have risen from 120.9 to 128.1 in the last year, the official said. Fees for house visits have risen from an index figure of 124.1 to 133.3.

August 19, 1966

MEDICARE BILLS PAID IN 3 WEEKS

By HAROLD M. SCHMECK Jr.
Special to The New York Times

WASHINGTON, June 14 — For most of the nation, physicians' bills under Medicare are now being processed in less than three weeks, Robert M. Ball, commissioner of the Social Security Administration, said today.

In the early days of Medicare last year, the average time lag rose to almost eight weeks. But it has been dropping steadily since then, Mr. Ball said at a news conference in which he gave a first anniversary assessment of the health insurance program for the elderly.

Medicare will be a year old at the end of this month. In its first year the program will have paid about $2.4-billion to provide hospital care and services for about 4 million Americans who have passed their 65th birthdays.

The program has also paid $640-million for physicians' bills and other medical services that are not directly related to hospital care. The figures are virtually up to date, but include conservative projections through the end of June, to round out the year, Mr. Ball said. He repeated what he has repeatedly said in the past — Medicare is a success.

Lives Have Been Prolonged

"The lives of many elderly people have been improved and, in some instances, prolonged because of this program," he said. "It is hard to measure the great improvement in the quality of life for an older person brought about by the removal of a cataract, the repair of a hernia, or other surgery or corrective therapy, but it is there, and, in substantial amount, and attributable to Medicare."

Older Americans have received, roughly, 15 per cent more in-patient hospital services during the year than would have been the case without Medicare, he said. There have been 5 million hospital admissions under the program, involving 4 million patients.

Physicians have arranged Medicare home health care for more than 200,000.

The upgrading of health care because of standards established under Medicare has been a benefit to patients of all ages, Mr. Ball said. The civil rights requirements of the program have opened many previously segregated hospitals so that, in many communities, "minority group members now have access to high-quality care for the first time," he declared.

59 Insurance Carriers

Among Medicare's problems, Mr. Ball mentioned the delays in processing reimbursement claims for physicians' services. This processing is done by 59 insurance carriers covering the entire nation.

In 51 of these areas, where 90 per cent of the Medicare beneficiaries live, the bills are being processed in less than 21 days, on the average. In only two areas does processing take longer than a month—35 days on the average for Maryland outside the Washington metropolitan area, and 50 days in Iowa.

Another problem is that of physician refusal to take Medicare case assignments. If a physician accepts such an assignment, he must agree to accept as full payment for his services the fee determined as reasonable under Medicare.

If the physician does not accept assignment, the patient must pay the bill and submit a claim for reimbursement himself.

"We are studying whether there are ways in which the patient can be relieved of the hardship arising from his physician's refusal to take an assignment without increasing inflationary pressures on the size of physicians' fees," Mr. Ball said.

June 15, 1967

BOOM UNDER WAY IN NURSING HOMES

By FRANKLIN WHITEHOUSE

An unparalleled boom in nursing home construction over the last five years has produced an industry with an estimated annual income of $2-billion that can thank the Federal Medicare program for much of its growth.

"It's mushroomed like the motel industry after World War II, both in buildings and the quality of their administrators," one Federal official said last week.

About half of the 600,000 beds in the country's 13,600 licensed nursing homes were added in the five-year period ending in June, 1966, according to the most recent figures of the United States Public Health Service and the American Nursing Home Association.

The rate of construction growth in the last three years has been about 12 per cent a year, said the Federal official, Dana Doten of the Public Health Service. Although no authoritative projections for 1967 are available, he added, "there is no evidence that the rate has slackened."

Between 85 and 90 per cent of all licensed homes fall into the proprietary category, that is, they are built and operated for a profit unlike voluntary and government-run institutions. Proprietary homes contain more than 70 per cent of all beds.

Homes 90 Per Cent Full

Nursing homes of all types in the country are 90 per cent full on average, Mr. Doten said. Many have long waiting lists of persons 65 years old or more who can qualify for Medicare.

Medicare will pay all expenses for qualifiers for the first 20 days. The patient, who must have spent at least three days in a hospital prior to admission in an extended-care home, is required to pay $5 a day for the next 80 days.

The cost of nursing home care ranges from $150 a month to as much as $1,000 for each patient.

Medicare, which has prompted a greater market for nursing homes, has also laid down standards of operation and profitability for qualifying institutions that has separated the skilled-care home with 24-hour nursing service from "the boarding house and the old folks' home."

Only about 4,000 of the 13,600 licensed homes have the services of professional dieticians and occupational therapists needed, in addition to 24-hour nursing care, to qualify as a Medicare institution.

These institutions now contain about 285,000 beds.

One of the Largest

Perhaps the largest Medicare qualified institution in the country is the DeWitt Nursing Home, a $6.5-million, 17-story building that is about to open on East 79th Street here.

The DeWitt was built by a Venezuelan realty concern, the Kalanco Corporation and leased for 21 years to Dr. A. Lee Lichtman, a Manhattan surgeon, who said his own investment in the home came to more than $1-million. He said he would pay an aggregate rent of more than $45-million over the term of the lease and its 21-year option.

Before opening, the DeWitt's 500 beds have been "totally committed" with a waiting list of between 700 and 800 patients, Dr. Lichtman said.

The New York architectural firm of Wechsler & Schimenti designed the DeWitt with a nursing station for every 40 beds, rooms with between one and four beds each and six elevators large enough to accommodate stretcher cases. The rooms are furnished with Italian Provincial furniture.

Dr. Lichtman said the per-patient rates would range from $150 to $350 a week, well above the national average of $250 a month reported by the Public Health Service.

Medicare reimburses participating proprietary homes for "reasonable costs" in addition to 1.5 per cent for profit and an additional 7.5 per cent on net equity, the investment less accumulated depreciation and debt.

A Big Business

That nursing homes have become a big business is reflected in the increasing size of the facilities. In 1954 the average size of a nursing home was 25 beds, according to the American Nursing Home Association. In 1961, the average size had increased to 31 beds and to 42 in 1965.

An association spokesman said that it is no longer efficient to build homes with less than 50 beds because Medicare-required services such as occupational therapy cannot be performed economically for so few.

As the business gets larger, the professionalism of management increases in quality, Mr. Doten said. The new homes, many of which are affiliated with hospitals, are being "dominated" by local doctors.

Five years ago, Mr. Doten added, the average nursing home administrator had completed the second year of high school. Now the average educational level "is a little better than a high school graduate."

July 2, 1967

Spiraling Medical Costs Reflect Deficiencies in U.S. Health Care

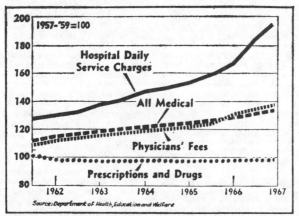

Medical care cost trends are indicated in percentage, with the 1957-59 cost in each category being 100%.

By HAROLD M. SCHMECK Jr.
Special to The New York Times

WASHINGTON, April 27—A patient in Massachusetts found to his dismay that his hospital clinic had raised its fee for visits from $6.50 three years ago to $12.

In Washington, a workman who had been badly burned in an accident was sent home recently after 85 days in the hospital. The bill was just over $30,000, but the patient did not seem to mind.

A schoolteacher in West Virginia went to a hospital emergency room with a pain in the right side of his chest. He emerged later with no clear diagnosis and a bill for $62.

In rural Mississippi a mother and 11 young children have grits for breakfast, pecans for lunch, rice, beans and greens for supper. One of the children has periodic blackout spells, but, until recently, had never seen a doctor in her life.

While each of these cases illustrates the rapidly rising cost of health in America, each gives a different aspect of this complicated problem. The patient in Massachusetts complained to the National Council of Senior Citizens about the steadily rising cost of routine health care.

So far as is known, the burn patient at the Washington Hospital Center has not complained to anyone. He has survived burns that covered 70 per cent of his body. Workmen's compensation insurance is expected to pay the costs for massive and expensive treatment that would have been unavailable 10 years ago at any cost.

The teacher in West Virginia thought he was given a lot of expensive tests to no purpose except that to relieve him of money. A doctor whom he consulted afterward agreed.

The family in Mississippi illustrates a different aspect of the problem. The cost of medical care does not have to be astronomical to be too high for the poor. A few dollars and a few miles can put a medical center out of reach. Medical problems in these cases might be largely solved by some decent food.

Dr. H. Jack Geiger of the Tufts-New England Medical Center cited the Mississippi family to show that "the health of the poor in the United States is an ongoing national disaster."

"The poor are likelier to be sick, the sick are likelier to be poor," he said during a Lowell Institute lecture. "Without intervention, the poor get sicker and the sick get poorer."

Millions of Needs

Altogether the nation's health care problem is a mosaic of millions of individual needs and difficulties. In this the clearest pattern is one of rising costs for almost everyone and a relative decline in health manpower to deal with the growing demand for health care.

These trends are expected to continue for the next several years.

The situation has generated books, Government - sponsored conferences, surveys and reports, bills before Congress and hearings before Congressional subcommittees.

Throughout this week such hearings were held by the Subcommittee on Executive Reorganization of the Senate Government Operations Committee. At one of these hearings Wilbur J. Cohen, Secretary-designate of Health, Education and Welfare,

said there were serious deficiencies in the organization, financing and delivery of health care in the United States.

He named three areas of high-priority need: child and maternity health programs, deployment of health manpower and facilities and continued investment in medical research as the source of future improvements in health.

Since 1961, Mr. Cohen said, personal expenditures for health care have increased from $24.7-billion annually to $41.5 billion. He said that more than a third of this could be attributed to increases in medical care costs and that 15 per cent resulted from a population increase of 16 million persons between 1961 and last year.

The remaining portion of the increase—almost half—results from the greater utilization of services, improvements in quality and the introduction of new medical techniques, he said.

Broad Spectrum of Ideas

Mr. Cohen's department is generating a broad spectrum of ideas for coping with the cost problem and improving the quality of care. Included are experiments in group medical practice on a prepayment basis, community health centers that are available to the poor, and new ways of rewarding hospitals for efficiency and penalizing inefficiency.

Nonetheless, experts say it is inevitable that the costs will continue to climb in the next several years.

Medical care costs have been rising for years, but there has been an acceleration recently.

Dr. Victor R. Fuchs of the National Bureau of Economic Research has estimated that the nation's total expenditures for medical care rose from $4-billion in 1929 to $10-billion 20 years ago, to $40-billion in 1965 and close to $50-billion last year. Medicare and Medicaid brought steep rises in 1966 and part of 1967.

Last year, one day's care in a general hospital cost an average of $58.06. Figures from the American Hospital Association show this was a 15.4 per cent increase over the previous year.

Many experts believe that a day's care will cost $100 before long—except that it will not be the same kind of care. At some hospitals, in some cases, the $100 figure has been reached already.

A little more than a year ago a report to the President on medical care costs described the upward trend as a cause for concern.

Large increases "cause severe hardship to individuals in need of medical care, whether they pay the prices directly or indirectly through higher insurance premiums," the report said.

"Medical price increases make Government - financed

medical care programs more expensive for the taxpayer."

Demand Increasing

Price rises were attributed to several factors. These included the increasing demand for medical services, the relatively slow increases in physicians and other health workers, the rising wage costs in hospitals without commensurate increases in productivity and the increasing complexity of the medical care the patient received.

All these factors are still in force. Costs in most aspects of medical care continue to rise.

The chief architect of the 1967 report to President Johnson was William Gorham, Assistant Secretary for Program Coordination in the Department of Health, Education and Welfare.

In a recent interview, he predicted that medical costs would continue to rise faster than the rest of the economy for the next several years at least.

Many experts agree that this is inescapable simply because of hospitals' rising labor costs. For decades hospitals paid their employes at rates far below industry's scales for the same level of skills. In recent years, government action and labor troubles have forced the hospitals to catch up.

Some hospitals are finding that doing so raises their efficiency because higher wages attract higher skills and better performance, but this is by no means translated into lower costs.

There are several reasons for this, according to Ray E. Brown, professor of hospital administration at the Harvard Medical School and executive vice president of the affiliated hospital center that encompasses Harvard's teaching hospitals in Boston.

"In the last five years hospitals have made great strides in raising wages," Professor Brown said in a telephone interview.

"They are now within 20 per cent of general wage levels," he said. That means, he said, that they have been rising more steeply than wages in general, with a corresponding effect of the institutions' costs.

Furthermore labor usually accounts for more than 60 per cent of a hospital's operating expenses as compared with only about 30 per cent in industry, he said.

In consequence, Professor Brown said, a rise in labor costs has a greater effect on a hospital than it would, for example, on a manufacturing plant.

There is another important disparity. In industry, new technology usually brings greater efficiency with a resultant increase in productivity for each employe.

In the economy of a hospital, the effect is sometimes the opposite. New technology means more things that can be done for the patient, but these new possibilities often call for more and higher paid technicians, and nursing care and expensive new equipment. Costs and prices go up again.

Also, there is much evidence that hospital administration is often inefficient and that many hospitals are too small to be efficient.

"I don't think this reflects an attempt to fleece the public," Mr. Gorham said. "They are not crooks, but they have a long way to go in improving management."

In this effort some major hospitals are finding new technology coming to their aid.

It costs a lot of money to rent a big computer, for example, but this expense can sometimes be translated into important savings. The computer can show the hospital management what is going on in detail and with immediacy that was out of the question in the past.

Insurance Poses Problem

Another problem for hospitals is the medical insurance policy that will pay for services rendered for a patient in a hospital but will not pay for the same services for the same person as an outpatient.

A recent report to the Secretary of Health, Education and Welfare made this point strongly.

The lack of community and regional planning has also produced an unhappy situation, the report said, in which two new hospitals, both half-empty, stand within blocks of each other in one city.

In another city, a committee found a half-dozen hospitals each equipped and staffed to do open heart surgery—one of the most expensive of all surgical specialties—yet there were barely enough cases to keep one of the centers busy.

The committee said that empty beds were the rule rather than the exception in obstetric and pediatric services across the nation. It found "aged, chronically ill patients lying idle in $60-a-day hospital beds because no nursing home beds are provided, overloaded emergency rooms and underused facilities and services that have been created for reasons of prestige rather than need."

The committee, under the chairmanship of John A. Barr, dean of the Graduate School of Business at Northwestern University, said that the remedy started with planning, "to be applied in massive doses over the entire surface of the health service economy."

There are dissents, however.

At a national conference on medical costs last year, Dr. Eli Ginzberg, Hepburn professor of economics at Columbia University, said he doubted that a medical crisis confronted the nation.

No Crisis Seen

"This is the third conference on an alleged medical crisis that I have attended in the city of Washington," he said. "I don't believe that any of the conferences deal with a crisis."

What they have dealt with, he said, is a clash between reality and expectation, which stems from radically changed health goals.

Dr. Ginzberg told his colleagues at the meeting that they had presented a series of speakers who said, in effect: "Everybody has a right to quality medical care, received in a dignified way, as a personalized service, without wasting his time and without jeopardizing his personal budget."

"To me," Dr. Ginzberg said, "this is all nonsense. We have never had such a system for anybody in this country, except possibly professors of surgery who know how to get their families treated by the professors of medicine. And I am not sure of that."

Another kind of dissent from the hospital report's basic philosophy was made by a member of the committee.

Scott Fleming of the Kaiser Foundation health plan in Oakland, Calif., said that the planning recommendations could be a straitjacket in situations where the need was for change. The potential result, he said, is "planning of, by and for the status quo and serious potential for stifling innovation."

Other critics of the health system as it works today ascribe a measure of the blame to the new big federally sponsored programs.

Government-sponsored care programs such as Medicare and Medicaid have been criticized for making payments on a cost-plus basis. This is an open invitation to inefficiency and rising costs, some experts say.

The Department of Health, Education and Welfare is sponsoring studies and experiments to find more effective reimbursement plans but no one expects a simple answer to the problem.

Planning Essential

Kenneth Williamson, associate director of the American Hospital Association, agreed in an interview that planning was essential.

He suggested that there must be a tighter incorporation of doctors into the business of hospital management. Physicians are the primary users of the hospital, yet often they are almost completely isolated from the economic realities of hospital functioning, he said.

The way the American doctor practices medicine has also been coming under increasing scrutiny. Many experts believe major changes must lie ahead if serious shortages and dislocations of the system are to be avoided.

Partly, these changes are related directly to the fees doctors charge. At the national conference on medical costs last year, one speaker cited the case of a radiologist in New York City who made $100,000 a year and paid his senior technician $185 a week.

Some doctors in large group practice arrangements provide their own laboratory services for patients and make large profits from the laboratory tests. This raises questions, among patients and cost experts alike. Is the doctor tempted to call for more tests than are really needed?

If so, it is a situation against which the patient is defenseless. No sick person or parent of a sick child is likely to haggle with a doctor over the things that need to be done to make the sick person well.

This kind of situation, potential or actual, is a worry to insurance carriers considering broadening their policies to cover more medical treatments outside the hospital.

Within the hospital there are at least some external controls over what the doctor does and prescribes. Outside the hospital there are virtually none.

Some professional observers believe that minor reforms will not be enough. They think major changes are needed in the very fabric and essence of American health care.

As one doctor put it, "It is just no use to build a better mousetrap when the problem is elephants."

April 28, 1968

DRUG STUDY FINDS COSTS EXCESSIVE, A BURDEN ON AGED

U.S. Panel Also Criticizes Research, Marketing and Prescription Practices

By HAROLD M. SCHMECK Jr.
Special to The New York Times

WASHINGTON, Sept. 12 — A Government study group has found that the drug industry makes exceptional profits without exceptional risk and that the elderly bear the brunt of high drug costs, probably suffering more illness as a result.

"The exceptionally high rate of profit which generally marks the drug industry is not accompanied by any peculiar degree of risk, or by any unique difficulties in obtaining growth capital," said the report of the Department of Health, Education and Welfare study group on prescription drugs.

The report, released today, said that the elderly had far greater need for prescription drugs than any other population group and that many could not meet their needs with income, savings or insurance coverage.

'Needless Sickness'

"Their inability to afford the drugs they require may well be reflected in needless sickness and disability, unemployability and costly hospitalization which could have been prevented by adequate out-of-hospital treatment," the report said.

It predicted that the problem would become increasingly serious.

The study group has been at work since May, 1967. Its 110-page document is described as a second interim report. The first, a less comprehensive one, was released in March.

The new report made more than 20 recommendations for improving such diverse matters as drug quality control and pharmacology education in medical schools.

It had some criticisms for almost all facets of the complex system by which drugs are developed, marketed and prescribed throughout the nation.

Report Is Criticized

C. Joseph Stetler, president of the Pharmaceutical Manufacturers Association, said that the study group had made a serious attempt to deal with a complex subject, but he criticized some parts of the report severely.

"The text, especially in the economic and research areas, contains inaccuracies and assumptions that simply do not square with the real world of the pharmaceutical industry," he said.

He said that the report suggested overly simple and premature conclusions based largely on unsupported opinions and secondary source information.

In a statement accompanying the report, Wilbur J. Cohen, Secretary of Health, Education and Welfare, said that the study group had assembled a large amount of basic information, much of it never before available. Volumes will be published periodically.

The head of the group is Dr. Philip R. Lee, Assistant Secretary for Health and Scientific Affairs.

The report said that the department should make a continuing survey of drug costs, average prescription prices and drug use. It recommended continuing, on a high-priority basis, the studies comparing the biological effectiveness of different brands of drugs that are chemically the same.

Research has disclosed cases in which such drugs are not biologically equivalent, but the study group said that the significance of this as a public health hazard had been grossly exaggerated.

The report advocated publishing a national drug compendium listing all lawfully available drugs, their uses and effects, good and bad.

It recommended the publication of objective, up-to-date guidelines for doctors on the use of drugs in treating patients and extra aid to medical schools so that they could improve the teaching of pharmacology.

The group described the teaching area as one in which there had been "much debate but little change."

The report said that the physician was the target of a barrage of advice, information, guidance and promotion of drugs and their use, and that this could be confusing.

"We find that few practicing physicians seem inclined to voice any question of their competency in this field," the report said.

"We have noted, however, that the ability of an individual physician to make sound judgements under these quite confusing conditions is now a matter of serious concern to leading clinicians, scientists and medical educators."

136 Member Companies

The report said that 95 per cent of prescription drug sales were made by the 136 member companies that make up the Pharmaceutical Manufacturers Association. It said that these concerns conducted essentially all of the industry's research and controlled the overwhelming proportion of drug patents.

The drug industry's research and development program was said to total nearly $500-million a year, almost all of it done by about 70 members of the association.

The report said that new drugs developed through research had given physicians remarkable weapons for the improved treatment of infections, metabolic disorders, arthritis, heart disease, high blood pressure and other crippling or deadly illnesses.

Based on the percentage of sales, the industry's investment in research was found to be about three times that of any other major industry.

The study group called the number of new drug products "impressive" — 311 important new single drug entities from 1957 to 1968.

But the report also asserted that a far larger number of drugs put on the market during that period represented minor modifications of existing drugs or new combinations of old ones.

The panel deferred detailed recommendations on providing out-of-hospital prescription drug payment for Medicare patients. These recommendations are expected before the year's end.

September 13, 1968

PATHOLOGISTS BAR LAB PRICE FIXING

In a Pact Ending Trust Suit, They Reject Practice but Admit No Wrongdoing

By EILEEN SHANAHAN
Special to The New York Times

WASHINGTON, June 14 — The College of American Pathologists, an organization of doctors who own and operate almost all of the nation's medical laboratories, agreed today not to attempt to fix uniform prices for laboratory tests they perform.

The agreement brought an end to an antitrust suit filed against the organization three years ago by the Department of Justice. The suit charged the pathologists with illegally conspiring to overcharge the public for medical tests and to keep everyone but themselves out of the medical laboratory business.

Under the agreement, which was filed today in Federal District Court in Chicago and announced here, the pathologists did not admit that they had ever done any of the things they were accused of. But they agreed not to do any of them in the future.

Group Makes Pledges

The organization agreed, among other things:

¶Not to attempt to prevent any person from owning or operating a medical laboratory.

¶Not to attempt to keep the advertising of laboratories not owned by its members out of medical publications.

¶Not to attempt to have the exhibits of such nonmember laboratories barred from medical or scientific meetings.

¶Not to attempt boycotts against physicians using nonmember laboratories.

¶Not to try to fix the salaries that must be paid to directors of medical laboratories in hospitals.

The consent agreement also requires the pathologists' organization to notify all of its own members and organizations representing virtually every doctor in the nation of the terms of the agreement. Organizations of potential competitors of the pathologists, such as the American Chemical Society, must also be notified.

Policing Right Retained

The pathologists retain under the agreement the right to police medical laboratories, to make sure they conform to high professional standards, providing the policing is done "upon an impartial basis."

Insofar as such activities do not conflict with other aspects of the agreement, the pathologists will be permitted "to adopt reasonable and nondiscriminatory technical or performance standards for the operation of laboratories."

The organization can also "maintain a program of inspection and accreditation of laboratories, which program shall be made available upon an impartial basis to all laboratories desiring to participate."

The organization will also be permitted to continue to discipline members who are shown, after investigation, to have been "deficient in moral character or professional competence, or guilty of professional misconduct."

In addition, rules forbidding members of the organization to report the results of their tests to anyone but other doctors will be permitted to continue in effect.

$3-Billion Total Bill

According to the Justice Department's original complaint in the case against the pathologists, the total bills of all the nation's 20,000 medical laboratories in July, 1966, amounted to more than $3-billion annually.

The department did not attempt to estimate how much smaller it believed that figure might have been if prices for medical tests had not been fixed at what it called "artificially high levels."

The department said that the alleged conspiracy to fix prices had slowed the adoption of advanced technology and equipment in laboratories and that large, automated laboratories were required to charge the same high fees as less modern laboratories.

The suit did not allege that prices for laboratory tests were fixed on a nationwide basis but rather that they were fixed regionally.

The consent agreement will go into effect in 30 days, unless either party withdraws its consent, which is rare.

June 15, 1969

A 'Gold Mine' for Some Doctors

On the eve of Medicare's becoming the law of the land three years ago, 238 physician-politicians of the American Medical Association's policy - making House of Delegates convened at the Palmer House in Chicago. The A.M.A. had lost its 25-year-long fight against the Federal medical payment plan and the speeches and resolutions of the doctors reflected their anger and disappointment. A few called for a boycott of the new program, some castigated the Washington bureaucracy, while others complained about Medicare's methods of payment for professional services.

In the wings a member of the A.M.A.'s own staff looked on morosely and said, "The fools. It's a gold mine for most of them and they haven't realized it yet."

His point was that in their bitterness at having a Federal program forced upon them, the doctors had lost sight of some of the facts. Under Medicare they would be getting paid for some professional services that previously had been rendered free to the elderly; that payment of "reasonable and customary fees" for 20 million persons enrolled in Medicare would be guaranteed by the Government; and that many elderly and retired persons who had hesitated to see a doctor because they didn't have the money, now would do so, thus increasing the number of fees.

Unforeseen Dividends

Medicare allowed two methods of payment. The patient could either pay his physician in cash when a bill was presented and then send the receipt to reimbursement offices designated by Medicare, or the doctor sent the bill and the payment was sent directly to him. An important point that was overlooked by doctors when the program went into effect was that in either case a record was kept by the Medicare apparatus.

In the past three years many doctors have found out that the Federal legislation they had fought bitterly for years was indeed yielding professional fees beyond their expectations.

Some doctors were immediately wise enough to sense the financial possibilities of Medicare, such as a general practitioner who was clearing $25,000 a year in his Brooklyn practice. He moved to Miami Beach, started catering to the Medicare generation and his after tax income shot to $75,000 a year. He did complain, however, that the constant round of house calls to the aged was getting him down.

In recent months Federal and state investigators have begun turning up many cases—though still a small minority of the profession—in which doctors and other health care professionals, such as dentists and pharmacists, have been receiving enormous fees from Medicare and another Federal medical payment program called Medicaid which is for the benefit of the poor and the disabled. Medicaid payments are made directly to medical professionals by city or county health or welfare agencies in the 40 states that have programs. The comprehensiveness and administration of the programs vary from state to state.

A Miami osteopath, for example, solved the house call problem by having the patients come to the clinic and hospital he opened. Federal records showed he took in $286,866 in Medicare fees in 18 months.

Last year a spot check of dental work billed to New York State under the Medicaid program showed that 18 per cent either had not been performed or was "very poorly" done. Earlier this year, one Harlem dentist was suspended from participation in the Medicaid program after it had been found that he had been taking in $300,000 a year for himself and the nine dentists he had hired to help him.

Last week at Senate Finance Committee hearings Senator Russell B. Long, Democrat of Louisiana, cited examples of a general practitioner who had billed Medicare for $58,000 in 1968 for house calls to 49 patients, and of another G.P. who had been paid $42,000 by Medicare for administering 8,275 injections to 149 patients in a year.

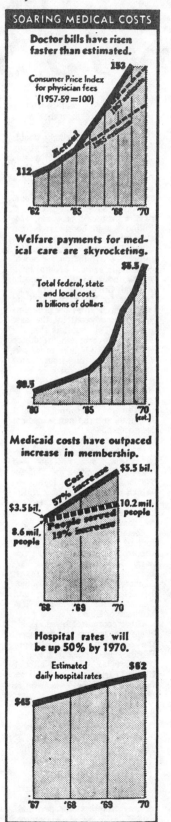

SOARING MEDICAL COSTS

Doctor bills have risen faster than estimated.

Consumer Price Index for physician fees (1957-59 = 100)

Welfare payments for medical care are skyrocketing.

Total federal, state and local costs in billions of dollars

Medicaid costs have outpaced increase in membership.

Cost 57% increase — $5.5 bil.
$3.5 bil. — 10.2 mil. people
8.6 mil. people — People served 19% increase

Hospital rates will be up 50% by 1970.

Estimated daily hospital rates $62 / $45

Senator Long said cases such as these had helped push the voluntary program covering doctors' fees under Medicare to $1-billion a year more than had been originally estimated. The hospital insurance program for the aged under another section of Medicare is costing $3-billion a year more than was foreseen in 1965.

The Senators spilled out reams of statistics: The cost of Medicaid has tripled in four years; cost increases are triple the increased number of Medicaid patients; the average daily cost of hospitalization has risen 25 per cent in the past two years, while physicians' fees since Medicare started have risen at a rate that is double the increases of the years before the program started.

Because of the computerized medical records kept by Medicare, Federal overseers are beginning to find out which doctors and which hospitals are charging unexpectedly large fees or treating unusually large numbers of patients. Armed with better records, state and local investigators of the Medicaid program, which is paid for by a blend of Federal, state and city money, also are starting to check into not only the cost of the medical care being paid for but also the quality of the services.

Pressures Build

Wilbur Cohen, the former Secretary of Health, Education and Welfare who was the architect of Medicare, warned that if doctors don't hold down fees "we are going to see pressures for some kind of control."

Last week these pressures started building. The Internal Revenue Service began checking the tax returns of medical professionals getting large sums from Medicare, Medicaid, Blue Cross and Blue Shield. A decade ago it was almost impossible to check a doctor's income against his tax return because most payments were made in cash by individuals. Today, however, the check-writing computers of Medicare, Medicaid and other health plans pay most bills—and the machines have long memories.

Some of the doctors who warned of "governmental interference in medicine" three years ago now may have cause for alarm, but for reasons they never anticipated. Doubtful doctors have been told for years that computers were going to revolutionize medical care—soon they are going to know why. —RICHARD D. LYONS

July 6, 1969

National Health Insurance Proposed by 15 Senators

By RICHARD D. LYONS
Special to The New York Times

WASHINGTON, Aug. 27—A bipartisan bill that would create a comprehensive health insurance program for all Americans at an estimated cost of $40-billion a year was introduced in Congress today by 15 Senators.

As envisioned by its sponsors, the plan would cover three-quarters of all personal health expenses. It would be an expanded Medicare program for people of all ages, not just those 65 or over.

While half a dozen similar concepts have been introduced in Congress, the bill offered today, unlike most of the others, includes detailed proposals on financing.

A Health Security Trust Fund, similar to the Social Security Trust Fund, would be set up. Into it would go special income and payroll taxes that would cover 60 per cent of the system's cost. The remaining costs would be met from general tax revenues, to which all taxpayers contribute.

The Health Security Act, as the bill is titled, deals not only with financing but also with reforming the organization and delivery of health care services. Public health experts have long contended that disorganization has substantially contributed to driving up medical costs, which in the last decade have risen twice as fast as consumer prices in general.

Senator Edward M. Kennedy, Democrat of Massachusetts, who introduced the bill, said in a Senate speech, "Until we begin moving toward national health insurance, neither Congress nor the medical profession will ever take the basic steps that are essential to reorganize the system."

Thirteen Democrats and two Republicans are sponsoring the measure, and several other Senators are expected to join them. Three other Senators have introduced or will introduce national health insurance plans of their own.

While it is extremely doubtful that this bill, or anything like it, will be passed by this session of Congress, supporters of a national health insurance program say that such a system will be created in this decade.

Of the $40-billion total cost of the proposed program, $24-billion would be derived from the special payroll and income taxes. The remainder of the $40-billion — $16-billion — would come from general Federal revenues. About $6-billion that the Federal Government now contributes to Medicare, Medicaid and other health-care programs would be covered by the new program. The result is that the Federal Government would be investing $10-billion more out of general revenue than it now spends for health care.

The total Government expenditures for all health costs is $20-billion, but part of this is used to train personnel, to build hospitals and to finance medical research.

Reuther Played Role

The bill stems from spadework done over the last year by the Committee of 100 for National Health Insurance, which was organized by Walter P. Reuther, the late president of the United Automobile Workers.

Members of the committee include Senator Kennedy and the three principal co-sponsors, Senator Ralph W. Yarborough, Democrat of Texas; Senator John Sherman Cooper, Republican of Kentucky; and Senator William B. Saxbe, Republican of Ohio.

Other committee members include Dr. Michael E. DeBakey, the Houston heart surgeon; Whitney M. Young Jr., executive director of the National Urban League; and Mrs. Albert D. Lasker of New York, who is prominent in medical affairs.

Details of the bill were prepared mainly by another committee member, Dr. I. S. Falk, professor emeritus of public health at Yale University, who is an authority in the field of health economics.

Would Start in 1973

Benefits, which would start in mid-1973, would cover all services "required for personal health" with the exception of long-term institutional care, psychiatric and dental care, and some drugs and medical appliances. "The four exceptions are dictated by inadequacies in existing resources or in management potentials," Senator Kennedy said.

Other areas that would not be covered include the cost of personal items such as toothbrushes and nonprescription drugs such as aspirin.

No fees would be charged to those persons taking advantage of the system, which would be called the Health Security Program. Providers of services, such as doctors and hospitals, would be directly compensated by the program. The system would be flexible to allow compensation either on a fee-for-service, a per-capita or a retainer basis.

Mr. Kennedy emphasized that the bill would not set up a national health service of Government-owned facilities and federally employed doctors, as is the rule in Europe. He said the bill sought a "working partnership" between the public and private sectors of the economy.

All residents of the United States would be eligible for benefits. The program would not require a means test; that is, proof that the prospective user of the program is unable to afford adequate medical care. This test is an unpopular feature of the Medicaid program of health care for the needy in some states.

One significant benefit would be the plan's coverage of what is referred to as preventive medicine—the early detection, through physical examinations, of disease before it becomes serious. Such coverage is a major omission from the Medicare program and from many private health insurance plans.

The program would set national standards of performance for professionals and institutions. It would supplement existing health manpower training programs. It would create a Health Security Board under the Secretary of Health, Education and Welfare—which would set national health policy.

Hospitals would be paid on the basis of budgets approved by the new system's supervisors. This one item could force hospitals, many of which are considered inefficiently run, to institute economies and management changes.

Up to 5 per cent of the money in the health trust fund would be earmarked for innovations and improvements in the nation's health delivery system. These might include modern food service and laundry systems in hospitals.

Under today's proposal, Medicare, Medicaid and other existing and sometimes conflicting Federal health programs would be scrapped and some state programs would be superseded by the Health Security Program.

The bill would impose a 3.5 per cent tax on employers' payrolls. The percentage paid by employers and employes is left open. In addition, a 2.1 per cent tax would be assessed on individual income up to $15,000 a year.

Estimate on Cost

Mr. Kennedy said, "Had the program been in existence in 1969 it would have paid approximately 70 per cent of the $53-billion in total personal health expenditures," or $37.1 billion. If current statistics were used the amount would be about $40-billion.

Other national health insurance proposals before Congress are less sweeping than that introduced today. The American Medical Association, for example, has a Medicredit plan calling for negative income taxes that would cost an estimated $15.5-billion. Most of this money would be used to pay the medical expenses of low-income families.

The Nixon Administration has proposed a Part C to Medicare and Medicaid that would cover more comprehensive services for the elderly and the poor. This is being studied by the House Ways and Means Committee.

The other sponsors, all Democrats, are George S. McGovern of South Dakota, Walter F. Mondale of Minnesota, Claiborne Pell of Rhode Island, Philip A. Hart of Michigan, Alan Cranston of California, Harold E. Hughes of Iowa, Birch Bayh of Indiana, Lee Metcalf of Montana, Eugene J. McCarthy of Minnesota, Edmund S. Muskie of Maine and Stephen M. Young of Ohio.

August 28, 1970

Myth and Reality: Problems of Health Care

By ELLIOT L. RICHARDSON

WASHINGTON — Social issues are often shrouded in myth and misconception. As an example, for too long it was popularly believed that fathers of welfare families irresponsibly abandoned their wives and children to live carefree, devil-may-care lives financed by the public's largesse. But careful analyses by social scientists revealed that, in fact, able-bodied men on welfare were often forced by the system to leave their families.

Health care in the United States is a current example of a vast social issue encrusted with a layer of invention and illusion. We all know there is something wrong with the current health care system, and it is commonly held that too few doctors, greedy insurance companies, and an apathetic government are at fault. But are these the real problems? Does such conventional "wisdom" mislead us to propose inadequate solutions to complex problems? Let us examine some of the nation's health myths in order to see the Administration's health proposals in light of the true problems behind them.

Myth: The United States is the only major industrial nation in the world that does not have a national health service or a program of nationalized health insurance. This claim was made last month on the floor of Congress, and the idea is widely shared, even among some health "experts." Those who hold this view seem to have in mind the British and Eastern European model in which health services are paid for out of general tax revenues.

But the British model is not the typical Western European model. In fact, continental health-insurance schemes are predominantly financed by employer-employe contributions and operate within the framework of national standards. This is basically the route the President has proposed that we travel—national health insurance, not nationalized health insurance.

Myth: There is a gross shortage of doctors in America. In fact, we have one of the highest ratios of doctors per capita in the world—and the number of physicians is growing at a rate faster than the population. The basic problem is maldistribution. There are too few doctors in the ghettos, in rural America and in the primary care disciplines, such as general practice and pediatrics, while there is no real shortage of doctors in suburban practices or in certain specialties like surgery. To meet this paradox of scarcity amid plenitude, the Administration has proposed incentives to bring doctors to the areas and types of practice where they are most needed.

Myth: It is better doctoring that is making us a healthier nation. In fact, infant mortality rates have declined and longevity has increased due largely to better nutrition and sanitation, higher income, and improved education. For example, when we replaced the horse and buggy, the death rate of infants and children fell because of an accompanying decline in fatal diarrhea caused by animal filth. In recognition of these interrelationships, the Administration has proposed efforts to clean our environment, provide a basic income for poor families, provide adequate nutrition, and make education available to more people. In truth, the Administration is concerned about health and not only medical care. That is one reason why we feel that very expensive federally financed health insurance schemes may, in fact, preempt too large a share of Federal tax revenues for medical care, when a more balanced approach would better achieve health goals.

Myth: Insurance companies are getting fat on health insurance. In reality, these companies on the average have retained less than 6 per cent of premiums for administrative overhead and profit on group health insurance. The Administration's choice to build upon the present strengths of our system was based on a desire to reform, not dismantle, our health care institutions. We see no need to create another mammoth bureaucracy in response to the misconception that we are making the rich richer.

An Old Saying: "An ounce of prevention is worth a pound of cure." Not all ancient wisdom is myth. Prevention is a more satisfactory solution than cure. It can be demonstrated that significant improvements in our health status will come about more through prevention of accidents and chronic disease than through improvements in curative medicine. The President's proposed health education, accident prevention, and biomedical research programs are targeted at those areas of prevention where we can hope to have the greatest success.

With our health program we have attempted to eschew the simple, grant solution, which often turns out to be both expensive and misdirected. A hallmark of a responsible government is the ability to distinguish between sound reasoning and chimeras.

April 2, 1971

All-Embracing Health Care or Band-Aids?

To the Editor:

Secretary Elliot L. Richardson in "Myth and Reality: Problems of Health Care" does indeed dispel some myths, but he also obscures some issues. [Op-Ed April 2.] Western European financing mechanisms do display great variety. But they have one characteristic in common—everyone is entitled to care as a matter of right. The Nixon Administration proposals fall far short of this goal.

Yes, we do have a high ratio of doctors to population; and maldistribution, both in geographic and functional terms, is a major problem. We have shortages of physicians both in cities and rural areas. We have shortages of primary-care physicians and gross excesses of surgeons.

But to suggest that the Nixon proposals will significantly effect a redistribution in our lifetime is illusory. This is not to suggest that the problem is an easy one to solve.

For the Russians, the British and the Swedes, with much more "control," have been only marginally successful. But we can do much better than the Administration proposes. Better incentives are possible.

Yes, most of the progress which has been made in reducing mortality and morbidity has been through means other than doctoring. Prevention is indeed better than cure. But where are the preventive efforts even under existing legislation and Congressional appropriation?

Why are we seeing more measles in 1971 than in preceding years when it is a wholly preventable disease? The Family Planning Services and Population Research Act of 1970 authorized the President to spend $225 million for family planning services and $145-million for research over a three-year period. This was to be in addition to more than $100 million being spent in these areas. President Nixon described this as "landmark legislation." This money is not being spent.

How can we accept Mr. Richardson's assertion that "the Administration is concerned about health and not only medical care"? Where is the balance? What are the priorities?

Yes, Mr. Richardson is right. The insurance companies are not getting fat on health insurance. But the insurance industry has largely been concerned only with paying the bills, not with what they might do to improve the system.

Their posture and their mode of action have been major contributors to the horrible inflation in the costs of medical care. The Administration proposes to give them a larger role, more money and little constraint.

What the United States needs now is a firm and well-defined health policy, a national health program which asserts the right of every citizen to prevention, to treatment, to rehabilitation, to access, to availability, to quality of care to the best of our capability in knowledge and in application, at a cost which is acceptable to our society.

What this Administration is doing and proposes to do falls far short of that. A box of Band-Aids just won't do it.

SIDNEY S. LEE, M.D. Associate Dean
Harvard Medical School
Boston, April 2, 1971   April 10, 1971

Nixon Assails Liberal Plan For National Health Care

By RICHARD D. LYONS
Special to The New York Times

ATLANTIC CITY, June 22— President Nixon for the first time today strongly attacked a bipartisan liberal proposal for national health insurance, telling the American Medical Association that it "would tear apart" the present health care system.

Mr. Nixon told an approving audience of several thousand doctors and guests that a national health insurance plan like that proposed by Senator Edward M. Kennedy would cost too much and would burden the doctor "with the dead weight of more bureaucracy, more forms, more red tape."

The President did not refer specifically to the Kennedy proposal, which the Massachusetts Democrat has introduced into Congress with bipartisan liberal support as well as that of organized labor. A White House spokesman later made it clear, however, that Mr. Nixon had been speaking of the Kennedy plan when he said:

"I believe that the most expensive plan that has been offered in the current discussion on health care in America — a plan for nationalized compulsory health insurance — is the plan that would actually do the most to hurt American health care."

Mr. Nixon referred to his own health legislation, which is aimed at solving what he has called a "massive crisis in health care," but he did not comment on the A.M.A.'s own proposal.

The President's program would rely heavily on private enterprise by mandating that every employed American and his family members be given a private health insurance policy whose premium costs would be shared by the employer and employe. In addition, a family health insurance program would use Federal funds to buy policies for the poor. About 15 million people who are neither employed nor poor would not be covered.

The A.M.A. proposal would have a similar plan for the poor but would give income tax credits for the purchase of private health policies.

The Kennedy plan—the most comprehensive of all proposals to date—would pay almost all the costs of medical services and would cover everyone. It would be operated by the Federal Government and financed by the Government through general tax revenues and a payroll tax on employers and employes that would be earmarked for health care.

Elliot L. Richardson, Secretary of Health, Education and Welfare, who accompanied the President here today, told the Senate Finance Committee in April that the A.M.A.'s "medicredit plan" would not go far enough in bringing about reform of the health care system. He also challenged the Kennedy plan as too expensive.

Mr. Nixon also indicated, in remarks that were not included in his prepared text, that the national health insurance issue probably would not be resolved soon. He said that the debate on the subject "will be one that will command the attention of the country in the weeks and months and perhaps for years ahead."

During his 35-minute address to the A.M.A.'s 120th annual convention at the Chalfonte-Haddon Hall, the President also appealed for support from the doctors for the Administration's drive against drug abuse.

"The best way to end drug abuse is to prevent it, and America's doctors are the indispensable front-line soldiers for success in this all-important battle," he declared.

U. S. 'Character' Involved

"The health of America is in your hands, and by its health I speak not just of its physical health — its mental health, its moral health, its character. Meet this challenge."

Mr. Nixon noted that he was the fourth President of the United States to address the A.M.A. and the first since President Eisenhower, in 1959. None of the men have been Democrats. According to association records, the others were Calvin Coolidge in 1927 and William McKinley in 1897.

The last four Democratic Presidents were at odds — sometimes bitterly — with the association over social legislation that they desired, such as Medicare, but that the association opposed.

Mr. Nixon's relations with the association have been cordial. He even went to the extent of not appointing as the nation's top medical officer a physician whom the association leadership opposed, Dr. John Knowles of Boston. The man subsequently given the post, Dr. Roger O. Egeberg, and his successor-designate, Dr. Merlin K. Duval, accompanied Mr. Nixon here today.

After his speech, Mr. and Mrs. Nixon met socially for about 20 minutes with association leaders, including the current president, Dr. Walter C. Bornemeier of Chicago; the president taking office tomorrow, Dr. Wesley W. Hall of Reno, and Dr. Max H. Parrott of Portland, Ore., the chairman of the association's board of trustees.

Dr. Parrott commented later that the nation's doctors "will be more than glad to join" in the Administration's campaign against drug abuse.

He added: "We would like to second the President's objections to health care programs that might lead to complete Federal domination. We agree that such a health system would be almost prohibitively expensive and unworkable."

Of the national health insurance plans before Congress, the A.M.A. proposal has drawn the widest support — that of about 140 Congressmen.

The Senate Finance Committee has already held hearings on national health insurance. Representative Wilbur D. Mills, Democrat of Arkansas who heads the House Ways and Means Committee, has announced that he will start hearings next month.

The potential cost of national health insurance has been paramount in the debate on the issue thus far, and Mr. Nixon was quick to bring the subject up today.

He said that if the Kennedy proposal were passed "by fiscal year 1974 it would cost the Federal Government over $77-billion—It will drive the health share of the Federal budget to nearly 25 per cent." The President went on:

"Our present Federal health programs, if continued, would cost the average family in America an estimated $405 per year by 1974. My plan would increase that cost, but increase it only to $466 per year. Under the nationalized compulsory health insurance program, the average household's, the average family's American Federal tax bill for health programs alone would be tripled to $1,271 a year.

He also said the Kennedy plan would lead to "complete Federal domination of our medical system."

"The Administration's health insurance partnership would build on the strength of the present health care system. Nationalized health insurance would tear that system apart," Mr. Nixon said.

In recent months the Kennedy forces and the Committee for National Health Insurance have taken issue with the numbers used by the Administration in attacking their proposal. They have contended that it would cost $68-billion, rather than $77-billion, but more importantly, that much of either amount would be money already being spent on health care through Blue Cross, other private insurance, Medicare and Medicaid.

After the appearance here today Mr. Nixon returned to Washington. He flew up at midmorning from the Florida White House in Key Biscayne.

June 23, 1971

Americans Now Favor A National Health Plan

By RICHARD D. LYONS
Special to The New York Times

WASHINGTON, Aug. 8 — Subtly but unmistakably, Americans from all strata of society and all economic classes are swinging over to the idea that good health care, like a good education, ought to be a fundamental right of citizenship.

It was less than a generation ago that proposals for national health insurance put forward again and again by President Harry S. Truman were bitterly resisted as a form of socialism and repeatedly smothered in Congress.

Today, programs that are similar though not necessarily as broad have won the support of a majority in Congress. In addition, they are backed by labor unions, chambers of commerce, hospital administrators, insurance executives and doctors.

Even the American Medical Association, which in the nineteen-forties was publicly characterizing national health insurance as "socialistic" and "pink-tinged," has now come forward with its own version of such a program.

What lies behind this shift in national attitudes is widespread frustration — especially in the middle class—over higher taxes for ever more costly governmental health programs, the failure of Blue Cross and other forms of private health insurance to control soaring medical costs, and the inability of millions to get health services when and where they want them.

But whether national health insurance would satisfy the nation's unmet medical needs or bankrupt the Federal Treasury is still a major question mark. According to a Federal study released last week, cradle-to-the-grave coverage might cost taxpayers $100-billion a year.

Nonetheless, proponents of national health insurance insist that it is an idea whose time has come.

In Congress, for example, a poll conducted by The New York Times shows that as of today no less than 57 Senators and 243 Representatives—clear majorities of both houses—favor one of the major national health insurance plans offered for enactment. At least a score more Congressmen say they will support some form of federally directed health insurance.

President Nixon, who has called for a "new era in American medicine" because the nation faces a "massive crisis" in health care, says his own national health insurance plan is "of the highest priority."

Senator Edward M. Kennedy, the Massachusetts Democrat who is both a potential political threat to Mr. Nixon as well as the leading Congressional proponent of national health insurance, says his more comprehensive program is needed "because the health needs of the American people in the 20th century can no longer be met by the country's horse and buggy medical care system."

And Representative Wilbur D. Mills, another potential White House aspirant who, as chairman of the House Ways and Means Committee, is the fulcrum on which all financial legislation turns, says: "There will be a national health insurance bill through the House this year."

Congress has been flooded with health-related bills. There have been 2,000 in the last session alone, or quadruple the number of six years ago. This session is sure to see more, with at least 45 bills containing combinations of the words "national," "health," and "insurance." But the bills that have

received the most support in brief, are these:

¶The Health Insurance Partnership Act, introduced by the Nixon Administration, would require employers to provide health insurance with a uniform level of benefits to all employes while a companion family health insurance plan would use general tax revenues to underwrite policies for low income families with children.

¶The Health Security Act introduced by Senator Kennedy with the backing of organized labor would pay almost all the health expenses of all Americans through a combination of general tax revenues and payroll levies.

¶Medicredit, an American Medical Association proposal, would have the Federal Treasury cover the health insurance premiums of the poor while income tax credits would be given the more affluent toward the purchase of the insurance.

¶Health Care, backed by the Health Insurance Association of America, would provide both tax credits and policies for the poor, but have the states play a major role in the program's administration.

¶Ameriplan, which the American Hospital Association is having drafted, would set up 4,000 local health care corporations to dispense medical care to everyone, paid for from Federal funds and private health insurance.

¶National Health Insurance, introduced by Senator Jacob K. Javits, would extend the benefits the elderly receive under Medicare to all Americans over a period of years.

The extra cost of these plans to Federal and state taxpayers, if they were enacted in 1974, range from as little as $4.5-billion a year for the A.M.A. plan to as much as $60-billion a year for the Kennedy plan, according to the Government study made public last week. The Nixon plan would cost $11-billion extra, the Javits plan, $48-billion extra, and the Health Insurance Association plan, $15-billion extra. There was no estimate for the Hospital Association plan. These amounts would be in addition to the $33-billion a year that Federal and state governments would be spending on health programs by then.

Compromise Emerging

The huge discrepancy between $4.5-billion and $60-billion is accounted for by the wide variations in who pays for the health insurance. Private health insurance, for which the taxpayer would pay premiums, is the main financial mechanism in some bills. Others would have the Federal Government collect most of the money and pay the medical bills. Ultimately, it is the tax-

payer who pays; the central issue is from which pocket.

A compromise is shaping up between the widely differing proposals, with the basis sure to be cost. Senator Russell B. Long, chairman of the Senate Finance Committee, who has drawn up one insurance proposal, has speculated that the costs of a cradle-to-the-grave health program might rise to $200-billion a year in the near future.

"We might not have anything else, but we sure would be healthy," he commented dryly.

Yet money is no guarantee of results. In 1967, for example, the life expectancy of American men actually dropped while health expenses continued to rise. Federal committees continue to turn out massive reports documenting the fragmentation of the nation's health delivery system and the lack of quality results.

Many public health specialists foresee even worse times ahead for the American health care system, especially the delivery of services to the urban slums and rural areas.

"True reform of the medical system is not going to happen in my lifetime," says Dr. Sidney Lee of the Harvard School of Public Health. "Practical reforms are available, but they're not being pushed."

Paul D. Ward, a health planner in San Francisco, put it this way: "I'm pinning my hopes on chaos — only when conditions become sufficiently chaotic will there be genuine reform."

Backed 2 to 1, in Poll

Both men and most other experts believe, however, that national health insurance — a means of reforming the financing of care though not necessarily its quality or quantity— is both inevitable and near. A Louis Harris poll conducted last February found public support for such a plan running at almost two to one.

Behind the resurgence of interest in health insurance as a political issue there is a pervasive feeling, among experts and laymen alike, that the nation has failed to provide quality medical care to all its citizens.

In the simpler world of the nineteenth century, good, even adequate, medical care went to the rich, the privileged and the lucky. But the twentieth century has brought with it not only a vast expansion of medical knowledge and capabilities but also a far more intricate system of delivering services. In place of the doctor and his black bag are platoons of medical specialists, vastly intricate machines, and sprawling medical centers that can provide far better health care but at a far greater price.

Consumers have thus had to pay large increases in doctors'

fees, hospital bills and insurance payments, and this in turn has led to an enormous growth in health insurance. A generation ago only 12 million Americans were covered by health insurance; today, the number is 180 million.

The number is impressive but shallow, for coverage does not necessarily mean low medical costs. Beneficiaries pay about twice as much in out-of-pocket expenses for health care as is covered by their policies. This has led to considerable bitterness among members of the middle class who have believed that they were "covered" only to find that they were financially liable for large medical bills.

A Long Island insurance salesman, mindful of the potential costs of serious illness, bought what he considered the best possible health insurance policy for his family. Yet when his son was seriously injured in a football accident, the father found that he was liable for medical bills of over $50,000.

The wife of a Manhattan hotel employe was hospitalized for diabetes for seven weeks at a cost of $5,895.95. Blue Cross and Medicaid picked up all but $986.12 of the bills, but how was the husband going to pay the remainder with take-home pay of $84.33 a week?

Going from doctor to doctor is impossible for many residents of urban ghettos and rural areas because doctors are so hard to find. According to some estimates, between 35 million and 45 million Americans — mainly members of minority groups living in ghetto and rural settings—are not receiving adequate medical care. This is most dramatically displayed in the life expectancy of American Indians, 42 years, a full quarter of a century less than whites.

To further complicate the list of grievances against the health care system, there may at times be too much health care, rather than too little. Surveys have found that the United States has twice as many surgeons per capita as England and Wales, and that these American doctors perform twice as many operations as their British counterparts.

These examples and millions of other complaints combine to underline the depth and complexity of the troubles besetting the American system of health care. Remedies such as the Medicare and Medicaid programs, which were enacted in 1965, were supposed to provide medical care to the two groups in American society that needed it most—the elderly and poor. Medicare has been a qualified success, but Medicaid, it is generally agreed, is a catastrophe.

Medicaid Benefits Reduced

Dr. Jeoffry B. Gordon, head of outpatient services at University Hospital in San Diego, said increasing demands by the county and state that the poor pay for their medical care have drastically reduced Medicaid benefits there. "Many people who need care are voting with their feet and staying away—they can't afford it," he said, adding that some cross to Mexico for treatment, while others patronize faith healers.

According to Dr. Ray E. Trussell, a former New York City hospitals commissioner, Medicaid benefits have been repeatedly reduced there because "we started too big a program overnight, one that could not be supported by the local tax base."

Hospital officials in Phoenix say the main reason that Arizona—along with Alaska one of the two states without Medicaid—did not adopt a program was the fear of the "Anglo" politicians that the state's share of providing medical services to large Chicano and Indian populations would have bankrupted Arizona's treasury.

In addition to the complaints of the poor, labor is angered with rising medical costs that erode fringe benefits won at the bargaining table; the powerful medical lobbies are wrestling over who and what would control a national health insurance program, and private industry has become aware that there might be money to be made in such a system.

'Sweepstakes Is On'

The result, says a Congressional aide who has watched the emergence of the health insurance issue, is that "the great health care sweepstakes is on. Congressmen are trying to get all the political mileage they can out of the issue. It's pure political cynicism, but every Congressman has to have a bill with his name on it to show to the voters."

Since the first batch of insurance bills was introduced

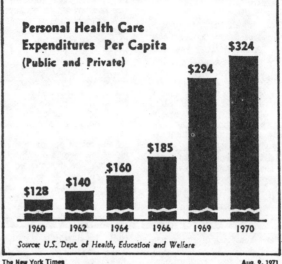

Personal Health Care Expenditures Per Capita (Public and Private)

$128 — 1960
$140 — 1962
$160 — 1964
$185 — 1966
$294 — 1969
$324 — 1970

Source: U.S. Dept. of Health, Education and Welfare

The New York Times   Aug. 9, 1971

in January, there has been a tremendous amount of lobbying, bickering and criticism of the plans. The Nixon proposal has been attacked for being too complicated and for not offering the same benefits to the poor and the middle class. The Kennedy concept is faulted as being too expensive, the A.M.A. idea as not containing cost controls, and the Health Insurance Association program as pandering to the greed of the insurance interests.

Congressional party lines have become blurred over the issue. In general, however, conservatives tend to support the A.M.A. and Health Insurance Association bills, liberals the Kennedy and Javits ideas, and centrists the Administration's concept.

The shopping list of major insurance bills has one significant omission, which might be the most important proposal of all. This is the bill that Mr. Mills says he will introduce "with my name on it."

Mr. Mills says his bill will "obviously be some kind of

compromise, but I'm not sure what it will contain," although he adds that benefits would "be pretty nearly equal" for the poor and the middle class.

Dr. Russell B. Roth, a leader and spokesman of the American Medical Association, says health services for the poor should be paid for by tax dollars, rather than payroll deductions. "We think this is a nonnegotiable point," he said.

Dr. Roth raised another issue —who would oversee a national health insurance system? The A.M.A. wants panels of doctors to act as watchdogs under a "peer review system." A.M.A. critics are wary of the idea, insisting that independent surveilance would be necessary. But Dr. Roth foresees a compromise.

Compromise was also predicted by Senator Clinton P. Anderson, Democrat of New Mexico, who is a member of the Finance Committee and was a cosponsor of the Medicare bill. "A lot of people are going to start asking the tough ques-

tions in the next few months which I'm sure will lead to some kind of compromise in which the best features of each bill are picked up," he says.

"The potential costs scare the hell out of me because I pay taxes, but I wouldn't worry too much about money," he adds. "It might be possible to put in $10-or $15-billion of Federal money, but it might be less than that." Mr. Anderson believes that Senator Abraham A. Ribicoff, Democrat of Connecticut, "might act as the catalytic force between the right and the left in getting a bill out."

Ribicoff Has Hopes

Mr. Ribicoff, who has a staff at work examining the main pieces of health legislation, says: "I hope to come out with something meaningful, but I'm not going to be in a hurry. Too much time is being spent talking about money, rather than discussing reform of the health system that would benefit the people."

President Nixon said five months ago that he would "soon" be sending to Congress additional legislation to regulate the health insurance industry as a companion to his health insurance partnership act. The time lag, in addition to the lack of fanfare over the introduction into Congress of the Administration's main bill, has led to speculation that the President really is not pushing a health program. Some have suggested that Mr. Nixon was merely trying to head off Senator Kennedy, politically.

Whatever the political nuances, Mr. Ribicoff says that Congress and the Administration "will have to take our time to make sure that whatever we pass will be worthwhile."

"As with Medicaid," Mr. Ribicoff said, "the greatest tragedy would be to pass something that ends up as a catastrophe."

August 9, 1971

Six Major Health Plans

Following are summaries of the major national health insurance proposals under consideration. All but Ameriplan are currently before Congress.

The Administration

The Nixon Administration's plan, called the National Health Insurance Partnership Act, provides mandatory insurance for the employed and federally financed coverage for the poor. Private insurance companies would underwrite and administer the plan, subject to Government regulation. Subscribers to the working man's plan would receive unlimited hospital and physician services and laboratory and X-ray services, subject to deductibles and co-insurance. There are provisions for catastrophic coverage. Insurance for the poor is limited to 30 hospital days, all in-patient doctors' services and eight outpatient visits a year. Employes and employers would pay for the general plan; insurance for the poor would be paid out of general tax revenues. Federal officials estimate the Government's

share of the cost at $5.5-billion. Employer-employe premiums would rise, they say, from the present voluntary $13-billion to a compulsory $20-billion by 1974.

The Javits Plan

The National Health Insurance and Health Services Improvement Act, sponsored by Senator Jacob K. Javits, Republican of New York, would make health insurance universally available by expanding Medicare to include the general population. Like Medicare, the Federal Government would collect monies and provide coverage through private carriers. But subscribers could choose approved private or employer plans. Subscribers would be entitled to 90 days' hospital care, post-hospital care, all physician-related services, with appropriate deductibles and co-insurance. Drugs for chronic illness would be available in 1973 and annual check-ups and dental care for children under 8 years old in 1975. All citizens and permanent residents would be eligible over a two-year period. The insurance would be paid for through employer-employe contributions and through general tax revenues. The Government's share of the cost has been estimated at $10.5-billion the first year, rising to $68.1-billion by the fifth year.

Medicredit

Under Medicredit, a plan endorsed by the American Medical Association, the Federal Government would pay insurance premiums for the poor and would allow income tax credits to all others toward the purchase of approved private insurance. Benefits would include 60 days' hospitalization, all emergency and outpatient services, all physician services, dental and ambulance services, drugs, blood, psychiatric and physical therapy, subject to deductibles and co-insurance. Catastrophic illness coverage would also be available. Everyone under the age of 65 would be eligible, based on their tax liability. Those who pay no income taxes would receive certificates redeemable for 100 per cent of the cost of approved basic coverage. The A.M.A. estimates the cost at $4.5-billion.

The Kennedy Plan

The Health Security Act, sponsored by Senator Edward M. Kennedy, Democrat of Massachusetts, seeks to establish "cradle-to-grave" nationalized insurance coverage for every United States resident. The plan would provide all physician and institutional services without limits and dental care, drug treatment, nursing-home care, and private psychiatric care with some limitations. Fifty per cent of the cost of the plan would be paid from general tax revenues. The rest would come from a series of payroll taxes. Cost estimates vary from $53-billion to $60-billion by the fiscal year 1974.

Insurance Companies' Plan

The National Health Care Act, the plan of the Health Insurance Association of America, would provide a standard of health insurance through private carriers paid by direct payments to insurance companies, income tax deductions and Government contributions. The poor and previously uninsurable would be covered by state-assigned risk pools. Medicaid and Medicare would remain. Benefits would initially be greater for state pools, with private and group plans offering the same levels of protection by 1976. By then, everyone would be entitled to 120 days' hospitalization, six outpatient doctor visits a year, all in-patient physician services, nursing-home care and well-baby care and dental services for children, subject to deductibles and co-insurance. The insurance association estimates the cost to the Government at $3.3-billion in the first year.

Ameriplan

Ameriplan has not been completely formalized by its sponsor, the American Hospital Association. It is based on the formation of health care corporations. Each corporation would cover a particular area and together they would supervise and oversee health care delivery for the entire population. Benefits have not been clearly defined but they would include a health maintenance benefit package for all short-term care and a catastrophic illness benefit package for chronic, long-term illnesses. The gaps between the two plans would be filled by supplemental, prepaid plans and by private insurance for those who wished to buy it. Cost has not been estimated.

August 9, 1971

Physician, Heal Thyself: I

By ANTHONY LEWIS

LONDON, Oct. 1—Wesley Hall, M.D., the president of the American Medical Association, visited Britain last summer and went away distressed. He observed the National Health Service in a small mining town in Scotland and found it so bad that Americans would never tolerate it.

"The people over there don't know any better," Dr. Hall told the National Press Club in Washington on his return. "It is tragic."

Before Americans shed too many tears for the health of their British friends, it seemed wise to look at a statistic or two. The result of this check shows that Dr. Hall is faithfully maintaining the A.M.A.'s well-known reputation for accuracy and fair-mindedness.

Infant mortality is one widely accepted test of a society's standard of health. In 1969 the rate in Britain per 1,000 live births was 18 infant deaths; in the United States, 20.7.

Then there is the maternal death rate. In Britain the 1969 figure per 100,000 births was 19, the American 27.4.

Not only are those British figures significantly better today. They were achieved, over one generation, from a starting point much worse than America's. In 1945 the infant mortality rate was 46 in Britain, 38 in the U.S. The maternal death rate was an appalling 1,260 in Britain, 207 in the U.S.

That generation is the one during which the British National Health Service, the system of tax-supported medicine for all, was created and grew up. Of course that is not the only reason for the spectacular changes in the figures. But it is certainly not irrelevant that the British standard of infant and maternal survival caught up with America's, and passed it, precisely during the years of the Health Service's development.

Outside the maternal-infant area, Britain publishes death rates for men and women from a number of diseases. A table published in Social Trends, a statistical annual, uses the 1950-52 average as a base of 100. If the rate is up by 10 per cent in a later year, for example, the table would show 110.

Seven leading causes of death were chosen completely at random for comparison with American trends: respiratory tuberculosis, diabetes, arteriosclerotic heart disease including coronary, hypertensive heart disease, influenza, pneumonia and bronchitis. With the same 1950-52 base as 100, these were the U.S. and British death rates for men in 1967, the last year available:

	U.S.	Britain
Tuberculosis	25	15
Diabetes	150	112
Arterio.	160	158
Hyperten.	55	40
Influenza	20	9
Pneumonia	135	118
Bronchitis	253	91

In every one of those randomly selected categories, then, the British figure is lower: the death rate has risen less since 1950-52 than the American, or fallen farther. A similar table for women shows exactly the same phenomenon, except that the British figures are comparatively even better.

Now there naturally may be many causes for the comparative death rate trends. American pollution could be growing worse faster, or family tensions increasing. But not even the sophists of the A.M.A. could read those figures to prove that Britons get inferior medical care.

Dr. Hall should stop shedding tears for the British and start worrying about the real problem. That is the inadequate medical care provided in the richest nation on earth.

At its best American medicine is superb, as British doctors often admiringly remark. But too few Americans get the best. That is why the United States is down farther than might be expected in world health tables, not only in comparison with Britain. In infant mortality, for example, a 1969 United Nations report showed 22 countries with a lower rate than ours.

The characteristic, generous answer to such evident national failings is to spend more money. But we know by now that in the medical field that alone is no solution. The United States spends about 6.9 per cent of its gross national product on health and medical care, Britain only 4.9.

What needs to be changed is the system of delivering medical care to the individual American. It is, as a British medical writer put it, "a desperately inefficient as well as a heartless way of bringing the benefits of modern medicine to the population: despite its wealth the health of America is poor."

October 2, 1971

Physician, Heal Thyself: II

By ANTHONY LEWIS

LONDON, Oct. 3—Robert Deindorfer, a New York writer, was here with his family last summer in Lower Slaughter, a Cotswold village. His four-year-old son, Scott, became seriously ill and spent three nights in a hospital, having numerous tests and intravenous feeding. Scott was in a private room, and Mr. and Mrs. Deindorfer were given a room near him. The hospital's bill at the end was $7.80—for the parents' meals.

That is not a unique experience for Americans in Britain. A fair number have discovered, to their amazement, that in emergencies they can receive free hospital care under the National Health Service.

The experience of Britons taken ill while visiting the United States is not exactly the same. A year ago Reginald Forrester, a businessman, was rushed to a hospital in New York in desperate condition. The hospital would not admit him until it obtained a financial guarantee. He died sixteen days later, and Mrs. Forrester was given a bill for $12,000.

Many horror stories of that kind have been told here—of humiliating terms for admission to American hospitals, of bills beyond British imagination. The general advice is that given in the title of a B.B.C. television program: "Don't get sick in America."

The president of the American Medical Association, Dr. Wesley Hall, recently renewed the A.M.A.'s warning against adoption by the United States of anything like the British Health Service. Americans, he said, must have the freedom to choose their own doctor. But that argument gets the realities in the two countries backward.

Many Americans have no family doctor. The poor rely mainly on char-ity treatment in clinics or hospital outpatient facilities. And there is a geographical factor as well; Five thousand small towns are said to be without any doctor. It is estimated that 40 per cent of Americans have no regular access to medical care. Dr. Hall's freedom is a middle-class myth.

In Britain, by contrast, nearly everyone does have a family doctor. Senator Edward Kennedy remarked on it when he was here last month to look into the Health Service. He asked factory workers and all sorts of people questions about their medical care; among other things, he asked each person the name of his doctor. To his astonishment, everyone came up with a name.

The reason is that everyone in Britain is entitled to be on the panel of a general practitioner in his area. Once he is on that list, he may go to the doctor's office or receive a house call —yes, a house call—without fee and without the slightest red tape, not even a signature. Relations between patient and doctor can in fact be quite personal and old-fashioned in this country.

Money is the more likely reason for A.M.A. opposition to anything like the National Health Service. A British G.P. is not paid fees per visit. He gets a flat Government salary plus additional amounts for special reasons, such as a large list of patients. He has a professional standard of living, but unlike his American counterpart he has no chance of becoming a millionaire.

The Health Service has faults, as British medical people are the first to say. It is underfinanced in many ways; its facilities are often outmoded; remote and poor areas inevitably tend to be short of doctors.

But there are qualities in the British system that ought to commend them-selves to Americans. One is universality. Everyone knows that he is entitled to medical and hospital care, without favor or explanation. Since that is the rule, forms and other red tape are seldom necessary.

Of course the middle-class or the well-to-do still have advantages: They subscribe to private health insurance to assure earlier hospital admission in non-urgent cases or to get private rooms. But almost any G.P.'s office will demonstrate that access to medicine is now as close to a classless affair in Britain as in any Western society.

Another vital quality is the subordination of money as a value in the medical profession. Many American doctors are motivated by traditional idealism, but the system of private practice seems to have turned too many others into grasping businessmen. The American public senses that, and so do many young doctors repelled by the image of their profession. It is a sick society that has doctors as its highest-paid workers.

The National Health Service has had practical results that are readily measurable. There have been dramatic improvements in British health standards in the generation since the service began.

But the psychological benefits may be as great as the medical. In matters of life and death, any civilized society should strive for equal treatment. That is an advantage to the privileged as well as the deprived. It is really a moral advantage.

The Roman Catholic Primate of England, Cardinal Heenan, was speaking last year about contemporary morals. He worried about challenges to decency, but then he said:

"We have made great moral progress. Anyone who sneers at our welfare state needs to live in such a highly sophisticated country as the United States, where a family can be reduced to misery by the cost of medical treatment."

October 4, 1971

Britain Plans Remedies for Health Service Failings

Special to The New York Times

LONDON, Aug. 1—The Government today proposed sweeping administrative reforms in Britain's system of socialized medicine to meet growing criticism of bureaucracy and shortcomings in the service.

The reforms, the first since the National Health Service came into being 24 years ago, amount to a complete structural shake-up of a system cited often as one of the finest examples of socialized medicine.

In recent years that service has come under increasing criticism. There have been complaints about the neglect of the aged, handicapped and mentally ill, the long waiting time for major operations, the refusal of some doctors to visit patients' homes and the lack of adequate medical facilities in many areas.

"The changes are administrative," Sir Keith Joseph, Secretary of State for Social Services, said today. "But the purpose behind the changes proposed is a better, more sensitive service to the public." His ministry was responsible for drawing up the changes, which appeared in a white paper.

The proposals, which will undoubtedly be approved by Parliament, are aimed mainly at decentralization of the vast health service, assuring that regional and local authorities have a stronger voice in policy and planning. "The public will have a vigorous local voice in the remodeled N.H.S.," Sir Keith said.

One of the main recommendations in the white paper—an official statement of Government policy—was the appointment of an ombudsman to deal with specific complaints by patients. Other major proposals called for an entire revamping of the administrative setup.

Community Units Planned

Fourteen new regional health authorities would be created, and under them would be 90 new local health authorities. On a local level, community health councils would be appointed representing districts with populations of 200,000 to 500,000.

"The community health coun-cils will be entirely devoted to representing the patients' interest and would be able to bring tremendous pressure on neglected areas of community health," Sir Keith said. He added that the councils would be able to "demand entry to hospitals and carry out investigations."

All of the recommendations are designed to answer criticisms leveled at the health service that it has become in many instances a corporate body insensitive to individual needs. While each employe contributes about 20 cents a week, it is financed mainly from general taxation. Last year it cost about $4.4-billion to run the service, or about 12.5 per cent of the national budget.

Despite the criticisms, Britons in general, especially those who have traveled abroad and come under the expensive care of private foreign medical services, are grateful for the health service.

It is used by the rich as well as poor, and it is generally true that everyone is accorded equal treatment. No one is denied even the most costly treatment or operation because he lacks the means to pay for it.

But often the comprehensiveness of the service offered causes shortcomings. Patients sometimes have to wait months for major operations because of the shortage of beds in hospitals. These delays, coupled with difficulties in getting specialized treatment, have prompted many persons to join private medical health insurance plans.

Another shortcoming has been the long waiting time in doctors' offices because of a shortage of full-time health service doctors. Many doctors deal with both private and national health patients.

Doctors in the health service are permitted to have 3,500 patients on their rolls and their waiting rooms are often packed.

Criticisms of treatment are mainly directed at the care given to the aged, mentally ill and handicapped. In addition, there have been complaints about the placement of elderly people with physical infirmities into mental homes because the hospitals could not spare beds.

The recommendations are an outgrowth of consultations between the Ministry of Social Services and professional and voluntary medical bodies. They incorporate many of the proposals put forth by the former Labor Government and they are unlikely to stir much partisan criticism.

August 2, 1972

Social Security Rise Becomes A Nightmare for Many Elderly

By DAVID K. SHIPLER

Like millions of other aged Americans, Marie Nashif of Denver will receive a 20 per cent increase in her Social Security check this month. But unlike most, she will not welcome the extra cash.

Mrs. Nashif is among the 187,000 or so elderly for whom Congressional election-year generosity has become a nightmare. The Social Security rise, voted by Congress June 30, has pushed her income just high enough to make her ineligible for the welfare and Medicaid benefits that she needs so desperately.

Mrs. Nashif, a small, alert, 74-year-old woman, suffers badly from arthritis. Until now, her heavy medical bills have been paid fully by Medicaid. But when her monthly Social Security check rises from $138.40 to $166.10, it will surpass the $147 figure that Colorado uses to divide those who are eligible from those who are not.

In exchange for her $27.70 additional from Social Security, Mrs. Nashif will have to pay $5.80 a month in medical insurance premiums, 20 per cent of all doctors' bills, the first $68 a year in hospital expenses, $17 a day after 60 days in the hospital, and the total amount of prescription drugs.

Further, she will lose $7 a month in welfare payments, she will probably become ineligible for food stamps, and her rent will rise, since she lives in Federally subsidized housing where rents are tied to income.

"When I take all this into consideration," she said, "I'll be a darn sight worse off than I am now."

Congressional action could eliminate such hardships, and several bills addressed to the problem are now pending. Last Friday, the Senate voted a solution for welfare recipients by passing a measure that would force states to raise the eligible income limits for welfare by the same dollar amount as the Social Security increases. Prospects for the bill in the House are uncertain.

Even if the bill becomes law, it will not help people who now collect Medicaid and are not welfare recipients, and there are thousands of those in New York City alone who risk losing their medical benefits. The bill addresses itself only to welfare recipients.

Action by States

Some states have already taken action on their own. Gov. William T. Cahill of New Jersey has ordered Medicaid benefits continued for 4,000 elderly who would otherwise become ineligible.

Delaware has allocated $1-million to raise the eligibility income maximums. Gov. Winfield Dunn of Tennessee has changed administrative regulations to keep 7,500 people on the welfare rolls. Nebraska, Missouri, Iowa, Florida and Wyoming are among the states that have increased the income levels that determine eligibility.

No action has been taken in New York. The state's Department of Social Services contends that it has no power to make the necessary changes without approval from the Legislature, whose regular session begins in January.

New York City has already sent letters informing 6,000 elderly people that their welfare benefits will be halted. This means that they will have to begin paying 20 per cent of their medical expenses.

In addition, many aged New Yorkers who are not on welfare and are not addressed by the Senate bill will be hurt by the Social Security increases.

The city's Office For the Aging estimated that 14,696 persons who now receive 80 per cent of their medical expenses from Medicaid will be cut off altogether. In addition, 22,434 who are not on welfare but are fully covered by Medicaid will have until they have spent all their income above the welfare maximum on medical bills. At that point Medicaid will pick up the full burden again. This totals about 43,000 elderly affected adversely in New York City alone.

The figures elsewhere are smaller, ranging from about 10,000 in California to 400 in Vermont. The United States Department of Health, Education and Welfare calculates that nationwide, 187,000 people will become ineligible for welfare and 93,000 will lose Medicaid.

Even many who do not lose will not gain from the Social Security increase, since some states apply Social Security income against welfare payments. As Social Security rises, welfare decreases; the beneficiary is not the individual, but the state.

"I'm all for the increase," said John Maros, administrator of the Wyoming Division of Public Assistance. "The more Social Security they get the less public assistance is needed."

The State of Washington estimates that it will save $2.3-million in welfare payments by next June 30.

"The average pensioner in Alabama won't gain a dime as a result of the increase," said Ruben K. King, Alabama director of pensions and security.

Ban Under Senate Bill

"This is a form of psychological deceit practiced upon senior citizens," said C. Christopher Brown, head of the law reform unit of the Baltimore Legal Aid Bureau. "The Government is giving with one hand and taking away with the other."

This cannot happen if the bill passed by the Senate is approved by the House and signed by President Nixon. Under the measure states would be prohibited from reducing welfare payments in response to the Social Security increase.

The bill would also cost the states additional money by requiring them to raise the income limits for eligibility, not merely for those welfare recipients who are on Social Security, but for all disabled, aged and blind. In New York, many in the disabled category are narcotics addicts.

In most states, elderly people on Social Security receive only small amounts of money from welfare, and their removal from the rolls is less of a hardship in terms of direct welfare payments than it is in terms of the services that are corollaries to a welfare status.

In many states, for example, Medicaid—whose cost is shared by the Federal and state governments—is available only to those whose incomes are low enough to qualify them for welfare, even though the Federal guidelines allow Medicaid benefits for those with incomes up to 133 per cent of the welfare maximum.

Other benefits, such as food stamps, legal help and home-making services, are also often tied directly to welfare.

Bronx Woman Hit

Mrs. Elesabeth Miles of 1365 Finley Avenue, the Bronx, for example, faces the loss of a valuable homemaker because the Social Security rise will make her ineligible for welfare. She is 62.

"The letter came last Wednesday," she said, "and now I have nothing. I have been a widow for 29 years and am completely blind in the right eye and partially blind in the left eye. My son is unable to take of me because he has eight children of his own."

Her monthly Social Security check, to rise from $133.10 to $159.70, will have to cover her $70.40 a month rent, as well as her food and other expenses.

"They say that they are giving me a 20 per cent increase, but they been taking back everything back and all I get is nothing," Mrs. Miles said. "We worked hard to take care of ourselves and they just don't care if we live or die."

In a small, sad room on West 86th Street, Joseph Wolfson, 80, a frail, asthmatic man, spoke with fear. "Most of the time I am in the hospital because of asthma," he said. "I feel all right now, but who knows what can happen next week? I just can't live with that little amount of money and no Medicaid."

Eva Estelle Jackson, 70, lives alone in Montgomery, Ala., and has suffered from tuberculosis and ulcers. She now receives $132 a month in Social Security and $24 in wel-

361

fare, but she has been told that the Social Security increase will raise her a few dollars above the welfare maximum. She will therefore lose Medicaid, which paid several thousand dollars for three weeks she spent in hospitals last year.

"It's gonna hit me hard," Miss Jackson said. "If they'd just left me with a pension of $1 or $2, and Medicaid, I'd have been a lot better off. If I had some illness, I just don't know what I'd do. I'd just be in bad shape, because I've got nobody to fall back on."

Miss Jackson discovered that she will also have to pay a $2-a-month garbage collection fee to the City of Montgomery. Only those on welfare are exempted from the fee.

Another Montgomery resident, Emily Shepherd, 75, is now in the hospital, being treated for emphysema. When her $137-a-month Social Security check rises to $164, she will lose $66 in welfare from the state, ending up with $39 less a month than now, and no Medicaid.

At that point, her choices will

be "either to go into a convalescent home or just go back to my apartment and die," she says. "It's the most ridiculous thing I ever heard of. They should have had a little forethought. They're just a bunch of meatheads in Congress."

In Las Vegas, the Social Security check of Henrietta G. Oberg, 78, will rise from $153 to $183 a month, but her $23 welfare payment will be eliminated as a result, leaving her $7 ahead, but without Medicaid. She is being treated for cancer. "What am I going to do?" she asked.

In Cedar Rapids, Iowa, Mary Wright also lost Medicaid. "It will take it all away from me," she said of the Social Security increase. "I can't afford it. I'm having it all canceled. I got to pay my rent, clothes and feed myself. There's nobody else to do it for me. You can't get any glasses, can't get any teeth—anything you need you can't get."

The difficulties have also affected some younger people. Lennell Frison, 40, a father of

10 in Portland, Ore., is a former foundry worker whose arthritis put him out of a job two years ago. He and his wife, who has diabetes, were told recently that the Social Security rise would mean the end of welfare and the end of medical payments.

"Without that aid to the doctor, man, I don't know how we're going to make it." His wife, he says, works sometimes as a janitor at night, making about $100 a week. They had planned to try to buy the six-room house they now rent, he said, "but we're probably gonna lose it."

Mr. Frison has considered sending his 17-year-old son to work, but he is torn by powerful doubts. "I hate to take my oldest boy out of school, because then he'd be where I am. I think I'd go back to work and punish myself instead. I can't stand up too long. My legs won't hold me. But it gets you. A man ain't nothing if he can't feed his children."

In Hazelwood, Mo., a suburb

of St. Louis, Mr. and Mrs. Russell French face similar difficulties. Mr. French suffers from heart disease and diabetes, she from arthritis and rickets. Two of their children, Charles, 15, and Lorraine, 12, have rickets, and a third, Russell, is diabetic.

"It's the Medicaid that counts," said Mrs. French. "I figure it would cost us $100 a month just to keep my husband supplied with medicine." Neither she nor her husband can work; their Social Security comes to about $400 a month.

The family's physician, who asked not to be identified, confirmed that the French family needed constant medical attention. "Of all my families, this is the one that is probably the most in need," he said.

When Mrs. French was 10 years old and living in Corning, Ark., she recalled, her mother died because she could not get medical help. "If anyone thinks things have changed, they haven't," she said, "because the same thing probably will happen to us."

October 3, 1972

Health Maintenance Program Hurt by Lack of Action

By NANCY HICKS

Despite its promotion by the Nixon Administration almost two years ago, there is growing evidence that the so-called health maintenance organization will not become a major alternative to the current method of delivering the nation's health services in the near future.

While the number of health maintenance organizations — prepaid group medical services —is increasing, the failure of Congress to enact legislation, the growing opposition of organized medicine and the seeming disaffection with the idea by the Administration that proposed it are hampering widespread development.

The prepaid group practice became popular after President Nixon's health message to Congress in January, 1971. In that speech, he applied the term health maintenance organization to the 40-year-old prepayment concept and said that his Administration would support the expansion of this type of practice to reach about one-fifth of the American population.

Although there is no one model, basically a health maintenance organization is set up so that a patient pays one fee each year to a group of physicians for all of his family's

medical services — physician, hospital, emergency and prevention—regardless of how often he uses them.

The method is considered by many health specialists to be an efficient and economical way of pooling resources and organizing health services. In addition, studies have shown that since the group's financial stability is dependent on the health of the enrolled patients, hospitalization and surgery rates are much lower than those of patients with other types of insurance coverage.

The Kaiser-Permanente plans are the largest with about a million-and-a-half enrolled patients. The second larges group is the Health Insurance Plan of Greater New York, which is experiencing financial difficulties.

About six million persons are enrolled in all plans. An additional two million are served through prepayment to private physicians, who may not be in one center and who probably serve other patients on a fee-for-service basis. These cooperating physicians make up medical foundations.

New health maintenance organizations have begun to operate in the last two years, including one that opened in Minnesota last week. The Blue Cross Association, the nonprof-

it health insurance plan, is also heavily involved in developing health maintenance organizations around the country, as are other profit - making insurers.

Yet the systematic development of prepaid group practices has been hampered by slow Federal legislative activity, which would provide grants, or more probably loans, to start new health maintenance organizations.

Late last month, the Senate passed a health maintenance organization bill sponsored by Senator Edward M. Kennedy, Democrat of Massachusetts. The House has not yet voted on a different bill, sponsored by Representatives Paul G. Rogers, Democrat of Florida and William R. Roy, Democrat of Kansas. Congress is scheduled to adjourn within the next 10 days, leaving only that period for the House bill to be passed and a compromise worked out in conference. Many see this as unlikely.

A Health Maintenance Organization office has been set up in the Department of Health, Education, and Welfare, and it has distributed about $15-million to aid groups who need funds for planning or development.

About 80 individual projects are being helped now, though no new projects will be con-

sidered until after a bill has been passed, according to the director, Dr. Gordon K. MacLeod.

Of projects receiving grants, seven are now operating. About 12 will begin to serve patients within a year, Dr. MacLeod predicts.

The American Medical Association, which lobbied against the Kennedy bill, says it wants to see how these programs run before the association will support expansion.

Dr. MacLeod feels this position is uncalled for.

Meanwhile, the Administration seems to be backing away from the concept of health maintenance organizations. Secretary Elliot L. Richardson of H.E.W. has said in speeches that the idea was never meant to be the answer to health reform but one of several "interesting alternatives."

But despite these setbacks, the health maintenance organization will continue to grow, Dr. MacLeod said.

"The Administration did not invent the idea. Many health specialists had come to the conclusion that H.M.O.'s should be expanded before the President's speech. Even without legislation, much has happened and will happen, just because the country is aware of them," he said.

October 10, 1972

Medicare Aid Is Extended To Major Kidney Patients

By HAROLD M. SCHMECK Jr.
Special to The New York Times

WASHINGTON, June 26—The Federal Government announced regulations today extending Medicare coverage to persons of any age who need kidney transplants or regular periodic treatment with artificial kidney machines.

The coverage, which goes into effect next Sunday, is expected to cost the Government nearly $250-million the first year and much more thereafter. Some estimates have indicated it could cost as much as $1-billion a year within a few years.

The new Medicare coverage is of crucial importance to thousands of patients with advanced incurable kidney disease. In the past, many have died primarily because they lacked funds for the high cost of treatment.

The artificial kidney treatments—known as dialysis — cost between roughly $4,000 and $25,000 a year depending on the circumstances and must be continued for the rest of the patient's life unless a transplant is involved. The total cost of a transplant often is estimated at about $20,000.

Now, most of the cost of dialysis and transplantation will be paid for under Medicare regardless of the age of the patient. An amendment to the Social Security law calling for this coverage was signed by President Nixon late last year to become effective July 1.

The rules announced today are interim regulations. Because the type of coverage is unprecedented and because the issues involved are extremely complicated, the Department of Health, Education and Welfare needs more time to work out final regulations. These are expected before the end of this year.

"For the first time, persons with chronic kidney disease who need dialysis or a kidney transplant will not have to face financial ruin in order to prolong their lives in a useful manner," said Dr. Charles C. Edwards, Assistant Secretary for Health in the Department of Health, Education and Welfare, at a news conference.

Dr. Edwards noted that the extension of Medicare to persons of any age who have been disabled for as long as two years, also becomes effective Sunday and said the two provisions are among the most significant additions made to the Medicare program since its creation in 1965.

He said they marked the first time that Medicare had been used to pay the costs of health care for persons other than the elderly and the first time a Medicare benefit has been linked to a specific medical condition.

Because of these circumstances, the kidney regulations are widely considered a test case for Government coverage of catostrophic illness in general.

Training Covered

The interim regulations cover training and equiment for dialysis at home, as well as for the treatments themselves; and also cover alternative dialysis arrangements such as treatment in a hospital center or in a separate commercial facility set up specificially for dialysis. These are sometimes called "free standing" dialysis centers.

Even including cost of equipment, home dialysis is by far the least expensive method, and many specialists also consider it best for the patient. Dialysis in a hospital is most expensive while treatment in a center is intermediate.

Basically, the interim regulations call for Medicare to pay 80 per cent of a "reasonable" cost of dialysis. For administrative purposes they have put this "reasonable" figuure at a maximum of $150 for a single dialysis.

Spokesmen for the department said today this was not a ceiling, but that centers charging more would be asked to justify the higher charges. Centers charging less will not automatically be able to raise fees. Most of the costs of visits to doctors and care for any episodes of acute illness will also be covered.

To prevent a sudden proliferation of dialysis centers and transplant teams, the interim regulations establish a freeze that will be in effect at least until final regulations are drafted.

Under the terms of the freeze, only hospitals and other facilities that are already active in dialysis or transplant work will be eligible for reimbursement under Medicare.

The department said there are 750 facilities in the United States providing dialysis services now and about 235 hospitals performing kidney transplants. Some of these hospitals do only a few such operations a year.

Records of Patients

A registry operated by the National Institute of Arthritis, metabolism and digestive diseases, has records of 8,321 patients on dialysis as of April 1, but estimates that this is only about 85 per cent of the total.

Roughly 8,000 to 10,000 patients a year reach the stage at which they must have regular dialyses two or three times a week, or have a transplant or die. As each new yearly group of these patients is accepted for dialysis under the new program, the number of patients covered by the Government will rise rapidly for the next several years.

An estimated 2,900 kidney transplants were done last year.

The law requires a 90-day waiting period between the time of first dialysis and the patient's entitlement to Medicare coverage, but the regulations permit payment for a tarnsplant without such a waiting period.

Dr. E. Lovell Becker, professor of medicine at Cornell Medical Center-New York University Hospital, who is president of the National Kidney Foundation, called the interim regulations "enlightened" and said the foundation was pleased with them, particularly the lack of a 90-day waiting period for transplants. The foundation campaigned actively for passage of the amendment to Medicare last year.

June 27, 1973

Swedish Medicine Is Troubled

By LAWRENCE K. ALTMAN

Sweden's medical system, often cited as a paragon of sophisticated, socialized health care in a free enterprise setting, is suffering from serious economic strains.

With taxes frozen at the saturation level, concerned officials are wondering how long Swedish taxpayers, the most heavily taxed in the world, can continue to meet the steadily rising costs of their "cradle-to-grave" health services.

Reforms in recent years have not only failed to check the spiral but have also led to widespread complaints of a burgeoning bureaucracy, impersonality in the doctor-patient relationship and disruptions in the continuity of patient care.

Few Swedish experts would suggest that their health care system was unsound in any essential way or that its high standards were declining. Yet few, too, would suggest that other countries try to copy the Swedish blueprint.

As Dr. Bror A. Rexed, Sweden's top health official, told a group of medical educators in Washington last month: "It is not possible to move an organizational structure and a special type of planning process from one country to another. There are too many differences in the general organizations of two societies."

Nonetheless, with the cost of medical care rising in the United States and other developed countries, there is an increasing interest in the Swedish experience, a feeling among medical authorities that whatever its problems, something of value can be learned from it.

Swedish hospitals have traditionally been run by county governments, but it was common until about two decades ago for an individual to choose his own doctor and finance his own medical care through voluntary health insurance.

Since then Swedish medicine has evolved stepwise into a compulsory, tax-based system in which each citizen is assigned to a government hospital where duty physicians treat everything from minor complaints to catastrophic illnesses.

In the process, costs have risen almost nine-fold from

363

$305-million a year in 1960 to $2.77-billion a year in 1972.

To one who spent five months observing Swedish medicine both in vast urban complexes and tiny Arctic villages, there is a striking similarity in the way economics underlies the criticisms that both Swedes and Americans direct at their fundamentally different health care systems.

Indeed, many of the complaints that surface in newspapers and private discussions in Stockholm seem familiar to an American—delays in seeing the doctor for routine appointments or in getting hernias or gallbladder conditions repaired surgically, insufficient attention to preventive medicine, inadequate facilities for old people and for those needing psychiatric care and, above all, costs, soaring costs.

In 1970 major reform legislation was enacted, primarily to hold down costs, but the escalation continued so rapidly that earlier this year the ruling Social Democratic party — despite upcoming national elections—was forced to nearly double a patient's out-of-pocket costs for a doctor's visit.

The reforms of 1970 and other changes since then have had a profound effect on the practice of medicine in Sweden. Among other things, they have done the following:

¶Put most doctors on fixed work-week schedules, equalizing salaries regardless of sex, medical or surgical specialty and stopping salaried physicians from practicing privately in outpatient departments of government hospitals.

¶Attempted to correct a shortage of physicians, particularly in rural areas, by vastly expanding medical school classes so that one in 115 20-year-old Swedes is becoming a doctor.

¶Simplified payment of doctor bills, eliminating the physician's role in collecting fees, stimulating more outpatient care in hopes of cutting down on needless costly hospitalizations, raising costs to patients for the services of the declining numbers of private practitioners, and eliminating private rooms in government hospitals. The rare private Swedish hospitals are confined to Stockholm and Goteborg.

How much of all this could be—or should be—borrowed by the United States? Authorities in both countries tend to become more cautious the more familiar they become with their counterparts' circumstances.

As one Swedish doctor said: "So much of a nation's personality is built into a medical system that you cannot export the blueprint of one system to deliver health care universally."

Delivery of health care is a deceptively simple phrase. It covers the diagnosis and treatment of all known diseases—

A Profile of Two Health Systems

		SWEDEN	UNITED STATES
Population		8,000,000	208,000,000
Life Expectancy (in years)	Men	75.44	67.4
	Women	79.42	74.9
Infant Mortality (per 1,000 population)		13	18.5
Doctors (per 100,000 population)		135	172
Hospital Beds (per 1,000 population)		18	7.4
Average Length Hospital Stay (in days)		11.9	7.9
Health Expenditures (as % of G.N.P.)		8	7.6
Total Tax Burden (as % of G.N.P.)		41.4	30.2

The New York Times/Dec. 23, 1973

the few that can be cured and the many that cannot — as well as the fuzzy margins between emergency, elective and luxury medicine.

Moreover, the design of an effective health care delivery system does not come straight off a drawing board. Rather, culture, history and politics are just as influential as economics in shaping the pattern.

Life-styles, too, are important. Swedes, who live in a highly organized society and stress equality tend to be more patient and disciplined and less individualistic than Americans, which perhaps helps explain why many Swedes have so easily abandoned the free choice of doctor.

Though the need for extensive reforms in the last four years indicates that it was never really a paragon, the Swedish health care system is nonetheless widely admired.

By all the evidence, the competence among Swedish physicians and surgeons—most of whom got their training under the old system—is high, comparing favorably with that in the United States. Like most Americans, most Swedes die from diseases that have been properly diagnosed and treated to the best of their doctors' abilities.

In addition, Sweden produces some of the best health care statistics in the world. For example, the Swedish infant mortality rate of 13 for every 1,000 born is matched by only a few other countries and is much lower than the 18.5 per thousand in the United States.

Moreover, the Swedish welfare system underwrites most of the economic hardships as-

sociated with sickness. Each person who misses work because of illness or disability is guaranteed an income and, for a week, the Government will take the patient's own word that he is ill.

A Swede is also secure in the knowledge that his financial condition will not be ruined by catastrophic illness.

For each visit to a doctor's Government office or to a Government hospital clinic, a Swedish patient pays 12 crowns ($3), the Government health insurance company reimburses 48 crowns ($12) and the local county contributes an estimated 32 crowns ($8). The price includes costs of necessary laboratory and X-ray tests and fees for additional medical consultations.

For each return visit to the Government doctor, the patient pays 12 crowns ($3), whether the appointment is for a complicated diagnostic evaluation or simply for removal of surgical stitches.

However, the Government does not pay for preventive medical care like annual physical check-ups or for birth control pills and contraceptive devices.

Ambulance Service Free

Private practitioners, who treat about one-fourth of outpatients in Sweden, are allowed to set their own fees, with the patient paying the extra costs beyond what the Government will reimburse for the services rendered.

If hospitalization is required, the patient pays 10 crowns ($2.50) each day. The Government pays the remainder, which according to the Swedish Insti-

tute, a Government information unit, is 350 or more crowns ($87.50) for each day's hospitalization.

Ambulance service is free. Taxi costs are reimbursed if the patient needs such transportation. But doctors complain that the Government is apathetic toward checking abuse of taxi privileges—when, for example, patients take taxis to see doctors about nonemergency problems.

Obstetrical care and drugs for some chronic diseases are free.

Insulin for diabetes, factor eight blood concentrate for hemophilia, digitalis for heart failure, anticonvulsants for epilepsy and thyroid extract for hypothyroidism are also provided at no additional cost to the patient. But patients must pay for drugs for high blood pressure, among other conditions.

Drugs not included on the Government's free medication list cost the patient no more than 15 crowns ($3.75) for each prescription. Doctors say that this policy has led to a wastage of drugs because patients often demand the largest possible supply to minimize the out-of-pocket cost.

Problems Within System

Before the 1970 reforms, the patient paid the doctor's entire fee. Then officials reimbursed three-fourths of the fee according to a Government approved schedule. The patient paid additionally for laboratory tests as an outpatient. But inpatients received all such tests free as part of hospitalization benefits

As a result, doctors said, they admitted patients who needed laboratory tests that could have been done on an outpatient basis. Though such hospital admissions reduced the costs to the individual patient, the practice raised the over-all costs to the Government. A similar problem has existed in the United States as an outgrowth of Blue Cross-Blue Shield and other private health insurance plans.

Although the Government has not conducted a follow-up evaluation of the reforms, there are signs of serious problems. Indeed, the Swedes themselves, while generally proud of their health-care accomplishments, are the first to point out that Sweden is still far from a medical utopia, that no one there, to put it another way, has yet cured death.

The price of Swedish medicine to the individual Swede is very high, as is at least indicated by the high taxes that he must pay. Exact comparisons are impossible because of the differing social and economic structures in Sweden and the United States, but this rough approximation can be made:

A Swedish family of four earning 50,000 kroner ($12,500)

a year pays, not counting property taxes, about 55 per cent of its income in national, local, Social Security and value-added taxes. (About one-fourth of Sweden's total tax revenue comes from the 17.65 per cent value-added tax that is imposed on all consumer items.) An American family of four earning $13,000 a year pays, again excluding property taxes, about 20 per cent of its income in Federal, state, local, Social Security and sales taxes.

Earlier this year, the Government almost doubled the basic cost to a patient for each visit to a doctor from 7 to 12 crowns ($3), partly to avoid raising taxes and to finance more resources for outpatient care. For some patients, out-of-pocket costs for chronic care for aftereffects of a heart attack or for flareups of arthritis have risen substantially.

As the young doctors trained at high cost by the Swedish Government begin to flood the labor market, local politicians are concerned whether the counties can afford their salaries. The attitude that it is wrong to profit from treating sick people, coupled with the reforms, has created an atmosphere that has discouraged younger doctors from entering private practice. As a result, Swedes are discussing the possibility of physician unemployment.

A Fatalistic Attitude

Such a prospect elicits a fatalistic attitude from young Swedish doctors whose education has been state-financed and anger from their older colleagues who not only paid for their own schooling but also have vivid memories of the nineteen-thirties when they could not find a job.

Swedes, whose patience is world famous, are often frustrated by long waiting periods to see doctors — several weeks, if not months, for routine medical appointments or years for gall bladder, hernia or other elective surgery in some cities.

Also many are irritated that they often cannot see the same doctor on a return visit, wasting both the doctor's and their own time when the lengthy details of a medical history must be repeated.

Doctors, in turn, complain about the same problem — the lack of continuity and impersonal nature of patient care.

"It's purely accidental if you see a patient the second time," Dr. Peter Reizenstein, a blood disease specialist at the Karolinska Hospital, said in a tone of frustration. He went on: "I can pull out any chart and you will see no more than two visits to any one doctor. Sick patients do mind that."

Indeed, the reforms have been more popular among younger Swedes, for whom lack of continuity and depersonalization have little meaning, perhaps, because so few of them have ever been truly sick.

To physicians, "the fun" of medicine is the satisfaction of following a patient's progress and in evaluating the success of a prescribed therapy. Because more than one way exists to treat many diseases, each physician tends to have his particular solution to the myriad disorders affecting his patients.

Many Swedish doctors feel their intellectual curiosity and medical competence declines when they know the chances are great that they will not see the patients they are examining on the next visit.

"The doctor has lost the little kick he had before to improve his efforts and see more patients," said Dr. Krestin Magard, a surgeon in the Arctic mining town of Kiruna.

Swedish doctors also say they have lost some incentive due to the fixed work-week and salary arrangement. Many acknowledge they would be busier if it were not for the tax system, which discourages working longer than the prescribed period. Further, practitioners say frankly that they are not rewarded for efficiency and that under such circumstances they see no reason to work hard to see 40 patients a day instead of 25 at a more leisurely pace.

Though senior doctors earn about $30,000 a year for their 48-hour work weeks, taxes take such a huge bite — at least 75 per cent — from overtime work that physicians say they are inclined to take time off, not money, in compensation. The net effect, seemingly, is a decrease in productivity.

Doctors formerly would often work up to 80 hours a week, earning from $50,000 to $100,000 a year.

The Swedish medical system permits practitioners complete professional freedom in treating patients without any worry about the individual patient's bill.

Instead, such decisions seem to be made on a broader basis. In the United States, 57,200 open-heart operations were done last year. Swedish cardiac surgeons, who are among the world's leaders, did just 500. This means that about one-fifth the number of such operations were done in Sweden compared with the United States when the statistics are corrected for population differences. Swedish doctors agree economics is the apparent explanation.

A Matter of Atmosphere

Some Swedish medical authorities are concerned that the new atmosphere created by the reforms may eventually undermine the quality of Swedish medicine.

Swedish researchers have contributed more to medicine than might be expected from an Artic country the size of California with the population of New York City.

Swedes have helped develop drugs like heparin, prostaglandins, lidocaine and dextran; devices like artificial kidneys and cardiac pacemakers; sophisticated techniques like ultracentrifugation and electrophoresis; advanced specialties like radiology; and general knowledge of protein chemistry, to cite just a few examples that apply to everyday medical care internationally. Accordingly, Swedes have won their share of the Nobel prizes in physiology or medicine awarded here each fall.

With such a heritage, a booming economy and popular support for science, few were surprised a decade ago when a study found that Sweden, unlike other European countries, was not losing scientists in the brain drain to the United States.

But now 10 years later Swedish leaders are beginning to talk of a threatened brain drain that may affect the supply of researchers and practitioners.

December 23, 1973

Swedish Health Care

By LAWRENCE K. ALTMAN

When Americans with an interest in medicine get together to discuss ways to improve the health care system in their country, they inevitably mention Sweden's system as a model to emulate.

Doctors praise the quality of Swedish medical research. Administrators point to the benefits of regional planning. Medical students envy an education provided free by the Government. Epidemiologists cite a system of centralized medical records that facilitates tracing disease patterns. Journalists quote the favorable statistics of infant mortality and longevity.

News Analysis

However, each group tends to see the Swedish system through binoculars focused on a special field. Few seem aware that Sweden's socialized health system is beset with such problems as soaring costs, long waits to see the doctor, a proliferating bureaucracy and a maldistribution of doctors.

Meanwhile, the Swedish experience appears to be growing more relevant every year as demands mount for fundamental changes in the American system. Already this year, eight major health programs have been introduced in Congress, with two more to come. They cover a broad spectrum of ideas ranging from increased use of privately financed medical insurance plans to the establishment of a national health care system that would be as comprehensive, for all practical purposes, as the Swedish system.

Key Questions Raised

All of this raises several fundamental questions. How much, to begin with, can the United States learn from the Swedish health care system?

There are two things that attract the attention of Americans observing Swedish medicine — protection of the individual against economic disaster from catastrophic illness and regional planning to reduce the costs of treatment that depends on sophisticated technology.

Most Americans are covered by Blue Cross-Blue Shield and other health insurance plans. But some have none, and for the rest, gaps exist in the extent of coverage.

The cost of hospitalization treatment for, say, injuries suffered in an automobile accident can be so staggering as to completely drain a middle class savings account. While Americans can purchase major medical insurance policies to protect against such a catastrophe, many do not. And while some American health insurance plans cover care of birth defects or illnesses associated with the first few weeks of infancy, many do not.

By contrast, the Swedes are secure in the knowledge that their system uniformly protects against the costs of a major, lengthy illness.

As biomedical researchers develop better therapies, health leaders say there is little evidence that care will cost less. Accordingly, they urge more regional planning to avoid wasteful duplication of costly equipment and to concentrate patients needing complex operations like open heart surgery or kidney transplants in centers where specialists can best develop the techniques that maximize a patient's chances for survival.

The Swedish reliance on regional planning to avoid wasteful duplication has helped that

365

small country of 8 million people to make the most of its resources and become an international leader in health care.

One example of such planning is the hospital system. Swedish hospitals, the core of Swedish health care, are structured on a tier. At the base are nonspecialized general hospitals and chronic care nursing homes. At the next level are general hospitals that provide basic medical services according to community size. At the top are the regional university hospitals where the most complex cases are diagnosed and patients requiring unusual methods of care are treated.

Referrals within the system are made by doctors solely on the basis of medical considerations; a patient cannot seek a consultation from a Government specialist without such a referral.

Any assessment of the Swedish health system would have to deal with a series of recent Government reforms.

Sweden, like most other developed countries, has been hit by inflation in medical costs. This has led, among other things, to a decision to freeze the taxes that pay for health care and to introduce priorities and economies in a field where expenditures were rarely questioned in the past.

Swedes agree that it is difficult to answer what impact these major reforms have had because Swedish officials have not yet made any comprehensive evaluation.

Little effort has been made, for example, to run cost-effectiveness studies or to institute formally structured peer review systems like the P.S.R.O.'s (Professional Services Review Organizations) already under way in the United States.

Dr. Bror A. Rexed, Sweden's top health official, says: "I wouldn't advise introducing such a system in Sweden because I don't know how we could manage it. The methodology isn't there."

Another question, basic to Sweden's socialized system, is how equitable is health care there.

Swedes are hospitalized on a need-for-care basis and they take pride in saying that money cannot buy private rooms in the Government institutions. Because of the Swedish emphasis on equality, it is not unusual to see a millionaire sharing a four-bed room and the same staff of doctors and nurses with three laborers or welfare recipients.

However, strong hints that inequalities of care exist within geographic regions came from a study made by Dr. Erik Allander and his colleagues at the Karolinska Institute's department of social medicine.

That study—one of the rare independent evaluations of Swedish medical consumption —found that residents of Borlange, which is not served by a central hospital, had an underconsumption of medical services compared to their neighbors in Falun, which has a central hospital. Dr. Allander said that the gap between services provided and services needed amounted to about $7-million a year and challenged the fundamental concept that all citizens had equal access to care.

Though similar studies could be made to measure medical consumption elsewhere in Sweden, officials have chosen not to do so. Dr. Allander says: "Great inequalities of access to care exist in Sweden."

Equality of care also depends on a balanced distribution of doctors. Swedes, like Americans, complain about the shortage of doctors in rural areas, a situation that results because young doctors and their wives in Sweden generally prefer the urban life.

Signs of Change Seen

The Swedish doctor, like his American colleague, is free to practice where he can find a job. The Swedish Government cannot order a physician to practice in a particular locality. However, signs of change exist as Government health officials are setting priorities on vacancies according to the need for doctors on a geographic basis.

Among the fears many doctors have of practicing in the tundra is that in isolation from their professional colleagues they will not be able to keep up with the rapid advances being made in their fields. Young doctors fear the lack of daily discussion about the fine points of medicine because their older colleagues constantly remind them how important such intellectual discussions, combined with the experience of practice, are to keep a doctor's diagnostic skills finely tuned.

Sweden offers refresher courses for general practitioners and other specialists on a voluntary basis. But Dr. Rexed says that "continuing medical education is a big problem" in Sweden and that "we are really deficient—it is the next job we have in the reform of medical education."

One of the most significant questions about the Swedish health care system, at least insofar as it is relevant to the American health care system, concerns private practice.

Though the Swedish health care program is socialized, much of the country's business is conducted on a free-enterprise basis. Many Swedes own their homes. A few send their children to the dwindling number of private schools.

Private medical practice exists in Sweden but its future is uncertain as fewer younger doctors seem to choose to replace their older colleagues who are retiring as private practitioners. Because private hospitals are rare, private physicians are limited to office practices where they treat about 25 per cent of Swedish outpatients.

Most private doctors practice in Sweden's bigger cities. In Stockholm, for example, private doctors treat 60 per cent of out-patients whereas the private practitioners care for less than 10 per cent of out-patient visits in the northernmost county.

The extent of private practice seems to reflect several factors—the chronic shortage of Government doctors and outpatient facilities; the unwillingness of many Swedes to give up personalized care, and the desire for an independent second opinion about a troubling medical problem.

Further, doctors who have private practices say that many patients come just to talk about problems that they seem unable to discuss with the duty doctor in Government hospitals.

Some Swedes, while supporting the basic health care system, complain that the Government went too far too fast in restricting the options of people willing to pay out-of-pocket for services not otherwise readily available. Cosmetic surgery, for example, may not be offered in a Government hospital, or some types of elective operations like hernia repairs may have long waiting lists.

Indicated by all of this is an uneasiness among the Swedes over how far private practice should be preserved in a collectivized health care system, indeed how far the institution of individual fee-for-service practitioners can be preserved.

And that question, given the fact that private practice seems even more deeply ingrained in the United States than it was in Sweden, is critical to any effort to make a major overhaul of the American health care system.

December 25, 1973

Mr. Nixon and His Doctors

To the Editor:

Among various sweeping assertions and dubious homilies in support of private, profit-oriented medical care which President Nixon offered at the dedication of the Cedars of Lebanon Hospital Center in Miami on Feb. 14, he proclaimed: "When I go to a hospital, or when I call a doctor, I want that doctor to be working for the patient and not for the Federal Government."

He said this one day after his annual physical checkup at Bethesda Naval Medical Hospital, a thorough and expensive procedure carried out by a team of six physicians, every one of whom is on the public payroll and paid by our tax monies.

JAMES MATLACK Amherst, Mass., Feb. 16, 1974

February 26, 1974

The Real Health Issue

The public debate which was supposedly to lead to the enactment of an effective national health insurance program has turned into a sputtering contest of irrelevant and misleading information. After initial signs that an acceptable compromise might emerge from a variety of proposals, the chances of such a rational outcome have been greatly reduced by the tug o' war between those who insist that nothing is needed versus those who demand all or nothing.

Against Big Labor's insistence that only its proposal for a virtually total Federal underwriting of all medical bills is acceptable, now stands the charge by Dr. Russell B. Roth, president of the American Medical Association, that the entire issue is nothing but a politicians' ploy to deceive the American people about such real issues as inflation and unemployment.

Adding to the controversy, the Rand Corporation recently released a study concerning the potential cost of national health insurance, both in dollars and physicians' time, that could easily be misused as anti-health insurance propaganda. The report warned that any plan that covers costs of most medical bills would swamp doctors' offices and outpatient clinics, might add between $8 and $16 billion, exclusive of drugs, to the amounts now spent on health care, and could lead to long lines and even higher bills in local doctors' offices.

*   *   *

All of these threats to the enactment of a workable measure need to and can be answered. The organized medical profession's conservative posture—not necessarily representative of the majority of physicians—will not impress those who in their everyday lives face the high and at times disastrous cost of medical care, let alone those who cannot afford or obtain such care at all.

While the Rand study has performed a valuable service in presenting all the financial options, a careful reading of the data shows that the swamping of medical services can readily be averted by means of reasonable "deductibles" for all but the most indigent potential patients, as provided for in both the Administration and the Kennedy-Mills bills.

Missing from the discussion, however, has been what ought to be at the top of the agenda: the question of how the delivery of health care can be fundamentally improved by reforming the total approach to these vital services, instead of simply debating how to pay for the existing, inadequate and outmoded services. The inevitable move toward national health insurance ought to be seized as a unique opportunity to expand preventive health care. One obvious need is a revision of the recruiting and training of health personnel in order to reduce the use of physicians for the many tasks that can be performed as efficiently and more economically by a variety of health professionals.

The rigidities that have crept into the debate over national health insurance and the deliberate misinterpretation of available facts by vested interests may be doing more than postponing enactment of a necessary measure. They threaten to sabotage essential reform of a deficient and obsolete approach to the nation's health.

June 25, 1974

Medicare and Medicaid After Decade: A Mixed Picture of Gains and Excesses

By NANCY HICKS
Special to The New York Times

WASHINGTON, July 29—Ten years ago tomorrow, President Johnson signed into law the amendments to the Social Security program that created Medicare and Medicaid.

The event, held in Independence, Mo., in the presence of former President Harry S Truman, culminated half a century of political compromise and established the nation's first Government - sponsored health insurance programs.

Ten years later, reports on both Medicare and Medicaid are mixed.

Medicare set as its goal the elimination of the financial catastrophe that illness often meant for older Americans and their families. The program is generally considered a success, —though not without problems —for the 21.8 million elderly and three million disabled people who are currently enrolled.

Medicaid, a joint Federal-state program to subsidize health services for the poor, is not considered a success because of the abuses it has generated. Yet one in five Americans has at some point used it for medical services they could not otherwise afford. Most beneficiaries have been older people with such expenses as that of long-term nursing home care, which Medicare does not cover.

$31-Billion in 1975

The two programs, which are spending a total of $31-billion this year, have had a tremendous impact. Because of this, they will have a major influence on future Federal health programs, most experts agree.

"Medicare was a breakthrough," said Wilbur J. Cohen, who drafted health legislation that was unsuccessfully proposed in 1952 by President Truman, as well as the 1965 package that became law. "In its 10 years, it has broken the back of the ideological opposition to the public role in health insurance" he said.

Mr. Cohen, who is dean of the school of education at the University of Michigan, was Secretary of Health, Education and Welfare in the Johnson Administration.

Federally sponsored health insurance was first proposed by former President Theodore Roosevelt in his unsuccessful 1912 campaign to be elected again. The American Medical Association advocated such insurance in 1916 but later opposed it.

Federal health insurance was almost included in the 1935 act that established Social Security, but was withheld by President Franklin D. Roosevelt, who thought it might jeopardize passage of the program.

Health insurance legislation was introduced but did not pass in 1952, 1960, 1962 and 1964. It was finally enacted in 1965 in the wake of Mr. Johnson's landslide victory over Barry Goldwater.

At the time, the A.M.A. called such programs "incitement to revolution" and "communism." Now doctors overwhelmingly support them. One reason is that Medicare and Medicaid have proved profitable for doctors.

Today Medicare is criticized in much the same way that many other government programs proved profitable for doctors are: as insensitive to those it is supposed to serve and as inadequate in benefits. It is said to have caused inflation of health costs, which it does not completely absorb, and some people say it is too passive in regulating payments to physicians.

Voluntary Aspect

Medicare provides coverage of hospital bills and voluntary insurance for doctors' services. An estimated 95 per cent of those who receive hospital coverage buy the doctor insurance, which costs $6.70 a month. That amount is matched by the Government.

Only about 40 per cent of all health costs of the elderly are covered by Medicare. This represents a decrease in proportion in recent years. Most hospital charges are covered it an illness lasts two months or less. Only about half the doctors' fees are covered, although the program will pay if an illness lasts two months up to 80 per cent of what it considers "reeasonable charges."

A 1970 report of the Senate Special Committee on Aging showed that half of all Medicare recipients were paying $500-million a year in additional premiums for nongovernment insurance to supplement Medicare.

In Medicare's first year, Americans 65 or older paid an average of $236 of the total per capita medical expenditure of $445—Government and private—for their age group. In the fiscal year that ended June 30, 1974, the average individual paid $415 of a per capita expenditure of $1,217.

Nelson H. Cruikshank, the 73-year-old president of the National Council of Senior Citizens, tells of a recent illness of his brother, who accumulated $28,000 in bills in a series of complicated operations. All

but $2,000 was paid by Medicare, Mr. Cruikshank said.

It is this type of illness — short-term, hospital based — that is most completely covered by Medicaire.

Medicaid, meanwhile, is administered by the states. Patient eligiblity, services and payment levels are determined at the state level. As a result, benefits and services are uneven across the country and the program has been riddled with fraud.

The program received very little public attention in its initial years. Then its costs began to soar, legislators took notice and, in 1968, many states began cutting back benefits.

In New York, a watchdog group called Medicaid a "health Christmas" for poor families. A family of four with an income of $5,000 or less had all its health expenses covered in full.

Many Won't Take Part

Medicaid has spawned abuses by some doctors who specialize in Medicaid patients and cut corners or pad costs. Because the program pays physicians about 30 per cent less for their services than Medicare does, many will not participate.

This defeats the primary goal of Medicaid: to increase the access of the poor to health

services.

"Every day I live I see that programs designed for poor people are poor programs," said Robert M. Ball, who was commissioner of the Social Security Administration from 1962 to 1973.

Mr. Cohen agrees. The only social programs that work over a period of time, he says, are those that help primarily the middle class, such as Social Security and Medicare.

Lucille Reitman, associate commissioner for planning in the medical services administration of H.E.W., does not agree. Medicare could not work as well as it does without Medicaid, she said.

"The two programs could not exist without one another," she said, explaining that Medicare provides basic coverage for the elderly and that Medicaid, in addition to providing basic health care for the indigent young, insure the elderly against financially catastrophic illnesses.

Long-term nursing home care is not covered by Medicare. But 40 per cent of the medicaid budget is spent on such care. Seventy per cent of the 25 million recipients are elderly, nmmost of them women, accor ing to Federal statistics.

Medicaid and Medicare have been criticized severely in Congress as inflating the cost of

hospital care. The average daily hospital rate increased 138 per cent from 1965 to 1973, the consumer price index shows.

One reason given was that the legislation had been written with basically no guidelines to control spending. The legislation would never have been passed if such restrictions had been spelled out, Mr. Cohen and Mr. Ball agree.

In 1972, Congress amended the Social Security Act to require panels of doctors to review services covered by Medicaid and Medicare to make certain that they were necessary and consistent with the medical diagnoses. This program is not scheduled to become fully effective, however, until next year.

Medicare and Medicaid reforms have been proposed by Senator Herman E. Talmadge, Democrat of Georgia. He is chairman of the health subcommittee of the Senate Finance Committee, which oversees for the two programs.

The Senator has proposed a new department of health financing to coordinate regulations among various programs that often affect the same hospital or doctor, to monitor fraud and to increase the efficiency of administration. He also would set a minimum level of payment to doctors.

July 30, 1975

Rationing Medical Care

By Harry Schwartz

Vice President Rockefeller has created a ministorm by asserting that government cannot afford to give everyone first class medical care. Mr. Rockefeller's critics feel particularly betrayed because as Governor of New York he was an outspoken advocate of national health insurance and a decade ago sponsored the most generous state Medicaid law in the nation.

The Vice President's critics seem unaware that his present position almost echoes the official stand of the British Labor Government toward the demands on the National Health Service, Britain's generation-old "free" — that is, tax-supported—medical system.

The Wilson Government's position was put this way earlier this year by Dr. David Owen, the man directly in charge of the National Health Service: "The health service is a rationed service. There will never be a government or a country that has enough resources to meet all the demands any nation will make on a national health service."

Last month the editor of the respected British magazine, New Scientist, gave this description of the bitter

reality behind Dr. Owen's words: "The plight of Britain's Health Service conflicts desperately with the avowedly utopian ideals of its founders. Yet the myth persists—the myth that the NHS not only can but does offer a high and unvarying level of medical care to all members of the community. For most of us, it is only when we join a year-long hospital waiting list, or have to take an injured child to a hospital casualty department on Saturday afternoon, that we realize just how threadbare and starved financially the service really is."

But even before Dr. Owen or Mr. Rockefeller had spoken, many medical economists realized that "free medical care"—that paid for by the government rather than the recipient—is a bottomless pit. No society can supply all the medical care consumers could want and that doctors, hospitals and others might provide if there were no limits on resources. Potential demand for "free" medical care is infinite; human resources are finite and there is severe competition for these resources from many quarters.

This conclusion is a bitter one, especially for those Americans captured by the idea that the "right to health care" necessitates "free" medical care for all. Efforts to escape the

conclusion range from those who see salvation in more emphasis on health education and prevention to those who think it's all the fault of greedy entrepreneurs like those exposed in the nursing home industry and finally those who think the need for rationing can be averted by getting more efficiency through reorganizing the medical system.

Unfortunately in this increasingly permissive United States there is little evidence that health education has done very much to curb such sources of disease as smoking, promiscuity, alcoholism and drug abuse. The British don't have any Bernard Bergmans but they find demand for "free" health care outstrips their resources. Moreover, Washington's efforts these past two years to push health maintenance organizations as a cheaper form of medical care have had rather disappointing results so far for those who urged this solution.

There can, of course, be economies and improvements in American medicine but there is growing realization among American health care specialists that the gains from these sources are unlikely to avoid the need for hard, even tragic, choices, if medical care is made "free" for all. A major culprit is medical progress, the advanced technology that permits today's medicine to do so much more than was ever possible for seriously sick people, but at an ever increasing cost with no end in sight.

The other day a New Jersey father petitioned a court to allow him to have doctors disconnect a respirator that has kept his comatose daughter alive since last April. The father's lawyer said the suit was necessary because the law has never addressed the question of "When is enough enough?" in the use of complex and expensive modern medical technology.

When, as and if we have "free" medical care the problem will be solved very quickly by bureaucratic fiat as part of the rationing system that will inevitably accompany any national health insurance scheme. The machinery for imposing this rationing is already being put into place by the recently enacted laws requiring national planning of medical facilities and imposing utilization controls through the Professional Standards Re-

view Organizations now being formed nationwide. These mechanisms will permit government officials a few years from now to dole out all the national health insurance medical care the budget will allow, a very much smaller amount than the patients of that time will want.

Harry Schwartz is a member of the Editorial Board of The Times.

September 16, 1975

LIFE AND DEATH DECISIONS

MOST DOCTORS LET A DEFECTIVE LIVE

At the hearing of the Coroner's jury in Chicago on Friday, when Health Commissioner Robertson assailed Dr. Haiselden for not attempting to operate upon the Bollenger baby, Dr. Haiselden interrupted the witness with: "Don't you know that this is done in Chicago every day?"

The Medical Review of Reviews in a forthcoming issue will publish the views of forty-five prominent American obstetricians on this subject. "One day," writes the editor of this symposium, "I was sitting at an obstetrical clinic in Chicago waiting for the baby to be born. A famous surgeon was presiding over the clinic. In the course of his talk he remarked casually that when a hopelessly malformed child is born in his practice he 'neglected' to tie the umbilical cord, and thus the child escaped from a world into which it never should have been born." The baby slowly bled to death.

The medical magazine then decided to institute an inquiry to decide what the representative obstetricians thought about the problem. Forty-five of the leading obstetricians in the United States expressed their views. Most of them are unqualifiedly opposed to Dr. Haiselden's stand, but others warmly support his attitude.

Eugene W. Belknap, professor of obstetrics at Syracuse University, writes:

"We have no right to sacrifice any life except to save another. The world undoubtedly would be better off if we could do away with the imbeciles, the hopelessly insane, the habitual criminals, &c., but that is not what we, as medical men, have the right to determine. Let society at large decide that question. Our duty as medical men is, first, to prolong life, and, secondly, to make that prolonged existence as comfortable and as useful as possible. There is but one ground to take in this question without opening the door to shameful abuses."

Professor Stricker Coles of Jefferson Medical College fortifies his argument by citing an interesting case. "I have now under my care," he says, "a woman without arms, only a stump on the left side. She has been married twice and has raised a family of five normal children. Would it have been justifiable to kill this child?"

Professor Colie's Views.

Professor Edward Martin Colie, Jr., associate in clinical obstetrics at Columbia University, thinks the time has not yet arrived for the profitable discussion of such a question. He says: "The physician has no right under the laws as they exist to terminate the life of a newborn infant, no matter how horrible the deformity, for no one shall be deprived of life without the process of law. There exists at the present time no process of law by which this, however desirable, can be accomplished.

"While it is true," he continues, "that in a large number of cases the deformity is not compatible with life and the babe survives but a few precarious hours, there are, we must admit, a large group of cases where the span of life—if life it can be called—is spun over a period of days, months, or even years."

Professor Colie believes that the question is mainly an economic one, "and the ethical questions involved ultimately arise from the economic facts." Personally he condemns as most rash "any assumption upon the part of any person of the power of life and death, however clear cut may seem the particular case, as being a usurpation of a very dangerous power."

Professor Carey Culbertson of the obstetrical department of the University of Chicago has similar beliefs. "This whole matter should be put on a legal basis," he writes, "not only relative to monsters, but to children of defectives. Until such a basis for scientific elimination is established, however, no physician, alone or with consultation, is justified (nor can he defend himself legally) in being the judge as to which individuals shall live and which perish. It were certainly better for society that monsters should not live, but I personally cannot be, and do not desire to be, the executioner."

"No physician can assume to correct the mistakes of the Creator, unless he be definitely appointed," writes Professor Walter Lewis Croll, a well-known obstetrician of Pittsburgh. "No one can tell with absolute certainty just how great the deformity is, or how well the child, by subsequent development, may overcome it, or compensate for it by greater capacities in other respects."

Says Human Life Is Sacred.

Professor Joseph Bolivar De Lee of Northwestern University, one of the most famous obstetricians in the country, feels that human life is too sacred to permit even the most deformed baby to perish. "We have no right to take human life It is a matter for the State," he writes. "Fortunately, a monster seldom survives. In the milder deformities surgical art often helps a great deal."

Professor De Lee wonders if the war in Europe has not depreciated our ideals of the sacredness of human life. His conclusion is emphatic: "No, my feeling and opinion are that we have no right to let a deformed baby succumb through negligence or intent."

Professor Charles Sumner Bacon of the University of Illinois, another celebrated obstetrician, discusses the matter almost wholly from the standpoint of medical jurisprudence.

In the first place, he argues, the baby will not always, or indeed not usually, die from hemorrhage from an untied cord. "Hence," he says, "if one sets out to kill the deformed child he cannot rely upon this method. The usual methods of killing a new-born are by smothering, strangling, or dividing. I cannot see that these methods are more objectionable than the one suggested."

Secondly, Professor Bacon points out, there are many kinds of deformities. Some are compatible with a fairly normal life. Another class of monsters who might live would always remain freaks. "These might be of great financial value to the parents, and their destruction might lead to extensive damage suits. They are, moreover, of considerable scientific interest and value."

Finally, there are the hopelessly malformed children who will not survive long in any event. "Generally the parents wish these children destroyed,"

says Professor Bacon, "and not only consent to any measure, but beg the physician to interfere. Of course, they have no right to beg this act of the physician. If he consents he may feel that he is doing a humane act by relieving the parents of a horrible burden. This is a dangerous ground, and in general the path of safety from moral and legal difficulties is to avoid the appearance of evil and resist the importunities of relations."

However, leading obstetricians in the United States are by no means united in opposition to the principle that Dr. Haiselden would establish.

Allowed to Perish at Birth.

"I fully sympathize with the views of those who advocate that the child with great congenital deformity should better perish at birth, and in the few cases of extreme deformity or monstrosity where I have been accoucheur I have cut without ligating the cord," writes Professor David Monash of the Northwestern University Medical School at Chicago. "I fully realize that the obstetrician cannot well preside as judge and arbitrarily decide what grade and degree of deformity he will grant the child. There is a wide border line of deformities between the two extremes. The physician cannot constitute himself, in all fairness to his ethical attitude, and to the rights of others interested, the sole arbiter of the life of the unfortunate child. One parent should share the responsibility."

Another well known obstetrician, Dr. William Rausch, Jr., of Albany, writes as follows:

"It has always been my opinion that all children who are born with a congenital abnormality are a detriment to society. I sincerely believe that it is humane to cut off their future suffering by one means or another, preferably 'forgetting' to tie the cord. It must be remembered, however, that very often parental love and religious principles have more sway than the laws of medical ethics."

"I have never been able to bring myself deliberately to kill any kind of a baby, however deformed, which has been born alive," says Professor W. H. Rubovits of Chicago. At the same time I would not criticise any one who would do so under certain conditions. The subject is a very difficult one to decide, but it would be easier if some definite conclusion could be arrived at by the profession and the practice could be sanctioned by law."

Professor George H. Washburn of Boston, a well-known New England obstetrician, says:

"Fortunately, so far I have never had to decide the question of allowing a monstrosity to live. I have always thought that the general opinion of the profession was in favor of letting them die if they were born alive."

"I believe that a child with congenital malformation of an extent to distinctly oppose the mental development to a degree necessary to a self-reliant individual should be permitted to die," writes Dr. Robert Hale Ellis of Portland, Ore. "This applies also to the physical deformities of the severer type —condemning the individual to an early death, or life as the ward of private or public charity."

Professor Henry D. Fry of Washington would permit a malformed child to die after birth under two conditions. First, if it be the wishes of the parents; second, according to the degree of abnormality. He does not discuss what constitutes the degree of abnormality that would justify the physician in taking such action.

November 21, 1915

UNFIT IMPERIL US, ROOSEVELT IS TOLD

Georgia Tech Committee Says Prolonging of Lives of Weak Is National Decadence.

CALLS IT 'HUMAN EROSION'

War, Land Erosion, Industrial Specialization Also Classed as Destructive Forces.

Special to THE NEW YORK TIMES.
ATLANTA, Ga., Dec. 17.—"Prolonging the lives of the weak and even physically unfit is, in a very real sense, undermining the physical well-being of future generations," says a report prepared for President Roosevelt and made public tonight by a special faculty committee of the Georgia School of Technology.

The report was made in response to a recent Presidential inquiry sent to engineering colleges. It will be condensed and forwarded to the President by Dr. M. L. Brittain, president of Georgia Tech.

The committee declared that advances in medical science were bringing about one major form of "human erosion," the "decadence of our national health."

"This type of human erosion," the committee's report says "is now fully recognized by authorities in biology and medicine.

"No less an authority than Dr. Alexis Carrel, in his recent book, 'Man the Unknown,' demonstrates this phenomenon quite forcibly."

The report adds:

"The term 'human erosion' may be considered to include those dislocations of body, mind and spirit produced by the vast social forces to which a modern nation is exposed. The causes of such erosion are many and only a few can be mentioned here.

"That war is the most powerful of these erosive factors has become definitely apparent."

In addition to medical science advances and war, the committee lists as "destructive natural and social forces" the following:

"Land erosion, which produces a shifting agricultural population or an impoverishment of agricultural workers, and industrial specialization, which renders workers highly vulnerable to economic changes."

The report suggests that "our institutions of higher learning must abandon the traditional worship of unrelated knowledge for itself alone and begin the work of developing leaders of thought and action who may be better able to guide this country toward a solution of its difficulties."

The committee was headed by Professor Montgomery Knight of the Aeronautics Department of Georgia Tech, and included Professor Count D. Gibson, head of Georgia Tech and included Professor Franklin C. Snow of the Civil Engineering Department.

December 18, 1936

SANCTION IS SOUGHT FOR 'MERCY DEATHS'

New Group Formed to Fight for Legalization of Ending Agony of Incurably Ill

---

DR. POTTER IS FOUNDER

Members Include Leaders in Various Fields—Opposition Expected to Be Strong

---

A National Society for the Legalization of Euthanasia, commonly known as "mercy killing," has been formed here, it was announced yesterday.

Among the directors of the society, subscribing to the belief that, with adequate safeguards, it should be made legal to allow incurable sufferers to choose immediate death rather than await it in agony, are the following:

Dr. Harry Elmer Barnes, historian.
Rabbi Sidney E. Goldstein of the Free Synagogue, New York.
Dr. Frank H. Hankins, Professor of Sociology at Smith College.
Mrs. F. Robertson Jones, honorary president of the American Birth Control League.
Dr. Clarence Cook Little, managing director of the American Society for the Control of Cancer.
Dr. George H. Parker, Professor of Zoology in Harvard University.
Dr. Oscar Riddle of the Department of Eugenics, Carnegie Institution of Washington.
Dr. Walter F. Willcox, Professor of Economics in Cornell University.

The Advisory Board

The Advisory Board, in addition to the above, includes:
Sherwood Anderson, author.
Dr. Henry H. Goddard, Professor of Abnormal and Clinical Psychology, Ohio State University.
Dr. Truman Lee Kelley, Professor of Education, Harvard University.
Dr. Foster Kennedy, Professor of Neurology, Cornell University Medical College.
Dr. William McDougall, Professor of Psychology, Duke University.

Dr. Horatio H. Newman, Professor of Zoology and Embryology, and dean in the Colleges of Science, University of Chicago.
Leon F. Whitney, biologist, executive secretary, American Eugenics Society.

The American society also has on its advisory board a number of prominent Englishmen who are likewise members of a society which has already introduced a euthanasia bill in the House of Lords. They include Havelock Ellis, Julian Huxley, the Earl of Listowel and H. G. Wells.

The announcement of the formation of the National Society for the Legalization of Euthanasia was made by Dr. Charles Francis Potter, leader of the First Humanist Society. He said he was the founder and president of the new organization, which will have offices at 1,775 Broadway.

He explained that it was "not a part" of his Humanist Society but "a definite outgrowth of its policy, which fosters all projects for human betterment."

"We have for years been active in the birth-control movement," Dr. Potter said, "and since that fight is largely won we feel free to transfer some of our efforts to the euthanasia enterprise.

Opposition Expected

"The Christian church, especially the Roman Catholics, I have been told, will bitterly oppose euthanasia; the legal profession may say there are insuperable obstacles to the passing of laws, and medical men may bring up their Hippocratic oath (dated 400 B. C.).

"But common men and women, faced with the practical problems of whether or not they will let their loved ones suffer torment for months before death, will cut through all this ancient red tape and somehow make it possible to do the decent and right thing.

"There is sure to be some one who says it is against the Ten Commandments of Moses, who said 'Thou shall not kill.' Perhaps the time has come to forget Moses and listen to the words of Jesus, 'Blessed are the merciful.'"

Dr. Potter concluded that most of the arguments against euthanasia were founded on emotion rather than on reason. He considered separately, however, the possibility that unscrupulous and impatient heirs might use it to hasten the death of a wealthy person. "Our laws," he added, "will prevent that possibility."

He said the purpose of the new society was to conduct a national campaign of education so that bills might be introduced in State Legislatures and in Congress with hope of eventual passage.

January 17, 1938

CLERGYMEN BACK BILL FOR 'MERCY' KILLINGS

Fifty-four prominent Protestant clergymen in New York have signed a statement approving voluntary euthanasia under careful safeguards, the Euthanasia Society of America, Inc., announced yesterday.

The statement, prepared by the society, declared that "mercy" killing, with proper safeguards, could not be regarded as "contrary to the teachings of Christ or the principles of Christianity."

Among those listed as signing the statement were Dr. Henry Sloane Coffin, president-emeritus of Union Theological Seminary; the Rev. Dr. Harry Emerson Fosdick, pastor-emeritus of the Riverside Church; the Rev. Dr. George Paull T. Sargent of St. Bartholomew's Church; the Rev. Dr. Guy Emery Shipler, editor of The Churchman, and the Rev. Dr. Ralph W. Sockman of Christ Church.

The statement said:

"A proposal has been put forward to legalize voluntary euthanasia, i. e., painless death for persons desiring it, who are suffering from incurable, fatal and painful disease. A bill has been drafted to give effect to this, and the proposal is receiving encouragement and support from many thinking people. Such a proposal raises important issues on ethical, legal and medical grounds.

"As regards the ethical issue, after giving the matter careful consideration, we wish to state that, in our opinion, voluntary euthanasia, under the circumstances mentioned above, should not be regarded as contrary to the teachings of Christ or to the principles of Christianity."

September 28, 1946

1,000 DOCTORS URGE 'MERCY DEATH' LAW

Petition Sent to Every Member of Legislature—Humane Motives Stressed

A petition urging that voluntary euthanasia, or "mercy death" for an incurable sufferer, be permitted by law has been signed by 1,000 physicians in the state and sent to every member of the Legislature. This was announced yesterday by the Committee of 1776 Physicians for Legalization of Voluntary Euthanasia in New York State and the Euthanasia Society of America.

The petition was signed by members of the committee, of which Dr. Robert L. Dickinson, senior gynecologist and obstetrician at Brooklyn Hospital and former president of the American Gynecologists Society, is chairman. Vice presidents of the committee are Dr. George M. Mackenzie of Cooperstown, N. Y., and Dr. H. A. Pattison of Livingston, N. Y.

The petition says that the proportion of the aged subject to painful, chronic and degenerative diseases is increasing rapidly; that the cancer death rate reached a new high in 1946; that "many incurable sufferers, facing months of agony, attempt crude, violent methods of suicide, while in other cases distraught relatives of hopeless incurables who plead for merciful release secretly put them out of their misery and thereby render themselves liable to prosecution as murderers," and that to permit the termination of useless, hopeless suffering at the request of the sufferer is in accord with the humane spirit of this age.

It urges that "voluntary euthanasia should be permitted by law, brought out into the open and safeguarded against abuse rather than, as at present, practiced illegally, surreptitiously and without supervision or regulation."

It also urges that the Legislature amend the law "to permit voluntary euthanasia for incurable sufferers, when authorized by a Court of Record, upon receipt of a signed and attested petition from the sufferer and after investigation of the case by a medical committee designated by the court."

Among the other signers were: Dr. Albert F. R. Andresen, Professor of Clinical Medicine, Long Island College of Medicine; Dr. Frank L. Babbott, former president, Long Island College of Medicine; Dr. George P. Berry, Professor of Bacteriology, University of Rochester; Dr. Siegfried Block, chief neuro-psychiatrist, Brooklyn Hebrew College; Dr. Russell L. Cecil, Professor of Clinical Medicine, Cornell University Medical College; Dr. John F. Erdmann, surgeon; Dr. William Sargent Ladd, former dean of Cornell University Medical College; Dr. Herbert Willy Meyer, surgeon and member of American Cancer Research Society; Dr. Alan deF. Smith, orthopedic surgeon-in-chief of New York Orthopedic Hospital; Dr. William St. Lawrence, pediatrician, and Dr. Thomas A. C. Rennie, psychiatrist.

December 15, 1947

Pius Gives View on Saving Dying; Tells When Doctors May Give Up

By PAUL HOFMANN
Special to The New York Times.

ROME, Nov. 24—Human life may linger after the heart stops, and medical science has the right to struggle with all its means to bring a seemingly dead person back to life, Pope Pius XII said today.

The Pontiff made a pronouncement on "reanimation" before an international audience of physicians. He referred specifically to heart massage by hand and to artificial respiration through the administration of oxygen.

These modern resuscitation techniques "contain in themselves nothing that is immoral," the Pope said. However, he made clear that when life was ebbing hopelessly physicians might abandon further efforts to stave off death, or relatives might ask them to desist "in order to permit the patient, already virtually dead, to pass on in peace."

The Pope said "considerations of a general nature permit the belief that human life continues as long as its vital functions — as distinct from the simple life of organs — manifest themselves spontaneously or even with the help of artificial proceedings."

He cited the tenet of Roman Catholic doctrine that death occurs at the moment of "complete and definitive separation of body and soul." In practice, the Pope added, the terms "body" and "separation" lack precision. He explained that establishing the exact instant of death in controversial cases was not the task of the Church but of the physician.

He mentioned the opinion of modern medicine that death takes place "only when the circulation has come to a complete standstill despite prolonged artificial respiration."

Speaking in French, the Pope set forth the Church's views on the religious and moral aspects of reanimation in answer to a questionnaire submitted to him some time ago by Dr. Bruno Haid of Innsbruck, Austria, on behalf of Catholic anesthetists in several countries.

Vatican officials recalled that an oxygen tent was kept in readiness in the Apostolic Palace three years ago when the Pope was critically ill. Physicians who saw the Pope today said he looked healthy and vigorous. He will be 82 years old next March.

In his address, the Pontiff acknowledged that advanced reanimation techniques had shaved lives. He mentioned cases of asphyxia caused by drowning or in surgery, chest injuries, polio myelitis, tetanus, gas and alcohol poisoning and hypnotic coma.

Replies To Questions

Replying to specific queries of the anesthetists, the Pontiff said:

¶Even in seemingly desperate cases modern apparatus for artificial respiration may be used. But the physician "has no obligation to do so unless it were the only way of fulfilling another certain moral duty." The Pope did not give an example of such moral duty.

Relatives of a patient are generally under moral obligation to insure only conventional medical treatment. If artificial respiration or other advanced techniques in seemingly hopeless cases "represent for the family such a burden as one could not in conscience impose upon them, they may lawfully ask the doctor to end his efforts and the doctor may lawfully comply." In such cases there is no question of euthanasia, or mercy killing, "which would never be lawful," the Pope said.

¶The Church allows the administration of extreme unction to patients while artificial respiration is being applied. If physicians are in doubt whether the soul has already left the body, the Church permits conditional administration of the last sacrament with the ritual Latin formula "si capex est" (if he is capable of receiving sacramental grace).

¶If the blood circulation and the life of a patient in a state of deep unconsciousness following a central paralysis are maintained only by artificial respiration without any improvement during some days, the Church leaves to science the verdict when death has taken place.

In many such cases there will be "insoluble doubt" and the Church accepts the presumptions that jurisprudence provides in this matter.

Elaborating on the three questions put to him, the Pontiff stressed that a person had the right and duty in a case of serious illness to take necessary measures to save life and health. This duty to defend God given life necessitates only treatment of the standard type for the person, area, epoch and civilization in question, the Pope explained. However, he added, "it is not forbidden to do more than what is strictly necessary to conserve life and health" unless higher duties are neglected.

Artificial respiration in seemingly hopeless cases and other advanced reanimation techniques go beyond generally accepted medical standards, the Pope said. It is, therefore, "not obligatory" to adopt them or to authorize the physician to adopt them.

"The physician," the Pope declared, "with regard to the patient has no separate or independent right" to use such treatment. The physician may resort to it when he has been expressly authorized to do so by the patient's family, the Pope said.

As for euthanasia, the "gentle death," the Pope reiterated his former condemnations.

November 25, 1957

The Patient's Right to Live—And Die

Britons wage a periodic debate on a sensitive issue: 'mercy killing' and a doctor's moral responsibilities toward a dying patient. Many find they favor euthanasia.

By JOHN BEAVAN

LONDON.

ONE day last spring Maurice Millard, a 58-year-old family doctor practicing in Leicester, gave a talk on euthanasia at what he thought was a private meeting of the Burton-on-Trent Rotary Club. He told the story of a devout Christian lady who asked her family physician to give her a "fatal dose" if ever she contracted a painful and deadly disease. She did, in fact, develop an incurable cancer and three months later she told her doctor that she had discussed the matter with her only relations, her sister and brother-in-law, and had her worldly affairs in order. Would he now give her the dose which would end her suffering?

The doctor, this Rotary lecturer continued, had no backing from state or church for such an action, but out of compassion he finally decided to give what help he could. The patient went into a coma and died in peace. "The story I have told you," said the lecturer, "is true. It happened to me. I was the doctor."

To his astonishment the next day, Dr. Millard found that every morning paper carried the story in a prominent position, and that Britain had begun one of its periodic debates on the rights and wrongs of "mercy killing" or "easy death," with himself the center of the debate. Dr. Millard explained that he had told the story for one reason only: to rebut arguments that there was no

need of legislation giving doctors and their patients the right to reach an understanding in such tragic circumstances. Dr. Millard is a fervent advocate of such legislation; he is also a member of the Euthanasia Society, which his father, the late C. Killick Millard, founded twenty-five years ago.

In a further interview Dr. Millard explained that he had not sought to kill the patient nor, in fact, did he kill her. "She had a bedside service with some relatives and she asked me to read a prayer. Then she asked me to give her something that would make her sleep. From that time I had no intention that she would come round again * * *. I had no indication of exactly what effect a drug would have on someone in such a weak condition. It was possible that a very small dose

JOHN BEAVAN is a British editor and writer on political and sociological topics.

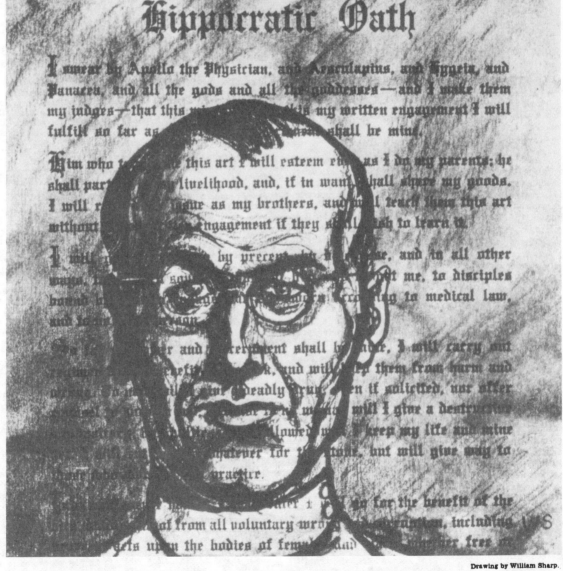

Pledge—The Hippocratic Oath reads, in part, "To none will I [the doctor] give a deadly drug, even if solicited * * *."

Drawing by William Sharp.

would put her into a coma, and that was what I intended. I think it is what many doctors do. It is not deliberate killing. One knows one takes a risk and one probably hopes it will be the end."

Since then, Dr. Millard has received many letters and messages praising his courage and compassion, and medical correspondents in the British press have pointed out that he acted in accordance with the best ethics of his profession. The only difference between Dr. Millard and the average doctor is that the average doctor does not talk about such things.

But this does not mean that there is widespread support for mercy killing, which is quite different from the action Dr. Millard took. Dr. Millard gave his patient ease from pain, but he had no intention of killing her. She was dying and he was prepared to go on giving her ease until she died. What he could not do and what he did not do was to give her a lethal dose deliberately. Dr. Millard would like the law to be changed so that in such circumstances a patient who asked for it could be given a fatal dose.

IF a British doctor complied with a dying patient's plea and deliberately shortened the patient's life, he would be technically guilty of murder. Since, as Dr. Millard made clear, there was no intent to kill but only the intent to ease, no legal proceedings were taken against him or could be.

The leading case on the subject is an American one, that of the Commonwealth of Massachusetts v. Bowen, which was heard as long ago as 1816. A prisoner in a cell next to that of a condemned man urged him to destroy himself and thus disappoint the sheriff and the crowd. The condemned man hanged himself and his neighbor was charged with murder. The judge directed the jury to find him guilty and explained that the offense was not diminished because justice was thirsting for a sacrifice and only a small proportion of the deceased's earthly existence remained to him. The jury took a common-sense view and acquitted the man, but the judge's direction accurately represented the law.

American precedents, incidentally, often are cited in English courts because the common law of America had its origin in English common law. American precedents are not binding on English judges, but they may have considerable persuasive authority. The Massachusetts case is frequently quoted because it shows in a striking way that even to accelerate in such an indirect fashion the almost certain natural death of a person is murder, according to law.

BUT the question arises: does the British doctor stand in peril from what is standard practice? For when a patient is suffering from a highly painful and incurable disease, the doctor gives him a narcotic, and as the patient becomes habituated the dosage must be constantly increased. Inevitably there comes a time when a dose proves fatal.

The doctor's legal position in these circumstances

is uncertain, because it has never been tested in a court of law. Prof. Glanville Williams of Cambridge University has given a good deal of thought to the matter. He argues that once you admit that a doctor may shorten a patient's life, then he may, in certain circumstances, knowingly end a patient's life immediately. The legal justification of his act would rest upon the doctrine of necessity; the doctor would have to show that there was no way of relieving pain except by measures which imperiled the patient's life.

But, says Professor Williams, it is extremely doubtful whether a judge would accept a doctor's right to anticipate matters—say, by doubling the previous dose of morphine—in order to save the patient from dragging out a numbed and useless existence. That is why he advocates a change in the law.

A CHANGE in the law is what the Euthanasia Society is working for. For years it has had ready the draft of a bill to make euthanasia legal in certain narrowly defined cases. This does not appear to be an opportune time, how-

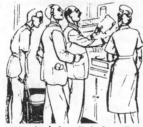

ever, to bring it before Parliament, although it has been eight years since the House of Lords debated the subject, and twenty-three years since the society's proposals first came before them.

The society believes that the problem is one of public concern since more people today live to an age at which they are likely to contract cancer. It says that Dr. Millard's story has increased interest in reform enormously and, in fact, that in the past year or two it has frequently been asked for an outline of its arguments by speakers taking part in debates on the subject. Usually when a debating society has voted on a motion in favor of euthanasia, it has been approved or just failed to carry.

Nevertheless, indications are that the times are less propitious than they were before the war. For one thing, British intellectuals are less rationalistic than they were in the Marx-Freud-dominated Thirties, and are more susceptible to religious ideas of the spiritually creative value of suffering.

FOR another, memories are still strong of what the Nazis did to the old and feeble, the useless mouths who could never be of use to the state. In fact, the world's doctors, outraged by what Nazi medical men had done during the war, drew up a new code of medical ethics re-emphasizing the sanctity of human life. Then in 1950 the World Medical Association agreed that euthanasia was contrary to public interest as well as to natural and civil rights; the British Medical Association approved that resolution.

But the Euthanasia Society goes on, and its efficacy or hopes of success must not be written off because it has merely three or four hundred members, an income of a few hundred pounds a year and a desk in a shared office in Kensington. This is the traditional way of British reform societies, some of which have achieved their aims against what seemed to be impossible odds.

The president of the Euthanasia Society is the Earl of Listowel, now Governor-General of Ghana. Vice presidents include the Very Rev. W. R. Matthews, the dean of St. Paul's; Sir Julian Huxley, Sir Harold Nicolson, and Lord Woolton, who is still high in the councils of the Conservative Government.

The society argues that a person suffering from an incurable, fatal and severely painful illness should have the right to ask that his life be painlessly terminated. He should be at least 21 years old, of sound mind, and make his application for death on a prescribed form to a euthanasia referee—an official appointed for the purpose.

THE applicant also would present two medical certificates, one from his own and the other from an independent doctor, setting out the medical facts. The euthanasia referee would then visit the sufferer and satisfy himself that the case was a proper one and that the applicant knew what he was doing. The referee would finally issue an official permit for the sufferer to receive euthanasia, which might be administered only by a person specially licensed for the purpose.

These cool and rational proposals have sent shivers down the spines of a number of ordinary, rational British people with whom the writer has discussed them—though they were vaguely sympathetic to the idea. Professor Williams, though a vice president of the society, thinks that it might be easier to get a bill passed saying that a doctor who intentionally accelerates the death of a patient should not be convicted unless it is proved that the act was not done in good faith, that is, with the consent of the patient and for the purpose of saving him from severe pain in a fatal and incurable illness.

It is often argued against euthanasia that nobody can say a disease is incurable. But it is not the disease which would be held incurable but the particular illness from which the individual was suffering. There is, of course, the possibility of doctors being wrong about a particular illness, but this, say the advocates of euthanasia, is a risk the patient has to balance against the prospect of continuing and increasing suffering.

Another argument against it is that voluntary euthanasia, if legalized, would destroy the incentive of medical research. The answer given this is that it is untrue; the first objective of the medical profession is to prevent disease and save life.

DOCTORS opposed to legalized voluntary euthanasia argue that it would put too great a responsibility upon them, and that it is a doctor's business to cure, not to kill. Against this is the new conception that it is part of a doctor's duty to relieve suffering.

The freest debate on the subject in recent weeks was held on a B. B. C. television program. Participants included the chairman of the society, a Church of England clergyman who supported him, and the Roman Catholic Bishop of Leeds, the Rt. Rev. George P. Dwyer, who, of course, was strongly opposed. Dr. Dwyer put the theological point that we have no dominion over our own life and that no suffering is "useless" if offered to Christ our Lord. But he also had some practical arguments—that legalized euthanasia, no matter what the safeguards, would lead people to fear doctors and shatter the confidence of the poor in hospitals.

Dr. Dwyer's case on this last ground is a powerful one; there is a strong folk belief still extant in Britain's mean streets that hospitals practice euthanasia by exposing dying patients to drafts that will accelerate death by

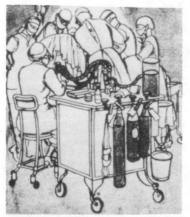

pneumonia. His argument on theological grounds is perhaps less strong. As the late Pope made clear only two years ago, the Roman Catholic Church accepts the fact that drugs which have the unintended effect of shortening life may be given to relieve pain.

THE Church of England has made no pronouncement on euthanasia and eminent Anglican clerics differ widely in public. While some have given their support, others fear that giving a "license to kill" would be the first step on a slippery slope. What argument would there be then against killing off the feeble-minded, those so physically crippled that they could be of no service to the nation, people in mental asylums or babies born with gross deformities? And what, a former Archbishop of York once asked, would be the effect on old people with incurable infirmities who are already suspicious that those around them want to get rid of them?

The highest view of the British medical profession paraphrases a dictum of the late Lord Horder, George VI's physician. The doctor knows, Lord Horder said, how to distinguish between prolonging life and prolonging the act of dying.

What the average doctor, having made the distinction, will not say—for very good legal and professional reasons—is exactly how he feels called

upon to act. An anonymous doctor wrote, in a comment on the Millard story:

"I would guess that the average family doctor does this thing perhaps half a dozen times a year. Usually it is done in the last stage of cancer when death is only a few days away and often he knows the amount of drug that is sufficient to relieve pain may be more than his exhausted patient can stand."

WHAT weakens the case for legal reform is that there appears to be no desire on the part of doctors for change. Nor has any quantitative, factual evidence been produced that doctors are deliberately withholding drugs and allowing dying people to suffer lest their lives be curtailed.

Doctors I have spoken to feel that they have no real difficulty in behaving in a compassionate and moral way, and need have no fear of legal consequence. Some of them say that legislation purporting to widen their professional freedom might actually reduce it, and would certainly diminish their personal responsibility to do what they think best for dying patients.

There has been a change in the attitude of doctors toward their responsibility to a dying patient. It was best expressed by another leader of the profession, the late Lord Dawson of Penn:

"If one goes back fifty years I think it will be true to say that the medical profession concentrated all its endeavors on the maintenance of life despite the nature of the illness and even despite sometimes the imminence of death. It was an accepted tradition that it was the duty of the medical man to continue the struggle for life right up to the end.

"With time that has changed. There has gradually crept into medical opinion, as there has crept into lay opinion, the feeling that one should make the act of dying more gentle and more peaceful even if it does involve curtailment of the length of life."

August 9, 1959

VATICAN SEES 'CRIME' IN FINKBINE ABORTION

Special to The New York Times.

ROME, Aug. 19 — "A crime has been committed," the Vatican radio said today in comments on Mrs. Robert Finkbine's abortion in Stockholm.

Mrs. Finkbine underwent surgery yesterday to prevent the birth of a malformed child as the result of taking thalidomide pills in the first weeks of her pregnancy. The Vatican radio said:

"Crime is the only possible definition of what happened yesterday at Caroline Hospital in Stockholm, Sweden. Morally, objectively, it is a crime, and all the graver because it was committed legally.

"Motives brought forward to justify it do not escape the falsity and captiousness of pretexts. There is no doubt that the victim was a human being. . . .

It was killed as though it were an assailant against whom legitimate defense is more than justified.

". . . It is not his fault if his existence and the ways of his existence cause danger to another person, even to his mother. He has not even desired life and still less has he asked for it. It is therefore arbitrary to consider him an intruder and condemn him to death."

August 20, 1962

Averting Deformed Births

TO THE EDITOR OF THE NEW YORK TIMES:

I am grateful to you for reporting the Rev. Dr. Israel Margolies's sermon upholding the idea that "a truly civilized mind would be hard put to devise a greater sin than to condemn a helpless infant to the twilight world of living death . . ."

If it is the will of society that science is to be encouraged to experiment with drugs whose effects we cannot be sure of, then it is the duty of society to permit parents who have unwittingly submitted to the use of such drugs to refuse to bear or rear children who have been denied that measure of human form and likeness that will permit them to grow and live in the dignity that we presume to be every human's right.

If "sin" is involved in this process, then it is society that is the sinner and should take measures to relieve the parent of guilt when faced with the necessity for such tragic but morally justifiable decisions.

MRS. LEWIS MUMFORD.
Amenia, N. Y., Nov. 28, 1962.

December 8, 1962

UnbornChild'sRight UpheldOverReligion

By United Press International

TRENTON, June 17—The state's highest court ruled in an emergency decision today that the right of an unborn child to live overrode its mother's religious convictions.

The Supreme Court, acting within a few hours after receiving the case, ordered the 29-year-old mother to receive a blood transfusion that physicians say is necessary to save the child's life, and possibly hers, too.

"We are satisfied that the unborn child is entitled to the law's protection," the court said.

Mrs. William Anderson, a former Roman Catholic who is studying to become a Jehovah's Witness, refused to take a blood transfusion, although complications developed in her seven-and-one-half month pregnancy. Physicians warned her that she might die at any minute, and take the life of her child as well.

Hospital attorneys asked the high court to clarify an unborn child's right to live.

Chief Justice Joseph Weintraub said that, in view of the emergency, there was not time for a sweeping decision.

The court ordered a "special guardian" appointed for the child, and directed that the guardian "consent to such blood transfusions as may be necessary to preserve the lives of the mother and the child."

The order also directed Mrs. Anderson to consent to the transfusions, and forbade her husband from interfering.

The court said it had "no difficulty" in making its decision to protect the child, since it had ruled in 1962 that the state concern for the welfare of an infant justified blood transfusions notwithstanding the objections of parents.

An Undecided Question

"The more difficult question is whether an adult may be compelled to submit to such medical procedures when necessary to save his life," the court said.

But it said that there was no need to decide this question at this time because, in the present case, "the welfare of the child and the mother are so intertwined and inseparable that it would be impracticable to attempt to distinguish between them. . . "

Mrs. Anderson left the Fitkin Memorial Hospital yesterday and went home against her doctor's advice. She and her husband, Stewart, live over a store in Asbury Park with their two children, Scott, 4, and Mark, 3.

On June 2 Mrs. Anderson's husband, an electrician and a member in the Jehovah's Witness congregation that his brother heads, had taken her to the hospital when she began hemorrhaging.

She refused to have a transfusion. The hospital went to court, and judge Leon Leonard of the Chancery Division of Superior Court refused to grant an order forcing her to take a transfusion.

Eugene W. Landy, attorney for the hospital, appealed, arguing that Mrs. Anderson "does not have the right to choose to die."

She is represented by Glenn How, a Toronto, Ont., lawyer, who also is a Jehovah's Witness.

Mr. How asked the Supreme Court to grant a 72-hour stay to give him time to appeal to the United States Supreme Court to grant a 72-hour stay Court.

"I doubt whether I could give you five minutes, Chief Justice Weintraub replied. "I would feel pretty badly if I consented to a stay and had this woman die in the meantime."

June 18, 1964

SOME DRUG TESTS ON PEOPLE SCORED

Professor at Harvard Hits Ethics of Experiments

By JANE E. BRODY

A Harvard Medical School professor has charged that some medical experiments in humans are ethically unsound—performed without the patients' full knowledge and consent and without promise of benefit to them or to other patients.

In a special article in the current issue of The New England Journal of Medicine, published yesterday, Dr. Henry K. Beecher cited 22 examples of what he called "unethical or questionably ethical" human experiments to support his charges

He wrote, "It is evident that in many of the examples presented, the investigators have risked the health or the life of their subjects."

One example described additional tests of the drug chloramphenicol, already known to reduce by half the death rate from typhoid fever. Of 408 charity patients with typhoid fever, 251 were treated with the drug and 20, or 8 per cent of the test group, subsequently died. Chloramphenicol was withheld in the control group of 157 patients, of whom 36, or 23 per cent, died.

According to Dr. Beecher's interpretation of this study, 23 patients died who would not have if they had received the proper drug therapy.

Dr. Beecher, who is Henry I. Dor Professor of Research in Anesthesia at Harvard, had submitted 50 examples to the journal, of which only 22 were printed for reasons of space. All the examples were authenticated by the editors of the journal, a spokesman said.

Dr. Beecher said the examples came from "leading medical schools, university hospitals, private hospitals, Governmental military departments and institutes, Veterans Administration hospitals and industry."

Dr. Beecher also examined "100 consecutive human studies published in 1964, in an excellent journal."

He said "12 of these seemed to be unethical," but even if only three were "truly unethical, this still indicates the existence of a serious situation."

He said a physician in England had collected more than 500 papers based upon unethical experimentation, concluding from this that "unethical or questionably ethical procedures are not uncommon."

According to the American Medical Association's Code of Medical Ethics, there are three requirements for clinical, or human experimentation: The voluntary consent of the person must be obtained, the danger of such experiment must be previously investigated in animals, and the experiment must be performed under proper medical protection and management.

Interpretation Varies

The interpretation of these principles varies, an A. M. A. spokesman said, but "voluntary consent" means the person should be told all that the experiment entails, what the known or possible risks are and what previous experiments have shown.

Dr. Beecher said that of the 50 examples compiled, only two studies actually mentioned that consent had been obtained before the experiments, and it was not known to what extent test subjects were informed of risks involved.

In one case where consent was obtained, skin cancer was transplanted from a girl to her mother "in the hope of gaining a little better understanding of cancer immunity and in the hope that the production of tumor antibodies might be helpful in treatment of the cancer patient," the researchers had written.

However, Dr. Beecher noted, the hope expressed "seems to have been more theoretical than practical" since the girl was a terminal patient and died the day after transplantation.

The transplant was removed from the mother 23 days later, but had already spread too far and the woman died a year and three months later.

June 17, 1966

A.M.A., in Reversal, Favors Liberalizing Of Abortion Laws

By DONALD JANSON
Special to The New York Times

ATLANTIC CITY, June 21—The American Medical Association took an unequivocal stand today in favor of liberalizing abortion laws.

The action by the A.M.A.'s policy-making House of Delegates is expected to speed a slowly developing trend toward the liberalization of state laws.

It marked the association's first policy change on the subject since 1871.

The 242-member House adopted the statement by a voice vote. The presiding officer, Vice Speaker Russell B. Roth, said there was "significant but inadequate opposition." The 216,-000-member association is the chief spokesman for organized medicine.

In the discussion preceding the vote, a spokesman for the opposition. Dr. Joseph P. Donnelly of Jersey City. asserted that "what you are doing here is opening up vast new changes in American medicine."

Dr. Edward C. Hughes of Syracuse, a past president of the American College of Obstetrics and Gynecology, said that the change would not "open the door to misuse."

He said it was "timely" for the association to lay down guidelines for changes in state laws because change was on the horizon anyway and association guidelines would help insure that "changes will be made properly."

The new association policy condones abortion under the following conditions:

To safeguard the health or life of the mother.

To prevent the birth of a child with a physical or mental defect.

To terminate pregnancies resulting from rape or incest.

The policy statement follows recommendations in the model penal code of the American Law Institute. It distinguishes between therapeutic and criminal abortion by insisting that abortions be induced only in an accredited hospital by a licensed physician, in consultation with two other qualified doctors who have examined the patient and concurred in writing on the need for the operation.

"It is to be considered consistent with the principles of ethics of the American Medical Association," the statement said, "for physicians to provide medical information to State Legislatures in their consideration of new legislation regarding therapeutic abortions."

Most state laws permit abortion only to save the mother's life. The opposition of the Roman Catholic Church to abortion for any reason has been instrumental in blocking liberalization in all parts of the country.

This year, however, California, Colorado and North Carolina modified their statutes in line with the recommendations of the model penal code.

A similar bill has been passed by the Florida Senate. Legislation was introduced this year for changes or study commissions in 19 other states.

A national public opinion poll last year found that a majority approved the kind of change now advocated by the A.M.A.

"There is unmistakable evidence of restiveness in all segments of the population regarding our current therapeutic abortion practices," said the report of the association committee recommending liberalization. "It is clear that change and reform in this area is inevitable."

The report called the new policy "a reasonable and conservative approach to the problem."

The report followed an 18-month study that the committee said confirmed that the association's 96-year-old policy intended to guide doctors had been vague and "antiquated."

The policy adopted by the House of Delegates in 1871 held it "unprofessional for any physician to induce abortion or premature labor" without consultation with another physician "and then always with a view to the safety of the child."

The new policy endorses therapeutic abortion when the doctor has "documented medical evidence" that the pregnancy could threaten the life or mental or physical health of the patient or could produce a mentally or physically defective infant.

The statement was modified in floor debate to take note that "there are many physicians who on moral or religious grounds oppose therapeutic abortion under any circumstances."

In 45 states, abortion is legal only to save the life of the mother. As many as half the therapeutic abortions performed in the United States are recommended by psychiatrists to preserve the mother's mental health.

The action was taken before more than 1,000 doctors in the crowded Pennsylvania Room of Haddon Hall. Ten thousand physicians are attending the annual convention. The total registration, including guests and industrial exhibitors, is 33,000.

The House chose Dr. Dwight L. Wibur of San Francisco as the association's president-elect by acclamation. His term will begin next June. His election marked the first time the son of a former president of the association had been elevated to the presidency of the 120-year-old organization.

Dr. Wilbur, a 63-year-old internist, is the son of Ray Lyman Wilbur, who was Secretary of the Interior in the Cabinet of President Herbert Hoover and later chancellor of Stanford University.

June 22, 1967

Britain's Health Ministry Bars Automatic Ban on Resuscitation

By ALVIN SHUSTER
Special to The New York Times

LONDON, Sept. 23—The Ministry of Health told hospitals today that patients should not automatically be denied the prospect of resuscitation because of their age or the nature of their illness.

The Ministry thus tried to abate a controversy stirred up this week over a directive posted at one Northwest London hospital that excludes certain patients from resuscitation if their hearts have stopped.

The notice, posted at Neasden Hospital for more than a year before it was reported to hospital authorities, said that no effort should be made to resuscitate anyone over 65 who had suffered cardiac arrest.

It also excluded as a matter of hospital policy those with malignant diseases or chronic chest or kidney disease.

Those patients, the notice to doctors and nurses said, were to have medical treatment cards labeled "NTBR" (not to be resuscitated).

The Ministry of Health began an inquiry and received a report from the hospital management board saying it agreed with Dr. William McMath, the hospital's medical superintendent, in the general idea of providing some guidance to his medical staff.

Today Sir George Godber, the Ministry's chief medical officer, issued his guidance to the country5s 2,500 hospitals.

"No patient should be excluded from consideration for resuscitation by reason of age or diagnostic classification alone, and without regard to all the individual circumstances," he said. "Any form of general instruction is wholly unacceptable."

Sir George noted that only a "very small number of patients" in hospitals suffered cardiac arrest — cessation of effective heartbeat—under circumstances that would enable doctors to resume the heart's action.

But, he continued, the "nature of the decision to be taken is no different in principle from that required in other grave circumstances, and a decision to operate on a patient or to refrain from intervention may often be of similar importance."

But there should be no automatic exclusion, he said. The decision to attempt resuscitation, he continued, "must be the decision of the responsible doctor" in each case.

"While age is a factor which may properly be taken into account," he added, "it is only one of many factors involved and these must include—in any individual case—both the nature of the underlying disease and the doctor's assessment of the likelihood that any attempt to resuscitate will be successful."

Some Sick Humor Results

The controversial notice, posted by Dr. William McMath, Neasden Hospital's Medical Superintendent, was recently seen by a patient. It was withdrawn immediately. The British reacted with shock to the disclosure, but not without a little sick humor as well.

A cartoon in The Evening Standard shows one hospitalized elderly man in a wheelchair asking another: "Is this one of those hospitals where one daren't stop breathing?"

There have also been letters to the editors of newspapers here in which the writers contended they had "died" in a hospital only to be revived by the heroic efforts of their doctors.

In its report to the Ministry of Health, the hospital management board said that it believed that during the months the directive was posted, no patient who might have benefitted from resuscitation efforts failed to receive it.

It found "particularly unfortunate" the wording of the notice, but said it agreed with Dr. McMath in the general idea of providing some guidance to his medical staff. It said some advice was necessary to insure the proper use of resources and "protection of some patients from distressing and unprofitable procedures."

Basis of the Directive

The report thus touched on the apparent reasoning behind Dr. McMath's directive. The superintendent has declined to answer all questions on the matter, but medical experts have pointed out that to have any chance of success heart action must be started within three minutes after it stops.

Thus the decision on whether to attempt to restore life must be made within seconds after cardiac arrest. This would require doctors to be at the ready all the time to man the high-powered resuscitation units needed to attempt heart beat resumption. And, as one doctor noted, Neasden is a small hospital without resources to deploy manpower in this way.

Another reason for Dr. McMath's action presumably lies in what the hospital board's report called "distressing and unprofitable procedures" — instances where incurably ill patients have been revived only to survive one or two more days in agony.

But the board made it clear that it was against arbitrary categories of patients to be excluded from resuscitation efforts, adding that "the decision on each patient should be taken at the highest medical level available in the particular circumstances."

September 24, 1967

Ethics Debate Set Off By Life Science Gains

This article was prepared by Jane E. Brody, a science writer, and Edward B. Fiske, religion editor.

Scientists and doctors, theologians and legislators and a host of other professionals around the country are showing an intense new interest in the moral issues created by innovations in the life sciences.

The growing ethical concern, which amounts to a movement, arises from such recent developments as heart transplants and new drugs to alter emotions and behavior. It is also prompted by such future possibilities as the creation of test-tube babies and the manipulation of genes to "improve" the human race.

Unless thought is given to such matters now, said James Watson, the Nobel Prize-winning geneticist, "the possibility of our having a free choice will one day suddenly be gone."

Last week Senator Walter F. Mondale, Democrat of Minnesota, and 17 bipartisan cosponsors introduced a bill in the Senate to establish a two-year National Advisory Commission on Health Science and Society to explore the moral, social and legal implications of developments in biology and medicine.

The new interest has already given rise to a number of institutions that are investigating the ethics of biology and medicine, a rapidly proliferating literature on the subject and a burgeoning number of scientific conferences on ethical issues:

Under attack are many of the traditional assumptions that underlie not only biology and medicine but all science and technology. Among them are the beliefs that scientific progress is automatically good, that what is medically beneficial to the individual is necessarily good for society, and that scientists are the best judges of the direction in which their research should go.

At this point "agreement is far greater on the questions than the answers," said Dr. J. Russell Elkinton, editor of the Annals of Internal Medicine. But. he added, at least a responsible debate is under way.

The debate is focused upon discoveries capable of radically affecting the quality of life, altering the structure of society and even changing the very nature of man himself.

Doctors have already developed drugs and elaborate machinery capable of prolonging the lives of countless millions of people suffering from terminal illnesses.

When should the plug be pulled? Does a person have the right to ask that he be left untreated to die in peace? Should the physician, in some cases, speed the end to the patient's suffering? Where do the rights of society come in when physicians, funds and hospital beds used to keep terminal patients alive are in short supply?

Similarly. the first transplant of a human heart in December, 1967, created a host of still

Life and Death Decisions

unresolved ethical questions. When is a person dead? How can a limited organ supply be fairly used in face of an overwhelming need and demand? Can society justify the costly treatment in view of other pressing medical needs?

As the American Friends Service Committee put it in a recent report: "A single heart transplant costs $20,000 to $50,000. How many individuals could be rehabilitated with glasses, hearing aids, or dental care for the cost of one heart transplant?"

A Broader Menace

Dr. René Dubos, bacteriologist and scientific humanist at Rockefeller University, sees a broader question of social commitment than simply the either-or questions within traditional medicine.

"Why become excited about a few hundred organ transplants when every day in New York City 30,000 children are exposed to the possibility of permanent handicaps from lead poisoning and no one is doing anything about it?" he asks.

On the horizon are science-fiction sounding discoveries that would create a vast array of brand-new ethical issues. Scientists have already been able to take a cell from an adult frog and, by placing its nucleus into a frog egg, create a new frog that is a genetic carbon copy of the original adult. Although the same feat in mammals is technically far more difficult, some geneticists expect it to become a human reality within a decade or two.

This process, known as cloning, has already raised questions. Does an individual have a right to his uniqueness? What would be the psychological effects of seeing one's genetic blueprint played out in advance if, for example, the person one was cloned from developed muscular dystrophy at age 35?

Beethoven Multiplied

For musical reasons, it might be nice to have a whole conservatory of Beethovens, but the societal effects of so many persons with Beethoven's temperament might be disastrous. What would be the effect on family structure if scores of American men could order their own copy of Raquel Welch? And what if cloning had been a reality when Hitler was in power?

Other future ethical problems are expected to grow out of the increasing ability of neurologists to define precisely the areas of the brain that control certain aspects of behavior. Questions will clearly arise, too, from a rapidly growing array of potent drugs that can change behavior, raise or lower intelligence, enhance or impair memory and affect specific kinds of learning.

Should criminals be forced to accept rehabilitation that would involve direct electrical or chemical stimulation of their brains, or even brain surgery? Such techniques are already being tested in man.

Would the use of a drug that raised the general level of intelligence create a society of persons unwilling to do essential menial chores? Would man twice as smart as he now is still be human?

On a Narrow Base

Until now consideration of such ethical and social questions has generally been confined to a few isolated individuals in science and religion.

Recently, however, a number of institutes have sprung up to pursue such issues on a formal interdisciplinary basis and in anticipation of scientific advances wherever possible.

Set in the tranquil beauty of Hastings-on-Hudson, N.Y., the Institute of Society, Ethics and the Life Sciences, now two years old, has recruited 70 persons in fields ranging from philosophy to biochemistry to serve on task forces in the areas of population control, genetic engineering, death and dying, and behavior control.

In dealing with population problems, said the institute's director, Daniel Callahan, a Roman Catholic philosopher, "our job is not to provide easy answers but to spell out the ethical acceptability of various approaches — such as mandatory abortion or birth control incentives — that might be adopted as government policy."

A second major organization, the Institute of Religion, operates in the midst of Houston's huge Texas Medical Center. The institute promotes interdisciplinary discussions of ethical problems that arise out of medicine and research, including the heart transplants for which the center is famous.

Buses to Poor Delayed

Kenneth Varrett, an economist at the Xerox Center for Health Care Research in the Houston complex, noted in an interview that largely as a result of discussion with the Rev. Kenneth L. Vaux of the institute staff, his center had postponed plans to put experimental diagnostic equipment on buses and send them out into poor areas.

"We realized that it would be unethical to screen people for illnesses and raise expectations of their being helped until we were also prepared to offer them treatment," he explained.

Several smaller institutes recently created include the Center for Human Values in the Health Sciences in San Francisco and the Institute for Theological Encounter with Science and Technology at St. Louis University. Dr. Leon Kass is heading a new 15-member committee on Life Sciences and Social Policy, a part of the National Academy of Sciences.

Some theologians specializing in ethics are trying to acquaint themselves with the facts and future of biology and medicine. Paul Ramsey, professor of religion at Princeton University, for instance, recently spent a sabbatical year studying genetics and ethics at Georgetown Medical School and has since written widely on the ethical problems of genetic engineering.

Panels in Centers

In the last few years committees have been set up at virtually all medical centers to review proposed human experiments.

Such panels, which would, for example, prevent an experiment that would involve injecting cancer cells into persons incapable of understanding the nature of the experiment, are now mandatory for federally financed research.

And medical schools throughout the country, often under pressure from students, have started to set up courses on ethical issues.

Dr. Willard Gaylin, a 46-year-old psychiatrist who is helping to develop an ethics program at Columbia College of Physicians and Surgeons, recalls that in his medical school days, "ethics meant what size shingle a doctor should hang outside his office." "Today's students," he says, "are grappling with such sticky questions as whether to let a 10-year-old girl with a terminal illness die in peace as her mother requested or whether to try to prolong her life."

Who Will Decide

Underlying the new ethical concern is a conviction that the authority of science, like that of universities, the churches and the military, must increasingly come into question.

Scientists and others are now asking whether scientific progress necessarily serves the good of man and, in cases where it obviously does, whether scientists should be the only ones to determine the direction it takes. There is, in short, a growing consensus that the consequences of science are too important to be left to the scientists.

"We're talking about changing the bodies and minds of men," remarked Dr. Kass, himself a biochemist. "Scientists are not peculiar repositories of wisdom on these matters."

He and other individuals and institutions concerned with the new ethics would like to see critical scientific questions, such as whether to create carbon copies of people—posed on an interdisciplinary basis.

Dr. Robert Francoeur, an embryologist at Fairleigh Dickinson University and a married Roman Catholic priest, favors an "international consortium of scientists, physicians, sociologists, economists, lawyers, theologians and others" to deal with such matters.

The Mondale proposal would set up a 15-member committee appointed by the President from the areas of medicine, law, theology, biology, sociology, physics, the humanities, government, public affairs and health care.

How can the ethical questions they discuss ever be resolved? There is a consensus that some problems—the definition of death, perhaps, or the use and distribution of organs for transplants—might be best dealt with through legislation. Others, however, such as policies governing euthanasia, may be more appropriately handled through professional guidelines and the evolution of a public consensus.

Among the new ethicists there is general agreement that some way must be found to involve the public. Dr. Ramsey would like to see the public represented even on fairly technical interdisciplinary boards.

"Some people might be simply stunned and overwhelmed," he said, "but their symbolic presence would put the professions on notice that society does have a concern."

Yet many scientists on the firing line are nervous about having the public looking over their shoulders. One fear is that the public is antiscience and will inhibit research.

Scientists' Fears

When Senator Mondale first introduced a resolution to establish a national commission on medical ethics three years ago, he expected scientists to welcome it.

Instead, "I was disappointed and appalled by the almost unexplainable fear on the part of some scientists about the public being involved. Their attitude was, 'It's none of the public's business.' Others said, 'Do it, but keep it within the profession'."

The senator said: "Research has more to gain from the public process than to lose. Secrecy could do a lot of harm."

Dr. Kass said: "Instead of raising the bogy man of interference, scientists should help legislators and the public discriminate between the technology we should scrutinize and that we should leave alone."

Another fear of scientists is that the long process of public deliberation might grind scientific research to a halt.

Dr. Robert White, a neurosurgeon at Western Reserve University who studies brain and body transplants in dogs and monkeys, said he welcomed the new sensitivity to

378

ethical concerns. But he added: "If we were starting now, open heart surgery would take two or three times longer to develop than it actually did because universities, hospitals and doctors themselves are very much more sensitive to what they're doing to patients."

Terms It Cheap

Implementing the ideas of the biomedical ethicists presents a number of difficulties. "For one thing, there's no lobby group," said Robert Veatch, a pharmacologist, theologian and medical ethicist at the Hastings Institute. "No one organizes around the fact that he's sick. What we really need is a Ralph Nader for medical ethics."

Another serious limitation is money. Dr. Callahan's group found that few foundations that support research have thus far shown interest in the area and have difficulty fitting requests for funds for medical ethics into their traditional categories.

Dr. Kass noted, however, that "the kind of research and thought needed is cheap compared to the cost of what produces these problems" and suggested a routine budgeting of 1 per cent of research funds for study of the ethical consequences of the research.

A third difficulty is that there are no real answers to ethical questions, and in most cases the choice is not between good and evil but between relative goods.

"We're not dealing with solvable problems in the usual sense of the word," said Dr. Kass. "In a fragmented, pluralistic society, you're not going to come to agreement on matters that have divided the best of human minds since antiquity."

Yet the growing consensus is that the thinking must be done and done now. "What man can do is becoming more obvious," said Dr. Elkinton. "What man ought to do is yet a dark enigma."

March 28, 1971

Dignity in Dying Is Goal of New Studies

By JANE E. BRODY

ROCHESTER, May 1 — A growing league of professionals is trying to throw new light on a long-taboo subject that sooner or later touches every human being—death.

Their interest, as shown at a two-day conference, is neither morbid nor academic. It is intended, rather, to make dying more dignified in a day when it most often occurs in harsh institutional settings amid strangers and elaborate medical equipment. It is designed to make death less fearful in a time when fewer people believe in afterlife.

In short, it is directed at making death easier to take for the person who dies, the professionals who attend him and the survivors who loved him.

Care of the dying patient has become increasingly important now that swift deaths from acute illnesses like pneumonia are rare and many if not most people die over months or years from chronic, degenerative diseases like cancer. Can their passing be made less dehumanizing, less psychologically painful?

Another impetus to the new interest in the subject of death has been the finding that the survivors of the deceased are far more likely than other people their age to suffer physical illness and death during the period of bereavement. Is there a way to soften the blow?

The conference this week on "The Patient, Death and the Family," which brought together a score of experts from a wide range of disciplines, reflects the new interest in death and dying that has been evolving with increasing rapidity during the last decade.

Participants included psychologists, sociologists, philosophers, clergymen, psychiatrists, nurses and physicians who commonly treat fatally ill patients.

As demonstrated at the conference, which was sponsored by Rochester General Hospital in cooperation with the University of Rochester Medical School, the current interest in death has already resulted in a new understanding of the psychological challenges to the dying person and his family.

It has revealed, for example, that many dying patients pass through five distinct psychological stages as their death approaches. With a little help from the professionals who attend him, one expert told the conference, the dying person and his family can be guided through these stages together, making the death more acceptable and "healthier" for all concerned.

Dr. Elisabeth Kubler-Ross, then a psychiatrist at the University of Chicago, formulated the five-stages theory two years ago as a result of extensive videotaped interviews with some 500 dying persons. Dr. Ross is currently medical director of the Mental Health Center of South Cook County in Flossmoor, Ill.

The Stage of Denial

The first stage is denial— "No, not me." The patient cannot accept the fact that he has a fatal illness. Sometimes patients are unable to pass out of this stage and, as a result, die with much unfinished business. Other times it is the family that cannot accept the fatal prognosis.

In most people, however, Dr. Ross found, denial quickly give way to anger and rage—the "Why me?" stage. The patient becomes hard to handle, overtly critical, nasty and uncooperative. The people around him react by making visits shorter and less frequent, by jabbing in the needle just a little harder. The result, said the Illinois psychiatrist, is to make the patient feel even more deprived, isolated and rejected.

Following anger, there often comes a period of bargaining—"Yes, me, but . . . ." "If you give me one more year, God, I promise you I'll be a good Christian." Dr. Ross told the conference about a terminally ill woman who was in intense pain nearly all the time. The woman asked for only one day without pain so that she could leave the hospital and attend her son's wedding. Through self-hypnosis, her wish was granted. On returning to the hospital she said, "Don't forget now, I have another son."

A Time of Mourning

The next stage is usually depression, a time of mourning over things already lost and of grieving over impending losses. This is when the patient psychologically separates himself from his loved ones.

"The worst thing you can do at this stage is call in a psychiatrist," Dr. Ross said. "That implies that the patient is not behaving properly, that he should shape up—'Cheer up, things are not so bad.' Not so bad for whom? A widow is encouraged to grieve and she has suffered the loss of only one person. A dying person is suffering the loss of everyone and everything he has ever loved. His grief is a thousand times greater. He should be told, 'I admire you for crying. It takes a man to cry.'"

Finally, the dying person enters the last stage, acceptance—"My time is very close now and it's all right," Dr. Ross said, "This is not a happy stage, but neither is it unhappy. It's devoid of feelings but it's not resignation, it's really a victory."

The psychiatrist emphasized that not all patients go through this orderly progression. Sometimes they skip stages or they return to a previous stage. And not everyone, she pointed out, wants to die in a state of acceptance.

"Some want to go out fighting," she said, "and they should. We should not try to impose our will on them. If you listen to the patient, he will tell you how he wants to die."

The study of dying has also

revealed the importance of honesty and openness in dealing with the dying patient, both for his sake and his family's.

The Pain of Deception

Robert Anderson, the playwright, described the pain of deception at the meeting here. "I was advised not to tell Phyllis the truth," he said of the protracted, ultimately fatal illness of his first wife. "It would have been easier, far, far less lonely, if she had known. I would want to

know. The complicated ruses, deceptions, explanations, were incredible. The heartbreak of watching her thinking she was improving, while I knew that any improvement was temporary. I remember her saying as we woke up one morning, 'I've decided that I am not going to make slow improvement. I am just going to wake up one morning completely well.'"

Sometimes the physician recognizes the importance of dealing truthfully with his

fatally ill patients but the family thwarts him.

Sixteen-year-old Fred was dying of leukemia. His doctor wanted to discuss his illness with him but Fred's parents refused and circumvented the boy's questions. Finally Fred asked the same questions of his doctors and nurses, then confronted them all with the discrepancies in their replies. He told his parents that he no longer believed them, that he knew he was going to die and how he wanted his

favorite belongings disposed of.

Dr. Ross said there was a need for teaching young students and even young children about death so that death can be a more beautiful and ennobling experience for more people—both the dying and their survivors. In the last two years, she said, seminars on dying have been started at more than 50 institutions around the country. The death taboo is beginning to die.

May 3, 1971

The Right to Die With Dignity

By DEBORAH JOSEPHS

Few people ever think about their own death. Some occasionally may joke about "going" this way or that but it is a rare person who can truly contemplate a world without him in it. However, there are some who can envision such a world. People who are desperately sick often are forced by circumstances to such contemplation. Over the last year, we have lived with someone forced to that kind of self-awareness. My husband's brother, Flip, died of cancer on June 23, 1971, at the age of 23.

Flip was a tall, handsome, perenially healthy boy of 22 when he first became ill in June of 1970. After a relatively cheerful diagnosis of a deformed kidney, he was admitted to a Brooklyn hospital and operated on the following day. The new diagnosis was cancer. When a family is faced with a crisis such as this, there is a terrible feeling of helplessness. The decision as to what is the best thing to do is difficult. We made two crucial decisions. The first was to refrain from telling Flip the true nature of his condition and the second was to move him to another hospital, one specializing in cancer research and care. We never regretted that first decision: the word cancer is very chilling and generally brings on a feeling of helplessness and finality. But we did, in most ways, regret our second decision because it served to postpone, torturously, the inevitable.

A second operation, at the new hospital in New York, proved to be more heartbreaking than the first. After five hours of surgery, doctors told us that there was no chance for Flip, that the cancer was already, incredibly, too widespread to treat. He lived for 11 months after that—never once out of pain, never once feeling good, and, in the end, telling us that he was more afraid of living than dying. In those months, he was an inpatient six different times and was also treated as an outpatient. He had other opera-

tions, received both chemotherapy and cobalt treatments, and was more or less treated as a research specimen for the remainder of his life.

If there had been some possibility of a cure, then we would have had little cause to object to the treatment of Flip. But we were told after that second operation that there was no hope, there was no cure, and we accepted that fact. We were also told, when we asked if he would be in much pain, that pain was the one thing the hospital could take care of. That was very far from the truth. In the 11 months it lasted, Flip had not a day without pain and most of his pain was created by doctors continuing in their efforts to help him. He and many others were and are forced to die this way because they are not permitted by doctors and by society itself to die with dignity.

There must be a point where a patient is left alone and permitted to die. People with terminal illnesses should not be seen as threats to hospitals and doctors. There should be a time when operations, when radiation, when everything is stopped so that patients can die in relative comfort.

During our months with Flip, visiting him at the hospital, we saw people an hour away from death being taken out on stretchers to be X-rayed. We saw dying patients who had contracted pneumonia treated rigorously so that they would not die of pneumonia but live a few days longer until their inevitable death from cancer. We were told, at one point, that Flip could receive no stronger pain killers because of the danger of addiction.

On a hospital level, there should be better communication with doctors. Many times, during our ordeal with Flip, we were made to feel that our questioning a doctor was a blatant infraction of their rules. When Flip's operations and treatments were decided we were never consulted but told that Flip, as he was not a minor, could make his own decisions. A terminal patient, especially one in constant pain, may not be capable of making

his own decisions no matter what his age and that fact should be recognized.

Toward the end Flip was put on more chemotherapy that made him very uncomfortable. One result of radiation is to make a patient lose his hair. We were determined that now, with so little else left him, this one vanity would not be denied him. We decided to have the treatments stopped. The doctor in charge of these treatments told us that Flip would have to leave the hospital if treatments were stopped. As it was the tubes and instruments to which Flip was attached that were keeping him alive we didn't think he should be moved.

Money is a problem that everyone faces when they enter a hospital, whether they are in for a couple of days or a couple of months. Hospitals and doctors are terribly expensive, especially when a doctor prescribes surgery, lengthy hospital stays, radiation, and so forth. Never, in all that time, were we asked if we could afford continued hospital expenses. If there had been any possibility that Flip could be cured, money would have been of very little importance to us. But there was no hope for him and never any concern for our ability or desire to pay for what we considered to be futile and excessive.

We would suggest, then, that upon entering a hospital, the administrative offices do more than simply ask for your Blue Cross card or proof of hospitalization coverage. They should discuss with you the possibilities of long-term care and expenses and help arrange financing if needed.

Last we would suggest and hope that Congress finally go about the business of creating a national healthcare plan coupled with the promised funding for the fight against cancer.

But, until the answers are all in, people are entitled to die as they are entitled to live—with love, compassion and dignity.

Deborah Josephs is a secretary in New York.

September 25, 1971

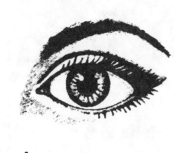 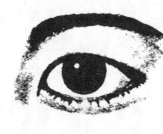 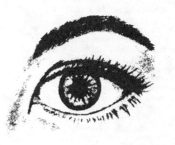

A   B   C

FIG. 5–3 MEDICAL BLUNDER in the description of the eye folds of the so-called "mongoloid" patient. The mongoloid patient has a distinct skin fold in the inner corner of the eye (C). The eye of the Oriental person is distinguished by a curved, overlapping eyelid (B). Except for the skin fold, the eye of the mongoloid patient is formed in the same way as that of any Caucasian person (A).

From "Human Heredity and Birth Defects" (Pegasus) by E. Peter Volpe.

'Doctor, do we have a choice?'

The baby is a mongoloid. If he is to live, surgery will be necessary. A surgeon tells how he allows parents to make the life-or-death decision.

By ANTHONY SHAW

IN the grim drama of surgery the pediatric surgeon's lot is usually a happy one. He operates on critically ill newborn infants and gives them the 70 years' life expectancy of which nature would have deprived them.

A common script for practitioners of my specialty: Baby is born with a portion of his intestines missing; his food and intestinal juices swell his little belly; he vomits repeatedly and will die if nothing is done. Enter the pediatric surgeon. He performs a 45-minute operation; the intestine is rejoined; digestion proceeds unimpeded, and a healthy infant goes home with his happy parents. Events unfortunately do not always follow this cheerful script. Sometimes a baby with this new gift of years has a digestive tract that is superior in potential to that of his brain. He is a mongoloid.

About 1 in 600 births in the United States is a baby with Down's syndrome — mongolism. John Langdon Haydon Down, who

Anthony Shaw, M.D., is associate professor of surgery and pediatrics at the University of Virginia Medical Center.

described this form of mental retardation about 100 years ago, thought that the Oriental appearance common to children with mongolism proved an ancient link between the Caucasian and Oriental races. We don't know much more about why mongoloid children look the way they do than Down did, but we tend to reject the simple notion that these severely retarded youngsters are throwbacks to a more primitive race of man. Geneticists have found that mongoloids have an extra chromosome inside the cell nucleus. They should have 46, like you and me; instead, they have 47. The chromosomes carry the genes which determine all our characteristics from the color of our eyes to the potential size of our brain. Why that 47th chromosome causes a baby to have slanted eyes, a broad nose, a protruding tongue, a single crease running the breadth of his palm, and an I.Q. of 30, we don't know yet.

Most mongoloid infants survive the traumas of birth and proceed into infancy, but many are born with lethal defects, such as congenital heart disease and obstructed intestines. Not very many years ago such babies were not

salvageable, and physicians and parents alike were relieved when a merciful God prevented the survival of what was then called a "mongolian idiot." But we have learned how to operate on the intestines and even the hearts of newborns.

As women get deeper into middle age their chances of bearing a mongoloid child increase. Miss H, a busy attorney, was well into her 30's when she married her law partner, Mr. G. Three years later their efforts to have a baby were finally rewarded by a four-and-one-half pound premature infant, unmistakably mongoloid. Happiness dissolved into grief, shock, rage and disbelief. "How could this happen to us? Why did this happen to us?" Then—"Are you sure, doctor?" We *were* sure. An examination of the nuclear material of the baby's blood cells showed the extra chromosome. The G's were faced with a difficult choice: take home this bitter fruit of their years of dreaming or place him in an institution and banish him from home and mind. But at age two days, Baby G changed the options. He vomited every feeding, spitting up a combination of formula and bile. He

had an intestinal obstruction. Surgery was necessary.

Twenty-five years ago a newborn with a blocked intestinal tract stood less than a 50-50 chance of surviving surgery. Many surgeons would have considered such surgery in an obviously mongoloid infant not worth the risk and effort. With the development of pediatric surgery and the better understanding of the differences between newborns and adults, surgery and anesthesia have improved to the point where operations on tiny infants are routine. An instance of intestinal surgery on a newborn mongoloid, which would have been considered heroic surgery a few years ago, was described in a recent newspaper article as a "simple operation."

Baby G's pediatrician expected me to perform this "simple operation." The internes and residents were eager to assist; the anesthetist was standing by. Then Mr. G asked, "Don't we have any choice?" And, indeed, I felt they did.

The choice they made was—no surgery. They had no intention of raising a human being whose maximum achievement might be

381

the ability to write his own name. Furthermore, they did not wish to sentence their child to an institutional existence. "If I knew the baby would be mongoloid," Mrs. G said, "I would have had an abortion." This argument allowed the G's to live with their decision. When Mr. G called me a year later on the anniversary of their baby's death and asked me if I thought they had made the right decision, I said, "Yes, I think you did."

Another parent who opted for no surgery was a physician who called me a few hours after we had diagnosed intestinal obstruction in his newborn mongoloid son. The first thing Dr. L asked was, "What would you do if he were your son?"

I am asked this frequently by parents of terribly deformed or severely retarded infants who need surgical attention in order to survive. In many cases, if it were my own child I would refuse to allow any measures other than simple procedures to relieve terminal suffering. But in the case of other people's children, I feel that as a physician I must reserve more of a sense of objectivity. I told Dr. L that he and his wife must make the decision, but that we would help them arrive at a decision and support them in whatever they decided.

There are many people who can help parents like the L's to reach a decision—pediatricians, genetic counselors, social workers, psychologists, psychiatrists, clergy, representatives of institutions for the retarded, family or friends with similar problems, and, of course, their own family physician. A decision need not be made hastily. By feeding the baby intravenously and by keeping his stomach and intestines from becoming distended by the use of a stomach tube attached to a suction pump, we can keep him alive and relatively comfortable for at least a few days.

My colleague, Dr. N, envies Mr. G. and Dr. L. Dr. N has two mongoloid children, both in a private institution, costing him $1,000 a month. Dr. N had originally placed the youngsters in a state institution after he and his wife had made an unsuccessful effort to raise them with their two normal children. While in the ancient, understaffed state building the children were constantly dirty and required hospitalization for one infection after another. This was more than the N's could stand. Paying $1,000 a month allows them to sleep at night.

I know many physicians with mongoloid children. Almost all have placed them in institutions. Couples who are success-oriented and have high expectations for their children are likely to institutionalize their mentally deficient offspring rather than

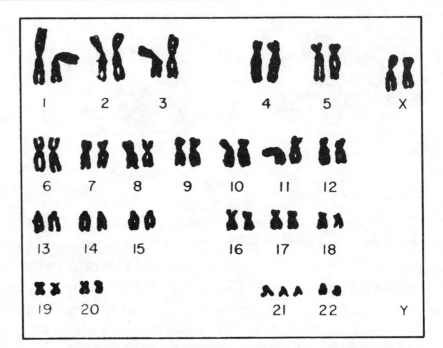

ONE TOO MANY—Mongoloids have an extra chromosome in the cell nucleus—giving them 47 instead of the normal 46. In this chromosomal picture of a mongoloid girl, the extra chromosome is in group 21.

keep them at home. The argument that mongoloids raised in the home perform better than those raised in an institution is rarely persuasive with such parents.

On the other hand, I operated on the mongoloid child of a farm couple who had several other children working in their fields. They were far from well-to-do but they were a happy family. The parents viewed this mongoloid baby as a child who would stay with them on the farm when the others had gone their ways. Such parents as these, with lesser expectations, are more likely to insist that everything be done for their mongoloid baby and to welcome it into their homes.

SOME of my surgical colleagues have unyielding philosophical positions that enable them to take a consistent stand with respect to each mongoloid infant they see in consultation. These positions enable them to keep their emotional involvement minimal. One surgeon feels that the infant's mongolism is not relevant to his need for surgery. He cites Article II of the Declaration of General and Special Rights of the Mentally Retarded, which was adopted by the Assembly of the International League of Societies for the Mentally Handicapped in 1968: "The mentally retarded person has a right to proper medical care and physical restoration . . . as will enable him to develop his ability and potential to the fullest possible extent, no matter how severe his degree of disability." To this surgeon not to operate is a basic violation of the right of a person to live—it is murder.

The problem is equally simple to another colleague. He will not operate on any mongoloid infant. He feels that the burden inflicted on the family and on society by the emotional and financial costs involved are too great to justify the procedure. He is particularly irked by parents who insist that everything be done to save their mongoloid infant and then place the baby in an institution to be supported by the taxpayers.

I find it impossible to adopt a rigid view one way or the other. I have seen families emotionally and financially drained by mongoloid children whose congenital heart defects and extraordinary susceptibility to infection bring them repeatedly to death's door. I have seen marriages destroyed by the inability of the partners to deal with the guilt and mutual recriminations stirred up by a mongoloid child. Although most parents allow the necessary surgery, many of them would be relieved to have their mongoloid die. Some have strong guilt feelings which are not dispelled by our sophisticated knowledge of genes and chromosomes. Such parents do not consider a lethal birth defect as a second chance to "abort" a mongoloid baby but feel their guilt would be increased if they did not grant the infant the chance of life.

As a decision with respect to surgery is delayed, the baby himself becomes a major spokesman in his own behalf. Even individuals firmly committed to an active eugenic policy may weaken when confronted with the pink, crying, kicking, gurgling infant despite its slanty eyes and big

tongue. The attitudes of the G's and the L's were unusual, since most of the couples I know who have actually seen their mongoloid babies and held them rarely decide to withhold life-saving surgery. Of course, once the parents make the decision that the baby should survive, my team and I will work on that baby with every tool and skill in our surgical armamentarium to pull him through, as we did when the middle-aged wife of a wealthy executive gave birth to a mongoloid on whom I operated within hours after its birth. This couple had looked forward to having a baby for years. The nursery was decorated. The road to college and success was plainly marked. In spite of their disappointment they were willing to accept this infant and asked that everything be done. The surgery went well, but subsequently heart failure developed in an irreparably defective heart. This story had a happy ending. One year later the couple adopted a normal little girl, rescuing a bright youngster from institutional life. It is a dilemma for our society: the emotional and financial resources of many families are poured out for helpless retardates while children with real potential are stunted in institutions or a series of foster homes.

PARENTS of mongoloids have the legal (and, I believe, the moral) responsibility of determining if their child with a potentially deadly but surgically correctible defect should live or die. The surgeon's responsibilities to the parents include being completely honest; allowing them to make a decision based on fact with respect to the child's ultimate capabilities; and providing sustained emotional support. Should the surgeon undertake responsibility for operating on the baby he must, despite any philosophical reservations, go all out to achieve the same results he would strive for in a normal infant. Where surgery is denied he must try to keep the infant from suffering while natural forces sap the baby's life away. As a surgeon whose natural inclination is to use the scalpel to fight off death, standing by and watching a salvageable baby die is the most emotionally exhausting experience I know. It is easy at a conference, in a theoretical discussion, to decide that such infants should be allowed to die. It is altogether different to stand by in the nursery and watch as dehydration and infection wither a tiny being over hours and days. This is a terrible ordeal for me and the hospital staff—much more so than for the parents who never set foot in the nursery.

The science of genetics combined with effective counseling will ultimately lead to a downward spiral of the mongoloid birth rate. Geneticists have already made significant progress by using a highly accurate technique called amniocentesis. Some of the fluid which continually bathes the fetus in the uterus is drawn off through a needle inserted into the womb. Living fetal cells floating in this fluid can be grown in the laboratory and their chromosomes inspected. Amniocentesis cannot be performed safely prior to the 13th or 14th week of pregnancy and it takes an additional few weeks to grow the cells for chromosome analysis. We would prefer to detect mongolism earlier in pregnancy when abortion is simpler and safer. The few geneticists who have had a large experience with amniocentesis, however, feel that the technique can be of significant benefit right now. Women who might choose to have their pregnancies interrupted if they knew they were nurturing a mongoloid fetus would include those over the age of 40 whose chances of having an infant with a serious chromosome abnormality is about 1 in 40 and a mongoloid infant in particular is 1 in 100. It would also include those younger women who have already given birth to a mongoloid infant and the rare young woman who, though normal herself, has a chromosome abnormality which predisposes a high proportion of her offspring to mongolism.

In the meantime, mongoloids are still being born at the rate of about 1 in 600. Perhaps society should assume more of the decision-making responsibility for those who require surgery for survival. And if the decision is in favor of life, society must provide the necessary funds and facilities to meet the continuing medical and psychological needs of these unfortunate children. It seems to me that a society which does not provide for its defectives is less than humane.

In the absence of some sort of uniform social philosophy, we physicians who deal with mongoloid children must view each one and its family as unique and try to react with a combination of sound judgment and compassion for the parents and the baby and the society in which they live. ◼

January 30, 1972

Syphilis Victims in U.S. Study Went Untreated for 40 Years

By JEAN HELLER
The Associated Press

WASHINGTON, July 25—For 40 years the United States Public Health Service has conducted a study in which human beings with syphilis, who were induced to serve as guinea pigs, have gone without medical treatment for the disease and a few have died of its late effects, even though an effective therapy was eventually discovered.

The study was conducted to determine from autopsies what the disease does to the human body.

Officials of the health service who initiated the experiment have long since retired. Current officials, who say they have serious doubts about the morality of the study, also say that it is too late to treat the syphilis in any surviving participants.

Doctors in the service say they are now rendering whatever other medical services they can give to the survivors while the study of the disease's effects continues.

Dr. Merlin K. DuVal, Assistant Secretary of Health, Education and Welfare for Health and Scientific Affairs, expressed shock on learning of the study. He said that he was making an immediate investigation.

The experiment, called the Tuskegee Study, began in 1932 with about 600 black men, mostly poor and uneducated, from Tuskegee, Ala., an area that had the highest syphilis rate in the nation at the time.

Four hundred of the group had syphilis and never received deliberate treatment for the venereal infection. A control group of 200 had no syphilis and did not receive any specific therapy.

Some subjects were added to the study in its early years to replace men who had dropped out of the program, but the number added is not known. At the beginning of this year, 74 of those who received no treatment were still alive.

As incentives to enter the program, the men were promised free transportation to and from hospitals, free hot lunches, free medicine for any disease other than syphilis and free burial after autopsies were performed.

Could Have Been Helped

The Tuskegee Study began 10 years before penicillin was found to be a cure for syphilis and 15 years before the drug became widely available. Yet, even after penicillin became common, and while its use probably could have helped or saved a number of the experiment subjects, the drug was denied them, Dr. J.D. Millar says.

Dr. Millar is chief of the veneral disease branch of the service's Center for Disease Control in Atlanta and is now in charge of what remains of the Tuskegee Study. He said in an interview that he has serious doubts about the program.

Dr. Millar said that "a serious moral problem" arose when penicillin therapy, which can cure syphilis in its early stages, became available in the late nineteen-forties and was withheld from the patients in the syphilis study. Penicillin therapy became, Dr. Millar said, "so much more effective and so much less dangerous" than pre-existing therapies.

"The study began when attitudes were much different on treatment and experimentation," Dr. Millar said. "At this point in time, with our current knowledge of treatment and the disease and the revolutionary change in approach to human experimentation, I don't believe the program would be undertaken."

Members of Congress reacted with shock to the disclosure today that the syphilis experimentation on human guinea pigs had taken place.

'A Moral Nightmare'

Senator William Proxmire, Democrat of Wisconsin, a member of the Senate Appropriations subcommittee that oversees Public Health Service budgets, called the study "a moral and ethical nightmare."

Syphilis is a highly contagious infection spread by sexual contact. If untreated, it can cause bone and dental deformations, deafness, blindness, heart disease and deterioration of the central nervous system.

No figures were available as to when the last death in the program occurred. One official said that no conscious effort was apparently made to halt the program after it got under way.

A 1969 study of 276 untreated syphilitics who participated in the Tuskegee Study showed that seven had died as a direct result of syphilis. The 1969 study was made by the Atlanta center, whose officials said they could not determine at this late date how many additional deaths had been caused by syphilis.

However, of the 400 men in the original syphilitic group, 154 died of heart disease that officials in Atlanta said was not specifically related to syphilis. Dr. Millar said that this rate was identical with the rate of cardio-vascular deaths in the control, or non-syphilis, group.

Dr. Millar said that the study was initiated in 1932 by Dr. J. R. Heller, assistant surgeon general in the service's venereal disease section, who subsequently became division chief.

Of the decision not to give penicillin to the untreated syphilitics once it became widely available, Dr. Millar said, "I doubt that it was a one-man decision. These things seldom are. Whoever was director of the VD section at that time, in 1946 or 1947, would be the most logical candidate if you had to pin it down."

'Never Clandestine'

The syphilis study "was never clandestine" and 15 scientific reports were published in the medical literature, Dr. Millar said in a telephone interview yesterday from Atlanta.

Officials who initiated the study in 1932 had informed the syphilis victims that they could get treatment for the infection at any time, Dr. Millar said.

"Patients were not denied drugs," Dr. Millar stressed. Rather, they were not offered drugs.

When the study began, doctors could offer only what is now regarded as poor therapy—injections of metals like bismuth, arsenic and mercury. Such treatments were known to be toxic.

Many doctors, Dr. Miller said, then thought "it better not to treat syphilis cases because of the mortality from" the metal therapies.

The critical period in ethics was in the late nineteen l forties and early nineteen-fifties when antibiotics could have been but were not prescribed for the syphilis patients.

July 26, 1972

383

Few Mercy Killers Draw Full Penalties

By LESLEY OELSNER

Robert Waskin's mother was in a Chicago hospital dying of leukemia. One day in 1967, just before he was to graduate from college, he went to her room and fired three shots. He made no attempt to hide his action, saying: "She's out of her misery now. I shot her."

He was indicted for murder, but a jury found him not guilty.

William R. Jones was also indicted for murder, charged with — and admitting to — the electrocution of his wife in 1953. His wife, an amputee and a diabetic who was in constant pain, had asked to be killed.

Jones was convicted. But on sentencing day in a Detroit court the judge wept. And Jones, who could have spent decades in prison, got a year and a day.

Mercy killers do not always get such treatment. In 1952, for instance, Charles M. Collins of Belfast, Me., was sentenced to life imprisonment after pleading guilty to the fatal shooting of his son, an often violent youth who was about to be sent to the state mental hospital.

But Mr. Collins is the exception. Mercy killing, classified as homocide, is illegal in every state in the union. Yet according to Sidney D. Rosoff, legal adviser to two groups developing policies on euthanasia (the Euthanasia Education-

al Council, which disseminates information, and the Euthanasia Society of America, which suggests legislation), few defendants in recent years have been subjected to the full penalties the law seems to allow.

The law on the subject, technically at least, is clear. But in practice the rules differ and the general area of euthanasia is mired in legal as well as ethical, religious and medical problems. In the history of the prosecution of mercy killers, as Mr. Rosoff puts it, there are "some very strange things."

Varieties of Homicide

Homicide statutes generally set up different degrees of homicide. The most serious is premeditated murder, involving "malice aforethought"—a deliberate plan to kill someone. The least serious is manslaughter—a killing that can be either accidental or a result of some immediate provocation.

Statutes in a few other countries state that mercy killings merit lighter sentences than do less charitable types of murder, Mr. Rosoff said, but American statutes do not.

In mercy killing, Mr. Rosoff said, "every one of these cases is premeditated." But he said only a handful of defendants were ever found guilty of that offense. He and other lawyers say this comes about for a variety of reasons.

For example, the judge may simply dismiss the charges. Such was the outcome in the case of Anne Eldredge of Philadelphia, a 71-year-old retired schoolteacher who in 1958 helped her sister commit suicide by giving her a glass of water with which to take an overdose of sleeping pills.

Or the defendant may be ruled insane; the jury may acquit him as "not guilty by reason of temporary insanity." In 1953, Albert J. Sell Jr. killed his 5-year-old son, a cerebral-palsy victim. According to the Passaic County Prosecutor's office, Mr. Sell was found insane was put in a mental institution for a year and was then released.

Sometimes the jury may find the defendant guilty of a lesser charge, such as manslaughter, which carries a lesser penalty.

Or the jury may simply acquit the defendant altogether, feeling that the prosecutor did not prove that the defendant matched the jury's conception of a murderer.

One of the most notorious mercy-killing cases of recent times involved Dr. Herman N. Sander of Manchester, N. H., who was accused in 1949 of killing a female patient who had incurable cancer by injecting air into her veins.

Dr. Sander had noted the injection on the hospital records. But at the trial a witness testified that the patient had died before the injection.

To many observers it was a dubious argument. As one lawyer said yesterday: "Why would he have bothered if she were already dead?" But the jury acquitted nevertheless.

Over the years, relatively few such cases have even been prosecuted—a paucity lawyers explain by saying that prosecutors often do not hear of such cases and that mercy killing is a difficult and traumatic crime to commit.

Nor has there been much agitation for legislative change. Lately, some reform proposals have been made in a few states, but they generally have involved lesser degrees of the general area variously called euthanasia, mercy killing or the "right to die with dignity."

In addition to the actual killings that capture headlines, as Mr. Rosoff sees it, the field breaks into these areas or degrees of complicity in death: terminating treatment needed to keep someone alive, refraining from initiating necessary treatment (an operation on a newborn baby, for example) and actively inducing death through a "painless" method (unplugging a necessary machine, for instance).

The second of these is generally thought to involve a medical rather than legal decision. Proposals have been made to allow euthanasia in the first type of case in Florida Oregon, and West Virginia. Proposals regarding the third type have been made in Idaho and Montana.

June 26, 1973

High Court Rules Abortions Legal the First 3 Months

By WARREN WEAVER Jr.
Special to The New York Times

WASHINGTON, Jan. 22 — The Supreme Court overruled today all state laws that prohibit or restrict a woman's right to obtain an abortion during her first three months of pregnancy. The vote was 7 to 2.

In a historic resolution of a fiercely controversial issue, the Court drafted a new set of national guidelines that will result in broadly liberalized anti-abortion laws in 46 states but will not abolish restrictions altogether.

Establishing an unusually detailed timetable for the relative legal rights of pregnant women and the states that would control their acts, the

majority specified the following:

¶For the first three months of pregnancy the decision to have an abortion lies with the woman and her doctor, and the state's interest in her welfare is not "compelling" enough to warrant any interference.

¶For the next six months of pregnancy a state may "regulate the abortion procedure in ways that are reasonably related to maternal health," such as licensing and regulating the persons and facilities involved.

¶For the last 10 weeks of pregnancy, the period during which the fetus is judged to be capable of surviving if born, any state may prohibit abortions, if it wishes, except where they may be necessary to preserve the life or health of the mother.

Today's action will not affect existing laws in New York, Alaska, Hawaii and Washington, where abortions are now legally available in the early months of pregnancy. But it will require rewriting of statutes in every other state.

The basic Texas case decided by the Court today will invalidate strict anti-abortion laws in 31 states; a second decision involving Georgia will require considerable rewriting of more liberal statutes in 15 others.

Justice Harry A. Blackmun wrote the majority opinion in which Chief Justice Warren E. Burger and Justices William O. Douglas, William J. Brennan Jr., Potter Stewart, Thurgood Marshall and Lewis F. Powell Jr. joined.

Dissenting were Justices Byron R. White and William H. Rehnquist.

Justice White, calling the

decision "an exercise of raw judicial power," wrote that "the Court apparently values the convenience of the pregnant mother more than the continued existence and development of the life or potential life which she carries."

The Court's decision was at odds with the expressed views of President Nixon. Last May, in a letter to Cardinal Cooke, he opposed "liberalized abortion policies" and spoke out for "the right to life of literally hundreds of thousands of unborn children."

But three of the four Justices Mr. Nixon has appointed to the Supreme Court voted with the majority, with only Mr. Rehnquist dissenting.

The majority rejected the idea that a fetus becomes a "person" upon conception and is thus entitled to the due process and equal protection guarantees of the Constitution. This view was pressed by opponents of liberalized abortion, including the Roman Catholic Church.

Justice Blackmun concluded that "the word 'person,' as used in the 14th Amendment, does not include the unborn," although states may acquire, "at some point in time" of pregnancy, an interest in the "potential human life" that the fetus represents, to permit regulation.

It is that interest, the Court said, that permits states to prohibit abortion during the last 10 weeks of pregnancy, after the fetus has developed the capacity to survive.

In both cases decided today, the plaintiffs had based their protest on an assertion that state laws limiting the availability of abortion had circumscribed rights and freedoms guaranteed them by the Constitution: due process of law, equal protection of the laws, freedom of action and a particular privacy involving a personal and family matter.

In its decision on the challenge to the Georgia abortion law, the high court majority struck down several requirements that a woman seeking to terminate her pregnancy in that state would have to meet.

Decision for Doctors

Among them were a flat prohibition on abortions for out-of-state residents and requirements that hospitals be accredited by a private agency, that applicants be screened by a hospital committee and that two independent doctors certify the potential danger to the applicant's health.

The Georgia law permitted abortions when a doctor found in "his best clinical judgment" that continued pregnancy would threaten the woman's life or health, that the fetus would be likely to be born defective or that the pregnancy was the result of rape.

The same Supreme Court majority, with Justice Blackmun writing the opinion again, emphasized that this medical judgment should cover all relevant factors—"physical, emotional, psychological familial and the woman's age."

In some of the 15 states with laws similar to Georgia's, doctors have tended to take a relatively narrow view of what constituted a woman's health in deciding whether an abortion was legally justified.

The Texas law that the Court invalidated entirely was typical of the criminal statutes passed in the last half of the 19th century prohibiting all abortions except those to save a mother's life. The Georgia law, approved in 1972 and altered by the Court today, was patterned after the model penal code of the American Law Institute.

In the Texas case, Justice Blackmun wrote that the constitutional right of privacy, developed by the Court in a long series of decisions, was "broad enough to encompass a woman's decision whether or not to terminate her pregnancy."

He rejected, however, the argument of women's rights groups that this right was absolute "and she is entitled to terminate her pregnancy at whatever time, in whatever way and for whatever reason she alone chooses."

"With this we do not agree," the Justice declared.

"A state may properly assert important interests in safeguarding health in maintaining medical standards and in protecting potential life," Mr. Blackmun observed. "At some point in pregnancy, these respective interests become sufficiently compelling to sustain regulation of the factors that govern the abortion decision."

The majority concluded that this "compelling" state interest arose at the end of the first three months of pregnancy because of the "now established medical fact" that until then, fewer women die from abortions than from normal childbirth.

During this three-month period, the Court said, a doctor can recommend an abortion to his patient "without regulation by the state" and the resulting operations can be conducted "free of interference by the state."

The "compelling state interest" in the fetus does not arise, however, until the time of "viability," Justice Blackmun wrote, when it has "the capability of meaningful life outside the mother's womb." This occurs about 10 weeks before delivery.

In reading an abbreviated version of his two opinions to the Court this morning, Justice Blackmun noted that most state legislatures were in session now and would thus be able to rewrite their states' abortion laws to conform to the Court's decision.

Both of today's cases wound up with anonymous parties winning victories over state officials. In the Texas case, "Jane Roe," an unmarried pregnant woman who was allowed to bring the case without further identity, was the only plaintiff after the Supreme Court disqualified a doctor and a childless couple who said that the wife's health would be endangered by pregnancy.

In the Georgia case, the surviving plaintiff was "Mary Doe," who, when she brought the action, was a 22-year-old married woman 11 weeks pregnant with her fourth child.

January 23, 1973

The Right to Die

Renewed discussion of euthanasia has been aroused by two recent dramatic incidents. In one, a young man was accused of fatally shooting his brother who had been paralyzed in a motorcycle accident and who had begged for death; in another, a physician has been charged with the "wilful" murder of a cancer victim who was in a comatose state and was believed to have two days at most to live.

The traditional ethical imperative is that everything possible be done to help the sick and prolong their lives. But a growing movement now asserts that there is a right to die as well as a right to live, and that the former right is violated often by officious, prolonged, excruciating and expensive medical interventions that keep people alive who would be better off dead since they are in agony or are living vegetables without hope of recovery. As Prof. O. Ruth Russell asserted in an Op-Ed page article published earlier this year: "Surely it is time to ask why thousands of dying, incurable and senile persons are being kept alive — sometimes by massive blood transfusions, intravenous feeding, artificial respiration and other 'heroic' measures — who unmistakably want to die."

It is no great secret that euthanasia is frequently practiced here and abroad. Normally, this takes the form of cessation of "extraordinary measures" when all rea-

sonable hope seems gone; it is the decision, for example, not to put the comatose patient in a respirator when he develops breathing difficulties.

But even such a passive response to the problem involves the physician in subjective judgments on the probability of recovery that should not be left to one individual acting alone. In any event, practice varies widely from case to case, doctor to doctor, and hospital to hospital. "Unofficial" euthanasia is obviously open to abuse since it is normally unperceived for what it is and unreviewed by independent parties.

Dr. Malcolm C. Todd, president-elect of the American Medical Association, is quite correct in arguing that physicians should not have to make the decisions on mercy killings — even if they are merely decisions to refrain from medical intervention — by themselves. He suggests that boards made up of diverse kinds of people make the needed determinations.

A long-overdue first step might be creation of a committee to study the problem of euthanasia. Such a committee could first assemble some badly needed basic facts. To what extent is euthanasia practiced unofficially now? What is the cost—both in human suffering and in money—of the present continued legal bans against euthanasia? With such data available, the stage would be set for formulating a sensible national policy on one of life's most difficult and poignant problems: the right to die.

July 3, 1973

Euthanasia vs. the Right to Live

To the Editor:

Your July 3 editorial "The Right to Die" is at best misguided and at worst extremely dangerous. The two cases cited, rather than supporting the argument for euthanasia, reveal its inherent risks.

The patient with terminal cancer in a comatose state who had two days to live was certainly not suffering. In addition, the saving of two days hardly seems to justify legalization of overt acts in the destruction of life. It seems that the only gain in the induction of this patient's death was the convenience of both the physician and the family.

With regard to the young man who was quadraplegic as a result of a motorcycle accident, it is obvious to anybody who has looked after the health of these patients that they are extremely depressed immediately after the accident, but I would suggest that the editors of The Times visit the Rusk Institute and discuss with Dr. Rusk (a former member of The New York Times) the rehabilitation of these patients and the remarkable strides toward creative life that can be achieved for them. Certainly, blowing out his brains with a shotgun does not represent a tenable solution to this patient's problem in a civilized society.

Certainly, Professor Russell's criteria for mercy killing are too vague to be useful and vague enough to be vicious. I would like to know who is senile enough to be killed by these criteria and who is not.

In these days of wiretapping, erosion of civil rights, invasion of privacy and, most recently, ill-informed sterilization of adolescent black girls in the South, I think that we should be standing up for protection of our most basic civil right, which is the right to live. Diluting the decision by delegating it to a panel and involving the state in decisions regarding continuation of life is a very certain step toward tyranny. There has been enough historical experience in both past and contemporary totalitarian states to establish the fact that there is no moral protection in numbers or bureaucracy.

I believe that your editorial is one of the most poorly thought out pieces I have ever seen published in The Times and I would hope that more sensitive and less hysterical thought would be applied to this problem in the future.

MELVIN RUBENSTEIN, M.D.
Westfield, N. J., July 5, 1973

July 23, 1973

Euthanasia Backed In Terminal Illness By 53% in a Poll

Most Americans now favor mercy killing for people who have incurable diseases, according to a Gallup Poll released yesterday.

Fifty-three per cent of those interviewed said that doctors should be allowed by law to painlessly end the life of a person with an incurable disease if the patient and his family request it.

Only about one-third of Americans (36 per cent) said they approved of such a practice when a similar poll was taken in 1950.

The biggest change in views on euthenasia has occurred in adults under 30 years old, the Gallup analysis showed. Thirty-nine per cent of this age group favored mercy killing in 1970; 67 per cent do now.

The question asked of 1,544 adults in the period July 6-9—the same question asked 23 years ago—read as follows:

"When a person has a disease that cannot be cured, do you think doctors should be allowed by law to end the patient's life by some painless means if the patient and his family request it?"

A spokesman for the Gallup organizations said the phrasing of the question paralleled that used in 1950. In 1973, as a result of medical advances, "terminal illness" is more commonly used than "a disease that cannot be cured"; the Gallup spokesman said those questioned appeared to relate their answers to terminal illnesses.

August 2, 1973

To Decide What Dead Means

By ALEXANDER M. CAPRON

The questions sound like law school hypotheticals. One man shoots another in the head. The victim is rushed to the hospital and hooked up to modern life-support systems. Although his heart and lungs are functioning, the doctors decide his brain is dead. His heart is removed and transplanted. Is the assailant guilty of murder? A man has an automobile accident that causes severe brain damage to a young girl whose still beating heart is given to a waiting cardiac patient. Can he be convicted of manslaughter, or only of felonious drunken driving?

But these cases are real. Both are in the courts in California. And practicing doctors and lawyers there, and across the country, have found themselves faced with many questions and few answers. When is a person legally and medically dead? Can there be, or should there be, any difference between the medical and legal definitions? And who should decide?

California Attorney General Evelle Younger has appointed a "blue ribbon" committee of physicians, clergymen and lawyers, chaired by the eminent cardiologist Dr. George C. Griffith, to assess the impact of the recent cases and to formulate a new legal rule. The premise of the committee, Deputy Attorney General Joel Moscowitz says, is that the definition of death is a matter for resolution by public bodies, and not merely by the medical profession.

At issue is the application of the traditional legal definition of death—the cessation of all vital bodily functions, including circulation and respiration — to new medical capabilities. In the shooting and accident cases, doctors determined the victims had suffered "brain death," and transplant procedures followed. In one of the cases, now on appeal, trial court judges have disagreed about the actual cause of death.

Uncertainty about the legal definition has "scared hell out of doctors and coroners" in California, according to Dr. Folkert Belzer, chief of the transplant service at the University of California Medical Center. There's been a "precipitous decline" in kidneys available for transplant as a result of these cases, he added.

The Doctors' Dilemma

The difficulty with the "complete cessation of all vital functions" test presently applied in the courts is that so long as a patient is supported by an artificial respirator, doctors cannot tell if his heart is beating naturally. As Dr. Alfred P. Fishman, director of the Cardiovascular-Pulmonary Division at the hospital of the University of Pennsylvania, has put it: "If we turn off the machine to find out, we may prejudice the survival chances of a weak patient who still has some chance of recovering. The deterioration of the patient's organs is also accelerated, which is bad if he's slated as a donor." The dilemma is not unique to transplant cases. The question "Is this person dead?" arises even more frequently in the routine care of terminal patients whose general condition is too poor for their organs to be used.

In the past, many doctors have held that deciding when a person is dead is entirely a medical matter, in which the courts and legislatures ought not to meddle. The American Medical Association, meeting in Anaheim, California, in December, 1973, reaffirmed its opposition to any "inflexible" statutory definition. But other physicians, including Dr. Griffith, argue that the medical profession must respond to the fact that public bodies are going to have a hand in deciding how death will be defined legally.

Another issue is whether it should be the courts or the legislatures that frame a new general standard. The present definition is the result of judicial decisions taken over the years as new cases arose. Alameda County Deputy District Attorney Albert W. Meloling plans to urge the judge in one of the cases to rule that determining death should be left to the doctors, but under proper guidelines set by either the courts or the legislature.

To reach a definition favorable to "brain death," however, the courts will have to go against precedent. As recently as 1968, a California appellate court rejected the notion that new transplant techniques should lead to abandonment of the current definition. And some doctors fear that a court ruling might be slow in coming, and not be definitive.

Legislative Answers

One resolution of both the legal and medical problems in the present rule would be a statute or precedent recognizing that in cases in which artificial means of support preclude reliance on the traditional life signs (heartbeat and breathing), a patient may be declared dead on the basis of a permanent and irreversible cessation of spontaneous activity in his brain, including cessation of those faculties that control respiration and circulation.

Dr. Thomas V. Byrne of the Los Angeles County-University of Southern California Medical Center says that transplant physicians in California have been seeking such legislation for the past year, but with no success. Deputy Attorney General Moscowitz has distributed to the California committee charged with formulating a new rule a model statute proposing such a definition.

Mr. Moscowitz has also considered the statute "relating to and defining death" adopted in Kansas in 1970, and the similar legislation enacted in Maryland in 1972. Both measures provide two definitions of death. In the first, death is considered to have occurred if a doctor determines "there is the absence of spontaneous respiratory and cardiac function and . . . attempts at recuscitation are considered hopeless." In the second, death is defined by the absence of spontaneous brain function, if it appears that "further attempts at resuscitation or supportive maintenance will not succeed."

Both the Kansas and the Maryland statutes have been criticized for setting forth two "alternative" criteria but not stipulating when they are to be applied. Professor Ian Kennedy of University College, London, has argued, too, that the Kansas statute "is bound [to create] popular misunderstanding," since it suggests that a person could be dead under one definition, but alive under the other. Rather than use the Kansas statute, Mr. Moscowitz has drawn up and circulated a proposal of his own.

Dr. Griffith expects the California Attorney General's committee to consider the proposals, and other suggestions from its members. "I hope it will arrive at agreement fairly quickly," he says, "so a law could be adopted this spring."

Alexander M. Capron teaches law at the University of Pennsylvania.

February 24, 1974

DEFINING DEATH HELD DOCTOR ROLE

PORTLAND, Ore., Dec. 3 (UPI) — The American Medical Association adopted a resolution today urging that physicians—not legislators—decide when death occurs.

The resolution was one of two dozen adopted by the policy-making body of the 170,000-member association as it began work on reports from nine committees.

The only resolution drawing more than perfunctory debate was one aimed at obtaining legislative limits on the practice of acupuncture. Also approved were statements opposing use of a popular hormone weight-reducing program, encouraging establishment of emergency rural medical services programs, urging continued imposition of a 55-mile-an-hour speed limit on the nation's highways and defining cosmetic surgery.

The delegates adopted without discussion a substitute resolution on the definition of death presented by its reference committee.

"At present," it said, "statutory definition of death is neither desirable nor necessary." It asked that state medical associations urge legislatures to postpone enactment of legislation defining death by statute, and said death should "be determined by the clinical judgment of the physician."

Brain Function Cited

Listed among the criteria that physicians may use to determine that death has occurred is "permanent and irreversible cessation of function of the brain." The resolution proposed earlier had listed specific criteria for determining whether death had occurred.

The action by the A.M.A. is designed to broaden the medical definition of death, which in the past had been determined in most cases by heart function. However, heart transplant cases have weakened that definition.

The A.M.A. wants to preserve the existing criteria of cause of death, including heart malfunction, as well as allow attending physicians to cite other criteria, especially the cessation of brain function.

The acupuncture resolution finally adopted states that "acupuncture in the United States is an experimental medical procedure" and "should be performed in a research setting by a licensed physician or under his direct supervision and responsibility."

December 4, 1974

California Court Limits Doctor-Patient Privilege

By ANDREW H. MALCOLM
Special to The New York Times

SAN FRANCISCO, Dec. 24— The California Supreme Court has ruled that doctors who believe one of their patients intends to hurt or kill someone must notify the potential victim, his relatives, friends or the authorities.

The decision, which was handed down here late yesterday, aroused immediate criticism from psychiatrists concerned that the requirement would inhibit treatment of patients and force the doctor to violate the confidential doctor-patient relationship.

But in the 5-to-2 ruling, Chief Justice Mathew O. Tobriner wrote, "The protective privilege ends where the public peril begins."

Dissenting View

In a dissent, Justice William P. Clark Jr. said that the decision would have a "devastating impact in the field of mental health."

The case stemmed from the murder on Oct. 27, 1969, of Tatiana Tarasoff, a 20-year-old student at the University of California at Berkeley, by Prosenjit Poddar, a 26-year-old graduate student who was a rejected suitor of Miss Tarasoff's.

Mr. Poddar had been receiving outpatient psychiatric treatment at a campus hospital. Two months before Miss Tarasoff was slain with a carving knife on her family's front porch Mr. Poddar confided to his doctor that he intended to kill the girl.

According to testimony, the doctor, Lawrence Moore, notified the campus police, who briefly detained Mr. Poddar. He was released, however, when he appeared rational. And a hospital supervisor, Dr. Harvey Powelson, ordered no further action against him.

The victim's parents have sued the university for $200,000 for failing to warn them or Miss Tarasoff. Originally, the Alameda County Superior Court found no grounds for the suit. But this view is overturned now by the state's highest court, which sent the case back to Superior Court for a trial.

Freed and Deported

Mr. Poddar was convicted of murder but later freed by the high court, which said he suffered from diminished mental capacity and could not have harbored malice toward the victim, a necessary element for a murder conviction. Last summer Mr. Poddar was deported to his native India.

In his decision, Chief Justice Tobriner wrote, "A patient with severe mental illness and dangerous proclivities may, in a given case, present a danger as serious and as foreseeable as does the carrier of a contagious disease or the driver whose condition or medication affects his ability to drive safely."

The Justice also said: "Our current crowded and computerized society compels the interdependence of its members. In this risk-infested society we can hardly tolerate the further exposure to danger that would result from a concealed knowledge of the therapist that his patient was lethal."

The court said that doctor-patient confidentiality had not been violated because California's Evidence Code listed a specific exception when disclosure was necessary to prevent the danger.

After the ruling, Dr. David Allen, former president of the Northern California Psychiatric Association, said, "If it's publicly known that psychiatrists are required to report these things, then the patient will be less likely to talk about it."

Dr. Morris Grossman, a Stanford University professor who is an expert on doctor-patient confidentiality, said: "The soundest practice is to try to defuse a person's homicidal urges through treatment. The minute you report them, they drop out of therapy."

And Dr. Grossman added, "If you locked up everybody who made a threat, there wouldn't be enough room in the hospitals."

Little Change Seen

The decision of the California Supreme Court apparently does little to change what has long been a general practice in psychiatry: warning appropriate individuals and law enforcement authorities if a patient presents a distinct and immediate threat to someone.

"The doctor must act in such cases," according to Dr. Alfred Freedman, chairman of psychitry at New York Medical College and immediate past president of the American Psychiatric Association. "An immediate threat to someone overrides the necessity of confidentiality in the doctor-patient relationship," he added.

A dilemma may arise, however, Dr. Freedman said, if a patient makes an ide or remote threat that the doctor interprets as not serious or not directed at anyone in particular. It was not clear from the California decision, he said, how liable a doctor would be if he failed to report a vague threat that the patient eventually acted upon.

December 25, 1974

Doctor Guilty in Death Of a Fetus in Abortion

By LAWRENCE K. ALTMAN
Special to The New York Times

BOSTON, Feb. 15—Dr. Kenneth C. Edelin was found guilty today of manslaughter in the death of a male fetus after a legal abortion that he performed at the Boston City Hospital on Oct. 3, 1973.

The jury, which had heard evidence for six weeks, reached its decision at 1:25 P.M. on the second day of its deliberation in a case that had become the focus of medical, religious and political controversy. The nine men and three women had been considering uncharted legal areas following the landmark decision on abortion by the United States Supreme Court on Jan. 22, 1973.

The verdict was widely regarded as a victory for anti-abortion and "right-to-life" groups.

Dr. Edelin's lawyer, William P. Homans Jr., said the case would be appealed because of the decision's importance to everyday medical practice and because "the verdict was against the weight of the evidence."

The verdict is expected to make obstetricians much more cautious in performing abortions during the second trimester, or the fourth through sixth months, of pregnancy. The abortion was performed by Dr. Edelin on a woman during her sixth month of pregnancy.

Dr. Edelin, composed but drawn, told newsmen, after the verdict, "We are not through with the battle yet."

"I just hope that this decision today will not throw us back where [women] will have to continue to put their lives and their health on the line," he said.

"I did nothing that was illegal, immoral or bad medical practice. Everything was in accordance with good medical practice."

Dr. Edelin also said he was uncertain how he would practice now that he had been found guilty of manslaughter. The answer, he said, would depend on consultations with his attorneys and decisions by the state medical licensing board.

Dr. Carl Goldmark Jr. of New York, a spokesman for the American Medical Association, said the verdict "probably will please the right to life committees, but I think it will soon be forgotten—I hope," The Associated Press reported.

Nellie J. Gray, speaking for a Washington, D.C., right to life committee, told the A.P. the verdict "starts America back on the road to respect for the dignity of human life,"

After the verdict, Judge McGuire ordered Dr. Edelin freed, pending an unspecified sentencing date, on his own recognizance and a $100 bond posted earlier. The maximum sentence is 20 years in jail.

In its case, the prosecution said that Dr. Edelin, after having ended the pregnancy in the abortion, killed the fetus by depriving it of life-sustaining oxygen while it was still in the womb.

The defense maintained that Dr. Edelin, who is 36 years old, could not have committed manslaughter because the fetus was not a person and therefore no person ever existed. Further, the defense maintained, the law had never given rights to the unborn.

Protective Clause Cited

Yesterday, Judge James P. McGuire said in his charge to the jury that Dr. Edelin could be found guilty only if the jurors considered the fetus a person and, then, if Dr. Edelin had shown wanton and reckless conduct.

He also told the jury that "you must be satisfied beyond a reasonable doubt that the defendant caused the death of a person alive outside the body of the mother."

The jury deliberated more than four hours yesterday. Shortly after it resumed deliberations this morning, the foreman sent a note to Judge

McGuire requesting a copy of the closing portion of the judge's charge. This portion dealt with the specifics of the laws concerning manslaughter, definitions of a person and fetus, and Judge McGuire's instructions.

In the charge, Judge McGuire also said that the Supreme Court abortion ruling protected Dr. Edelin from criminal conduct during the abortion he performed.

But because Massachusetts had not taken legislative action to regulate or proscribe abortion in accordance with the decision, the judge said that in Dr. Edelin's case "the law of manslaughter is inextricably intertwined in the Supreme Court decision."

In that decision the Supreme Court barred states from interfering with a woman's right to an elective abortion before the fetus became viable—able to survive outside the womb. The Court also issued new guidelines for the relative legal rights of pregnant women and of the states that would control their acts.

At 11:45 this morning, the jurors—all stern and stiff-lipped — walked in and were told by Judge McGuire that "I decline to give you a copy of the charge" unless the jury "cares to be more specific" about the sections it wishes to see.

Some Shocked by Verdict

In the closing portion of his 90-minute charge, Judge McGuire said he cited conflicts in the testimony "for purposes of illustration and example only." In rejecting the jury's request, the judge told the jury that it was "your memory on the facts that governs."

After a luncheon recess, the jury walked into the high-ceilinged, chilly courtroom on the ninth floor of the Suffolk County Courthouse in downtown Boston.

"Guilty," Vincent Shea, the foreman, responded in a loud voice when Judge McGuire asked him what verdict the jury had reached.

Exclamations of displeasure from shocked members of Dr. Edelin's family and from spectators sounded through the court-

room. As some spectators asked each other "How could they do that?", Dr. Edelin walked over to comfort his family.

His lawyer, Mr. Homans, expressed displeasure by saying:

"The vehemence with which the foreman shouted out the word 'guilty' says something about the temper of the populace."

Sixteen jurors heard all testimony given at the trial, but four of them, chosen by lot, were made alternate jurors after the judge's charge yesterday. The four included two of the youngest members of the original jury and an engineer, believed to be the only college graduate in the group.

Francis E. McLaughlin, a juror, said the first vote, taken two hours after the deliberations began, was eight to four. Then it stood 11 to 1 on a series of votes until shortly after noon when the last juror, a man, changed his mind on the secret ballot.

Mr. McLaughlin told reporters that the jurors believed the fetus was a person on the basis of the pattern of evidence rather than on the basis of

specific testimony. Though the jurors agreed that the abortion was legal, Mr. McLaughlin said, "I don't think he [Dr. Edelin] did a thorough job once it [the fetus] was removed."

The jurors generally felt that the defense witnesses were "too cocky" in their answers and that the doctors were too callous in their concern about possibility that the fetus might be alive, Mr. McLaughlin said.

Some observers said that the charge might have encompassed broader questions about Dr. Edelin's obligation, if any, to use all possible means to save the fetus after he had performed the abortion.

Now, Dr. Edelin's conviction on a charge of manslaughter in a legal abortion may lead to further cases challenging such points.

Some legal observers said they were surprised by the decision. Earlier, they had said they regarded the judge's charge as narrowing the case to the legal definition of "a person" from the broader issues of deciding viability of a fetus and determining when life begins.

February 16, 1975

Court Rules Karen Quinlan's Father Can Let Her Die By Disconnecting Respirator if Doctors See No Hope

By JOSEPH F. SULLIVAN
Special to The New York Times

TRENTON, March 31 — The New Jersey Supreme Court ruled today that the mechanical respirator that was keeping Karen Anne Quinlan alive might be disconnected if her attending physicians and a panel of hospital officials agreed that there was "no reasonable possibility" that she would recover.

The 7-to-0 decision, written by Chief Justice Richard J. Hughes, also ruled that there would be no civil or criminal liability if the mechanical device was removed following the guidelines laid down in the 59-page opinion.

The court appointed Miss Quinlan's father her guardian and empowered him to seek physicians and hospital officials who would agree to remove the respirator.

The 22-year-old woman has been in a coma for almost a year, and her parents petitioned last September for court approval for removal of "artifi-

ficial" life-sustaining procedures so she might die "with grace and dignity." Their request was denied in a lower-court ruling.

Paul W. Armstrong, the attorney for the Quinlan family, said the young woman's parents "wept" when he informed them of today's opinion. He added: "The court has advanced a right of privacy on the part of the father to act in Karen Quinlan's best interests."

He said the opinion would allow the young woman's parents to "return their daughter to her natural life processes, and if those processes fail, she will die."

Medical experts who testified at the lower-court hearing in October said the young woman could not survive for very long without the mechanical respirator and other around-the-clock medical procedures.

When asked who would turn off the respirator if that decision was approved by the attending physicians and concurred in by the required

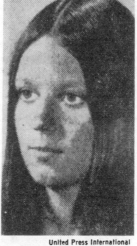

United Press International
Karen Anne Quinlan

medical panel, Mr. Armstrong said: "That decision will be a familial one, and any action will be taken in private."

Meeting with newsmen at Our Lady of the Lake Church in Mount Arlington, Mr. and Mrs. Quinlan expressed joy and relief at the court decision and said they would begin consultations with doctors tomorrow as

the first of a series of steps that could lead to the removal of their daughter's life-support system.

"This decision showed courage and the will of God," declared Mr. Quinlan, who said he had been "shocked and overwhelmed" by the ruling.

"This is the decision we've been praying for," said Mrs. Quinlan.

The high court quickly dispensed with Mr. Armstrong's novel constitutional arguments that Miss Quinlan's parents had a right to seek removal of the respirator under constitutional amendments that guarantee freedom of religion and ban cruel and unusual punishment.

But the court asserted a right of privacy for Miss Quinlan to make life-sustaining medical decisions and said that since the young woman was incompetent to make the decision herself, it belonged to her father, acting as her guardian.

"The magic of the common law has overcome the problems posed by technological advances in medicine," Mr. Armstrong said in commenting on the Supreme Court decision.

In ruling on the existence of Miss Quinlan's right of privacy, the court said: "We have no doubt, in these unhappy circumstances, that if Karen were herself miraculously lucid for an interval and perceptive of her irreversible condition, she could effectively decide on discontinuance of the life-support apparatus, even if it meant the prospect of natural death."

The court added: "If a putative decision by Karen to permit this noncognitive, vegetative existence to terminate by natural forces is regarded as a valuable incident of her right of privacy, as we believe it to be, then it should not be discarded solely on the basis that her condition prevents her conscious exercise of the choice.

"The only practical way to prevent destruction of the right is to permit the guardian and family of Karen to render their best judgment, subject to the qualifications here and after stated, as to whether she would exercise it in the circumstances.

"If their conclusion is in the affirmative, this decision should be accepted by a society, the overwhelming majority of whose members would, we think, in similar circumstances exercise such a choice in the same way for themselves or for those closest to them. It is for this reason that we determined that Karen's right of privacy may be asserted in her behalf, in this respect, by her guardian and family under the particular circumstances presented by this record."

William F. Hyland, the State Attorney General, who was one of the defendants in the case, said this evening that he agreed with many points of the ruling, especially the naming of Mr. Quinlan as guardian for his daughter, but he said no final decision on possible appeal had been made pending further review of the decision.

Mr. Armstrong said no final decision to remove the respirator would be sought until other parties to the case had an opportunity to file an appeal.

Near the end of its 59-page opinion, the court stated that "the exercise of a constitutional right, such as we here find, is protected from criminal prosecution."

"We do not question the state's undoubted power to punish the taking of human life," the ruling said, "but that power does not encompass individuals terminating medical treatment pursuant to their right of privacy."

In bolstering its recognition of an individual's right to privacy regarding life-sustaining

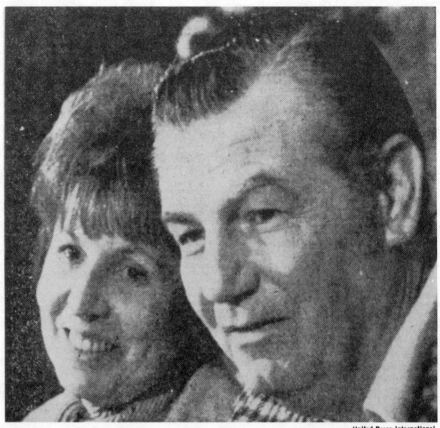

United Press International

Julia and Joseph Quinlan talking to reporters in Mount Arlington, N.J., after court ruled

medical decisions, the court referred to the United States Supreme Court decision in Griswold v. Connecticut, in which a woman's right to privacy in deciding whether to have an abortion was asserted.

"Presumably this right is broad enough to encompass a patient's decision to decline medical treatment under certain circumstances, in much the same way as it is broad enough to encompass a woman's decision to terminate pregnancy under certain conditions," the court said.

The high court also balanced the state's interest in preserving the sanctity of human life with the newly asserted right of privacy and found that in cases involving medical procedures, "the state's interest weakens and the individual's right to privacy grows as the degreee of bodily invasion increases and the prognosis dims."

"Ultimately there comes a point at which the individual's rights overcome the state's interest," the court said.

The opinion also gave the guardian the stronger voice in deciding what constitutes the best interest of an incompetent, even in the face of an opposing opinion by attending physicians. In fact, the court authorized the Quinlans to change

physicians, if they wished, in the event the present physicians failed to reconsider their opposition to the request to remove the respirator.

The court said, however, that Superior Court Judge Robert Muir Jr. was correct in denying the Quinlans' original request for removal of the respirator "under the law as it then stood," and it said the attending physicians, Dr. Robert Morse and Dr. Arshad Javed, were supported in their decision by proof offered at the trial "as to the then existing medical standards and practices."

But the court denied the existence of such uniform medical standards and put the blame for some of the reticence of physicians to give their best judgment in medical situations such as Miss Quinlan's on "the modern proliferation of substantial malpractice litigation and the less frequent, but even more unnerving possibility, of criminal sanctions."

The New Jersey Supreme Court sought to lay these fears to rest through its insertion of the protected right of privacy.

In its decision, which took the form of a declaratory judgment, the court said: "Upon the concurrence of the guardian and family of Karen, should the responsible attending phy-

sicians conclude that there is no reasonable possibility of Karen's ever emerging from her present comatose condition to a cognitive, sapient state and that the life-support apparatus now being administered to Karen should be discontinued, they shall consult with the hospital 'ethics committee,' or like body of the institution in which Karen is then hospitalized.

"If that consultant body agrees that there is no reasonable possibility of Karen's ever emerging from her present comatose condition to a cognitive, sapient state, the present life-support system may be withdrawn and said action shall be without any civil or criminal liability thereafter on the part of any participant, whether guardian, physician, hospital or others."

The Supreme Court invited the medical profession to use these guidelines without the necessity of seeking similar declaratory judgments from the courts in the future.

The high court also said its guidelines might be used in other types of terminal cases, without the necessity of applying the "hopeless loss of cognitive or sapient life" test as a prerequisite for action.

April 1, 1976

Suggested Reading

General

Babbie, Earl R. *Science and Morality in Medicine. A Survey of Medical Educators.* Berkeley: University of California Press, 1970.

Galdston, I. *Medicine in Transition.* Chicago: University of Chicago Press, 1965.

Gregg, Alan. *Challenges to Contemporary Medicine.* New York: Columbia University Press, 1957 [?].

Lerner, Monroe and Anderson, Odin W. *Health Progress in the United States, 1900-1960.* Chicago: University of Chicago Press, 1963.

Rosenberg, Charles E., ed. *Medicine and Society in America.* A reprint series of 47 titles. New York: Arno Press, 1972.

Sigerist, Henry E. *American Medicine.* New York: Norton, 1934.

Biography

Benison, Saul. Tom Rivers: *Reflections on a Life in Medicine and Science.* Cambridge, Mass.: The M.I.T. Press, 1967.

Cassedy, James H. *Charles V. Chapin and the Public Health Movement.* Cambridge, Mass.: Harvard University Press, 1962.

Cushing, Harvey. *The Life of Sir William Osler.* Oxford: Clarendon Press, 1926, 2v.

Flexner, Abraham. *An Autobiography.* New York: Simon and Schuster, 1960.

Flexner, Simon and Flexner, James T. *William Henry Welch and the Heroic Age of American Medicine.* New York: Viking, 1941.

Heiser, Victor. *An American Doctor's Odyssey.* New York: Norton, 1936.

Marshall, Helen E. *Mary Adelaide Nutting: Pioneer of Modern Nursing.* Baltimore: Johns Hopkins Press, 1972.

Institutions

Chapman, Carleton B.: *Dartmouth Medical School. The First 175 Years.* Hanover: University Press of New England, [1972].

Corner, George W. *A History of the Rockefeller Institute, 1901-1953.* New York: The Rockefeller Institute Press, 1974.

Corner, George W. *Two Centuries of Medicine. A History of the School of Medicine,* University of Pennsylvania. Philadelphia: Lippincott, 1965.

Curran, Jean A. *Founders of the Harvard School of Public Health, 1909-1946.* New York: Josiah Macy, Jr. Foundation, 1970.

Forbush, Bliss. *The Sheppard & Enoch Pratt Hospital, 1853-1970. A History.* Philadelphia: Lippincott, 1971.

Gifford, James F., Jr. *The Evolution of a Medical Center. A History of Medicine at Duke University to 1941.* Durham: N.C.: Duke University Press, 1972.

Shryock, Richard. *The Unique Influence of the Johns Hopkins University on American Medicine.* Copenhagen: Munksgaard, 1953.

Diseases

Etheridge, Elizabeth W. *The Butterfly Caste. A Social History of Pellagra in the South.* Westport, Conn.: Greenwood Publishing Co., 1972.

Paul, John R. *A History of Poliomyelitis.* New Haven: Yale University Press [1972?].

Education, Licensure, Research

The American Foundation. *Medical Research: A Midcentury Survey.* Boston: Little, Brown, 1955. 2v.

Derbyshire, Robert C. *Medical Licensure and Discipline in the United States.* Baltimore: Johns Hopkins Press, 1970 [?].

Evans, Frank B. and Pinkett, Harold T., eds. *Research in the Administration of Public Policy.* National Archives Conferences, vol. 7. Washington: Howard University Press, 1975.

Evans, Lester J. *The Crisis in Medical Education.* Ann Arbor: University of Michigan Press, 1964.

Henry, Robert S. *The Armed Forces Institute of Pathology. Its First Century, 1862-1962.* Washington: Office of the Surgeon General, Department of the Army, 1964.

Lynch, Kenneth M. *Medical Schooling in South Carolina, 1823-1969.* Columbia, S.C.: R.L. Bryan Co., 1970.

Richmond, Julius B. *Currents in American Medicine. A Developmental View of Medical Care and Education.* Cambridge, Mass.: Harvard University Press [1969].

Shryock, Richard H. *Medical Licensing in America, 1650-1965.* Baltimore: Johns Hopkins Press, 1967.

Medical Profession, Medical Care, Social Welfare

Burrow, James G. *AMA; Voice of American Medicine.* Baltimore: Johns Hopkins Press, 1963.

Freeman, Allen W. *Five Million Patients.* New York: Scribner, 1946.

Glaser, William A. *Paying the Doctor. Systems of Remuneration and Their Effects.* Baltimore: Johns Hopkins Press, 1970 [?].

Malmberg, Carl. *140 Million Patients.* New York: Reynal and Hitchcock, 1947.

Shryock, Richard H. *National Tuberculosis Association, 1904-1954; A Study of the Voluntary Health Movement in the United States.* New York: National Tuberculosis Association, 1957.

Skidmore, Max J. *Medicare and the American Rhetoric of Reconciliation.* University, Ala.: University of Alabama Press, 1970.

Stevens, Rosemary. *American Medicine and the Public Interest.* New Haven: Yale University Press, 1973?.

Taylor, Lloyd C. *The Medical Profession and Social Reform, 1911-1945.* New York: St. Martin's Press, [1973?].

Trattner, Walter, I. *From Poor Law to Welfare State: A History of Social Welfare in America.* New York: Free Press, 1974.

Drugs

Bonnie, Richard J. and Whitebread, Charles H., II. *The Marihuana Conviction: A History of Marihuana Prohibition in the United States.* Charlottesville: University Press of Virginia, 1974.

Caldwell, Anne E. *Origins of Psychopharmacology: From CPZ to LSD.* Springfield, Illinois: Thomas, 1970.

Fixx, James A., ed. *Drugs.* New York: Arno Press, 1971.

Jackson, Charles O. *Food and Drug Legislation in the New Deal.* Princeton: Princeton University Press, 1970.

Talalay, Paul, ed. *Drugs in Our Society.* Baltimore: Johns Hopkins Press, 1964.

Other Subjects

Burnham, John C. *Psychoanalysis and American Medicine: 1894-1918.* New York: International Universities Press, 1967.

Carlson, Eric T., ed. *Classics in Psychiatry.* A reprint series of 46 titles. New York: Arno Press, 1976.

Gardner, Howard, and Gardner, Judith, eds. *Classics in Psychology.* A reprint series of 42 titles. New York: Arno Press, 1973.

Grob, Gerald, ed. *Mental Illness and Social Policy: The American Experience.* A reprint series of 41 titles. New York: Arno Press, 1973.

Kaufman, Martin. *Homeopathy in America. The Rise and Fall of a Medical Heresy.* Baltimore, Johns Hopkins Press, [1972?].

Ludmerer, Kenneth M. *Genetics and American Society.* Baltimore, Johns Hopkins Press, 1972 [?].

May, Jacques, M. *A Physician Looks at Psychiatry.* New York: Day, 1958.

McNeil, Donald R. *The Fight for Fluoridation.* New York: Oxford University Press, 1957 [?].

Pickens, Donald. *Eugenics and the Progressives.* Nashville: Vanderbilt University Press, 1968.

Smith, Robert L. *At Your Own Risk: The Case Against Chiropractic.* New York: Trident, 1969.

Stone, Eric. *Medicine Among the American Indians.* New York: Hoeber, 1932. Paperback reprint, New York: Hafner, 1962.

United States. War Department. Surgeon-General's Office. *The Medical Department of the U.S. Army in the World War.* Washington: Government Printing Office, 1921-29. 15 vols. in 17.

Whorton, James C. *Before Silent Spring. Pesticides and Public Health in Pre-DDT America.* Princeton: Princeton University Press, 1976.

Wilson, Charles M. *Ambassadors in White; The Story of American Tropical Medicine.* New York: Holt, 1942.

Young, James H. *The Medical Messiahs. A Social History of Health Quackery in Twentieth-Century America.* Princeton: Princeton University Press, 1968.

Index